Operative Techniques in Joint Reconstruction Surgery

SECOND EDITION

Also Available In This Series

OPERATIVE TECHNIQUES IN FOOT AND ANKLE SURGERY, Second Edition
Editor: **Mark E. Easley**
Editor-in-Chief: **Sam W. Wiesel**

OPERATIVE TECHNIQUES IN PEDIATRIC ORTHOPAEDIC SURGERY, Second Edition
Editors: **John M. Flynn & Wudbhav N. Sankar**
Editor-in-Chief: **Sam W. Wiesel**

OPERATIVE TECHNIQUES IN ORTHOPAEDIC TRAUMA SURGERY, Second Edition
Editors: **Paul Tornetta III**
Editor-in-Chief: **Sam W. Wiesel**

OPERATIVE TECHNIQUES IN SHOULDER AND ELBOW SURGERY, Second Edition
Editors: **Gerald R. Williams, Jr., Matthew L. Ramsey, & Brent B. Wiesel**
Editor-in-Chief: **Sam W. Wiesel**

OPERATIVE TECHNIQUES IN SPORTS MEDICINE SURGERY, Second Edition
Editor: **Mark D. Miller**
Editor-in-Chief: **Sam W. Wiesel**

OPERATIVE TECHNIQUES IN HAND, WRIST, AND ELBOW SURGERY, Second Edition
Editor: **Thomas R. Hunt III**
Associate Editor: **Brian D. Adams**
Editor-in-Chief: **Sam W. Wiesel**

OPERATIVE TECHNIQUES IN SPINE SURGERY, Second Edition
Editors: **John M. Rhee & Scott D. Boden**
Editor-in-Chief: **Sam W. Wiesel**

OPERATIVE TECHNIQUES IN ORTHOPAEDIC SURGICAL ONCOLOGY, Second Edition
Editors: **Martin M. Malawer, James C. Wittig, & Jacob Bickels**
Editor-in-Chief: **Sam W. Wiesel**

Operative Techniques in

Joint Reconstruction Surgery

SECOND EDITION

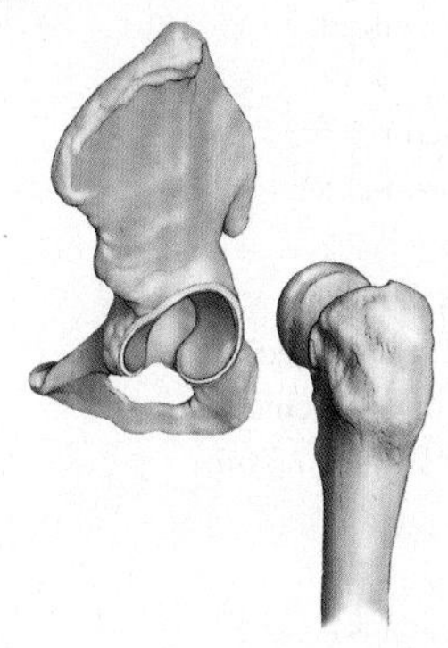

Javad Parvizi, MD
James Edwards Professor of Orthopaedic Surgery
Sidney Kimmel School of Medicine
Rothman Institute at Thomas Jefferson University
Philadelphia, Pennsylvania

Richard H. Rothman, MD
Founder, Rothman Institute
The James Edwards Professor of the Department of Orthopaedic Surgery
Jefferson Medical College, Thomas Jefferson University
Philadelphia, Pennsylvania

Sam W. Wiesel, MD
EDITOR-IN-CHIEF
Chairman and Professor
Department of Orthopaedic Surgery
Georgetown University Medical School
Washington, DC

With select chapters from:

Sports Medicine edited by
Mark D. Miller, MD

Pelvis and Lower Extremity Trauma edited by
Paul Tornetta III, MD

Shoulder and Elbow edited by
Gerald R. Williams, Jr., MD
Matthew L. Ramsey, MD
Brent B. Wiesel, MD

Pediatrics edited by
John M. Flynn, MD
Wudbhav N. Sankar, MD

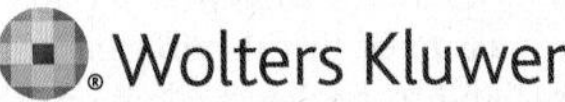

Philadelphia • Baltimore • New York • London
Buenos Aires • Hong Kong • Sydney • Tokyo

Acquisitions Editor: Brian Brown
Product Development Editor: Dave Murphy
Marketing Manager: Daniel Dressler
Production Project Manager: Bridgett Dougherty
Design Coordinator: Holly McLaughlin
Manufacturing Coordinator: Beth Welsh
Prepress Vendor: Absolute Service, Inc.

2nd edition

9 8 7 6 5 4 3 2 1

Printed in China

Library of Congress Cataloging-in-Publication Data

Names: Parvizi, Javad, editor. | Rothman, Richard H., 1936- , editor. | Wiesel, Sam W., editor.
Title: Operative techniques in joint reconstruction surgery / [edited by] Javad Parvizi, Richard H. Rothman ; Sam W. Wiesel, editor-in-chief.
Other titles: Operative techniques in adult reconstruction surgery
Description: Second edition. | Philadelphia : Wolters Kluwer, [2016] | Preceded by Operative techniques in adult reconstruction surgery / [edited by] Javad Parvizi, Richard H. Rothman ; Sam W. Wiesel, editor-in-chief. c2011. | Contained in Operative techniques in orthopaedic surgery / Sam. W. Wiesel, editor-in-chief. Second edition. 2016. | Includes bibliographical references and index.
Identifiers: LCCN 2015040260 | ISBN 9781451193060 (hardback)
Subjects: | MESH: Joint Diseases—surgery. | Arthroplasty—methods. | Hip—surgery. | Knee--surgery. | Orthopedic Procedures—methods. | Reconstructive Surgical Procedures—methods.
Classification: LCC RD686 | NLM WE 312 | DDC 617.4/720597—dc23 LC record available at http://lccn.loc.gov/2015040260

LWW.com

Dedication

To my mentor and great friend, Richard Rothman MD, PhD, who is a symbol of wisdom, humility and dedication. My sincere gratitude to him for his guidance and friendship.

—JP

Contents

Contributors

Farshad Adib, MD
Assistant Professor
Department of Orthopaedics
University of Maryland School of Medicine
Baltimore, Maryland

Yasushi Akamatsu, MD
Assistant Professor
Department of Orthopaedic Surgery
Yokohama City University School of Medicine
Yokohama, Japan

Pouya Alijanipour, MD
Postdoctoral Research Fellow
Rothman Institute
Thomas Jefferson University Hospital
Philadelphia, Pennsylvania

Derek F. Amanatullah, MD, PhD
Lower Extremity Reconstruction Fellow
Department of Orthopedic Surgery
Mayo Clinic
Rochester, Minnesota

Matthew S. Austin, MD
Associate Professor
Department of Orthopaedic Surgery
Rothman Institute
Thomas Jefferson University Hospital
Philadelphia, Pennsylvania

B. Sonny Bal, MD, JD, MBA
Professor
Department of Orthopaedic Surgery
University of Missouri
Columbia, Missouri

Christopher P. Beauchamp, MD
Associate Professor
Department of Orthopedics
Mayo Clinic
Phoenix, Arizona

Michael J. Beebe, MD
Surgeon
Department of Orthopaedics
University of Utah Hospitals and Clinics
Salt Lake City, Utah

Hari P. Bezwada, MD
Adult Reconstruction
Princeton Orthopaedic Associates
Princeton, New Jersey

Patrick M. Birmingham, MD
Clinical Professor
University of Chicago
Orthopaedic Surgery and Sports Medicine
NorthShore University HealthSystem
Chicago, Illinois

Diana Bitar, MD
Orthopaedic Surgeon
Research Fellow
Rothman Institute
Thomas Jefferson University Hospital
Philadelphia, Pennsylvania

Scot Brown, MD
Rothman Institute
Philadelphia, Pennsylvania

Brian D. Busconi, MD
Associate Professor
Department of Orthopaedic Surgery
University of Massachusetts Medical School
Chief of Division of Sports Medicine
UMass Memorial Medical Center
Worcester, Massachusetts

J.W. Thomas Byrd, MD
Nashville Sports Medicine Foundation
Nashville, Tennessee

Rajit Chakravarty, MD
Chief Resident
Department of Orthopaedic Surgery
Drexel University College of Medicine
Philadelphia, Pennsylvania

Anikar Chhabra, MD, MS
The Orthopedic Clinic Association, PC
Lead Orthopedic Consultant
Arizona State University
TOCA/BGS Sports Medicine Fellowship
Director
Phoenix, Arizona

Young Soo Chun, MD, PhD
Associate Professor
Department of Orthopaedic Surgery
Center for Joint Diseases and Rheumatism
Kyung Hee University Hospital at Gangdong
Seoul, Korea

Gregory Deirmengian, MD
Assistant Professor
Department of Orthopaedic Surgery
Rothman Institute
Philadelphia, Pennsylvania

Craig J. Della Valle, MD
Professor of Orthopedic Surgery
Adult Reconstructive Surgery of the Hip and Knee
Rush University Medical Center
Chicago, Illinois

Derek J. Donegan, MD
Assistant Professor of Orthopaedic Surgery
Hospital of the University of Pennsylvania
Philadelphia, Pennsylvania

Michael Dunbar, MD, FRCSC, PhD
Professor of Surgery
Professor of Biomedical Engineering
Professor of Community Health and Epidemiology
Director of Orthopaedic Research
Dalhousie University
Halifax, Nova Scotia, Canada

Kostas Economopoulos, MD
Attending Orthopaedic Surgeon
The Orthopedic Clinic Association
Phoenix, Arizona

Thomas C. Emmer, MD
Resident
Marshall University Medical Center
Huntington, West Virginia

Jill Erickson, PA-C
Physician Assistant
Department of Orthopaedics
University of Utah
Salt Lake City, Utah

Robert P. Good, MD
Clinical Associate Professor
Orthopaedic Surgery
Thomas Jefferson University
Philadelphia, Pennsylvania

Mark A. Hartzband, MD
Hartzband Center for Hip and Knee Replacement
Paramus, New Jersey

Philipp Henle, MD
Co-Chair Knee Surgery and Sports Traumatology
Sonnenhof Orthopaedic Hospital
Berne, Switzerland

Matthew S. Hepinstall, MD
Department of Orthopaedic Surgery
North Shore/LIJ Lenox Hill Hospital
New York, New York

MaCalus V. Hogan, MD
Assistant Professor
Division of Foot and Ankle Surgery
Assistant Residency Program Director
Department of Orthopaedic Surgery
University of Pittsburgh Medical Center
Pittsburgh, Pennsylvania

Colin R. Howie, MBChB, FRCS(Edin), FRCS(Glasg), FRCS(Orth)
Consultant Orthopaedic Surgeon
Royal Infirmary of Edinburgh
Honorary Senior Lecturer
University of Edinburgh
Edinburgh, Scotland

William Hozack, MD
Professor of Orthopaedics
Department of Orthopaedic Surgery
Rothman Institute
Thomas Jefferson University Hospital
Philadelphia, Pennsylvania

Adeel Husain, MD
Fellow, Adult Reconstruction
Department of Orthopaedic Surgery
University of Pennsylvania
Philadelphia, Pennsylvania

Julio J. Jauregui, MD
Orthopaedic Research Fellow
Rubin Institute for Advanced Orthopedics
Baltimore, Maryland

Lisa A. Kafchinski, MD
Resident
Department of Orthopaedic Surgery
University of Utah
Salt Lake City, Utah

Michael Kalisvaart, MD
Fellow
Orthopaedic Sports Medicine
Stanford University
Redwood City, California

Patrick Kane, MD
Rothman Institute
Thomas Jefferson University Hospital
Philadelphia, Pennsylvania

Bhaveen H. Kapadia, MD
Rubin Institute for Advanced Orthopedics
Center for Joint Preservation and Replacement
Sinai Hospital of Baltimore
Baltimore, Maryland

Bryan T. Kelly, MD
Codirector
Center for Hip Preservation
Hospital for Special Surgery
New York, New York

Kang-Il Kim, MD, PhD
Professor and Chairman
Department of Orthopaedic Surgery
Center for Joint Diseases and Rheumatism
Kyung Hee University Hospital at Gangdong
Seoul, Korea

Winston Y. Kim, MBChB, MSc, FRCS(Orth)
Consultant Orthopaedic Surgeon
Spire Manchester Hospital
Manchester, England

Young-Jo Kim, MD
Associate Professor of Orthopaedic Surgery
Department of Orthopaedic Surgery
Harvard Medical School
Boston Children's Hospital
Boston, Massachusetts

Scott King, DO
Orthopedic and Spine Specialists
York, Pennsylvania

Brian A. Klatt, MD
Assistant Professor of Orthopaedic Surgery
Division of Joint Reconstruction
University of Pittsburgh Medical Center
Pittsburgh, Pennsylvania

Gregg R. Klein, MD
Vice Chairman
Department of Orthopaedic Surgery
Hackensack University Medical Center
Hackensack, New Jersey

Ken Kumagai, MD, PhD
Lecturer
Department of Orthopaedic Surgery
Yokohama City University
Yokohama, Japan

Christopher M. Larson, MD
Physician
Minnesota Orthopedic Sports Medicine Institute at Twin Cities Orthopedics
Edina, Minnesota

Claudio Diaz Ledezma, MD
Clinical Fellow in Adult Reconstruction
Rothman Institute
Thomas Jefferson University Hospital
Philadelphia, Pennsylvania
Clinica Las Condes
Santiago, Chile

Gwo-Chin Lee, MD
Assistant Professor of Orthopaedic Surgery
Presbyterian Medical Center of Philadelphia
Philadelphia, Pennsylvania

Eric A. Levicoff, MD
Assistant Professor of Orthopaedic Surgery
Jefferson Medical College of Thomas Jefferson University
Philadelphia, Pennsylvania

Frank A. Liporace, MD
Associate Professor
Department of Orthopaedic Surgery
NYU Langone Medical Center
New York, New York

Jess H. Lonner, MD
Attending Orthopaedic Surgeon
Rothman Institute
Associate Professor
Department of Orthopaedic Surgery
Thomas Jefferson University
Philadelphia, Pennsylvania

Bassam A. Masri, MD, FRCSC
Professor and Chairman
Department of Orthopaedics
University of British Columbia
Vancouver, British Columbia, Canada

Travis H. Matheney, MD
Assistant Professor
Department of Orthopaedic Surgery
Harvard Medical School
Staff Physician
Department of Orthopedic Surgery
Boston Children's Hospital
Boston, Massachusetts

Paul B. McKenna, MB, BCh, MSc, FRCS(Tr & Orth)
Adult Reconstruction Clinical Fellow
Rothman Institute
Philadelphia, Pennsylvania

Sean McMillan, DO
Chief of Orthopedics
Director of Orthopedics Sports Medicine and Arthroscopy
Department of Orthopedics
Lourdes Medical Associates and Lourdes Medical Center
Burlington, New Jersey

R. Michael Meneghini, MD
Associate Professor of Orthopaedic Surgery
Adult Reconstruction Fellowship Director
Indiana University School of Medicine
Indianapolis, Indiana

Michael B. Millis, MD
Professor of Orthopaedic Surgery
Harvard Medical School
Boston Children's Hospital
Boston, Massachusetts

Peter N. Misur, MBChB, FRACS
Department of Reconstructive Orthopaedics
Vancouver General Hospital
Vancouver, British Columbia, Canada

Michael A. Mont, MD
Director, Center for Joint Preservation and Replacement
Rubin Institute for Advanced Orthopedics
Sinai Hospital of Baltimore
Associate Professor of Orthopaedics
The Johns Hopkins University School of Medicine
Baltimore, Maryland

Aaron Nauth, MD, MSc
Assistant Professor
Division of Orthopaedic Surgery
University of Toronto
Toronto, Ontario, Canada

Danyal H. Nawabi, MD, FRCS(Orth)
Attending Orthopaedic Surgeon
Sports Medicine and Shoulder Service
Hospital for Special Surgery
New York, New York

Charles L. Nelson, MD
Chief
Adult Reconstruction Section
University of Pennsylvania Health System
Associate Professor of Orthopaedic Surgery
Hospital of the University of Pennsylvania
Philadelphia, Pennsylvania

Ali Oliashirazi, MD
Professor and Chairman
Department of Orthopaedic Surgery
Chief, Division of Total Joint Replacement
Joan C. Edwards School of Medicine
Marshall University
Huntington, West Virginia

Alvin Ong, MD
Rothman Institute
Assistant Professor of Orthopaedic Surgery
Thomas Jefferson University Hospital
Philadelphia, Pennsylvania
Director of Orthopaedic Surgery
Atlanticare Regional Medical Center
Hammonton, New Jersey

Fabio Orozco, MD
Assistant Professor
Orthopaedic Surgeon Specialist in Hip and Knee Replacement
Department of Orthopedics
Rothman Institute
Thomas Jefferson University Hospital
Philadelphia, Pennsylvania

Patrick O'Toole, MD, FRCS (Tr & Orth)
Hip and Knee Arthroplasty Fellow
Rothman Institute
Philadelphia, Pennsylvania

Mark W. Pagnano, MD
Professor of Orthopaedic Surgery
Chairman
Department of Orthopedics
Mayo Clinic
Rochester, Minnesota

Javad Parvizi, MD
James Edwards Professor of Orthopaedic Surgery
Sidney Kimmel School of Medicine
Rothman Institute at Thomas Jefferson University
Philadelphia, Pennsylvania

Christopher L. Peters, MD
Professor
Department of Orthopaedic Surgery
University of Utah
Salt Lake City, Utah

Danielle Y. Ponzio, MD
Department of Orthopaedic Surgery
Rothman Institute
Thomas Jefferson University Hospital
Philadelphia, Pennsylvania

Robert J. Ponzio, DO
Ponzio Orthopedic
Sewell, New Jersey

Vishnu Prasad, MBBS, FRCS(Glasg), FRCS(Tr & Ortho)
Clinical Fellow
Department of Orthopaedics
QEII Health Sciences Centre Foundation
Dalhousie University
Halifax, Nova Scotia, Canada

Luis Pulido, MD
Clinical Fellow
Adult Reconstruction
Mayo Clinic
Rochester, Minnesota

James J. Purtill, MD
Associate Professor
Vice Chairman
Department of Orthopaedic Surgery
Rothman Institute
Thomas Jefferson University Hospital
Philadelphia, Pennsylvania

R. Lor Randall, MD, FACS
The L.B. and Olive S. Young Endowed Chair for Cancer Research
Director
Sarcoma Services
Chief
SARC Lab
Professor of Orthopaedics
University of Utah, Huntsman Cancer Institute
Salt Lake City, Utah

José A. Rodriguez, MD
Director
Center for Joint Preservation and Reconstruction
Lenox Hill Hospital
New York, New York

Craig M. Roberto, DO
Orthopaedic Sports Medicine Fellow
University of Massachusetts
Boston, Massachusetts

Marc Safran, MD
Professor
Department of Orthopaedic Surgery
Stanford University
Redwood City, California

Tomoyuki Saito, MD, PhD
Professor and Chairman
Department of Orthopaedic Surgery
Yokohama City University School of Medicine
Yokohama, Japan

Jonathan Salava, MD
Chief, Revision Joint Arthroplasty Service
Chief, Hip Arthroplasty Service
Assistant Professor of Orthopedic Surgery
Department of Orthopedic Surgery
Joan C. Edwards School of Medicine
Marshall University
Huntington, West Virginia

John P. Salvo, MD
Clinical Associate Professor
Orthopaedic Surgery
Rothman Institute
Thomas Jefferson University Hospital
Philadelphia, Pennsylvania

Wudbhav N. Sankar, MD
Assistant Professor of Orthopaedic Surgery
Director
Young Adult Hip Preservation Program
The Children's Hospital of Philadelphia
Assistant Professor of Orthopaedic Surgery
Perelman School of Medicine at the University of Pennsylvania
Philadelphia, Pennsylvania

Emil H. Schemitsch, MD, FRCSC
Professor of Surgery
Term Chairman in Fracture Care
St. Michael's Hospital
University of Toronto
Toronto, Ontario, Canada

Chloe E.H. Scott, MD, BSc, MSc, MRCS
Senior Registrar
Orthopaedic Surgery
Royal Infirmary of Edinburgh
Edinburgh, Scotland

Peter F. Sharkey, MD
Professor
Department of Orthopaedic Surgery
Rothman Institute
Riddle Hospital
Media, Pennsylvania

Klaus A. Siebenrock, MD
University of Bern, Inselspital
Department of Orthopaedic Surgery
Bern, Switzerland

Rafael J. Sierra, MD
Professor
Department of Orthopedic Surgery
Mayo Clinic
Rochester, Minnesota

Eric B. Smith, MD
Assistant Professor of Orthopaedic Surgery
Rothman Institute
Thomas Jefferson University Hospital
Philadelphia, Pennsylvania

Matthew D. Smith, MBChB, MRCS(Edin)
Specialist Registrar
Aberdeen Royal Infirmary
Aberdeen, Scotland

Mark J. Spangehl, MD, FRCSC
Associate Professor of Orthopaedics
Mayo Clinic College of Medicine
Phoenix, Arizona

Matthew A. Stanich, MD
Valley Anesthesiology and Pain Consultants
Phoenix, Arizona

Iain Stevenson, MBChB, FRCS (Tr & Orth)
Consultant Surgeon
Department of Orthopaedics and Trauma Surgery
Aberdeen Royal Infirmary
Aberdeen, Scotland

Moritz Tannast, MD
University of Bern, Inselspital
Department of Orthopaedic Surgery
Bern, Switzerland

Emmanuel Thienpont, MD, MBA
University Hospital Saint Luc
Brussels, Belgium

A. John Timperley, FRCS, DPhil(Oxon)
Princess Elizabeth Orthopaedic Centre
Exeter, United Kingdom

Frazer A. Wade, MBChB, FRCS(Edin), FRCS(Tr & Orth)
Consultant Orthopaedic Surgeon
Royal Infirmary of Edinburgh
Edinburgh, Scotland

Bas Weerts, MD
Arthroplasty Fellow
QEII Health Sciences Centre Foundation
Halifax, Nova Scotia, Canada

Matthew J. Wilson
Consultant Orthopaedic Surgeon
Exeter Hip Unit
Princess Elizabeth Orthopaedic Centre
Exeter, United Kingdom

Daniel P. Woods, MD
Orthopedic Sports Medicine Fellow
Rothman Institute
Thomas Jefferson University Hospital
Philadelphia, Pennsylvania

Preface

The purpose of the second edition of *Operative Techniques in Orthopaedic Surgery* remains the same as the first: to describe in a detailed, step-by-step manner the technical parts of "how to do" the majority of orthopaedic procedures.

It is assumed that the surgeon understands the "why" and the "when," although this information is covered in outline form at the beginning of each procedure.

Each of the nine major sections has been carefully reviewed and updated in both its content and artwork. The second edition has given each section editor the ability to include additional procedures and has also placed more emphasis in creating online content which is easily accessible and fully searchable.

The section editors and chapter authors have done an excellent job. Each has specific expertise and experience in their area and has given their time and effort most generously. It has again been stimulating to interact with these wonderful and talented people, and I am honored to have been able to play a part in this rewarding experience.

I also would like to thank all of the people at Wolters Kluwer. Dave Murphy has been especially helpful and had a great deal of input into this edition, as with the first edition. I would like, as well, to acknowledge Bob Hurley, who was a driving force for the first edition and has been a great resource for this second one as well.

Finally, special thanks goes to Brian Brown, the new acquisitions editor. It has been a wonderful experience to work with Brian who has done an excellent job of bringing this text to completion.

Sam W. Wiesel, MD
Washington, DC
January 2, 2015

Preface

to the First Edition

When a surgeon contemplates performing a procedure, there are three major questions to consider: Why is the surgery being done? When in the course of a disease process should it be performed? And, finally, what are the technical steps involved? The purpose of this text is to describe in a detailed, step-by-step manner the "how to do it" of the vast majority of orthopaedic procedures. The "why" and "when" are covered in outline form at the beginning of each procedure. However, it is assumed that the surgeon understands the basics of "why" and "when," and has made the definitive decision to undertake a specific case. This text is designed to review and make clear the detailed steps of the anticipated operation.

Operative Techniques in Adult Reconstruction Surgery differs from other books because it is mainly visual. Each procedure is described in a systematic way that makes liberal use of focused, original artwork. It is hoped that the surgeon will be able to visualize each significant step of a procedure as it unfolds during a case.

Each chapter has been edited by a specialist who has specific expertise and experience in the discipline. It has taken a tremendous amount of work for each editor to enlist talented authors for each procedure and then review the final work. It has been very stimulating to work with all of these wonderful and talented people, and I am honored to have taken part in this rewarding experience.

Finally, I would like to thank everyone who has contributed to the development of this book. Specifically, Grace Caputo at Dovetail Content Solutions, and Dave Murphy and Eileen Wolfberg at Lippincott Williams & Wilkins, who have been very helpful and generous with their input. Special thanks, as well, goes to Bob Hurley at LWW, who has adeptly guided this textbook from original concept to publication.

SWW
January 1, 2010

- However, careful assessment is necessary to ensure that the snapping is clearly the source of the patient's symptoms and also to evaluate other associated conditions, especially concomitant intra-articular pathology.
- Perhaps, most important is a careful assessment of the patient's motivation, understanding, and goals of recovery.
- It is important to bear in mind that coxa saltans often is encountered in asymptomatic individuals.
- Surgery is considered only if the patient has exhausted efforts at conservative treatment and demonstrates sufficient motivation for the postoperative recovery.

Positioning

- Iliopsoas tendon
  - Endoscopic release of the iliopsoas tendon is performed in conjunction with routine arthroscopy of the joint.
  - Arthroscopy can be performed with the patient in either the supine or lateral position, with each having their advantages.
- Iliotibial band
  - Open procedures employ the lateral decubitus position, and this also has been the preferred orientation for endoscopic methods (**FIG 4**).

Approach

- Iliopsoas tendon
  - Most endoscopic reports have described releasing the tendon from its insertion on the lesser trochanter within the iliopsoas bursa.[3,15]
  - This is the endoscopic counterpart to the open method described by Taylor and Clarke.[19] For the occasional case of a snapping iliopsoas tendon associated with a total hip arthroplasty, it clearly is the preferred approach.
  - Another endoscopic technique, in which the iliopsoas tendon is approached from the peripheral compartment, seems to provide a comparable effect of releasing the tendon.[15] The method is analogous to the open method described by Allen et al.[1] Theoretically, it may have an advantage of reduced morbidity and can be performed without traction.
  - Endoscopic release of the iliopsoas at the central compartment has been recently reported and demonstrated excellent results.[6] This technique is performed while viewing with a 70-degree arthroscope under traction.
- Iliotibial band
  - The various open approaches use a common, lateral, longitudinal incision over the greater trochanter.
  - Endoscopic methods employ laterally based portals, approaching the tendon from its superficial subcutaneous surface.

A

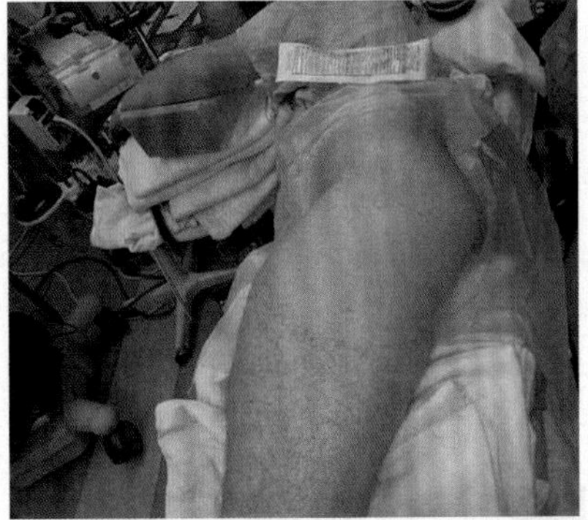

B

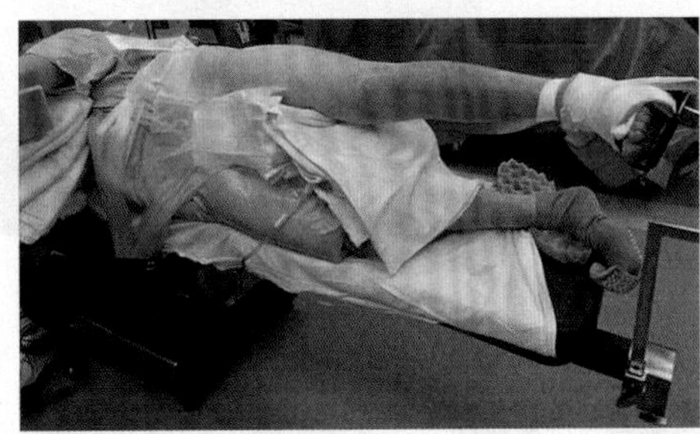

FIG 4 • **A.** Depiction of lateral decubitus positioning. **B.** Lateral decubitus position with beanbag on standard fracture table. Axillary roll and padded pressure points. Protect peroneal nerve on contralateral leg. Hip is slightly abducted, flexed, and externally rotated; position relaxes capsule. Well-padded perineum. (Courtesy of Brian Busconi, MD.)

TECHNIQUES

Endoscopic Iliopsoas Release

Lesser Trochanter (Iliopsoas Bursa)

- After completing routine hip arthroscopy, including intra-articular and peripheral compartments, traction is removed and the leg is repositioned in 20 degrees of flexion and full external rotation.
- Slight flexion partially relaxes the tendon but maintains some tension.
- External rotation brings the lesser trochanter more anterior for access from the laterally based portals (**TECH FIG 1A**).
- A portal is established distal to the standard anterolateral hip portal at the level of the lesser trochanter using fluoroscopic guidance (**TECH FIG 1B**).
  - This exposes the tendon within the iliopsoas bursa, which is the largest bursa in the body.
- Another portal is then placed distally, converging toward the lesser trochanter (**TECH FIG 1C**).
- The arthroscope and instruments are switched between these two portals for thorough visualization and instrumentation of the iliopsoas tendon (**TECH FIG 1D**).
- Adhesions within the bursa can be cleared, providing excellent visualization of the iliopsoas tendon.
- The tendinous portion of the iliopsoas is transected adjacent to its insertion on the lesser trochanter (**TECH FIG 1E**).
  - This is facilitated with the use of a flexible radiofrequency (RF) device.
- For safest technique, the medial side of the tendon is fully visualized, and the tendon is then released from medial to lateral. Its fibers will separate 1 to 2 cm.
- Muscular attachments of the iliacus muscle are preserved.

Peripheral Compartment

- After completing arthroscopy of the intra-articular compartment, traction is released, hip is flexed to 45 degrees, and standard portals are established in the peripheral compartment (**TECH FIG 2**).

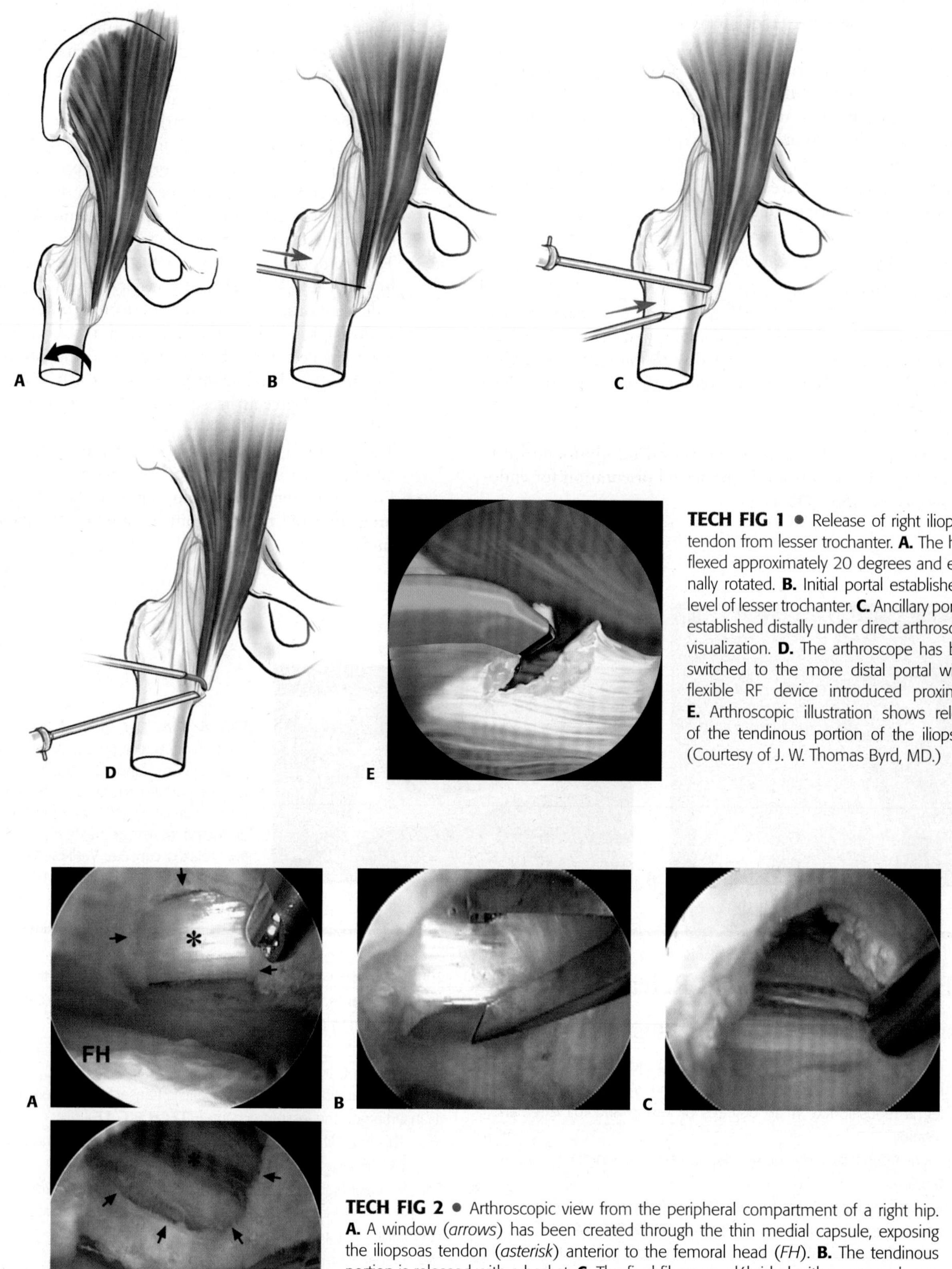

TECH FIG 1 • Release of right iliopsoas tendon from lesser trochanter. **A.** The hip is flexed approximately 20 degrees and externally rotated. **B.** Initial portal established at level of lesser trochanter. **C.** Ancillary portal is established distally under direct arthroscopic visualization. **D.** The arthroscope has been switched to the more distal portal with a flexible RF device introduced proximally. **E.** Arthroscopic illustration shows release of the tendinous portion of the iliopsoas. (Courtesy of J. W. Thomas Byrd, MD.)

TECH FIG 2 • Arthroscopic view from the peripheral compartment of a right hip. **A.** A window (*arrows*) has been created through the thin medial capsule, exposing the iliopsoas tendon (*asterisk*) anterior to the femoral head (*FH*). **B.** The tendinous portion is released with a basket. **C.** The final fibers are débrided with a power shaver. **D.** Through the capsular window (*arrows*), the tendon has been completely released, preserving the muscular fibers (*asterisk*). The relation between the capsular window and the acetabular labrum (*AL*) and femoral head (*FH*) is identified. (Courtesy of J. W. Thomas Byrd, MD.)

- An anterior hip capsulotomy is performed between the labrum and zona orbicularis, establishing a communication between the capsule and the iliopsoas bursa.
- The iliopsoas tendon is identified at this level and released via a thermal device, hand biter, or power shaver, being sure to leave the iliacus muscle intact just beyond the tendon.
- The muscular portion separates the tendon from the femoral nerve, which is the most lateral of the femoral neurovascular structures.

Central Compartment

- This technique is performed under traction with a 70-degree arthroscope.
- A capsulotomy is performed anteriorly between the anterior labrum and anterior femoral head at the 2 to 3 o'clock position of the labrum, via the direct anterior portal.
- The iliopsoas tendon is exposed through this capsulotomy and released at that level while the fibers of the iliacus are preserved.

Tendoplasty of the Iliotibial Band

Open Technique

- A straight, lateral longitudinal incision is centered over the greater trochanter (**TECH FIG 3**).
  - The length is dictated by the amount of exposure needed to precisely accomplish the tendoplasty.
  - A smaller incision is more cosmetic and can be accomplished with dissection of the subcutaneous tissues and selective retraction but should not compromise visualization for the procedure.
  - Several authors have described variations of a similar method for relaxing the tendon. These are based on an 8- to 10-cm longitudinal incision just posterior to the mid part of the greater trochanter in the thickest portion of the iliotibial band.
- Relaxation of the tendon is completed with paired or staggered 1- to 1.5-cm transverse incisions.
- The field is relatively bloodless, but meticulous hemostasis should be maintained and the subcutaneous tissues closed in layers to avoid formation of a hematoma.

Endoscopic Technique

- With the patient in lateral decubitus, care is taken to drape the patient to allow for free range of motion of the extremity; this is to ensure snapping phenomenon can be recreated intraoperatively.
- Traction is not required.
- Two portals are used: one just proximal to the tip of the greater trochanter and one distal to the greater trochanter, with area of snapping between both portals (**TECH FIG 4A**).
- The space under the iliotibial band can then be infiltrated with 40 to 50 mL of saline.
- The distal trochanteric portal is established with standard arthroscopic cannula introduced subcutaneously and directed proximally toward proximal trochanteric portal, using the blunt obturator to establish a working space above the iliotibial band.
- Then, with arthroscopic visualization, the proximal portal is established for dissection to release the subcutaneous tissue from the superficial surface of the tendon, maintaining careful hemostasis throughout (**TECH FIG 4B–D**).

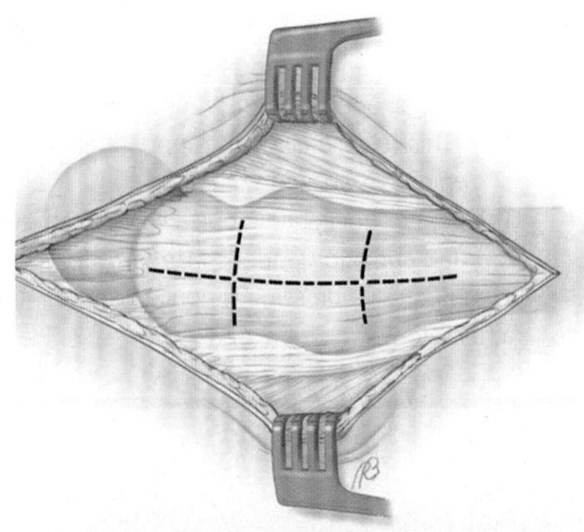
A

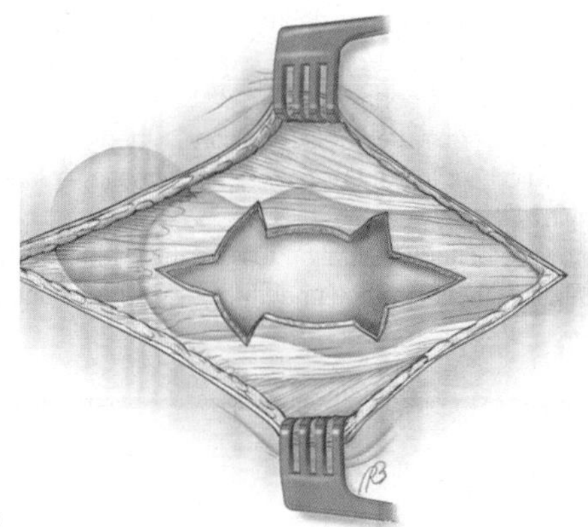
B

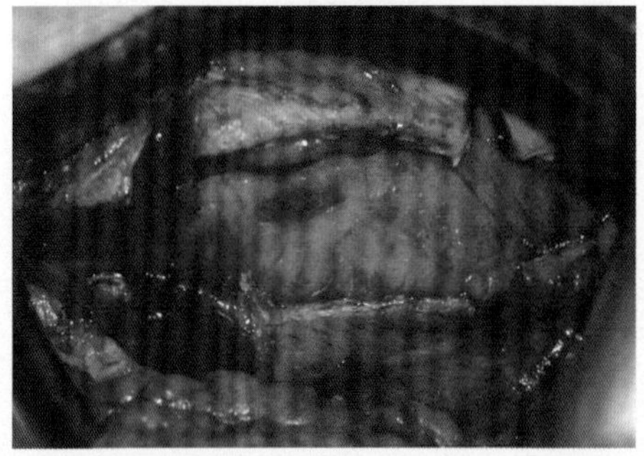
C

TECH FIG 3 • Our preferred approach includes an 8- to 10-cm longitudinal incision, posterior to the midpoint of the greater trochanter, with two pairs of 1- to 1.5-cm transverse incisions. This relaxes the iliotibial band, eliminating the snapping, without creating any suture repair lines that would necessitate prolonged convalescence. **A.** Incision pattern. **B.** Relaxing response to incision. **C.** Appearance at surgery. (Courtesy of J. W. Thomas Byrd, MD.)

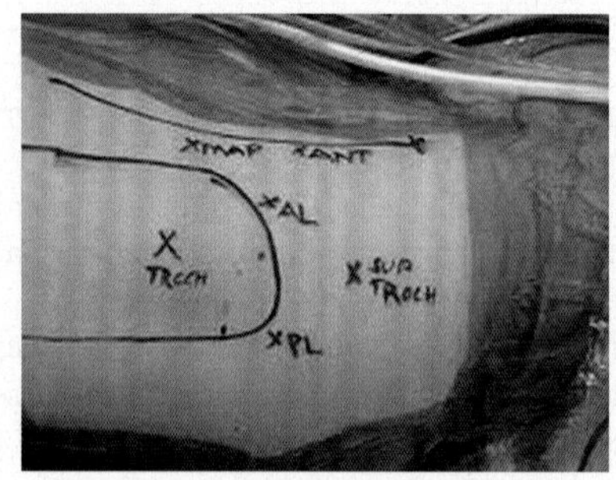

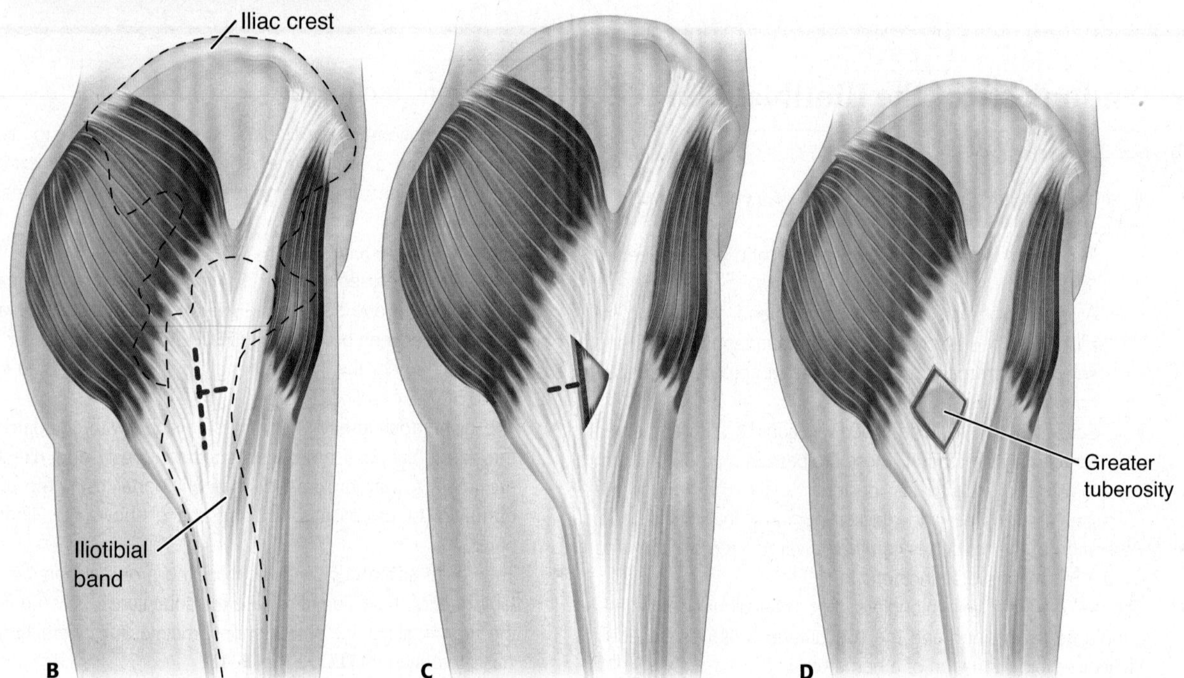

TECH FIG 4 • A. Portal sites marked for endoscopic iliotibial band tendoplasty. Illustrated as *troch* and *sup troch* for distal and proximal trochanteric portals, respectively. **B–D.** Endoscopic method of iliotibial band tendoplasty, shown in the right hip. **B.** After creating the longitudinal incision, the anterior limb is created by a perpendicular incision. **C.** Resecting the edges creates a triangle that aids in visualization of the underlying structures. **D.** The posterior limb is then created, and resection completes the diamond pattern of the tendoplasty. (**A:** Courtesy of Sean McMillan, DO; **D:** Adapted from Ilizaliturri VM Jr, Martinez-Escalante FA, Chaidez PA, et al. Endoscopic iliotibial band release for external snapping hip syndrome. Arthroscopy 2006;22:505–510.)

- A 4- to 5-cm longitudinal retrograde incision within the tendon is created using a shaver and/or an RF probe, beginning at the level of the distal viewing portal.
- An anteriorly based 2-cm transverse incision is then made at midpoint of vertical cut and the flaps resected, creating a long, obtuse triangle.
  - This provides better visualization to determine the relation of the iliotibial band and the underlying greater trochanter.
- Lastly, a posterior transverse incision is made at the same level as the anterior incision and the flaps excised, creating a diamond-shaped pattern of resection.
  - This release is most important and performed until snapping has ceased.
- The greater trochanteric bursa can be removed through the defect and abductor tendons inspected for tears.
- A compressive dressing is applied to minimize the formation of a hematoma.

PEARLS AND PITFALLS

Visualization	■ With any endoscopic technique, good visualization is essential. Poor visualization will result in a poorly performed procedure. Visualization is facilitated by use of a high-flow fluid management system and control of hemostasis by keeping the systolic blood pressure below 100 mm Hg, adding diluted epinephrine to the fluid, and judicious use of cauterization.
Violation of iliopsoas tendon	■ Surgical violation of the iliopsoas tendon carries the risk of heterotopic ossification in either an open or arthroscopic procedure. It is prudent to use pharmacologic prophylaxis for this condition.
Failure to fully release tendon	■ The iliopsoas tendon forms from the psoas and iliacus muscles. The tendon sometimes may remain bifid all the way to its insertion on the lesser trochanter. Whether addressing the tendon from the peripheral compartment (**FIG 5A–G**) or from its insertion within the iliopsoas bursa (**FIG 5H,I**), if the tendon looks inordinately small, search for a separate portion of the tendon. Failure to fully release the tendon fibers may result in incomplete resolution of the snapping.

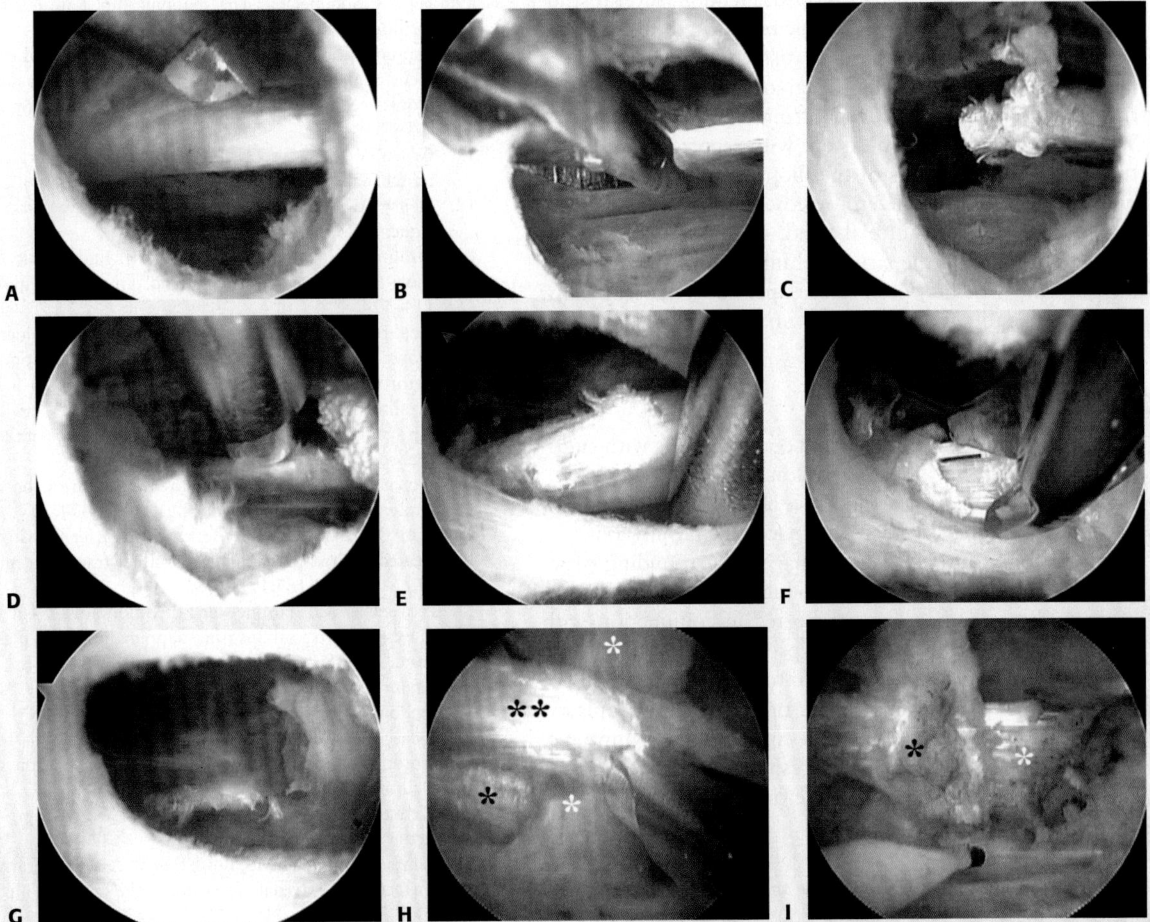

FIG 5 • **A–G.** The iliopsoas tendon of the right hip is exposed from the peripheral compartment. **A.** The initial tendon viewed through a capsular window is fully identified but is abnormally small. **B.** This tendon is released with a basket. **C.** A stump remains. **D.** This is resected with a shaver. **E.** Further dissection exposes a more substantial portion of the iliopsoas tendon. **F.** This is released as well. **G.** Complete release of the bifid tendon is documented. **H,I.** Viewing the iliopsoas tendon of a right hip at its insertion on the lesser trochanter within the iliopsoas bursa. **H.** A bifid iliopsoas tendon is identified with medial (*black asterisk*) and lateral (*two black asterisks*) bands separated by a vessel (*two white asterisks*) coursing perpendicularly. **I.** The lateral band (*black asterisk*) has been released with a flexible RF device, revealing the medial band (*white asterisk*) which subsequently is released. (Courtesy of J. W. Thomas Byrd, MD.)

Inadequate tendoplasty	■ Inadequate tendoplasty of the iliotibial band can result in incomplete resolution of symptoms, but excessive release can compromise the functional integrity of the abductor mechanism, rendering it virtually unsalvageable.
Proper diagnosis	■ With proper diagnosis, the surgical results for snapping of the iliopsoas tendon and the iliotibial band are highly predictable and finite in terms of resolution of the snapping. ■ However, the subjective response to surgery is highly dependent on the patient's expectations and motivations, which are equally essential in the evaluation process.

POSTOPERATIVE CARE

- After these procedures, the patient is capable of full weight bearing, but crutches are used for about 2 weeks until the gait pattern is normalized.
- Gentle range-of-motion, closed-chain, and stabilization exercises are introduced as symptoms allow.
- For iliopsoas release, aggressive hip flexion strengthening is avoided for the first 6 weeks; for the iliotibial band, aggressive stretching generally is not necessary.
- The patient should not anticipate returning to vigorous activities for at least 3 months.

OUTCOMES

- For endoscopic release of the iliopsoas tendon, several studies have reported highly predictable results in terms of eliminating the snapping and patient satisfaction.[3,13]
- Heterotopic ossification has been observed following arthroscopic release of the iliopsoas from the lesser trochanter.[13]
- These observations are consistent with reports in the literature on open techniques of the iliopsoas tendon that have noted a propensity for heterotopic bone formation.[18]
- For snapping of the iliotibial band, tendon-relaxing procedures that maintain the structural integrity of the abductor mechanism, whether performed open or endoscopically, have predictably corrected the snapping with minimal morbidity.[5,9,20]

COMPLICATIONS

- No reports have been published of complications with endoscopic release of the iliopsoas tendon.
- Cases of heterotopic ossification have been observed, for which Ilizaliturri has recommended pharmacologic prophylaxis.[13]
- Potential complication due to damage to surrounding structures (eg, femoral neurovascular bundle)
- No complications have been reported in conjunction with the less extensive tendon-relaxing procedures for a snapping iliotibial band. Careful attention to the precision of the release can help avoid inadequate or excessive tendoplasty. Inadequate release could result in residual symptoms, whereas excessive release could result in a virtually unsalvageable compromise of the abductor mechanism.

REFERENCES

1. Allen WC, Cope R. Coxa saltans: the snapping hip revisited. J Am Acad Orthop Surg 1995;3:303–308.
2. Brignall CG, Stainsby GD. The snapping hip, treatment by Z-plasty. J Bone Joint Surg Br 1991;73B:253–254.
3. Byrd JWT. Evaluation and management of the snapping iliopsoas tendon. Instr Course Lect 2006;55:347–355.
4. Byrd JWT. Evaluation and management of the snapping iliopsoas tendon. Tech Orthop 2005;20:45–51.
5. Byrd JWT. Snapping hip. Oper Tech Sports Med 2005:13:46–54.
6. Contreras ME, Dani WS, Endges WK, et al. Arthroscopic treatment of the snapping iliopsoas tendon through the central compartment of the hip. A pilot study. J Bone Joint Surg Br 2010;92:777–780.
7. Dobbs MB, Gordon JE, Luhmann SJ, et al. Surgical correction of the snapping iliopsoas tendon in adolescents. J Bone Joint Surg Am 2002;84A:420–424.
8. Faraj AA, Moulton A, Sirivastava VM. Snapping iliotibial band. Report of ten cases and review of the literature. Acta Orthop Belg 2001;67:19–23.
9. Fery A, Sommelet J. The snapping hip. Late results of 24 cases. Int Orthop 1988;12:277–282.
10. Flanum ME, Keene JS, Blankenbaker DG, et al. Arthroscopic treatment of the painful "internal" snapping hip: results of a new endoscopic technique and imaging protocol. Am J Sports Med 2007:35: 770–779.
11. Gruen GS, Scioscia TN, Lowenstein JE. The surgical treatment of internal snapping hip. Am J Sports Med 2002;30:607–613.
12. Henry AK. Extensile Exposure, ed 2. New York: Churchill Livingstone, 1973.
13. Ilizaliturri VM, Camacho-Galindo J. Endoscopic release of the iliopsoas tendon and iliotibial band. Oper Tech Sports Med 2011;19: 114–124.
14. Ilizaliturri VM Jr, Martinez-Escalante FA, Chaidez PA, et al. Endoscopic iliotibial band release for external snapping hip syndrome. Arthroscopy 2006;22:505–510.
15. Ilizaliturri VM Jr, Villalobos FE Jr, Chaidez PA, et al. Internal snapping hip syndrome: treatment by endoscopic release of the iliopsoas tendon. Arthroscopy 2005;21:1375–1380.
16. Jacobson T, Allen WC. Surgical correction of the snapping iliopsoas tendon. Am J Sports Med 1990; 18:470–474.
17. Kim DH, Baechler MF, Berkowitz MJ, et al. Coxa saltans externa treated with Z-plasty of the iliotibial tract in a military population. Mil Med 2002;167:172–173.
18. Provencher MT, Hofmeister EP, Muldoon MP. The surgical treatment of external coxa saltans (the snapping hip) by Z-plasty of the iliotibial band. Am J Sports Med 2004;32:470–476.
19. Taylor GR, Clarke NMP. Surgical release of the "snapping iliopsoas tendon." J Bone Joint Surg Br 1995;77B:881–883.
20. Velasco AD, Allan DB, Wroblewski BM. Psoas tenotomy and heterotopic ossification after Charnley low-friction arthroplasty. Clin Orthop Relat Res 1993;291:93–95.
21. Wettstein M, Jung J, Dienst M. Arthroscopic psoas tenotomy. Arthroscopy 2006;22:907.e1–e4.
22. White RA, Hughes MS, Burd T, et al. A new operative approach in the correction of external coxa saltans: the snapping hip. Am J Sports Med 2004;32:1504–1508.

Athletic Pubalgia and Adductor Injuries

2

CHAPTER

Kostas Economopoulos and Anikar Chhabra

DEFINITION

- Although the term *sports hernia* is commonly used in the media, *athletic pubalgia* is a more appropriate term to describe the constellation of injuries causing chronic groin pain in athletes.
  - Diagnosis of the cause of groin pain is difficult due to the complex anatomy of the groin and the fact that two or more injuries may coexist.
  - Intra-abdominal pathology, genitourinary abnormalities, referred lumbosacral pain, and hip joint disorders must first be excluded.
- Adductor strains are the most common cause of groin pain in athletes.
  - The adductors are usually strained during eccentric contraction of the muscles. The injury often occurs at the myotendinous junction, but the strain also can occur in the tendon itself or its bony insertion.
  - Other muscles in and around the groin region also can be strained, including the rectus femoris, the sartorius, abdominal muscles, and the conjoint tendon.
- *Sports hernia* is a condition of chronic groin pain that is caused by a tear in the inguinal floor without a clinically obvious hernia.[7,11]
  - Sports hernias result in an occult injury that usually is not identified by most examiners. However, with increasing experience, the examiner can feel an abnormal inguinal floor and appreciate abnormal tenderness inside the external ring.
  - In contrast, indirect and direct hernias involve easily palpable defects in the inguinal canal or through the anterior abdominal musculature, respectively.
  - Duration of symptoms typically is months, and pain is resistant to conservative measures.
- *Osteitis pubis* is characterized by symphysis pain and joint disruption and occurs commonly in distance runners and soccer players.
  - It may be difficult to distinguish from adductor strains, and the two conditions may coincide.
- Stress fractures are rare injuries that result from repetitive cyclic loading of the bone.
  - The pubic rami are the most common location for stress fractures in the pelvis. These fractures are most common in long-distance runners.

ANATOMY

- The anatomy in and around the groin is complex (**FIG 1**), and a thorough understanding of it is crucial in diagnosing the various groin injuries.
- In terms of athletic pubalgia, the pelvis is considered to contain two joints: the commonly known ball-and-socket of

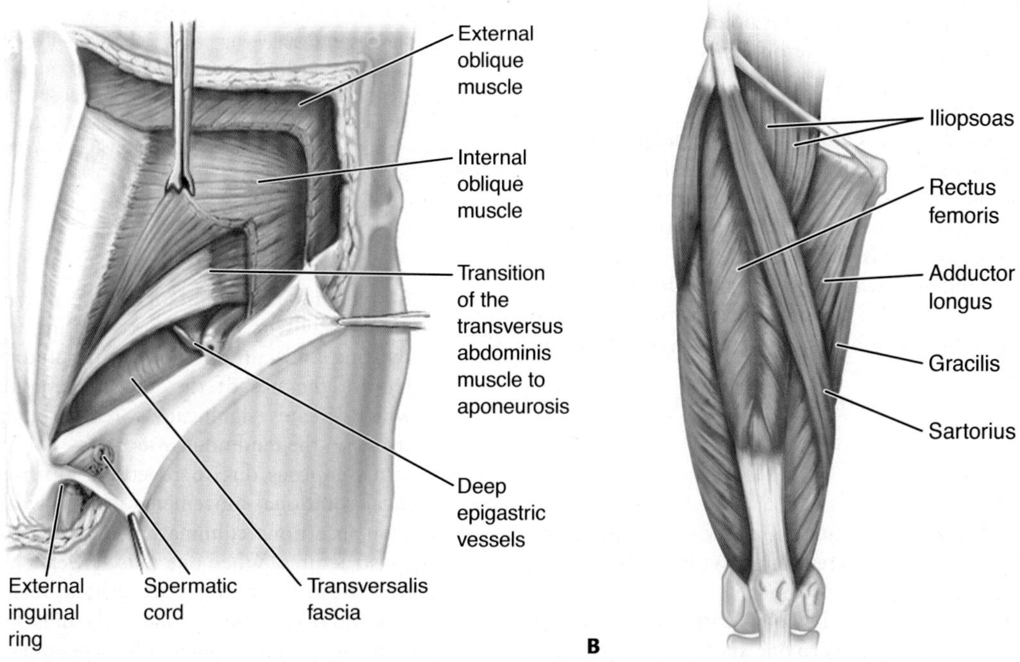

FIG 1 • Anatomy of the abdominal (**A**) and groin (**B**) musculature.

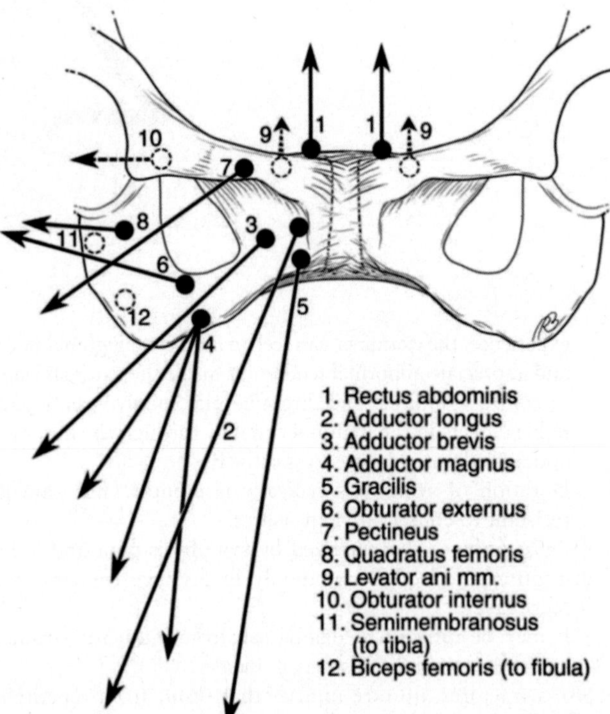

FIG 2 • Pubic bone joint. The pubic bone joint is made up of the anterior bone structures of the pelvis and all of the soft tissue attachments to the pubic bones. This diagram shows the many structures which attach to the anterior pelvis and the forces that are placed on the pubic bone joint. (Reprinted with permission from Meyers WC, Greenleaf R, Saad A. Anatomic basis for evaluation of abdominal and groin pain in athletes. Oper Tech Sports Med 2005;13:55–61.)

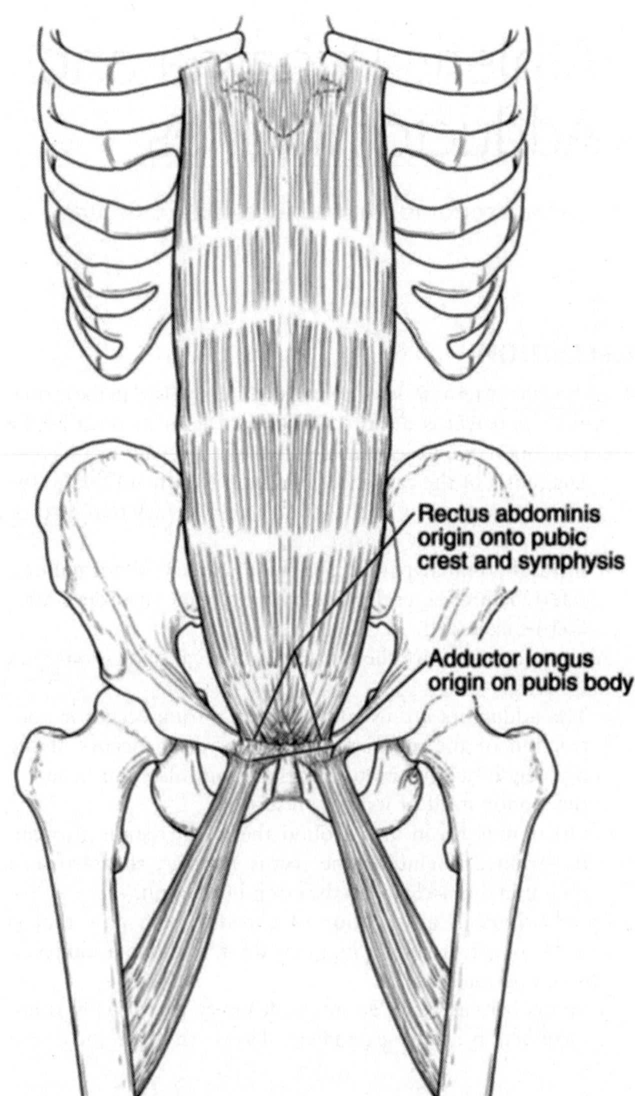

FIG 3 • Abdominis rectus and adductor attachments. The most important muscles in maintaining pelvis stability are the abdominis rectus and adductor muscles. These structures have a common attachment site on the anterior pubis and pull the pelvis in opposite directions. (Reprinted with permission from Meyers WC, Greenleaf R, Saad A. Anatomic basis for evaluation of abdominal and groin pain in athletes. Oper Tech Sports Med 2007;15:165–177.)

the hip joint and the second, less well known "pubic bone joint."
  - The pubic bone joint consists of a large, complex rotational joint that involves both pubic bones and all the soft tissue attachments on either side of the pubis (**FIG 2**).
  - The pubic symphysis is the center point of the pubic bone joint and is the site of numerous musculotendinous attachments that act to dynamically stabilize the position of the anterior pelvis.
  - The abdominal muscles attaching to the pubic symphysis consist of the external and internal oblique muscles, transversus abdominis, and rectus abdominis. The thigh adductors attaching to the pelvis include the pectineus, gracilis, adductor longus, brevis, and magnus.
- The posterior inguinal wall consists primarily of the transversalis fascia, along with the conjoint tendon, made up of the internal abdominal oblique and transversus abdominis aponeuroses.[7]
- The conjoint tendon inserts onto the pubic tubercle and along the iliopubic tract.

PATHOGENESIS

- The most robust and important muscles for maintaining stability of the anterior pelvis are the rectus abdominis and the adductor longus muscles.
  - These muscle groups pull the pelvis with opposite vectors and function as antagonists to one another during flexion, extension, and rotation of the pelvis (**FIG 3**).
  - A tremendous amount of torque is created at the level of the pelvis in athletes participating in sports requiring twisting and cutting. The cutting and twisting activities require the use of the abdominal and pelvic muscles, which creates significant force through the pelvis and stress on the tendinous insertions.
- Overuse injuries due to repetitive hip hyperextension and truncal rotational movements lead to wear and tear of the tendon insertions culminating in partial or full tearing of these structures. When one muscle weakens or its associated tendon torn, the result is an unequal distribution of pelvic forces and overpulling of one of the muscles leading to more anterior or posterior pelvic tilt, depending on which muscle or tendon is injured.

NATURAL HISTORY

- A majority of acute adductor strains will improve with appropriate conservative treatment over a course of 2 to 6 weeks. However, if not properly rehabilitated, an adductor injury may progress to chronic strains or tendinopathy.
- Recovery from athletic pubalgia varies greatly from athlete to athlete. Although many athletes will get improvement with rest and conservative treatment, recurrent symptoms are common after returning to play. A small subset of patients will improve with nonoperative treatment; however, most patients who have been accurately diagnosed with athletic pubalgia will eventually require surgical repair.[7,13] A hallmark of sports hernias is that patients have less pain when they are inactive and more pain when active.
- Osteitis pubis is self-limited but may take, on average, about 9 months to heal.[5]

PATIENT HISTORY AND PHYSICAL FINDINGS

- Patient history is the most important aspect of the evaluation of athletic pubalgia.
- The patient must be asked for duration of symptoms, any inciting events, relieving and exacerbating factors, and timing of pain.
- A thorough hip examination must be performed to rule out intra-articular hip sources of pain such as labral tears and femoroacetabular impingement (FAI).
  - Flexion, adduction, and internal rotation of the hip are used to identify anterior FAI. The FABER test (flexion, abduction, and external rotation of the hip) is used to identify posterior impingement.
  - Decreased hip internal rotation is common in patients with cam-lesion FAI. Internal rotation of less than 25 degrees is considered abnormal.
  - Hip flexion against resistance: tests the strength of the iliopsoas and may detect a strain or tear of this muscle.
- Groin examination:
  - Palpation of the insertion of the rectus and origin of the adductors can identify partial tears, inflammation, or injury to these tendons.
  - Palpation of insertion of conjoint tendon: Tenderness may increase, and a bulge may be felt by having the patient perform a Valsalva maneuver.
  - Straight-leg raise: In patients with radicular low back pain, this will reproduce the pain they are having.
  - Groin adduction resistance: helps to diagnose an adductor strain or tear
  - Palpation of the pubic symphysis: characteristic of osteitis pubis
  - Ober test: Patient's inability to lower the upper leg completely to the examination table is pathognomonic of a tight iliotibial band.

IMAGING AND OTHER DIAGNOSTIC STUDIES

- Three views of the affected hip should be obtained including anteroposterior (AP), lateral, and Dunn view to evaluate for possible FAI.
- Radiographs can be helpful in excluding fractures or avulsions.[4]
  - Stress fractures usually are not evident on radiographs.
- Magnetic resonance imaging (MRI) can be used to confirm muscle strain or tears and partial or complete tendon tears (**FIG 4A**).
  - MRI has been used to detect sports hernias, although it is not always successful.[4]
  - MRI can also be used to evaluate for possible hip labral tears.
- Dynamic ultrasound has been found, in certain cases, to detect posterior wall defects but is highly operator dependent.[17]
- Herniography, which involves an intraperitoneal injection of contrast dye followed by fluoroscopy or radiography, has been shown to identify sports hernias but has limited sensitivity and a substantial risk of perforation in up to 5% of patients.[2]
- Osteitis pubis has characteristic radiologic findings, including bone resorption, widening of the pubic symphysis, and irregular contour of articular surfaces or periarticular sclerosis (**FIG 4B**).
  - A bone scan may show increased uptake in the area of the pubic symphysis in osteitis pubis; however, not all patients who have symptoms show an abnormality.[12]
  - MRI has become increasingly useful in the diagnosis of osteitis pubis. Findings can include bone marrow edema or symphysial disc extrusion.[16]

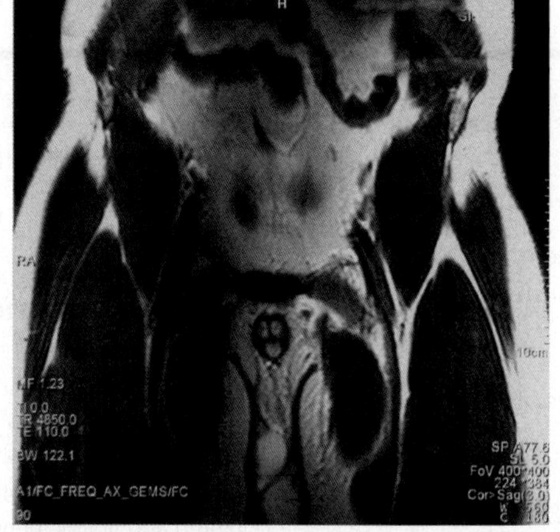

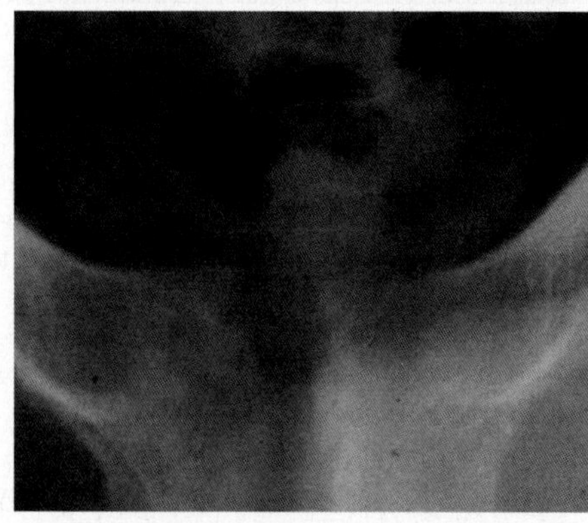

FIG 4 • **A.** MRI of an adductor tear in a hockey player. There is increased signal at the origin of the adductor tendon near the pubis. **B.** Characteristic radiograph of osteitis pubis. Notice the bone resorption, widening of the pubic symphysis, and irregular contour of articular surfaces.

DIFFERENTIAL DIAGNOSIS

- Groin disruption or strain
- Labral tear of the hip
- Cam or pincer FAI
- Osteitis pubis
- Pelvic stress fractures
- Indirect and direct hernia
- Avascular necrosis of the hip
- Hip osteoarthritis
- Abdominal muscle tear
- Lumbar radiculopathy
- Nerve entrapment
- Tumors
- Genitourinary problems
- Inflammatory bowel disease
- Endometriosis
- Pelvic inflammatory disease

NONOPERATIVE MANAGEMENT

- Initial treatment for lower abdominal strains or groin injuries consists of activity modification, anti-inflammatory medication, and physical therapy.
  - Core-strengthening exercises target the abdomen, lumbar spine, and hips.
  - Stretching focuses on the hip rotators, adductors, and hamstrings.
  - The goal of therapy is to correct the imbalance of the hip and pelvic muscle stabilizers.[18]
  - After 4 to 6 weeks, the athlete gradually returns to sport-specific activities as tolerated.
  - Acute treatment of adductor strain includes rest, ice, compression, and elevation.
  - The next goal is restoration of range of motion (ROM) and prevention of atrophy. Once the patient can tolerate this, the focus should be to regain strength, flexibility, and endurance.[8]
- Nonoperative management of athletic pubalgia includes physical therapy, anti-inflammatory drugs, and corticosteroid injections at the site of pain.[1,9]
- Osteitis pubis is a self-limiting condition; therapy should focus on hip ROM as well as adductor stretching and strengthening.
  - Corticosteroid injection in osteitis pubis is controversial but may be helpful in select populations of athletic patients.[10,16]
- Treatment in pelvic stress fractures is straightforward and involves 4 to 6 weeks of rest from the activities aggravating the area.

SURGICAL MANAGEMENT

- Surgical exploration and repair is indicated if nonoperative treatment fails and alternative diagnoses have been excluded.
- Three general categories of surgical repair are described, including pelvic floor repair with mesh, primary pelvic floor repair without mesh, and laparoscopic mesh repair.
- There is no consensus to which surgical approach is best.
- Some feel the use of mesh in athletes is not recommended due to the localized stiffness of the abdominal muscles and restricted movement caused by the mesh.[15]
- Our preferred management of adductor injuries that occur in conjunction with athletic pubalgia is to treat the underlying inguinal floor injury surgically and to manage the adductor component by therapy and rehabilitation.

Preoperative Planning

- Preoperative planning involves extreme care to ascertain that the patient truly has athletic pubalgia and not another disease process. This requires a complete history and physical examination performed by an examiner who understands the pathophysiology of this injury.
- The preoperative MRI can be used to plan the surgery. Evaluation of the rectus insertion can help in determining whether a formal rectus repair is necessary compared to simply tightening the muscle insertion.

Positioning

- The patient is positioned supine and draped with the affected groin exposed.

Anesthesia

- We use general anesthesia for our surgery.
- Preemptive analgesia is important to reduce postoperative pain and to make the anesthetic experience smoother. Also, local anesthesia is bactericidal, reducing the risk of infection.
- We suggest 0.25% Marcaine with epinephrine and sodium bicarbonate.

TECHNIQUES

The Minimal Repair Technique

Incision, Dissection, and Site Evaluation

- The incision is made along the path of the inguinal ligament, 1 cm medial and superior to the ligament. A length of 5 to 6 cm is adequate.
- Dissection is performed down to the external oblique fascia.
- The external oblique is incised to the external ring, and the fascia is mobilized both medially and laterally.
- The spermatic cord is carefully evaluated and mobilized.
- The strength of the posterior inguinal wall is evaluated by digital palpation.
- Typically, a circumscribed weakness is found in the posterior wall with the surrounding tissue being firm and intact (**TECH FIG 1A**).

Repair

- The transversalis fascia is split, starting in the area of the defect toward the deep internal ring (**TECH FIG 1B**).
- The transversalis fascia is only opened in the area where weakness is appreciated, and normal tissue is not opened.
- The genital branch of the genitofemoral nerve is assessed.
  - If the nerve is uninjured, it is retracted out of the zone of injury.
  - If the nerve is entrapped, a neurolysis is performed.
  - A severely injured and fibrotic nerve is resected.

- A continuous 2-0 Prolene suture (suture I) is performed from the medial toward the deep inguinal ring, creating a free fascial lip out of the iliopubic tract (**TECH FIG 1C**).
- The suture is then reversed and run toward the pubic bone (**TECH FIG 1D**).
  - The free lip is then included in the suture and brought to the inguinal ligament.
- A second suture (suture II) is used to stabilize or repair the rectus abdominis. If a tear is present, a primary repair back down to the pubis is performed. If the insertion of the rectus is attenuated but not torn, suture II is used to lateralize the rectus. This is accomplished by suturing the lateral edge of the rectus to the transversalis fascia (**TECH FIG 1E**).
  - This second suture is used to lateralize the rectus abdominis if no tear is present. This suture counteracts the increased tension at the pubic bone caused by the retraction of the rectus muscle in the upward and medial direction.
- Marcaine is injected thoroughly, and the external oblique, Scarpa fascia, and skin are closed with an absorbable suture.

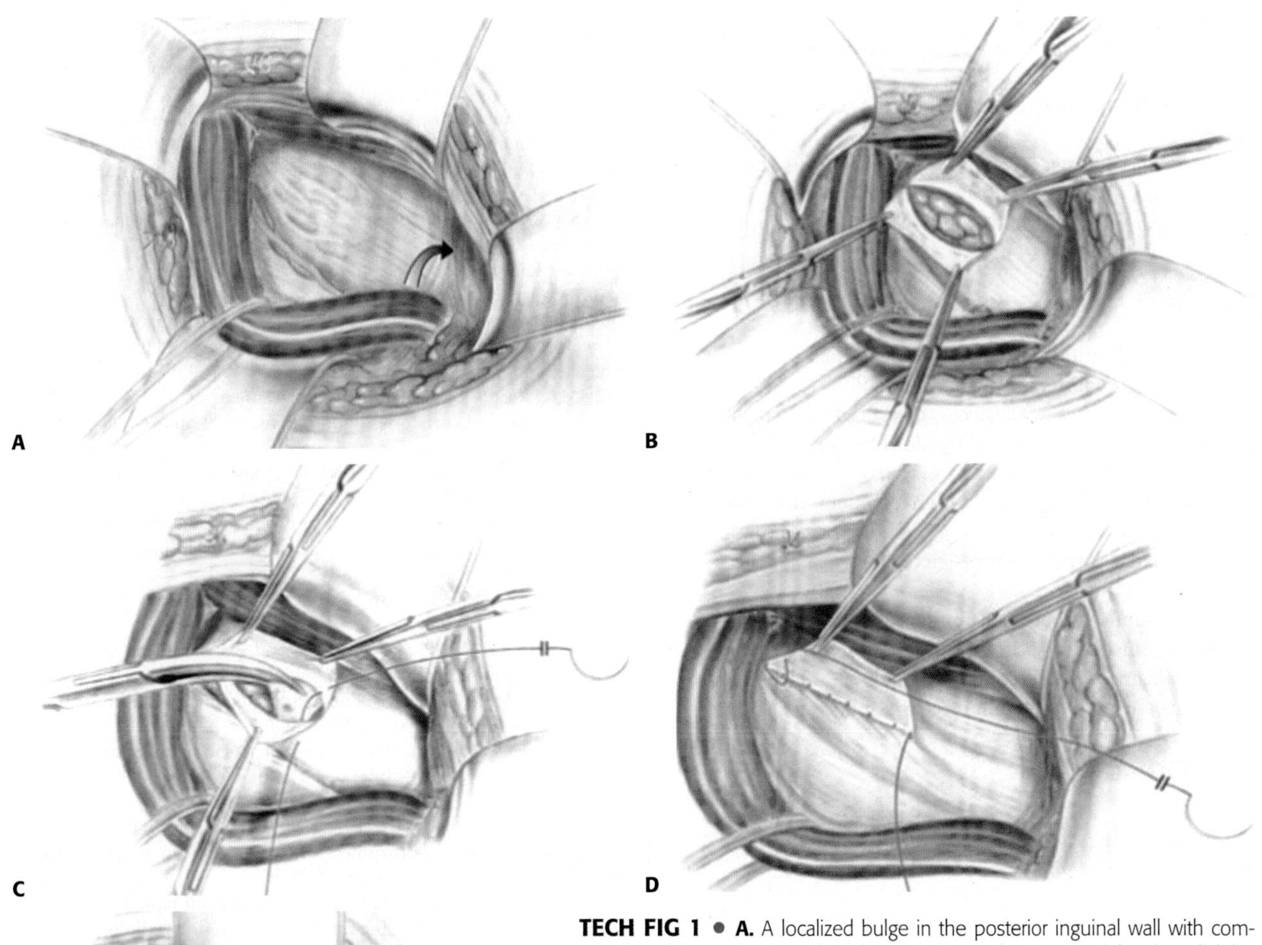

TECH FIG 1 • **A.** A localized bulge in the posterior inguinal wall with compression of the genital branch of the genitofemoral nerve. Cranial and medial displacement of the rectus abdominis muscle with increasing tension at the pubic bone. **B.** Only the defect is opened and, if necessary, resection of the genital branch of the genitofemoral nerve is performed. **C.** A continuous suture (suture I) is run from the medial toward the deep inguinal ring, creating a free lip. A Prolene 2-0 is typically used. **D.** Suture I is then reversed in its course toward the pubic bone and the free border is included in the suture and brought to the inguinal ligament. **E.** A second 2-0 Prolene (suture II) is used to repair a tear of the insertion of the rectus muscle or lateralize the rectus if the insertion is not torn. The 2-0 Prolene is run through the insertion of the rectus and run up and down the transversalis fascia lateralizing the rectus insertion. (Reprinted with permission from Economopoulos KJ, Milewski MD, Hanks JB, et al. Sports hernia treatment: modified Bassini versus minimal repair. Sports Health 2013;5:463–469.)

PEARLS AND PITFALLS

- Operate only if the patient has a good mechanism of injury, a good history, and clear indications on physical examination.
- Evaluation of the genital branch of the genitofemoral nerve is important. An injured nerve should be decompressed, or the injured section excised, to decrease groin pain.
- Rule out hip pathology such as FAI and labral tears as a source of the pain.
- Rectus repair or lateralization with a second suture is necessary for a good outcome.

POSTOPERATIVE CARE

- The goal of rehabilitation is to establish a full, normal ROM and flexibility followed by incremental increases in resistance for strength training.
- Athletes are permitted to lift up to 20 kg immediately after surgery.
- Biking with no resistance may be started on the second postoperative day.
- Runners should be running in 2 weeks and golfers golfing in 1 week.
- Contact athletes should be able to return to competition in 3 to 4 weeks.

OUTCOMES

- With appropriate indications and surgical technique, success rates in sports hernia repair have been as high as 97% to 100% in high-performance athletes, with success measured as a return to previous levels of performance and freedom from pain.[6,14]
- Using the minimal repair technique, 96.1% of patients resumed training at the 4-week point. The median time to return to training was 7 days. In a subset of professional athletes, 83.7% had returned to unrestricted sports activities at the 1-month follow-up.[15]
- Our own study found patients who underwent the minimal repair technique returned to sports at a median of 5.6 weeks, which was significantly faster compared with the modified Bassini repair group, with the median return of 25.8 weeks.[3]

COMPLICATIONS

- Recurrence
- Thigh pain in the early postoperative period
- Infection
- Hematoma
- Continued pain

REFERENCES

1. Ashby EC. Chronic obscure groin pain is commonly caused by enthesopathy: "tennis elbow" of the groin. Br J Surg 1994;81(11):1632–1634.
2. Calder F, Evans R, Neilson D, et al. Value of herniography in the management of occult hernia and chronic groin pain in adults. Br J Surg 2000;87(6):824–825.
3. Economopoulos KJ, Milewski MD, Hanks JB, et al. Sports hernia treatment: modified Bassini versus minimal repair. Sports Health 2013;5(5):463–469.
4. Ekberg O, Sjoberg S, Westlin N. Sports-related groin pain: evaluation with MR imaging. Eur Radiol 1996;6(1):52–55.
5. Fricker PA, Taunton JE, Ammann W. Osteitis pubis in athletes. Infection, inflammation or injury? Sports Med 1991;12(4):266–279.
6. Genitsaris M, Goulimaris I, Sikas N. Laparoscopic repair of groin pain in athletes. Am J Sports Med 2004;32(5):1238–1242.
7. Hackney RG. The sports hernia: a cause of chronic groin pain. Br J Sports Med 1993;27(1):58–62.
8. Holmich P. Adductor related groin pain in athletes. Sports Med Arthroscopy Rev 1997;5:285–291.
9. Holmich P, Uhrskou P, Ulnits L, et al. Effectiveness of active physical training as treatment for long-standing adductor-related groin pain in athletes: randomised trial. Lancet 1999;353(9151):439–443.
10. Holt MA, Keene JS, Graf BK, et al. Treatment of osteitis pubis in athletes. Results of corticosteroid injections. Am J Sports Med 1995; 23(5):601–606.
11. Joesting DR. Diagnosis and treatment of sportsman's hernia. Curr Sports Med Rep 2002;1(2):121–124.
12. Karlsson J, Jerre R. The use of radiography, magnetic resonance, and ultrasound in the diagnosis of hip, pelvis, and groin injuries. Sports Med Arthroscopy Rev 1997;5268–5273.
13. LeBlanc KE, LeBlanc KA. Groin pain in athletes. Hernia 2003;7(2): 68–71.
14. Meyers WC, Foley DP, Garrett WE, et al. Management of severe lower abdominal or inguinal pain in high-performance athletes. PAIN (Performing Athletes with Abdominal or Inguinal Neuromuscular Pain Study Group). Am J Sports Med 2000;28(1):2–8.
15. Muschaweck U, Berger L. Minimal repair technique of sportsmen's groin: an innovative open-suture repair to treat chronic inguinal pain. Hernia 2010;14(1):27–33.
16. O'Connell MJ, Powell T, McCaffrey NM, et al. Symphyseal cleft injection in the diagnosis and treatment of osteitis pubis in athletes. AJR Am J Roentgenol 2002;179(4):955–959.
17. Orchard JW, Read JW, Neophyton J, et al. Groin pain associated with ultrasound finding of inguinal canal posterior wall deficiency in Australian Rules footballers. Br J Sports Med 1998;32(2): 134–139.
18. Taylor DC. Abdominal musculature abnormalities as a cause of groin pain in athletes. Inguinal hernias and pubalgia. Am J Sports Med 1991; 19:239–242.

Hip Arthroscopy: The Basics

Marc Safran, Michael Kalisvaart, and Matthew A. Stanich

3

CHAPTER

DEFINITION

- The hip is increasingly recognized as a source of pain owing to heightened awareness of pathologies, recent research, enhanced imaging techniques, and greater popularity of hip arthroscopy as a diagnostic and therapeutic tool.
- Hip arthroscopy first was performed on a cadaver in the 1930s by Burman, but it was not performed regularly until the 1980s, serving mostly as a tool for diagnosis and simple treatments, such as loose body removal, synovial biopsy, and partial labrectomy.
- With improvements in instrumentation, indications for hip arthroscopy have expanded because surgeons now are able to do more in the hip with decreased risk of iatrogenic injury. Furthermore, enhanced imaging techniques have allowed noninvasive diagnosis, and research has led to increased understanding of hip pathologies, furthering interest in this procedure.
- Hip arthroscopy can be performed in the central compartment (femoroacetabular joint) and peripheral compartment (along the femoral neck), which also has expanded the indications and success of hip arthroscopy, propagating the popularity of this procedure.

ANATOMY

- The hip joint is a multiaxial ball-and-socket type of synovial joint in which the head of the femur (ball) articulates with the acetabulum (socket) of the hip.
- Articular cartilage covers the head of the femur and acetabulum but is not present at the fovea or cotyloid fossa.
  - The articular cartilage of the femoral head and acetabulum is relatively thin compared with that of the knee (**FIG 1A**).
- The acetabular labrum is a triangular fibrocartilage that attaches to the rim of the acetabulum at the articular cartilage edge, except at the inferior most region of the acetabulum, where the transverse acetabular ligament extends the acetabular rim.
- The hip joint is enclosed by a capsule that is formed by an external fibrous layer and internal synovial membrane and attaches directly to the bony acetabular rim.
- The fibrous layer consists of the iliofemoral, pubofemoral, and ischiofemoral ligaments, which anchor the head of the femur into the acetabulum (**FIG 1B,C**).
- The ligamentum teres is extracapsular and travels from the central acetabulum to the foveal portion of the femoral head (**FIG 1A**).
- The major arteries supplying the hip joint include the medial and lateral circumflex femoral arteries, which branch to provide the retinacular arteries that supply the head and neck of the femur (**FIG 1D**).
- The artery to the head of the femur also supplies blood and transverses the ligament of the head of the femur (ie, the ligamentum teres).
- The labrum has a relatively low healing potential because vessels penetrate only the outermost layer of the capsular surface.
- Pertinent extra-articular neurovascular structures near the hip joint include the lateral femoral cutaneous nerve, femoral nerve, superior gluteal nerve, sciatic nerve, and the ascending branch of the lateral circumflex femoral artery.
- The lateral femoral cutaneous nerve, formed from the posterior divisions of L2 and L3 nerve roots, supplies the skin sensation of the lateral thigh. It travels from the pelvis just distal and medial to the anterior superior iliac spine (ASIS) and divides into more than three branches distal to the ASIS.
- The femoral nerve and artery run together with the femoral vein. They pass under the inguinal ligament midway between the ASIS and the pubic symphysis, with the nerve being most lateral and the vein most medial but being mostly superficial at the level of the hip.
  - The femoral nerve is 3.2 cm from the anterior hip portal but slightly closer at the level of the capsule.
- The superior gluteal nerve, formed from the posterior divisions of L4, L5, and S1, passes posterior and lateral to the obturator internus and piriformis muscles, then between the gluteus medius and minimus muscles approximately 4 cm proximal to the hip joint.
- The sciatic nerve, formed when nerves from L4 to S3 come together, passes anterior and inferior to the piriformis and posterior to the deep hip external rotators to supply the hamstrings and lower leg, foot, and ankle.
  - The sciatic nerve is 2.9 cm from the posterior hip arthroscopy portal but is closest at the level of the capsule.
  - Internally rotating or flexing the hip prior to making the posterior portal brings the nerve dangerously close to the arthroscope.
- The lateral femoral circumflex artery is a branch of the femoral artery that, along with the medial circumflex artery, forms a vascular ring about the neck of the femur, providing arteriole branches to supply the femoral head (**FIG 1D**).
- The lateral femoral circumflex artery is 3.7 cm inferior to the anterior arthroscopy portal; it is much closer at the level of the capsular entry of the arthroscope.

PATHOGENESIS

- Loose bodies can be ossified or nonossified and can either appear after traumatic hip injury or be associated with conditions such as osteochondritis dissecans and synovial chondromatosis.[8]

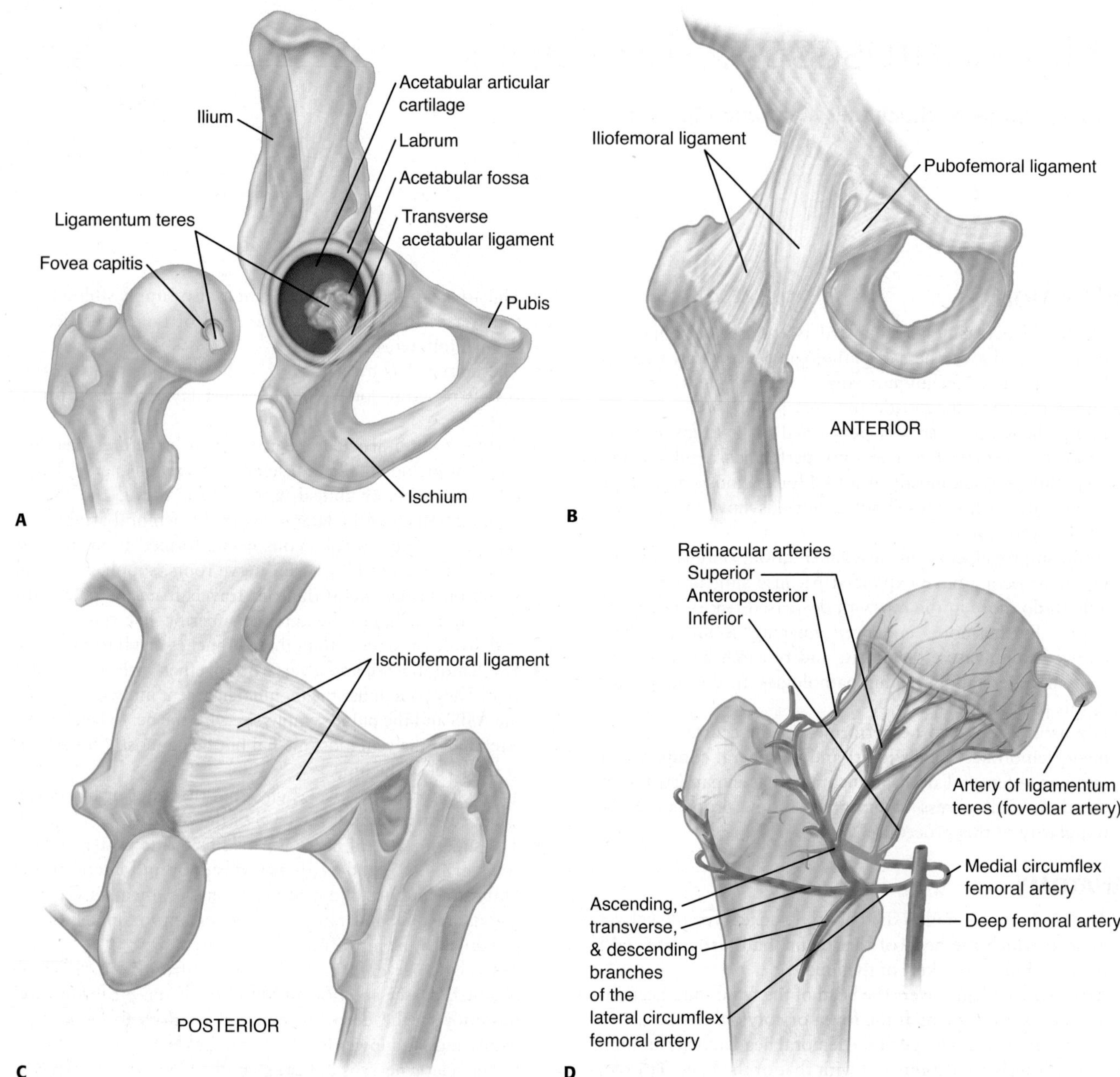

FIG 1 • Anatomy of the hip. **A.** Bony architecture of the hip joint with articular surfaces. Note the fovea and ligamentum teres. Also note the labrum does not continue along the inferior acetabulum and the lack of the articular cartilage on the inferior aspect of the acetabulum. **B,C.** Ligamentous anatomy. The iliofemoral and pubofemoral ligaments anteriorly and the ischiofemoral ligament posteriorly. **D.** Vascular anatomy. Note the medial and lateral circumflex arteries.

- Labral tear often results from hyperextension or external rotation of the hip and is more likely with hip dysplasia.
- Chondral (articular cartilage) damage can result from dislocation or subluxation of the hip or direct impact onto the hip and is associated with labral tears in more than half the cases.[9]
- Femoroacetabular impingement is a major cause of labral tears and chondral damage.
  - It usually occurs when there is loss of femoral head–neck offset (cam impingement), excessive acetabular coverage (eg, osteophytes, retroversion, overcorrection with pelvic osteotomy, protrusio acetabuli, or otto pelvis) (pincer impingement), or both.
  - The femoral head–neck junction abuts the acetabulum and labrum, resulting in tearing of the labrum, delamination of the articular cartilage, synovitis, and, eventually, arthritis.
- Ligamentum teres pathology may be due to ligament hypertrophy or partial or complete tearing and may be the result of trauma or degenerative joint disease (DJD).
  - Ligamentum hypertrophy or tearing may result in pain as a result of catching of a thickened or torn edge between the joint surfaces.
- DJD may be associated with loose bodies, labrum tears, chondral damage, ligamentum teres pathology, and synovitis.

- Avascular necrosis of the femoral head is primarily idiopathic but can be associated with corticosteroid use, alcohol consumption, fracture, and deep sea diving (caisson disease), among others.
- Synovial diseases such as pigmented villonodular synovitis, synovial chondromatosis, inflammatory arthritis, and osteochondromatosis can be sources of hip pain and joint damage.
- Hip instability, either traumatic or atraumatic, may be a cause of labral tears and chondral damage.
  - Hip instability may be traumatic (eg, acetabular posterior wall fractures) or atraumatic (eg, developmental dysplasia of the hip, connective tissue disorders, benign hypermobility) or as a result of microtrauma (repetitive external rotation).
  - Pathology exists as a spectrum from hip dislocation to subluxation to microinstability.

NATURAL HISTORY

- The natural history of most pathologies about the hip has not been studied; much of the purported natural history is therefore conjecture.
- Removal of loose bodies alleviates mechanical symptoms and reduces articular cartilage damage.
- Labral tears and chondral lesions that are débrided may result in degenerative arthritis.
- Untreated femoroacetabular impingement may result in degenerative arthritis.
- It has been proposed, but not proved, that labral repair or surgery for femoroacetabular impingement may lower the risk of developing DJD or slow the rate of degeneration.

PATIENT HISTORY AND PHYSICAL FINDINGS

- The patient history should include an investigation of the quality and location of pain, timing and precipitating cause of symptoms, and any referred pain.
- Patients with intra-articular pathology may have difficulty with torsional or twisting activities, discomfort with prolonged hip flexion (eg, sitting), pain or catching from flexion to extension (eg, rising from a seated position), and greater difficulty on inclines than on level surfaces.[2]
- Intra-articular pathology may be associated with groin pain extending to the knee and mechanical symptoms such as popping, locking, or restricted range of motion (ROM).[3]
  - The source of intra-articular pathology should be investigated in patients with continuous hip pain for longer than 4 weeks.
- Physical examination methods are summarized later.
  - It is important to follow a systemic approach to examination that includes inspection, palpation, ROM, strength, and special tests.[11]
- Intra-articular pathologies do not have palpable areas of tenderness, although compensation for long-standing intra-articular problems may result in tenderness of muscles or bursae.
- Motor strength and neurovascular examinations must be performed for the entire lower extremity.
- It is important to rule out other causes of pain referred to the hip.
  - Spinal pain usually is localized at the posterior buttock and sacroiliac region and may radiate to the lower extremity.
  - Injuries to the sacrum and sacroiliac joint are recognized by a positive gapping or transverse anterior stress test.
  - Abdominal injuries are recognized by basic inspection and palpation of the abdomen for a mass or fascial hernia, which can be evaluated by isometric contraction of the rectus abdominis and obliques.
  - Abdominal muscle injury is recognized by pain during contraction of the rectus abdominis and obliques.
  - Herniography may be used to rule out hernias.
    - Particularly difficult to diagnose is the sports hernia (Gilmore groin), which is not a true hernia.
  - Genitourinary tract
    - Injuries to the pelvic area, such as pubic symphysis and intrapelvic problems, are recognized by the gapping/transverse anterior stress test.
- Specific tests for the hip include the following:
  - McCarthy test: distinction of internal hip pathology such as torn acetabular labrum or lateral rim impingement
  - Stinchfield and Fulcrum test: diagnosis of internal derangements, primarily of the anterior portion of the acetabulum
  - Scour test: associated with microinstability or combined anterior anteversion, acetabular anteversion summation, hyperlaxity, or strain of the iliofemoral ligament
  - Thomas test: tests for flexion contracture. Extension to 0 degrees (in line with the body) without low back motion is normal. Less than full extension without rotating the pelvis or lifting the lower back is consistent with a flexion contracture.
  - Ober test: used to evaluate iliotibial band tightness. The test is positive when the upper knee remains in the abducted position after the hip is passively extended and abducted, then adducted, with the knee flexed. If, when the hip and knee are allowed to adduct while the hip is held in neutral rotation, the knee adducts past midline, the hip abductors are not tight; whereas if the knee does not reach to midline, then the hip abductors are tight.
  - Ely test: if on flexion of the knee the ipsilateral hip also flexes, then the rectus femoris is tight.
  - Trendelenburg test: indicative of hip abductor weakness and may indicate labrum pathology that affects neuroproprioceptive function. If the pelvis (iliac crest or posterior superior iliac spine) of the ipsilateral hip of the leg that is lifted elevates from the neutral standing position, this is normal. If the pelvis drops below the contralateral pelvis or from the starting position (ie, iliac crest/posterior superior iliac spine), this is considered a positive Trendelenburg sign and indicative of hip abductor weakness of the muscles on the extremity standing on the ground. If the pelvis stays level, then this is indicative of mild weakness and recorded as level.
  - Patrick test (FABER test): indicative of sacroiliac abnormalities or iliopsoas spasm. Pain may be felt with downward stress on the flexed knee. Pain in the posterior pelvis may be considered a positive finding that indicates the pain is coming from the sacroiliac joint.
  - Labral stress test: indicative of labral tear. The patient will note groin pain or a click in a consistent position as the hip is being rotated.
  - Piriformis test: Pain in the lateral hip or buttock reproduced by this maneuver is consistent with pain from the piriformis.

- Impingement test: Pain in the groin is a positive test and is consistent with intra-articular hip pain, not just femoroacetabular impingement.
- Hip extension and external rotation test: indicative of hip microinstability. The patient will note discomfort or apprehension in the anterior aspect of the hip.

IMAGING AND OTHER DIAGNOSTIC STUDIES

- Routine anteroposterior (AP) and lateral (usually cross-table lateral or Dunn view) radiographs should be obtained in all patients with hip pain to evaluate variations in bony architecture and visualization of areas that may present with hip pain such as the pubic symphysis, sacrum, sacroiliac joints, ilium, and ischium.
  - Radiographs help exclude degenerative joint changes, osteonecrosis, loose bodies, stress fractures, or other osseous pathology, and help assess for acetabular dysplasia and femoral neck abnormalities (bump or cam lesion) and femoroacetabular impingement (**FIG 2A,B**).
- Bone scan or radionuclide imaging is sensitive in detecting fractures, arthritis, neoplasm, infections, and vascular abnormalities but has low specificity and poor anatomic resolution.
- Magnetic resonance imaging (MRI) is used to detect stress fractures of the femoral neck and to identify sources of hip pain such as osteonecrosis, pigmented villonodular synovitis, synovial chondromatosis, osteochondromas, and other intra-articular pathology.
  - MRI arthrography can increase the ability to diagnose and describe labral pathology and articular cartilage loss (**FIG 2C**).
  - MRI combined with the use of intra-articular local anesthetic with gadolinium is used to assess pain relief and provide evidence that intra-articular pathology may be causing pain.
  - Recent studies have demonstrated a very high prevalence of asymptomatic labral tears in young, active people.
- Computed tomography (CT), MRI, and occasionally radioisotope imaging typically are required to help diagnose labral tears, hip instability, iliopsoas tendinitis, inflammatory arthritis, early avascular necrosis, occult fractures, psoas abscess, tumor, upper lumbar radiculopathy, or vascular abnormalities.
  - CT scan can be useful to measure ante- and retroversion of the femoral neck and acetabulum, to show the size and shape of the acetabulum and femoral head and neck, to elucidate bony architecture, to confirm concentric reduction after hip dislocation, and to rule out loose bodies.
  - CT scan has also been shown to be helpful in assessing the morphology of the AIIS (anterior inferior iliac spine), which has been implicated in subspinous impingement.
- Ultrasound is a nonirradiating way of evaluating intra-articular effusions and soft tissue swelling.
- Iliopsoas bursography is the choice imaging modality to detect iliopsoas bursitis and internal snapping hip.
  - Iliopsoas bursitis and internal snapping hip may be evaluated with real-time dynamic ultrasound.

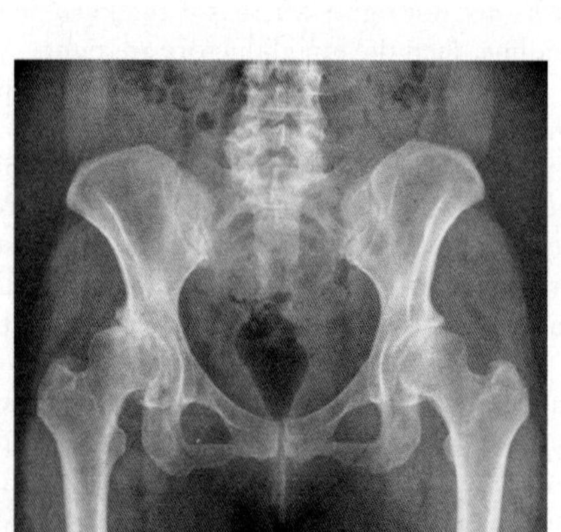
A

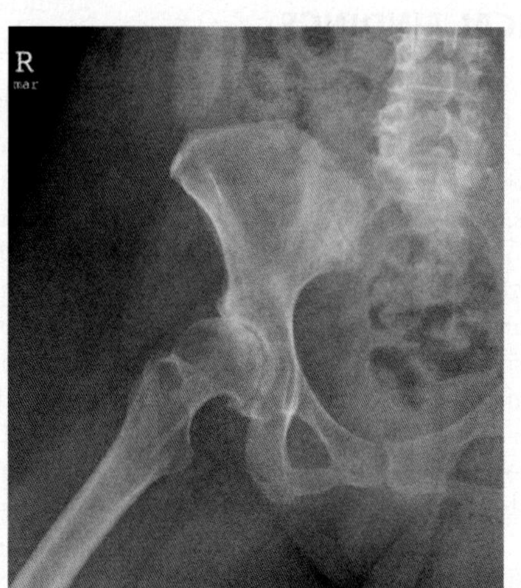

B

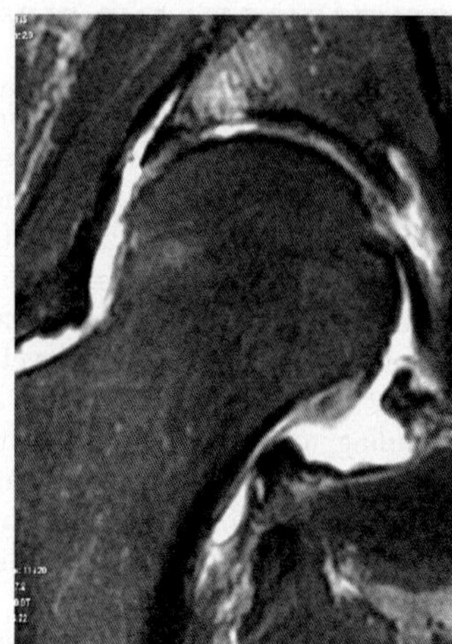
C

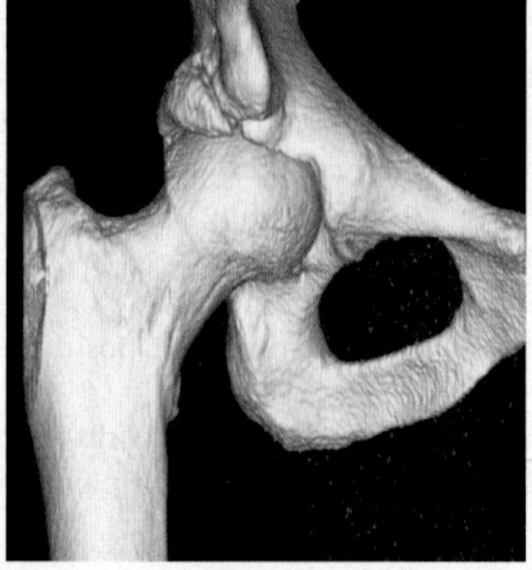
D

FIG 2 • AP radiographs of the pelvis (**A**) and lateral hip (**B**) of a patient with concomitant developmental dysplasia of the hip and DJD. **C.** MRI arthrogram of patient with femoroacetabular impingement. Note the subchondral edema and chondral lesion. **D.** Three-dimensional CT scan showing cam impingement with nonunion of a superior acetabular stress fracture in a 32-year-old athletic man.

- Three-dimensional CT is used to assess bony deformities, including osteophytes of the acetabulum and femoral neck bony lesions, which may cause impingement (**FIG 2D**).

DIFFERENTIAL DIAGNOSIS

- Labral tear
- Chondral delamination or degeneration
- Dysplasia
- Femoroacetabular impingement
- Synovitis
- Synovial chondromatosis
- Synovial osteochondromatosis
- Loose bodies
- Ligamentum teres tear
- Ligamentum teres hypertrophy
- Sepsis of the hip
- Arthritis of the hip
- Hip dislocation, subluxation, or microinstability
- Subspinous impingement (AIIS impingement)
- Avascular necrosis of the femoral head
- Sacroiliac joint pathology, including ankylosing spondylitis
- Trochanteric bursitis
- Athletic pubalgia
- Femur, pelvic, or acetabular fractures or stress fractures
- Myotendinous strains
- Piriformis syndrome
- Myositis ossification
- Neurologic irritation
- Hamstring syndrome
- Iliotibial band syndrome
- Iliopsoas tendon problems (eg, snapping and tendinitis)
- Tendinitis
- Tendon injuries (iliopsoas, piriformis, rectus, hamstring, or adductor)
- Benign tumors (eg, osteoid osteoma, osteochondroma)
- Occult hernia
- Lumbar spine (mechanical pain and herniated discs)
- Abdomen
- Osteitis pubis

NONOPERATIVE MANAGEMENT

- Conservative therapy includes rest, ambulatory support, nonsteroidal anti-inflammatory drugs, and physical therapy.
- Most pathologies about the hip usually are treated initially with conservative management, including relative rest, nonsteroidal anti-inflammatory drugs, and rehabilitation. Occasionally, protected weight bearing and use of ambulatory assist devices may be needed.
- However, several intra-articular pathologies do not resolve or heal with nonoperative management, including labral tears, loose bodies, articular cartilage lesions, and femoroacetabular impingement.

SURGICAL MANAGEMENT

- Proper patient selection is essential for a successful surgical outcome.
- Arthroscopy is most successful for patients with recent, symptomatic intra-articular hip joint pathology, particularly those with mechanical symptoms, and minimal arthritic changes.
- Arthroscopy should be considered if hip pain is persistent, is reproducible on physical examination, and does not respond to conservative treatment.
- Pain relief with intra-articular injection of local anesthetic also is a good predictive sign for success.
- Indications for arthroscopy include loose bodies, foreign objects, labral tears, chondral injuries, synovial disease, femoroacetabular impingement, mild degenerative disease with mechanical symptoms, osteonecrosis of femoral head, osteochondritis dissecans, ruptured ligamentum teres, snapping hip syndrome, impinging osteophytes, adhesive capsulitis, iliopsoas tendon release, iliopsoas bursitis, trochanteric bursectomy, iliotibial band resection, crystalline hip arthropathy, hip instability, subspinous impingement, joint sepsis, osteoid osteoma, osteochondroma, and unresolved hip pain.
- ROM should be evaluated before arthroscopy to determine the presence of contractures.
- Arthroscopy can be a means to delay total arthroplasty for DJD.
- Contraindications include systemic illness, open wounds, soft tissue disorders, poor bone quality (ie, unable to withstand traction), nonprogressing avascular necrosis of the femoral head, arthrofibrosis or capsular constriction, and ankylosis of the hip.
- Severe obesity is a relative contraindication that may be circumvented with extra-length instruments.
- Indications for labrectomy include relief of pain with intra-articular injection of anesthesia, no pain relief with physical therapy or nonsteroidal anti-inflammatory drugs, missed time due to delayed diagnosis, and symptoms for longer than 4 weeks.
- Arthroscopy for DJD should be considered for younger patients with mild–moderate disease who present with mechanical symptoms and no deformity.
- Microfracture is indicated for grade IV chondral lesions with healthy surrounding articular surface and intact subchondral bone.
- Treatment of sepsis involves drainage, lavage, débridement, and postoperative antibiotics, and requires early diagnosis.
  - Sepsis in the setting of joint arthroplasty requires prompt arthroscopic débridement, well-fixed components, a sensitive microorganism, and patient tolerance to and compliance with antibiotic therapy.[7]

Preoperative Planning

- A physical examination should be completed and radiographs and other imaging reviewed before arthroscopy.
- A three-dimensional CT scan may be obtained to further assess bony abnormalities (see **FIG 2D**).
- Arthroscopy usually is performed under general anesthesia.
- If epidural anesthesia is used, it also requires adequate motor block to relax muscle tone.
- Typical instrumentation includes a marking pen; no. 11 blade scalpel; 6-inch 17-gauge spinal needles; 60-mL syringe of saline with extension tubing; a Nitinol guidewire; 4.5-, 5.0-, and 5.5-mm cannulas with cannulated and solid obturators; a switching stick; a separate inflow adaptor; and a modified probe.
- Fluid used can be introduced by gravity or a pump.
- Specialized arthroscopy equipment for the hip is available that is extra-long and extra-strong to withstand the lever arm

due to the extra length. These instruments include shavers, burrs, biters, probes, curettes, and loose body retrievers.

Positioning

- The patient may be placed in either the supine or lateral decubitus position on a fracture table or attachment that allows for distraction of the hip joint.
  - The lateral decubitus position offers the benefit of directing fat away from the operative site.
- The involved hip joint is in neutral rotation, abducted at 10 to 25 degrees, and in neutral flexion–extension (**FIG 3A**).
- Flexion of the involved hip during distraction and portal placement increases the risk of injury to the sciatic nerve.
- The nonoperative hip also is abducted and is placed under slight traction to stabilize the patient and allow placement of the image intensifier between the legs and directed over the operative hip.
- A heavily padded perineal post is placed against the pubic ramus and ischial tuberosity, but lateralized against the medial thigh of the operative hip, with care taken to protect perineal structures (**FIG 3B**).
- It is important to lateralize the traction vector such that it is parallel to the femoral neck to minimize risk of pressure neurapraxia to the pudendal nerve and to optimize distraction of the joint.
- The surgeon, assistant, and scrub nurse stand on the operative side, facing the arthroscopic monitor on the opposite side of the patient (**FIG 3C,D**).
- The fluoroscopy monitor is placed at the foot of the fracture table.

Approach

- Portal placement and arthroscopic technique do not differ between the supine and lateral decubitus positions.
- Hip arthroscopy usually is performed through three portals: anterolateral, anterior, and posterolateral.
- A shortened bridge can accommodate the use of 4.5-, 5.0-, and 5.5-mm cannulas.
  - Although a 5.0-mm cannula is used for initial entry of the arthroscope, a 4.5-mm cannula permits interchange of the inflow, arthroscope, and instruments, and a 5.5-mm cannula allows entry of larger instruments (eg, shaver blades).

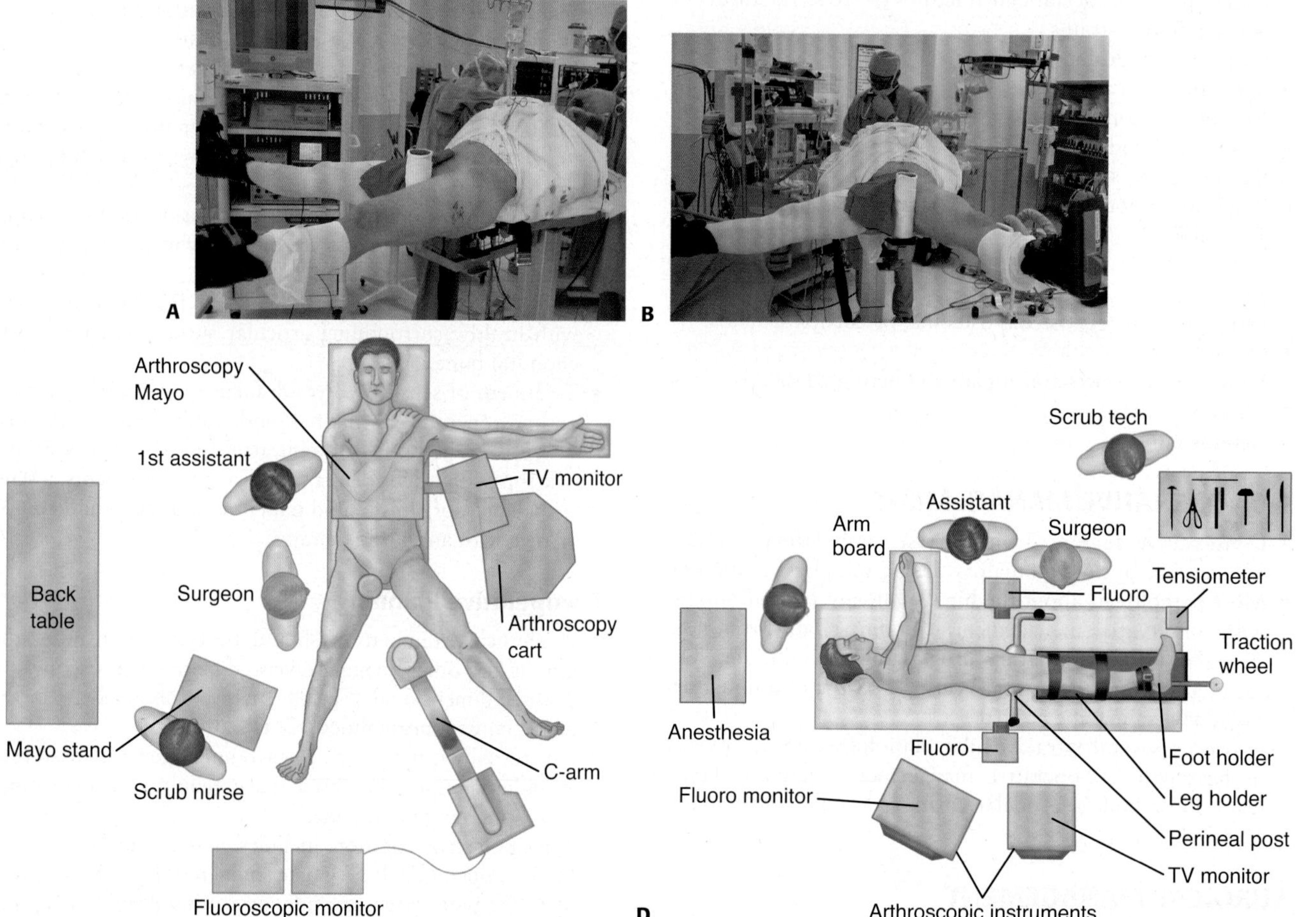

FIG 3 • **A.** Operating room setup for hip arthroscopy. The patient is supine on a fracture table, with the unaffected leg abducted approximately 60 degrees, and the hip to be operated on in neutral flexion–extension, neutral internal–external rotation, and 15 degrees of abduction. **B.** A well-padded peroneal post allows lateralization of the surgical hip in addition to distal displacement of the femoral head with distraction. **C,D.** Schematic representation of hip arthroscopy in the supine and lateral positions. The arthroscopic monitor is on the opposite side of the patient for hip arthroscopy. The fluoroscopic monitor is at the foot of the table; the fluoroscope is brought either between the legs or from the contralateral side of the patient for supine hip arthroscopy. For lateral hip arthroscopy, the fluoroscopic monitor is on the opposite side of the patient from the surgeon and the fluoroscope is next to the surgeon.

- A 30-degree videoarticulated arthroscope provides best visualization of the central portion of the acetabulum, the femoral head, and the superior aspect of the acetabular fossa.
  - A 70-degree video arthroscope provides optimal visualization of the periphery of the joint, the acetabular labrum, and the inferior aspect of the acetabular fossa.
- The radiofrequency device are used to ablate tissue and can offer increased maneuverability over shavers.
- Extra-length convex and concave curved shaver blades are used to remove tissue around the femoral head.
- Fragile, extra-length instruments designed for other arthroscopic procedures should be avoided because these have a greater tendency to break.

Hip Distraction

- The patient is prepared with chlorhexidine (Hibiclens) or povidone-iodine (Betadine).
- Traction is applied to distract the joint 7 to 10 mm.
- A tensiometer may be used to monitor traction force (typically 25 to 50 pounds).
- Traction time should be monitored. It is important to limit the time to less than 2 hours to prevent complications such as compression of the pudendal nerve or injury to other nerves.
- The spinal needle is introduced under fluoroscopy at the anterolateral position into the joint capsule to equilibrate the space with the ambient pressure (**TECH FIG 1A,B**).
- Pressure in the joint may be equilibrated with air or saline (**TECH FIG 1C**).
- Care should be taken to avoid penetrating the labrum and articular surfaces with the spinal needle.

A

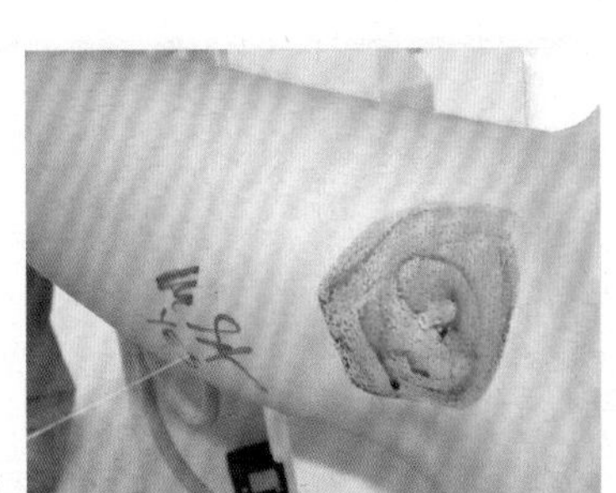

B

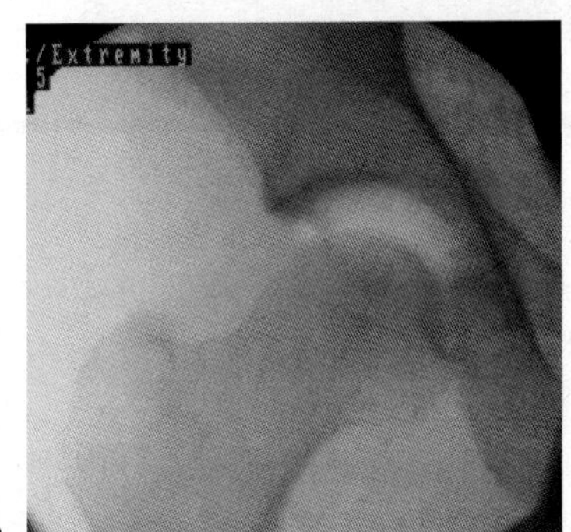

C

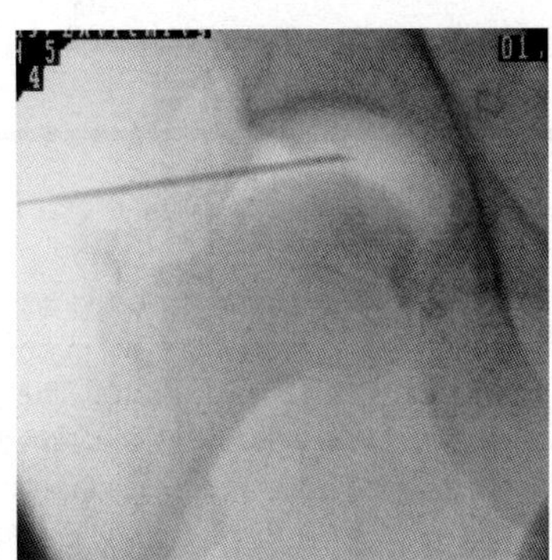

TECH FIG 1 • **A.** Equilibration of intra-articular pressure with ambient pressure. A spinal needle is introduced under fluoroscopic guidance in a prepped patient to relieve the suction cup effect of the negative intra-articular pressure to confirm adequate distraction prior to starting the hip arthroscopy. **B,C.** Fluoroscopic images taken during the initial stages of hip arthroscopy. **B.** The joint is distracted prior to introducing the spinal needle. **C.** Once the spinal needle has been introduced and the trocar removed, an air arthrogram is made, as evidenced by the air seen laterally in the joint and the increase in joint distraction without adding more traction force.

Making the Portals

- Portals are established by penetrating the skin with a 6-inch 17-gauge spinal needle and positioning the needle into the respective joint space.
- The trocar of the spinal needle is removed and a Nitinol guidewire (Smith & Nephew Endoscopy, Andover, MA) is run through the needle into the joint space (**TECH FIG 2A,B**).
- The needle is removed.
- A skin incision is made at the entry site, large enough to facilitate entry of a 5.0-mm cannula.
- A long cannula sheath with cannulated trocar is advanced over the guidewire into the joint space (**TECH FIG 2C,D**).
- The cannulated obturator should be kept off the femoral head to avoid articular damage.
- It is important to avoid cannula removal and reintroduction because this may damage cartilage.
- It may be necessary to release the capsule with an arthroscopic knife.
- The weight-bearing portion of the femoral head is visualized by using the arthroscope in all three central compartment portals with the 70- and 30-degree lenses or by internally and externally rotating the hip intraoperatively.
- The fossa and ligamentum teres typically are visualized from all three portals, particularly using the 30-degree lens.

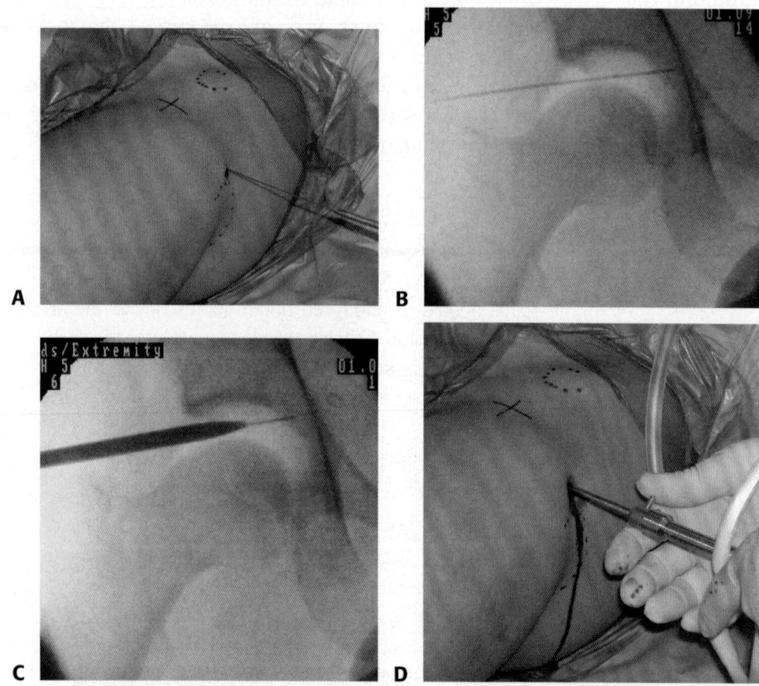

TECH FIG 2 • **A.** Guidewire in the anterolateral portal. The spinal needle has been exchanged for a guidewire which, in turn, is being used to guide the trocar and sheathed cannula. **B.** Fluoroscopic view of the guidewire in the distracted joint after removing the spinal needle. **C.** Fluoroscopic view of the trocar with sheathed cannula within the joint over the guidewire. **D.** The arthroscope placed in the anterolateral portal.

Anterolateral Portal

- The anterolateral portal is created first because it is the safest, being the most distant from and posing least risk of injury to the femoral and sciatic neurovascular structures.
- The portal penetrates the gluteus medius muscle and is positioned directly over the superior aspect of the greater trochanter at its anterior margin to enter the lateral capsule at its anterior margin (**TECH FIG 3**).
- When creating the anterolateral portal, it is important to introduce the spinal needle in the coronal plane by keeping it parallel to the floor (see **TECH FIG 2A**).
- As the cannula is positioned into the intra-articular space, care should be taken to avoid damage to the labrum or articular surfaces.
- The portal provides visualization of most of the acetabular cartilage, labrum, and weight-bearing femoral head within the central compartment, as well as visualization of the peripheral compartment, such as the non–weight-bearing femoral head, the anterior neck, the anterior intrinsic capsular folds, and the synovial tissues beneath the zona orbicularis and the anterior labrum.
- The superior gluteal nerve is the closest neurovascular structure and runs 4.4 cm posterior to the portal.

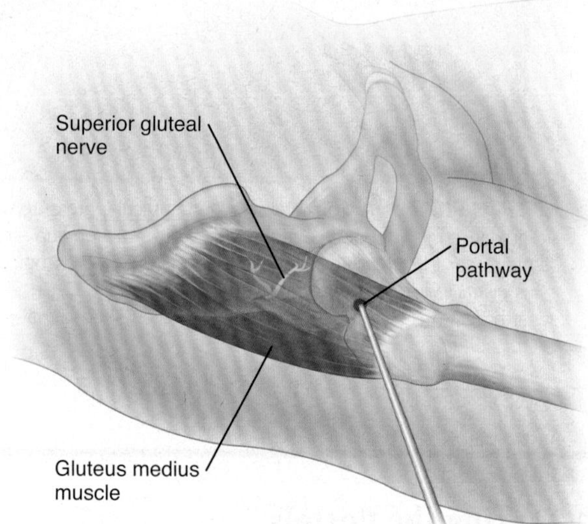

TECH FIG 3 • The anterolateral portal starts just anterior to the superior aspect of the greater trochanter and pierces the gluteus medius muscle.

Anterior Portal

- The senior author prefers to establish the anterior portal after the anterolateral portal, although some prefer to establish the anterior portal first.
- Arthroscopic visualization from the anterolateral portal and fluoroscopy facilitate correct portal placement, helping to avoid damage to the labrum or articular surfaces.
- Several different anterior portals have been described.
- One popular anterior portal enters at the junction of a line drawn distally from the ASIS and a transverse line across the superior margin of the greater trochanter (**TECH FIG 4A**).
- The portal penetrates the sartorius and rectus femoris muscles as it is directed 45 degrees cephalad and 30 degrees medially to enter the anterior capsule (**TECH FIG 4B,C**).

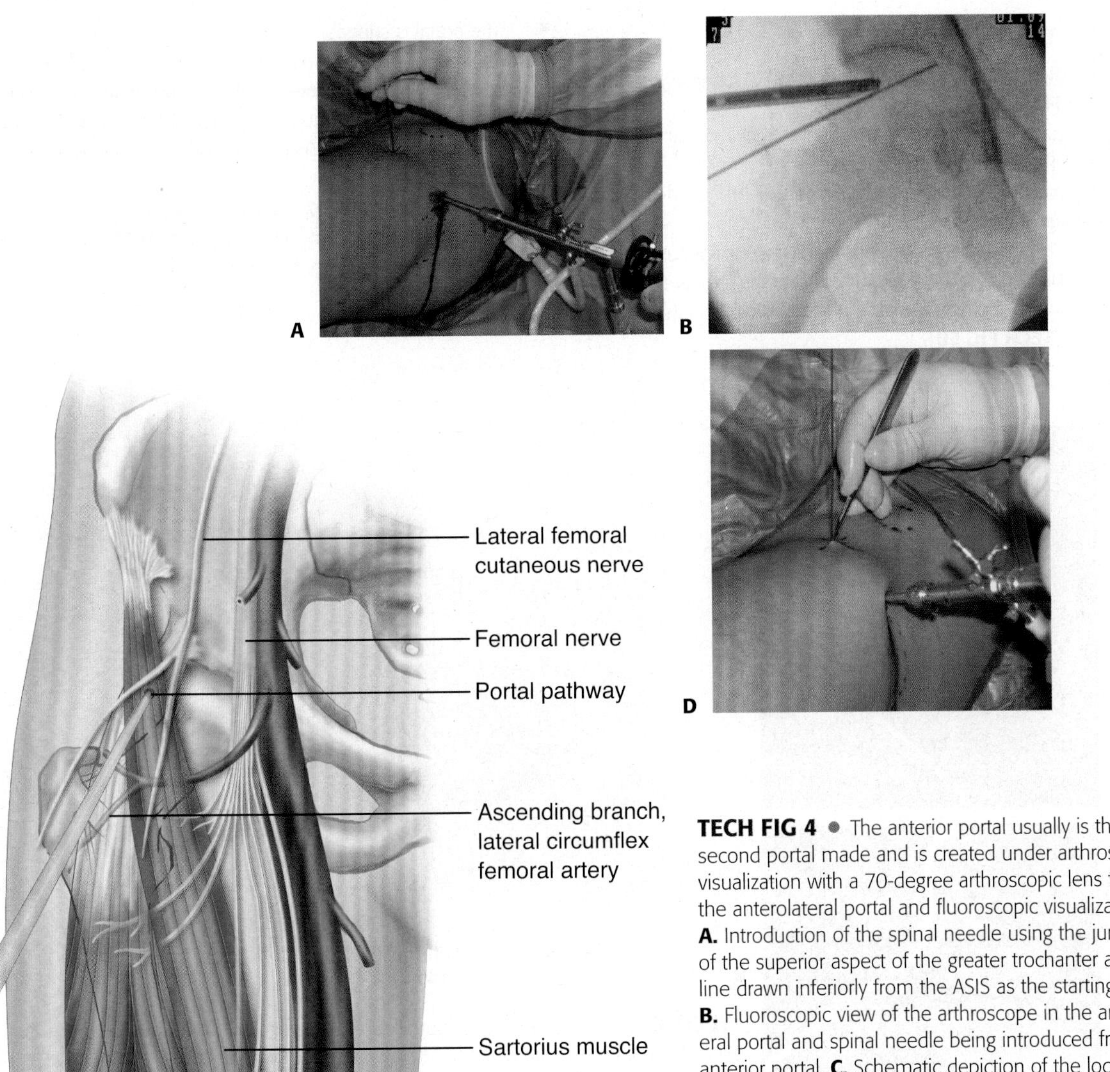

TECH FIG 4 • The anterior portal usually is the second portal made and is created under arthroscopic visualization with a 70-degree arthroscopic lens from the anterolateral portal and fluoroscopic visualization. **A.** Introduction of the spinal needle using the junction of the superior aspect of the greater trochanter and a line drawn inferiorly from the ASIS as the starting point. **B.** Fluoroscopic view of the arthroscope in the anterolateral portal and spinal needle being introduced from the anterior portal. **C.** Schematic depiction of the location of the portal adjacent to the branches of the lateral femoral cutaneous nerve, penetrating the sartorius and rectus femoris muscles. **D.** Care is taken only to cut the skin when making the anterior portal to help reduce the risk of laceration of the lateral femoral cutaneous nerve.

- As the cannulated obturator enters the joint space, it should be kept off the articular surface and directed underneath the acetabular labrum.
- The portal allows visualization of the anterior femoral neck, the anterior aspect of the joint, the superior retinacular fold, the ligamentum teres, and the lateral labrum.
- Care should be taken to minimize injury to branches of the lateral femoral cutaneous nerve by directing movement medially, avoiding deep cuts at the entry site, not using vigorous instrumentation, and using a 70-degree arthroscope at the anterolateral portal to guide entry (**TECH FIG 4D**).
- The femoral nerve is 3.2 cm medial and runs tangential to the portal.
- The ascending branch of the lateral femoral circumflex artery is 3.7 cm inferior to the portal, but terminal branches may be within millimeters of the portal at the capsular level.
- More recently, the anterior portal is made more distal (approximately 7 cm) and slightly lateral (1 to 3 cm) to the aforementioned anterior portal.
  - This position allows for easier access under the anterior acetabular rim in pincer impingement and provides a better approach for labral repair drilling and anchor placement.

Posterolateral Portal

- The posterolateral portal is established after the anterior portal (**TECH FIG 5A**).
- This portal is just posterior to the greater trochanter, at the same level as the anterolateral portal.
- Arthroscopic visualization and fluoroscopy are used to guide portal placement.
- The portal penetrates the gluteus medius and minimus muscles and is directed over the superior aspect of the greater trochanter at its posterior border to enter the lateral capsule at its posterior margin (**TECH FIG 5B**).
- The portal is superior and anterior to the piriformis.
- The portal allows visualization of the posterior aspect of the femoral head, the posterior labrum, the posterior capsule, and the inferior edge of the ischiofemoral ligament (**TECH FIG 5C**).
- The sciatic nerve is 2.9 cm posterior to the portal at the level of the capsule.
  - It is important to maintain the leg in neutral rotation and extension and to introduce the spinal needle horizontally to avoid injury to the sciatic nerve.

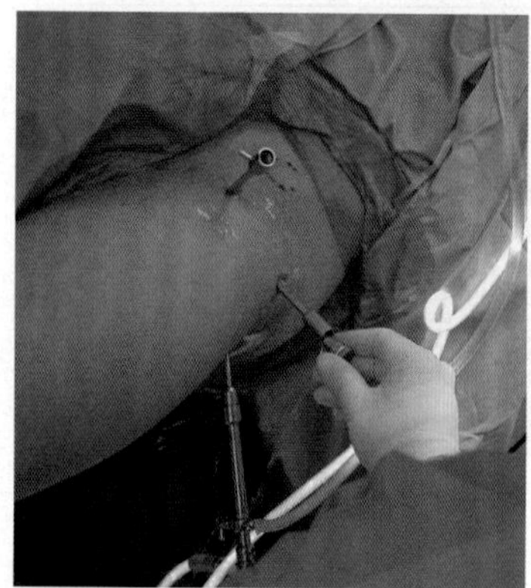

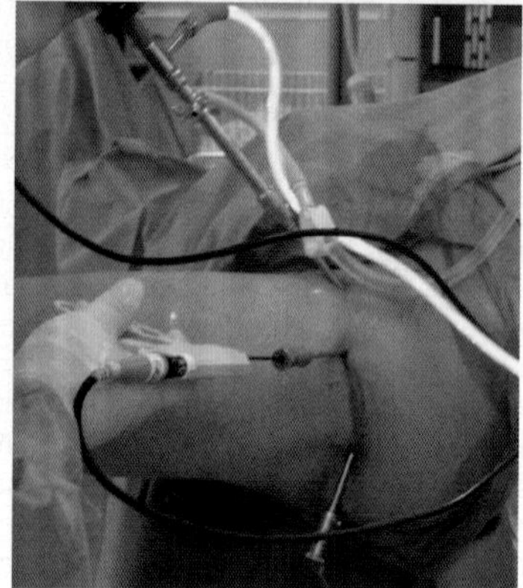

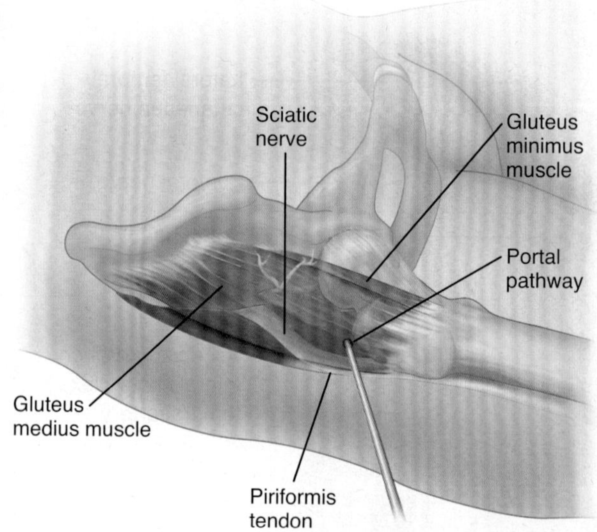

TECH FIG 5 • Posterolateral portal. The posterolateral portal usually is the last central portal made, although it can be made before the anterior portal. **A.** How the posterolateral portal is made, relative to the other portals. **B.** The posterolateral portal proceeds through the gluteus medius and minimus muscles. Note its relation to the superior gluteal nerve. **C.** View of obturators in all three central compartment portals to allow for complete central compartment hip arthroscopy. Both a 30- and a 70-degree lens are used in all the portals to allow for full visualization of the femoroacetabular joint to perform a complete hip arthroscopy of the central compartment.

Distal Anterolateral Portal

- To access the peripheral compartment–femoral neck region, two portals are used after traction is removed from the extremity.
- Peripheral compartment arthroscopy can be done in hip flexion to relax the anterior capsule or in neutral flexion extension.
- The anterolateral portal is used as one portal.
- A distal anterolateral portal is established 3 to 5 cm distal to the anterolateral portal, just anterior to the lateral aspect of the proximal femoral shaft and neck (**TECH FIG 6**).
- Fluoroscopy is used to guide portal placement.
- The portal penetrates the gluteus medius muscle and upper vastus lateralis.
- The spinal needle should enter the peripheral compartment laterally. The guidewire is brought through the spinal needle and can be gently advanced to the medial capsule—the easy passage until the medial capsule is reached helps confirm that one is in the peripheral compartment.
- The skin incision is made, and the trocar and the sheath are passed over the guidewire.
- The sheath and guidewire are exchanged for the arthroscope or instrumentation.
- Arthroscopy and fluoroscopy can be used together to perform surgery in the peripheral compartment.

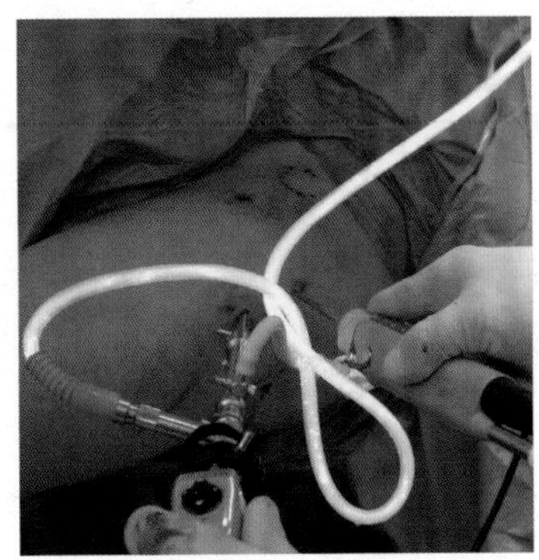

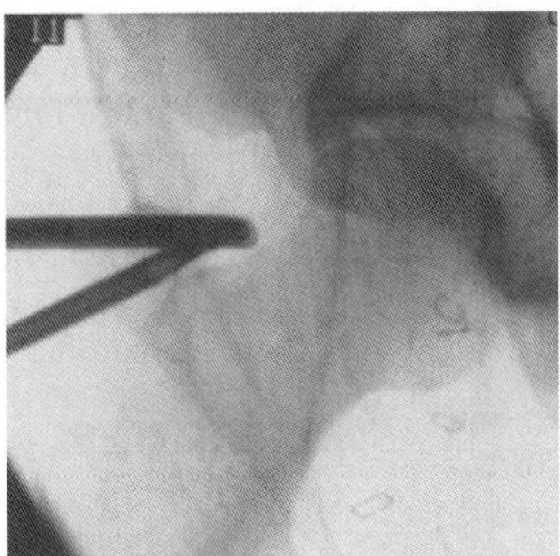

TECH FIG 6 • Distal anterolateral portal. The distal anterolateral portal allows a second portal for peripheral compartment arthroscopy. This portal is 2.5 to 5 cm distal to the anterolateral portal (**A**). This example shows the hip in neutral flexion–extension, which makes it easier to perform a cheilectomy or osteoplasty for cam-type femoroacetabular impingement to maintain orientation while using fluoroscopy to assist with the procedure (**B**). Alternatively, the hip can be flexed, relaxing the anterior capsule, making entry into the joint easier.

PEARLS AND PITFALLS

Patient selection	▪ A careful patient history, physical examination, and appropriate imaging should be performed. ▪ Distinguish intra-articular conditions that may require surgery from extra-articular problems that may only require conservative treatment. ▪ Patients should have clear expectations of outcomes.
Hip distraction	▪ Distract the hip with as much force as necessary to safely introduce instruments, typically 8–10 mm. ▪ Limit traction time to 2 hours or take a traction break if it is necessary to exceed this time. ▪ Too little traction may result in injury to the articular surfaces. ▪ Too much traction can result in nerve injury or injury to the perineum, knee, foot, or ankle.
Patient positioning	▪ Obtain the correct vector of joint distraction with minimal force necessary to distract the joint. ▪ The perineal post should be adequately padded and lateralized against the involved hip.
Portal placement	▪ Proper placement of the anterolateral portal is key to successful placement of other portals. ▪ It is important to avoid damaging the labrum or articular surfaces with either the spinal needle or cannula introduction. ▪ Use inflow from the secondary portal to improve fluid dynamics or use a pump. ▪ Use both 30- and 70-degree cannulas in each portal. ▪ Use specialized hip arthroscopy instruments and metal cannulas to reduce risk of instrument breakage and allow proper technique. ▪ Avoid inserting the cannula multiple times to reduce fluid extravasation and the risk of damage to labrum, cartilage, and neurovascular structures. ▪ Maintain systolic blood pressure below 100 mm Hg and use a radiofrequency device to minimize bleeding.

POSTOPERATIVE CARE

- Traction is released.
- Long-acting local anesthetic is injected into the joint.
- The portals are sutured, and a sterile dressing is applied to the wounds.
- Arthroscopy is an outpatient procedure and the patient typically leaves recovery room after 1 to 3 hours.
- If arthroscopy does not involve bony recontouring of the femoral neck, labral repair, or microfracture of the articular surfaces, then the patient is allowed to walk immediately, although weight bearing should be assisted with crutches for 3 to 7 days or until gait pattern is normalized.
- Rehabilitation should take into consideration soft tissue healing constraints, control of swelling and pain, early ROM, limitations on weight bearing, early initiation of muscle activity and neuromuscular control, progressive lower extremity strengthening and proprioceptive retraining, cardiovascular training, and sport-specific training.
- Swelling and pain are controlled by ice and nonaspirin, nonsteroidal anti-inflammatory drugs.
- The dressing is removed on the first or second postoperative day, and the wound is covered with adhesive bandages.
- Portal sutures are removed a few days after surgery.
- Patients who undergo labrum repairs on the anterior superior region and capsulorraphy should follow specific ROM and weight-bearing guidelines.
- Patients who undergo osteoplasty should limit impact activities that increase the risk of femoral neck fracture during the initial several weeks.
- Patients who undergo microfracture should adhere to 8 weeks of protected weight bearing on crutches.

OUTCOMES

- Record functional and prosthetic survivorship data, as applicable.
- Loose bodies are the clearest indication for arthroscopy, resulting in less morbidity and faster recovery than open surgery.[4]
- Labral débridement has been shown to result in successful outcomes in 68% to 82% of cases, with positive outcomes associated with isolated tears and poorer prognosis associated with arthritis.[2,5,12]
- Débridement of ligamentum teres, such as labral débridement, has shown best results when lesions are isolated and without associated acetabular fracture or significant osteochondral defect of either the acetabulum or femoral head.
- Treatment of hip DJD by arthroscopy has shown unpredictable results, with a range of 34% to 60% of patients reporting improvement of symptoms after arthroscopic débridement for DJD.[6,13]
- One study reported that 86% of patients treated for chondral lesions by microfracture showed a successful response at 2-year follow-up.[1]
- Arthroscopic synovectomy is palliative, and success is based on the integrity of the articular cartilage.
- Treatment of femoroacetabular impingement has shown better outcomes when there is less DJD.
- Treatment of avascular necrosis is controversial—the results are better when the articular surface is not disrupted or when treating mechanical symptoms.
  - O'Leary[10] reported 40% of patients improved at 30-month follow-up.
- More specifics are provided in the chapters describing specific techniques for the different processes treated about the hip.

COMPLICATIONS

- Traction neurapraxia
- Direct trauma to pudendal, lateral femoral cutaneous, femoral, and sciatic nerves
- Iatrogenic labral and chondral damage
- Fluid extravasation
- Vaginal tear
- Pressure necrosis to scrotum, labia and perineum, and foot
- Labia and perineum hematoma
- Knee ligament injury
- Ankle fracture
- Femoral head avascular necrosis
- Fracture of femoral neck
- Instrument breakage
- Portal hematoma and bleeding

REFERENCES

1. Byrd JWT, Jones KS. Microfracture for grade IV chondral lesions of the hip. Arthroscopy 2004;20:89.
2. Byrd JWT, Jones KS. Prospective analysis of hip arthroscopy with 2-year follow-up. Arthroscopy 2000;16:578–587.
3. Carreira D, Bush-Joseph CA. Hip arthroscopy. Orthopedics 2006; 29:517–523.
4. Epstein H. Posterior fracture-dislocations of the hip: comparison of open and closed methods of treatment in certain types. J Bone Joint Surg Am 1961;43A:1079–1098.
5. Farjo LA, Glick JM, Sampson TG. Hip arthroscopy for acetabular labrum tears. Arthroscopy 1999;15:132–137.
6. Farjo LA, Glick JM, Sampson TG. Hip arthroscopy for degenerative joint disease. Arthroscopy 1998;14:435.
7. Hyman JL, Salvati EA, Laurencin CT, et al. The arthroscopic drainage, irrigation, and débridement of late, acute total hip arthroplasty infections: average 6-year follow-up. J Arthroplasty 1999;14:903–910.
8. Kelly BT, Williams RJ III, Philippon MJ. Hip arthroscopy: current indications, treatment options, and management issues. Am J Sports Med 2003;31(6):1020–1037.
9. McCarthy JC, Noble PC, Schuck MR, et al. The role of labral lesions to development of early degenerative hip disease. Clin Orthop Relat Res 2001;393:25–37.
10. O'Leary JA, Berend K, Vail TP. The relationship between diagnosis and outcome in arthroscopy of the hip. Arthroscopy 2001;17:181–188.
11. Safran MR. Evaluation of the hip: history, physical examination, and imaging. Oper Tech Sports Med 2005;13:2–12.
12. Santori N, Villar RN. Acetabular labral tears: results of arthroscopic partial limbectomy. Arthroscopy 2000;16:11–15.
13. Villar RN. Arthroscopic debridement of the hip: a minimally invasive approach to osteoarthritis. J Bone Joint Surg Br 1991;73B:170–171.

Periarticular Arthroscopy

Danyal H. Nawabi and Bryan T. Kelly

4

CHAPTER

DEFINITION

- The periarticular sources of pain around the hip joint include, but are not limited to, disorders of
  - Peritrochanteric space (trochanteric bursitis, external coxa saltans, and abductor tears)
  - Iliopsoas musculotendinous unit (internal coxa saltans)
  - Rectus abdominis/pubic symphysis/adductor tendon (athletic pubalgia)
  - Proximal hamstring tendon (avulsion fractures and tendon tears)
  - Sciatic, ilioinguinal, obturator, and lateral femoral cutaneous nerves (LFCNs) (compression syndromes)
- Periarticular endoscopic procedures are capable of addressing pathology in all the aforementioned regions.
- The snapping/lateral hip (external and internal coxa saltans and trochanteric bursitis), athletic pubalgia, and proximal hamstring injuries have been covered in other sections of this book. This chapter will highlight the use of periarticular endoscopic techniques around the hip by providing a detailed overview of the repair of abductor tears.

ANATOMY

- The peritrochanteric space is located between the greater trochanter and iliotibial band. The boundaries of this space are formed by tensor fascia lata muscle anteriorly, the insertion of the gluteus maximus tendon to the femur just below the vastus lateralis inferiorly, and the gluteus medius and minimus tendons superiorly.
- The greater trochanter of the hip, much like the greater tuberosity of the humerus, has an osseous contour that reflects the attachments of the gluteal muscles.
- Four facets on the greater trochanter have been described[7]: anterior, lateral, superoposterior, and posterior facets (**FIG 1**).

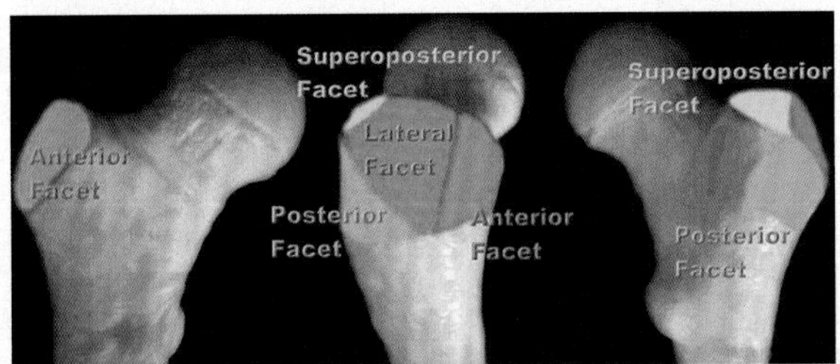

FIG 1 • From **left** to **right**: anterior, lateral, and posterior views of the greater trochanter showing the anterior, lateral, superoposterior, and posterior facets. (Reprinted from Dwek J, Pfirrmann C, Stanley A, et al. MR imaging of the hip abductors: normal anatomy and commonly encountered pathology at the greater trochanter. Magn Reson Imaging Clin N Am 2005;13[4]: 691–704, with permission from Elsevier.)

- The gluteus medius is a large, fan-shaped muscle consisting of three equal-sized segments—the anterior, middle, and posterior—that originates from the external surface of the ilium. Each segment is innervated by a separate branch of the superior gluteal nerve. Its tendon attaches at two distinct facets on the greater trochanter. The anterior and most of the central fibers are attached to the lateral facet, and the posterior fibers are attached to the superoposterior facet[16] (**FIG 2**).
- The anterior and central insertion of the gluteus medius tendon on the lateral facet is rectangular in shape, occupying an area of approximately[16] 440 mm^2. The portion of the tendon inserting into the superoposterior facet is more robust, with a circular shape, and a smaller surface area of approximately[16] 200 mm^2.
- The fiber orientation of the gluteus medius is thought to correlate with function during the gait cycle. The anterior and middle muscle segments are vertically oriented and aid in initiating hip abduction.[8] The anterior segment also externally rotates the pelvis during the swing phase of the contralateral limb.[8] The fibers in the posterior segment are more horizontal and act to stabilize the hip joint at heel strike.[8]
- The gluteus minimus also originates from the external ilium, running between the anterior inferior and posterior inferior iliac spines.[1]
- Distally, the gluteus minimus tendon attaches via two heads—the capsular head is fascial thickening that inserts into the

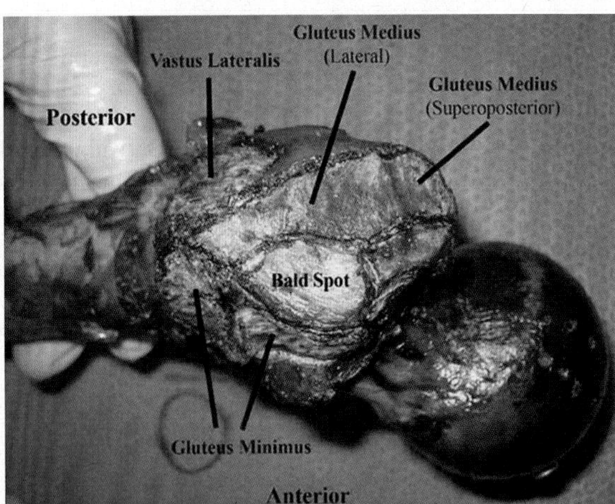

FIG 2 • Cadaveric specimen showing the insertional footprints of the gluteus medius at the lateral and superoposterior facets. A bald spot is present between the anterior aspect of the footprint of the gluteus medius and the attachment of the gluteus minimus at the anterior facet. (Reprinted from Robertson WJ, Gardner MJ, Barker JU, et al. Anatomy and dimensions of the gluteus medius tendon insertion. Arthroscopy 2008;24[2]:130–136, with permission from Elsevier.)

superior aspect of the hip capsule, just anterior to greater trochanter at the iliofemoral ligament.[1] The long head inserts on the inner aspect of the anterior margin of the greater trochanter at the anterior facet. The trochanteric insertion of the gluteus minimus is separated from the gluteus medius tendon footprint on the lateral facet by the trochanteric bald spot (**FIG 3**).

- The gluteus medius and minimus muscles have been likened to rotator cuff of the shoulder.[3,10] The gluteus medius has a moment arm similar to both supraspinatus and infraspinatus with its lateral and superoposterior insertion on the greater trochanter.[3] The gluteus minimus inserts on the anterior facet and has several different moments depending on the position of the femur relative to the pelvis—it can affect flexion, abduction, external, and internal rotation; and when these moments are counterbalanced, it acts as a primary stabilizer of the head in the socket.[1] Due to the strong internal rotation moment of the gluteus minimus in many functional positions, its action is also analogous to the subscapularis (**FIG 4**).
- When repairing tears of the gluteus medius, familiarity with the insertional anatomy is essential to prevent overestimation of the size of the true tendon footprint. Incorporation of the bald spot into an anatomic footprint repair of the medius tendon can occur if anchors are mistakenly placed in the bald spot of the trochanter—a situation that should be avoided.[17]

PATHOGENESIS

- Tears of the gluteus medius and minimus tendons were first described in the late 1990s and much like rotator cuff tendon tears in the shoulder, most likely result from a degenerative process.[3,10,16]

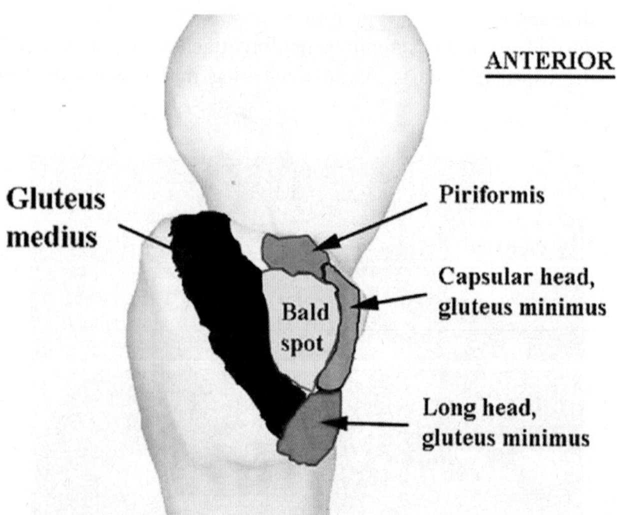

FIG 3 • Computer-generated replica of the cadaveric specimen seen in **FIG 2** showing a superolateral view of the right proximal femur. The soft tissue attachment sites of the gluteus medius tendon, the two heads of the gluteus minimus muscle, and the piriformis muscle are shown. The trochanteric bald spot is also labeled, located in between the anterior extent of the medius insertion on the lateral facet and the posterior extent of the minimus insertion on the anterior facet. (Reprinted from Robertson WJ, Gardner MJ, Barker JU, et al. Anatomy and dimensions of the gluteus medius tendon insertion. Arthroscopy 2008;24[2]:130–136, with permission from Elsevier.)

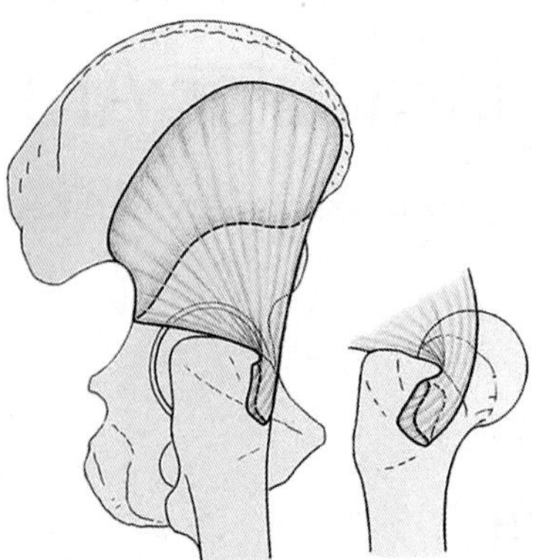

FIG 4 • A schematic diagram of gluteus minimus showing multiple fiber orientations in the muscle as it originates from the ilium and inserts on the anterior capsule and anterior facet of the greater trochanter. (Adapted with permission from Beck M, Sledge JB, Gautier E, et al. The anatomy and function of the gluteus minimus muscle. J Bone Surg Br 2000;82[3]:358–363.)

- Tears of the gluteus medius can be interstitial, partial thickness or full thickness, with full-thickness tears tending to be large in size.[16]
- Tears of the gluteus medius are significantly more common than those of the minimus. It follows that most tears occur in the anterior portion of the gluteus medius tendon as it attaches to the lateral facet of the greater trochanter.
- Tear propagation occurs by degeneration of the undersurface of the tear progressing posteriorly into a full-thickness tear.
- Tears were initially identified in the setting of open release of the iliotibial band for recalcitrant trochanteric bursitis,[10] total hip arthroplasty,[9] and femoral neck fracture treatment.[3]
- In performing iliotibial band release for trochanteric bursitis, Kagan[10] found a partial tear of the gluteus medius in seven patients that was picked up on magnetic resonance imaging (MRI) but not on physical examination. Tears were repaired with nonabsorbable suture through bone tunnels and all patients were pain free at a median follow-up of 45 months.
- In a series of 176 consecutive patients undergoing total hip arthroplasty for osteoarthritis, Howell et al[9] found that 20% of the patients had degeneration of the abductor muscles with majority occurring in elderly women.
- In a prospective study of 50 consecutive patients being treated for femoral neck fractures, Bunker et al[3] found rotator cuff tears of the hip in 22% of patients. The typical appearance was described as a circular or oval defect in the insertion of gluteus medius and minimus tendons. The tears had a rolled edge and were often associated with free fluid in the trochanteric bursa and an eburnated underlying surface of the greater trochanter.[3]
- A traumatic etiology in otherwise normal hips in the background of abductor tendinopathy is less common but can occur.[13,15]

NATURAL HISTORY

- Tendinopathy and tears of the abductor tendons are a common cause for intractable pain along the lateral side of the hip.
- In patients with greater trochanteric pain syndrome (GTPS) where conservative management has failed, a high index of suspicion should be maintained for an abductor tear.

- In keeping with a degenerative etiology, patients describe lateral-sided hip pain that is insidious in onset and is usually debilitating.
- Degenerative abductor tear states likely to represent a continuum of pathology with partial-thickness tears eventually progressing to full-thickness tears over time if left untreated, much like the rotator cuff of the shoulder.
- Tears are four times more common in women than men and the prevalence increases with age.[18] It is estimated that 25% of middle-aged women will develop a tear of the gluteus medius tendon. The increased incidence in women may partly be related to the wider female pelvis.[9]
- A full-thickness tear of the abductors is likely to cause severe lateral pain and a significant limp, resulting in a poor prognosis for those left untreated after failure of conservative management.

PATIENT HISTORY AND PHYSICAL FINDINGS

History

- Recalcitrant pain of insidious onset along the lateral side of the hip
- Pain may be exacerbated by walking, climbing stairs, lying on the affected hip, or resisted hip abduction.
- The patient may report a slight or moderate limp.
- The symptoms show minimal improvement with conservative forms of treatment for a presumed diagnosis of trochanteric bursitis.

Physical Examination

- The patient's gait should be observed for a limp, antalgia, or a frank Trendelenburg gait.
- If a Trendelenburg gait is suspected, a single-leg stance test should be conducted lasting 30 seconds or longer to look for a Trendelenburg sign—if positive, a distinct drop of the nonsupported pelvis is noted, indicating abductor weakness on the supported (single-leg stance) side. The Trendelenburg sign has been shown to be the most sensitive (73%) and specific (77%) physical sign for detection of abductor tears with an acceptable intraobserver reliability[2] of 0.68.
- The patient should then be examined in the supine position for range of motion of the hip. Range of motion is usually preserved in abductor tears but care must be taken to note positions that provoke pain, particularly to rule out intra-articular causes of hip pain.
- An abduction external rotation test is useful in suspected GTPS. Reproduction of pain with the hip flexed to 45 degrees, in abduction, and external rotation may draw attention to inflamed soft tissue structures and bursae over the posterior facet of the greater trochanter. This examination maneuver brings the posterior facet in close proximity to the ischium and posterior wall of the acetabulum resulting in a crushing over the interposed soft tissues.
- The resisted external derotation test is conducted with the patient lying supine, the hip flexed to 90 degrees and externally rotated to 30 degrees. The patient is then asked to internally rotate the hip to neutral against resistance. Reproduction of lateral pain when performing this maneuver has shown an 88% sensitivity and 97% specificity for detecting abductor tendinopathy.[12]
- The examination should then continue with the patient in a lateral decubitus position.
- Deep palpation over the greater trochanter may reproduce the lateral-sided pain.
- An abduction strength test may reveal abductor weakness indicative of tendinopathy or tear. This test is performed with the hip in neutral flexion/extension, stabilizing the pelvis with one hand and asking the patient to actively abduct the hip against resistance. The test can be performed with the knees both flexed and extended to allow relaxation and tension of the iliotibial band, respectively.
- Ober test can also be performed to evaluate the hip abductors for tightness or a contracture.

IMAGING AND OTHER DIAGNOSTIC STUDIES

- An anteroposterior (AP) radiograph of the pelvis and a Dunn lateral radiograph (90 degrees of hip flexion with 20 degrees of abduction and the beam centered on and perpendicular to the hip) are taken for the initial radiographic evaluation of all patients presenting with hip pain.
- Plain radiographs are usually normal in a patient with abductor tears in the setting of a nonarthritic hip, although enthesopathic calcifications may be seen in the region of the abductor insertions at the greater trochanter.
- High-quality MRI is the investigation of choice for diagnosing abductor tears and should be requested based on clinical suspicion.
- Both noncontrast MRI and gadolinium-contrast magnetic resonance arthrogram (MRA) can be used to evaluate the hip joint, using coronal inversion recovery and axial proton density sequences.
- Suspected gluteus medius tendon tears in patients with trochanteric bursitis may be confirmed with MRI.[11] MRI has a high sensitivity and specificity for the diagnosis of gluteus medius and minimus tendons tears (**FIG 5A–C**).
- MRI can differentiate between partial- and full-thickness abductor tears as well as identify calcific tendinitis and fatty atrophy within the muscle substance.
- MRI can also be used to assess the healing and quality of repair tissue after surgical repair of the abductor tendons (**FIG 6A–C**).
- Ultrasound can be used to evaluate gluteus medius and minimus tendinopathy and provide information about disease severity and tear size.[4]

DIFFERENTIAL DIAGNOSIS

- Greater trochanter bursitis
- Calcific tendinitis of the abductor tendons
- Greater trochanteric fracture
- Hip dysplasia
- External coxa saltans (external snapping hip secondary to thickened iliotibial band)
- Internal coxa saltans (internal snapping hip secondary to iliopsoas tendon pathology)
- Piriformis syndrome (sciatic nerve compression)
- Lumbar radiculopathy
- Sacroiliac joint pain

NONOPERATIVE MANAGEMENT

- Nonoperative treatment options can help alleviate pain and improve patient lifestyle.
- Conservative management begins with patient education regarding the diagnosis and natural history of the condition.

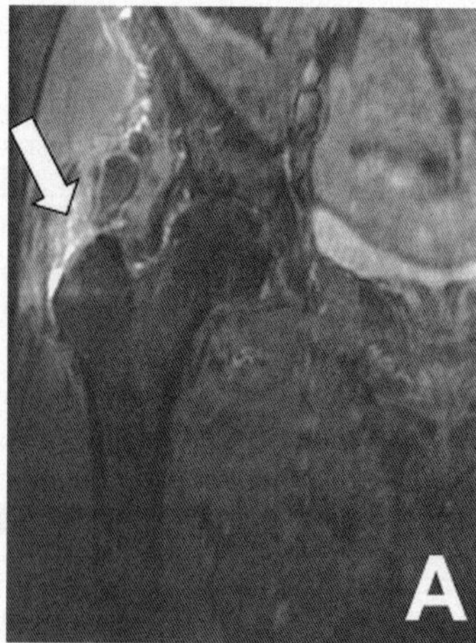

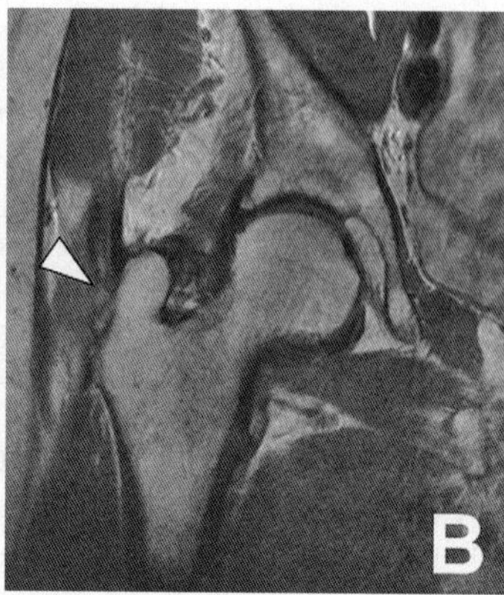

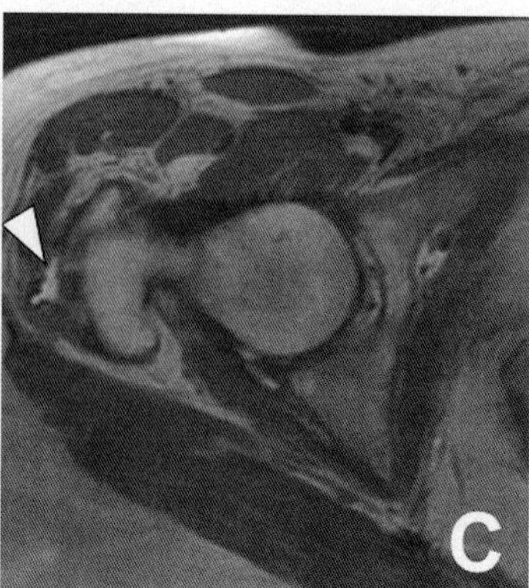

FIG 5 • **A.** Coronal inversion recovery image in a 55-year-old woman demonstrates soft tissue edema (*white arrow*) along the greater tuberosity in the region of the abductor insertions. **B.** Coronal and (**C**) axial fast spin echo (FSE) images demonstrate high-grade partial-thickness tear of the anterolateral fibers of the gluteus medius (*white arrowheads*) at their insertion on the lateral facet. (Courtesy of Alissa Burge, MD.)

All options are discussed, and a nonoperative approach is typically taken initially in treating abductor tears.

- This approach includes rest, ice, anti-inflammatory medication, and physical therapy focused on range-of-motion exercises, strengthening, and gait mechanics.
- If symptoms persist despite the previous interventions, we consider ultrasound-guided injections of local anaesthetic and platelet-rich plasma in MRI-confirmed abductor tears. Corticosteroid injections are reserved for patients with GTPS in the setting of a normal abductor insertion.

SURGICAL MANAGEMENT

- Surgical intervention is indicated for patients who have failed conservative treatment and remain symptomatic with lateral pain and weakness.
- Abductor repairs can be performed open or endoscopically.
- We reserve open repairs for complete avulsions of the abductor tendons from the greater trochanter with retraction on MRI. We believe that an open repair can afford a more durable repair in the setting of complete tendon avulsion with retraction but that repair of larger tears may be feasible endoscopically as techniques improve.
- Endoscopic repair of the abductor tendons can be performed reproducibly and results in resolution of pain and return to activity in a predictable manner in the short term.
- Entry into the peritrochanteric space typically follows routine evaluation and treatment of pathology in the central and peripheral compartments.
- Irrespective of technique, a working knowledge of the anatomy of the abductor tendon footprint on the greater

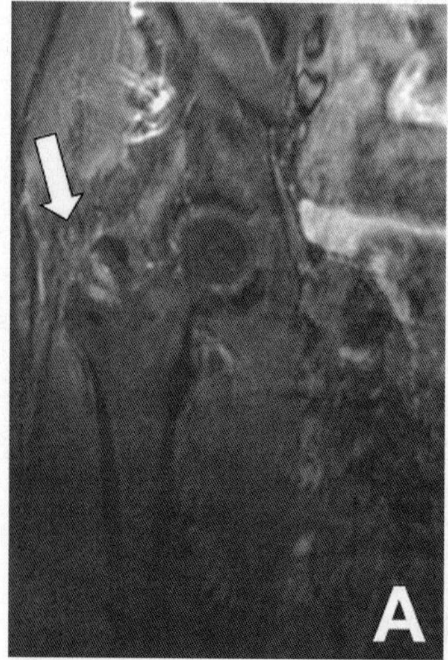

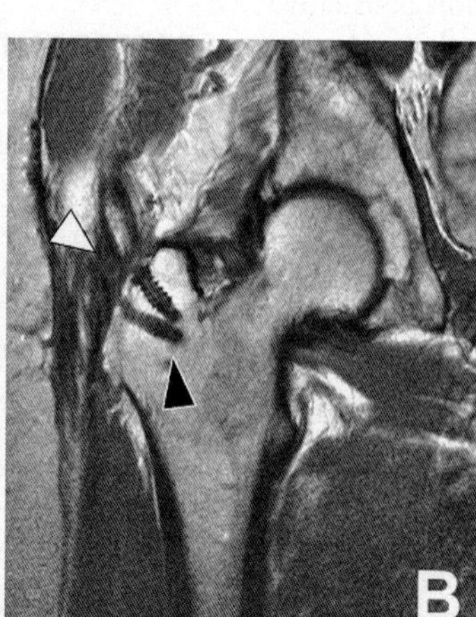

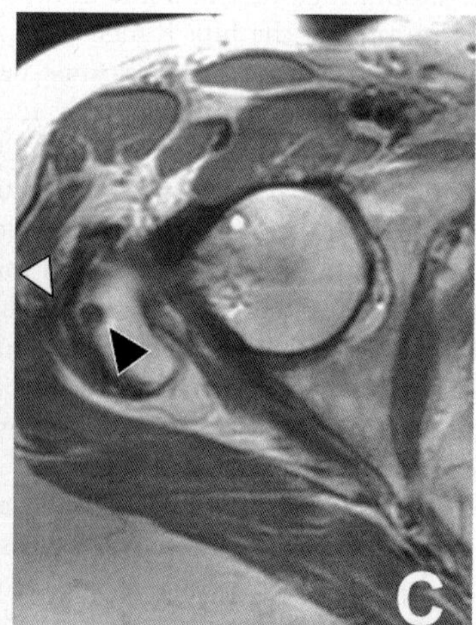

FIG 6 • **A.** Coronal inversion recovery image of the same patient in **FIG 5** following subsequent abductor repair demonstrates interval resolution of edema previously identified in the region of the greater trochanter (*white arrow*). **B.** Coronal and (**C**) axial fast spin echo (FSE) images demonstrate anchors (*black arrowheads*) within the lateral facet, with restoration of the previously torn anterolateral gluteus medius insertion (*white arrowheads*). (Courtesy of Alissa Burge, MD.)

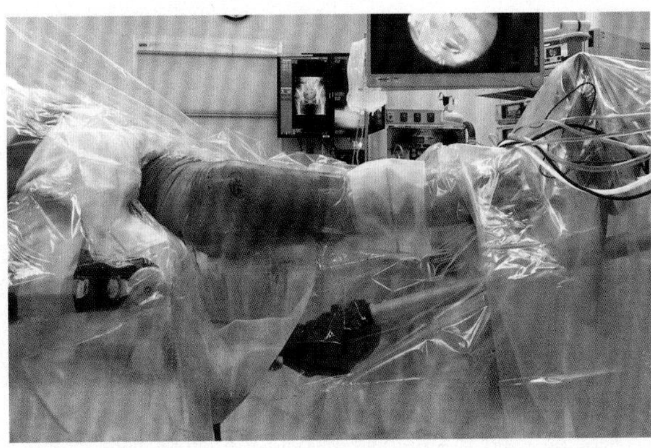

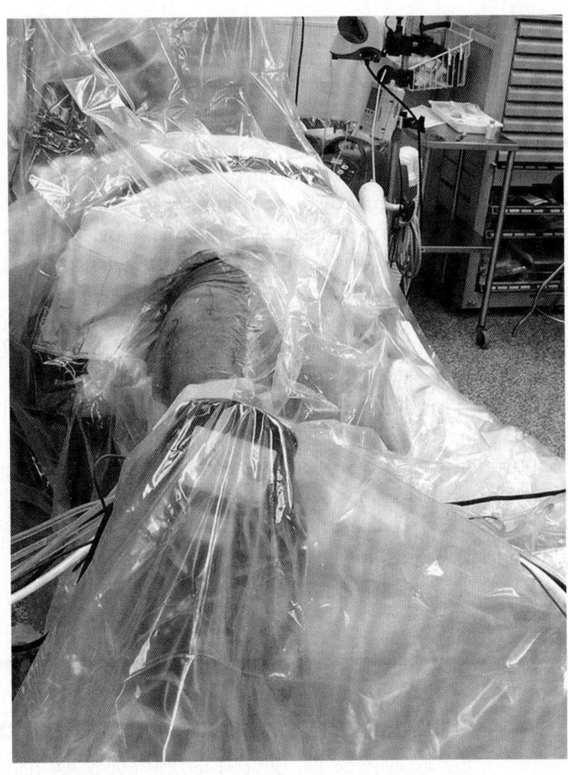

FIG 7 • **A.** Lateral view of a patient positioned on a standard OR table with a specialized lower extremity attachment. The operative leg is positioned in 0- to 20-degree flexion, 10 to 15 degrees of internal rotation, and 20 degrees of abduction to relax the iliotibial band and allow entry into the peritrochanteric space. **B.** "End of the table" view of a patient positioned on a standard OR table with a specialized lower extremity attachment. The operative leg is positioned in 0- to 20-degree flexion, 10 to 15 degrees of internal rotation, and 20 degrees of abduction to relax the iliotibial band and allow entry into the peritrochanteric space.

trochanter is critical to identify the site of injury at the time of endoscopy and to subsequently execute an anatomic repair.

Preoperative Planning

- Preoperative planning consists of a thorough history and physical examination confirming that the symptoms are originating from the lateral compartment of the hip.
- Any pathology in the central and peripheral compartments that can be treated arthroscopically has been identified and surgical intervention planned based on clinical and radiologic findings.
- A recent plain radiograph is available, as progressive joint space deterioration may contraindicate an arthroscopic procedure.
- A recent MRI scan is available, confirming the presence of an abductor tear that is amenable to endoscopic repair.

Positioning

- As a peritrochanteric space endoscopy typically follows routine arthroscopy of the central and peripheral compartments, the patient should already be set up on a standard operating room (OR) table with specialized lower extremity attachment.
- No distraction is required, and therefore, the perineal post is removed.
- Both feet are secured in well-padded boots.
- The nonoperative hip is placed in slight abduction, neutral extension, and full extension at the knee.
- The operative lower extremity is placed in 0 to 20 degrees flexion, 10 to 15 degrees internal rotation, and 20 degrees abduction to relax the iliotibial band and allow entry into the potential space between the greater trochanter and iliotibial band (**FIG 7A,B**).

Approach

- The anterior and midanterior (MA) portals can be both used to access the peritrochanteric space (**FIG 8**).
- Both these anterior portals are placed lateral to the anterior superior iliac spine (ASIS) to avoid injury to the LFCN and pass through the interval between the tensor fascia latae and sartorius.
- We routinely use the MA portal to enter the peritrochanteric space. This portal is 2 cm distal and lateral to the standard anterior portal.

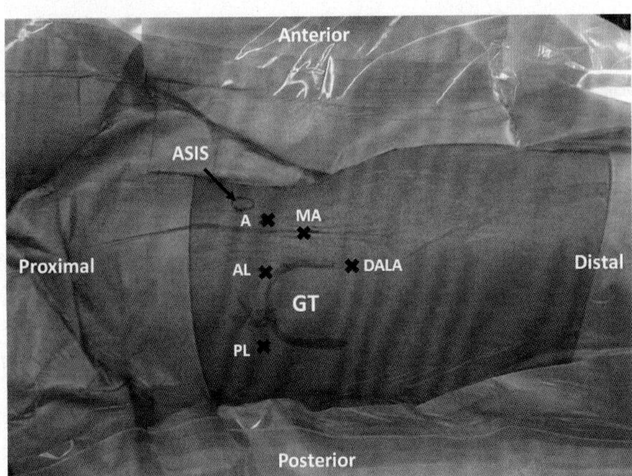

FIG 8 • The operative leg has been prepped and draped and the standard portals used for entry into the peritrochanteric space are marked. *A*, anterior; *AL*, anterolateral; *ASIS*, anterior superior iliac spine; *DALA*, distal anterolateral accessory; *GT*, greater trochanter; *MA*, midanterior; *PL*, posterolateral. (Courtesy of Bryan T. Kelly, MD.)

- The MA portal has two distinct advantages over the standard anterior portal:
  - It further reduces the risk of injury to the LFCN, as it is placed even more lateral to the ASIS compared to the standard anterior portal.[16]
  - It lies directly over the lateral flare of the greater trochanter and therefore is just distal to the gluteus medius muscle belly and proximal to the vastus lateralis. This position avoids injury to the abductor muscle mass when passing instruments to facilitate repair.
- Fluoroscopy is used to aid in proper placement of the MA portal by confirming placement directly over the lateral flare of the greater trochanter and proximal to the vastus ridge (**FIG 9**). This placement prevents inadvertent proximal gluteus medius and distal vastus lateralis muscular injury.
- Three portals are usually sufficient to complete an endoscopic abductor repair (MA, anterolateral, and distal anterolateral accessory [DALA]). Occasionally, the posterolateral portal is also used (see **FIG 8**).

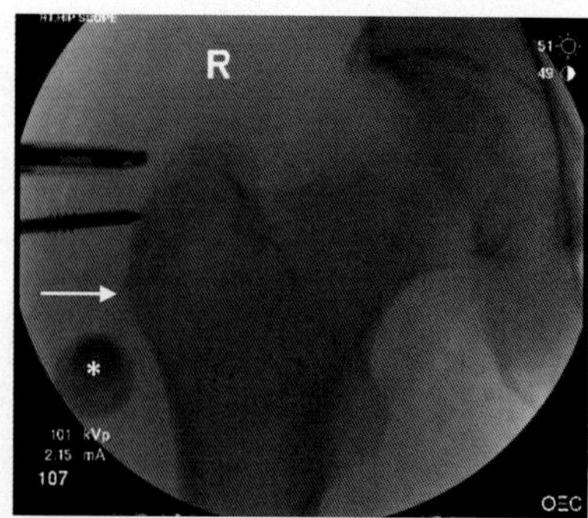

FIG 9 • Fluoroscopic image of a right hip. A metal cap (*asterisk*) is being used to externally palpate the lateral flare of the greater trochanter (*arrow*). The initial entry point using a trocar in an AP direction must be directed at this lateral prominence to avoid inadvertent injury to the gluteus medius fibers proximally and the vastus lateralis fibers distally. Fluoroscopy can also be used to confirm that the direction of entry of suture anchors is perpendicular to the lateral facet. (Courtesy of Bryan T. Kelly, MD.)

TECHNIQUES

Establishing Primary Viewing Portal

- After establishing the position for the MA portal under fluoroscopic guidance, a blunt plastic cannula is directed into the peritrochanteric space in an anterior to posterior direction.
- The cannula is swept back and forth between the trochanteric bursa and iliotibial band to release any adhesions in a fashion similar to that used when entering the subacromial space of the shoulder.
- Once the appropriate plane is identified, the space is distended with 50 mm Hg of fluid pressure and a 70-degree scope is introduced and locked into the plastic cannula.
- The light source and camera are oriented such that the light source is facing distally and the camera is parallel to the operative leg (**TECH FIG 1**).

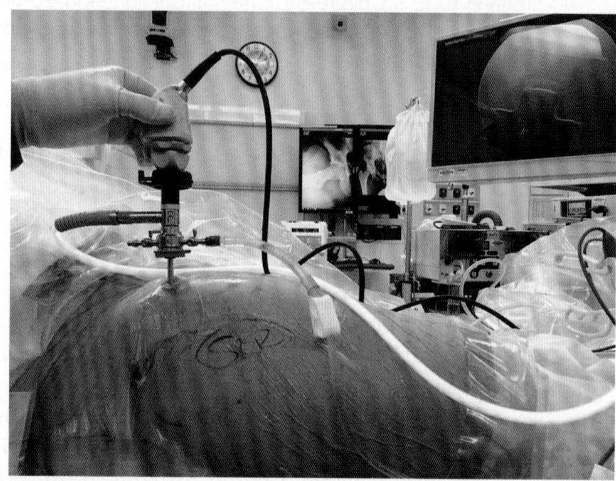

TECH FIG 1 • Upon entry into the peritrochanteric space, the camera is oriented parallel to the operative lower extremity and the light source is faced distally.

Bursectomy and Establishing Visualization

- Upon entry into the peritrochanteric space, the DALA portal is established using a standard Seldinger technique (see **FIG 8**). This portal is in line with the anterolateral portal, 4 to 5 cm directly distal to it.
- A motorized shaver is inserted into the peritrochanteric space through this portal, and the trochanteric bursa is thoroughly cleared (**TECH FIG 2**).
- The bursectomy begins distally at the gluteus maximus insertion into the femur and progresses proximally in a systematic fashion. This should allow easy visualization of the iliotibial band and greater trochanter, which define the lateral and medial borders of the peritrochanteric space, respectively.
- The standard anterolateral portal can then be used as a third working or viewing portal, improving proximal access or distal visualization.

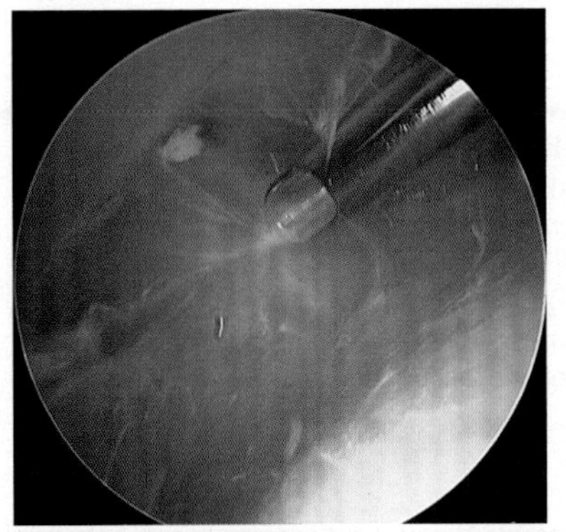

A

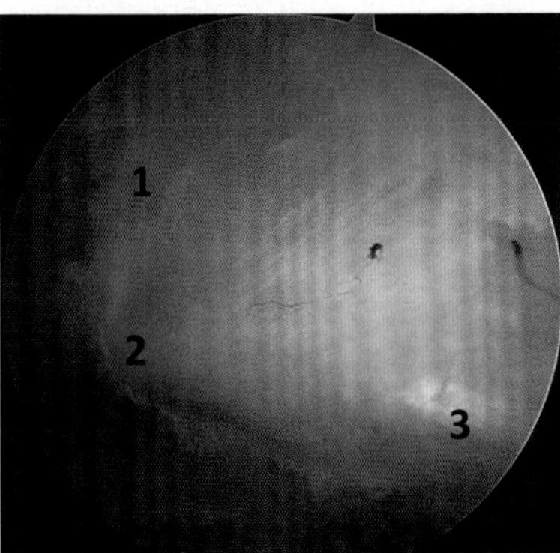

B

TECH FIG 2 • **A.** Endoscopic view of the peritrochanteric space upon initial entry with a 70-degree arthroscope in the MA portal with the light source directed distally. Visualization is facilitated by a thorough bursectomy, which is being performed in this photograph with a motorized shaver. **B.** Once the bursa is cleared, orientation is possible by identifying the gluteus medius (*1*), lateral facet (*2*), and vastus lateralis (*3*).

Establishing Orientation in Peritrochanteric Space

- The first structure that must be identified on establishing adequate visualization is the gluteus maximus tendon inserting on the femur just below the vastus lateralis (**TECH FIG 3A**).
- This is a reproducible landmark that establishes a safe zone—the sciatic nerve lies 3 to 4 cm posterior to the gluteus maximus insertion, and therefore, exploration posterior to the tendon should be avoided. Working distal to this tendon insertion is usually unnecessary.
- The light source is then directed to the lateral aspect of the femur where the longitudinal fibers of the vastus lateralis can be visualized and followed proximally to the vastus ridge. Proximal to the vastus ridge, the insertion and muscle belly of the gluteus medius is identified by directing the light source anterosuperiorly (**TECH FIG 3B**).

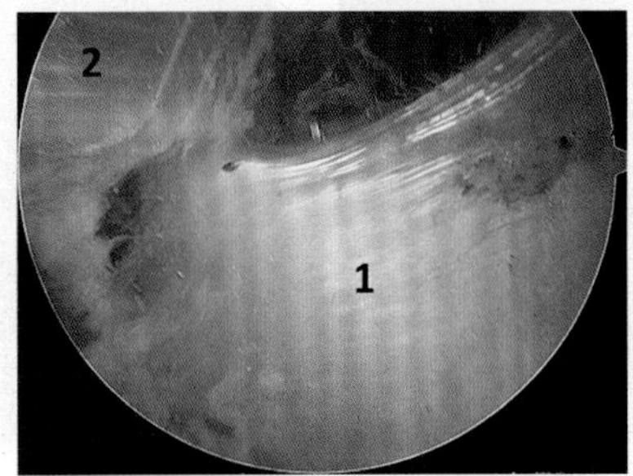

A

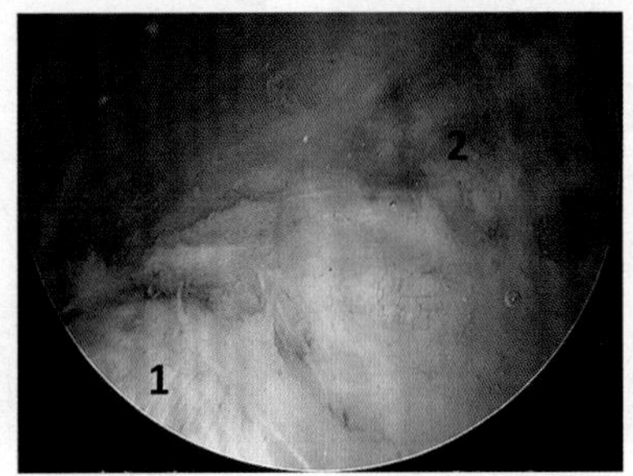

B

TECH FIG 3 • **A.** With the 70-degree scope in the MA portal, the most clearly identifiable landmark is the distal insertion of the gluteus maximus tendon into the femur (*1*). Visualization of this tendon establishes a safe zone for periarticular endoscopy and helps confirm that the sciatic nerve is not at risk during the procedure. Note the orientation of the gluteus maximus tendon posterior to the longitudinal fibers of the vastus lateralis (*2*). **B.** The longitudinal fibers of the vastus lateralis (*1*) can be visualized and followed proximally to the vastus ridge where the insertion and muscle belly of the gluteus medius (*2*) can be identified.

Evaluation of the Abductor Attachment

- The gluteus medius muscle and insertion are then evaluated at the lateral facet. The entire tendon should be inspected and carefully probed.
- The gluteus medius muscle and tendon are best visualized with arthroscope in the proximal anterolateral portal, which gives a global view of the abductors. The light source is rotated to visualize anterosuperiorly.
- The working instruments can then be placed in the MA and DALA portals.
- The gluteus minimus is often covered by the gluteus medius muscle and can be difficult to visualize. A switching stick can be used to gently retract medius muscle to see the tendinous insertion of the gluteus minimus onto the anterior facet (**TECH FIG 4**).
- Most commonly, the gluteus medius is degenerated and torn off its distal insertion on the lateral facet of the greater trochanter.
- Undersurface partial tears can also occur, but in case of significant thinning of the tendon insertion, the tear should be completed and repaired.

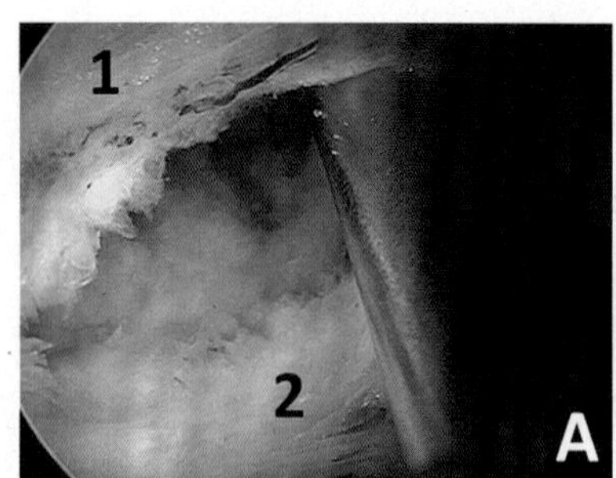

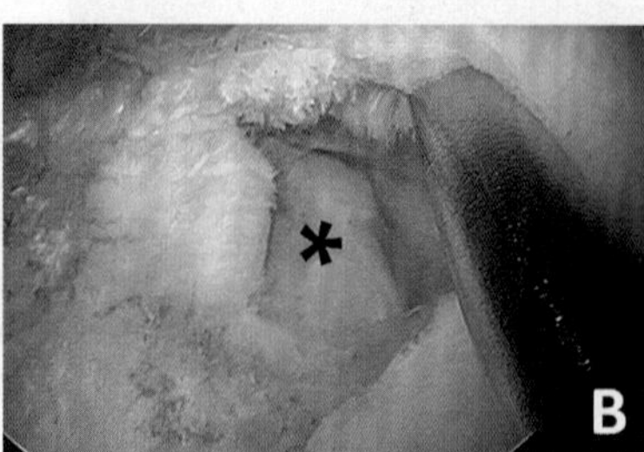

TECH FIG 4 • **A.** A plane is developed at the anterior margin of the gluteus medius (*1*), between the gluteus minimus (*2*) and medius, to allow visualization of the undersurface of the tendon. **B.** Upon elevation of the gluteus medius tear the footprint of the tendon at the lateral facet can be identified (*asterisk*). (Courtesy of Bryan T. Kelly, MD.)

Preparation for Endoscopic Abductor Repair

- If a tear in the gluteus medius is identified, it must be assessed for retraction and repairability similar to tears of the rotator cuff of the shoulder (**TECH FIG 5A,B**).
- A probe or grasper is used to manually reduce the tear to its anatomic position in the footprint in order to determine the tissue quality as well as the tendon mobility.
- A mechanical shaver is used to débride the edges of the tear to healthy, robust tissue.
- A motorized burr is used to decorticate the lateral facet of the greater trochanter and prepare a bleeding cancellous bone bed to facilitate healing (**TECH FIG 5C**).

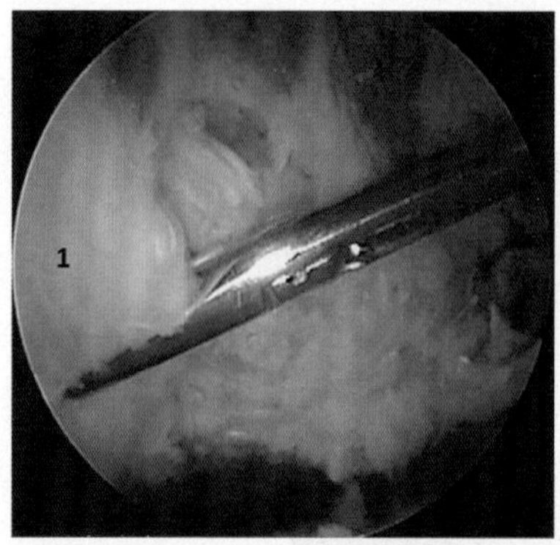

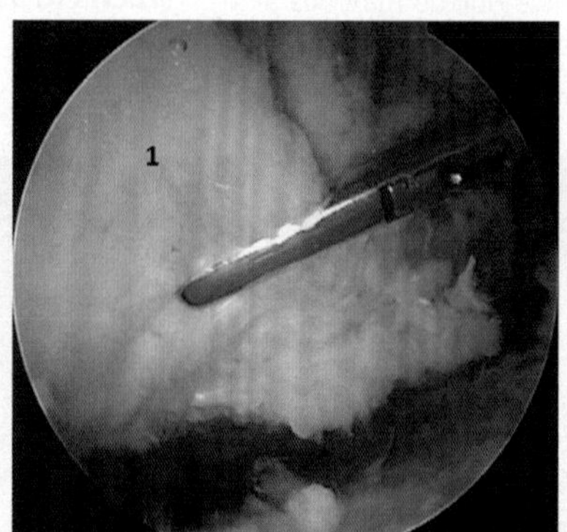

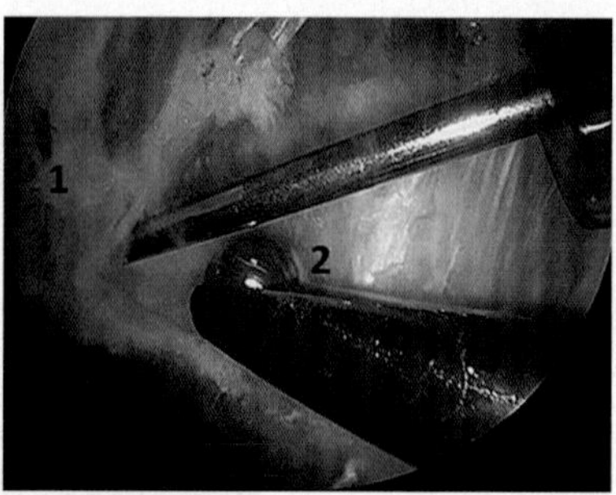

TECH FIG 5 • **A.** A grasper is being used to assess the mobility of the free edge of the gluteus medius tendon (*1*). **B.** In this case, the tear is reducible to its anatomic position at the footprint and the tissue is of adequate quality. **C.** The anterior edge of the gluteus medius tendon (*1*) is being retracted and a motorized burr is being used to decorticate the lateral facet of the greater trochanter (*2*) and prepare a bleeding cancellous bone bed to facilitate healing. (Courtesy of Bryan T. Kelly, MD.)

Endoscopic Rotator Cuff Repair of the Hip

- Due to the hard nature of bone in the greater trochanter, metallic or peek anchors are usually used for repair. The position of metallic anchors can be confirmed with fluoroscopy.
- Typically, two anchors will suffice to repair the anatomic footprint of a gluteus medius tendon tear off the lateral facet. Adequate spacing of anchors must be allowed for good bone stock to be present between anchors.
- To obtain the optimal trajectory for anchor placement, a spinal needle is placed first, and positioned with arthroscopic and fluoroscopic guidance. Anchors are then placed into the footprint through percutaneous stab incisions followed by confirmation of anchor position by fluoroscopy (**TECH FIG 6A**).
- After anchor placement, sutures are passed sequentially through the free tendon edge using a suture-passing device (**TECH FIG 6B,C**). The tendon edge can be captured with a needle-penetrating device placed through the DALA portal. Sutures are then parked in the MA portal.
- All sutures should be passed through long hip cannulas to avoid soft tissue entrapment.
- After all the sutures have been passed, arthroscopic sliding, locking knots are placed with a knot pusher to secure the gluteus medius and minimus back to their native footprint on the greater trochanter (**TECH FIG 6D**). We prefer to place two mattress stitches that are perpendicular to one another from a single suture anchor.
- Careful evaluation of the tendon repair should be performed to confirm anatomic restoration of the tendon footprint and security of repair.

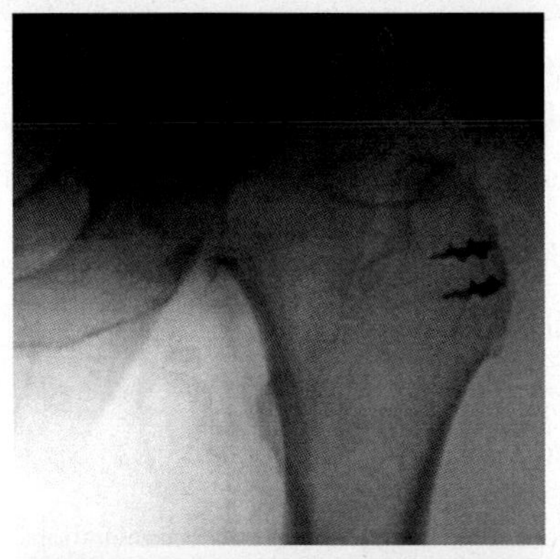
A

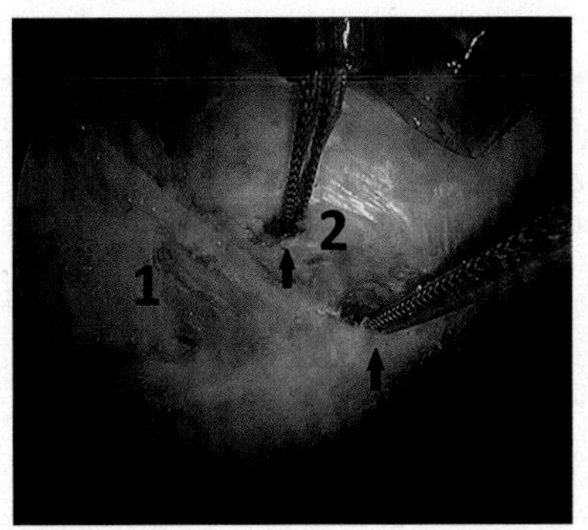

B

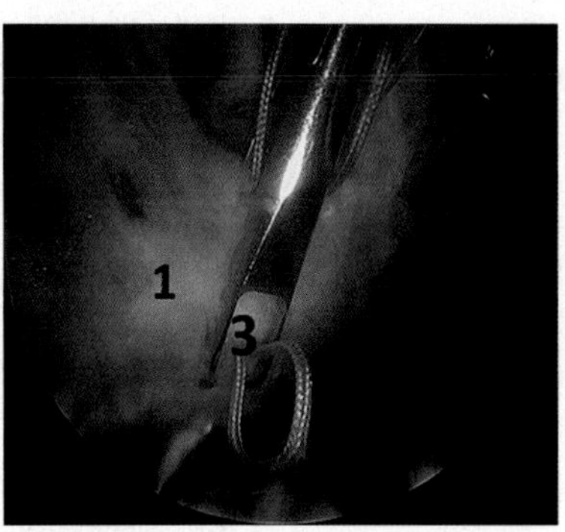

C

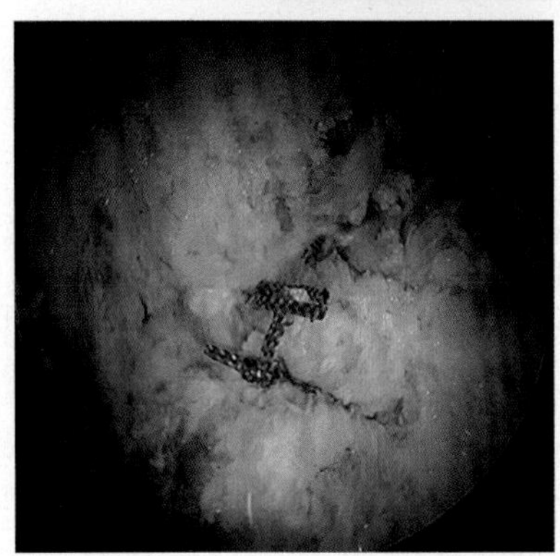
D

TECH FIG 6 • A. Fluoroscopic imaging is used during anchor placement to confirm that they are inserted perpendicular to the greater trochanter. **B.** Two anchors have been placed just distal to the torn edge of the gluteus medius (*1*), appropriately spaced to span the anatomic footprint in the lateral facet (*2*). **C.** The sutures are then passed sequentially through the free tendon edge using a suture-passing device (*3*). **D.** The abductor repair has been completed by tensioning and tying all sutures. A final inspection is then performed to ensure anatomic restoration of the tendon footprint and security of repair. (**A,C,D:** Courtesy of Bryan T. Kelly, MD.)

Surgical Management of Partial-Thickness Abductor Tears

- Partial-thickness undersurface tears that are seen on MRI are often difficult to see arthroscopically.
- These tears are analogous to an articular-sided rotator cuff tear of the shoulder, which extends posteriorly and may become a full-thickness tear.
- In contrast to rotator cuff tears of the shoulder, there is no space in the peritrochanteric compartment analogous to the intra-articular space of the shoulder from where the undersurface of a gluteus medius partial-thickness tear can be visualized.
- These tears may be better visualized by developing a plane at the anterior margin of the gluteus medius, between the gluteus minimus and medius.
- If they are high-grade lesions, they may be converted to a full-thickness tear and repaired using the previously described technique.
- A transtendinous repair is also possible and the technique has been described.[6]
    - A longitudinal split in the gluteus medius insertion at the lateral facet is made.
    - The undersurface tearing of the tendon is visualized through the split.
    - The arthroscope is inserted through the split to better visualize the undersurface tearing.
    - A shaver is used to débride pathologic tissue and a burr is used to decorticate the lateral facet.
    - Anchors are then placed through the tendon split under fluoroscopic guidance.
    - Suture-passing devices are used to pass one limb of each suture through the anterior and posterior parts of the tendon.
    - All sutures are tied down to effect a side-to-side repair of the tendon split while securing the tendon to the lateral facet.

PEARLS AND PITFALLS

Pearls	■ Use of the MA portal in conjunction with blunt dissection down the portal tract minimizes injury risk to LFCN. ■ Use of fluoroscopy to confirm that the initial entry point of the MA portal is adjacent to the lateral flare of the greater trochanter avoids injury to the gluteus medius proximally. ■ Fluid pressure should be titrated to visualization throughout the procedure to avoid fluid extravasation into the thigh and prevent injury to surrounding soft tissue structures. ■ Cannulas should be at least 90 mm in length to prevent soft tissue bridges between sutures while performing abductor repair. ■ Continuous passive motion for the first 4 weeks minimizes the development of postoperative adhesions.
Pitfalls	■ Large and irreducible abductor tears may result in inferior outcomes or fail early after endoscopic repair and therefore are better suited to open repair techniques. ■ Deep venous thrombosis (DVT) prophylaxis must be considered as the patient population is older than typical hip arthroscopy patients. ■ Early failure of abductor repair can be minimized by a graduated progression through postoperative rehabilitation.

POSTOPERATIVE CARE

- Twenty pounds of foot-flat weight bearing is permitted for the first 6 weeks with the aid of crutches.
- Abduction brace locked at 10 degrees of hip abduction
- Continuous passive motion initiated immediately for 4 hours per day and stationary biking for 20 minutes per day for the first 6 weeks to prevent adhesions.
- No active abduction and internal rotation or passive adduction and external rotation for the first 6 weeks to preserve repair integrity.
- Passive hip flexion to 90 degrees and passive abduction as pain allows are permitted for the first 6 weeks.
- Passive hip flexion beyond 90 degrees is permitted after the first 6 weeks.
- Sutures are removed in 10 to 14 days and scar massage of the portals is commenced thereafter.
- Isometric strengthening of the hip adductors, extenders, and external rotators is commenced after the first 2 weeks.
- Active strengthening is commenced at 6 weeks postoperatively, starting with isometric submaximal hip flexion and quadriceps strengthening.
- Progression to weight bearing as tolerated with crutches is permitted at 6 to 8 weeks postoperatively.
- Progressive hip range-of-motion exercises with passive internal and external rotation are commenced at 8 weeks postoperatively.
- After 10 weeks, lower extremity and core strengthening are progressed as tolerated.
- Between 3 and 6 months, patients should be pain free, demonstrate quadriceps and hamstrings peak torque strength within 15% of the contralateral extremity, and demonstrate a normal stepdown test.

OUTCOMES

- Outcomes data of endoscopic gluteus medius repairs are limited to small case series at short-term follow-up.
- Voos et al[18] reported on the outcomes of 10 patients (mean age 50 years) who underwent endoscopic repair of full-thickness gluteus medius tears, with a mean follow-up of 25 months. All patients had complete resolution of pain with mean modified Harris hip scores of 94 points and hip outcomes scores of 93 points at final follow-up.
- Domb et al[5] reported on 15 patients with an average age of 58 years at a mean follow-up of 28 months. Their series included six partial-thickness and nine full-thickness tears. Satisfaction with the surgery was good to excellent for 14 of 15 patients and outcomes scores improved by more than 30 points on four different hip-specific scoring scales.
- McCormick et al[14] studied 10 patients with an average age of 66 years at a mean follow-up of 23 months. All patients underwent endoscopic repair of full-thickness abductor tears. All patients had good to excellent outcomes with improved strength. They also noted that younger patients achieved better outcomes.

COMPLICATIONS

- In comparison to central and peripheral compartment hip arthroscopy, periarticular endoscopy of the peritrochanteric space has a lower complication rate.
- No serious complications have been reported in the literature.[14,18]
- Potential risks of LFCN neurapraxia and significant fluid extravasation into the thigh do exist, but the incidence is not known.

REFERENCES

1. Beck M, Sledge JB, Gautier E, et al. The anatomy and function of the gluteus minimus muscle. J Bone Joint Surg Br 2000;82(3):358–363.
2. Bird PA, Oakley SP, Shnier R, et al. Prospective evaluation of magnetic resonance imaging and physical examination findings in patients with greater trochanteric pain syndrome. Arthritis Rheum 2001;44(9):2138–2145.
3. Bunker TD, Esler CN, Leach WJ. Rotator-cuff tear of the hip. J Bone Joint Surg Br 1997;79(4):618–620.
4. Connell DA, Bass C, Sykes CA, et al. Sonographic evaluation of gluteus medius and minimus tendinopathy. Eur Radiol 2003;13(6): 1339–1347.
5. Domb BG, Botser I, Giordano BD. Outcomes of endoscopic gluteus medius repair with minimum 2-year follow-up. Am J Sports Med 2013;41(5):988–997.
6. Domb BG, Nasser RM, Botser IB. Partial-thickness tears of the gluteus medius: rationale and technique for trans-tendinous endoscopic repair. Arthroscopy 2010;26(12):1697–1705.
7. Dwek J, Pfirrmann C, Stanley A, et al. MR imaging of the hip abductors: normal anatomy and commonly encountered pathology at the greater trochanter. Magn Reson Imaging Clin N Am 2005;13(4): 691–704.

8. Gottschalk F, Kourosh S, Leveau B. The functional anatomy of tensor fasciae latae and gluteus medius and minimus. J Anat 1989;166:179–189.
9. Howell GE, Biggs RE, Bourne RB. Prevalence of abductor mechanism tears of the hips in patients with osteoarthritis. J Arthoplasty 2001;16(1):121–123.
10. Kagan A II. Rotator cuff tears of the hip. Clin Orthop Relat Res 1999;(368):135–140.
11. Lequesne M, Djian P, Vuillemin V, et al. Prospective study of refractory greater trochanter pain syndrome. MRI findings of gluteal tendon tears seen at surgery. Clinical and MRI results of tendon repair. Joint Bone Spine 2008;75(4):458–464.
12. Lequesne M, Mathieu P, Vuillemin-Bodaghi V, et al. Gluteal tendinopathy in refractory greater trochanter pain syndrome: diagnostic value of two clinical tests. Arthritis Rheum 2008;59(2):241–246.
13. Lonner JH, Van Kleunen JP. Spontaneous rupture of the gluteus medius and minimus tendons. Am J Orthop 2002;31(10):579–581.
14. McCormick F, Alpaugh K, Nwachukwu BU, et al. Endoscopic repair of full-thickness abductor tendon tears: surgical technique and outcome at minimum of 1-year follow-up. Arthroscopy 2013;29(12): 1941–1947.
15. Ozcakar L, Erol O, Kaymak B, et al. An underdiagnosed hip pathology: a propos of two cases with gluteus medius tendon tears. Clin Rheumatol 2004;23(5):464–466.
16. Robertson WJ, Gardner MJ, Barker JU, et al. Anatomy and dimensions of the gluteus medius tendon insertion. Arthroscopy 2008;24(2): 130–136.
17. Voos JE, Rudzki JR, Shindle MK, et al. Arthroscopic anatomy and surgical techniques for peritrochanteric space disorders in the hip. Arthroscopy 2007;23(11):1246.e1–e5.
18. Voos JE, Shindle MK, Pruett A, et al. Endoscopic repair of gluteus medius tendon tears of the hip. Am J Sports Med 2009;37(4): 743–747.

CHAPTER 5

Hip Arthroscopy

John P. Salvo and Daniel P. Woods

DEFINITION

- Hip arthroscopy is a minimally invasive technique to address a variety of painful hip conditions in the athletic and prearthritic population.
- A surge in technologic development since the mid-1990s has allowed surgeons to effectively and reliably treat a variety of painful hip conditions arthroscopically.
- The outcomes of hip arthroscopic techniques are equivocal to traditional, more invasive open techniques.[2]
- There is a tremendous learning curve when compared to knee and shoulder arthroscopy.

ANATOMY

- The hip is a constrained ball-and-socket joint, with the femoral head (ball) articulating with the acetabulum (socket) of the pelvis (**FIG 1**).
- The labrum is a pad of fibrocartilage attached to the acetabulum that deepens the acetabulum and provides stability to the

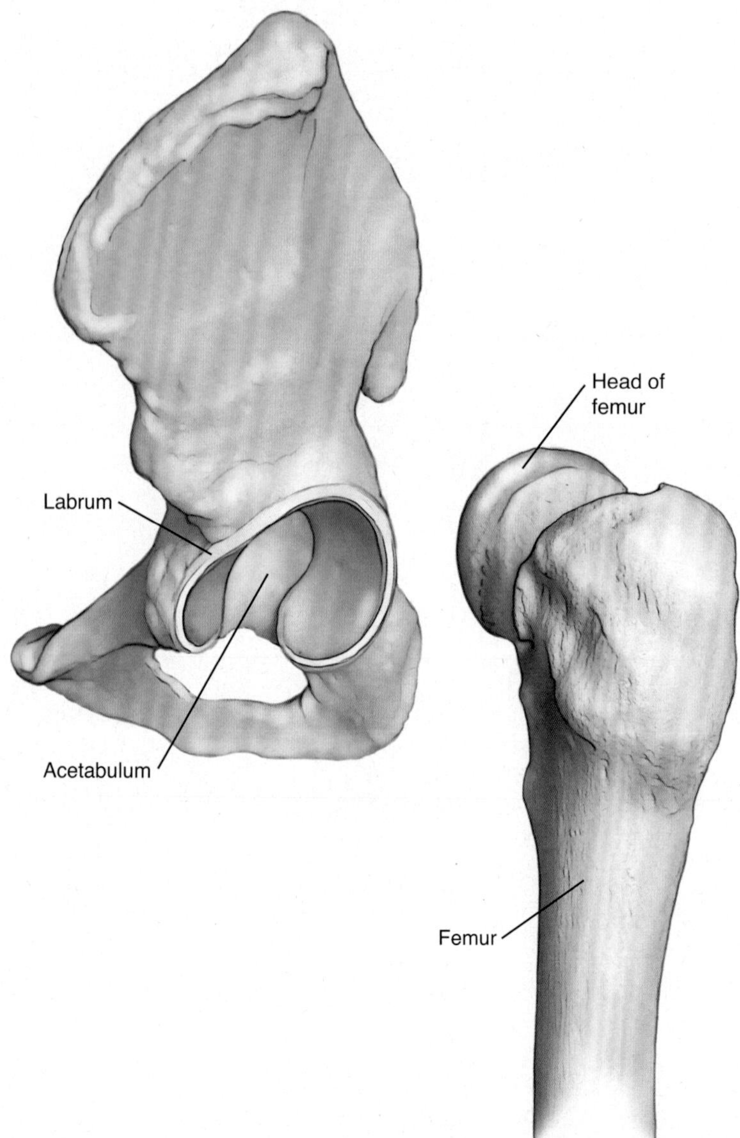

FIG 1 • Picture represents the bony and soft tissue anatomy of the hip joint. Femoral head, acetabulum, articular cartilage, and labrum are shown.

hip as well as a "suction-seal" effect around the femoral head, providing a secure environment for the articular cartilage and synovial fluid[6] (**FIG 2**).

- The alignment and shape of the hip is critical when determining the etiology of hip pain and thus proper treatment.
- Femoroacetabular impingement (FAI) refers to a bony over-constraint of the joint either from the femur (cam) or acetabulum (pincer) or both (combined)[11] (**FIGS 3** and **4**)
- Dysplasia refers to a shallow acetabulum, undercoverage of the femoral head, or both[12] (**FIG 5**).

PATHOGENESIS

- Hip and groin pain in athletic and prearthritic population has a wide variety of etiologies:
  - Labral tear
  - FAI
  - Loose bodies
  - Osteoarthritis
  - Core muscle injury (also known as *sports hernia*)
- Labral tear is the most common cause of hip pain and dysfunction in this population.
- Labral tears are usually secondary to FAI or dysplasia or both.

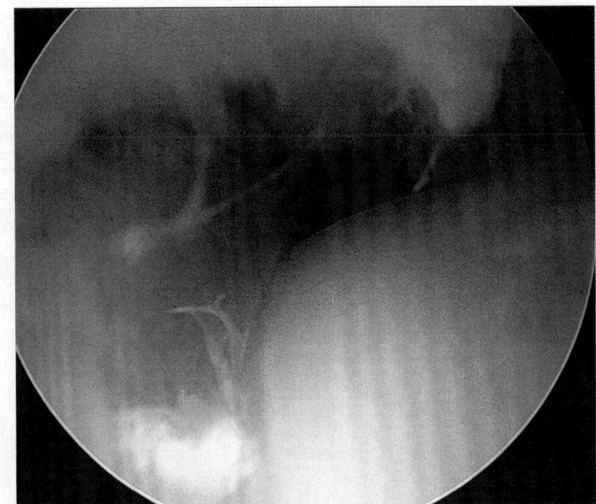

FIG 2 • Arthroscopic picture showing the femoral head (*right*) and the labrum (*left*) and the suction-seal effect of a normal labrum with the hip off traction.

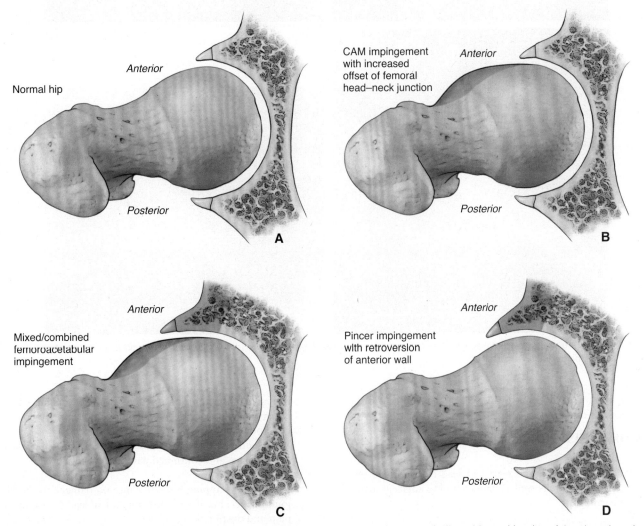

FIG 3 • FAI. Schematic diagram shows views of a normal hip, cam impingement with increased offset of femoral head–neck junction, pincer impingement with retroversion of anterior wall, and mixed/combined FAI.

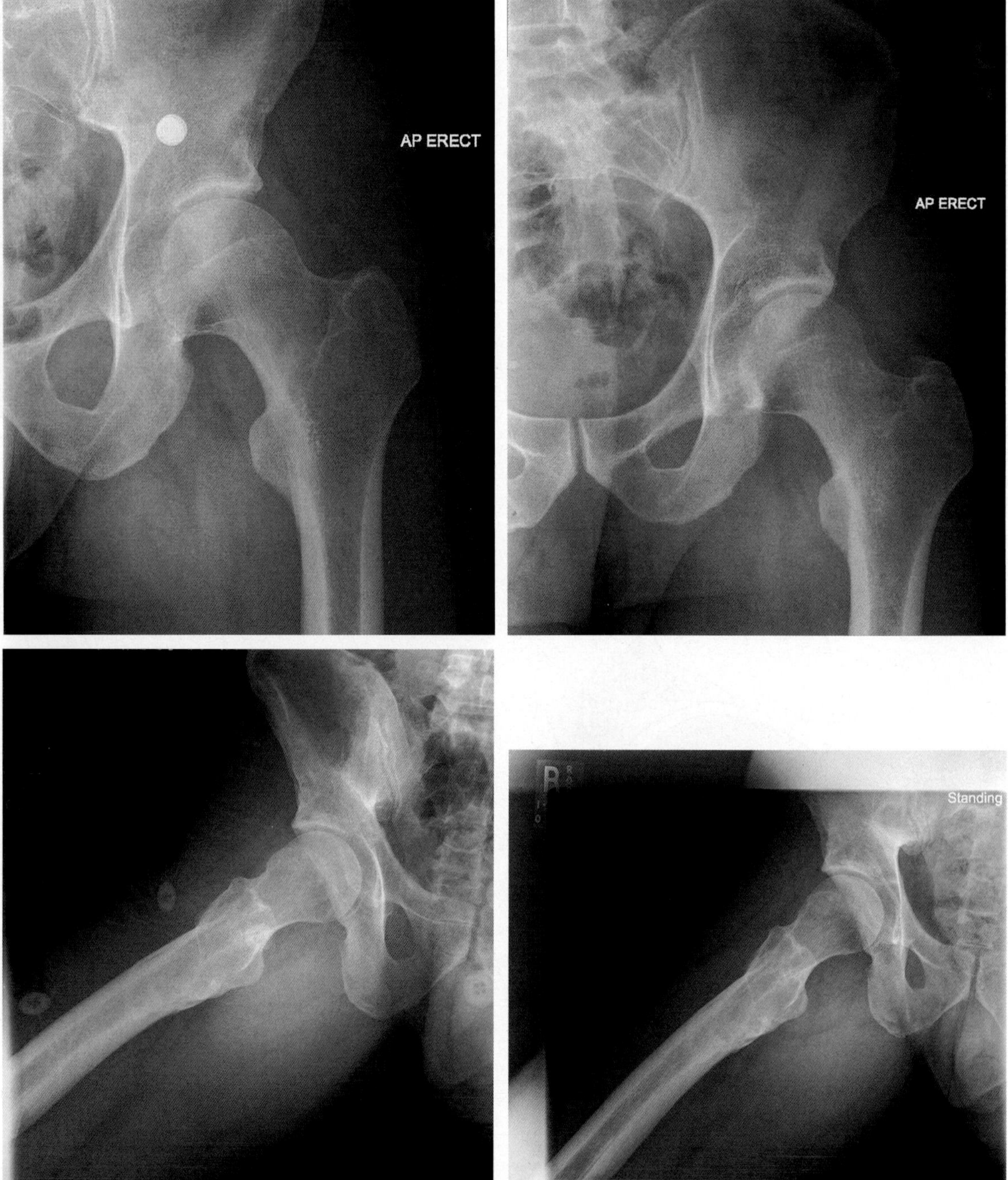

FIG 4 ● X-rays preoperative weight-bearing views AP and lateral of hip with mixed FAI. Postoperative AP and lateral views after femoroplasty and acetabuloplasty.

- If left unchecked, FAI may lead to early development of degenerative joint disease.[7]

NATURAL HISTORY

- Labral tear
  - If left untreated, labral tears can lead to continued pain and dysfunction as well as damage to the adjacent articular cartilage.
- FAI
  - If left untreated, many believe that FAI is a precursor to arthritis.
  - If treated at the appropriate time before irreversible articular cartilage damage occurs, the hip may be preserved.
- Loose bodies
  - If left untreated, loose bodies will lead to articular cartilage damage and continued pain and dysfunction.[9]
- Snapping hip
  - In general, snapping hip will cause no damage to the hip joint proper; but if left untreated, it can lead to continued pain and dysfunction.
  - Internal snapping hip can impinge on the anterior labrum, leading to tears in this area.

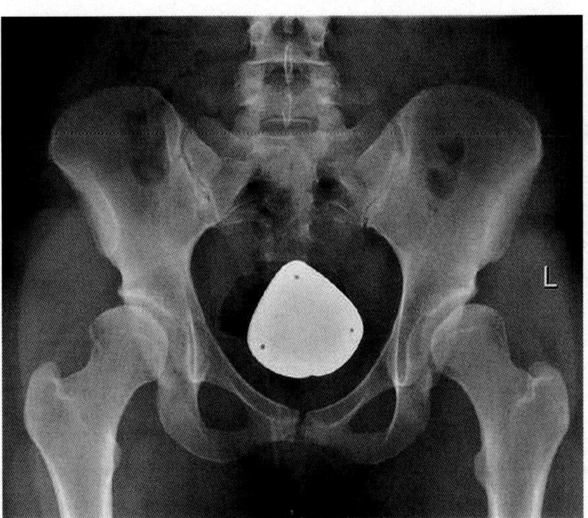

FIG 5 • X-ray of hip with acetabular dysplasia with decreased center-edge angle and lack of coverage of femoral head.

PATIENT HISTORY AND PHYSICAL FINDINGS

- A thorough and focused physical examination is essential.
- Observe gait, manual motor testing, palpation of bony prominences and tendons, range of motion (ROM), and provocative maneuvers for reproducing pain and symptoms.
- Perform the examination on the asymptomatic hip first to assess the ROM and stability of the normal hip when possible.

IMAGING AND OTHER DIAGNOSTIC STUDIES

- Weight-bearing x-rays (anteroposterior [AP] pelvis, frog lateral, false profile, and Dunn 45-degree views)[10]
- High resolution magnetic resonance imaging (MRI). Direct MRI arthrogram allows injection of lidocaine to determine if pain is generated from hip.
- Computed tomography (CT) scan allows the best detailed determination of FAI and alignment (dysplasia or version) and allows for detailed preoperative planning for decompression of FAI.[10]

DIFFERENTIAL DIAGNOSIS

- Labral tear
- FAI
- Loose bodies
- Synovitis
- Snapping hip
- Articular cartilage disease
- Arthritis

NONOPERATIVE MANAGEMENT

- Nonoperative management is always the first step in the treatment of painful hip conditions in the athletic and prearthritic population.
- Activity modification; physical therapy aimed at restoring strength, motion, and balance; and nonsteroidal anti-inflammatory drugs or other medications are the mainstays of nonoperative treatment.[11]
- The success of treatment depends on the etiology of the hip pain and the patient's activity level (college or professional athlete or "weekend warrior") and age.

SURGICAL MANAGEMENT

- The vast majority of patients treated with hip arthroscopy have a combination of labral tear and FAI.
- The goal of surgical treatment is to repair the labrum, treat any articular cartilage injury, and restore the normal biomechanics of the hip joint (ie, decompressing the FAI).

Preoperative Planning

- Weight-bearing x-rays (AP pelvis, frog lateral, false profile, and Dunn 45-degree views)
- Be sure to determine that the pain generates from the hip joint and is not referred (lumbar spine or sacroiliac joint) or from muscular pathology (core muscle injury or sports hernia).
- Be wary of other pathology such as dysplasia, connective tissue disorders, or myofascial pain syndrome.
- Make sure all appropriate equipment and personnel (eg, radiology technician) are available.

Positioning

- Distraction is required for hip arthroscopy as well as fluoroscopic visualization of the joint in all planes.
- Place the patient in the supine or lateral position on either a fracture table or commercially available distraction table to allow appropriate distraction of the hip (**FIG 6**).
- A well-padded perineal post, preferably with a lateralized post, should be used to allow distraction in the plane of the femoral neck.

Approach

- Standard portals (**FIG 7**)
  - Anterolateral
  - Anterior
  - Midanterior
  - Posterolateral
- Accessory portals
  - Modified anterior
  - Proximal midanterior
  - Distal lateral portal
  - Proximal lateral portal

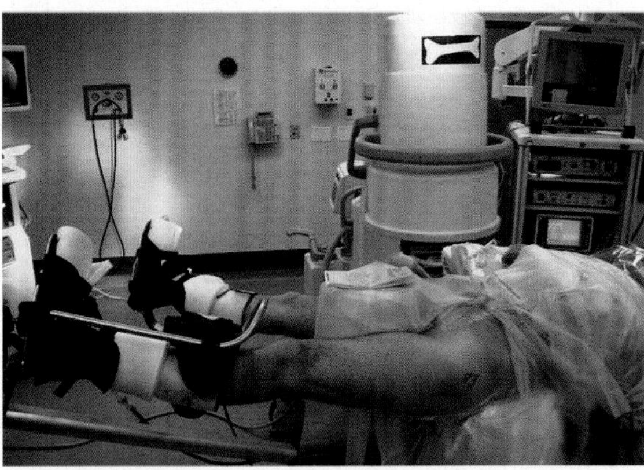

FIG 6 • Patient positioned supine on a hip distractor attached to operating room (OR) table. Full access for C-arm is noted.

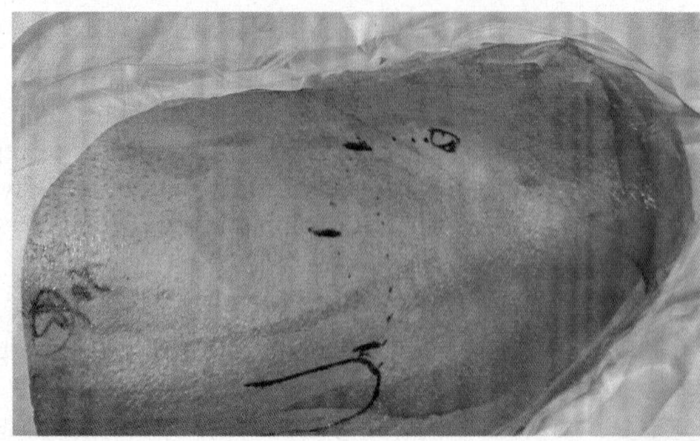

FIG 7 • Portals. Left hip demonstrating anterolateral, anterior, midanterior, and posterolateral portals.

TECHNIQUES

Positioning

- Allow free access around the hip with fluoroscopic access as well (see **FIG 6**).
- Use fluoroscopy to confirm appropriate distraction (**TECH FIG 1**).
- If appropriate distraction cannot be easily obtained, place a needle in the hip under sterile conditions to release the negative intra-articular pressure of the joint and allow distraction.[3]

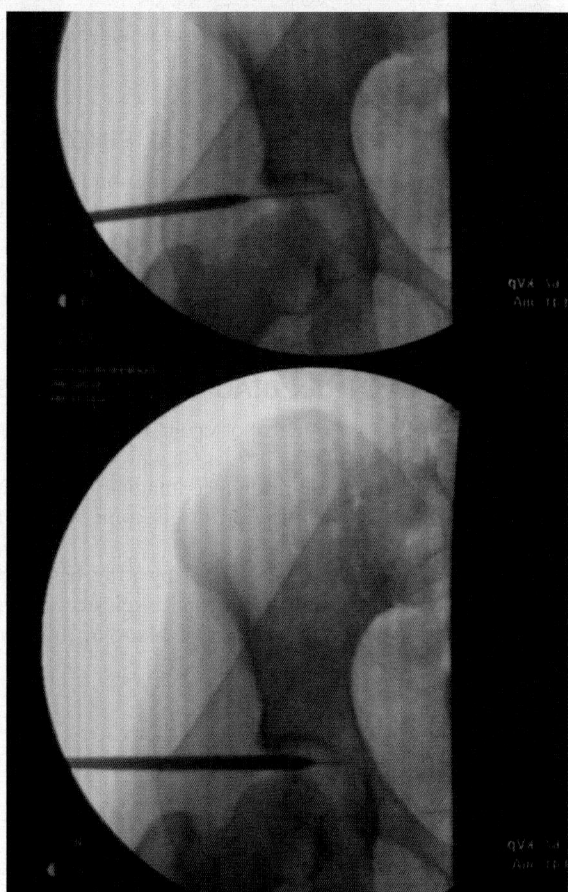

TECH FIG 1 • Fluoroscopic pictures of a right hip. Views show initial distraction of the hip followed by aeration of the capsule. Portals are created over flexible Nitinol guidewires with a metal cannula.

Portals

- Anterolateral (see **FIG 7**)
  - Initial portal established under fluoroscopic guidance
  - Start needle 1 to 2 cm proximal and 1 to 2 cm anterior to the tip of greater trochanter at a sufficient angle to enter the hip joint without damaging the cartilage.[3,5]
    - Removing the obturator from the needle releases the negative intra-articular pressure of the joint and allows increased distraction with the same amount of traction.
    - Some surgeons inject the hip with 20 to 40 mL of sterile saline prior to placing the guidewire through the needle.
  - After placing needle in hip, flexible guidewire is placed for creation of the portal.
  - Place cannula with gentle steady pressure and be careful not to bend or break the pin.
    - Use fluoroscopy as you are creating this portal.

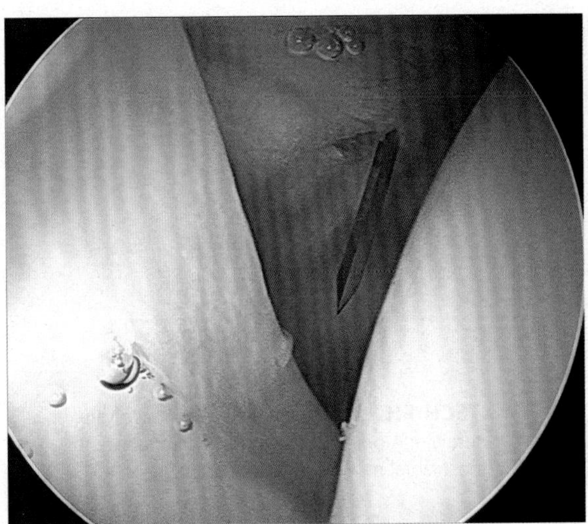

TECH FIG 2 ● Capsulotomies are created using a banana or beaver blade to connect portals. Exercise care with the blade to prevent iatrogenic cartilage damage.

- Anterior
  - Consists of the intersection of sagittal line from anterior superior iliac spine distal and line from tip of greater trochanter[3,5]
  - Placed after triangulation when viewing from the anterolateral portal
  - Most use a modified anterior portal, which is 2 cm more lateral than a standard anterior portal.
  - After establishing the anterior portal and performing appropriate capsulotomies (see next step), view initial anterolateral portal from anterior portal and complete capsulotomy.
- Capsulotomies
  - After entering the joint, perform capsulotomy with a banana blade or beaver blade under arthroscopic visualization (**TECH FIG 2**; **Video 1**).
  - Capsulotomies are required to allow sufficient movement of instruments in the hip.
  - Horizontal capsulotomy connecting the anterolateral and midanterior or modified anterior portal is generally required.
    - Try to keep a proximal flap of cartilage in case you want to close the horizontal capsulotomy at the end of the case.
  - "T capsulotomy" can be used for access to peripheral compartment for large cam lesions.
    - Must be repaired at the end of the case.
- Midanterior
  - Approximately 45-degree angle between anterolateral and anterior portals and starting distal[1,3]
  - Used for anchor placement or for access to peripheral compartment
  - Used for T capsulotomy when performed
- Accessory
  - See description of portal creation discussed earlier.
  - The steps are same for establishment of accessory portals.

Diagnostic Arthroscopy

- Perform a complete diagnostic arthroscopy of the hip in the same order as a routine arthroscopy (the order of structures inspected does not matter, but it is important to be consistent in your method).
- Perform diagnostic arthroscopy of the central compartment and complete repairs before removing traction and going on to the peripheral compartment.
- Inspect all structures in the central compartment with traction and peripheral compartment after traction released (list is not complete or comprehensive):
  - Central compartment (**TECH FIG 3A**)
    - Labrum, articular cartilage acetabulum, ligamentum teres, articular cartilage femoral head, and loose bodies
  - Peripheral compartment (**TECH FIG 3B**)
    - Medial synovial fold, medial head-neck, middle head-neck, lateral head-neck, labrum, lateral synovial fold, lateral gutter, and medial gutter
- Other areas are listed below but not covered in detail in this chapter:
  - Peritrochanteric space
  - Subgluteal space
  - Iliopsoas tendon

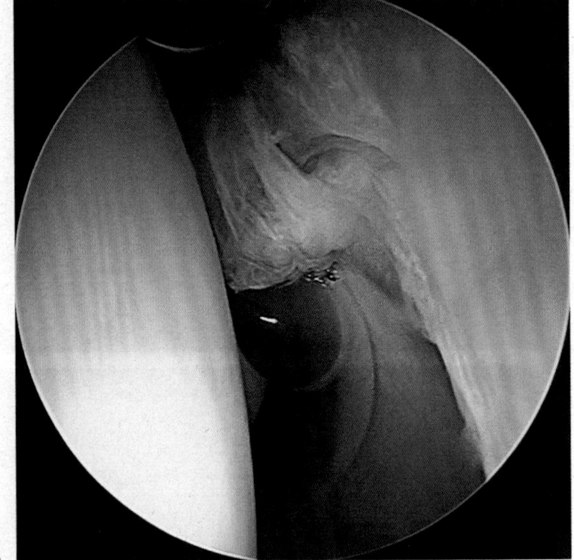

A

TECH FIG 3 ● **A.** Central compartment. Labrum with tear, femoral head, acetabulum with tear of articular cartilage. *(continued)*

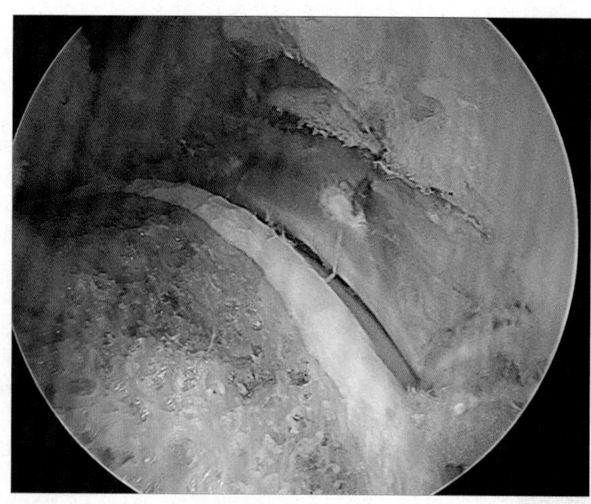

TECH FIG 3 • *(continued)* **B.** View of anterolateral portal of peripheral compartment post labral repair and femoroplasty.

Labral Repair or Débridement (Video 2)

- We prefer to repair the labrum to reestablish the suction-seal effect (**TECH FIG 4A**).
- If débridement is required, use a combination of shaver and radiofrequency device to remove pathologic tissue while preserving as much healthy and stable tissue as possible.
- Remove loose bodies, chondroplasty, and microfracture as indicated.
- Repair
  - Suture anchors or knotless device (according to surgeon preference)
  - The goal is to repair labrum to the edge of the articular margin of the acetabulum to restore the anatomy and the suction-seal effect of the labrum (**TECH FIG 4A**).
  - Vertical mattress or base stitch should be used when possible (tissue quality and size) because it gives the best restoration of the labral anatomy[8] (**TECH FIG 4B**).

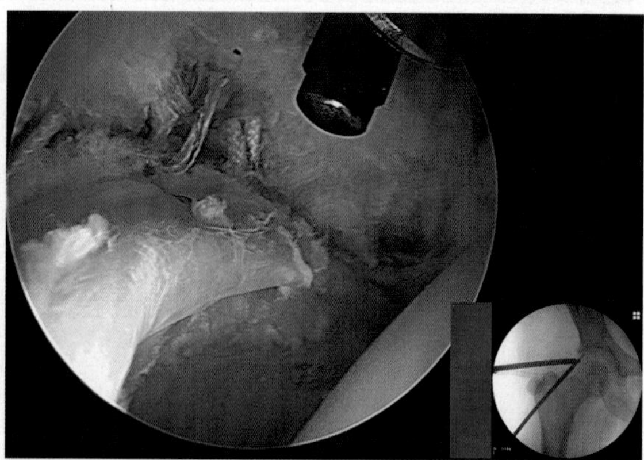

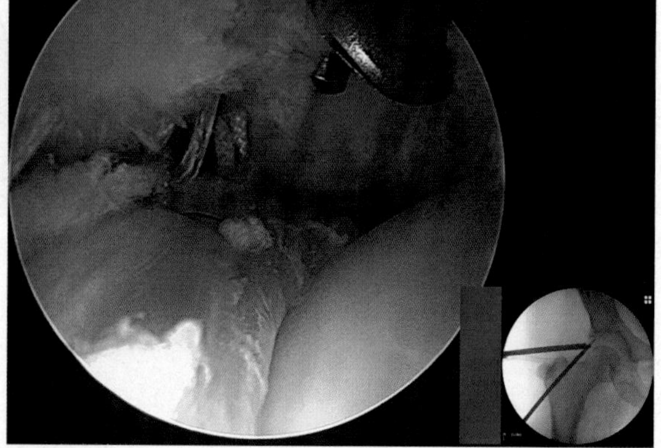

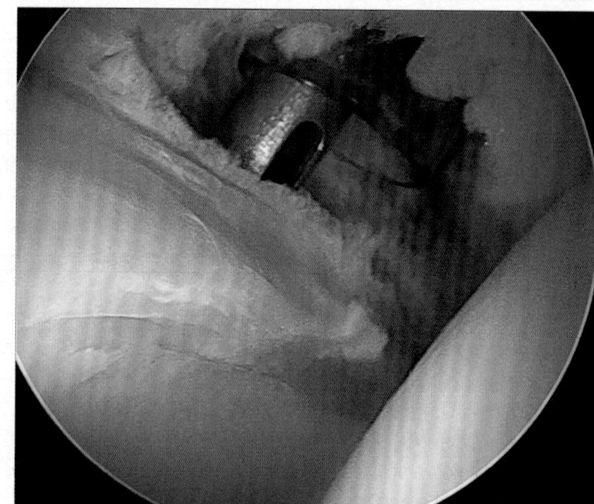

TECH FIG 4 • **A.** View from anterolateral portal after labral repair. Traction is removed and restoration of the suction-seal effect of the labrum is shown. **B.** Labral repair with vertical mattress base stitch restoring the labrochondral junction. Vertical mattress stitch avoids blunting of the labrum. **C.** Drill guide is placed from the midanterior portal at the edge of the acetabular rim. Care is taken not to medialize the labrum and also not to penetrate the subchondral plate.

- Elevate and mobilize labrum off acetabulum and try to preserve the labrocartilaginous junction.
- Perform acetabuloplasty/rim trimming when indicated or decorticate acetabular rim to provide a healing surface for labral repair.[8]
- Place anchors through the midanterior portal at a 30- to 45-degree angle relative to the edge of the acetabulum (**TECH FIG 4C**).
- Place anchors from anterior (medial) to anterolateral while viewing from anterolateral portal.
- Pass a single arm of suture under labrum at labrocartilagenous junction and retrieve the same suture through the labrum to create a vertical mattress stitch.
  - You may do a single pass around labrum in a "wrap around" fashion as well.
- Pass-retrieve-tie, move to next anchor, and repeat.
- Keep knots off articular surface (**TECH FIG 4B; Video 3**).

Acetabuloplasty/Rim Trimming

- Typically done as noted earlier during labral repair while under traction
- May also perform acetabuloplasty without labral detachment or repair
- Follow preoperative plan regarding location and amount of acetabulum to trim.
- Round burr (side cutting) or flat-top burr (end and side cutting) (**TECH FIG 5**)
  - Use combination of arthroscopic elevators, rasps, shaver, and a radiofrequency device to clear acetabular rim of periosteal coverage.
  - Use fluoroscopy to help guide resection (it is critical to obtain true AP of hip to allow appropriate resection).
- Can take down to edge of articular cartilage damage in small defects
- Preserve the labrum while performing acetabuloplasty.
- Exercise caution with resection to prevent overresection and subsequent iatrogenic instability.

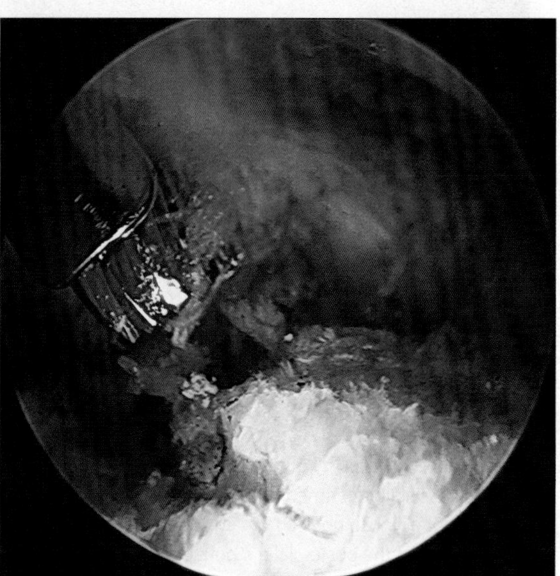

TECH FIG 5 • Arthroscopic view through anterolateral portal with flat-top burr performing acetabuloplasty. Femoral head on left and burr is on acetabular rim.

Femoroplasty

- Careful preoperative planning for location and amount of femoral resection for femoroplasty (**Video 4**)
- Allows access to peripheral compartment after completion of work in the central compartment and removal of traction
- Initially assess peripheral compartment through the capsulotomies.
- Flex hip to approximately 45 degrees and slight abduction to relax the capsule and allow access to peripheral compartment and head–neck junction.[4]
- Can access further lateral with internal rotation of the leg
- Begin with assessment and localizing the cam lesion and confirming access arthroscopically (**TECH FIG 6A**).
- Begin resection proximally with round burr slightly into the articular margin (usually in line with physeal scar but not always) (**TECH FIG 6B**).
- Work from anterior to anterolateral to lateral and proximal to distal, setting a proximal template and contouring distally in a gentle progression to the femoral neck.[4]
- Switch between anterolateral, midanterior, and anterior portals for viewing and working, depending on the area to be resected.
- Perform a dynamic examination at the end of femoroplasty, putting the hip in the impingement position to confirm resolution of the bony conflict.
- May need to perform a T capsulotomy to access large lesions or distal and lateral
  - Close the "T" with side-to-side sutures at end of femoroplasty (**Video 5**).

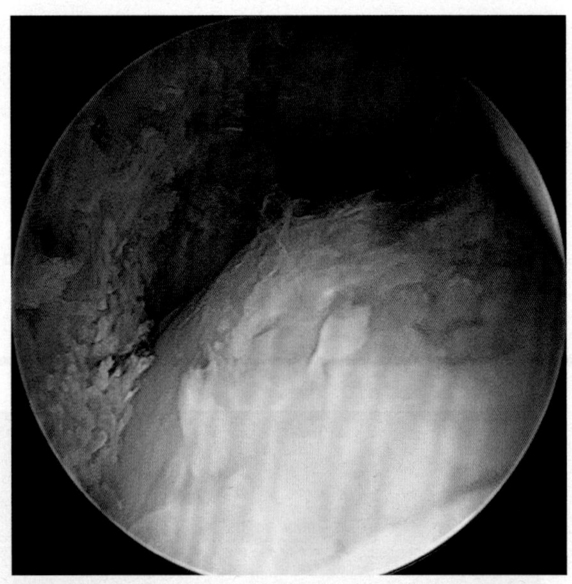
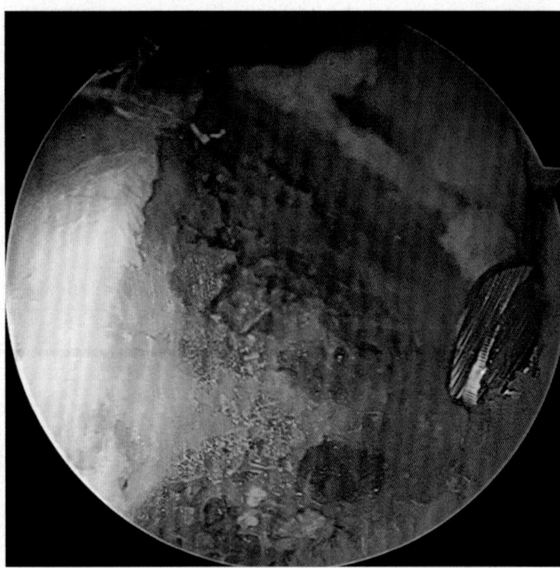

TECH FIG 6 • A. Arthroscopic view of cam lesion through anterolateral portal prior to femoroplasty. **B.** Arthroscopic view through anterolateral portal after femoroplasty showing resection of the cam lesion.

Loose Bodies

- Loose bodies that form in the hip can be located in the central and peripheral compartments.
- Removal of all loose bodies from central compartment typically requires use of the posterolateral portal.[9]
- Thorough examination of peripheral compartment is needed to remove all loose bodies.

Microfracture

- Typically used for acetabular cartilaginous defects
- Use curettes and a shaver to stabilize the edges of cartilage and remove calcified layers of cartilage in area of microfracture.
- Various angle picks are available.
  - However, you must be careful with the angle to avoid cutting off the acetabulum.

Iliopsoas Snapping (Internal Coxa Saltans)

- The iliopsoas tendon may snap or pop over the femoral head or iliopectineal line, causing pain.
- Tendon release can be done transcapsular at the level of the joint in the central compartment or extracapsular at the lesser trochanter.
- A radiofrequency device or beaver blade is used for release.

PEARLS AND PITFALLS

Confirm appropriate joint distraction prior to prep and drape and then release; replace traction after prep and drape. This will allow you to minimize traction time.	▪ After completion of work in the central compartment, remove traction and check status of labral repair viewing through the capsulotomy.
After placing initial needle into hip for anterolateral portal, remove under fluoroscopy and replace to ensure that it does not penetrate the labrum.	▪ View the peripheral compartment through the capsulotomy after flexion and slight abduction of the hip and confirm full access to cam lesion for femoroplasty.
Use fluoroscopy judiciously as needed, especially early in the learning curve, until you are comfortable with portal and instrument placement.	▪ If it is difficult to access the full cam lesion, then perform a T capsulotomy through the midanterior portal. This must be repaired with side-to-side stitches at the end of the procedure.
When placing anchors, get close to the edge of acetabulum without penetrating subchondral bone to prevent medialization of the labrum. Keep angle of drill guide at 30–45 degrees, relative to the acetabulum.	▪ Put hip through dynamic examination while viewing arthroscopically via anterolateral and anterior portals at the end of femoroplasty to confirm resection of the cam and resolution of the bony conflict.
Expose rim fully to allow appropriate anchor placement on edge of rim.	▪ Place all anchors through the midanterior portal and then pass sutures in vertical mattress fashion through labrum.

POSTOPERATIVE CARE

- Outpatient procedure and discharge with crutches and a hip brace
- Continuous passive motion is to be performed at home during the first week to 10 days.
- For labral débridement with or without FAI, crutches for 1 to 2 weeks.
- For labral repair, crutches and protected weight bearing for 2 to 4 weeks.
- Begin physical therapy 1 week after surgery.
- Advance to formal physical therapy and home programs throughout the recovery period.

OUTCOMES

- Multiple studies have reported good to excellent outcomes for hip arthroscopy used to treat FAI.
- A systematic review showed that 10 of 12 studies reported good to excellent outcomes in 75% or more of patients treated with hip arthroscopy.
- One of the keys to successful outcome is the stage of arthritis at the index surgery.

COMPLICATIONS

- Complication rates reported in the literature are low.
- Iatrogenic
  - Cartilage damage from cannulas or instrumentation
  - Damage from misplacement of anchors
  - Iatrogenic instability (overresection of acetabulum or capsular insufficiency or both)
- Neurologic
  - Positioning: perineal numbness/pudendal nerve
  - Traction: sciatic nerve
  - Portals: lateral femoral cutaneous nerve
  - Regional pain syndrome
- Procedure
  - Iatrogenic injury
  - Failure of fixation
  - Medialization of labrum with repair
- Postoperative
  - Deep vein thrombosis/blood clot
  - Fracture: overzealous resection of femoral neck for cam
- Other
  - Avascular necrosis
  - Stiffness

REFERENCES

1. Alwattar BJ, Bharam S. Hip arthroscopy portals. Op Tech Sports Med 2011:19(2):74–80.
2. Botser IB, Smith TW, Naser R, et al. Open surgical dislocation vs. arthroscopy for femoroacetabular impingement: a comparison of clinical outcomes. Arthroscopy 2011;27:270–278.
3. Byrd JW. Hip arthroscopy: applications and technique. J Am Acad Orthop Surg 2006:14(7):433–444.
4. Byrd JW, Jones KS. Arthroscopic femoroplasty in the management of cam-type femoroacetabular impingement. Clin Ortho Relat Res 2009;3:739–746.
5. Byrd JW, Pappas JN, Pedley MJ. Hip arthroscopy: an anatomic study of portal placement and relationship to the extra-articular structures. Arthroscopy 1995;12:603–612.
6. Fergunson SJ, Bryant JT, Ganz R, et al. The acetabular labrum seal: a poroelastic finite element model. Clin Biomech 2000;15:463–468.
7. Ito K, Leunig M, Keller I, et al. Impingement-induced damage of the acetabular labrum: a possible initiator of hip arthrosis. Eighth Annual Meeting, European Orthopaedic Research Society, 1998:55.
8. Kelly BT, Weiland DE, Schenker ML, et al. Arthroscopic labral repair in the hip: Surgical technique and review of the literature. Arthroscopy 2005;21:1496–1504.
9. Krebs VE. The role of hip arthroscopy in the treatment of synovial disorders and loose bodies. Clin Ortho Relat Res 2003;406:48–59.
10. Nepple JJ, Prather H, Trousdale RT, et al. Diagnostic imaging of femoroacetabular impingement. J Am Acad Orthop Surg 2013;21: S16–S19.
11. Parvizi J, Leunig M, Ganz R. Femoroacetabular impingement. J Am Acad Orthop Surg 2007;15:561–570.
12. Sanchez-Sotolo J, Trousdale RT, Berry DJ, et al. Surgical treatment of developmental dysplasia of the hip in adults: I. Nonarthroplasty options. J Am Acad Orthop Surg 2002;10:321–333.

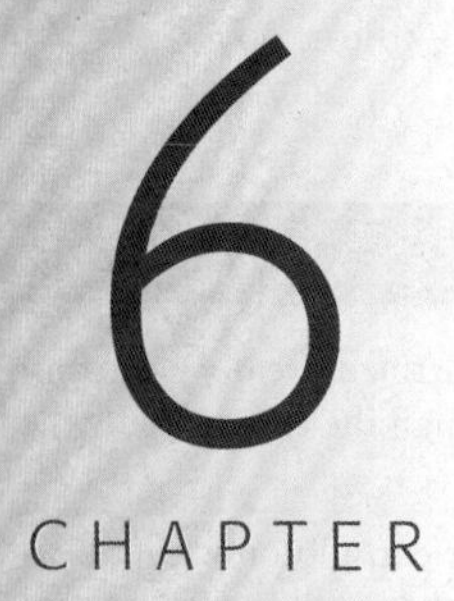

Scope for Femoroacetabular Impingement

Christopher M. Larson and Patrick M. Birmingham

DEFINITION

- Femoroacetabular impingement (FAI) is the result of abnormal contact between the proximal femur and the acetabular rim.
- Abnormalities can be identified on either the femoral or acetabular side but are more commonly seen on both sides.
- This abnormal contact can lead to acetabular chondral lesions and or labral lesions, leading to hip pain and the development of diffuse osteoarthritis of the affected hip if left untreated.[1,7,9]

ANATOMY

- The proximal femur and acetabulum normally articulate without abutment through a physiologic range of motion (ROM).
- Required ROM, however, is variable depending on the activities performed, with less range required for sedentary individuals and extreme range required for activities such as dance, ballet, and hockey goalies.
- The acetabulum normally is anteverted 12 to 16.5 degrees.
- The acetabulum normally covers the femoral head to a depth that avoids impingement (ie, overcoverage) and instability (ie, dysplasia or undercoverage) with a horizontal, thin sourcil (ie, the weight-bearing zone).
- The proximal femur normally has a spherical head–neck contour and appropriate offset that allows for impingement-free ROM.
- The normal femoral neck–shaft angle is 120 to 135 degrees; the femoral neck typically is anteverted 12 to 15 degrees.
- The acetabular labrum functions to create a fluid pressurization seal with the femoral head.[8]
- It is important to recognize and respect the location of the retinacular vessels that have been shown to enter the antero- and posterolateral portions of the femoral neck and supply the majority of the femoral head's blood supply.
- The capsule is an important hip stabilizer and should be preserved and repaired to maintain soft tissue stability, particularly in dysplastic variants, generalized hypermobility, and connective tissue disorders.[3]

PATHOGENESIS

- There are two primary mechanisms of FAI: pincer and cam-type impingement.[1,7,9]
- Pincer impingement is the result of contact between an abnormal acetabular rim and femoral head–neck junction (**FIG 1A**).
  - Pincer impingement typically is the result of a globally deep acetabulum (coxa profunda), focal anterior overcoverage (acetabular retroversion), or, less commonly, posterior overcoverage.
  - It leads to labral bruising and degenerative tearing and eventually may result in ossification of the labrum and contrecoup posterior acetabular chondral injury.

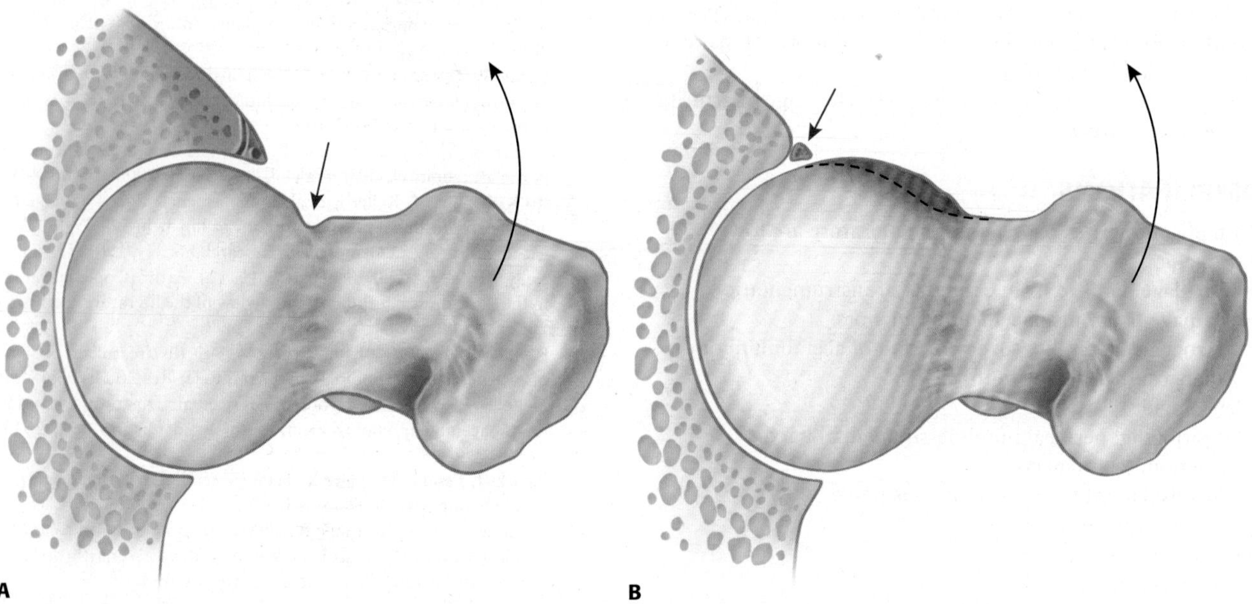

FIG 1 • **A.** Pincer impingement is the result of contact between an abnormal acetabular rim and a normal femoral head–neck junction. **B.** Cam impingement is the result of contact between an abnormal femoral head–neck junction and the acetabulum.

- Global overcoverage is more frequent in females, whereas acetabular retroversion is more common in males.
- Cam impingement is the result of contact between an abnormal femoral head–neck junction and the acetabulum (**FIG 1B**).
  - The abnormal femoral head–neck junction is typically secondary to an aspherical anterolateral head–neck junction but also can be secondary to a slipped capital femoral epiphysis, femoral retroversion, coxa vara, malreduced femoral neck fracture, and, less commonly, posterior femoral head–neck abnormalities.
  - Cam impingement results in a shearing stress to the anterosuperior acetabulum, with predictable chondral delamination and labral detachment or tearing in some cases.
  - Although cam impingement is reported to predominate in young athletic males and pincer impingement in middle-aged women, most patients with FAI have a combination of both cam and pincer impingement.
- Extra-articular sources of impingement have been recently described.
  - Anterior inferior iliac spine (AIIS) impingement is an increasingly recognized type of acetabular-based impingement.
  - The AIIS serves as the origin of the direct head of the rectus femoris, and impingement can be secondary to prior avulsion injury, pelvic osteotomy, or developmental as seen in the setting of acetabular retroversion.[12,18,26]
  - Ischiofemoral impingement is a rare type of proximal femoral-based impingement that occurs between the lesser trochanter and the ischial tuberosity.
  - The quadratus femoris occupies this space and may be compressed when this space is reduced.
  - The normal distance between the lesser trochanter and the ischial tuberosity is reported to be 20 mm. This space is reported to be reduced to around 13 mm in patients with ischiofemoral impingement.
  - In addition, women, as a result of the wider positioning of their ischial tuberosities, appear to be at greater risk.[30]

NATURAL HISTORY

- The likelihood of an individual with untreated FAI developing hip osteoarthritis is unknown because there have been no longitudinal studies prospectively following these patients before the development of symptoms.
- Clinical experience with over 600 surgical dislocations of the hip in patients with FAI has revealed a strong association of this disorder with progressive acetabular chondral degeneration, labral tears, and progressive osteoarthritis.[1,7,9]
- It is now well accepted that many patients with FAI will develop progressive chondral and labral injury, which can ultimately lead to end-stage hip osteoarthritis.
- One population study suggests that there is a 15% to 19% prevalence of deep acetabular socket and 5% to 19% prevalence of pistol grip deformity. This population had a relative risk ratio of developing hip osteoarthritis of 2.2 to 2.4.[11]
- FAI and, in particular, cam-type morphology has been reported in up to 90% of athletic male patients.[14,19]

PATIENT HISTORY AND PHYSICAL FINDINGS

- Patients typically are young to middle aged (second through fourth decade) at presentation with complaints of groin pain exacerbated by physical activity.
- Prolonged sitting, arising from a chair, putting on shoes and socks, getting in and out of a car, and sitting with their legs crossed often exacerbate the symptoms.
- We have found that patients may have a history of siblings, parents, and grandparents with hip pain or osteoarthritis of the hip, and patients may have milder or similar symptoms in the contralateral hip.
- Patients often have had pain for months to years with the diagnosis of chronic low back pathology, hip flexor strains, and sports hernias/athletic pubalgia and not infrequently have had other surgeries without relief of their pain.[28]
- Physical examinations should include the following:
  - Evaluation of hip ROM: Global ROM restriction indicates advanced osteoarthritis.
  - Anterior impingement test: Groin pain indicates anterolateral rim pathology.
  - Posterior impingement test: Groin pain or posterolateral pain indicates posterolateral rim pathology.
  - Extension/abduction and flexion/abduction indicates lateral-based pathology.
  - FABER test: FABER means *f*lexion, *ab*duction, and *e*xternal *r*otation of the hip. Increased distance from the lateral knee to the examination table can indicate femoroacetabular impingement.
  - For subspine impingement, there is pain with straight flexion, restricted flexion, and, often, tenderness to palpation of the AIIS that recreates the flexion-based discomfort.
  - For ischiofemoral impingement, the symptoms can be reproduced by a combination of extension, adduction, and external rotation (ER).

IMAGING AND OTHER DIAGNOSTIC STUDIES

- Plain radiographs including an anteroposterior (AP) pelvis, a frog-leg lateral, 45-degree modified Dunn lateral or a cross-table lateral, and false-profile view are obtained.
- The AP radiograph should have a coccyx to symphyseal distance of 0 to 2 cm, with the coccyx centered over the symphysis to properly evaluate acetabular version.
- The following are measured on the AP radiograph (**FIG 2A**):
  - A lateral center edge angle of 25 to 40 degrees distinguishes deep acetabulum from dysplasia.
  - The presence of a crossover sign represents retroversion and can indicate either local anterior overcoverage or superior posterior undercoverage.
  - The posterior wall sign indicates posterior undercoverage (retroversion).
  - Extension of the AIIS below the sourcil and cortical sclerotic change may be indicative of AIIS impingement.
- Decreased femoral head–neck offset and asphericity can be indicative of cam-type morphology.
  - A decreased femoral neck–shaft angle indicates coxa vara and may contribute to impingement.
- The frog-leg lateral, 45-degree modified Dunn lateral, and or cross-table lateral views with 15 degrees internal rotation (IR) should be evaluated for the following:
  - Alpha angle: normally less than 50 to 55 degrees (anterolateral prominence/aspherical femoral head–neck junction; **FIG 2B**).[25]
  - Femoral head–neck offset and offset ratio: Normal femoral head–neck offset is greater than 8 to 11 mm and the normal femoral head–neck offset ratio is greater than 0.15.
  - Femoral head–neck cystic changes and sclerosis

- The false profile is used to evaluate the following:
  - Anterior center edge angle: anterior over- and undercoverage
  - Excessive anterior and distal extension of the AIIS: Normally, the distal extent of the AIIS is proximal to the acetabular rim.
  - Anterior and posterior joint space
- A magnetic resonance imaging (MRI) arthrogram is useful to evaluate for the following:
  - Labral and chondral pathology, acetabular version, and deformity of the femoral head–neck junction, which is best seen on the axial cuts and, in particular, with radial imaging (**FIG 2C**).
  - Femoral neck version: Retroversion/torsion may contribute to impingement, whereas excessive anteversion/torsion can contribute to instability; measurements require additional cuts through the distal femoral condyles.
  - Synovial herniation pits/impingement cysts at the femoral head–neck junction are also indicative of FAI.
  - An anesthetic agent can be included with the gadolinium to verify the hip joint as the source of pain, which is indicated by temporary pain relief with provocative maneuvers in the first couple of hours after the injection. Occasionally, the high volume of such an injection can lead to capsular distention with increased pain. Alternatively, a lower volume (<5 mL) of anesthetic-only injections can be used for diagnostic purposes.
  - The normal distance between the lesser trochanter and the ischial tuberosity is said to be 20 mm. This space is said to be reduced to around 13 mm in patients with ischiofemoral impingement.[13]
- Three-dimensional computed tomography (CT) scanning can be invaluable and obtained in all or select cases:
  - The area of impingement can be more accurately mapped.
  - This may be done routinely in cases of subtle FAI or suspected unusual locations of FAI (eg, posterior femoral head/neck prominences) or for revision cases in order to better assess prior bone resection.
  - CT scan can also be used to evaluate femoral version/torsion (additional cuts through the distal femoral condyles required) and acetabular version.[5]

DIFFERENTIAL DIAGNOSIS

- Sports hernia/athletic pubalgia/core muscle injury
- Lumbar spine pathology
- Gynecologic or urologic pathology
- Intra-abdominal pathology
- Hip flexor pathology or iliopsoas snapping
- Iliotibial band pathology or snapping
- Other extra-articular myotendinous pathology
- Abductor/gluteus medius/minimus pathology
- Pelvic stress fracture
- Apophysitis or apophyseal injury in the developing skeleton
- Intra-articular pathology not related to FAI
- Extra-articular hip impingement
- Neurogenic disorders

NONOPERATIVE MANAGEMENT

- Nonoperative management of FAI consists of activity modification; avoiding painful activities such as deep hip flexion, aggressive hip flexion–based weight training, and other athletic activities that aggravate symptoms; and anti-inflammatories/analgesics and intra-articular injection in select cases.
- Intra-articular pathology often progresses without symptoms early in the disease, and there is concern that without surgical treatment, significant labrochondral injury and arthritis might eventually develop, particularly in large cam-type deformities.
- Nonoperative management may be best employed in the already degenerative hip with joint space narrowing prior to total hip arthroplasty or milder deformities in patients willing to modify activities and consists of activity modification, core trunk strengthening exercises, and occasional intra-articular corticosteroid or hyaluronic acid injections.

SURGICAL MANAGEMENT

- Physical examination and imaging studies consistent with FAI
- Pain despite activity modification
- Pain in patients who are unable or unwilling to modify activity
- Minimal to no degenerative changes
- Arthroscopic versus open procedure for FAI (Table 1)
- There are no strict indications for open versus arthroscopic management of traditional FAI, and decisions are typically made on the ability of the surgeon to correct the deformities with a given approach.
- Posteriorly based femoral deformities, extra-articular trochanteric–pelvic impingement, and cases of mixed FAI/dysplastic anatomy with a predominance of instability findings are better served with open corrective procedures.

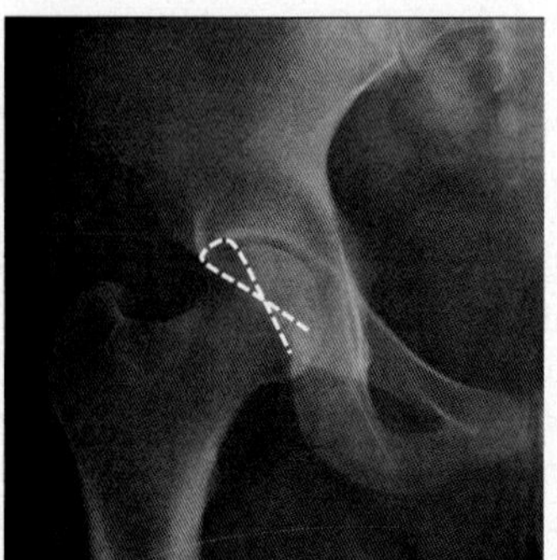

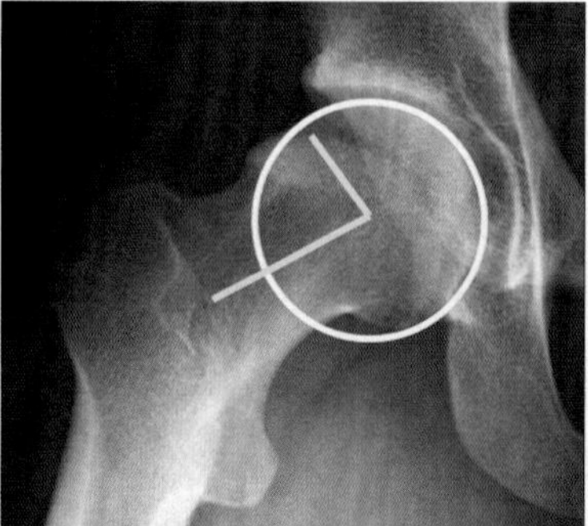

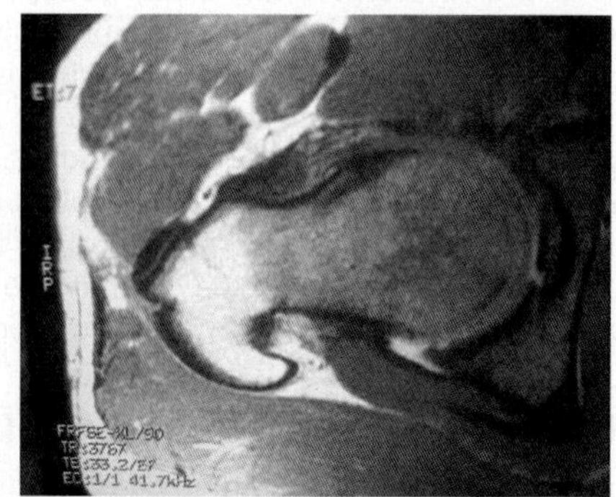

FIG 2 • **A.** Crossover sign (*white dashed line*) depicted in a hip with acetabular retroversion is depicted. **B.** Alpha (α) angle is elevated in cam impingement. **C.** Prominence of the anterolateral femoral head–neck junction is seen on axial MRI images.

Table 1 Guidelines for Arthroscopic versus Open Repair of Femoroacetabular Impingement

Pincer impingement
Lateral center edge angle
Typically correct to 30–35 degrees
>25 degrees: arthroscopic acetabular rim trimming
20–25 degrees: avoid rim trimming laterally
>16 to 20 degrees: consider corrective pelvic osteotomy
Anterior center edge angle
<20 degrees: avoid anterior rim resections
Moderate to severe acetabular retroversion
Consider corrective pelvic osteotomy
Cam impingement
If resection of >30% of the width of the neck is required to restore the alpha angle to normal, consider concomitant osteotomy (severe pistol grip deformity/slipped capital femoral epiphysis).
If significant femoral neck retroversion or coxa vara is present, a concomitant or staged osteotomy is considered if impingement is still present after femoral osteoplasty.
Posterior areas of femoral head–neck impingement can be more challenging and, depending on the surgeon's experience, may be better addressed with a surgical hip dislocation (SHD).
A high greater trochanter or excessive femoral neck anteversion (posterior impingement) or femoral neck retroversion (anterior impingement) can lead to extra-articular trochanteric/pelvic impingement, which should be managed with an SHD.

- Some higher level athletes may benefit from an arthroscopic approach with the possibility of an earlier return to sports compared to open corrective procedures.[29]

Preoperative Planning

- Initially, a fluoroscopic evaluation is done and the pelvis is leveled in order to recreate an image of the acetabulum that recreates a well-centered preoperative AP pelvis radiograph with respect to the relationship between the anterior and posterior acetabular walls. Next, a systematic evaluation of the femoral head–neck junction is performed with six specific views. Three views are taken in extension (ER, neutral, IR) in order to evaluate the lateral and medial head–neck junction and three views in 30 to 40 degrees of hip flexion (neutral, 30 degrees ER, 50 degrees ER) in order to evaluate the anterior and posterior femoral head–neck junction.
- Dynamic fluoroscopic evaluation by abduction of the hip in flexion, ER, and extension with IR and ER and abduction occasionally reveals impingement of the acetabulum on the proximal femur and results in a vacuum effect in the joint as the proximal femur is levered out of the acetabulum.

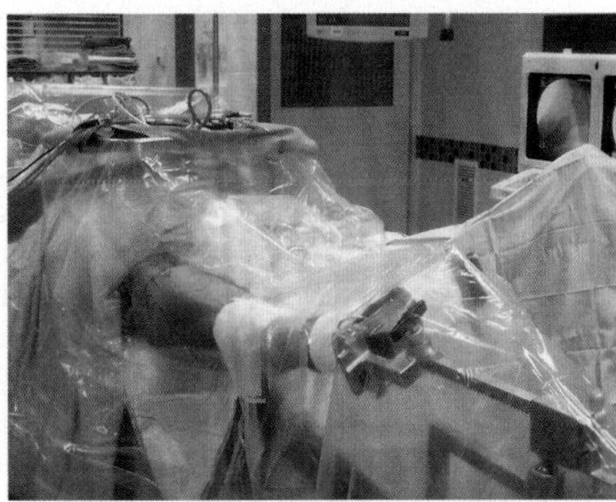

FIG 3 • The operative leg is placed in neutral abduction, slight flexion, and IR. The nonoperative leg is abducted with slight traction with a well-padded post in the peroneal region.

Positioning

- Arthroscopic management of FAI begins with standard hip positioning in either the supine or lateral position.
- We prefer the supine position with the hip in slight flexion, neutral abduction, and IR (**FIG 3**).

Approach

- Most cases can be performed using the standard anterior paratrochanteric and anterior or midanterior portals, with occasional use of the posterior paratrochanteric or accessory distal portal (**FIG 4**).

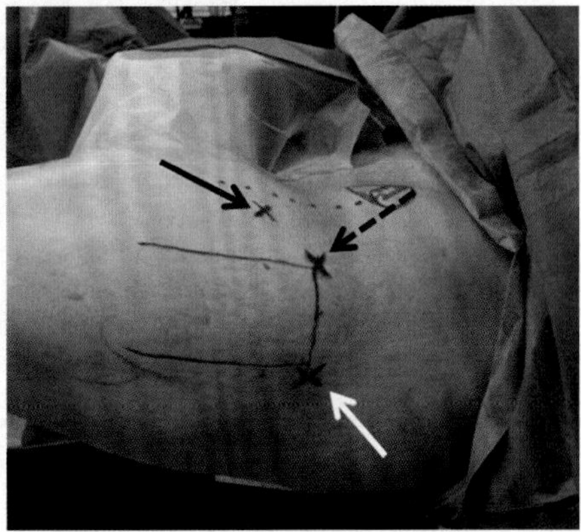

FIG 4 • Typical portals used for an arthroscopic FAI corrective procedure include the anterolateral portal (*black dashed arrow*), midanterior portal (*solid black arrow*), and occasionally a posterolateral portal (*white arrow*).

Diagnostic Arthroscopy

- Initially, the intra-articular portions of the hip are evaluated, including the acetabular labrum, acetabulum, and femoral head articular cartilage; fovea; ligamentum teres; transverse acetabular ligament; and capsular structures (**TECH FIG 1A,B**).
- The peripheral compartment is evaluated, including the femoral head–neck junction and femoral neck to the capsular reflection/peripheral capsular attachments, labrum, zona orbicularis, and medial and lateral synovial folds (**TECH FIG 1C**).
- The pathology present helps to define the pathomechanics at work, with chondral delamination in the anterior superior acetabulum often indicating cam-type impingement (**TECH FIG 1D**) and labral ecchymosis, tearing, and linear posterior acetabular chondral wear indicating pincer-type impingement. Focal labral and capsular bruising/synovitis in the region of the AIIS can be consistent with subspine/AIIS impingement. It is important to recognize that there are often a combination of pathomechanics at work and therefore a number of pathologic findings frequently coexist. In addition, these same findings can be seen in the setting of dysplasia as well (**TECH FIG 1E**).

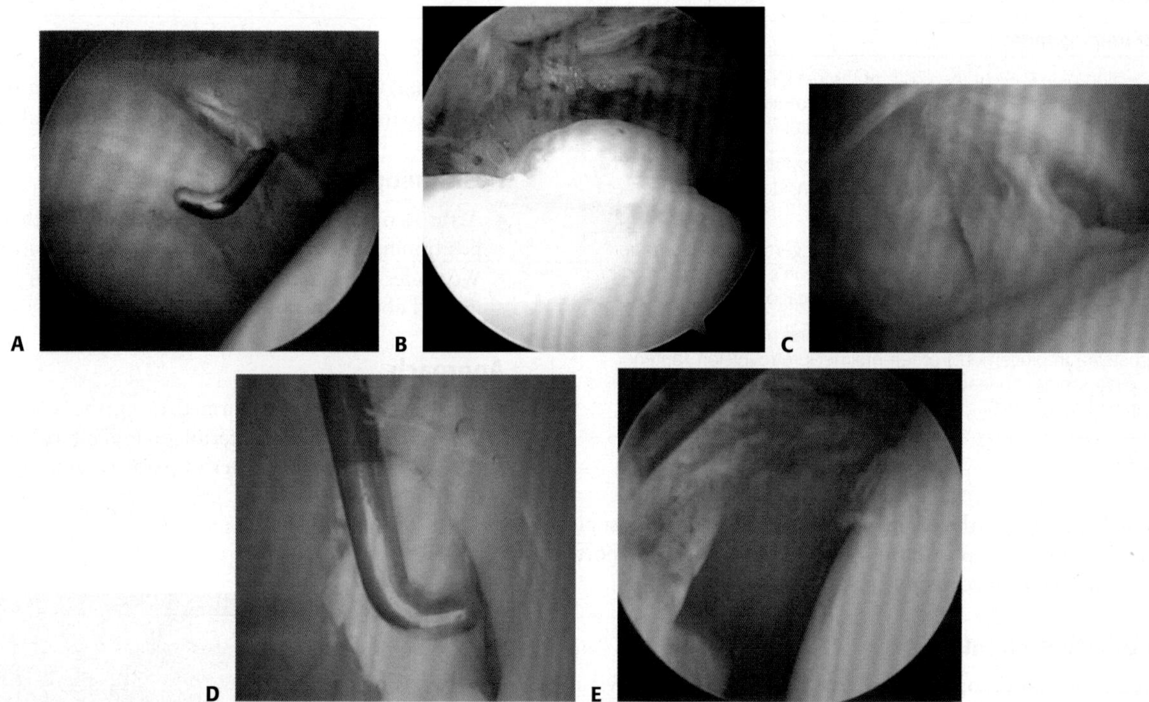

TECH FIG 1 • A. View from the anterior paratrochanteric portal reveals the anterolateral labrum, acetabulum (*left*), and femoral head (*right*). **B.** View of the fovea (*top*), ligamentum teres (*center*), and medial femoral head (*bottom*). **C.** View of the peripheral compartment through the anterior portal reveals the zona orbicularis (*top*), femoral neck and medial synovial fold (*center*), and femoral head–neck junction (*bottom*). **D.** Chondral delamination of the anterior superior acetabulum consistent with cam impingement. **E.** Diffuse labral ecchymosis (*left*) consistent with pincer impingement.

Pincer Impingement

- When pincer impingement is present, the labrum is assessed for ecchymosis (**TECH FIG 2A**), intralabral cyst, degenerative tearing, and ossification; regions of underlying rim prominence/rim fractures are identified.
- Attempts should be made to preserve the labrum when possible in order to preserve the potential sealing mechanism.
- If irreparable tearing of the labrum is present, the labrum is carefully/selectively débrided; however, the periphery of the labrum often remains intact and may be amenable to repair or refixation.
- If the labrum is amenable to repair or refixation, the current authors most frequently resect areas of acetabular overcoverage without labral detachment (**TECH FIG 2B,C**) and reserve labral detachment for cases of more severe focal or global overcoverage.
- The capsule is reflected away from the acetabular rim, and the labrum is left attached to the articular margin of the acetabular rim.
- Alternatively, the labrum can be carefully detached from the acetabulum using a Beaver blade and shaver, beginning at the periphery and extending to the articular side of the labrum.
- Care must be taken to detach as much of the labrum as possible without cutting too deep on the articular side, which could result in inadvertent delamination of the acetabular articular cartilage.
- The rim resection usually extends from the anterior portal to the 12 o'clock position for focal anterior overcoverage. Rim resection is quite variable and should be based on preoperative imaging studies and intraoperative findings consistent with pincer-type impingement.

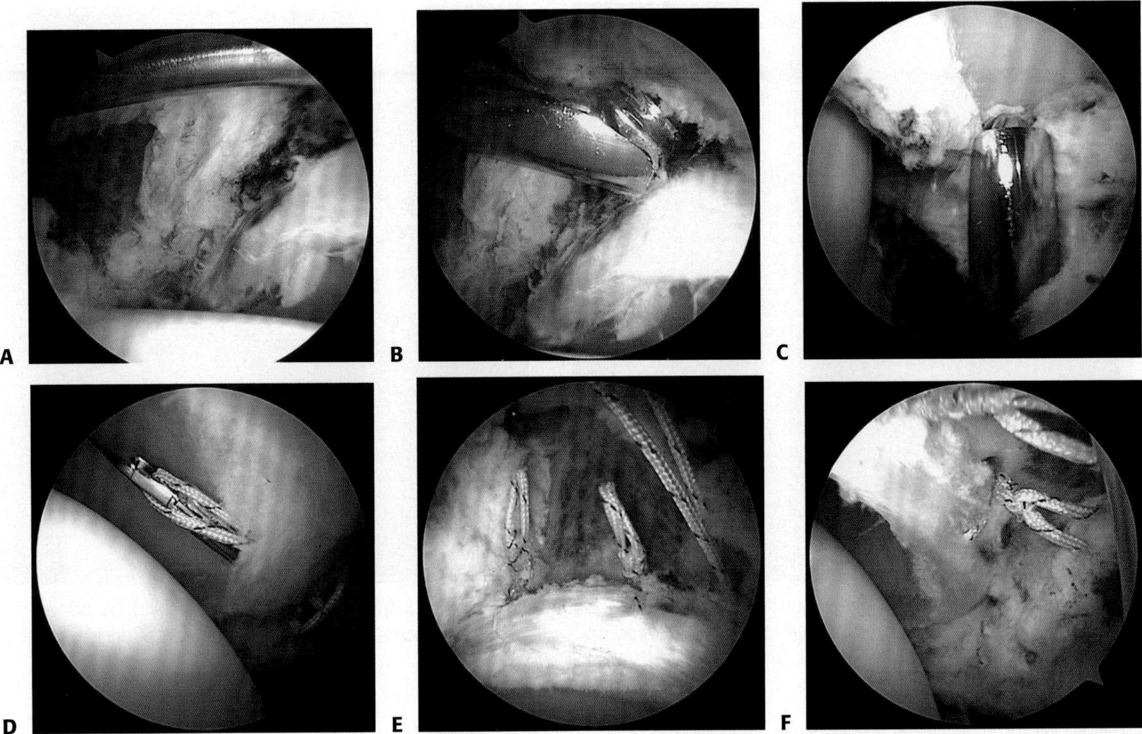

TECH FIG 2 • **A.** Peripheral labral ecchymosis for a left hip is noted consistent with pincer-type FAI. **B.** A burr is used to begin the rim resection via the midanterior portal. **C.** The burr is then introduced via the anterolateral portal in order to complete the rim resection without a formal takedown in this case. **D.** Suture anchors are placed in a mattress-type fashion, placing one limb of the suture through the labrochondral junction (figure) and retrieving the suture through the base of the labrum. **E.** View via the anterolateral portal after rim resection and labral repair with three suture anchors. **F.** Arthroscopic view via the midanterior portal reveals final labral repair.

- The current authors have become less aggressive with regard to rim resection, particularly in the setting of acetabular retroversion. The current authors try not to resect the rim beyond an lateral center edge angle of 30 to 35 degrees and typically leave 35% to 40% anterior and 40% to 50% posterior femoral head coverage. Again, the amount of resection is quite variable and should be based on preoperative imaging, intraoperative pathologic findings, and dynamic assessment.
- If areas of grade 4 chondromalacia remain after acetabular rim trimming, microfracture is performed on the exposed bone.
- Suture anchors (usually two to four anchors) are then placed 1 to 2 mm off the articular margin of the acetabulum with care to avoid intra-articular and anterior acetabular wall penetration. Up to five to eight anchors or more can be used for global labral refixation or reconstruction when indicated. The sutures are first passed under the labrum and then retrieved around or through the labrum, securing the labrum to the rim with standard knot-tying techniques (**TECH FIG 2D–F**).
- We generally prefer a mattress base stitch, which might better recreate the labral sealing function. In cases of minimal or poor tissue/hypoplastic labrum, a simple loop stitch can be used in order to avoid further labral compromise.
- Care is taken to place the knot on the capsular or medial side of the labrum to avoid damaging the femoral articular cartilage with prominent suture during weight bearing and ROM.

OS Acetabuli/Subspine and Ischiofemoral Impingement

- Occasionally, an os acetabuli or rim fracture is responsible for local anterior/posterolateral overcoverage and typically is attached to the acetabulum just peripheral to or behind the labrum.
- The os is exposed and excised using a burr beyond the fibrocartilage attachment of the native acetabulum with or without labral débridement or refixation (**TECH FIG 3**). Most often, the labrum is preserved. If the hip is dysplastic without the fragment, the fragment can be left alone (if stable) or stabilized with arthroscopic assisted cannulated screws after partial excision if necessary.[20] If AIIS impingement is present, the resection is carried further proximal at the anterior rim to identify and decompress the prominent AIIS.
- It is occasionally helpful to make an additional window through the medial capsule in order to perform a more proximal resection.

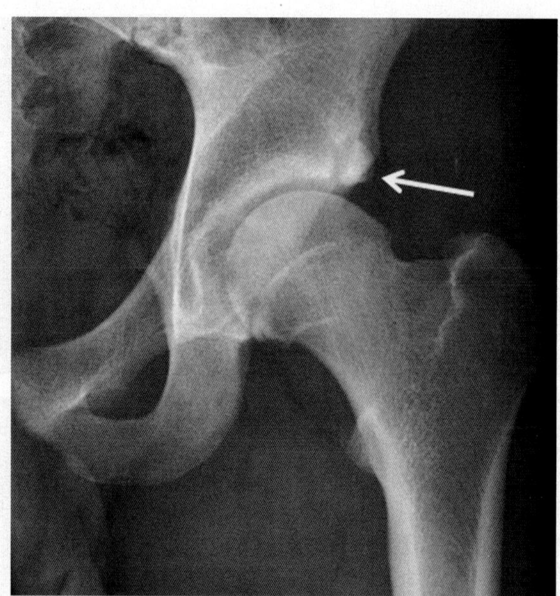

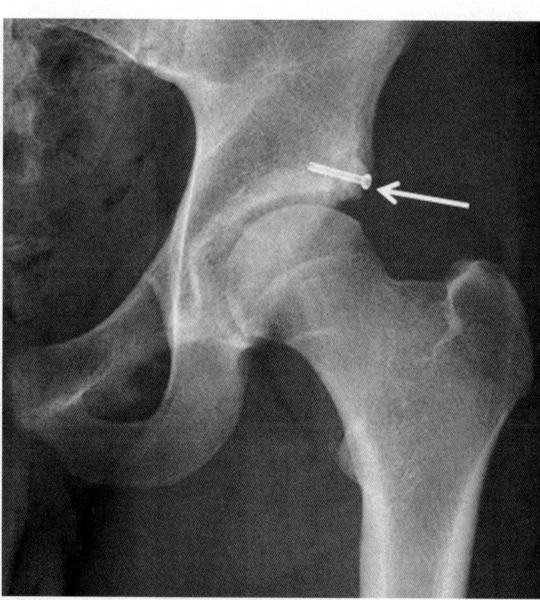

TECH FIG 3 • Although the majority of rim fractures/os acetabuli can be excised, if they contribute to hip stability (**A**, *arrow*), they can be left intact (if stable) or internally fixed with arthroscopic assisted cannulated screws (**B**, *arrow*) as part of an FAI corrective procedure.

This allows for greater resection for larger AIIS deformities with the ability to close the capsule at the conclusion of the case when deemed necessary.

- In severe cases of ischiofemoral impingement, the lessor trochanter can be burred down either open or arthroscopically to widen the ischiofemoral distance or, alternatively, the hamstrings can be detached from the ischial tuberosity followed by a lateral ischial decompression. The site of decompression depends on the degree and locations of ischiofemoral impingement.

Cam Impingement

- Exposure of the femoral head–neck junction can be performed using a generous capsulotomy, capsulectomy, or small capsular window.
- We prefer a generous capsulotomy beginning anterior to the anterior portal and extending to the posterolateral portal site (**TECH FIG 4A**).
- We find that with this technique and careful capsular exposure, the femur can be decompressed from the medial to lateral synovial folds, beyond the synovial folds staying proximal to the vessels, and distally to the level of the trochanter/capsular reflexion. In addition, a portion or all of the capsulotomy can be repaired or plicated at the conclusion of the procedure if deemed necessary.
- One alternative approach is to use a "T" capsulotomy to expose the cam, although we find this to be rarely necessary. This should be repaired at the end of the resection as it further compromises the capsule.
- At the conclusion of central compartment work, traction is released, and the hip is flexed/extended/abducted/adducted with varying degrees of IR and ER, allowing for visualization of the peripheral head–neck junction and the cam deformity.

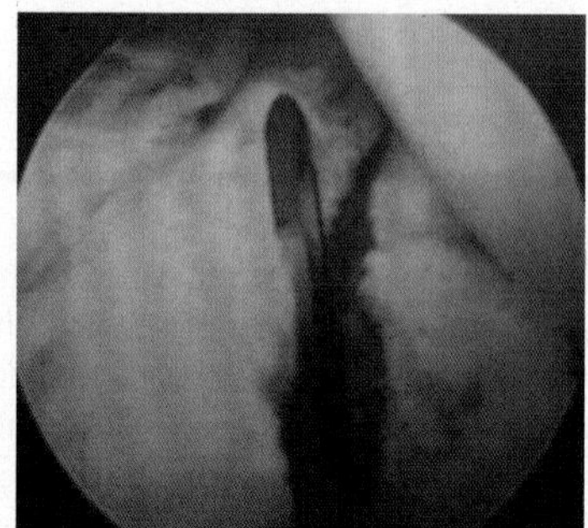

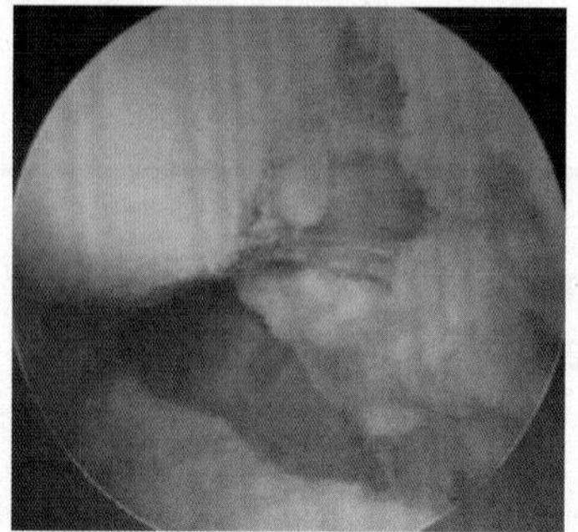

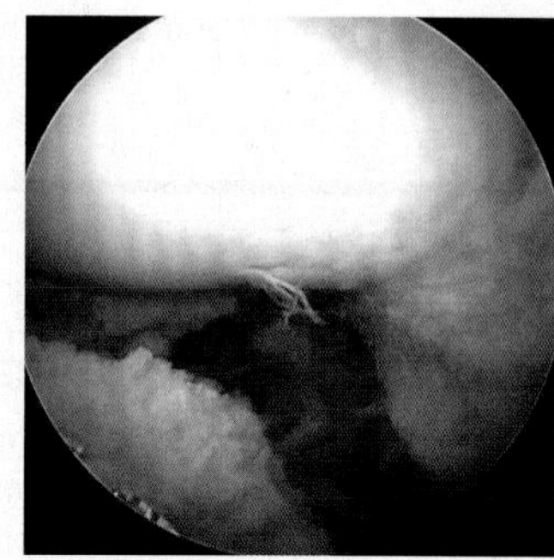

TECH FIG 4 • **A.** A generous capsulotomy is performed to allow exposure of the peripheral head–neck junction. The labrum (*left*) and femoral head (*right*) are seen. **B.** Arthroscopic view of the normal, spherical, femoral head–neck junction in the right hip. **C.** Cam impingement as indicated by a nonspherical, egg-shaped femoral head–neck junction in the right hip. *(continued)*

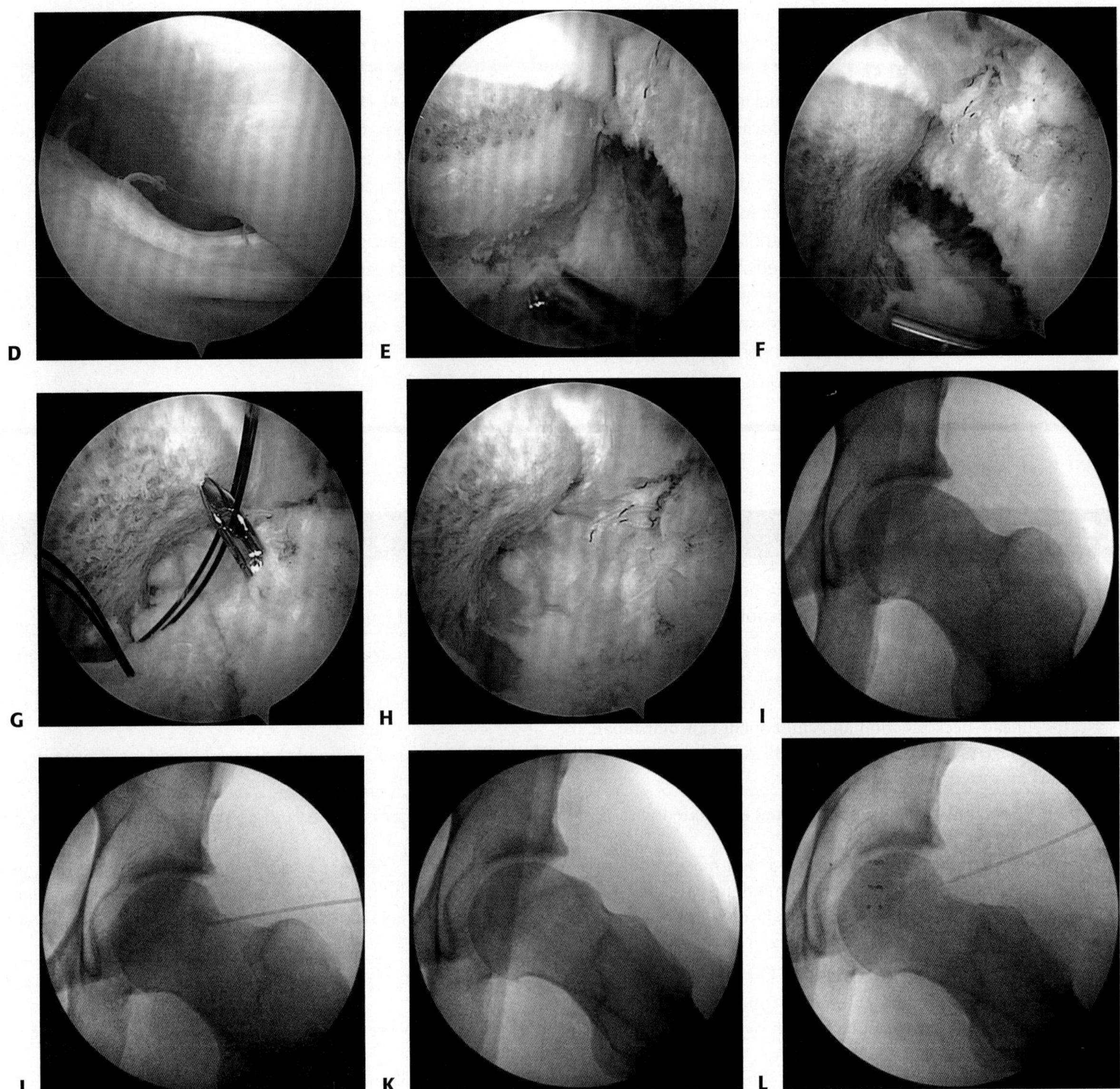

TECH FIG 4 • *(continued)* **D.** Arthroscopic image of the lateral synovial fold (site of the retinacular vessels) in the left hip. **E.** A burr is used to excise and recontour the femoral head–neck junction, seen here in the left hip. **F.** Completion of the osteoplasty restores normal femoral head–neck sphericity, seen here in the left hip. **G.** Passage of a looped suture for closure of the capsulotomy after femoral osteoplasty and acetabular rim trimming, seen here in the left hip. **H.** Final capsular closure with four sutures at the completion of the case. **I–L**. Pre- and postresection fluoroscopic AP and lateral images confirm appropriate cam decompression.

- The normal head–neck junction is relatively spherical (**TECH FIG 4B**), whereas in cam impingement, it appears egg-shaped, flat, or with a prominence at the head–neck junction (**TECH FIG 4C**).
- The cam deformity is covered with relatively normal-appearing articular cartilage with varying degrees of eburnation, which can progress to a more degenerative peripheral head–neck junction with clefts and intraosseous cysts in more advanced cases.
- The medial and lateral (**TECH FIG 4D**) synovial folds should be identified.
- Dynamic assessment confirms cam impingement and regions of impingement.
- A 5.5-mm burr is used to reshape the anterolateral prominence with the goal of improving sphericity and offset with impingement-free motion (**TECH FIG 4E**).
- Recontouring the femur and attempting to create a convexity into a concavity is ideal in an effort to preserve the labral sealing function through greater ROM than a concave resection (**TECH FIG 4F**).
- A recent cadaveric study recommended resecting no more than 30% of the thickness of the femoral neck in order to minimize the risk for pathologic fractures postoperatively.[21]
- The anterior head–neck junction is best recontoured in various degrees of flexion, and the lateral and medial head–neck junction are best recontoured in hip extension/IR with variable degrees of traction.

- Three views in extension and three views in flexion are used to confirm the resection medially/laterally (AP view) and anteriorly (lateral view) (**TECH FIG 4I–L**).
- Care is taken to keep resections proximal to the medial and lateral synovial folds for posterolateral and anteromedial resections in order to avoid damage to the retinacular vessels.
- The typical pattern of cam impingement extends down the neck on the anterolateral femoral head–neck junction and closer to the articular cartilage margin of the femoral head, more superiorly in the region of the lateral and medial retinacular vessels.
- Final confirmation of adequate resection is then verified arthroscopically with dynamic assessment in flexion/IR (anterior femur), extension/abduction, and flexion abduction (lateral femur).
- Capsular closure is then performed with two to six absorbable sutures passed through one side of the capsule with a looped suture passer and grasped through the other side of the capsule (**TECH FIG 4F–H**).
- A combination of absorbable and nonabsorbable sutures are considered for excessive capsular laxity, capsular incompetence in the revision setting, and connective tissue disorders such as Ehlers-Danlos syndrome.
- A knot is then tied blindly at the periphery of the capsule using standard arthroscopic knot-tying techniques.
- The hip is then infiltrated with an anesthetic, and the portals are closed in the usual fashion.

PEARLS AND PITFALLS

Indications	■ History, physical examination, and imaging studies should be consistent with FAI and hip joint–related pain. ■ Intra-articular anesthetic injection should confirm the hip as the source of pain.
Exposure	■ Care should be taken to preserve as much labrum as possible and avoid iatrogenic acetabular chondral damage in order to allow for labral preservation. ■ Adequate capsulotomy with preservation of capsular tissue should be performed to allow for exposure of the femoral head–neck junction and subsequent capsular repair. ■ Variable hip positions in hip flexion and extension allow for complete visualization of the femoral head–neck prominence in cam impingement.

Pincer	■ Acetabular retroversion is often associated with normal anterior acetabular coverage and no resection is indicated in this setting.
	  ■ If indicated, generally 3–5 mm of acetabulum is trimmed, with more removed based on preoperative imaging and arthroscopic confirmation, taking care not to create a dysplastic acetabulum based on preoperative center edge angles.
	  ■ Further, distal-based portals allow for a better angle for anchor placement close to the articular margin of the acetabulum with less risk for intra-articular penetration.

Cam	■ Adequate (usually 5–10 mm) but not overly aggressive femoral osteoplasty is confirmed by repeated dynamic arthroscopic ROM evaluation and fluoroscopic AP and lateral images.
	  ■ Resections should recreate a convexity into a concavity in order to preserve the labral sealing function through a greater hip ROM.
	  ■ Anterior resection is best achieved in flexion, whereas lateral/posterolateral resection is best achieved in extension/IR with variable degrees of traction.

Complications	■ More complex cases of FAI managed arthroscopically can be lengthy procedures, and alternating between traction and flexion or release of traction can help prevent traction-based neurapraxias. ■ Meticulous irrigation of all bony debris and postoperative use of nonsteroidal anti-inflammatories can help to minimize the incidence of heterotopic bone formation.

POSTOPERATIVE CARE

- Pre- and postoperative radiographs confirm adequate osteoplasty and rim trimming (**FIG 5**).
- Postoperative restrictions are not consistent from one surgeon to the next and are based on the procedures done.
- We recommend the following restrictions:
  - Proximal femoral osteoplasty is treated with protected weight bearing with crutches for 2 to 4 weeks depending on the quality of bone and no high-impact or running activities for 2.5 to 3 months.
  - Acetabular rim trimming with labral débridement requires no specific restrictions.
  - Acetabular labral repair and refixation is treated with toe-touch weight bearing for 2 weeks and avoidance of the extremes of external rotation for 2 weeks.
  - Significant capsular repairs should be protected against passive hip extension and extremes of ER for 2 to 4 weeks.
  - Microfracture procedures are treated with 4 to 8 weeks of toe-touch weight bearing depending on the size of the lesion.
  - There is no evidence to support or refute the benefit of hip braces, derotational boots, or continuous passive machines (CPMs).
- Passive ROM with circumduction, stationary bicycle, or CPM should be instituted the day of surgery or postoperative day 1.

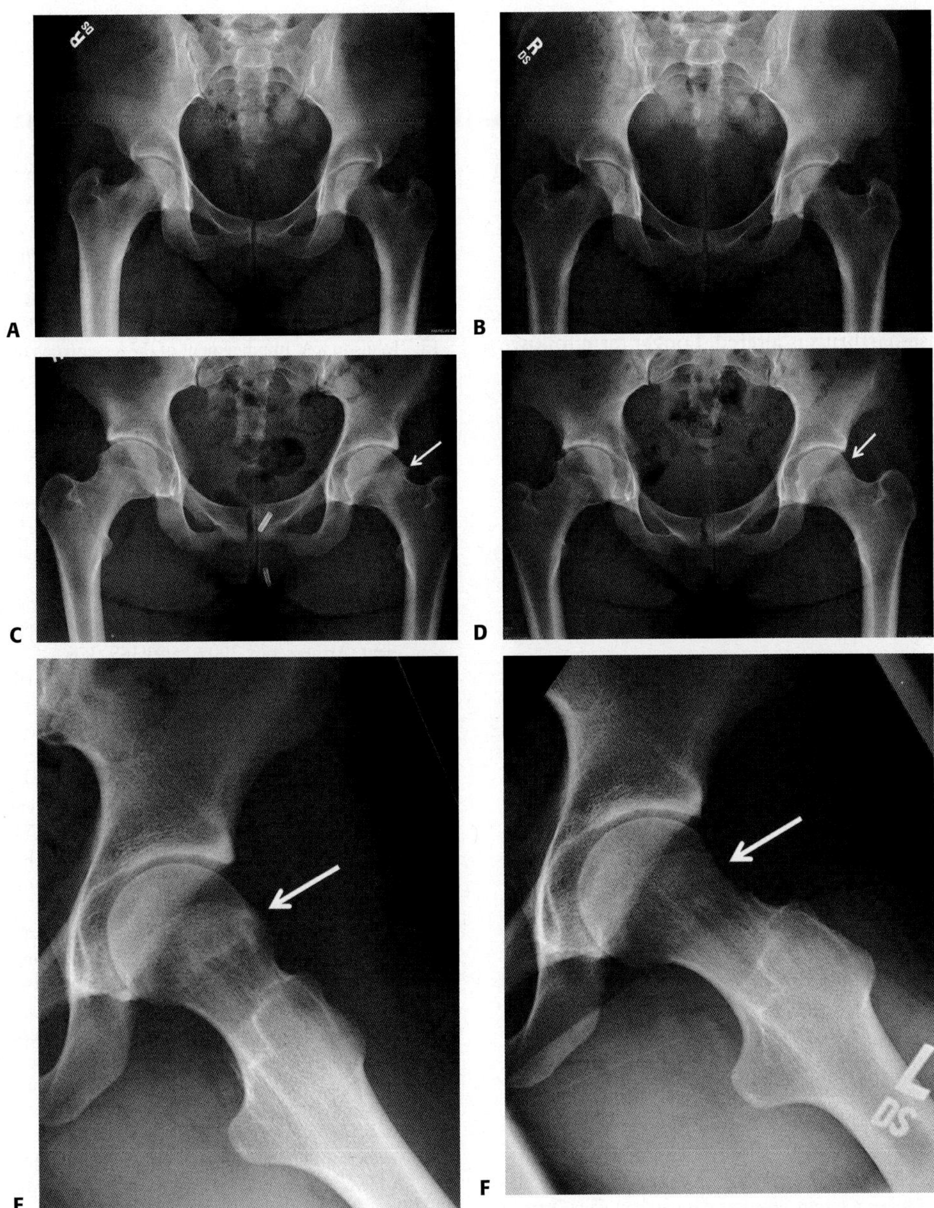

FIG 5 • **A.** Preoperative AP pelvic radiograph reveals left-sided acetabular retroversion with a low AIIS. **B.** Postoperative AP pelvic radiograph after rim resection, labral repair, and AIIS decompression. **C.** Preoperative AP pelvis radiograph shows cam-type morphology (*arrow*). **D.** Postoperative AP pelvis radiograph after cam decompression (*arrow*). **E.** Preoperative lateral radiograph reveals cam-type morphology (*arrow*). **F.** Postoperative lateral radiograph after cam decompression (*arrow*).

- The first 2 months focus on restoration of ROM, gait and pelvic alignment, and gentle core strengthening.
- At 2 months, more aggressive core strengthening is instituted, with resumption of full sporting activities at 3 to 6 months based on functional improvement.
- Further research is required to develop the optimal rehabilitation programs after the various procedures that have been discussed.

OUTCOMES

- Early and midterm results and systematic reviews for FAI indicate that pain and function are improved for the majority of patients and directly correlates with the degree of osteoarthritic changes found at the time of surgery.[1,2,4,6,7,22–24,27]
  - Studies looking at open and arthroscopic approaches found improvement in pain in 68% to 96% of patients regardless of approach.[2,4,6,22,24]
  - In a review of 45 professional and Olympic level athletes with FAI treated arthroscopically, all had symptomatic improvement and returned to play.[29]
  - In another series of 320 patients with FAI treated arthroscopically, 90% had elimination of the impingement sign and were reportedly satisfied with their results.[10]
- Some evidence indicates that repair or refixation of the labrum results in improved outcomes when compared to labral débridement or excision in a consecutive series.[7,17]
  - Larson and Giveans[16] prospectively followed 100 patients with FAI treated arthroscopically for a mean of 3.5 years,

with statistically significant better outcomes (Harris hip score, SF-12, and visual analogue pain scoring) with labral preservation versus excision with 92% good to excellent results versus 68%, respectively.
 - Krych et al,[15] in a randomized study, found better outcomes with labral repair for Activities of Daily Living and Sports subscale of the Hip Outcome Score than labral débridement in females at 32-month follow-up.
- No well-designed, long-term, or randomized studies have been done to evaluate outcomes after management of FAI to determine whether the natural history with regard to the development of osteoarthritis is altered. Longer term follow-up and studies after open versus arthroscopic treatment should better define the optimal indications and procedures for patients with FAI.

COMPLICATIONS

- Lateral femoral cutaneous nerve neurapraxia (common and typically resolves)
- Heterotopic bone or myositis ossificans formation
  - Three weeks of nonsteroidal anti-inflammatory drugs recommended
- Iatrogenic acetabular and femoral chondral damage
  - Careful surgical technique required to minimize
- Rarely postoperative femoral neck fracture
  - Osteopenic bone/overresections/early aggressive weight bearing
- Potential for sciatic or pudendal nerve neurapraxia
  - Minimize traction amount and time
- Potential for avascular necrosis
  - Not reported after femoral resections
- Uncommon: deep venous thrombosis/pulmonary embolism
  - Typically have risk factors
- Uncommon: fluid extravasation
  - Recommend avoiding prolonged high-pressure fluid systems

REFERENCES

1. Beck M, Leunig M, Parvizi J, et al. Anterior femoroacetabular impingement: part II. Midterm results of surgical treatment. Clin Orthop Relat Res 2004;418:67–73.
2. Bedi A, Chen N, Robertson W, et al. The management of labral tears and femoroacetabular impingement of the hip in the young, active patient. Arthroscopy 2008;24(10):1135–1145.
3. Bedi A, Galano G, Walsh, C, et al. Capsular management during hip arthroscopy: from femoroacetabular impingement to instability. Arthroscopy 2011;27(12):1720–1731.
4. Botser IB, Smith TW Jr, Nasser R, et al. Open surgical dislocation versus arthroscopy for femoroacetabular impingement: a comparison of clinical outcomes. Arthroscopy 2011;27(2):270–278.
5. Buller LT, Rosneck J, Monaco FM, et al. Relationship between proximal femoral and acetabular alignment in normal hip joints using 3-dimensional computed tomography. Am J Sports Med 2012;40(2):367–375.
6. Clohisy JC, St John LC, Schutz AL. Surgical treatment of femoroacetabular impingement: a systematic review of the literature. Clin Orthop Relat Res 2010;468(2): 555–564.
7. Espinosa N, Rothenfluh DA, Beck M, et al. Treatment of femoroacetabular impingement: preliminary results of labral refixation. J Bone Joint Surg Am 2006;88(5): 925–935.
8. Ferguson SJ, Bryant JT, Ganz R, et al. An in vitro investigation of the acetabular labral seal in hip joint mechanics. J Biomech 2003; 36(2):171–178.
9. Ganz R, Parvizi J, Beck M, et al. Femoroacetabular impingement: a cause for osteoarthritis of the hip. Clin Orthop Relat Res 2003;(417):112–120.
10. Glick JM, Sampson TG, Gordon RB, et al. Hip arthroscopy by the lateral approach. Arthroscopy 1987;3(1):4–12.
11. Gosvig KK, Jacobsen S, Sonne-Holm S, et al. Prevalence of malformations of the hip joint and their relationship to sex, groin pain, and risk of osteoarthritis: a population-based survey. J Bone Joint Surg Am 2010;92(5):1162–1169.
12. Hapa O, Bedi A, Gursan O, et al. Anatomic footprint of the direct head of the rectus femoris origin: cadaveric study and clinical series of hips after arthroscopic anterior inferior iliac spine/subspine decompression. Arthroscopy 2013;29(12):1932–1940.
13. Johnson KA. Impingement of the lesser trochanter on the ischial ramus after total hip arthroplasty. Report of three cases. J Bone Joint Surg Am 1977;59(2):268–269.
14. Kapron AL, Anderson AE, Aoki SK, et al. Radiographic prevalence of femoroacetabular impingement in collegiate football players: AAOS Exhibit Selection. J Bone Joint Surg Am 2011;93(19):e111(1–10).
15. Krych AJ, Thompson M, Knutson Z, et al. Arthroscopic labral repair versus selective labral debridement in female patients with femoroacetabular impingement: a prospective randomized study. Arthroscopy 2013;29(1):46–53.
16. Larson CM, Giveans MR. Arthroscopic debridement versus refixation of the acetabular labrum associated with femoroacetabular impingement. Arthroscopy 2009;25(4):369–376.
17. Larson CM, Giveans MR, Stone RM. Arthroscopic debridement versus refixation of the acetabular labrum associated with femoroacetabular impingement: mean 3.5-year follow-up. Am J Sports Med 2012;40(5):1015–1021.
18. Larson CM, Kelly BT, Stone RM. Making a case for anterior inferior iliac spine/subspine hip impingement: three representative case reports and proposed concept. Arthroscopy 2011;27(12):1732–1737.
19. Larson CM, Sikka RS, Sardelli MC, et al. Increasing alpha angle is predictive of athletic related "hip" and "groin" pain in collegiate NFL prospect. Arthroscopy 2013;29(3):405–410.
20. Larson CM, Stone RM. The rarely encountered rim fracture that contributes to both femoroacetabular impingement and hip stability: a report of two cases of arthroscopic partial excision and internal fixation. Arthroscopy 2011;27(7):1018–1022.
21. Mardones RM, Gonzalez C, Chen Q, et al. Surgical treatment of femoroacetabular impingement: evaluation of the effect of the size of the resection. Surgical technique. J Bone Joint Surg Am 2006;88(suppl 1) (pt 1):84–91.
22. Matsuda DK, Carlisle JC, Arthurs SC, et al. Comparative systematic review of the open dislocation, mini-open, and arthroscopic surgeries for femoroacetabular impingement. Arthroscopy 2011;27(2):252–269.
23. Murphy S, Tannast M, Kim YJ, et al. Debridement of the adult hip for femoroacetabular impingement: indications and preliminary clinical results. Clin Orthop Relat Res 2004;(429):178–181.
24. Ng VY, Arora N, Best TM, et al. Efficacy of surgery for femoroacetabular impingement: a systematic review. Am J Sports Med 2010;38(11):2337–2345.
25. Notzli HP, Wyss TF, Stoecklin CH, et al. The contour of the femoral head-neck junction as a predictor for the risk of anterior impingement. J Bone Joint Surg Br 2002;84(4):556–560.
26. Pan H, Kawanabe K, Akiyama H, et al. Operative treatment of hip impingement caused by hypertrophy of the anterior inferior iliac spine. J Bone Joint Surg Br 2008;90(5):677–679.
27. Peters CL, Erickson JA. Treatment of femoro-acetabular impingement with surgical dislocation and debridement in young adults. J Bone Joint Surg Am 2006;88(8):1735–1741.
28. Philippon MJ, Maxwell RB, Johnston TL, et al. Clinical presentation of femoroacetabular impingement. Knee Surg Sports Traumatol Arthrosc 2007;15(8):1041–1047.
29. Philippon MJ, Schenker ML. Arthroscopy for the treatment of femoroacetabular impingement in the athlete. Clin Sports Med 2006;25(2):299–308, ix.
30. Torriani M, Souto SC, Thomas BJ, et al. Ischiofemoral impingement syndrome: an entity with hip pain and abnormalities of the quadratus femoris muscle. AJR Am J Roentgenol 2009;193(1):186–190.

Proximal Femoral Osteotomy

Claudio Diaz Ledezma, Philipp Henle, Moritz Tannast, and
Klaus A. Siebenrock

7
CHAPTER

DEFINITION

- Varus intertrochanteric osteotomy involves the reorientation of the proximal femur in order to improve femoral head coverage and joint congruency. It may serve either as a reconstruction or salvage operation. Varus intertrochanteric osteotomy may be beneficial in treating the following conditions[1,2]:
  - Developmental dysplasia of the hip. Although it is most commonly used in conjunction with a pelvic osteotomy, it has also been reported as an isolated procedure.
  - Femoral head osteonecrosis. The osteotomy can remove a circumscribed necrotic lesion from the weight-bearing area.
  - Coxa valga, in particular when the fovea lies within the weight-bearing zone
  - Mild epiphyseal dysplasia of the femoral head with the lateral part of the head intact
  - Posttraumatic joint incongruence
  - Osteochondritis dissecans of the femoral head
- The ability to improve or maintain an adequate hip joint congruency is key to obtain satisfactory surgical results.
- Variations of the technique can be used for correction of the proximal femur in the coronal and sagittal plane,[3] as well as to improve the rotational alignment.

ANATOMY

- The hip joint is an enarthrodial, polyaxial joint between the pelvis and the femoral head. Adequate joint congruency is crucial for well-functioning and normal load transmission across the hip joint.
- The acetabular labrum increases the femoral head coverage and participates in normal load transmission. Considering the labrum, more than half of the femoral head fits within the acetabulum.
- The femoral head is covered with articular cartilage except for the fovea.
- The central and inferior part of the acetabulum, the acetabular fossa, does not participate physiologically in load transmission.
- The medial circumflex femoral artery is the main blood supply of the femoral head. It is mandatory to protect it during hip preservation procedures.

PATHOGENESIS

- Diverse pathologies, including congenital and acquired hip conditions, can alter joint congruency.
- Abnormal hip joint congruency produces high-contact stress on the articular cartilage, predisposing the patient to end-stage osteoarthritis.

NATURAL HISTORY

- If load transmission forces across the hip joint constantly exceed the physiologic limits of the articular cartilage, degenerative changes are inevitable. If untreated, this condition results in progressive osteoarthritis.

PATIENT HISTORY AND PHYSICAL FINDINGS

- A complete medical history should be taken. Groin pain is the most important symptom in hip-related disorders. The severity and duration of pain, stiffness, and altered physical function should be asked. Previous trauma, childhood hip disorders, and the use of corticosteroids must be inquired about as part of the relevant medical history.
- General examination of the hip should always include active and passive range of motion as well as gait inspection and leg length comparison.
- Specific physical examination also includes the following:
  - *Anterior impingement test.* The test is positive if passive movement provokes groin pain, relating to femoroacetabular impingement at the anterior wall or a labral tear.
  - *Apprehension test.* The test is positive if the patient complains of imminent joint luxation, which indicates insufficient coverage of the femoral head.

IMAGING AND OTHER DIAGNOSTIC STUDIES

- A plain, anteroposterior (AP) radiograph of the entire pelvis is needed to determine the type of pathology in the femoral head or the femoral neck. The patient is positioned with 15 degrees of internal rotation of the hip to compensate for the femoral anteversion.
  - Other helpful projections are (1) an axial view, (2) the false-profile view as a true lateral projection of the acetabulum, and (3) an oblique view on the acetabulum tangential to its superoanteromedial edge (**FIG 1**).
- An AP radiograph of the hip in maximal abduction also may be helpful to determine the optimal degree of correction.
  - It simulates the postoperative position of the femoral head and the expected joint congruency.
- Pelvic magnetic resonance imaging or computed tomography scans are optional. They may offer additional information on accompanying lesions on labrum or cartilage or the extent and stage of femoral head necrosis.
- A postoperative AP pelvis view as well as a cross-table view of the hip are useful to evaluate the surgical correction (**FIG 2**).

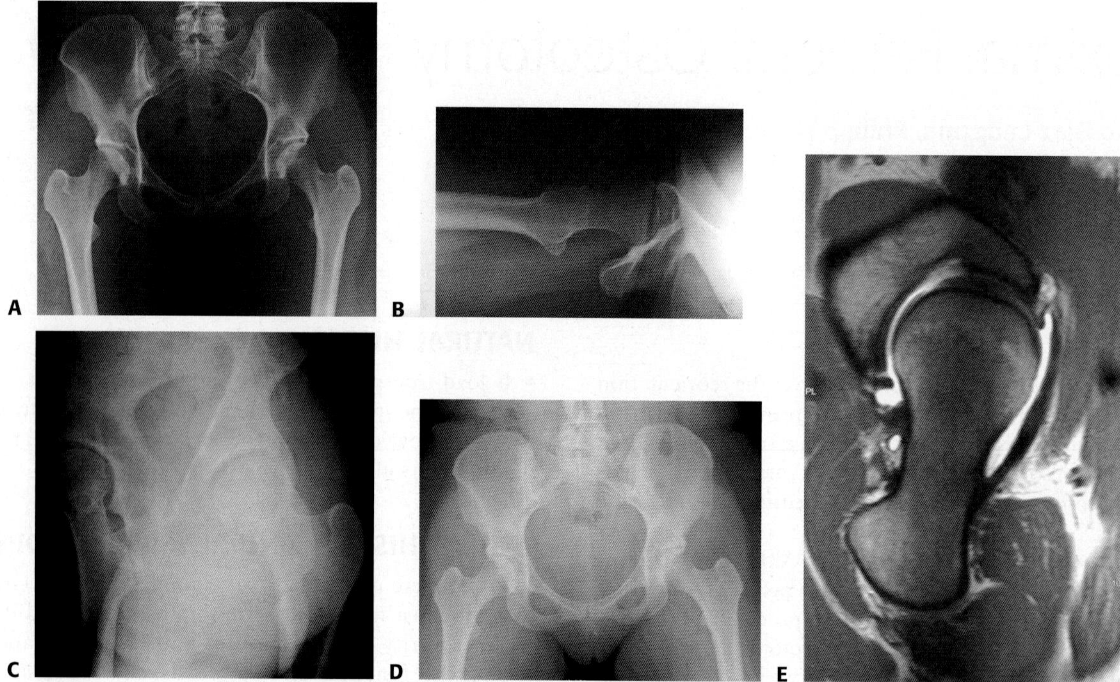

FIG 1 • Preoperative imaging. Standard AP radiograph of the pelvis (**A**), axial view (**B**), and false-profile view (**C**) of a patient with mild hip dysplasia. **D.** Radiograph of the pelvis with hips in maximum abduction to determine the optimal degree of varization and to simulate the expected head position and coverage. **E.** Magnetic resonance imaging (MRI) scanning of the hip can provide additional information on the joint cartilage, labrum, and possible associated femoral head necrosis.

SURGICAL MANAGEMENT

Preoperative Planning

- A preoperative drawing is mandatory. It serves to determine the level and localization of the osteotomy, as well as the entry point and direction of the implant in relation to reference points that can be identified intraoperatively.
- Because a preoperative drawing is a crucial part of the operative technique, it is described in the Techniques section.

Positioning

- A lateral decubitus position on the contralateral side is preferred, allowing unimpeded access to the operation field and free movement of the afflicted leg (**FIG 3**). However, some surgeons prefer the supine position.
- Intraoperative fluoroscopy is strongly recommended. Therefore, a radiolucent operating table must be used, and the position of the C-arm and image intensifier should be checked before draping.

Approach

- The standard procedure uses a lateral approach with an L-shaped detachment of the vastus lateralis muscle, thus increasing the gap medial to the abductors.
- Optionally, a transgluteal approach also can be used. It allows better visualization of the anterior joint capsule. However, this approach is not recommended when an osteotomy of the greater trochanter is planned.

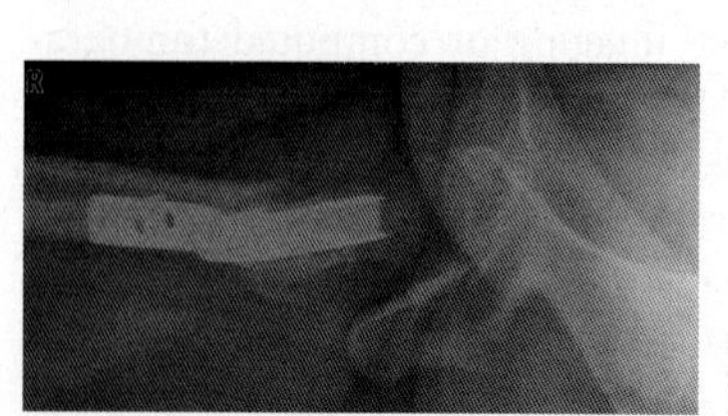

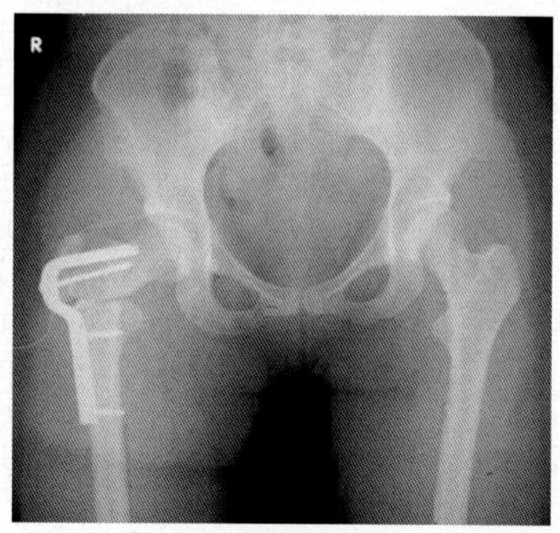

FIG 2 • **A,B.** Postoperative radiograph with the desired varus correction of the right hip. An additional distalization of the greater trochanter was performed in this patient.

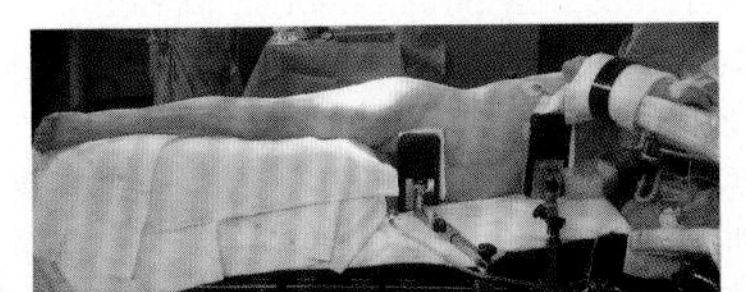

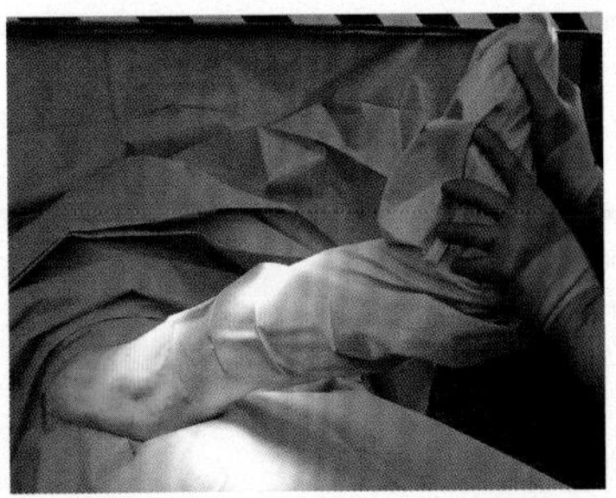

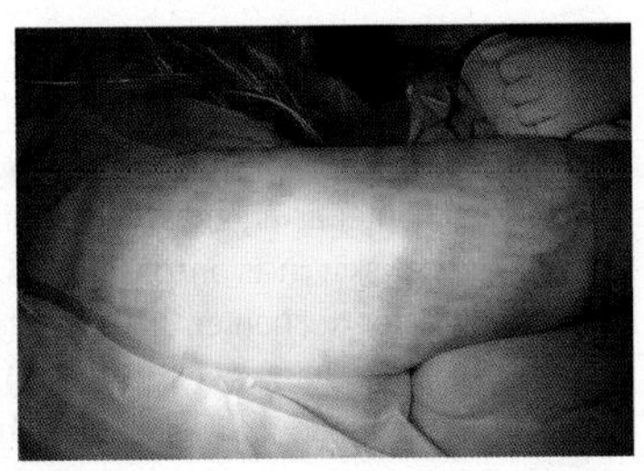

FIG 3 • **A.** A patient in the lateral decubitus position, stabilized with arm and side rests. A foam pillow is placed between the legs. **B.** The affected leg is draped separately in a bag to allow free movement of the hip joint. **C.** View of the prepared operating field, centered over the greater trochanter.

Preoperative Drawing

- Outlines of the femur and pelvis are transferred from the radiograph to drawing paper. Alternatively, some software allow preoperative planning directly on digital images. Magnification of the images should be considered when transferring the planning to the actual surgery. It applies for the measured distances and not for the angles.
- The drawing should focus on the following (**TECH FIG 1**):
  - Identification of the innominate tubercle as the most lateral, intraoperatively detectable point of reference
  - Drawing of the planned osteotomy perpendicular to the femoral shaft axis. The level of the osteotomy is determined by aiming at the cranial extension of the lesser trochanter.
  - Measurement of the distance between the osteotomy and the innominate tubercle
  - Determination of the point within dense bone trabeculae for optimal blade placement
  - Blade position is now determined by that point and the designated correction angle relative to the planned osteotomy.
  - The intersection point of the outlined blade position and the lateral cortex marks the entry point of the blade. Its distance to the innominate tubercle is measured so it can be reproduced intraoperatively.
- An additional trochanteric osteotomy is recommended in those cases with an intertrochanteric correction angle of more than 25 degrees.
  - The osteotomized trochanter should be at least 10 mm thick. The angle of the resected wedge should be equal to the resection angle to allow an accurate apposition of the trochanter fragment.

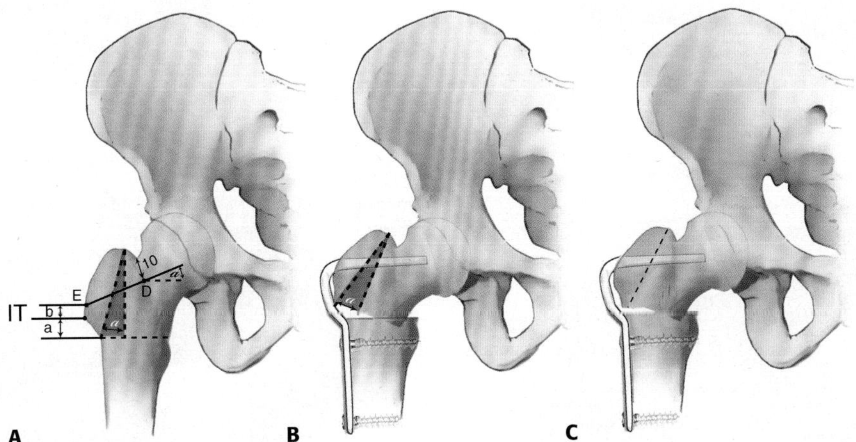

TECH FIG 1 • **A.** The osteotomy level is determined in relation to the innominate tubercle (*IT*), the point of dense bone trabeculae (*D*), and the blade position with the desired correction angle (α), after which the blade entry point (*E*) can be determined. The gray area represents the optional trochanteric osteotomy, which is recommended only when the correction angle exceeds 25 degrees. **B.** Final plate position after intertrochanteric adduction osteotomy without trochanteric osteotomy. **C.** Final plate position after an additional trochanteric osteotomy.

Approach

- The approach begins with identification and marking of the greater trochanter as an anatomic landmark.
- A longitudinal skin incision of 20 to 30 cm is made centered over the greater trochanter, starting 3 to 4 cm cranial to the tip of the greater trochanter (**TECH FIG 2**).
- Subcutaneous tissue, fascia lata, and the trochanteric bursa are split longitudinally to expose the insertion of the gluteus medius and the origin of the vastus lateralis.
  - To facilitate the exposure, the leg can be abducted to release the fascia lata.
- If the incision is placed too anteriorly, it may sever the tensor fasciae latae muscle. If placed too far posteriorly, the cranial part of the gluteus maximus may be erroneously incised.
- The vastus lateralis is detached at its origin in an L-shape, thus increasing the gap medial to the abductor muscles.
  - The muscle is detached from the fascia at the posterior border with a knife and broad periosteal elevator until the entire lateral aspect of the femur is exposed.

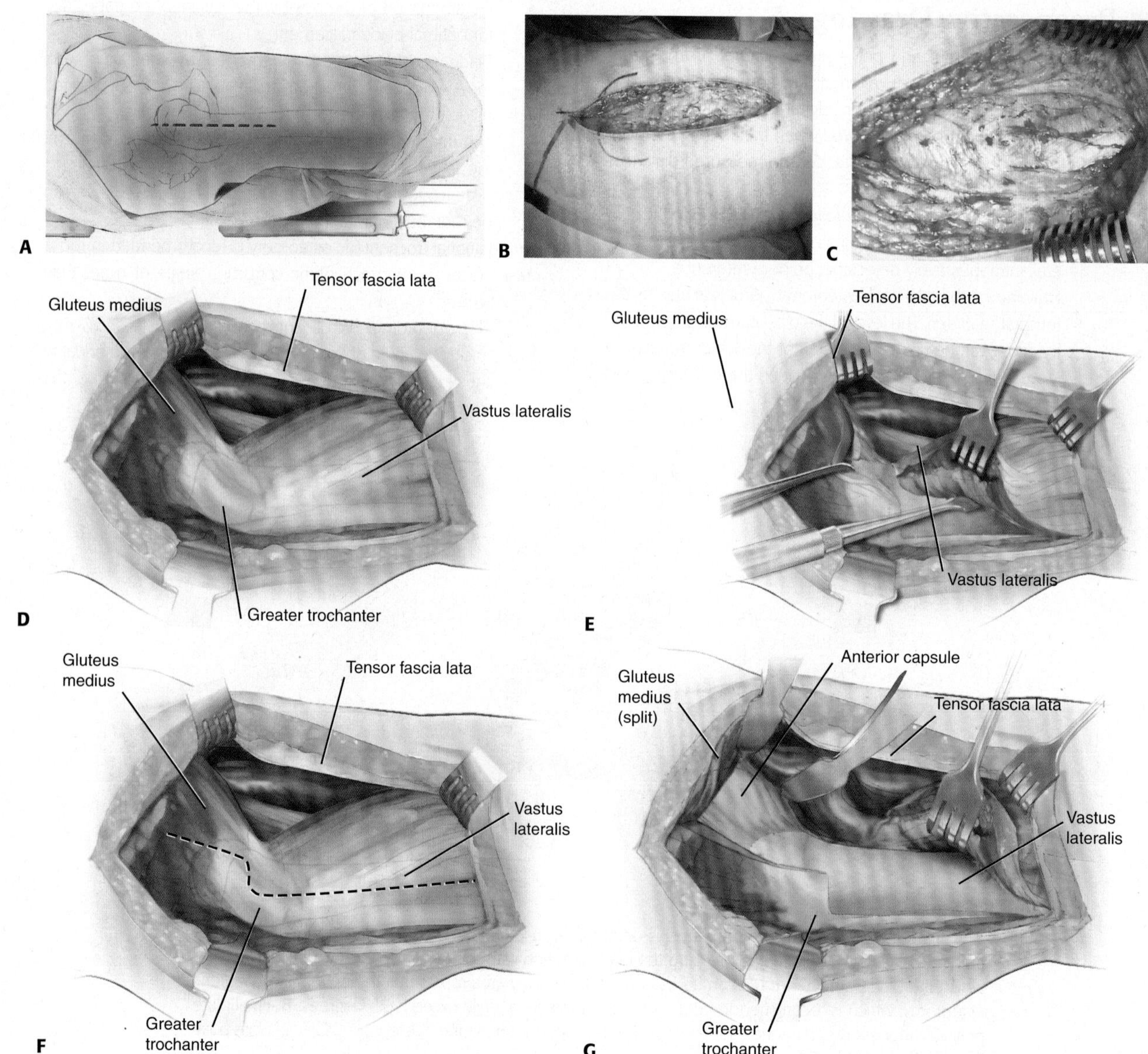

TECH FIG 2 • Approach. **A.** The skin incision is centered over the greater trochanter, starting 3 to 4 cm cranial of the tip of the trochanter and reaching 20 to 30 cm distally along the axis of the femur. **B.** Intraoperative view of the incision. The greater trochanter is marked as an anatomic landmark. **C.** The fasciotomy is performed longitudinal to the axis of the femur. **D.** After retraction of the fascia, the greater trochanter is exposed. **E.** L-shaped detachment of the vastus lateralis at its origin. **F.** Transgluteal approach as a variant. **G.** This approach allows a better view of the anterior capsule.

- The mobilized muscle is retracted anteriorly to expose the lateral aspect of the femur up to the first perforating arteries, which are usually found 8 to 10 cm distal to the innominate tubercle. The vessels are ligated.
- A transgluteal approach may be used as an alternative.
  - Here, the anterior part of the gluteus medius and the anterior insertion of the gluteus minimus are detached, and the incision is continued into the vastus lateralis.
  - A step is cut in the posterior direction between the two muscles, allowing continuity to be maintained between both glutei and the vastus lateralis.
  - During splitting of the gluteus medius, attention must be paid to the nerve branch supplying the tensor fasciae latae, which crosses 3 to 5 cm cranial to the insertion.

Blade Channel Placement

- The anterior capsulotomy is performed in line with the femoral neck and extended to the labrum, which is preserved (**TECH FIG 3**).
  - This approach does not affect blood supply to the femoral head.
- Capsulotomy and exposure of the femoral neck and head are facilitated by insertion of as many as three 8-mm Hohmann retractors, which are inserted on the acetabular rim just proximal to the labrum with the hip in a slightly flexed position.
- At this time, if the leg is externally rotated, direct visualization of the femoral anteversion and part of the articular cartilage is possible.
- At the level of the blade entry point, which was determined on the preoperative drawing in relation to the innominate tubercle, a cortical window measuring 15 × 5 mm is made.
  - It lies almost completely anterior to an imaginary line dividing the lateral aspect of the greater trochanter into two equal parts.
  - Previous marking of the window with a scalpel or an osteotome is recommended.
- The direction of the blade, which was also determined by the preoperative drawing, can now be measured with quadrangular positioning plates and marked with a K-wire inserted into the trochanter cranial to the cortical window.
- An additional K-wire is placed along the femoral neck and pushed into the femoral head to indicate the anteversion of the neck.
  - Measurement should not be done too close to the origin of the vastus lateralis because the diameter of the femur decreases significantly over a distance of 2 to 3 cm.
- The U-shaped seating chisel is inserted into the cortical windows with the direction defined by the two K-wires.
  - It is recommended that the chisel be introduced only after it has obtained some purchase.
  - The position is then checked in all planes and the chisel readjusted if necessary.
  - The seating chisel is advanced under continuous control of all three alignments into the femoral neck and head until the desired depth has been reached (generally 50 to 60 mm).
- Before the osteotomy is performed, the chisel is withdrawn slightly to make it easier to remove it later.

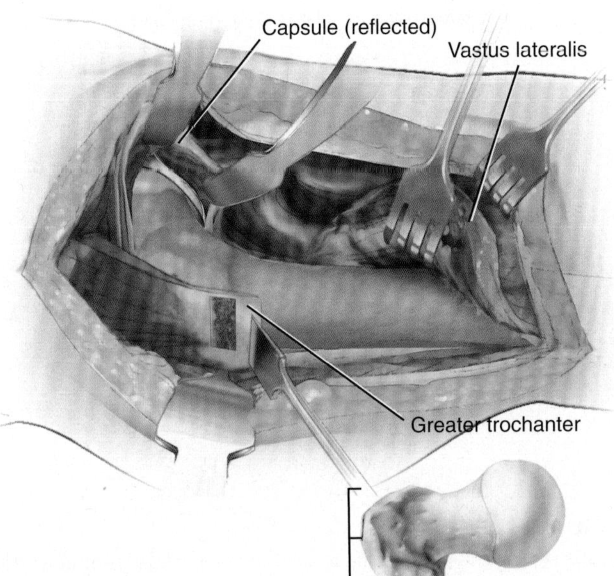

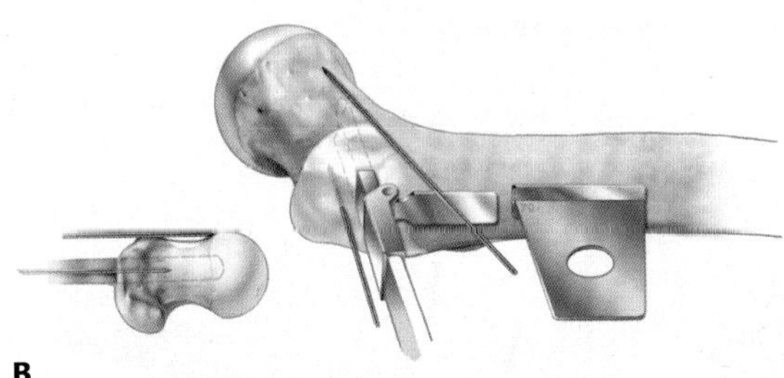

TECH FIG 3 • Blade channel placement. **A.** Anterior capsulotomy in line with the femoral neck. After visualization of the anteversion of the femoral neck, a cortical window is made at the blade entry point. **B.** Placement of two K-wires shows the desired direction of the blade, along which the seating chisel is inserted into the cortical window.

Osteotomy

- The level of the osteotomy is identified in relation to the innominate tubercle, according to the preoperative drawing.
  - An exact drawing obviates the need for palpation of the lesser trochanter.
- Two K-wires are placed into the femur in an anteroposterior direction, one proximal and one distal to the planned osteotomy to allow later rotational realignment (**TECH FIG 4**).
- The osteotomy is performed perpendicular to the long axis of the femur under continuous irrigation.
  - The surrounding soft tissues, in particular posteriorly, must be protected with blunt retractors.
  - The medial femoral circumflex artery runs approximately 15 mm proximal to the lesser trochanter, close to the bone, and can be easily injured.
- If an additional trochanteric osteotomy is performed, anastomoses from the internal iliac artery may be severed, invariably causing necrosis of the femoral head.
  - Therefore, it is recommended that the anterior cortex be osteotomized first and the osteotomy completed posteriorly thereafter.
- A broad chisel (20 mm) is inserted to spread the osteotomy gap.
  - The chisel and the patient's foot are used as levers to mobilize the fragments in opposite directions.
- Manipulation with the seating chisel in the femoral neck must be avoided because this could lead to loosening.

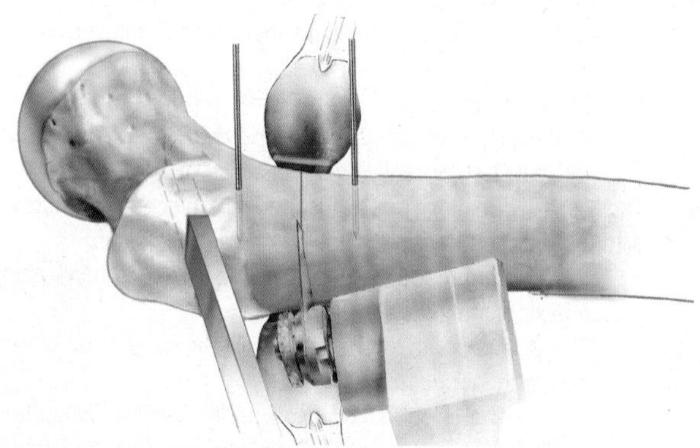

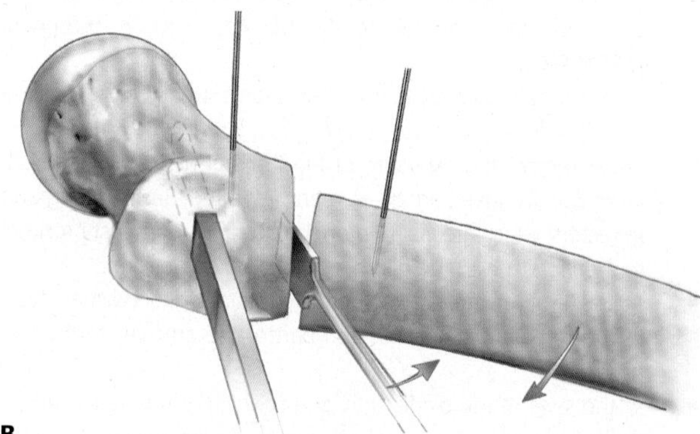

TECH FIG 4 • Osteotomy. **A.** After placing two parallel K-wires proximal and distal to the planned osteotomy for later rotational control, the osteotomy is performed under protection of the surrounding soft tissue. **B.** Insertion of a broad chisel to spread the osteotomy. The chisel and the patient's foot are used as levers to mobilize the fragments.

Blade Insertion

- Before the seating chisel is withdrawn, the blade plate must be readily mounted on the inserter. The blade and inserter must be in line with each other.
- For the first 2 to 3 cm, the blade is advanced manually with repeated pushes (**TECH FIG 5**).
  - As long as the blade follows the channel, easy advancement should be possible.
  - If the force necessary for insertion of the blade increases dramatically, the plate should be removed, the seating chisel should be reintroduced, the direction should be checked, and the plate insertion repeated.

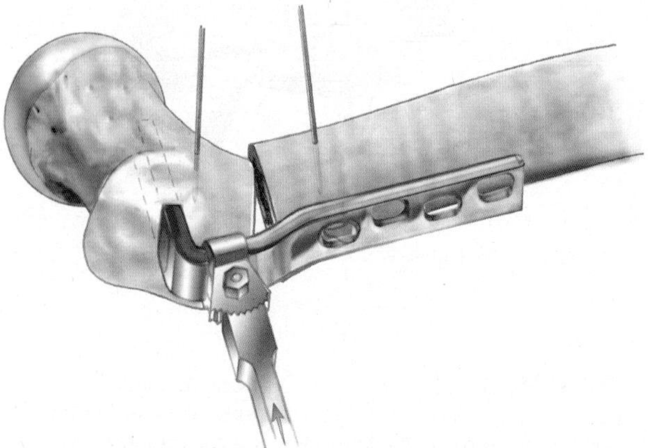

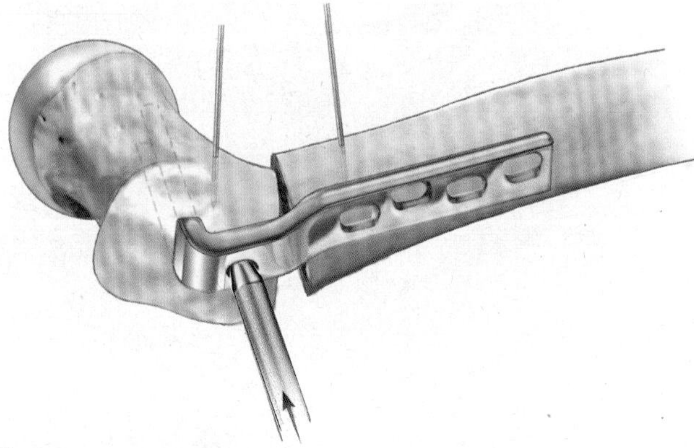

TECH FIG 5 • **A.** Insertion of the blade into the channel formed by the seating chisel. **B.** For the final 10 mm, the blade is advanced with the impactor.

- Hammer blows to advance the plate are allowed only after the direction of the blade has been confirmed. Otherwise, the blade can be pushed in the wrong direction or even perforate the femoral neck.
- During blade insertion, contact of the plate with soft tissue or the femoral shaft must be avoided because this might change the direction of the blade.
  - Such contact is best prevented by positioning the thigh in adduction until three-fourths of the blade has been introduced.
- Once the distance between offset of the plate and bone has reached 1 cm, the inserter is removed and the blade is further advanced with the impactor until full contact with the bone is achieved.
- If an additional trochanteric osteotomy has been performed, the trochanter fragment is flipped over the blade through an already prepared window. The blade with the trochanter is then pushed into the femoral neck.
  - Care must be taken not to split the trochanter fragment.

Correction and Plate Placement

- Achievement of the desired approximation between plate and lateral cortex of the femoral shaft can be facilitated by manipulation of the leg. For rotational realignment, the previously inserted K-wires are used as references.
- After the plate is positioned, it is held against the bone with a reduction forceps (Verbrugge forceps; **TECH FIG 6**).
- Fixation of the plate to the distal fragment can be achieved in three ways:
  - Without interfragmentary compression
  - With interfragmentary compression obtained by use of the gliding holes
  - With interfragmentary compression obtained with a plate tensioner
- The amount of compression depends on the degree of optimal stability as well as the surgeon's preference.
- When using a plate tensioner, compression must be applied judiciously because strong compression may cause a loss of correction, especially in cases of reduced bone quality.
- If no trochanteric osteotomy is performed, the use of gliding holes is recommended.
- If further stability is needed, an additional screw can be inserted through the hole in the offset and engaged into the proximal fragment.
- While the screws are being tightened, rotational alignment of the fragments must be closely observed.
  - External malrotation may occur when only the posterior rim of the plate is in contact with bone.
- The stability of the fixation is checked once the first screw has been tightened and the reduction forceps is still in place.
  - The hip is put through a full range of motion, with the hip in 90 degrees of flexion.
- If the fixation proves to be stable, the second screw is inserted.
- With good bone stock, two bicortical screws are sufficient.
- In cases in which an additional intertrochanteric osteotomy is performed, the removed bone wedge is inserted into the lateral gap between the two main fragments.
  - The use of a plate tensioner is preferable because its use reduces the risk of revalgization.

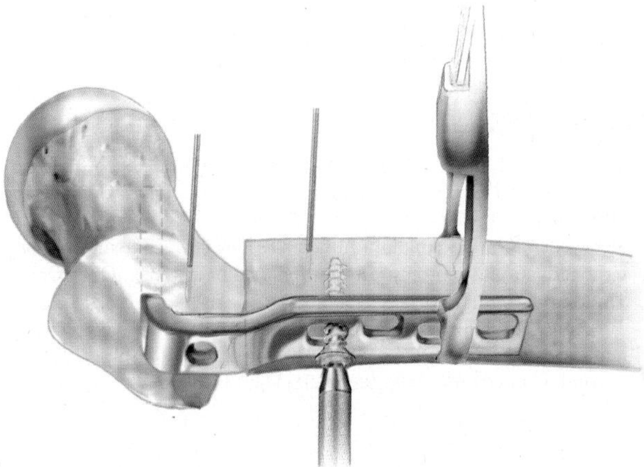
A

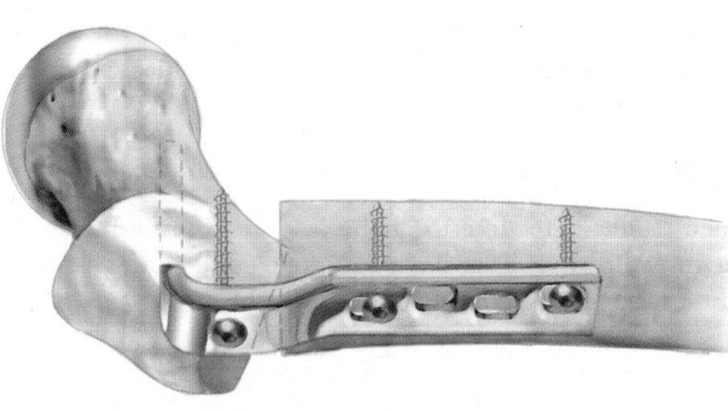
B

TECH FIG 6 • Correction and plate placement. **A.** After the desired correction is reached and full contact of the plate with the lateral femur is achieved, the plate is held in place with a reposition forceps, and the first screw is placed through the plate. **B.** With good bone quality, two screws distal to the osteotomy are sufficient. If bone quality is reduced, another screw can be inserted through the offset of the plate for additional stability.

PEARLS AND PITFALLS

Contraindications	■ Severe osteoporosis ■ Advanced osteoarthritis with marginal osteophytes ■ Spasticity or extensive loss of range of motion ■ Inflammatory arthritis
Unsatisfactory correction or unexpected leg length discrepancy	■ Meticulous preoperative planning is mandatory. ■ Intraoperative use of an image intensifier to check the resulting correction angle and change of leg length. ■ If the achieved correction angle does not reflect the preoperative goal, the seating chisel should be replaced.
Unstable placement or cutting out of the blade	■ Loosening of the blade is best avoided by a correct one-time placement of seating chisel and blade. ■ Under exceptional circumstances, augmentation of the blade with bone cement can be considered.
Incorrect blade length	■ If the blade is too short, the stability of the proximal fragment is reduced, which may cause tilting of the femoral neck and head. ■ If the blade is too long, perforation of the femoral head may result. ■ If intra- or postoperative radiographs show that an improper blade length was used, the implant must be replaced.
Endangered blood supply to the femoral head	■ Proper placement of the blade must be confirmed by visualization with the image intensifier. ■ If the blade is placed too far posteriorly, the deep branch of the medial femoral circumflex artery can be injured. ■ Heavy bleeding from posterior soft tissues should not be addressed by blind coagulation but by hemostasis under direct vision. The use of clips should be considered.

POSTOPERATIVE CARE

- The leg is positioned on a splint with the hip and knee in slight flexion.
- The patient is taken off bed rest on day 1 or 2, with partial weight bearing (15 kg) for 8 weeks.
- Non–weight bearing, which necessitates that the operated hip be held in flexion, leading to increased strain on the osteotomy, should be avoided.
- Physical therapy is required only for gait training using canes.
- Indomethacin (75 mg once daily) is given for 3 weeks for the prevention of heterotopic ossification.
- Radiographic follow-up is done after 6 weeks.
- At 6 weeks after the operation, strengthening exercises of the abductor muscles can be started.
- Final radiographic follow-up is done 1 year after surgery.
- The implant is removed only in case of symptoms such as soft tissue irritation or trochanteric bursitis and not before 1 year postoperatively.

OUTCOMES

- Published studies after intertrochanteric osteotomy for the treatment of hip dysplasia have reported good long-term outcomes, ranging from 63% to 87% after 21 to 26 years.[1]
- Treatment of femoral head osteonecrosis with an intertrochanteric osteotomy can be expected to achieve good results in 65% to 90% of cases, depending on the radiographic stage.
- Data are limited on patients with osteochondritis dissecans treated with an intertrochanteric osteotomy.

COMPLICATIONS

- Unsatisfactory correction
- Incorrect blade placement
- Malrotation
- Femoral head necrosis
- Delayed or nonunion
- Heterotopic ossification
- Femoral or sciatic nerve injury

REFERENCES

1. Santore RF, Kantor SR. Intertrochanteric femoral osteotomies for developmental and posttraumatic conditions. Instr Course Lect 2005;54:157–167.
2. Siebenrock KA, Ekkernkamp A, Ganz R. The corrective intertrochanteric adduction osteotomy without removal of a wedge. Oper Orthop Traumatol 2000;8:1–13.
3. Turgeon TR, Phillips W, Kantor SR, et al. The role of acetabular and femoral osteotomies in reconstructive surgery of the hip: 2005 and beyond. Clin Orthop Relat Res 2005;441:188–199.

Valgus Osteotomy of Proximal Femur

8 CHAPTER

Wudbhav N. Sankar

DEFINITION

- Valgus osteotomy of the proximal femur can be performed for a number of different conditions including (among others) congenital or acquired coxa vara, fracture nonunion, avascular necrosis (AVN), or Legg-Calvé-Perthes disease (LCPD).
- Coxa vara is a deformity of the proximal femur associated with a neck–shaft angle of less than 110 degrees.[11] It can be congenital or developmental in origin.
- Femoral neck fracture nonunions can result (in part) from a vertically oriented fracture plane. A valgus osteotomy can improve mechanical loading at the fracture site and aid in fracture healing.
- AVN of the femoral head typically affects the anterosuperior region of the femoral head while sparing the medial and posterior regions. In certain cases, a valgus osteotomy (with flexion) can rotate better parts of the femoral head into the weight-bearing zone.
- In LCPD, valgus osteotomy can help those hips in which the primary goal of containment is no longer possible owing to hinge abduction. Under these circumstances, a valgus osteotomy can relieve the hinging and improve congruency of the joint.

ANATOMY

- Valgus osteotomy creates an apex medial angulation in the proximal femur.
- In doing so, the medial aspects of the femoral head are rotated more centrally into the joint and, correspondingly, the lateral aspects of the head are rotated away from the joint.
- Adding flexion or extension at the osteotomy site similarly rotates the posterior (flexion) or anterior (extension) aspects of the femoral head into the joint.
- Valgus osteotomy increases a patient's effective hip abduction by the amount of correction and similarly reduces the patient's adduction by an equivalent amount.
- Length of the limb is increased by a valgus correction, which can be useful in cases of mild limb shortening (eg, LCPD).
- Valgus correction moves the greater trochanter distally, which improves abductor mechanics.

PATHOGENESIS

- The pathogenesis of the deformity to be treated by valgus osteotomy is specific to the underlying condition.
- The exact cause of developmental coxa vara is unknown, but one theory postulates that the varus deformity is due to a primary ossification defect in the medial femoral neck that results in a more vertical physis. The physiologic shearing stresses that occur during weight bearing fatigue the dystrophic bone in the medial femoral neck, resulting in progressive varus.[7]
- AVN of the femoral head is the final common pathway of a spectrum of disease processes that disrupt circulation to the femoral head including embolism from deep sea diving, alcohol use, corticosteroid use, hemoglobinopathies, chemotherapy, LCPD, and traumatic injuries to the hip.[1]
- Hinge abduction in LCPD can result from fragmentation and extrusion of the epiphysis, which can create coxa magna and/or a ridge of lateral bone. As a result, the lateral aspect of the deformed femoral head may impinge on the acetabulum with attempted abduction. Continued abduction creates a lateral hinge, which pulls the inferomedial portion of the head away from the acetabulum.[8]

NATURAL HISTORY

- As described by Weinstein et al,[11] the most reliable factor for progression of coxa vara is the Hilgenreiner–epiphyseal angle (HEA), measured between the line of Hilgenreiner and a line parallel to the proximal femoral physis (**FIG 1**).
  - Patients with HEAs more than 60 degrees will invariably progress, whereas those between 45 and 60 degrees have a less defined prognosis and must be followed for progression of varus deformity or increased symptoms.
- AVN of femoral head typically results in progressive collapse, pain, and stiffness often necessitating total hip arthroplasty.[1]
- At maturity, patients with LCPD and unrelieved hinge abduction would generally be classified as Stulberg category IV

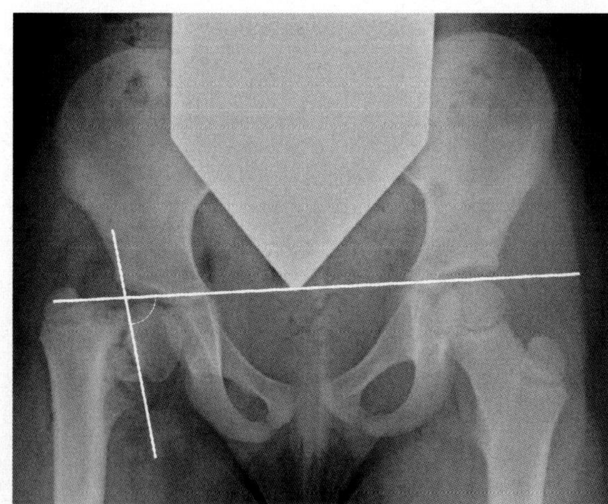

FIG 1 • AP radiograph of the pelvis demonstrates the classic appearance of developmental coxa vara on the right side. The HEA is formed by crossing Hilgenreiner line with a line parallel to the proximal femoral physis. This angle is thought to be the best predictor of progression and postoperative recurrence.

(flattened femoral head with congruent acetabulum) or category V (flattened femoral head with a round acetabulum), both of which have been found to be associated with early-onset osteoarthritis.[10]

PATIENT HISTORY AND PHYSICAL FINDINGS

- History and physical findings are specific to the underlying condition.
- Typically, patients who would benefit from a valgus osteotomy have pain with ambulation that is relieved by rest.
- There is generally 1 to 2 cm of limb shortening.
- Abductor weakness often causes a Trendelenburg gait.
- Limited abduction is common, and occasionally, patients have frank adduction contractures.

IMAGING AND OTHER DIAGNOSTIC STUDIES

- Plain radiographs are generally diagnostic for the conditions that may require a valgus osteotomy.
- Anteroposterior (AP) x-rays of the hip in coxa vara will demonstrate a reduced neck–shaft angle and a wider more vertically oriented proximal femoral physis. Classically, a triangular metaphyseal fragment will be seen in the inferior neck surrounded by physis, giving an inverted Y pattern[11] (see **FIG 1**).
- Femoral neck nonunions typically result in medial collapse and varus deformity. Subtle nonunions can be confirmed by computed tomography (CT) scan.
- On the AP view, AVN typically results in sclerosis and/or collapse of the lateral and superior regions of the femoral head. On the frog view, the anterior head is more commonly affected.
- Hinge abduction in LCPD is best diagnosed using dynamic arthrography. Although pooling of dye medially is often considered diagnostic for hinge abduction, this can simply reflect an area of flattening of the epiphysis. It is most accurate to determine whether the lateral edge of the femoral head is able to rotate underneath the lip of the acetabulum and labrum with abduction (**FIG 2**). Congruency is generally improved when the hip is adducted.
  - The arthrogram should also be studied in AP and lateral projections with abduction, adduction, and internal and external rotation to determine the position that maximizes congruency and relieves impingement.

DIFFERENTIAL DIAGNOSIS

- Congenital or acquired coxa vara
- Femoral neck nonunion
- AVN
- LCPD with hinge abduction or poor congruency
- Pathologic bone condition causing progressive varus deformity (eg, fibrous dysplasia, osteogenesis imperfecta, renal osteodystrophy)

NONOPERATIVE MANAGEMENT

- Mild forms of coxa vara, precollapse AVN, and early-stage LCPD may be managed conservatively.
- Depending on the circumstance, short courses of anti-inflammatory medications, protected weight bearing, and/or activity modification can be helpful.
- In LCPD, if hinge abduction is seen on radiographs but the patient is symptom-free, an osteotomy can still improve the prognosis. In that scenario, it would be reasonable to wait until the patient is symptomatic before proceeding with surgery.

SURGICAL MANAGEMENT

- The valgus osteotomy is indicated for unacceptable varus deformity, fracture nonunion, and certain cases of AVN among others.
- In LCPD, valgus osteotomy is considered a salvage operation for late cases in which the femoral head has developed a lateral ridge that can no longer be brought under the acetabulum (hinge abduction) or to improve congruency of an aspherical hip (**FIG 3**).

Preoperative Planning

- Clinically or radiographically assess limb lengths to determine if concomitant shortening is necessary.
- Carefully evaluate preoperative range of motion including flexion, extension, and rotation.
- Specifically evaluate a patient's adduction and abduction prior to surgery to guide the amount of correction. Keep in

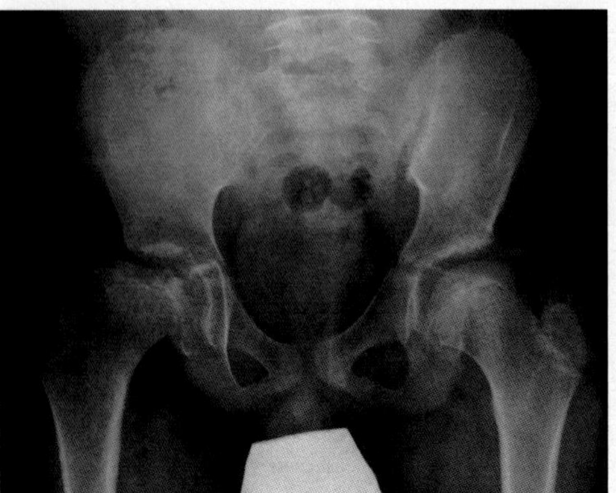

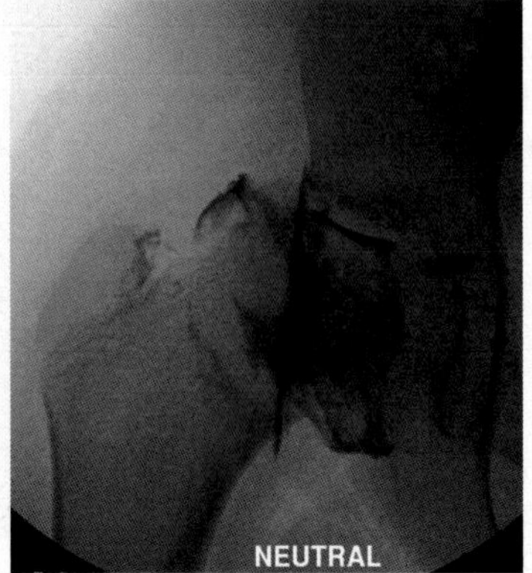

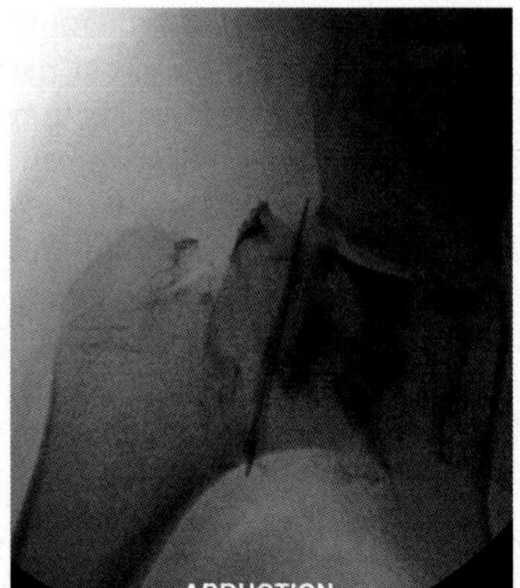

FIG 2 • **A.** AP radiograph of the pelvis demonstrates bilateral Perthes disease, worse on the right. **B.** Arthrogram of the right hip in neutral demonstrates poor congruence and a lateral ridge on the femoral head. **C.** As the hip is brought into abduction, the lateral aspect of the femoral head impinges on the edge of the acetabulum causing pooling of dye medially (hinge abduction). The head does not truly slip underneath the labrum/lateral aspect of the cartilaginous acetabulum in this position.

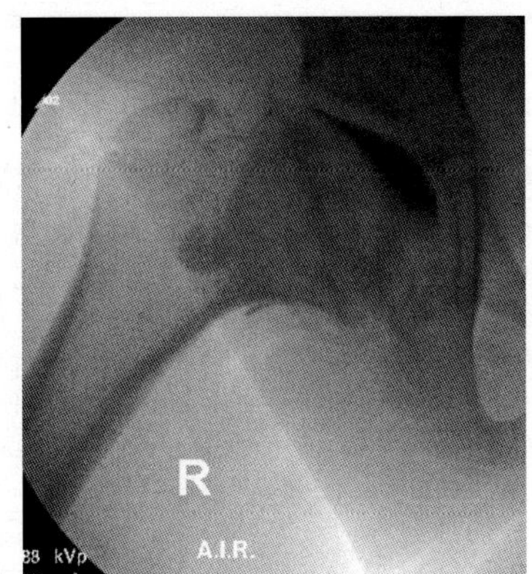

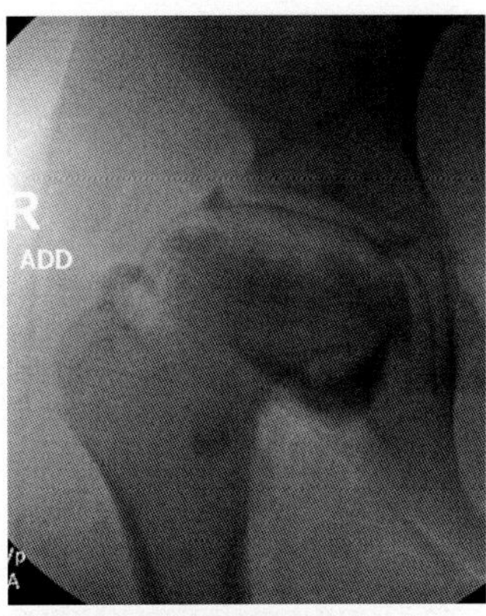

FIG 3 • **A.** Arthrogram of the hip in a patient with healed LCPD. Note the poor congruence in the neutral position. **B.** Congruence is improved when the hip is adducted.

mind that adduction will be decreased and abduction will be increased by the amount of osteotomy correction. Generally, it is preferable to achieve at least 20 degrees of abduction after surgery.

- If an arthrogram was performed, it should be reviewed carefully. In cases of hinge abduction, extension, flexion, or rotation may be required in addition to valgus to fully relieve impingement and maximize congruency.
- Review preoperative AP and frog lateral radiographs to determine the native neck–shaft angle and size of bone.
- Based on range-of-motion measurements and preoperative radiographs, one should determine the desired amount of valgus correction.
- Implant choice is critical as the placement and shape of the implant, rather than the saw cut, will determine the final position of the osteotomy.
- The author prefers a 130-degree nonoffset blade plate, which lateralizes the femoral shaft and preserves head–shaft offset (**FIG 4A**).
  - Using a standard blade plate or proximal femoral locking plate can medialize the femoral shaft excessively such that the limb resembles a "post" without any physiologic offset (**FIG 4B**).
- Depending on the size and weight of the patient, both 3.5- and 4.5-mm plate options exist for one particular manufacturer (Orthopediatrics, Warsaw, IN). The width of the 3.5-mm blade plate system is 11 mm. The width of the 4.5-mm blade plate system is 14 mm.
- The blade plate should occupy 50% to 75% of the width of the femoral neck on the lateral projection for optimum strength.
- To calculate the angle for insertion of the blade plate relative to the femoral shaft, the angle of the planned correction is subtracted from 130 degrees.
  - Example: For a desired 20 degrees of valgus correction, the blade is inserted at 110 degrees from the shaft. With the blade at 110 degrees, the shaft must come into 20 degrees of valgus to accommodate a 130-degree fixed-angle blade plate.

Positioning

- The patient is placed supine on a radiolucent surgical table with a small bump under the ipsilateral pelvis to facilitate access to the lateral femur. Too large of a bump can distort orthogonal imaging.
- The surgeon should check that sufficient AP and frog lateral radiographs can be obtained.
- The entire limb should be draped free to allow manipulation of the limb during surgery.

Approach

- The standard lateral approach to the proximal femur is used.

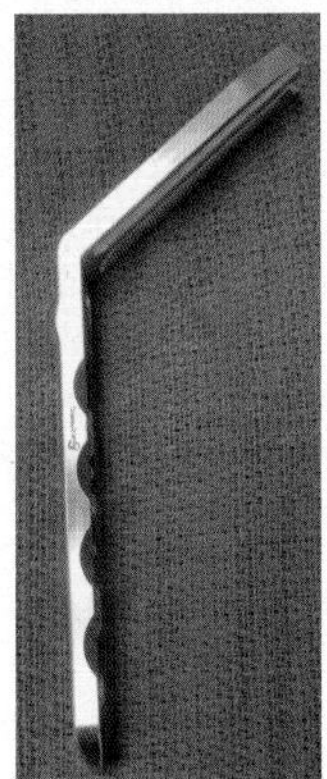
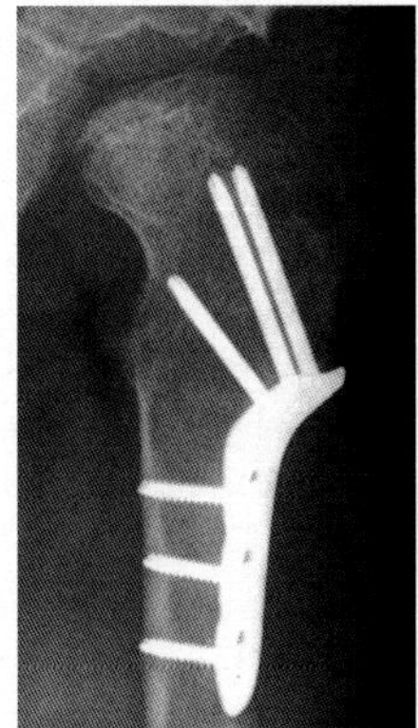

FIG 4 • **A.** A 130-degree nonoffset blade plate. **B.** AP of the left hip demonstrates a valgus osteotomy for a patient with LCPD using a proximal femoral locking plate designed for valgus correction. Note that the shaft is medialized excessively such that the limb resembles a post without any physiologic offset.

Exposure

- Skin incision is made in line with the proximal femur starting a few centimeter proximal to the vastus ridge and extending distally approximately 10 to 12 cm depending on the size of the patient and the intended implant.
- The fascia lata is split in line with the fibers over the palpated lateral border of the femur.
- The vastus lateralis fascia is incised longitudinally about 5 to 10 mm anterior to the intermuscular septum and is elevated atraumatically from the femur. Perforating vessels are identified and cauterized.
- Proximally, the fascia of the vastus lateralis is opened anteriorly with the electrocautery along the vastus ridge, creating an L shape (**TECH FIG 1A**).
- The periosteum is incised along the anterolateral femur, and subperiosteal dissection is performed circumferentially just proximal to the level of the lesser trochanter. The exposure should be extended sufficiently distal to allow shortening of the bone (if necessary) and application of the plate (**TECH FIG 1B**).

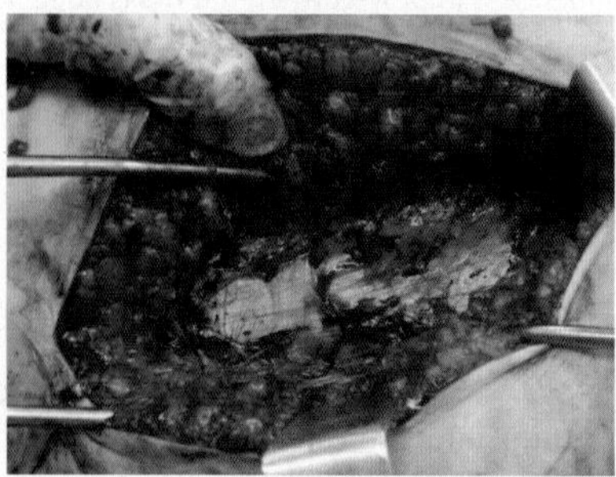

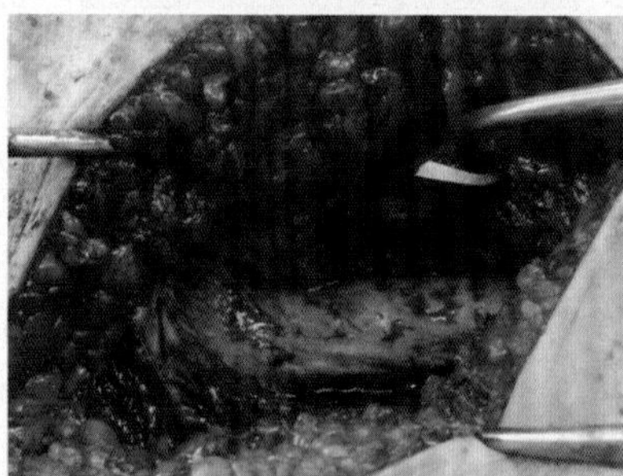

TECH FIG 1 • A. The vastus lateralis is opened in an L fashion (*purple*) with the vertical limb along the vastus ridge and the posterior limb 5 mm anterior to the posterior border of the muscle. **B.** The lateral femur is exposed in a subperiosteal fashion circumferentially.

Valgus Osteotomy of the Femur Using a Cannulated Blade Plate

Guidewire Placement

- In a cannulated blade plate system, the guidewire establishes the position of the chisel which in turn dictates the position and trajectory of the blade. Therefore, precise placement is critical.
- To provide a reference, a standard Kirschner (K) wire is inserted perpendicular to the femoral shaft at the intended osteotomy site (usually at the proximal aspect of the lesser trochanter).
- The entry site for the cannulated blade plate guidewire is proximal to the osteotomy site at a distance specified by the implant design. This typically ends up being just distal to the vastus ridge and trochanteric apophysis. The entry site should be centered on the lateral aspect of the femur in the sagittal plane (**TECH FIG 2A**).
- Using a triangle template to guide the trajectory (chosen based on the amount of intended correction), the guidewire is inserted into the femoral neck.
  - To use the previous example, if a 20-degree correction is desired and a 130-degree implant is being used, the guidewire should be placed 110 degrees from the shaft. A 110-degree angle with the shaft corresponds to a 20-degree angle compared to the perpendicular K-wire (90 + 20). Therefore, a 20-degree triangle is used to confirm the angle between the wires (**TECH FIG 2B,C**).
- In the lateral plane, the wire should parallel the proposed track of the blade plate (ie, centered in the femoral neck) (**TECH FIG 2D**).
- The guidewire is advanced short of the physis, and length is measured.
- The guidewire should be inserted bit further than the intended blade plate depth to prevent dislodgement during chisel placement.

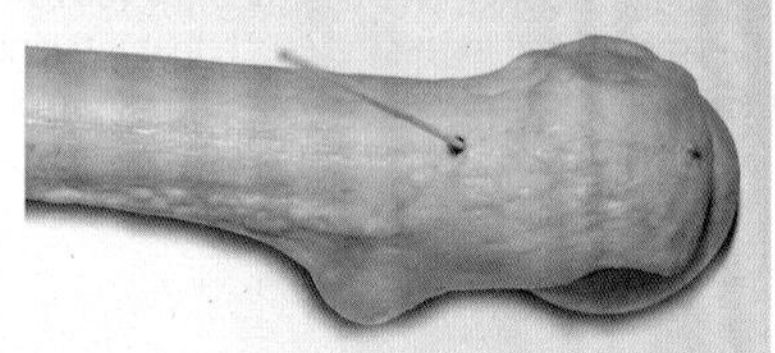

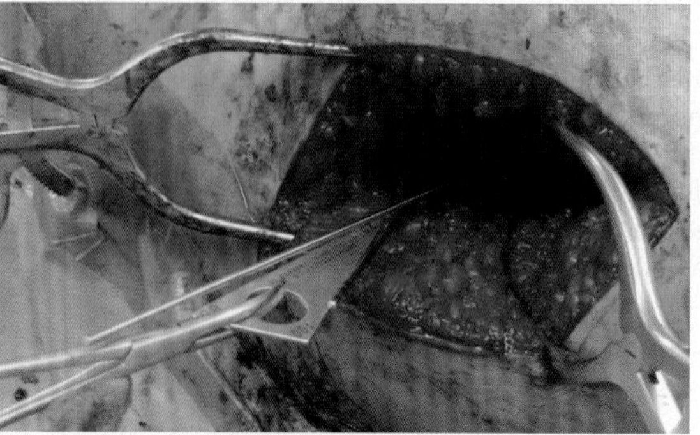

TECH FIG 2 • A. In the sagittal plane, the guidewire entry site is in the midpoint of the femur. A reference K-wire is inserted perpendicular to the femoral shaft. Depending on the amount of desired correction, the guidewire for the cannulated blade plate is then inserted up the femoral neck at a specific angle to the first K-wire. **B.** A triangle is used to judge the angle between the K-wires. *(continued)*

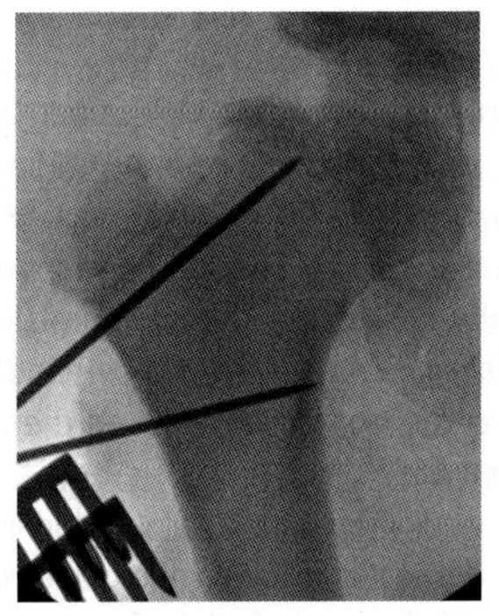
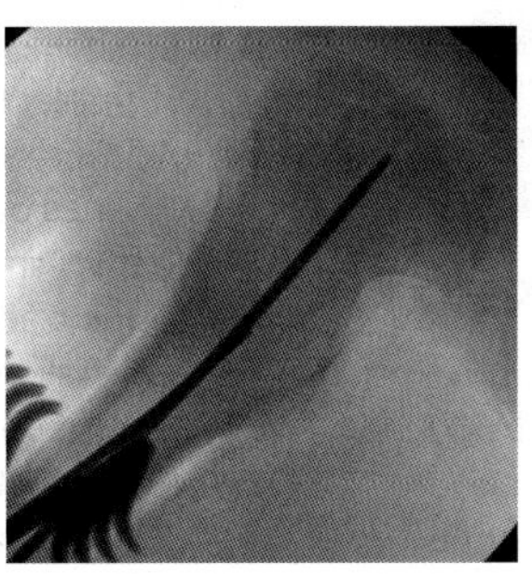
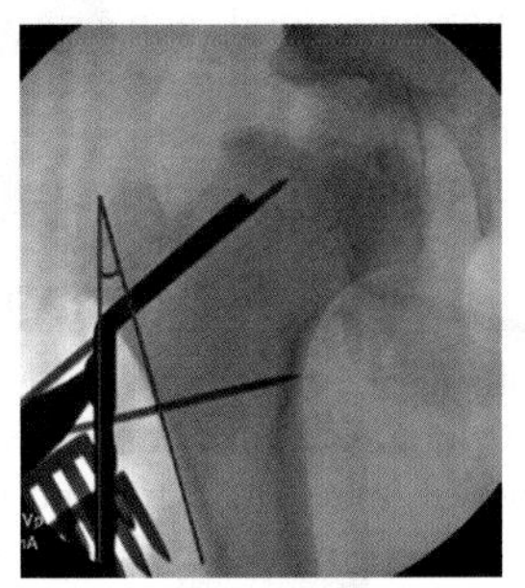

TECH FIG 2 • *(continued)* **C.** The angle between the two wires can also be confirmed using the C-arm. **D.** The position of the guidewire is confirmed in the frog lateral view. **E.** As a double check to confirm that the guidewire that was just placed will result in the desired correction, the 130-degree blade plate is laid over the skin of the patient in line with the guidewire and imaged using the C-arm. The angle created between the lateral aspect of the femoral shaft and the shaft of the plate will be the amount of correction.

- As a double check to confirm that the guidewire that was just placed will result in the desired correction, the 130-degree blade plate is laid over the skin of the patient in line with the guidewire and imaged using the C-arm. The angle created between the lateral aspect of the femoral shaft and the shaft of the plate will be the amount of correction. This can be estimated visually or measured using a goniometer (**TECH FIG 2E**).

Chisel Insertion

- The cannulated chisel is now inserted over the guidewire (**TECH FIG 3A**).
- For pure valgus, the chisel is rotated so that it is perpendicular to the lateral shaft of the femur.
- To add extension or flexion, the chisel is rotated posteriorly or anteriorly from perpendicular, respectively. The desired amount of flexion or extension should be marked on the bone (**TECH FIG 3B,C**).
  - A guide arm that can be slid over the chisel is helpful to visualize the amount of flexion or extension.
- The chisel should be frequently backed out a bit during insertion (using a slap hammer) to prevent incarceration.
- The path of the chisel is checked periodically with fluoroscopy.
- The chisel is backed up to loosen it before making the osteotomy. The surgeon should verify it has actually backed up by checking the depth measurement or by taking a C-arm image.

Making the Osteotomy

- Prior to making the cut, the bone is scored longitudinally with electrocautery or a saw across the osteotomy site, or K-wires can be placed proximal and distal to the osteotomy site to assess rotation after the osteotomy has been performed (see **TECH FIG 3A**).
- A transverse osteotomy is made using an oscillating saw at the site of the original, perpendicularly directed K-wire (generally at the proximal aspect of the lesser trochanter). The K-wire can be left in place to help guide the saw cut so that it is perpendicular to the femoral shaft or the trajectory can be confirmed using the C-arm.
  - A single transverse cut is the simplest means of performing the osteotomy and generally heals quite well, but it does

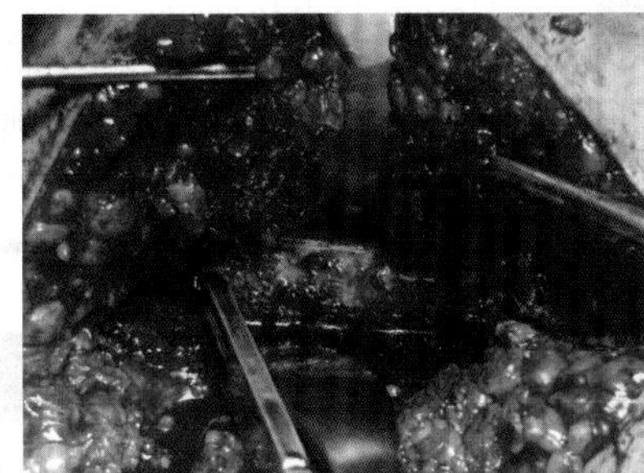

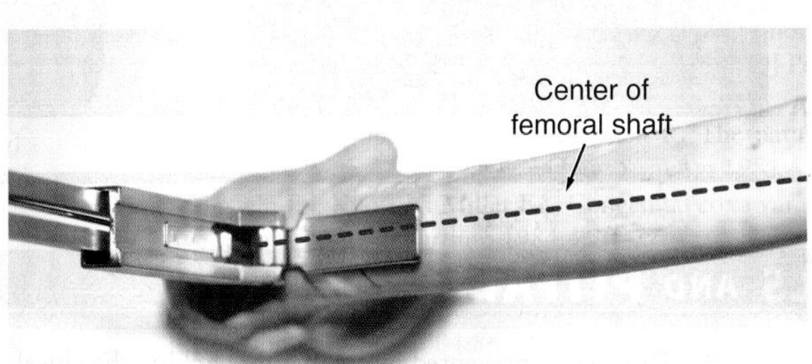

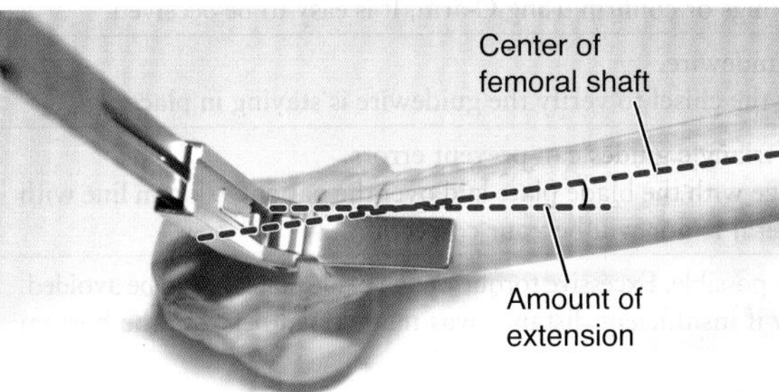

TECH FIG 3 • **A.** The cannulated chisel is now inserted over the guidewire. Prior to making the cut, the bone is scored longitudinally with a saw to assess rotation after the osteotomy has been performed. **B.** A guide arm can be slipped over the chisel. Placing this arm in line with the shaft will produce pure valgus. **C.** Rotating the guide arm posteriorly will add extension to the osteotomy (conversely, rotating the arm anteriorly will add flexion).

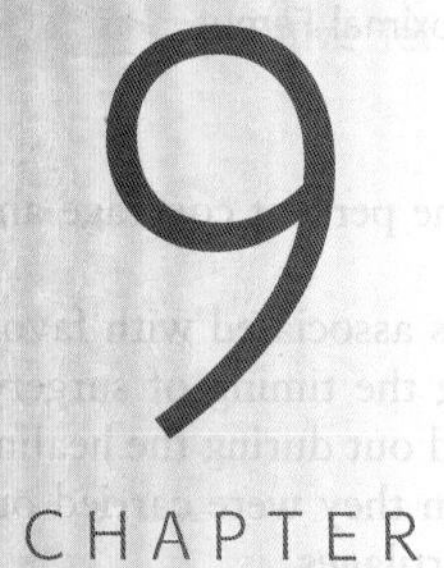

Flexion Intertrochanteric Osteotomy for Severe Slipped Capital Femoral Epiphysis

Young-Jo Kim

DEFINITION

- Pistol grip deformity after slipped capital femoral epiphysis (SCFE) can cause anterior impingement leading to pain, cartilage and labral damage, and eventual osteoarthritis.[1,2,8]
- Realignment of the proximal femur, as well as restoration of the anterior head–neck offset, has been shown to improve hip clinical outcomes.[7]
- This technique can be used to correct anterior impingement after an SCFE that has healed with residual posterior displacement.
- The first part of the procedure is a surgical hip dislocation approach with femoral head–neck osteoplasty.
- If additional deformity correction is needed, the flexion intertrochanteric osteotomy is performed.

PATHOGENESIS

- The true etiology of SCFE is unclear. However, because it occurs mainly in adolescent boys (80%), hormonal factors are thought to be involved.
- Additionally, the orientation of the growth plate becomes more vertical in adolescents compared to the juvenile hip, leading to increased shear stress across the physis.
- The transition from juvenile to adolescent is a period of rapid weight gain, leading to the stereotypical obese body habitus in the SCFE patient.

NATURAL HISTORY

- Undetected SCFEs can lead to hip arthrosis. Murray[4] suggests that up to 40% of hips with degenerative arthritis have a "tilt deformity" or other deformities that may be due to an undetected subclinical SCFE or other developmental problems.
- A review by Aronson[1] found that 15% to 20% of patients with SCFE had painful osteoarthritis by age 50 years. Additionally, 11% of patients with end-stage osteoarthritis had an SCFE.

PATIENT HISTORY AND PHYSICAL FINDINGS

- Patients will complain of insidious-onset groin or knee pain that may have previously been diagnosed as a sprain.
  - They may walk with a limp, but typically they walk with an externally rotated foot progression angle, which may indicate chronic SCFE or femoral retroversion.
  - Pain is elicited with hip flexion, adduction, and internal rotation stress (impingement test).
  - The physical examination should include flexion and internal rotation range-of-motion tests. Normal, physiologic hip flexion needed for activities of daily living is at least 90 degrees.
  - Patients with a chronic SCFE and anterior impingement will have less than 90 degrees of true hip flexion.
  - Patients with impingement secondary to SCFE will have less internal rotation in flexion than extension and may have a compensatory external rotation of the hip as it is flexed (obligate external rotation).

IMAGING AND OTHER DIAGNOSTIC STUDIES

- Plain radiographs include an anteroposterior (AP) and frog-leg lateral views of the pelvis or the involved hip (**FIG 1A,B**).
- Computed tomography (CT) scans with two- and three-dimensional reconstructions are helpful for preoperative planning (**FIG 1C,D**).

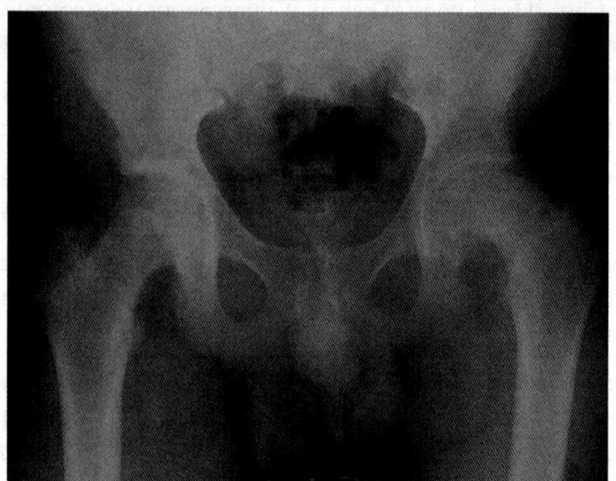

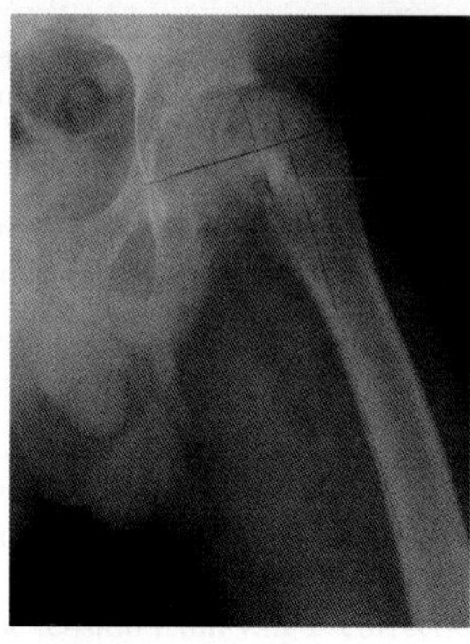

FIG 1 • Preoperative AP (**A**) and frog-leg lateral (**B**) radiographs of the left hip demonstrate a chronic, stable severe SCFE with greater than 70 degrees of posterior slippage. *(continued)*

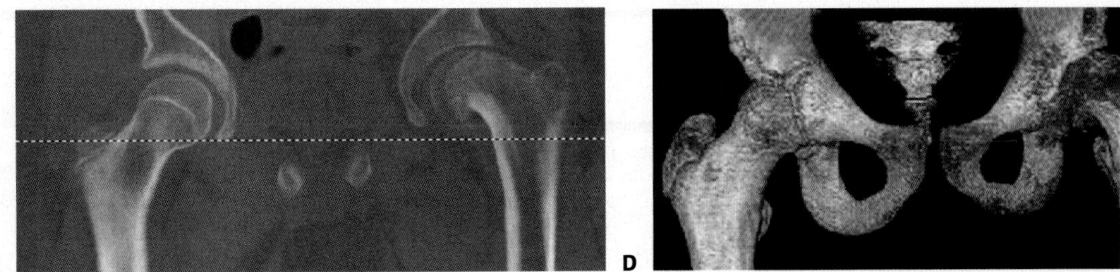

FIG 1 • *(continued)* Preoperative two-dimensional (**C**) and three-dimensional (**D**) CT reconstructions further define the severity of the deformity.

DIFFERENTIAL DIAGNOSIS

- Femoral or acetabular retroversion
- Idiopathic femoroacetabular impingement

NONOPERATIVE MANAGEMENT

- Nonoperative management includes cessation of aggravating activities and symptomatic treatment using nonsteroidal anti-inflammatories.
- Physical therapy to strengthen the hip musculature does not address the mechanical impingement associated with an SCFE.
- All SCFE should be stabilized surgically. Nonoperative management if for impingement symptoms.

SURGICAL MANAGEMENT

- A chronic slip may be pinned in situ to prevent continued slippage. Remodeling of the SCFE deformity has been described in long-term follow-up studies.
- Corrective osteotomies have been described through the femoral neck at the growth plate (cuneiform), at the base of the femoral neck, or intertrochantic or subtrochanteric.[6]

Preoperative Planning

- The anterior head–shaft angle is measured on the AP pelvis radiograph on both the affected and normal sides. The difference is the amount of varus deformity on the slip side that can be addressed with a valgus-producing intertrochanteric osteotomy (**FIG 2A**).
- The lateral head–shaft angle is measured on the frog-leg lateral view in a manner similar to that used on the AP view. The difference is the amount of posterior deformity present that is corrected with a flexion-producing intertrochanteric osteotomy (**FIG 2B**).

Positioning

- Because the first part of the procedure is done through a surgical hip dislocation, the patient is placed in the full lateral position secured on a pegboard, as shown in Chapter 13, Figure 3. A flat-top cushion placed beneath the operative side is helpful to stabilize the leg during the approach.
  - A hip drape with a sterile side bag is used, which will capture the leg during the dislocation maneuver.

Approach

- The incision from the surgical hip dislocation is extended slightly distal, along the lateral aspect of the thigh, in line with the femoral shaft.
- The lateral approach to the proximal third of the femur is required for the intertrochanteric osteotomy.

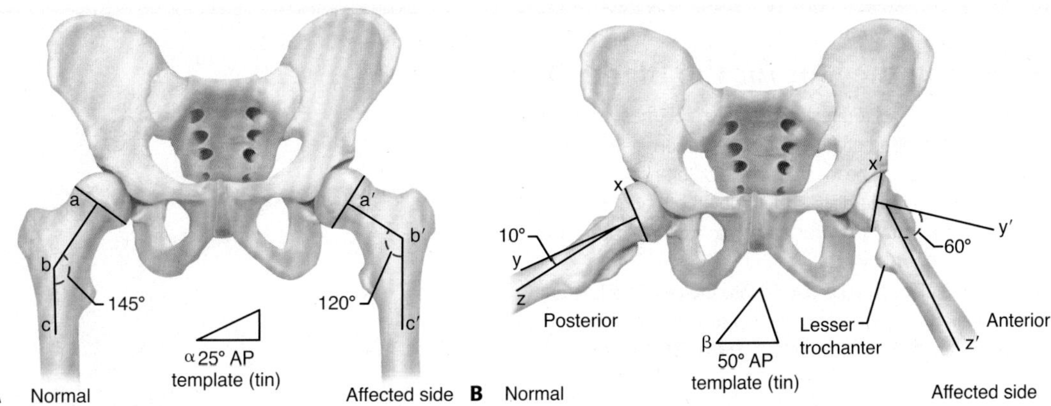

FIG 2 • Methods for determining the anterior head–shaft angle (**A**) and the lateral head–shaft angle (**B**). **A.** The difference in the angle determines the anterior osteotomy template. **B.** The posterior angulation of the affected side determines the angle of the lateral osteotomy template.

Approach to Proximal Femur

- The longitudinal incision from the surgical hip dislocation can be extended distally, in line with the lateral shaft of the femur (**TECH FIG 1A**).
- The vastus lateralis, supplied by the femoral nerve, is reflected anteriorly from the vastus ridge distally (**TECH FIG 1B**).
- Several perforating vessels from the profunda femoris artery to the vastus lateralis should be identified and coagulated before they are avulsed by blunt dissection.
- The anterolateral aspect of the femoral shaft is then exposed subperiosteally, and the lesser trochanter is identified.

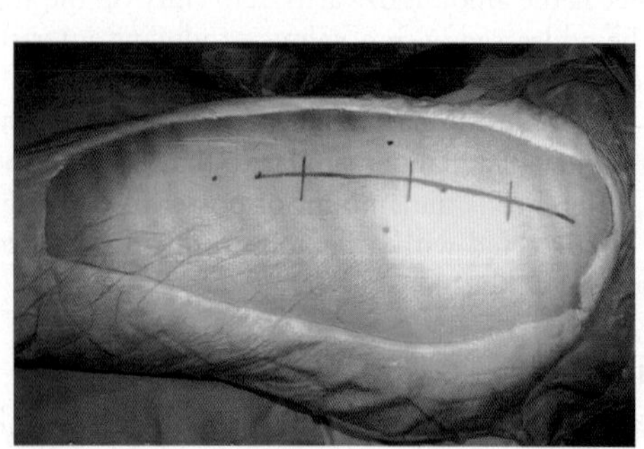

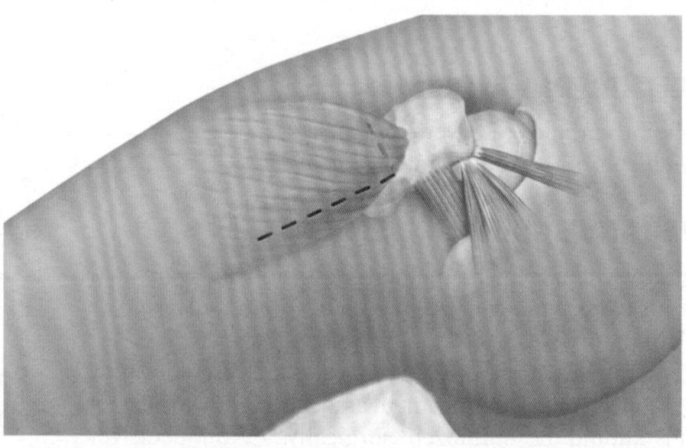

TECH FIG 1 • A. The proposed incision after the patient is prepared and draped. **B.** Approach to the intertrochanteric region of the femur. The vastus lateralis is reflected anteriorly from its origin at the vastus ridge.

Planning the Osteotomy

- A 2-0 Kirschner wire is placed just above the level of the lesser trochanter, beginning in the lateral cortex of the proximal femur. This is placed parallel to the floor in the axial plane and perpendicular to the shaft of the femur in the coronal plane. This is the reference for the level of the osteotomy.
- A second Kirschner wire is placed 3 cm proximal to the first. This is placed parallel to the first guidewire in the axial plane. In the coronal plane, the Kirschner wire is placed with an appropriate amount of valgus, determined from the anterior head–shaft angle difference on preoperative radiographs. In the Imhauser technique, addition of a valgus osteotomy is not necessary, hence, a pure flexion osteotomy is performed. This will act as the guidewire for the seating chisel for the blade plate.

Creating the Slot for the Blade Plate

- The seating chisel is directed parallel to the most proximal guide pin with the appropriate amount of flexion, as determined on the frog-leg lateral head–shaft angle difference.
- A slot for the blade plate should now be made in the trochanteric fragment to allow for anatomic fixation of the trochanter after the osteotomy.
- The blade plate chisel is placed into the proximal fragment after preparation of the trochanteric flip fragment and before cutting the intertrochanteric osteotomy (**TECH FIG 2**).

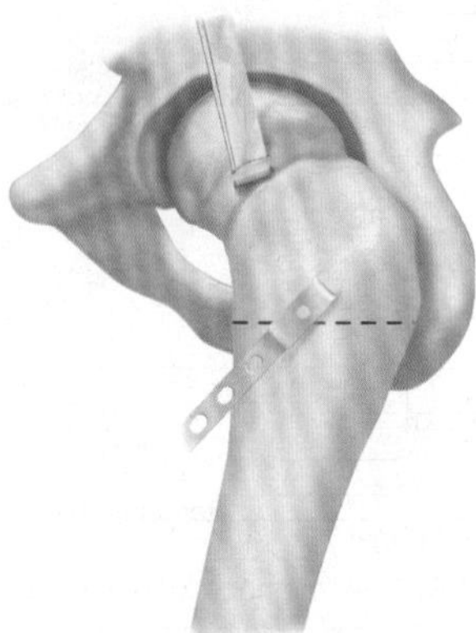

TECH FIG 2 • The blade plate is impacted into the proximal fragment through a slot created in the trochanteric wafer. The amount of flexion is based on the preoperative lateral head–shaft angle measurement.

TECHNIQUES

Osteotomy

- Before osteotomy, a rotational reference mark is made at the level of the osteotomy on both the proximal and distal fragments.
- Using an oscillating saw, the proximal femur is cut using the distal Kirschner wire as a guide. The cut should be made perpendicular to the shaft of the femur.

Blade Plate Placement

- The seating chisel is removed and the blade plate is impacted into the proximal fragment.
- The osteotomy is provisionally reduced and held with a Verbrugge clamp.
- Often, the distal fragment will need to be internally rotated to match the hip rotation of the normal side.
- After confirming reduction using an image intensifier, the plate is fixed to the shaft of the femur in standard fashion (**TECH FIG 3**).

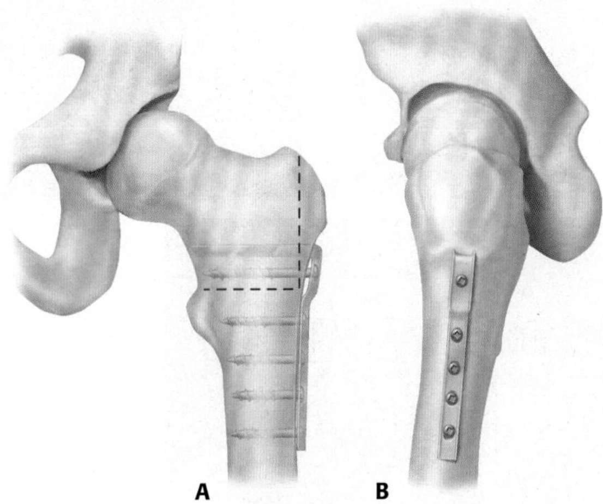

TECH FIG 3 • After the osteotomy, the distal fragment is reduced to the blade plate (**A**) and secured in standard fashion (**B**).

Closure

- The vastus lateralis fascia is closed with 2-0 absorbable running suture.
- The iliotibial band is closed using a running no. 1 absorbable suture.
- Skin is closed in routine fashion.

PEARLS AND PITFALLS

Indications	■ A complete history and physical examination should be performed. ■ All associated pathology should be addressed.
Osteotomy planning	■ Southwick's technique advises against needing a flexion osteotomy of greater than 60 degrees. If there is greater than 60 degrees of posterior slippage, the femoral head–neck osteoplasty performed through a surgical hip dislocation can reduce the amount of flexion needed to relieve anterior impingement.
Seating chisel removal	■ After fully inserting the seating chisel, the surgeon should remove and replace it by hand before making the osteotomy. This will allow easy removal after the proximal fragment is less stable.
Reduction of osteotomy	■ Control of the proximal fragment is gained with a Weber bone-holding clamp instead of using the inserted blade plate for fragment manipulation, which could weaken the fixation.
Nonunion	■ Any areas that lack bone-to-bone contact require bone graft.

POSTOPERATIVE CARE

- The hip is held flexed and in neutral rotation by placing two pillows under the leg and one under the greater trochanter.
- The patient is placed in a continuous passive motion machine for 6 hours a day, set from 30 to 80 degrees of flexion.
- Prophylaxis for deep venous thrombosis is individualized; however, all patients should be started on mechanical compression devices immediately.
- After the epidural is removed, out-of-bed ambulation is permitted with one-sixth body weight partial weight bearing.

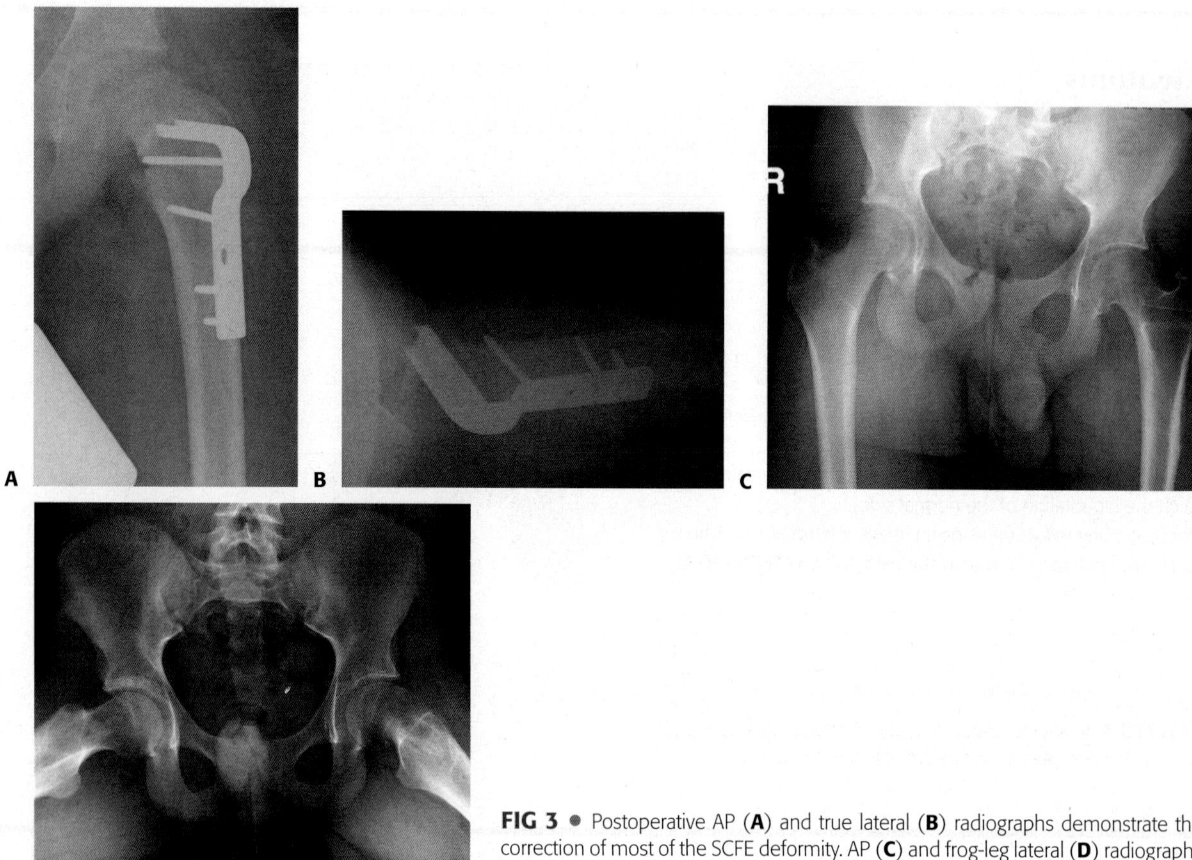

FIG 3 • Postoperative AP (**A**) and true lateral (**B**) radiographs demonstrate the correction of most of the SCFE deformity. AP (**C**) and frog-leg lateral (**D**) radiographs of the pelvis 4 months after removal of hardware. The patient has no symptoms.

- Range-of-motion exercises are started, but care is taken to protect the greater trochanter osteotomy by limiting adduction to midline and avoiding resisted abduction exercises for 6 weeks.
- AP and true lateral hip radiographs are obtained to evaluate healing of the osteotomy (**FIG 3A,B**).
- Prominent hardware may be removed after 6 months if radiographic evidence of a healed osteotomy is seen (**FIG 3C,D**).

OUTCOMES

- In Southwick's original article,[6] where he treated the deformity with a proximal femoral osteotomy without surgical hip dislocation, out of 28 hips (26 patients) with at least 5 years of follow-up, 21 were rated as excellent, 5 as good, and 2 as fair.
- In patients who had both osteoplasty and an intertrochanteric osteotomy, Western Ontario and McMaster Universities (WOMAC) pain and function scores improved in four of six patients.[7]
- Internal rotation in flexion improved from −20 to +10 degrees.[7]
- Long-term results of flexion osteotomy for SCFE shows 55% to 77% good to excellent results at ~20 year follow-up.[3,5]

COMPLICATIONS

- Avascular necrosis of the femoral head can occur if care is not taken to follow the technique and to preserve the retinacular vessels.
- Nonunion of the greater trochanteric osteotomy or the intertrochanteric osteotomy
- Sciatic or femoral nerve neurapraxia
- Heterotopic ossification

REFERENCES

1. Aronson J. Osteoarthritis of the young adult hip: etiology and treatment. Instr Course Lect 1986;35:119–128.
2. Goodman DA, Feighan JE, Smith AD, et al. Subclinical slipped capital femoral epiphysis: relationship to arthrosis of the hip. J Bone Joint Surg Am 1997;79(10):1489–1497.
3. Kartenbender K, Cordier W, Katthagen BD. Long-term follow-up study after corrective Imhäuser osteotomy for severe slipped capital femoral epiphysis. J Pediatr Ortho 2000;20:749–756.
4. Murray RO. The aetiology of primary osteoarthrosis of the hip. Br J Radiol 1965;38:810–824.
5. Schai PA, Exner GU, Hänsch O. Prevention of secondary coxarthrosis in slipped capital femoral epiphysis: a long-term follow-up study after corrective intertrochanteric osteotomy. J Pediatr Orthop B 1996;5:135–143.
6. Southwick WO. Osteotomy through the lesser trochanter for slipped capital femoral epiphysis. J Bone Joint Surg Am 1987;49(5):807–835.
7. Spencer S, Millis M, Kim Y. Early results of treatment for hip impingement syndrome in slipped capital femoral epiphysis and pistol grip deformity of the femoral head-neck junction using the surgical dislocation technique. J Pediatr Orthop 2006;26:281–285.
8. Wenger DR, Kishan S, Pring ME. Impingement and childhood hip disease. J Pediatr Orthop B 2006;15:233–243.

Modified Dunn Procedure for Slipped Capital Femoral Epiphysis

CHAPTER 10

Wudbhav N. Sankar

DEFINITION

- The modified Dunn procedure is an open realignment of the capital femoral epiphysis performed through a surgical dislocation approach.[18]
- Like the original Dunn osteotomy, the modified Dunn corrects a slipped capital femoral epiphysis (SCFE) at the site of maximal deformity (ie, the physis).[4]
- The procedure can be performed on both unstable SCFEs and stable SCFEs.

ANATOMY

- The main source of perfusion to the femoral epiphysis is the medial femoral circumflex artery (MFCA) (**FIG 1**).
- The deep branch of the MFCA runs posterior to the obturator externus and perforates the hip capsule just distal to the piriformis and proximal to the superior gemellus.[5]
- It ends in two to four retinacular branches that enter the superior aspect of the femoral head.
- The intact external rotator muscles, especially the obturator externus, protect the MFCA during surgical dislocation of the hip.
- To safely reduce a SCFE, which typically displaces posterior and inferior to the neck, tension must be minimized on the retinacular vessels.[18]

PATHOGENESIS

- The posteroinferior translation of the epiphysis relative to the femoral neck alters the resting position of the femoral head within the acetabulum.
- This altered position combined with the residual offset of the metaphysis can dramatically affect the motion of the hip joint.
- With flexion and internal rotation, the metaphyseal prominence can either enter the joint potentially causing damage to the acetabular cartilage or abut against the acetabular rim and the labrum[13] (**FIG 2**).
- In situ fixation, while effective for preventing further slippage, does not correct the deformity associated with SCFE.

NATURAL HISTORY

- Historically, the long-term outcome after in situ screw fixation has generally been considered to be good.[1,2]
- Recent studies, however, have established an association between the residual proximal femoral metaphyseal deformity left by in situ treatment and the development of femoroacetabular impingement, lost hip motion, and premature osteoarthritis.[6,9,11,17]
- Increasing slip severity has been associated with poorer outcome.[3]

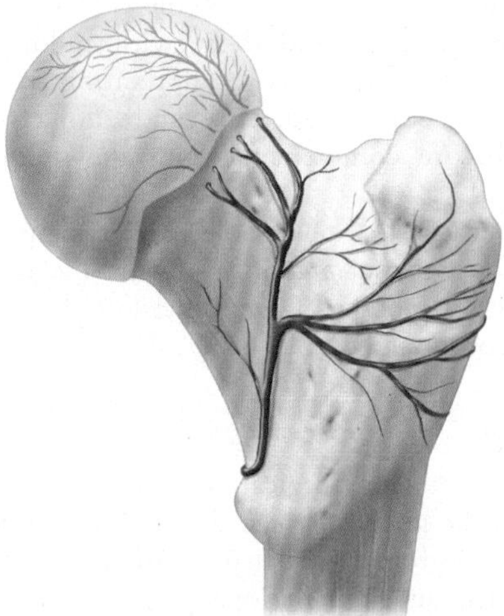

FIG 1 • Posterior view of the vascular anatomy of the proximal femur. Note the proximity of the terminal branches of the MFCA to the insertion of the piriformis tendon.

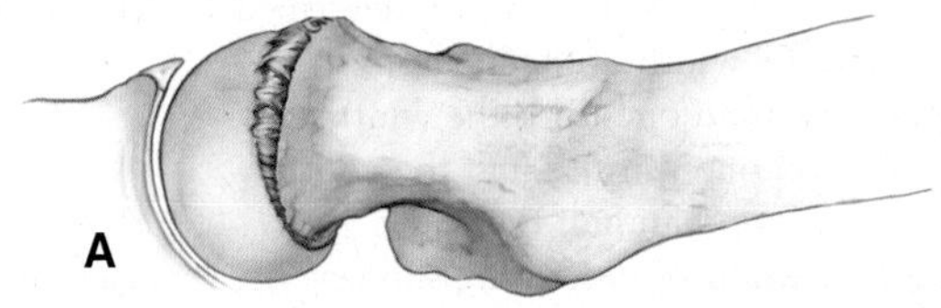

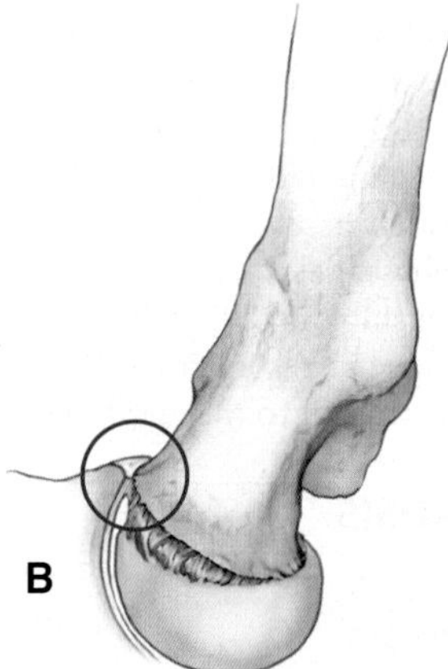

FIG 2 • Clinical implication of a residual SCFE deformity: With flexion and internal rotation, the metaphyseal prominence can either enter the joint potentially causing damage to the acetabular cartilage (**A**) or abut against the acetabular rim and the labrum (**B**).

PATIENT HISTORY AND PHYSICAL FINDINGS

- Patients with an unstable SCFE usually present acutely with an abrupt onset of symptoms.
  - Pain is intense and can be elicited even with simple logrolling of the affected extremity.
  - By definition, patients with unstable SCFE are unable to ambulate with or without walking aids.[10]
  - Further forced range of motion (ROM) of the affected hip is discouraged to minimize the risk of additional trauma to the femoral head blood supply.
- Patients with severe, stable SCFE can present with variable duration of symptoms.
  - Patients complain of hip or groin pain, thigh pain, or knee pain and usually occurs without a history of trauma.
  - By definition, patients are able to ambulate with or without walking aids and typically present with an antalgic gait and an external foot progression angle.[10]
  - Hip flexion, abduction, and internal rotation in the flexed position will be markedly decreased in a severe SCFE as a result of femoroacetabular impingement.
  - Many patients will also demonstrate obligate external rotation which is forced external rotation that results from passive hip flexion.

IMAGING AND OTHER DIAGNOSTIC STUDIES

- Plain radiographs of the pelvis, including anteroposterior (AP) and frog-leg lateral views, should be obtained in any pediatric patient with hip, thigh, or knee pain and are generally diagnostic of a SCFE.
  - The femoral epiphysis is typically displaced posterior (on the frog view) and slightly inferior (on the AP view) in relation to the femoral neck.
- A widened physis on AP or lateral views can be an early sign of SCFE.
- The severity of a SCFE can be described by displacement relative to the width of the metaphysis:
  - Mild: less than one-third the width
  - Moderate: one-third to half the width
  - Severe: more than half the width
- Another method of describing slip severity is measuring the difference between the epiphyseal shaft angle on each side[16]:
  - Mild: less than 30 degrees
  - Moderate: 30 to 50 degrees
  - Severe: 50 degrees or greater
- In cases with delayed presentation in which the modified Dunn is being considered, computed tomography (CT) scan can be used to more accurately assess the degree of displacement and the amount of physeal closure.
- In certain patients with unstable SCFEs who present late, bone scan or contrast magnetic resonance imaging (MRI) can be used to assess the perfusion to the epiphysis.

DIFFERENTIAL DIAGNOSIS

- SCFE
- Legg-Calvé-Perthes disease
- Hip labral tear
- Femoral neck fracture
- Septic arthritis of the hip
- Knee derangement
- Greater trochanteric bursitis

NONOPERATIVE MANAGEMENT

- Immobilization in a spica cast was the historical treatment but is no longer recommended for SCFE.
- Once SCFE is identified in any patient with an open physis, management is surgical to avoid further slippage and the possible development of femoral head avascular necrosis (AVN).

SURGICAL MANAGEMENT

- The modified Dunn procedure is indicated for unstable SCFEs and for certain stable SCFEs in which the residual deformity that would be left by in situ fixation is deemed unacceptable.
- It is most easily performed when the physis is still open.
- The modified Dunn procedure is a technically demanding procedure that requires familiarity with the surgical dislocation approach and the development of the retinacular flap.
- Alternative techniques for treating unstable SCFEs include (1) positional reduction followed by percutaneous screw fixation (with at least two screws) and capsular decompression[7] or (2) gentle manual open reduction performed via an anterolateral approach followed by Kirschner wire (K-wire) or screw fixation.[12]
- Alternative techniques for treating severe stable SCFEs include in situ fixation followed by osteoplasty of the femoral head–neck junction and/or proximal femoral osteotomy.

Preoperative Planning

- All imaging studies are reviewed.
- Both AP and frog views should be reviewed for the presence of posteroinferior callus. This finding implies some chronicity to the SCFE and its removal is necessary to achieve an anatomic reduction.
- Pure displacement (ie, angulation or translation) can be corrected via the modified Dunn, but some chronic changes such as femoral neck retroversion are more difficult to address.
- In chronic and severe stable SCFEs, CT scans can be used to assess the status of the physis and determine the indication for the modified Dunn procedure.
- The contralateral hip should be evaluated both clinically and radiographically to determine whether a SCFE is present.
- In younger patients, and those with endocrinopathies, prophylactic percutaneous screw fixation of the normal side should be considered. This can be done in the supine position before commencing with the modified Dunn procedure.
- Timing of surgery for an unstable SCFE is somewhat controversial. For cases that present overnight, the author prefers performing the modified Dunn procedure the next morning with an appropriately skilled surgical team.

Positioning

- As with a standard surgical dislocation of the hip (see Chap. 13), the patient is placed in full lateral position, secured on a pegboard. A flat-top cushion (with cutout for the down leg) supports the operative extremity during the procedure (**FIG 3**).
- A hip drape with a sterile side bag is used, which will capture the leg during the dislocation maneuver.

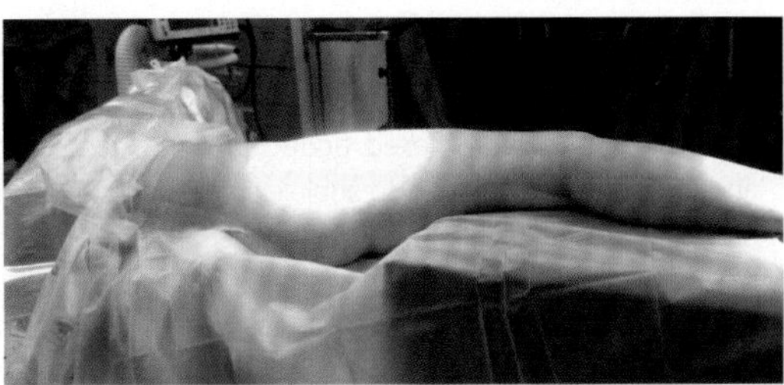

FIG 3 • As with a standard surgical dislocation of the hip, the modified Dunn procedure is performed with the patient placed in full lateral position, secured on a pegboard. A flat-top cushion (with cutout for the down leg) supports the operative extremity during the procedure.

Approach

- As with other surgical dislocations of the hip, the Kocher-Langenbeck or Gibson approach may be used.
- The Kocher-Langenbeck incision is followed by splitting of the gluteus maximus muscle. In obese patients, this approach does facilitate anterior exposure.
- The abductors and gluteus maximus muscles can be spared by performing a Gibson approach, which proceeds between the gluteus medius and maximus. This results in less hip extensor dysfunction but may make anterior exposure more difficult especially in obese patients.

Exposure

- For a detailed description of the surgical dislocation approach please refer to Chapter 13. The following technique for the modified Dunn procedure begins after the hip capsule has been fully exposed.

Hip Arthrotomy, Provisional Fixation, and Dislocation

- A Z-shaped capsulotomy is performed, with the longitudinal arm of the Z in line with the anterior neck of the femur (**TECH FIG 1A**).
  - The inferior limb extends along the intertrochanteric line toward but proximal to the lesser trochanter. A cuff of capsular tissue should be left for later repair.
  - Superior limb extends along the acetabular rim posteriorly toward the piriformis tendon. Care should be taken not to injure the labrum (**TECH FIG 1B**).
- It is helpful to tag the corners of the capsulotomy to help distinguish this layer from the retinacular flap which will be developed later in the procedure.

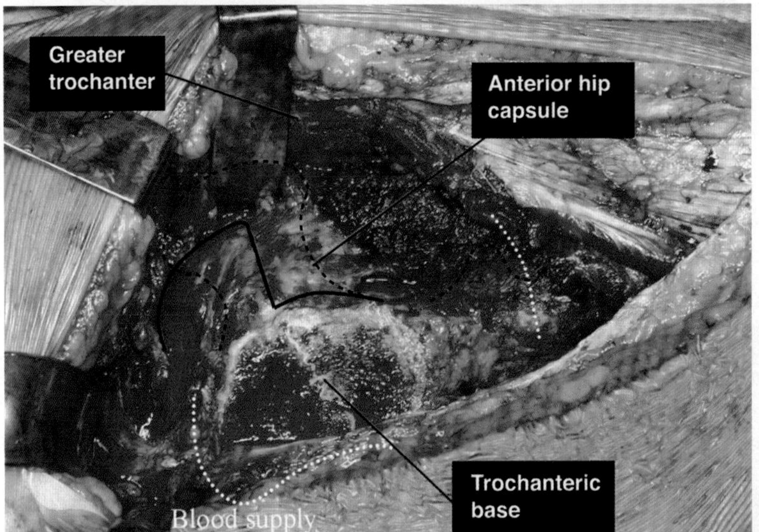

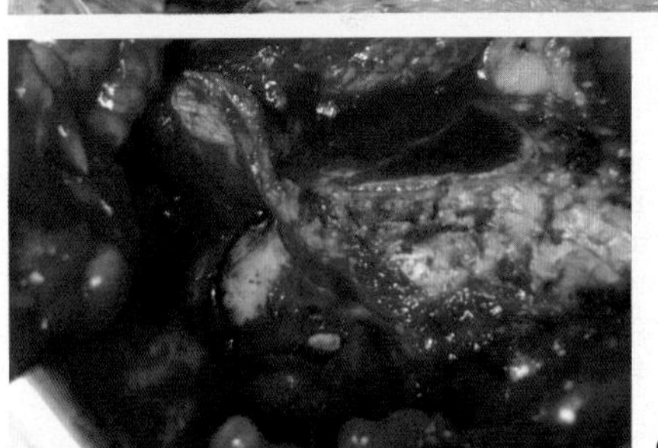

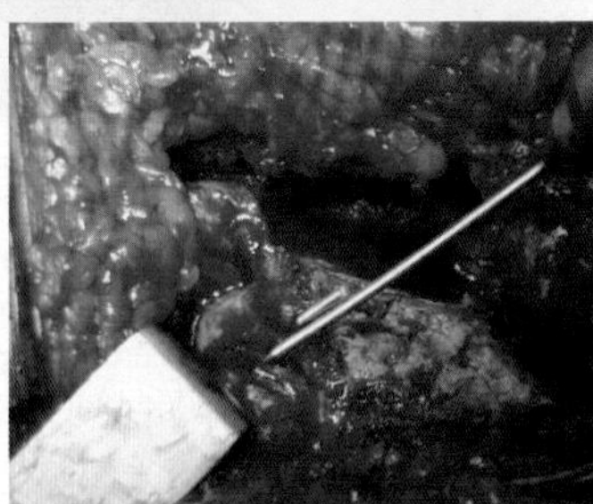

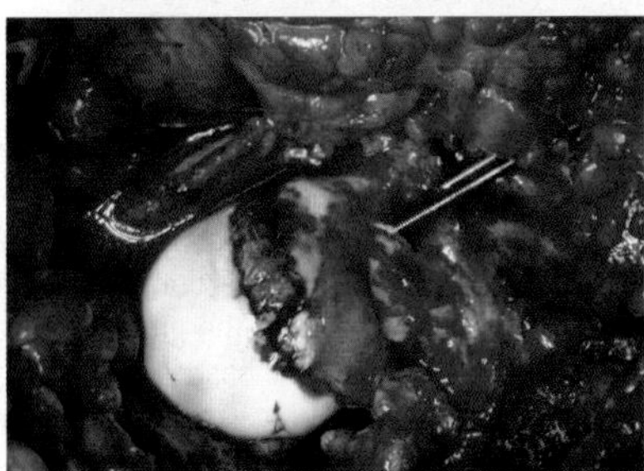

TECH FIG 1 • **A.** Path of the Z-shaped capsulotomy (*solid line*). The limb along the posterior aspect of the acetabulum protects the entry of the terminal branches of the MFCA (*white dashed line*) and allows access to the hip joint and the femoral head (*black dashed line*). **B.** Z-shaped capsulotomy. **C.** For unstable SCFEs, threaded K-wires are used to provisionally pin the epiphysis in situ in order to allow the hip to be dislocated without endangering the retinacular vessels. **D.** Once the hip is dislocated, the full SCFE deformity can be assessed. In this unstable SCFE, note the tearing of the periosteum.

- At this point, the hip should be gently manipulated to assess the intraoperative stability of the slip and the acuity of the injury.
  - Unstable slips characteristically have torn periosteum anteriorly with the epiphysis clearly disengaged from the metaphysis.
  - Stable slips move as a single unit.
- For unstable SCFEs, one to two threaded K-wires are used to provisionally pin the epiphysis in situ to allow the hip to be dislocated without endangering the retinacular vessels (**TECH FIG 1C**).
  - The wires are cut with approximately 2 cm out of bone to keep the fixation out of the way but still allow later removal.
- A bone hook is placed around the neck.
- The limb is then gently flexed, adducted, and externally rotated, and the bone hook is used to subluxate the hip. Curved scissors are inserted into the joint, and the ligamentum teres is transected to allow full dislocation of the hip.
- The full SCFE deformity can now be assessed. It is important to evaluate the acetabulum as well for chondral or labral pathology (**TECH FIG 1D**).

Retinacular Flap

- The retinacular flap is best developed with the hip located.
- The periosteum is split longitudinally on the femur distal to the trochanteric osteotomy site, and a periosteal elevator is used to start the periosteal flap posteriorly (**TECH FIG 2A**).
- Similarly, the periosteum on the anterior neck can be split in line with the capsulotomy and elevated.
- To reduce tension on the retinacular flap and allow the epiphysis to be safely mobilized, the posterosuperior third of the trochanteric base needs to be removed.
- The apophyseal cartilage in skeletally immature patients provides a useful landmark for the extent of trochanteric resection.
- The original technique uses an osteotome to perform the osteotomy (at the site of apophyseal cartilage) followed by careful peeling of the freed trochanteric fragment from the periosteal flap[18] (**TECH FIG 2B,C**).
- Alternatively, the subperiosteal flap can be carefully extended proximally around the tip of the greater trochanter and a Kerrison rongeur or standard rongeur can be used to "nibble" back the trochanteric base (**TECH FIG 2D**).
- As the trochanteric base is trimmed, the periosteal flap can be extended to the base of the femoral neck (**TECH FIG 2E**).

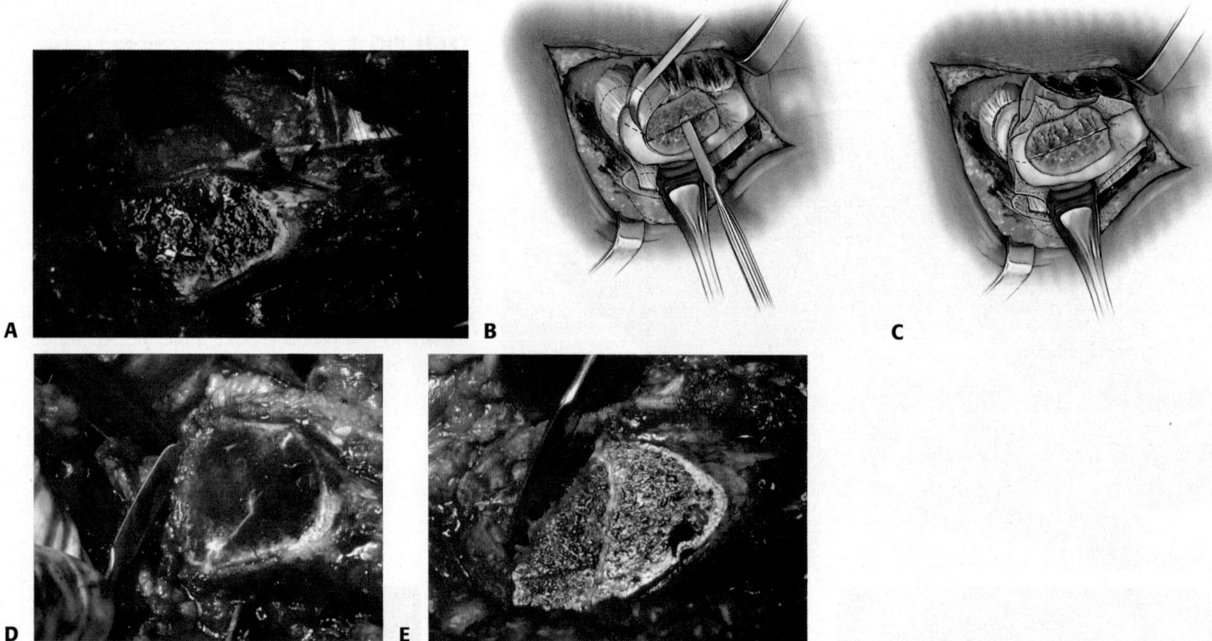

TECH FIG 2 • **A.** To develop the retinacular flap, the periosteum is first split longitudinally on the femur distal to the trochanteric osteotomy site and a periosteal elevator is used to elevate the periosteal flap posteriorly (*arrow*). **B,C.** The posterosuperior segment of the stable trochanter can be removed with an osteotome and peeled from the periosteal sleeve to allow access to the posterior periosteum of the femoral neck for further subperiosteal dissection. **D.** One technique for developing the retinacular flap involves careful elevation of the periosteal sleeve proximally around the tip of the greater trochanter; a Kerrison rongeur or standard rongeur can then be used to nibble back the trochanteric base. **E.** As the trochanteric base is trimmed, the periosteal flap can be extended to the base of the femoral neck. (*Note*: up is posterior on all panels.)

Mobilization of the Epiphysis

- The hip is dislocated to complete the retinacular flap.
- The periosteum over the anterior neck is split and elevated over the superior neck and the piriformis fossa to connect to the previously created periosteal sleeve (**TECH FIG 3A**).
- A sponge can be placed inside the acetabulum to prevent the femoral head from falling posteriorly as it is mobilized.
- While manually stabilizing the epiphysis, the provisional K-wires are removed.
- In unstable SCFEs, a small elevator placed into the slip site should be sufficient to mobilize the epiphysis. The remaining adhesions to the retinacular flap can be addressed (**TECH FIG 3B**).
- In stable SCFEs, the physis should be localized and an elevator or osteotome used to separate the epiphysis from the metaphysis.
- Once the epiphysis has been freed, any residual physis should be curetted to facilitate bone healing.

A

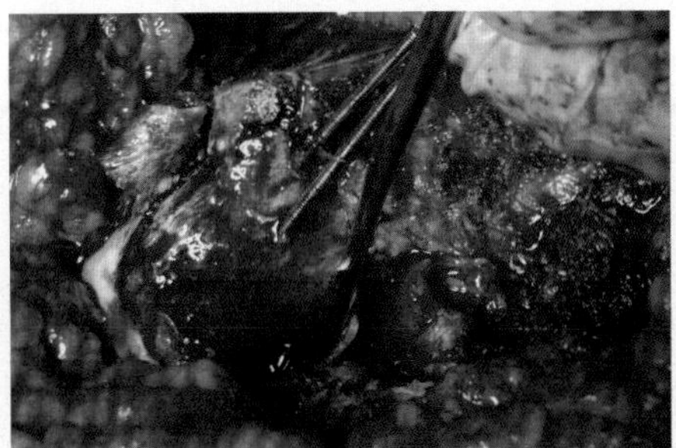

B

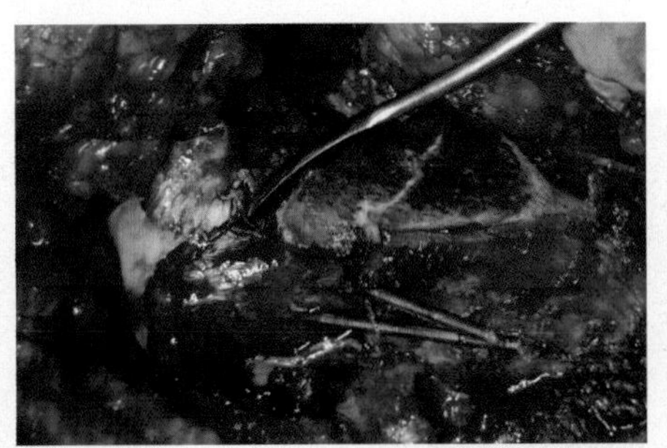

TECH FIG 3 • **A.** With the hip dislocated, the periosteum is elevated over the anterior neck as well as superiorly into the piriformis fossa to connect to the previously created periosteal sleeve. **B.** In unstable SCFEs, a small elevator placed into the slip site should be sufficient to mobilize the epiphysis. The remaining adhesions to the retinacular flap can be released.

Reducing the Epiphysis

- The fully exposed metaphysis/neck should be inspected for signs of chronic callus. This is typically located posterior and inferior. Removing this with an osteotome and rongeur helps facilitate epiphyseal reduction (**TECH FIG 4A**).
- The end of the neck should be trimmed slightly to provide a fresh bony surface for healing. Excessive shortening should be avoided as this can create postoperative instability (**TECH FIG 4B**).
- The epiphysis can now be manually reduced. There should be minimal tension on the retinacular flap during this maneuver. If excessive tension persists, the retinacular flap should be extended and the epiphysis and metaphysis should be revisited to be sure that all callus has been removed (**TECH FIG 4C**).

A

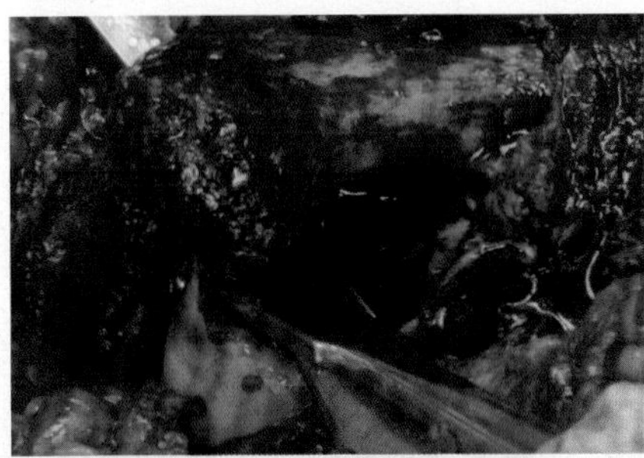

B

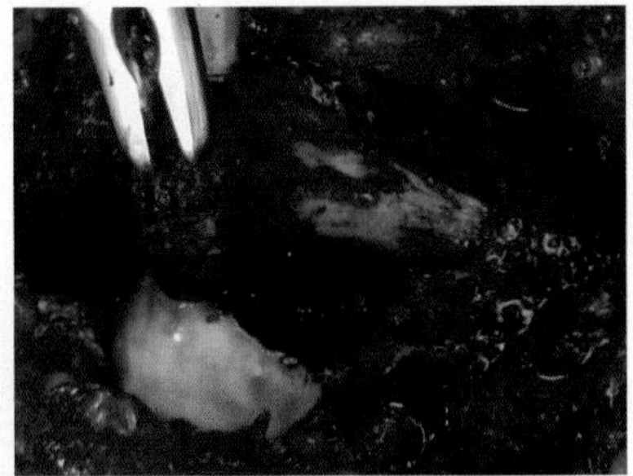

C

TECH FIG 4 • **A.** The fully exposed metaphysis/neck should be inspected for signs of chronic callus. This is typically located posterior and inferior. Removing this with an osteotome and/or rongeur helps facilitate epiphyseal reduction. **B.** The end of the neck should be trimmed slightly to provide a fresh bony surface for healing. Excessive shortening should be avoided, as this can create postoperative instability. **C.** The epiphysis can now be manually reduced.

Epiphyseal Fixation

- Initial fixation is achieved by inserting a threaded K-wire from proximal to distal through the fovea and exiting out the anterolateral femur (**TECH FIG 5A**).
- The hip is carefully relocated to allow assessment of reduction and placement of definitive fixation.
- To confirm adequate epiphyseal reduction, the C-arm can be brought underneath the table and rotated to provide an AP view of the hip. The limb can be manually frogged to achieve a lateral view of the proximal femur.
- If the reduction is acceptable, definitive fixation for the epiphysis should be placed distal or anterior to the trochanteric base to facilitate later removal if necessary.
- The author prefers using two 6.5-mm cannulated screws to minimize the risk of implant failure; however, two or three solid 4.5-mm screws or multiple threaded K-wires can also be used.[14]
- Implant position can be checked using the C-arm (**TECH FIG 5B,C**).
- The initial threaded K-wire can now be removed if desired.

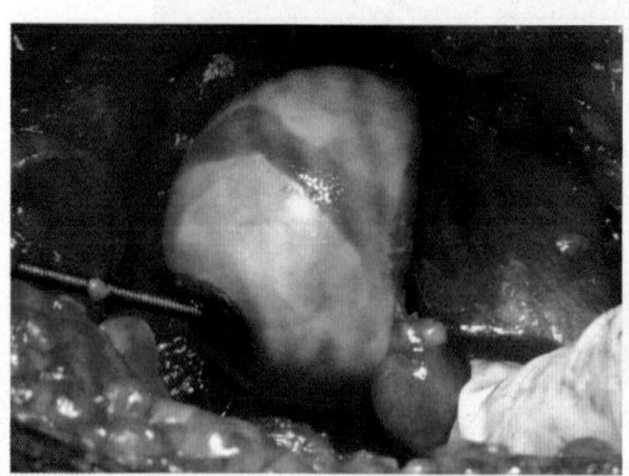
A

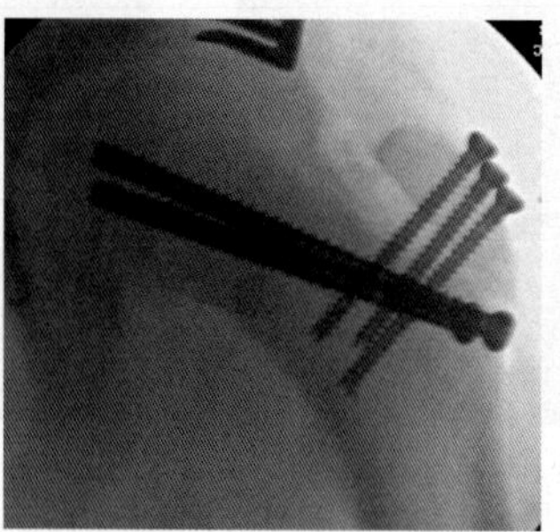
B

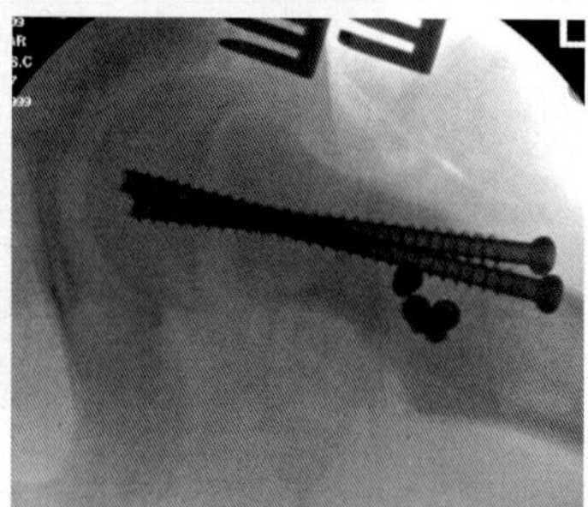
C

TECH FIG 5 • A. Provisional fixation is achieved by inserting a threaded K-wire from proximal to distal through the fovea and exiting out the anterolateral femur. **B,C.** AP and frog lateral fluoroscopic views demonstrating implant position (for both epiphyseal and trochanteric fixation).

Monitoring Perfusion

- Perfusion of the epiphysis can be monitored periodically throughout the case (eg, during development of the retinacular flap, after epiphyseal reduction, etc.) by placing a small 1.5-mm drill hole into the anterior head away from the weight-bearing surface. Fresh bleeding should be visualized from the head.
- A more objective means of perfusion monitoring involves placement of an intracranial pressure catheter into the small drill hole. A discrete waveform should be visualized (**TECH FIG 6**).
- If perfusion is lost after epiphyseal reduction, the tension on the retinacular flap should be checked. If necessary, the flap should be extended, the neck slightly shortened, and the epiphysis rereduced in a tension-free manner.

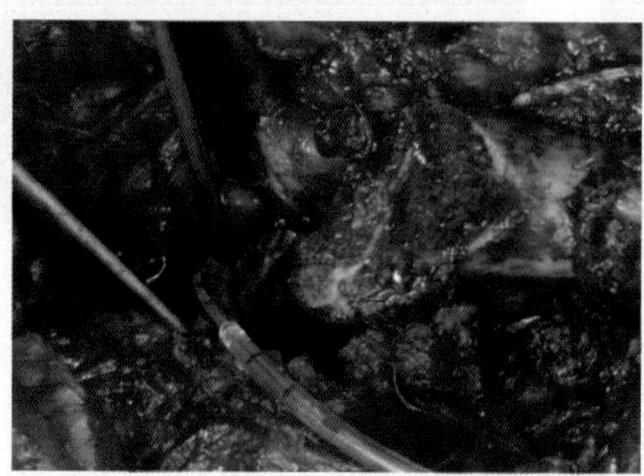
A

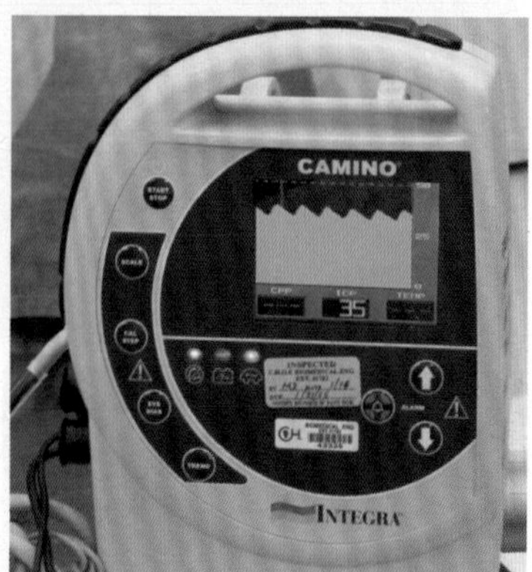

B

TECH FIG 6 • A. Perfusion can be monitored by placing an intracranial pressure catheter into a small drill hole. **B.** A discrete waveform should be visualized.

Deep Closure

- A few tacking sutures can be placed loosely in the anterior periosteum; but in general, the retinacular flap should not be repaired to avoid causing unnecessary tension.
- The capsule is loosely approximated with interrupted heavy (no. 1) absorbable sutures. Again, it is important to avoid creating unnecessary tension on the retinacular flap (**TECH FIG 7**).

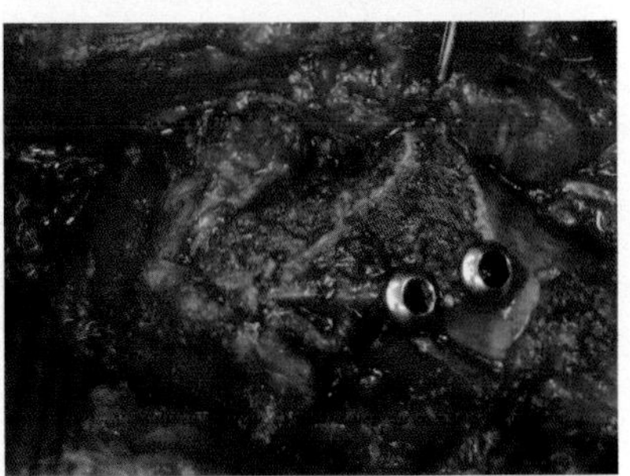

TECH FIG 7 • The capsule should be loosely approximated.

Trochanteric Osteotomy Fixation

- The trochanteric wafer is reduced to the same or slightly distal position and held in place using a ball spike probe.
- Three guidewires for a 4.5-mm cannulated screw system are inserted across the osteotomy site aiming slightly distal (toward the lesser trochanter) (**TECH FIG 8**).
- The reduction of the osteotomy and the wires can be confirmed with the C-arm.
- The wires are then measured and overdrilled. Fully threaded 4.5-mm cannulated screws are used to facilitate later removal if necessary.
- Alternatively, solid 3.5- or 4.5-mm screws can be used.

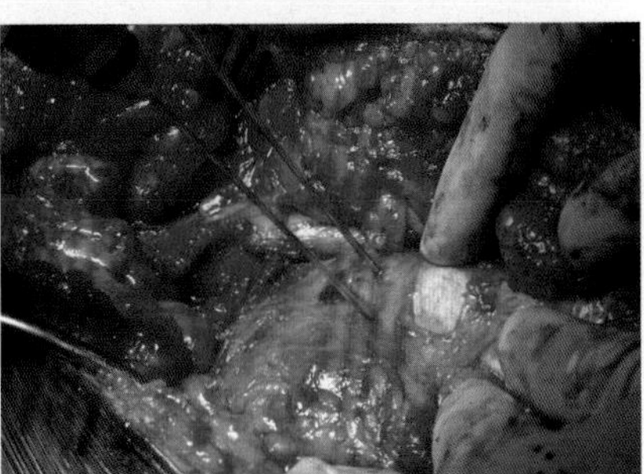

TECH FIG 8 • Placement of guidewires for trochanteric fixation with 4.5-mm cannulated screws.

Closure

- The vastus lateralis is repaired using a running absorbable suture (eg, 2-0 Vicryl).
- The fascia lata is closed in a watertight fashion using interrupted heavy absorbable suture (eg, no. 1 Vicryl), followed by layered closure of the dermis (2-0 Vicryl) and the subcuticular layer (4-0 Monocryl).

PEARLS AND PITFALLS

Difficulty distinguishing capsule from retinacular flap during closure	■ This can be prevented by tagging the capsule after performing the Z-shaped capsulotomy.
Excessive tension on retinacular flap during mobilization of the epiphysis	■ This happens if the flap has not been developed distal enough.
Excessive tension on retinacular flap during reduction of the epiphysis	■ This can be prevented by being sure the flap is developed distal enough, by trimming posteroinferior callus from the neck, and by shortening the neck slightly.
Implant failure	■ One study suggests that using larger implants (eg, 6.5-mm cannulated screws) for epiphyseal fixation may minimize the risk of hardware breakage.[14]
Tension on the retinacular flap during closure	■ This can be avoided by not repairing the retinacular flap and by loosely approximating the capsule.
AVN	■ The risk of this complication is best minimized by meticulous surgical technique and frequent monitoring of epiphyseal perfusion.

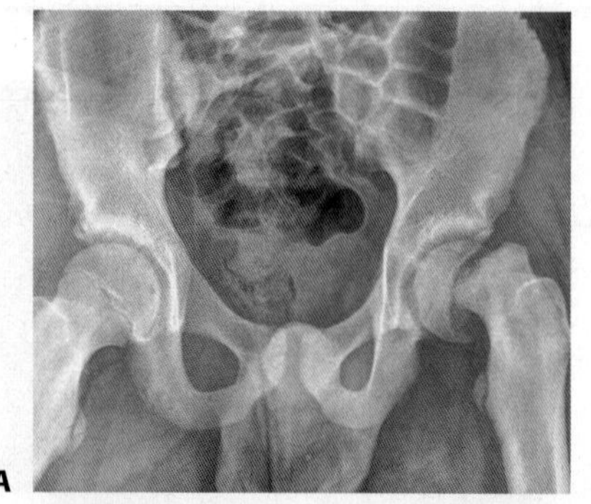

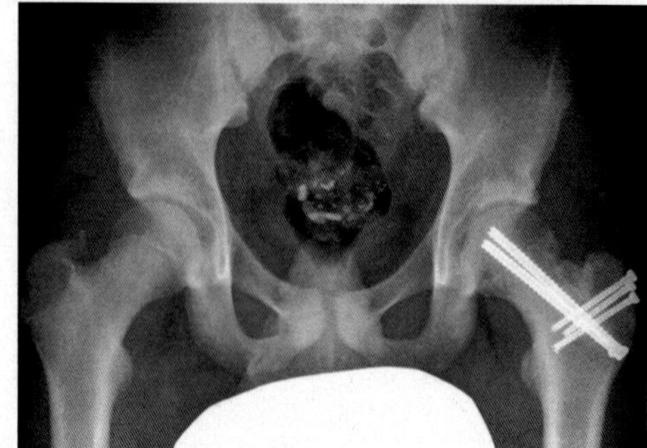

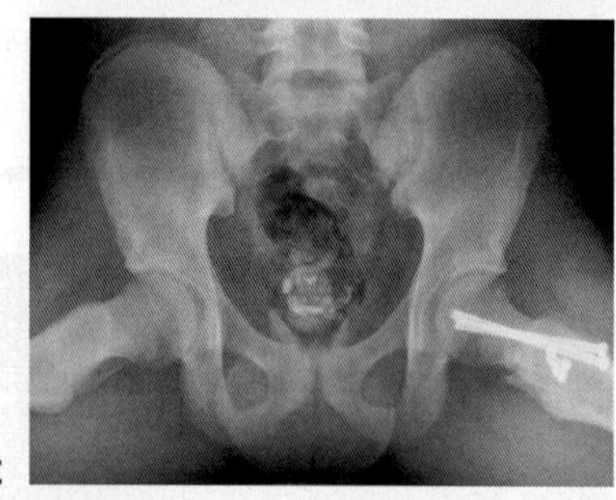

FIG 4 • **A.** Preoperative AP view of the hip reveals a severe left unstable SCFE. **B,C.** Postoperative AP and frog-leg lateral views, respectively, of the pelvis 18 months later demonstrate a well-reduced epiphysis with no signs of AVN.

POSTOPERATIVE CARE

- Patients are made toe-touch weight bearing with crutches. Weight bearing is generally advanced around 8 weeks based on early radiographic signs of healing at the physis.
- Physical therapy is then initiated for gait training and abductor strengthening.
- If radiographic healing progresses as expected, patients are generally cleared for sports around 6 months after surgery.
- After the immediate postoperative period, patients are followed every 2 to 3 months for at least a year with AP and frog lateral radiographs to monitor for the development of osteonecrosis.

OUTCOMES

- The initial series describing the modified Dunn procedure consisted of 40 patients followed for a minimum of 1 year and 3 years from two institutions.[18] The authors reported excellent functional outcomes, improved ROM, near-anatomic slip angles, and no cases of AVN.
- Two additional follow-up studies have also reported excellent functional scores and anatomic radiographic results following the modified Dunn procedure in both stable and unstable SCFEs.
  - One series of 23 patients reported excellent clinical and radiographic outcomes in 21 patients. The poor outcomes occurred in 2 patients who developed osteonecrosis and osteoarthritis.[15]
  - Another series of 30 SCFEs reported near-anatomic reduction in all cases. Twenty-eight patients had excellent clinical outcomes with one patient developing AVN. Failure of implants requiring revision surgery occurred in four hips.[8]
- A multicenter study of 27 unstable SCFEs treated with the modified Dunn procedure demonstrated higher rates of AVN (26%) and failed epiphyseal fixation (15%) than previous reports.[14] Patients that did not develop osteonecrosis had excellent clinical and radiographic results (**FIG 4**).

COMPLICATIONS

- Chondrolysis
- AVN (more common with unstable SCFEs)
- Nonunion
- Failed epiphyseal fixation

REFERENCES

1. Boyer DW, Mickelson MR, Ponseti IV. Slipped capital femoral epiphysis. Long-term follow-up study of one hundred and twenty-one patients. J Bone Joint Surg Am 1981;63(1):85–95.
2. Carney BT, Weinstein SL, Noble J. Long-term follow-up of slipped capital femoral epiphysis. J Bone Joint Surg Am 1991;73(5):667–674.
3. Castañeda P, Ponce C, Villareal G, et al. The natural history of osteoarthritis after a slipped capital femoral epiphysis/the pistol grip deformity. J Pediatr Orthop 2013;33(suppl 1):S76–S82.
4. Dunn DM. The treatment of adolescent slipping of the upper femoral epiphysis. J Bone Joint Surg Br 1964;46:621–629.
5. Gautier E, Ganz K, Krugel N, et al. Anatomy of the medial femoral circumflex artery and its surgical implications. J Bone Joint Surg Br 2000;82(5):679–683.
6. Goodman DA, Feighan JE, Smith AD, et al. Subclinical slipped capital femoral epiphysis. Relationship to osteoarthrosis of the hip. J Bone Joint Surg Am 1997;79(10):1489–1497.
7. Gordon JE, Abrahams MS, Dobbs MB, et al. Early reduction, arthrotomy, and cannulated screw fixation in unstable slipped capital femoral epiphysis treatment. J Pediatr Orthop 2002;22(3):352–358.
8. Huber H, Dora C, Ramseier LE, et al. Adolescent slipped capital femoral epiphysis treated by a modified Dunn osteotomy with surgical hip dislocation. J Bone Joint Surg Br 2011;93(6):833–838.
9. Leunig M, Casillas MM, Hamlet M, et al. Slipped capital femoral epiphysis: early mechanical damage to the acetabular cartilage by a prominent femoral metaphysis. Acta Orthop Scand 2000;71(4):370–375.

10. Loder RT, Richards BS, Shapiro PS, et al. Acute slipped capital femoral epiphysis: the importance of physeal stability. J Bone Joint Surg Am 1993;75(8):1134–1140.
11. Mamisch TC, Kim YJ, Richolt JA, et al. Femoral morphology due to impingement influences the range of motion in slipped capital femoral epiphysis. Clin Orthop Relat Res 2009;467(3):692–698.
12. Parsch K, Weller S, Parsch D. Open reduction and smooth Kirschner wire fixation for unstable slipped capital femoral epiphysis. J Pediatr Orthop 2009;29(1):1–8.
13. Rab GT. The geometry of slipped capital femoral epiphysis: implications for movement, impingement, and corrective osteotomy. J Pediatr Orthop 1999;19(4):41–424.
14. Sankar WN, Vanderhave KL, Matheney T, et al. The modified Dunn procedure for unstable slipped capital femoral epiphysis: a multicenter perspective. J Bone Joint Surg Am 2013;95(7): 585–591.
15. Slongo T, Kakaty D, Krause F, et al. Treatment of slipped capital femoral epiphysis with a modified Dunn procedure. J Bone Joint Surg Am 2010;92(18):2898–2908.
16. Southwick WO. Osteotomy through the lesser trochanter for slipped capital femoral epiphysis. J Bone Joint Surg Am 1967;49(5): 807–835.
17. Tannast M, Goricki D, Beck M, et al. Hip damage occurs at the zone of femoroacetabular impingement. Clin Orthop Relat Res 2008; 466(2):273–280.
18. Ziebarth K, Zilkens C, Spencer S, et al. Capital realignment for moderate and severe SCFE using a modified Dunn procedure. Clin Orthop Relat Res 2009;467(3):704–716.

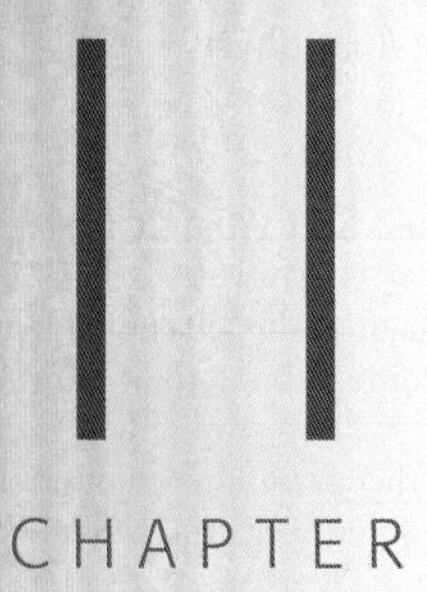

CHAPTER 11

Bernese Periacetabular Osteotomy

Travis H. Matheney and Michael B. Millis

DEFINITION

- Hip dysplasia is the most common etiology of coxarthrosis, often leading to arthroplasty long before joint replacement can be considered a lifetime solution.[3]
- Surgical realignment of the congruous dysplastic acetabulum can improve or eliminate symptoms for years, sometimes indefinitely, in a majority of appropriately selected patients, even in those with some degree of preoperative arthrosis.[1,3,4,6–8]
- Age limits for this procedure are adolescence (closed triradiate cartilage) to an indefinite upper age limit (limited by preoperative arthrosis and other considerations that might make arthroplasty a better choice).

ANATOMY

- The acetabulum lies between the anterior and posterior columns of the pelvis.
- The most common area of acetabular deficiency in developmental dysplasia of the hip (DDH) is anterior and lateral.
- The Bernese periacetabular osteotomy (PAO) differs from the triple osteotomy primarily by maintaining the integrity of the posterior column of the pelvis.
- The Bernese PAO uses up to five steps to divide the acetabular fragment from the remainder of the pelvis, allowing multiplanar reorientation.
- Important bony landmarks include the following:
  - Iliopectineal eminence (which marks the medialmost extent of the acetabulum)
  - Infracotyloid groove (just distal to the acetabulum, where the obturator externus tendon lies; this is the site of the anterior ischial osteotomy)
  - Anterior superior iliac spine (ASIS)
  - Apex of the greater sciatic notch
  - Ischial spine
- The posterior column is triangular and thickest just posterior to the acetabulum; it becomes much thinner closer to the sciatic notch. For this reason, the optimal plane for the posterior column is angled obliquely to the medial cortex and perpendicular to the lateral cortex of the ischium–posterior column.

PATHOGENESIS

- Genetic and developmental causes exist for "developmental dysplasia."
- Neuromuscular: Charcot-Marie-Tooth disease and spastic diplegia
- Posttraumatic: injuries to the triradiate cartilage and aggressive excision of the limbus in the infant hip

NATURAL HISTORY

- There is a clear correlation between acetabular dysplasia and osteoarthrosis of the hip.
- The more severe the acetabular dysplasia and any subluxation, the earlier the onset of symptoms from arthrosis.
- Murphy et al[5] found that every patient with a lateral center-edge angle less than 16 degrees developed osteoarthritis by age 65 years.

PATIENT HISTORY AND PHYSICAL FINDINGS

- Key portions of the history include the following:
  - Personal or family history or treatment of DDH
  - History of other hip disorders, including Legg-Calvé-Perthes
  - Trauma
  - Skeletal dysplasias
  - History of cerebral palsy
  - Birth order and weight
  - Description of pain or mechanical symptoms, including location, duration, activity limitation, giving way, "clicking," "catching," and "popping"
- Physical examination should include gait, limb length, assistive devices, and strength.
- Specific hip tests include the following:
  - Trendelenburg test: demonstrates weakness in abductors
  - Anterior apprehension test: A positive result is a subjective noting of "apprehension" or instability by the patient.
  - Anterior impingement test (pain with passive hip flexion, adduction, and internal rotation): test of anterior labral pathology, not just a tear
  - Bicycle test for abductor fatigability
- Range of motion (ROM): Dysplastic hips may demonstrate a relative increase in flexion due to anterior acetabular uncoverage. Decreased ROM with pain may indicate arthrosis.

IMAGING AND OTHER DIAGNOSTIC STUDIES

- Radiography includes weight-bearing anteroposterior (AP) views of bilateral hips (**FIG 1A**), false profile of hips (**FIG 1B**), and AP views of the hips in maximal abduction and internal rotation (von Rosen view; **FIG 1C**). These studies allow assessment of lateral and anterior coverage of the femoral head as well as congruency of the hip joint. Additionally noted will be the presence of hinge abduction, which is a relative contraindication to PAO.
- Radiographic parameters include the following:
  - Lateral center-edge angle of Wiberg measured from AP view of the hip (lower limits of normal about 25 degrees; see **FIG 1A**)

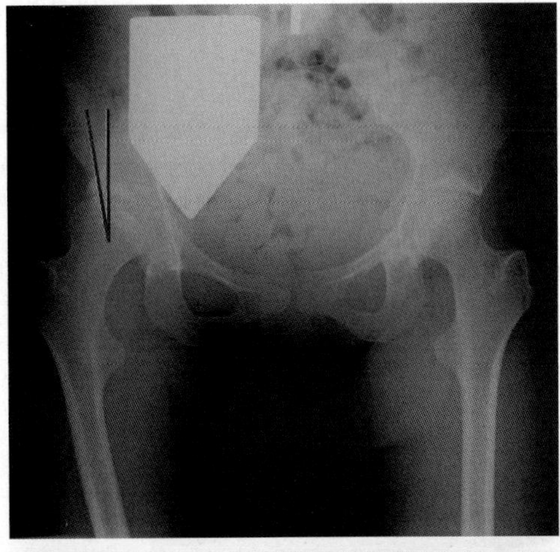
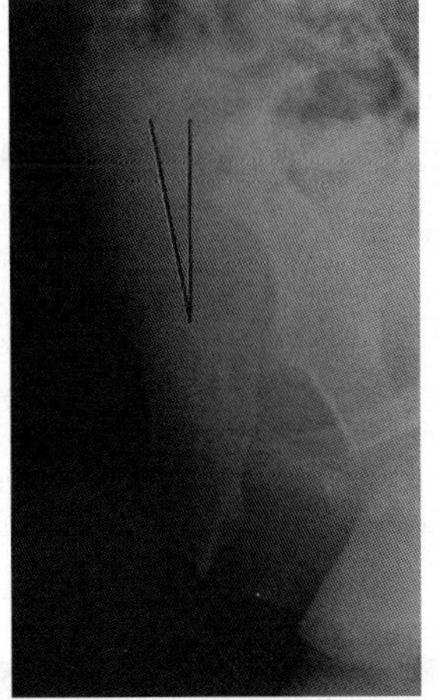
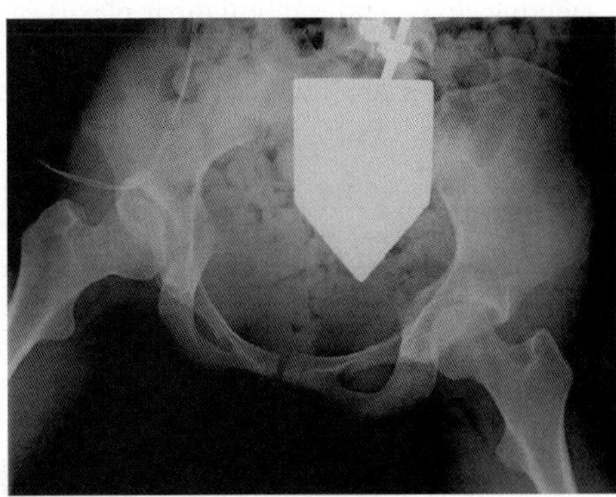
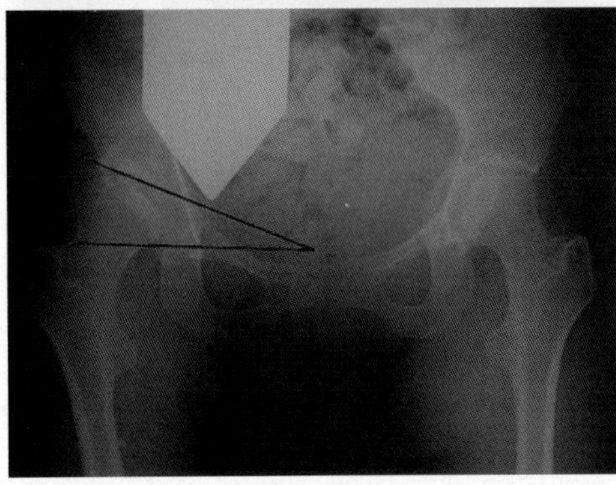

FIG 1 • **A.** AP view of pelvis and hips. Lateral center-edge angle of Wiberg is marked on right hip. **B.** False-profile view of right hip. Anterior center-edge angle of Lequesne and de Seze is marked. The anterior edge is marked to the edge of the sourcil. **C.** Von Rosen AP view of pelvis with hips in maximal abduction and internal rotation. This is used to assess congruency and mimic the appearance of the hip after reorienting acetabular osteotomy. **D.** AP view of pelvis and hips. The Tönnis acetabular roof angle is marked on the right hip.

  - Anterior center-edge angle of Lequesne and de Seze (lower limits of normal 20 degrees measured on the false-profile view; see **FIG 1B**)
  - Tönnis acetabular roof angle measured on the AP view of the hip (upper limits of normal 10 to 15 degrees; **FIG 1D**)
  - Crossover sign (anterior wall shadow crossing posterior wall shadow on AP view of the pelvis)
  - Assessment of the line of Shenton for breaks indicative of femoral head subluxation
- Computed tomography (CT) scan of both hips with three-dimensional reconstruction as well as with axial slices through the femoral condyles may be of assistance in preoperatively assessing the amount and direction of correction required as well as the potential need for proximal femoral osteotomy.
- Magnetic resonance imaging (MRI) of involved hips with radial sequences centered at the femoral head allows assessment of articular and labral cartilage.
  - Delayed gadolinium-enhanced MRI of cartilage (dGEMRIC) is a recently developed technique that assesses the mechanical damage to the articular cartilage. It has been demonstrated to be a better preoperative predictor than plain radiographs in determining outcome after PAO.[2]

NONOPERATIVE MANAGEMENT

- Activity and job modification may be of benefit in delaying or mitigating arthritic symptoms.
- Physical therapy may be of some benefit in increasing ROM and strength. To date, there are no data to suggest that a specific therapy regimen can affect the onset of arthritis in the dysplastic hip.

SURGICAL MANAGEMENT

- Indication: symptomatic, congruous acetabular dysplasia (closed triradiate cartilage) with lateral and anterior center-edge angles 18 degrees or less
- Contraindications: Tönnis osteoarthrosis grade 2 or more (subchondral cysts, significant joint space narrowing), severe limitation of motion secondary to arthrosis, active joint infection

Preoperative Planning

- Radiographs and MRI are evaluated to assess the following:
  - Degree and character of dysplasia
  - Amount and direction of correction required to normalize the Tönnis acetabular roof angle (0 to 10 degrees), correct subluxation, and improve mechanical stability
- Proximal femoral deformity may also require treatment at time of PAO.
- Presence of acetabular articular or labral lesions (seen on MRI) should also be taken into consideration, as treatment either arthroscopically (before the osteotomy) or intraoperatively through limited arthrotomy may be required for best long-term results.
  - Isolated treatment of a labral lesion in the presence of acetabular dysplasia is contraindicated. Simultaneous acetabular realignment must be considered.
  - The torn acetabular labrum is usually associated with other structural abnormality within the hip (femoroacetabular impingement or DDH), which may also require correction for best results.[9]

- Partial weight-bearing technique is taught preoperatively in preparation for postoperative mobilization.
- For perioperative pain management, we recommended considering either epidural or lumbar plexus catheter placement preoperatively as well as multimodal perioperative analgesia. Catheters are removed the morning of postoperative day 1 or 2.

Positioning

- The patient is positioned supine on a radiolucent table.
- The operative extremity is prepared and draped free up to the costal margin; the surgeon should be certain to prepare and drape posteriorly to at least the posterior third of the ilium and medially to the umbilicus.

Approach

- The standard longitudinal anterior Smith-Petersen incision and approach to the hip provides the appropriate access (**FIG 2A**).
- As an alternative, an ilioinguinal (bikini) incision may be used followed by a similar deep approach (**FIG 2B**). This incision typically provides a better cosmetic result but can limit access for the anterior ischial osteotomy. Therefore, we recommend the standard anterior incision for larger and more muscular patients.

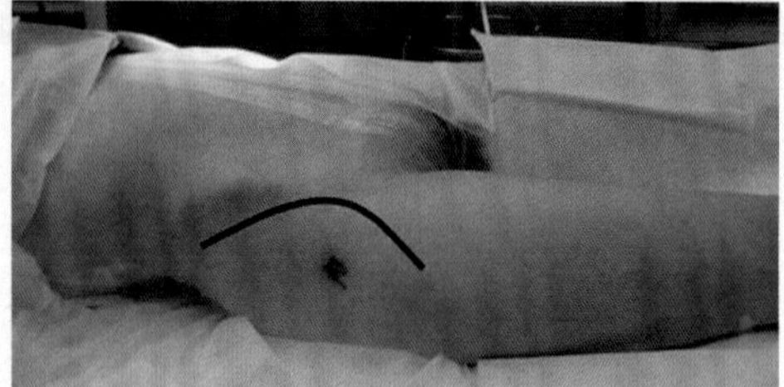
A

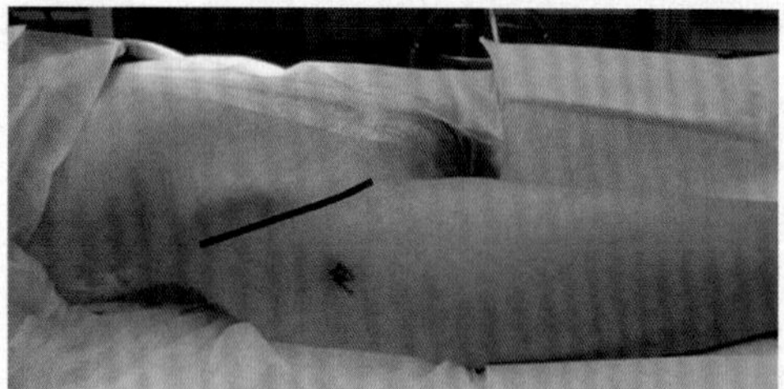
B

FIG 2 • **A.** Hip with traditional Smith-Petersen incision marked. **B.** Hip with bikini-type incision marked.

TECHNIQUES

Superficial Dissection

- The skin is incised into subcutaneous tissue.
- The fascia over the external oblique and gluteus medius is identified and incised posterior to the ASIS, and the plane between the two muscles is developed to expose the periosteum over the iliac crest.
- The periosteum is sharply divided over the iliac crest and subperiosteal dissection carried out over the inner table of the ilium. This space is packed with sponges for hemostasis.
- Entry into the tensor fascia lata–sartorius interval is initially accomplished via the compartment of the proximal tensor fascia lata to avoid injury to the lateral femoral cutaneous nerve. The tensor fascia lata is bluntly elevated off the intermuscular septum and the compartment floor is identified proximally until the anterior ilium is palpated.
- Once hemostasis is attained, the ASIS is predrilled with a 2.5-mm drill and the anterior 1- × 1- × 1-cm portion is osteotomized to facilitate the medial dissection and later repair.
  - Alternatively, the sartorius can be taken off with just a thin wafer of bone that will be sewn back in place at the end instead of with a screw.
- Subperiosteal dissection is continued to the anterior inferior iliac spine (AIIS).

Deep Dissection

- Before proceeding with the deep dissection, it is important to have determined preoperatively whether there is intra-articular pathology that will require performing an arthrotomy to address. Examples include labral tear, perilabral cyst, and femoral head–neck cam lesion. If so, the rectus femoris generally is detached (see in the following text). If however, no intra-articular work is needed, the rectus tendon can be left intact.
- Flexion and adduction of the hip facilitates the deep intrapelvic and superior ramus dissection.
- The reflected head of the rectus femoris is divided at its junction with the direct head (**TECH FIG 1A,B**).
- The direct head and underlying capsular iliacus are elevated as a unit and reflected distally and medially off the underlying joint capsule.
- If one is performing a rectus femoris-sparing PAO, identifying the interval between the capsular portion of the iliacus and the rectus femoris can be a challenge. To assist with this, it is recommended to start within the pelvis dissecting underneath the iliacus there, then following it over the pelvic brim onto the capsule.
- The iliacus, sartorius, and abdominal contents are reflected medially.
- The psoas sheath is opened longitudinally, and the psoas tendon is retracted medially to allow access to the superior pubic ramus medial to the iliopectineal eminence.
- The interval between the medial joint capsule and the iliopsoas tendon is created and sequentially dilated using the tip of a long-handled Mayo scissor, then further by Lane bone levers, with the tips of each palpating the anterior ischium at the infracotyloid groove.
  - Proper placement of the scissor and bone levers can be confirmed with the image intensifier (**TECH FIG 1C,D**).

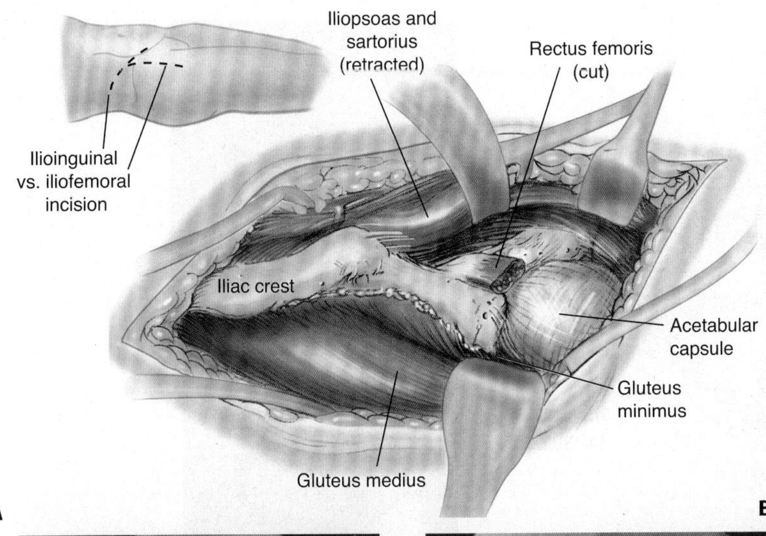

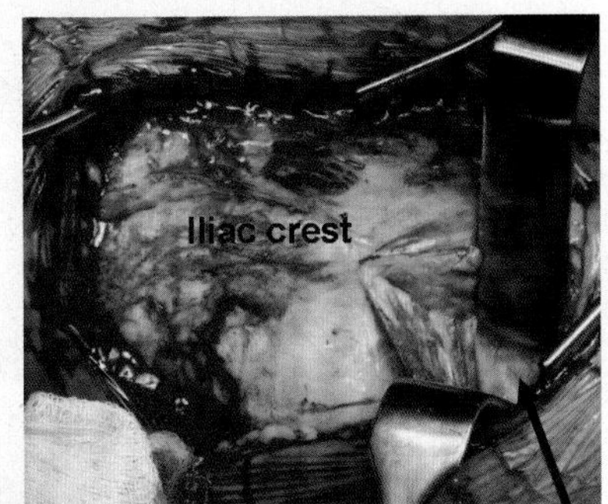

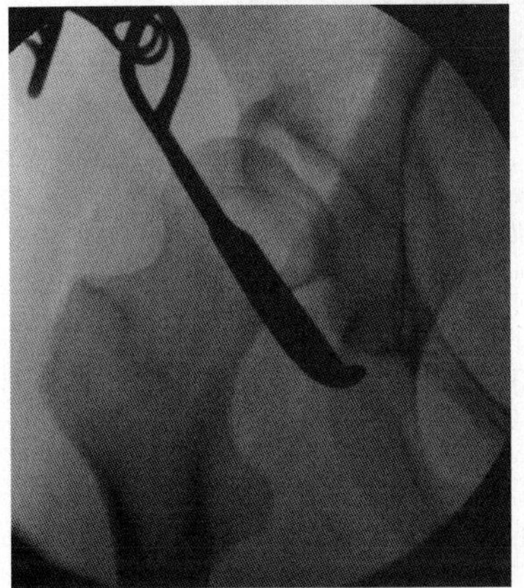

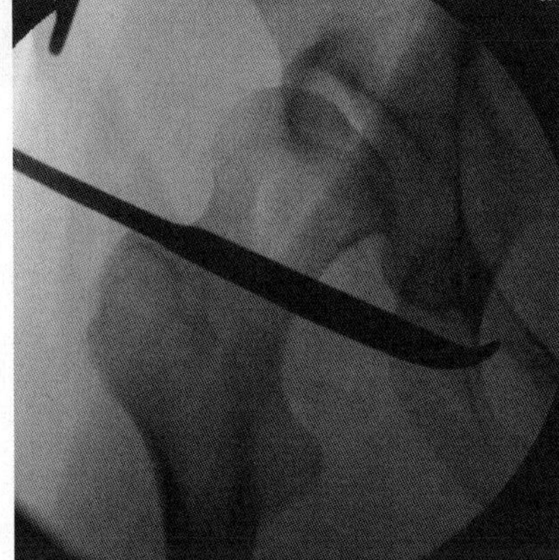

TECH FIG 1 • **A.** Deep dissection through anterior hip interval. The direct and indirect heads of the rectus femoris have been cut. **B.** Surgical exposure of the anterior hip capsule (*arrow*). The iliac crest is marked in the left half of the wound before subperiosteal dissection of the iliacus. **C,D.** Intraoperative fluoroscopic AP views of the right hip. Lane bone lever is used to first palpate the outer and inner aspects of the anterior ischium.

Osteotomies

Anterior Ischial Osteotomy

- Before performing the first osteotomy, it is recommended that one confirms with the anesthesia team that the patient is no longer paralyzed. Without paralytic, direct contact of the sciatic or obturator nerves during any of the osteotomies will elicit a muscular response, warning the surgeon of that they may be in harms way.
- With the hip flexed 45 degrees and slightly adducted, a 30-degree forked, angled bone chisel (Synthes USA, West Chester, PA; in 15- or 20-mm blade widths) is carefully inserted through the previously created interval between the medial capsule and psoas tendon to place its tip in contact with the superior portion of the infracotyloid groove of the anterior ischium, just superior to the obturator externus tendon (**TECH FIG 2A–C**).
- Staying proximal to the obturator externus tendon helps to protect the nearby medial femoral circumflex artery. The medial and lateral aspects of the ischium should be gently palpated with the chisel. Proper chisel placement (about 1 cm below the inferior acetabular lip) is confirmed on AP and oblique projections with the image intensifier (**TECH FIG 2D**).
- The osteotome is impacted in a posterior direction to a depth of 15 to 20 mm and through both medial and lateral cortices of the ischium (**TECH FIG 2E**).
- Care should be taken not to drive the osteotome too deeply out the lateral cortex, as the sciatic nerve is nearby.

Superior Pubic Ramus Osteotomy

- The hip is kept flexed and adducted to relax the anterior soft tissues.
- The psoas tendon and medial structures are gently retracted medially (**TECH FIG 3A**).
- After circumferential subperiosteal dissection of the ramus, either a spiked Hohmann retractor or a large-gauge Kirschner wire may be impacted into the superior aspect of the ramus at least 1 cm medial to the iliopectineal eminence (**TECH FIG 3B**).
- Blunt Hohmann retractors, Rang retractors, or Lane bone levers are placed anteriorly and posteriorly as well as inferior to the ramus to protect the obturator nerve and artery.
- The osteotomy is perpendicular to the long axis of the ramus when viewed from above but oblique from distal medial to proximal lateral when viewed from the front and may be carried out either by passing a Gigli saw around the ramus and sawing upward away from the retractors or by impacting a straight osteotome just lateral to the spiked Hohmann or Kirschner wire. In the former method, the Gigli saw is passed with the aid of a Satinsky vascular clamp.
  - The key to this osteotomy is to *stay medial* to the iliopectineal eminence and avoid entering the medial acetabulum (**TECH FIG 3C**).

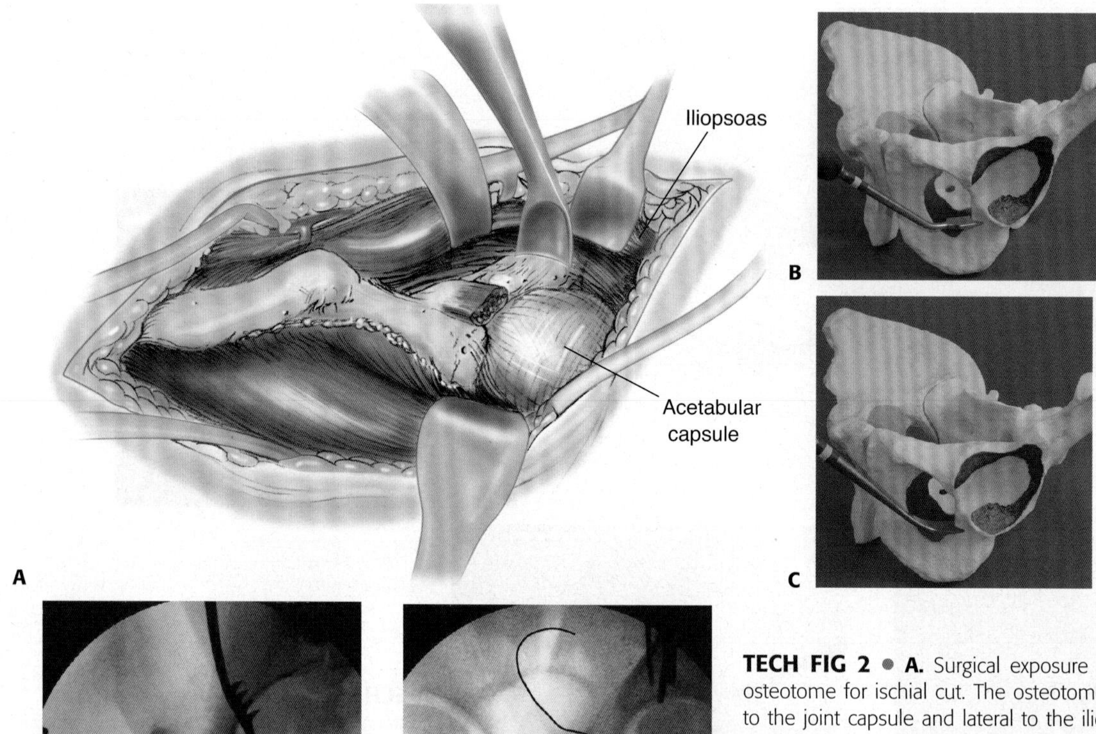

TECH FIG 2 • **A.** Surgical exposure and placement of osteotome for ischial cut. The osteotome is placed medial to the joint capsule and lateral to the iliopsoas. **B,C.** Bone models demonstrating the planned position of the osteotome for the ischial cut: Ganz angled chisel (**B**) and Mast curved chisel (**C**). **D,E.** Intraoperative fluoroscopic AP view of right hip with Ganz 30-degree osteotome (**D**) at the anterior ischium and false-profile view of right hip with Mast curved chisel (**E**) seated into anterior ischium. The sciatic notch and ischial spine are outlined in *black*. Proper direction of this cut should also be confirmed on fluoroscopic false-profile view.

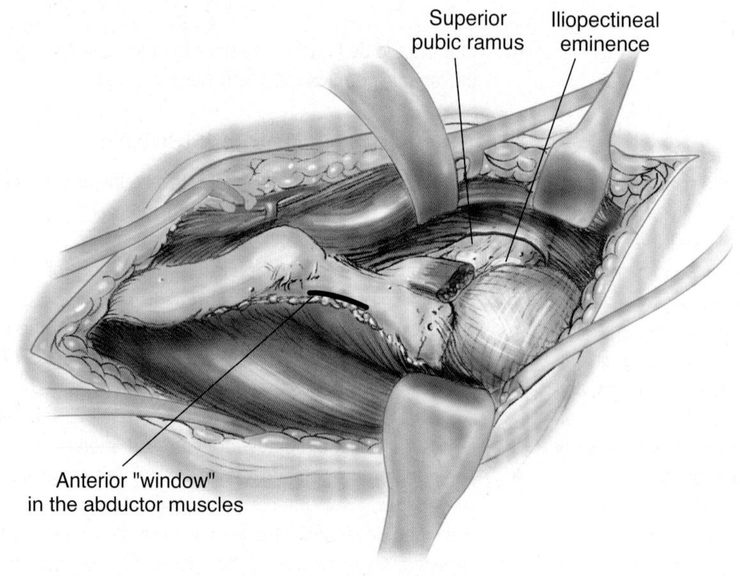

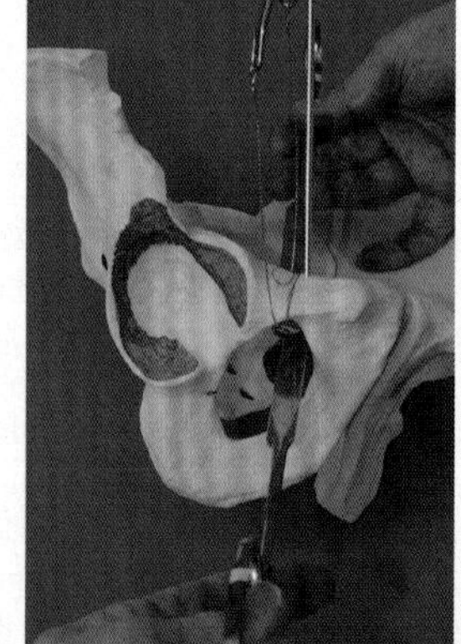

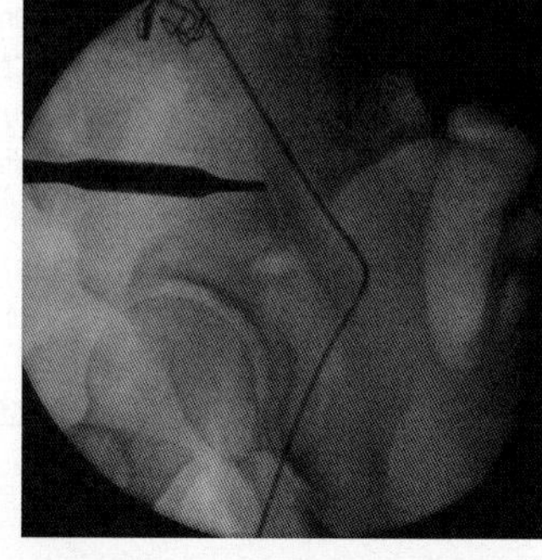

TECH FIG 3 • **A.** Anterior approach. The superior pubic ramus is exposed and the iliopsoas is retracted medially. **B.** Bone model demonstrating the superior ramus osteotomy. The Lane bone levers are placed on either side of the ramus and a Kirschner wire is placed as a retractor. The iliopectineal eminence is marked with a *circle*. **C.** Intraoperative fluoroscopic false-profile view of hip. A small Hohmann retractor is placed under the abductors aiming toward the apex of the sciatic notch.

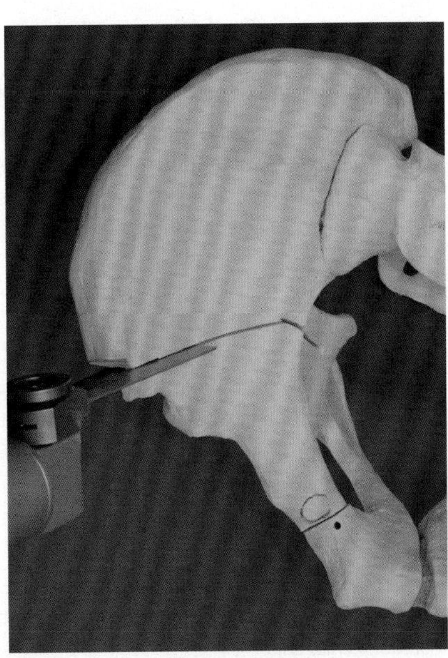

TECH FIG 4 • Bone model demonstrating the saw cut of the ilium aiming toward a point about 1 cm above the iliopectineal line.

- Arthrotomy and intracapsular inspection: At a point before all osteotomies are completed, an arthrotomy may be performed to identify and treat intra-articular lesions such as a torn labrum or impingement lesions of the femoral head and neck.
  - This is closed loosely with simple, interrupted absorbable suture before proceeding with the remainder of the osteotomies.

Supra-acetabular Iliac Osteotomy

- A 1.5- to 2-mm subperiosteal window is started beneath the anterior abductors just distal to the ASIS without disturbing the abductor origin.
- The leg is slightly abducted and extended to allow atraumatic subperiosteal dissection using a narrow elevator posteriorly toward, but not into, the apex of the greater sciatic notch.
- A narrow, long, spiked Hohmann retractor is placed in this window. Correct placement is confirmed with image intensifier; in the lateral projection, the spike of the Hohmann should point toward the apex of the sciatic notch (**TECH FIG 3C**).
- The iliacus and abdominal contents are retracted medially with a reverse Hohmann with its tip on the quadrilateral surface.
- Under direct vision, the iliac osteotomy is performed with an oscillating saw and cooling irrigation in line with the Hohmann retractor until reaching a point about 1 cm above the iliopectineal line (well anterior to the notch). This end point of the iliac saw cut represents the posterosuperior corner of the PAO. This corner is also the starting point of the posterior column osteotomy, which will be midway between the sciatic notch and posterior acetabulum (**TECH FIG 4**).
- At this point, a single Schanz screw on T-handled chuck is inserted into the acetabular fragment distal and parallel to the iliac saw cut, well above the dome of the acetabulum, into a hole predrilled with a 3.2-mm drill.

Posterior Column Osteotomy

- The leg is once again flexed and adducted to relax the medial soft tissues.
- A reverse blunt Hohmann retractor is placed medially with the tip on the ischial spine. Dissection into the sciatic notch is neither necessary nor recommended.
- The osteotomy is made through the medial cortex with a long, straight 1.5-cm osteotome. It extends from the posterior end of the iliac saw cut, passing over the iliopectineal line, through the medial quadrilateral plate, parallel to the anterior edge of the sciatic notch on iliac oblique fluoroscopy, and is directed toward the ischial spine (**TECH FIG 5A**).
- This osteotomy must extend at least 4 cm below the iliopectineal line to avoid entry into the acetabulum when completing the

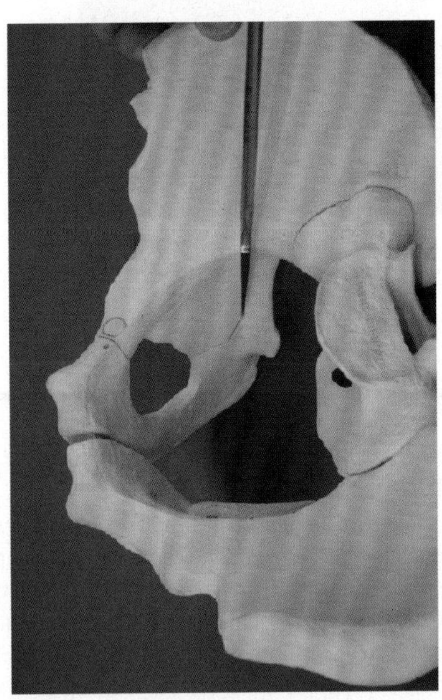

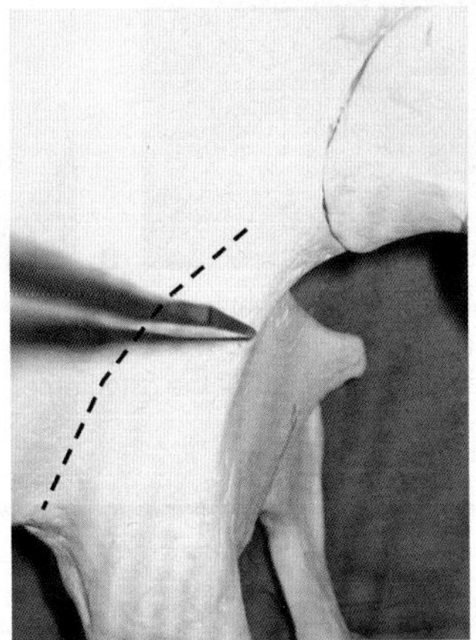

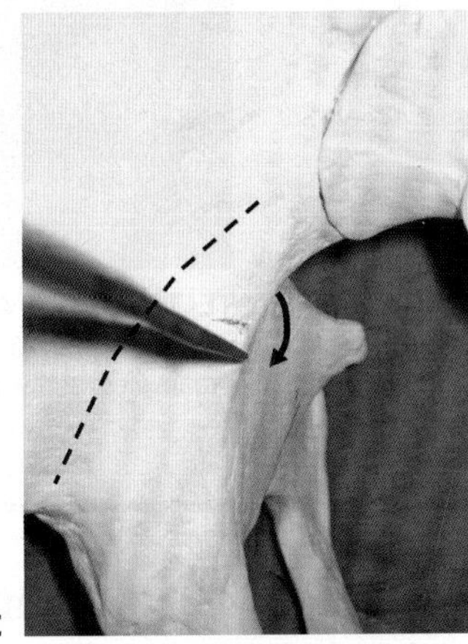

TECH FIG 5 • **A.** Bone model demonstrating the division of the posterior column. **B,C.** The incorrect (**B**) and the correct (**C**) angles of the osteotome for division of the posterior column. The *dotted line* indicates the relative position of the acetabulum and lateral aspect of the ischium. The proper angle of the osteotome is *away* from the sciatic notch about 10 to 15 degrees. *(continued)*

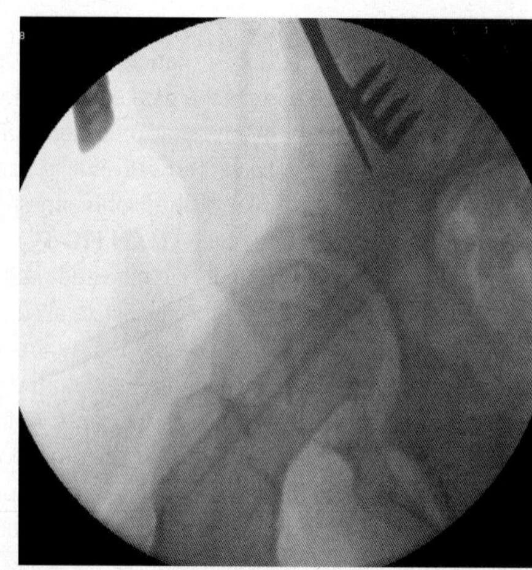

TECH FIG 5 • *(continued)* **D.** Intraoperative fluoroscopic false-profile view of the right hip. Division of the posterior column is performed here. The borders of the osteotomy (acetabulum anteriorly and sciatic notch posteriorly) should be clearly visible to avoid intra-articular or intranotch extension of the osteotomy.

final (posteroinferior) infra-acetabular osteotomy. This posterior cut is made first through the medial, then second through the lateral wall of the ischium.

- The ischium is wider here than at its anterior extent. If pictured from above, it resembles a triangle with the narrower apex at the anterior edge of the sciatic notch. Therefore, the surgeon should not place the osteotome perpendicular to the medial quadrilateral plate. Instead, the free medial edge of the osteotome should be tipped 10 to 15 degrees *away* from the sciatic notch to create a more true coronal plane osteotomy, perpendicular to the *lateral* cortex of the posterior column (**TECH FIG 5B,C**).

- Correct angulation and positioning are once again confirmed by the image intensifier (**TECH FIG 5D**).
  - If your initial anterior ischial osteotomy was placed sufficiently deep, it is possible to have this osteotomy propagate into your anterior osteotomy and potentially avoid the need for the "completion" osteotomy described in the next step.

Completion Osteotomy

- The final osteotomy is a completion osteotomy of the posteroinferomedial corner of quadrilateral plate connecting the anterior and posterior ischial cuts.
- A 30-degree long-handled chisel is used to connect these two prior osteotomies (**TECH FIG 6**).
- A key point: The blade is placed to connect the prior cuts, and the osteotome face should *not* be more than 50 degrees off the quadrilateral plate. This will prevent accidentally aiming anteriorly into the acetabulum.

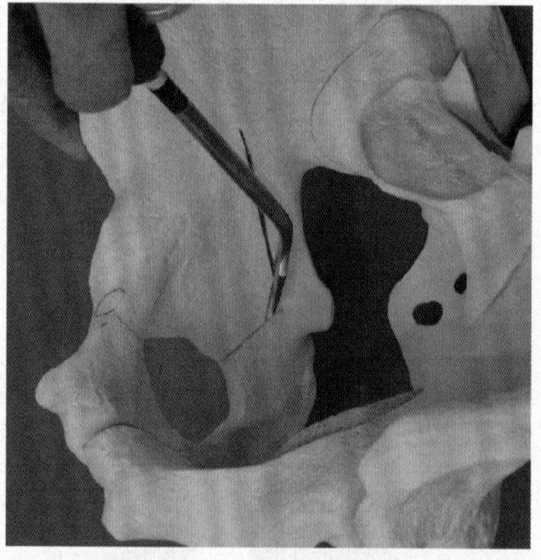

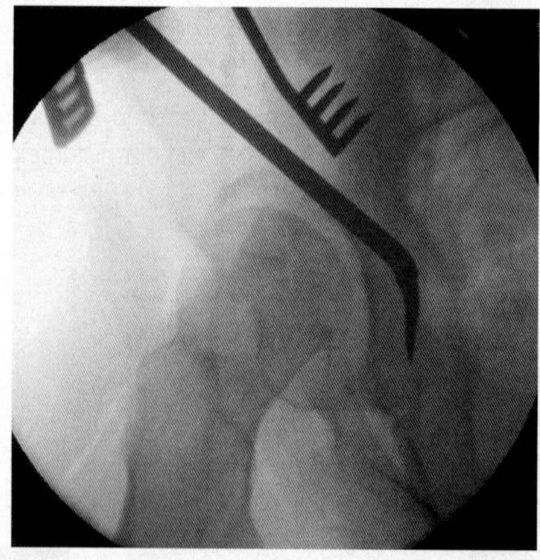

TECH FIG 6 • **A.** Bone model of right pelvis demonstrating the final cut with a bent osteotome to connect the anterior ischial and posterior column osteotomies. **B.** Intraoperative fluoroscopic false-profile view showing proper positioning of the osteotome.

Acetabular Displacement

- A 1-inch straight Lambotte chisel is placed into the supra-acetabular iliac saw cut to both confirm completion of the lateral cortex osteotomy and protect the cancellous bone above the acetabulum during displacement.
- The tines of a Weber bone clamp are placed onto the superior ramus portion of the acetabular fragment in such a way as to place its handle anterior and in contact with the Schanz screw (**TECH FIG 7A**).
- A lamina spreader is placed into the iliac osteotomy between the posterosuperior intact ilium and the Lambotte chisel anteriorly.
- While gently opening the lamina spreader, the Schanz screw and Weber clamp are used to mobilize the acetabular fragment. It is important to ascertain whether the posterior and anterior osteotomies are complete; otherwise, the fragment will not

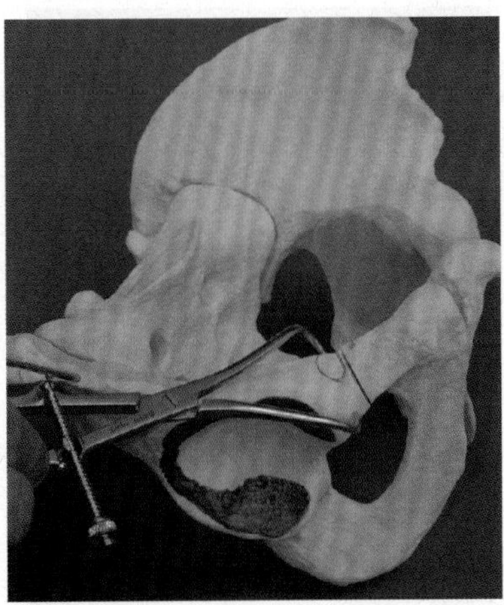
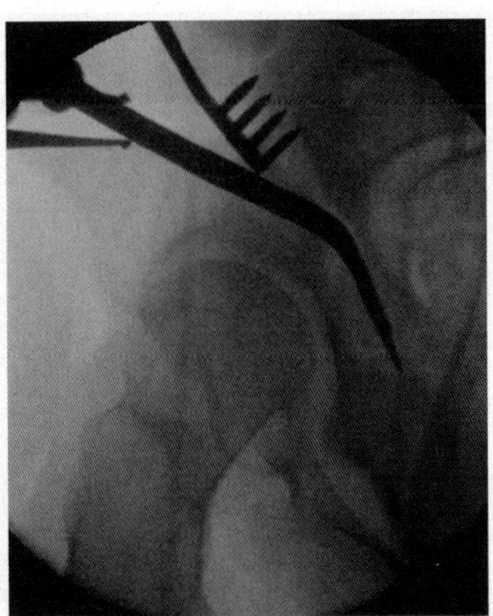
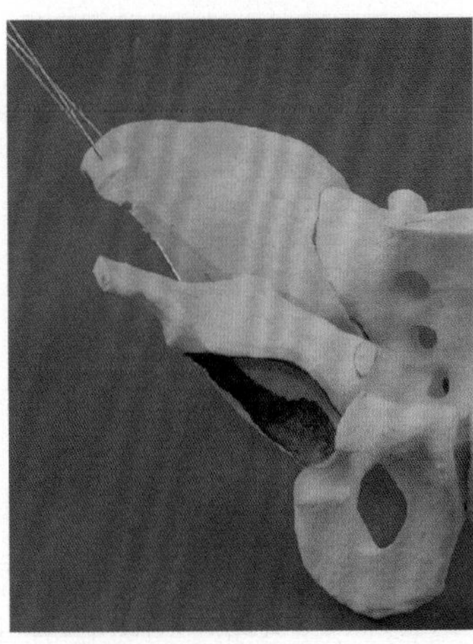

TECH FIG 7 • **A.** Bone model showing placement of Schanz screw (*far left*) and large bone-holding clamp for manipulation of acetabular fragment. The bone clamp is placed anterior to the Schanz screw. **B.** Intraoperative fluoroscopic false-profile view of right hip. Seen here is displacement of the acetabular fragment with a lamina spreader (*top*) and use of an angled chisel from medial to lateral to find areas where the osteotomies are not complete. **C.** Sawbones model showing acetabular fragment placement. The posteroinferior corner of the fragment is impacted into the superior iliac wing and its prominent anterior spike is roughly in line with the intact iliac crest.

freely rotate and the common outcome will be distal and lateral displacement as you hinge on the lateral, intact cortices. These cuts can be inspected with a narrow or broad 30-degree chisel (**TECH FIG 7B**).

- Once the fragment is completely free, it may be positioned to obtain the desired correction. As previously noted, the most common deficiency is anterior and lateral. Therefore, the most commonly used maneuvers are to lift the acetabular fragment slightly toward the ceiling, creating an initial displacement, followed by a three-step movement of lateral, distal, and internal rotation.
  - When performed properly, the posteroinferior corner of the acetabular fragment should be impacted slightly into the superior intact iliac cut and the prominent superior tip of the acetabular fragment should be roughly in line with the superior intact iliac crest (**TECH FIG 7C**).
- The radiographic "teardrop" and its relation to the femoral head after fragment positioning should be elevated and tilted laterally commensurate with the amount of lateral correction.
  - It is commonly necessary to medialize the acetabular fragment a little once the desired anterolateral coverage is obtained to recreate the proper position of the femoral head in relation to the medial pelvis. This will maintain proper biomechanical position of the femur in relation to the pelvis.

Acetabular Fixation

- Once the desired acetabular position is obtained, 3/32- or 7/64-inch smooth Kirschner wires (the approximate diameter of a 2.5- and 3.5-mm drill bits) are placed proximal to distal through the ilium and into the fragment in a divergent pattern.
- At this point, we perform a final fragment position check in the AP and false-profile views (**TECH FIG 8A,B**).
  - Importantly, in the false-profile view, we check the anterior femoral head coverage in full extension and at 100 degrees of flexion (**TECH FIG 8C**). In the former view, the sourcil should be roughly horizontal, the femoral head should be well covered, and the line of Shenton should be intact. The false-profile view is to confirm that we have neither overcovered the femoral head nor created impingement from a femoral-sided deformity.
  - If there is less than 90 degrees of flexion on palpation or radiograph, it may be necessary to either reposition the fragment or address femoral-sided deformity.
- The Kirschner wires are measured for depth and length and then replaced with either 3.5- or 4.5-mm cortical screws.
- The image intensifier is used to confirm extra-articular placement of all screws (**TECH FIG 8D,E**).
- An additional "home-run" screw may be placed anterior to posterior from the AIIS posteriorly into the inferior ilium if required for stability (especially in patients who are ligamentously lax or have a neuromuscular condition or poor bone quality). We prefer not to use this screw unless necessary, as it is our practice to remove these screws once bony healing is confirmed for screw head irritation or in case MRI is to be performed at a later point.
- The anterior iliac prominence of the acetabular fragment is trimmed and used for bone graft.
- Gelfoam may be placed along osteotomy sites to assist with hemostasis.

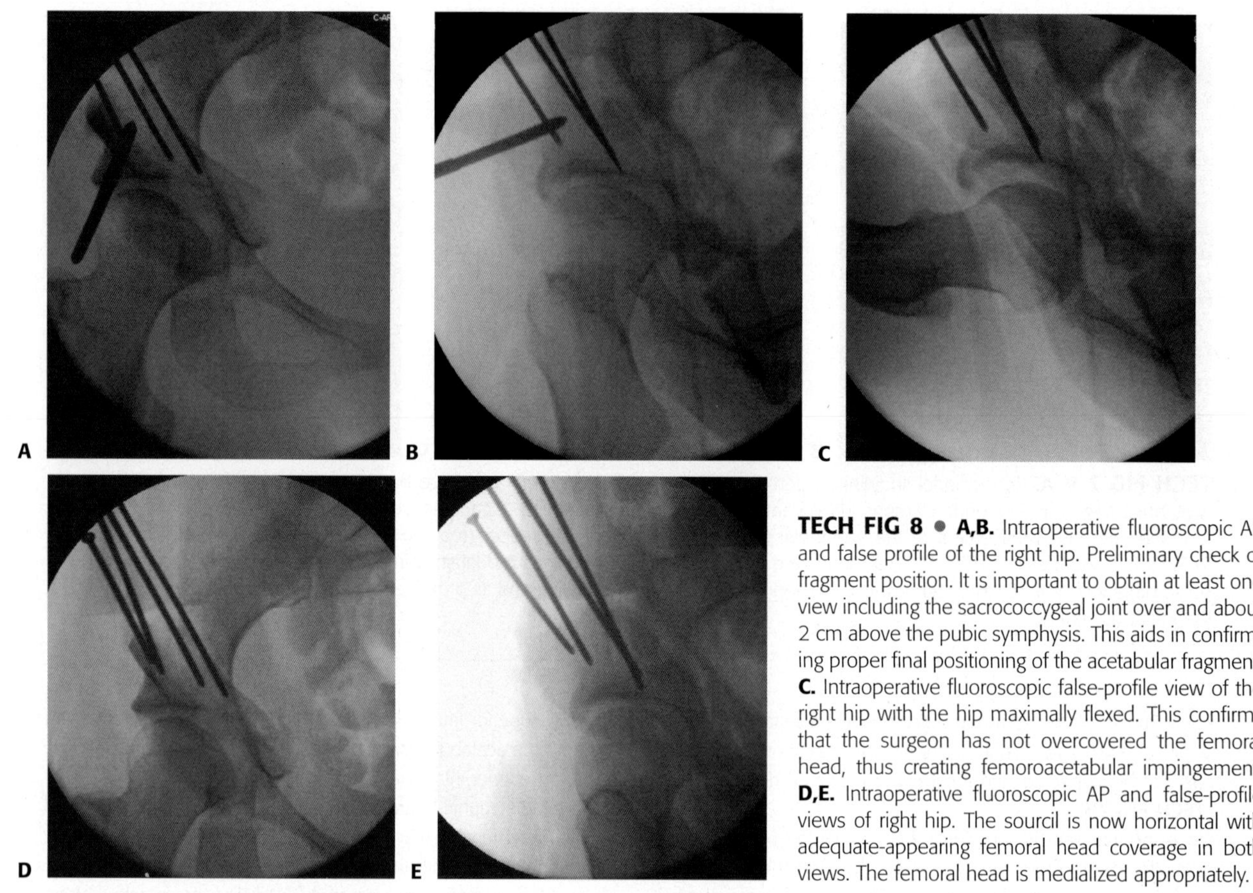

TECH FIG 8 • A,B. Intraoperative fluoroscopic AP and false profile of the right hip. Preliminary check of fragment position. It is important to obtain at least one view including the sacrococcygeal joint over and about 2 cm above the pubic symphysis. This aids in confirming proper final positioning of the acetabular fragment. **C.** Intraoperative fluoroscopic false-profile view of the right hip with the hip maximally flexed. This confirms that the surgeon has not overcovered the femoral head, thus creating femoroacetabular impingement. **D,E.** Intraoperative fluoroscopic AP and false-profile views of right hip. The sourcil is now horizontal with adequate-appearing femoral head coverage in both views. The femoral head is medialized appropriately.

Wound Closure

- All sponges are removed, and wounds are irrigated copiously.
- Suction drains are placed under the iliacus.
- The ASIS osteotomy (if performed) is reattached either by using a 3.5-mm, partially threaded cancellous screw and washer or by being sewn back with heavy, absorbable suture passed through the thinner wafer.
- Careful attention is paid to proper, tight closure over the iliac crest. This is accomplished by predrilling holes in the iliac crest to facilitate passage of heavy, absorbable sutures to reattach the abductor, iliacus, and external oblique musculature.
- The remainder of the wound is closed in layers.

PEARLS AND PITFALLS

Patient selection	■ Appropriate patient selection is paramount. ■ Risk factors for failure include older age, poor congruency, decreased joint space (<2 mm), and advanced arthrosis. ■ Presence of a labral tear preoperatively may also be an indicator of degeneration, more than may be apparent on plain radiographs.
Pubic osteotomy	■ The hip should be flexed 40–50 degrees for making the pubis osteotomy, which takes tension off the iliopsoas and improves access to the brim of the pelvis.
Ischial osteotomy	■ If the medial joint is entered while attempting to gain access for the ischial cut, the surgeon can open the psoas sheath and try a second approach dissecting through the floor of the sheath. This technique can be helpful in reestablishing an extra-articular dissection to the ischium. ■ Straying too medial risks injury to the neurovascular bundle.

Iliac osteotomy	■ In general, given true supine positioning of the pelvis and patient, the iliac wing osteotomy will be roughly directed perpendicular to the floor. This sighting technique gives a second visual reference, which, in combination with intraoperative imaging, will aid in proper positioning of the osteotomy.
Incomplete osteotomies	■ Connecting the inferior ischial (infracotyloid) osteotomy and the posterior ischial cuts may require a medial to lateral osteotome cut through their medial junction. This is most commonly necessary when the lateral portion of these osteotomies is incomplete and the finding is an inability to freely move the acetabular fragment at the initial completion of all planned osteotomies.
Schanz screw placement	■ The Schanz pin (screw) should be placed nearly in line with and 1–1.5 cm below the iliac wing osteotomy. In poorer quality bone, it may be necessary to place the screw closer to the acetabular subchondral bone. Additionally, the acetabular fragment should be mobilized by using both the Schanz pin and the bone clamp holding the pubic portion of the free fragment.

POSTOPERATIVE CARE

- Partial weight bearing is reviewed by a physical therapist.
  - Out-of-bed mobilization is permitted on the first postoperative day if a lumbar plexus block is used; day 2 or 3 if an epidural catheter is used.
- Weight bearing is progressed from partial to full, typically by 4 to 6 weeks with radiographic healing and return of abductor strength.
- ROM is limited to 90 degrees of flexion; 10 degrees from full extension; and 10 degrees of adduction, abduction, and rotation for the first 4 to 6 weeks.
- Resistive exercises are avoided for 3 months.
- Patients older than 16 years are given either low-molecular-weight heparin or warfarin for 4 to 6 weeks.
- Nonsteroidal anti-inflammatories are avoided.

OUTCOMES

- Outcomes are generally good to excellent in the appropriately selected patient.
- Hips with minimal arthrosis (more than 2 mm of joint space and no significant subchondral changes) in younger (younger than 35 years old) patients have demonstrated significant improvement in Harris hip and Merle D'Aubigne scores that can last at least 20 years.[1,3,4,6–8]
- Hips with moderate to advanced arthrosis in older patients can still show significant improvement in symptoms. However, their symptom relief may be shorter lived, requiring conversion to either a surface replacement or total hip arthroplasty.

COMPLICATIONS

- Sciatic or lateral femoral cutaneous nerve palsy
- Postoperative wound hematoma requiring return to operating room
- Wound infection
- Nonunion of pubic ramus
- Heterotopic ossification
- Vascular injury
- Intra-articular osteotomy
- Malalignment of fragment leading to insufficient correction or overcorrection

REFERENCES

1. Clohisy JC, Barrett SE, Gordon JE, et al. Periacetabular osteotomy for the treatment of severe acetabular dysplasia. J Bone Joint Surg Am 2005;87(2):254–259.
2. Cunnigham T, Jessel R, Zurakowski D, et al. Delayed gadolinium-enhanced magnetic resonance imaging of cartilage to predict early failure of Bernese periacetabular osteotomy for hip dysplasia. J Bone Joint Surg Am 2006;88(7):1540–1548.
3. Ganz R, Leunig M, Leunig-Ganz K, et al. The etiology of osteoarthritis of the hip: an integrated mechanical concept. Clin Orthop Relat Res 2008;466:264–272.
4. Millis MB, Kim YJ. Rationale of osteotomy and related procedures for hip preservation: a review. Clin Orthop Relat Res 2002;(405): 108–121.
5. Murphy SB, Ganz R, Muller M. The prognosis in untreated dysplasia of the hip. A study of radiographic factors that predict the outcome. J Bone Joint Surg Am 1995;77(7):985–989.
6. Peters CL, Erickson JA, Hines JL. Early results of the Bernese periacetabular osteotomy: the learning curve at an academic medical center. J Bone Joint Surg Am 2006;88(9):1920–1926.
7. Steppacher SD, Tannast M, Ganz R, et al. Mean 20-year followup of Bernese periacetabular osteotomy. Clin Orthop Relat Res 2008; 466:1633–1644.
8. Trousdale RT, Ekkernkamp A, Ganz R. Periacetabular and intertrochanteric osteotomy for the treatment of osteoarthrosis in dysplastic hips. J Bone Joint Surg Am 1995;77(1):73–85.
9. Wenger DE, Kendell KR, Miner MR, et al. Acetabular labral tears rarely occur in the absence of bony abnormalities. Clin Orthop Relat Res 2004;(426):145–150.

12

CHAPTER

Pelvic Osteotomy

Michael J. Beebe, Jill Erickson, and Christopher L. Peters

DEFINITION

- This chapter's focus is the use of pelvic osteotomies for acetabular reorientation for the treatment of symptomatic acetabular dysplasia, including acetabular retroversion.
- The Bernese periacetabular osteotomy (PAO) is a major progression from previously described triple innominate osteotomies (TIO).
  - The TIO was originally described by Le Coeur[30] in 1965. In his technique, the pubis and ischium are osteotomized through a single incision near the symphysis. The ilium is then osteotomized just above the sourcil through a Smith-Petersen approach.
  - In 1973, Steel[46] described his technique for the TIO, in which an incision is made just proximal the gluteal crease and the ischium is divided at the tuberosity. An ilioinguinal approach is then used to divide the ilium, followed by division of the pubis medial to the pectineal tubercle.
  - In 1981, Tönnis modified Steel's TIO by changing the location of the ischial cut so that it runs immediately inferior to the acetabulum and ends proximal to the sacrotuberous and sacrospinous ligaments, improving acetabular mobility.[51] The ischial osteotomy is performed in the prone position, requiring an intraoperative flip to the supine position, where the pubic and iliac osteotomies are performed similar to those described by Steel.
  - In 1982, Carlioz introduced a modification to Steel's technique in which the ischial osteotomy starts just below the acetabulum and runs horizontally, ending between the sacrospinous and sacrotuberous ligaments, leaving the sacrospinous ligament attached to the mobile fragment and the sacrotuberous ligament attached to the stable fragment.[4] The benefit of the Carlioz technique is that it does not require an intraoperative flip.
- *Periacetabular osteotomy* is a general term that describes a series of bony cuts involved in mobilizing the acetabulum from the surrounding innominate bone to allow reorientation but is often used eponymously in reference to Ganz technique for the Bernese PAO.
  - In 1975, Eppright[13] described a barrel-shaped PAO oriented along an anteroposterior axis. This osteotomy allows for increased lateral coverage but limits the amount of achievable anterior coverage.
  - In 1976, Wagner described three separate types of PAO (types I, II, and III).[43]
    - In a type I PAO, a hemispherical cut is made around the acetabulum down to the obturator foramen using a specifically designed chisel. The loosened acetabular fragment is then redirected to allow anterolateral coverage of the femoral head.
    - In a type II PAO, a cut is made similar to type I and autologous bone graft is inserted between the ilium and the acetabular osseous fragment to distalize the acetabular fragment and correct superior subluxation of the femoral head.
    - The type III PAO combines a type I osteotomy with a Chiari-like innominate osteotomy to allow realignment and medialization.
  - The Bernese PAO, originally described by Ganz, uses four or five straight osteotomies to separate the acetabulum from the surrounding innominate bone.[15] It has a number of benefits over other techniques, including the following:
    - It can be performed through a single incision in the supine position.
    - The posterior column of the innominate bone remains intact, greatly improving stability and allowing for immediate postoperative mobilization without a cast or brace.
    - The bone cuts are performed very close to the acetabular center of rotation, facilitating correction of the acetabular fragment.
    - The Bernese PAO reliably results in medialization of the acetabular center of rotation, improving the biomechanics when compared to previously described techniques.[6]
    - The vascularity of the acetabular fragment is preserved via the inferior gluteal artery, allowing simultaneous hip arthrotomy without concern for devascularization of the mobile fragment.

ANATOMY

- The hip differs from most other joints in the body in that it is deep and nonpalpable from the surface, enforcing the importance of understanding the surface anatomy when planning surgical intervention.
  - The anterior landmarks consist of the prominent anterior superior iliac spine (ASIS), anterior inferior iliac spine (AIIS), and the medial aspect of the superior pubic rami.
    - The ASIS serves as the origin of the sartorius.
    - The AIIS serves as the origin of the direct head of the rectus femoris.
    - The medial aspect of the superior pubic ramus serves as insertion for the inguinal falx, rectus abdominis, and pyramidalis.
  - The lateral and posterior landmarks consist of the iliac crest, posterior superior iliac spine (PSIS), and the greater trochanter of the femur.
    - The PSIS serves as the attachment of the oblique portion of the posterior sacroiliac ligaments and the multifidus muscle.

- The greater trochanter serves as the attachment of the gluteus medius (superolateral), gluteus minimus (anterior), vastus lateralis (inferolateral), and short external rotators (medial).
- The iliac crest serves as insertion for multiple abdominal muscles, erector spinae, and the tensor fascia lata (TFL).

- During childhood, the articular cartilage of the acetabulum is continuous medially with the triradiate cartilage, lying between the ilium (superiorly), ischium (inferiorly), and pubis (anteriorly).[41]
  - Triradiate cartilage closure occurs at the halfway point on the ascending limb of the pubertal growth curve, corresponding to an approximate bone age of 12 years for girls and 14 years for boys.[10]
  - The acetabulum is oriented at approximately 48 ± 4 degrees caudal tilt and in 21 ± 5 degrees anteversion.[28] It is hemispherical in shape and covers 170 degrees of the femoral head.[40]
- The hip joint is a highly constrained and inherently stable enarthrodial (ball and socket) diarthrosis (synovial joint), formed by the confluence of the acetabulum with the femoral head.
  - Normal hip range of motion can be highly variable[48] (**FIG 1**).
    - Flexion: 110 to 140 degrees
    - Extension: 10 to 30 degrees
    - Abduction: 40 to 50 degrees
    - Adduction: 25 to 30 degrees
    - Internal rotation: 30 to 50 degrees
    - External rotation: 30 to 60 degrees
  - The cartilage surface of the acetabulum is horseshoe-shaped with an ovoid depression inferomedially, known as *cotyloid fossa*, from which the ligamentum teres arises.
    - The ligamentum originates in the cotyloid fossa and inserts in the fovea capitis femoris, a depression in the femoral head slightly posteroinferior to center.[2]

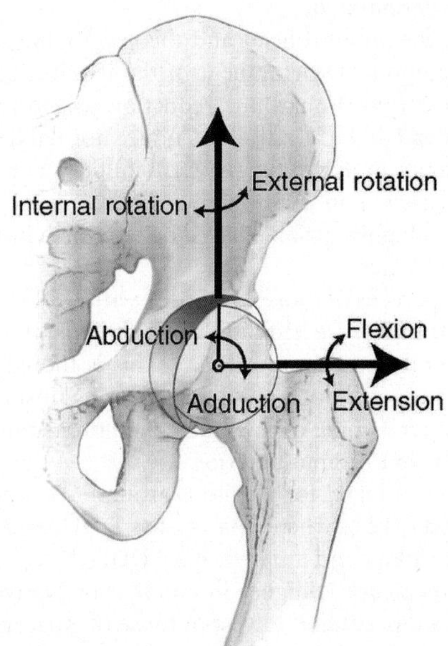

FIG 1 • Axis and movements of the hip joint.

    - The ligamentum teres has been shown to contain small vessels, originating from the obturator artery and ranging from only 0.02 to 0.05 cm. These vessels are able to supply only a small portion of the subfoveal femoral head.[57]
  - Coverage of the acetabulum is increased by the labrum, a fibrocartilaginous ring running circumferentially around the rim and varying in width from approximately 3 to 8 mm (mean, 5.3 ± 2.6 mm). The labrum increases the surface area of the acetabulum, on average, by more than 25% (36.8 vs. 28.8 cm^2) and the volume by more than 30% (41.1 vs. 31.5 cm^2).[49]
    - The fibrocartilaginous labrum attaches to the acetabular articular cartilage through a 1- to 2-mm zone of transition, marked by a zone of calcified cartilage with a well-defined tidemark.[44]
    - The labrum is supplied by radial branches of a periacetabular vascular ring derived from the superior and inferior gluteal arteries, with lesser contributions from the medial and lateral circumflex femoral arteries.[26]
    - The transverse acetabular ligament connects the anteroinferior and posteroinferior horns of the labrum as well as the inferior cotyloid fossa.
- The articular capsule consists of strong and dense collagen fibers arranged in a cylindrical sleeve, connecting the margins of the acetabulum to the proximal femur.[55] Distinct thickening of the articular capsule forms four reinforcing ligaments:
  - The iliofemoral ligament, also known as the *Y-ligament* or the *ligament of Bigelow*, lies anteriorly and has an inverted Y shape. The lateral limb restricts internal and external rotation in extension. The medial limb restricts external rotation in extension.
  - The pubofemoral ligament resembles a sling covering the inferior and medial aspect of the hip joint capsule and tightens with hip extension and abduction. The pubofemoral ligament's main restriction is external rotation in extension.
  - The ischiofemoral ligament lies posteriorly. Its two horizontal bands spiral upward to blend with the zona orbicularis. The ischiofemoral ligament's major contribution to the stability of the hip is in internal rotation.[33]
  - The zona orbicularis is a circumferential ligament surrounding the femoral neck at the lateral edge of the capsule. The fibers of the zona orbicularis are most abundant at the inferoposterior aspect of the capsule and anteriorly blend with the deep surface of the iliofemoral ligament. The zona orbicularis contributes to stability in distraction.[23]
- The hip joint is surrounded by 23 muscles divided into five groups based on function:
  - The flexors are the iliacus, psoas, iliocapsularis, pectineus, rectus femoris (direct and indirect heads), and sartorius muscles.
  - The extensors are the gluteus maximus, semimembranosus, semitendinosus, biceps femoris (long head), and posterior part of the adductor magnus (ischiopubic ramus origin).
  - The abductors are the gluteus medius, gluteus minimus, and TFL.
  - The adductors are the adductor brevis, adductor longus, gracilis, and anterior part of the adductor magnus muscle (ischial tuberosity origin).
  - The external rotators are the piriformis, quadratus femoris, superior gemellus, inferior gemellus, obturator internus, and obturator externus.

- The acetabulum receives its blood supply from the superior gluteal, inferior gluteal, and obturator arteries.[24]
  - The obturator artery, a branch of the internal iliac artery, passes anteroinferiorly across the inner table of the pelvis, where pubic branches supply the quadrilateral plate. After exiting through the upper border of the obturator foramen, the artery splits into anterior and posterior branches. The posterior branch gives off an acetabular branch, which supplies the acetabulum ascending through the cotyloid fossa.
  - The largest branch of the internal iliac artery, the superior gluteal artery, heads posterior between the lumbosacral trunk and the first sacral nerve, passes above the superior edge of the piriformis as it exits the greater sciatic notch, then divides into superficial and deep branches. The deep branches descend to supply the superior rim of the acetabulum.
  - The inferior gluteal artery descends on the sacral plexus before passing below the inferior border of the piriformis, exiting the inferior portion of the greater sciatic notch. Outside the pelvis, a transverse branch runs inferiorly to supply the inferior and posterior region of the acetabulum.
- The corona mortis, an anastomosis between the obturator and external iliac vascular systems traversing cranial to the superior ramus, is present in 83% to 84% of hemipelvis according to two cadaveric studies.[9,52] The anastomosis is found, on average, 6.5 cm lateral to the symphysis (range, 3.0 to 9.0 cm). Thirty-four percent to 36% of hemipelvis have an arterial connection, whereas 60% to 70% have a venous connection and 20% to 27.5% have both.
- The major pelvic innervations of the lumbar plexus originate from the L1, L2, L3, and L4 roots:
  - The femoral nerve (L2–L4) courses through the psoas and emerges on the inferolateral aspect of the psoas. It then travels between the psoas and iliacus, behind the iliac fascia until it passes under the inguinal ligament, before bifurcating into anterior and posterior branches.
  - The lateral femoral cutaneous nerve (LFCN) (L2–L3) emerges from the lateral border of the psoas major and crosses the iliacus muscle toward the ASIS. It then passes under the inguinal ligament medial to the ASIS and over the sartorius in the thigh, where it divides into an anterior and a posterior branch.
    - In two cadaveric studies assessing a total of 63 limbs, the LFCN was always found medial to the ASIS and deep to the inguinal ligament.[19,54] On average, the LFCN was 3.25 cm medial to the ASIS (range, 0.6 to 9.2 cm).
  - The obturator nerve (L2–L4) pierces the psoas major, emerging from its medial border near the brim of the true pelvis. It travels posterior to the common iliac artery, then descends lateral to the internal iliac artery and ureter. It then travels along the lateral wall of the lesser pelvis, superior and anterior to the obturator artery, before exiting through the superior edge of the obturator foramen.
- Major pelvic innervations of the lumbosacral plexus originate from the L4, L5, S1, S2, and S3 roots:
  - The sciatic nerve (L4–S3) exits the greater sciatic foramen and most commonly courses anterior (deep) to the piriformis before crossing posterior (superficial) to the superior gemellus, inferior gemellus, and obturator internus. It then travels down the posterior thigh, crossing below the long head of the biceps femoris.
    - Approximately 17% of limbs have an anomalous path to the sciatic nerve.[45]
      - Type B anomaly, where the common peroneal branch passes through the piriformis and the common tibial traverses below, is present in 80.9% of anomalous specimens.
      - Type C, where the common peroneal branch passes above the piriformis and the common tibial traverses below, is present in 7.6% of anomalous limbs.
      - Type D, in which the entire sciatic nerve passes through the piriformis, is present in 3.1% of anomalous gluteal regions.
      - Type E, in which the common peroneal branch traverses above the piriformis and the tibial passes through the piriformis, and type F, where the entire sciatic nerve passes above the piriformis, are each present in 0.5% of anomalous hindquarters.
  - The superior gluteal nerve leaves the pelvis through the greater sciatic notch above the piriformis, accompanied by the superior gluteal artery and the superior gluteal vein. The superior gluteal nerve provides innervation to the gluteus medius, gluteus minimus, and TFL.
  - The inferior gluteal nerve exits through the greater sciatic notch below the piriformis, accompanied by the inferior gluteal artery and the inferior gluteal vein. The inferior gluteal nerve provides innervation to the gluteus maximus.

PATHOGENESIS

- Developmental dysplasia of the hip (DDH) describes a spectrum of disorders ranging from a shallow acetabulum to a subluxated hip joint to complete dislocation of the hip joint.
- During embryonic development, the limb buds first appear at approximately 4 weeks' gestation.[56] As early as 6 weeks, an area of densely packed cells between the femoral head and triradiate cartilage mark the area of the future hip joint. By 11 weeks, the basic structures of the hip joint are completely differentiated.
- At birth, the femoral head and the acetabulum are primarily cartilaginous. Development of the femoral head and acetabulum requires anatomic reduction as the forces of the femoral head in the acetabulum induce normal development.
- DDH occurs in approximately 10 children per 1000, with approximately 1 in 1000 having a frank dislocation; however, this is highly variable based on sex, birth history, family history, and race.[20]
  - Eighty percent of those diagnosed with DDH are female.[59]
  - The left hip is affected in 60% of patients, the right hip in 20%, and both hips in 20%.[12] This is thought to be due to the adducted position of the left leg against the mother's lumbosacral spine in the most common intrauterine position, the left occiput anterior.
  - The risk of DDH for a child is around 6% when a sibling has DDH, 12% when a parent has DDH, and 36% when both a sibling and a parent have DDH.[60]
  - The prevalence is higher in children of Native American or Sami descent and lowest in those of African descent.[20]
  - Conditions such as oligohydramnios or breech position predispose patients to DDH.[5]

- Changes in DDH vary in severity, but in general, patients considered for a PAO in adolescence or early adulthood will have mild symptoms of DDH. The acetabulum is typically shallow, lateralized, anteverted, and deficient along the anterosuperior rim.[37] The femoral head is usually small and the neck generally has excessive anteversion with an increased neck–shaft angle. The intramedullary canal of the femur is also generally narrow.
  - These changes result in a decrease in contact area between the femoral head and acetabulum as well as increased shear at the cartilage interface.

NATURAL HISTORY

- DDH appears in 29% of primary total hip arthroplasties (THA) in people up to the age of 60 years and 7.7% of THA overall.[14]
- In 1939, Wiberg[58] published on a series of 18 patients (19 hips) with a center edge angle (CEA) less than 20 degrees whom he followed for 4 to 29 years, all of whom developed osteoarthritis. He showed a linear relationship between decreased CEA and the rate of appearance of arthritis.
  - In 1983, Cooperman et al[8] followed 20 patients (32 hips) (mean age, 43 years) with a CEA of less than 20 degrees for an average of 22 years. All hips developed arthritis; however, the authors found no correlation between the rate of arthritis development and CEA, acetabular angle of Sharp, percentage of the femoral head covered by the acetabulum, acetabular depth, or Tönnis angle. Furthermore, they reevaluated Wiberg's[58] data and found that 7 of the 19 hips were subluxated on initial presentation. When these patients were excluded, they found no correlation between the rate of osteoarthritis development and the aforementioned values.
- Murphy et al,[35] in a study of the natural history of DDH, found several criteria that predicted significant arthritis in the hip (Kellgren-Lawrence grade 3 or 4) by the age of 65 years. Poor prognostic factors included the following:
  - CEA of less than 16 degrees
  - Acetabular depth-to-width ratio of less than 38%
  - Tönnis angle of more than 15 degrees
  - Uncovering of the femoral head of more than 31%
  - An acetabulum in which the most cranial point of the dome was at the lateral edge of the acetabulum (peak-to-edge distance)
- In 2005, Jacobsen et al[25] reviewed the upright pelvis radiographs of 4151 adults living in Copenhagen as a subanalysis of the Copenhagen City Heart Study. They excluded patients with off-angle radiographs, previous hip fracture, inflammatory arthritis, treatment of childhood hip disorder, or previous hip surgery other than THA, leaving 3859 patients with an average age of 61 years (range, 22 to 93 years) and a CEA ranging from 6 to 67 degrees. The incidence of dysplasia was 3.3% for men and 3.5% for women using a criterion of CEA less than 20 degrees. Risk factors for joint space narrowing (osteoarthritis) included increasing age, in women only, or a CEA of less than 20 degrees.
  - In 2010, Gosvig et al[18] reported a very similar study on the same group of 4151 patients with slightly altered exclusion criteria of THA, Legg-Calvé-Perthes disease, childhood hip disease, rheumatoid arthritis, and unreadable radiographs. The overall prevalence of acetabular dysplasia was 4.3% in men and 3.6% in women. Using a cutoff CEA of less than 20 degrees, they found a very strong trend toward osteoarthritis in patients with dysplastic hips; however, this did not reach significance ($P = .053$). Age was a significant risk factor for arthritis in both sexes (relative risk = 1.02/year, 95% confidence interval [CI] = 1.007 to 1.02).

PATIENT HISTORY AND PHYSICAL FINDINGS

- A thorough history, including a family history of hip problems, is of particular importance.
- Patients with mild to moderate dysplasia may have a painless hip for three or more decades before developing symptoms.
  - Most often, patients present between their mid-teens to late 40s, with an average age of 25 to 30 years.
  - The duration of pain ranges from months to years.
  - Most patients have seen multiple prior health care providers before an appropriate diagnosis is made, with as many as 15% of the patients having undergone prior surgery for their hip pain.[38]
- In 1991, Klaue et al[27] described acetabular rim syndrome associated with hip dysplasia.
  - Symptoms include knife-sharp pain in the groin and a sensation of locking of the hip that most often occurred after a period of sitting or sometimes after walking.
  - Symptoms could be quickly relieved by repositioning and normal walking could be resumed.
  - Common inciting factors were activities where forced movements of adduction in combination with rotation in either direction occurred, such as pivoting sports.
- Nunley et al[37] reviewed the history and physicals of 57 patients and found that the majority (97%) presented with hip pain of insidious onset, localized to the groin in 72% of patients and to the lateral aspect of the hip in 66%.
  - An increase in pain is associated with walking in 81%, running in 80%, standing in 70%, impact activities in 55%, pivoting on the affected side in 45%, and prolonged sitting in 44%.
  - Eighty percent of patients report catching, clicking, popping, or locking, whereas 48% report a limp and 35% report a limitation in walking distance because of their pain.
- Location and description of the symptoms must be fully delineated as patients may have symptoms related to confounding pathology such as trochanteric bursitis or sacroiliac joint pain, even when the imaging supports a diagnosis of acetabular dysplasia.
- During the physical exam, it is important to assess both the affected limb as well as the normal or less affected limb. A general exam of range of motion, strength, tenderness, and visualization of the landmarks and musculature is paramount. Specific tests include the following:
  - *Gait*—a Trendelenburg gait, when the pelvis falls during the stance phase of the affected side, suggests abductor weakness or hip discomfort. A coxalgic, or antalgic, gait is nonspecific and occurs during any cause of hip pain, represented by a shortened swing phase on the affected side. A short limb gait may be present with DDH, usually occurring through pronation of the long leg and supination and a pelvic drop of the short leg. An abnormal gait is seen in 85% of patients, even when walking a short distance.
  - *Leg length (both apparent and true)*—a leg length discrepancy of less than 1 cm is normal. Patients with severe DDH often have shortening of the affected limb.

- *Anterior impingement test*—also known as the *flexion, adduction*, and *internal rotation test*, the examiner simultaneously flexes (90 to 100 degrees), adducts (10 to 20 degrees), and internally rotates (5 to 20 degrees) the hip. This brings the anterior femoral neck in contact with the anterosuperior rim of the acetabulum, which is the usual site of overload in DDH. A positive test elicits hip pain and reproduces symptoms. Nearly all patients with DDH will test positive for impingement.[37]
- *Apprehension test*—the hip is extended past neutral and then externally rotated. Pain does not indicate a positive test. The test is positive if the patient complains about the feeling of joint subluxation or instability. A positive test indicates an insufficient coverage of the femoral head.
- *Trendelenburg test*—the examiner observes and palpates the pelvis from behind while the patient performs a single-legged stance. A level pelvis in single-legged stance is normal, and dropping of the contralateral hemipelvis indicates abductor weakness of the symptomatic hip. Abductor weakness is found in more than one-third of patients with DDH.[37]
- *Logroll*—the lower extremity is rolled side to side at the proximal thigh with the leg in neutral position. The test is positive if it elicits pain in the groin. Logrolling moves only the femoral head in relation to the acetabulum and the surrounding capsule without significant excursion or stress on the surrounding myotendinous structures or nerves, making it the most specific, but not sensitive, test for intracapsular hip pathology.[3]

IMAGING AND OTHER DIAGNOSTIC STUDIES

- Initial x-ray radiographs should include the standing anteroposterior (AP) pelvis and false-profile views. Optional views include a supine, cross-table lateral, frog-leg lateral, or 90-degree Dunn view. Additionally, a supine AP pelvis with the hip in maximum abduction and internal rotation can be useful to demonstrate hip congruence.
  - Proper positioning of the patient during radiograph procurement is of paramount importance as improper positioning may result in false-positive findings.
  - The standing AP image can be taken with the feet in 15 degrees of internal rotation to offset femoral anteversion.
  - Although the beam will generally be near parallel to the floor, on the AP radiograph, physiologic increase in lumbar lordosis and pelvic tilt must be accounted for so that the tip of the coccyx is within 1 to 3 cm from the superior edge of the pubic symphysis.
  - The false-profile view, originally described by Lequesne and de Sèze[31] in 1961, is a lateral view of the acetabulum taken with the patient standing with the affected hip against the cassette, the pelvis rotated 65 degrees from the AP, and the ipsilateral foot parallel to the cassette.
  - The Dunn view is an AP view of the hip with the patient supine, the hips and knees flexed at 90 degrees, the legs abducted 15 to 20 degrees from the midline, and the femur in neutral rotation, similar to the position a patient would be on the exam table in stirrups.[11]
  - The frog-leg lateral view is obtained with the patient in a standing position. The foot ipsilateral to the affected hip is rested on a step and the affected hip and ipsilateral knee are each flexed approximately 30 degrees. The leg is then externally rotated and abducted.
- The first assessment of any radiograph of a patient being considered for a PAO should evaluate for preexisting osteoarthritis as patients with preexisting degenerative joint disease may not be a candidate for hip preservation surgery, which will be discussed later in this chapter.
- The following should be assessed on the standing AP radiograph:
  - The interrelationship between the anterior and posterior rims of the acetabulum should be evaluated to determine anterior and posterior coverage along with acetabular version. Presence of a crossover sign, where the anterior acetabular rim crosses the posterior rim on the AP radiograph, may represent retroversion of the acetabulum, although this view is sensitive to lumbar lordosis of the patient.[42]
  - The visible edge of the posterior wall should descend through the center point of the femoral head or lateral to it. A medial position, or posterior wall sign, may represent posterior dysplasia.
  - The lateral CEA is traditionally measured using the angle formed by a line drawn perpendicular to a baseline that passes through the center of both femoral heads and a line connecting the center of the femoral head and the edge of the sourcil.[58] A CEA of less than 20 degrees or greater than 39 degrees may be indicative of lateral acetabular dysplasia or relative over coverage of the femoral head, respectively.
    - Anderson et al[1] proposed a more reproducible method for determining the center of the femoral head rather than visual estimation as used by Wiberg.[58] In this method, a computer-generated circle is superimposed over each femoral head, ignoring lateral asphericity, and the center of this circle is used as the basis for the lines used for calculation of the CEA.[1]
  - The Tönnis angle of inclination, also known as the *acetabular index* or *horizontal toit externe* (HTE), is also assessed on the AP radiograph and measures the slope of the weight-bearing region of the acetabulum, or the sourcil.[50] The HTE is assessed by the angle formed by a line drawn horizontally through the medial aspect of both sourcils and a line extending from the medial to lateral edges of the sourcil on either side. Normal values range from 0 to 10 degrees, with those higher and lower values indicating relative dysplasia and overcoverage, respectively (**FIG 2**).
- The false-profile view allows assessment of anterior acetabular coverage through evaluation of the anterior CEA, also

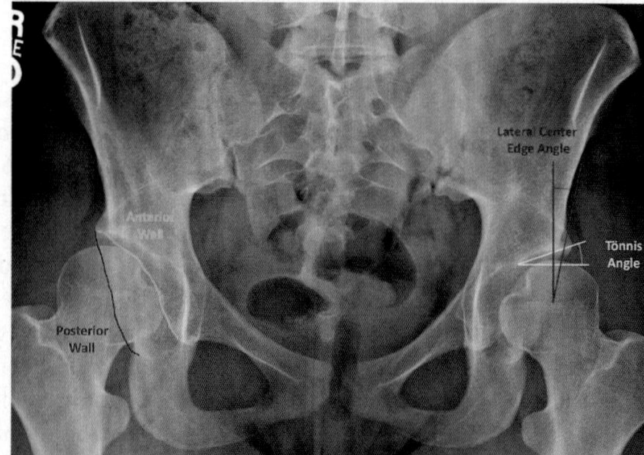

FIG 2 • An AP pelvis radiograph displaying the lateral CEA (*red*) and Tönnis angle (*yellow*) on the left hip and the lateral edge of the anterior (*green*) and posterior (*blue*) walls on the right.

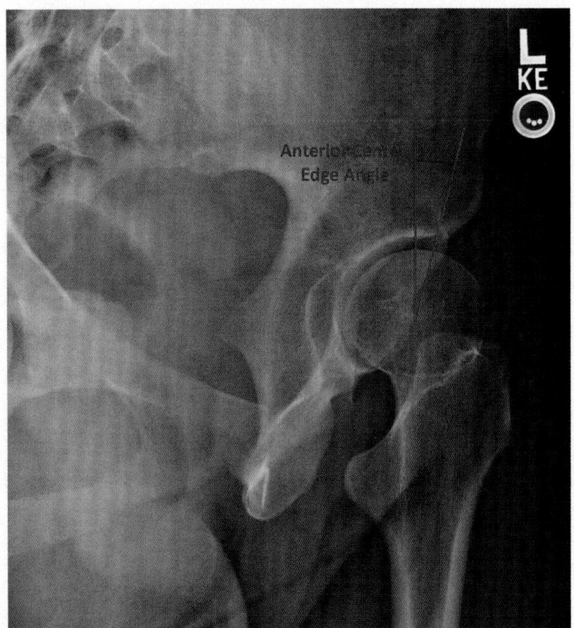

FIG 3 • A false-profile radiograph of the left hip displaying the anterior CEA.

known as the *vertical-center-anterior* (VCA) *angle*. The VCA angle is measured similar to the CEA using the angle formed by a line drawn perpendicular to a baseline that passes through the center of both femoral heads and a line connecting the center of the femoral head to the anterior edge of the dense shadow of the subchondral bone slightly posterior to the anterior edge of the acetabulum.[31] A normal value is that greater than 20 degrees, with lesser values representing anterior dysplasia (**FIG 3**).

- In hip dysplasia, anterolateral femoral head–neck morphology, which is often characterized by a reduced head–neck offset but not necessarily a true cam deformity, can be evaluated on the frog-leg lateral or 90-degree Dunn view.
  - Failure to recognize a decrease of femoral head–neck offset or increased alpha angle preoperatively can cause postoperative anterior femoroacetabular impingement (FAI) through increased anterior acetabular coverage.[36] This potential problem should be anticipated preoperatively and managed intraoperatively when present (**FIG 4**).
- When preoperative radiographs show reason to be concerned for preexisting degeneration of the chondral surface or significant labral pathology, magnetic resonance imaging (MRI) with or without arthrography (MRA) may be useful.
  - MRA is more valuable in delineating pathologic changes to the labrum but less sensitive in evaluating articular cartilage.
  - For evaluation of the chondral surfaces, delayed gadolinium-enhanced MRI of cartilage or T1 and T2 relaxation in the rotating frame (T1 rho, T2 rho) are more sensitive.[17]
- Computed tomography (CT) scans may help the surgeon appreciate acetabular version but are rarely necessary.
  - CT angiogram may be used to assess the integrity of the labrum if an MRA is contraindicated.

DIFFERENTIAL DIAGNOSIS

- Avascular necrosis of the femoral head
- Bursitis
- FAI

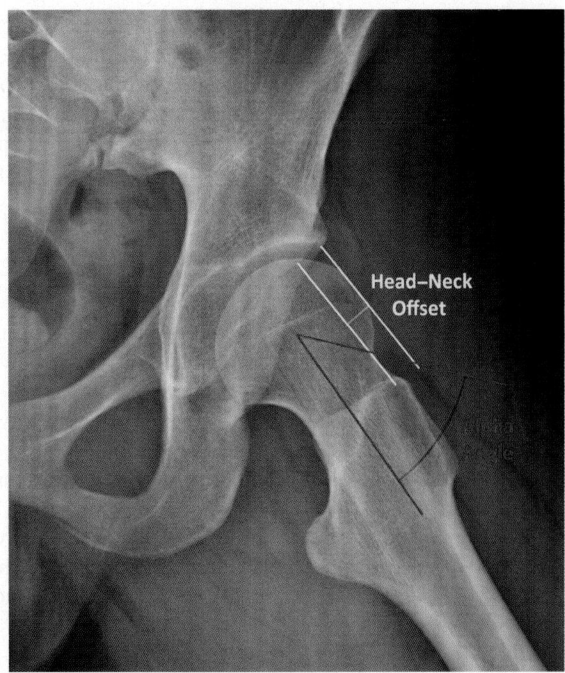

FIG 4 • A Dunn lateral radiograph of the left hip displaying the head–neck offset (*yellow*) and alpha angle (*red*).

- Hernia (inguinal or femoral)
- Infection (eg, septic arthritis)
- Isolated labral tear
- Lumbar spine pathology (eg, disc herniation)
- Malignancy
- Muscle strain/tear
- Pelvic pathology (eg, endometriosis or ovarian cysts)
- Sacroiliac joint pathology (eg, ankylosing spondylitis)
- Femoral neck stress fracture

NONOPERATIVE MANAGEMENT

- Patients who have radiographic findings of dysplasia with no or minimal symptoms should be treated nonsurgically but followed closely and seen in the clinic every 1 to 2 years to evaluate for early signs of joint arthrosis.
- Nonsteroidal anti-inflammatory agents should be used as needed for intermittent symptoms.
- High-impact activities such as running should be avoided as these may induce further strain across the hip joint.
- Steroid injections may be employed but should not be used on a regular basis in young individuals.
- Physical therapy, including hip abductor and core strengthening, may be used with some success.

SURGICAL MANAGEMENT

- Indications for performance of a PAO include a patient with closed triradiate cartilage and symptomatic acetabular dysplasia without preexisting arthrosis.
- Although there is an apparent association between dysplasia and secondary arthrosis, there is potential but no strong evidence that correction of the dysplasia will decrease the development of future arthritis. Thus, a PAO should be a pain-relieving surgery first and a joint-preserving surgery second, not vice versa.

- Although the lower age limit for PAO is dictated by closure of the triradiate cartilage, the upper age limit is more ambiguous. Any patient with dysplasia without arthrosis may be considered, but in North America, most patients are younger than the age of 40 to 45 years, as those with significant dysplasia will often show signs of significant arthritis by the fifth or sixth decade and may be better served by a THA.[16]

Preoperative Planning

- Using imaging obtained prior to surgery, the surgeon should have a plan regarding the amount of correction needed as well as the direction of correction.
- Labs are performed on the day of surgery, including a type and crossmatch for 2 units of packed red blood cells.
- Tranexamic acid can be considered to decrease postoperative bleeding.
  - Tranexamic acid is an antifibrinolytic that competitively inhibits the activation of plasminogen to plasmin, thus preventing degradation of blood plasma proteins, most notably fibrin clots.
  - Although no studies have been performed in patients undergoing PAO, a meta-analysis of the total knee literature has shown that tranexamic acid reduces the amount of blood loss and the number of blood transfusions per patient while showing no difference in the number of deep vein thrombi or pulmonary emboli.[61]
  - Dosing can be weight-based (a single dose of 20 mg/kg intravenously preoperatively) or 1 g intravenously at incision and 1 g intravenously at wound closure.
- General endotracheal anesthesia is often combined with a supplemental epidural, which is continued for 48 hours postoperatively.
- A cell saver is used during the surgery because intraoperative blood loss from the bony cuts is variable but often quite rapid, making blood loss significantly high in some patients, even in the hands of an experienced surgeon (**FIG 5**).

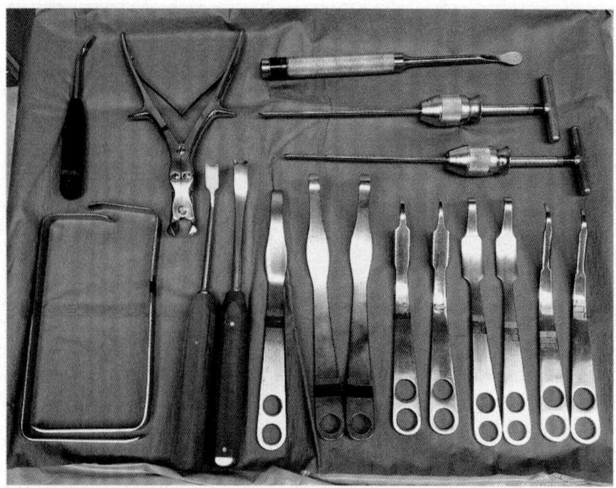

FIG 5 • Common instruments used in completion of a Bernese PAO including wood-handled Ganz osteotomes.

Positioning

- The patient is placed in the supine position on a radiolucent flat-top table for isolated DDH or on a traction table if intracapsular osteochondroplasty is planned in conjunction. The hip is then prepped and draped in a sterile fashion.

Approach

- Five approaches have been described for the Bernese PAO[21]:
  - Classic Smith-Petersen
  - Modified Smith-Petersen
  - Ilioinguinal
  - Direct anterior
  - Two-incision
- The modified Smith-Petersen approach is the most common approach and thus will be described in this chapter.

TECHNIQUES

Approach

- The planned incision begins approximately 3 cm posterior to the ASIS along the iliac crest, extends to a point just lateral to the ASIS, and curves down in line with the lateral border of the sartorius to end approximately 10 cm inferior to the ASIS (**TECH FIG 1**).
- Subcutaneous flaps are raised medially and laterally, aiming to identify the fascia over the TFL muscle belly.
- The interval between the sartorius and the TFL is identified distally and traced proximally, incising sharply in line with the fibers while taking great care taken to identify and avoid direct trauma to the LFCN, which courses through the fascia.
- The inner table of the ilium is exposed at the proximal portion of the incision by reflecting off the abdominal musculature from the iliac crest to a point just lateral to the ASIS.
- The ASIS is osteotomized using an oscillating saw in order to keep the attachment of the sartorius and inguinal ligament in continuity. The ASIS fragment is retracted medially using a Hohmann retractor. Further dissection along the inner iliac wing brings the surgeon to the AIIS and insertion of the direct head of rectus femoris muscle.
- Angled retractors are placed for exposure, the rectus femoris is tagged, and both the direct and indirect heads are reflected off the AIIS and anterior acetabulum, respectively, leaving a stump for future repair.
- A plane over the anterior hip capsule and under the psoas tendon is developed by reflecting off the iliocapsularis muscle fibers using a Cobb elevator.

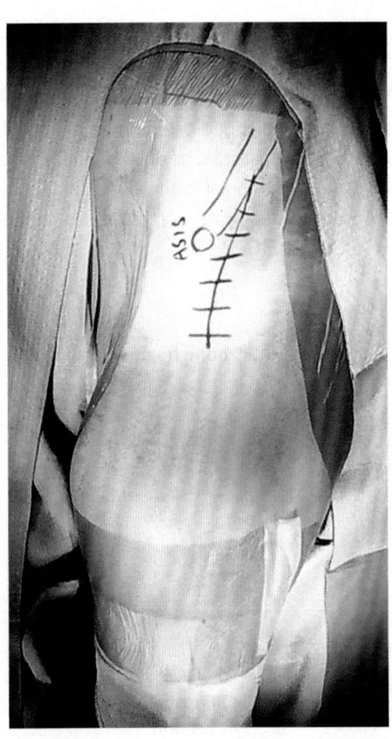

TECH FIG 1 • The planned incision drawn with anatomic landmarks.

Ischial Osteotomy

- Under two-plane image intensification, an angled Ganz osteotome is placed into the infracotyloid groove between the hip capsule (superiorly), obturator foramen (medially), and the hamstrings musculature (laterally).
- The ischial osteotomy most often takes multiple passes. The first two passes of the osteotome are on the inner and outer cortices of the ischium, followed by a central pass to complete the cut.
  - All passes of the osteotome should be visualized using a two-plane image intensification and should end approximately 1 cm anterior to the posterior cortex of the posterior column.
  - The cut on the lateral column is often only 2 to 3 cm in depth. Extreme care should be taken with this cut as the sciatic nerve is in close proximity to the lateral aspect of the ischium (**TECH FIG 2**).

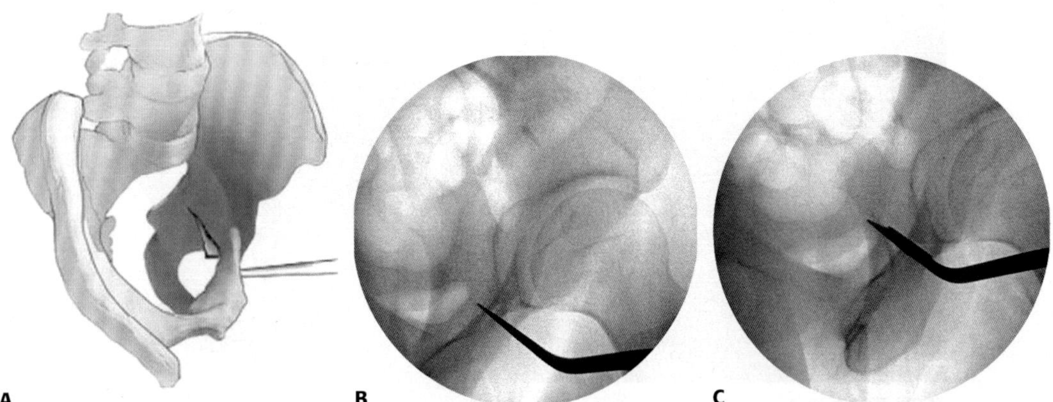

TECH FIG 2 • An illustration of osteotome placement for the ischial cut (**A**). Intraoperative fluoroscopic images of the beginning (**B**) and end (**C**) of the ischial cut. Complete separation of the inner and outer tables often takes three passes.

Pubic Osteotomy

- The hip is flexed and the interval along the pubic ramus is further developed through subperiosteal dissection, retracting the psoas tendon and the femoral neurovascular bundle medially with gentle retraction.
- Curved rami retractors are placed anterior and posterior to the pubic ramus, subperiosteally, to protect from entering the obturator foramen too deeply and injuring the obturator neurovascular bundle.
  - A Hohmann retractor can be malleted into the ramus 1 cm medial to the planned osteotomy site for better exposure.
- A pencil-tip burr is used to begin the osteotomy of the pubis approximately 1 cm medial to the iliopectineal eminence, and a half-inch curved osteotome is employed to complete the pubic osteotomy (**TECH FIG 3**).

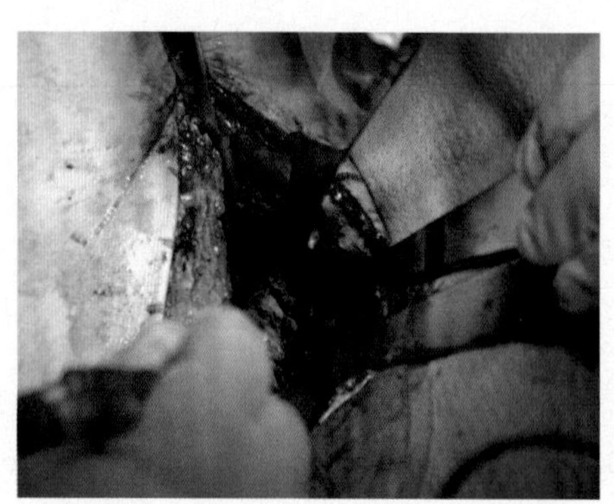

A

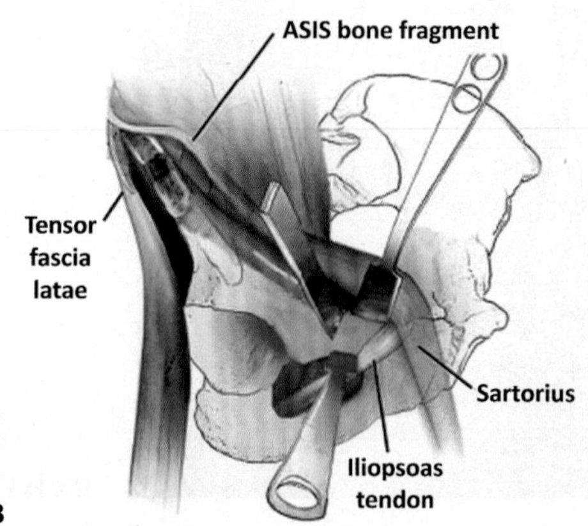

B

TECH FIG 3 • **A.** An intraoperative image of retractor placement prior to the pubic cut. **B.** An illustration of osteotome placement for the pubic cut and surrounding tissues. The pubic cut is often started with a burr prior to completion with an osteotome.

Iliac Osteotomy

- The inner table of the ilium is further exposed through subperiosteal elevation of the iliacus muscle to the level of the greater sciatic notch, where a Hohmann retractor is placed.
- The anterior 1 to 2 cm of the TFL origin are reflected from the outer table of the ilium to allow a Hohmann retractor to be placed for protection of the abductor musculature.
- An oscillating saw is used to make the transverse, posteriorly directed, supra-acetabular cut across the ilium, starting proximal to the AIIS and stopping 1 cm short of the pelvic brim. Two passes are often necessary, one each on the inner and outer table of the ilium.
  - The leg should be extended and slightly abducted for the outside cut and slightly flexed for the inside pass (**TECH FIG 4A,B**).

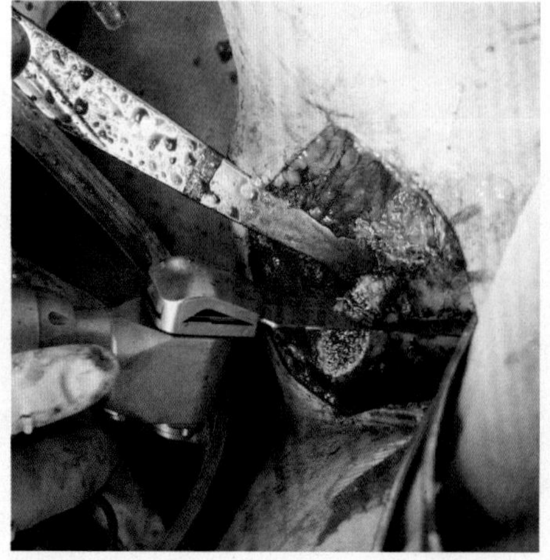

A

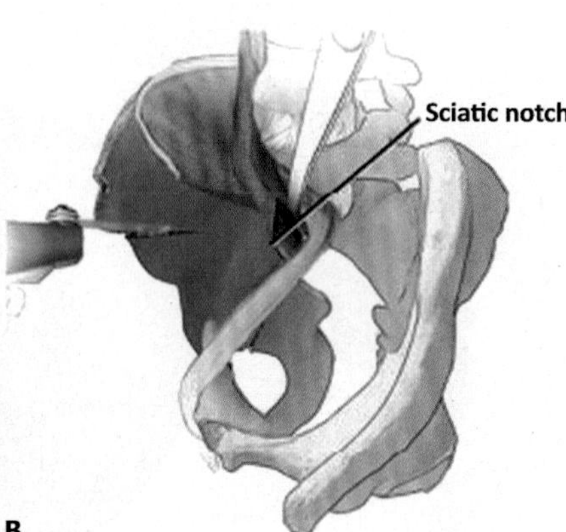

B

TECH FIG 4 • **A.** An intraoperative image of the first iliac osteotomy, a transverse, posteriorly directed cut performed with an oscillating saw. **B.** An illustration of the same cut. Two passes are often necessary, one each on the inner and outer table of the ilium. *(continued)*

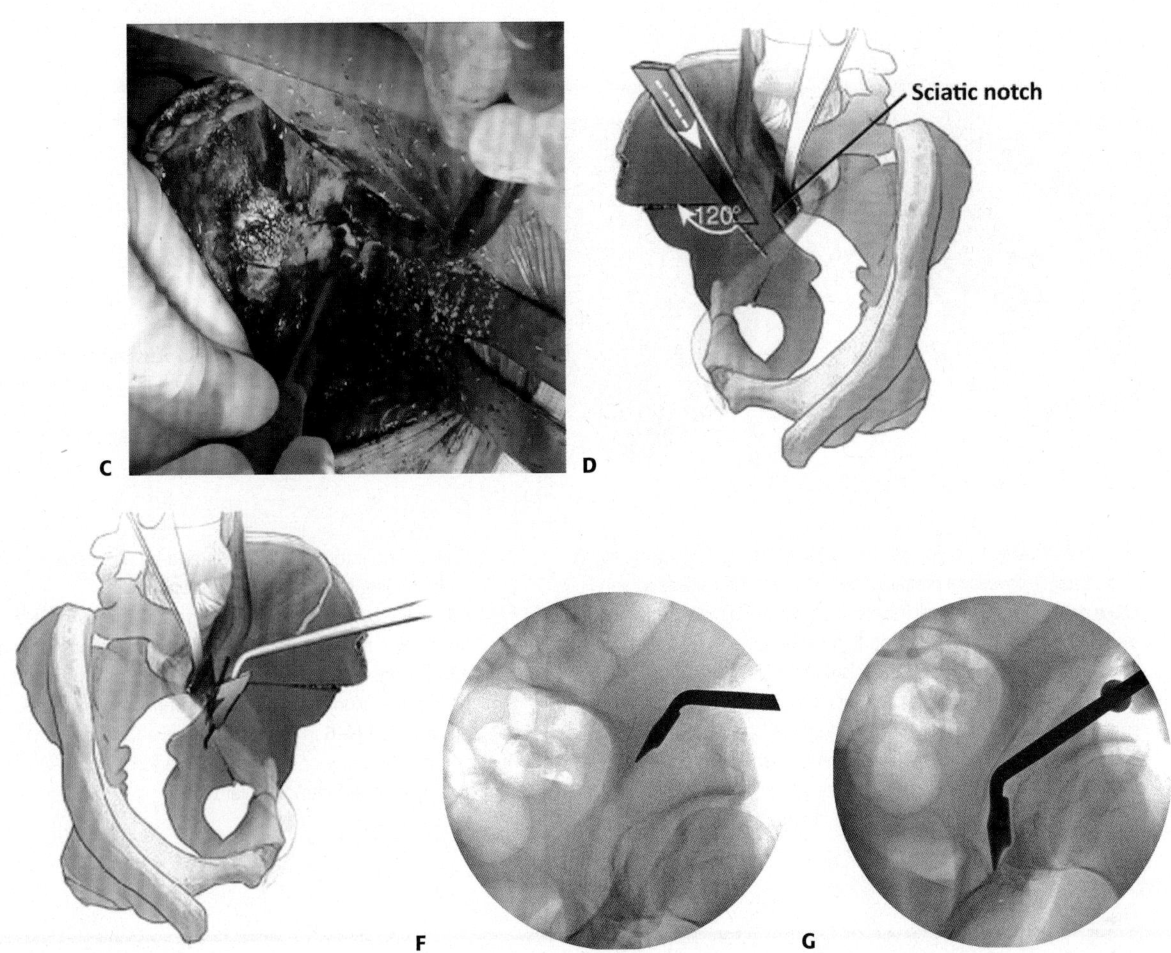

TECH FIG 4 • *(continued)* **C.** An intraoperative image of the burr being used to create a groove at the posterior aspect of the supra acetabular osteotomy for placement of the Ganz osteotome before the second iliac osteotomy. **D.** An illustration of the orientation of the first and second iliac osteotomies. **E.** An illustration of osteotome placement for the second iliac cut between the posterior column and posterior surface of the acetabulum. **F.** Intraoperative fluoroscopic images of the beginning and end (**G**) of the second iliac osteotomy.

- A round-tip burr is used to create a groove angled at approximately 120 degrees, starting from the posterior aspect of the supra-acetabular osteotomy and heading inferiorly toward the ischial spine (**TECH FIG 4C,D**).
- An angled Ganz osteotome is then placed into the grove and passed along the inner table of the quadrilateral plate, under two-plane image intensification, with care taken to stay between the posterior column and posterior surface of the acetabulum. The same osteotome is used to complete the cut through the outer table in a similar fashion. Some surgeons prefer the use of a straight osteotome for the posterior column cut (**TECH FIG 4E–G**).

Mobilization, Correction, and Fixation

- Two Schanz pins are placed into the supra-acetabular region of the mobile fragment for directional control.
  - A circular motion on the Schanz pins can be used to work free any small remaining bony connections between the mobile fragment and stable pelvis.
  - If the osteotomies have been completed, the fragment should mobilize relatively easily. Difficulty in mobilizing the fragment should hint at an incomplete osteotomy. In this situation, it is better to revisit the other osteotomies as loosening of the Schanz pins will result in forced mobilization of the fragment with incomplete osteotomies (**TECH FIG 5**).
- Final positioning of the acetabular fragment is unique to each patient. However, general lateral coverage and anteversion are achieved by a combination of internal rotation and slight adduction of the fragment. This maneuver in turn medializes the acetabular fragment and can be verified by the teardrop moving medial to the ilioischial line. After first ensuring a good quality, a nonrotated AP image of the pelvis and hip with two-plane image intensification is used to verify the final position of the acetabulum, with the goal of a horizontal sourcil and lateral CEA of 20 to 30 degrees.

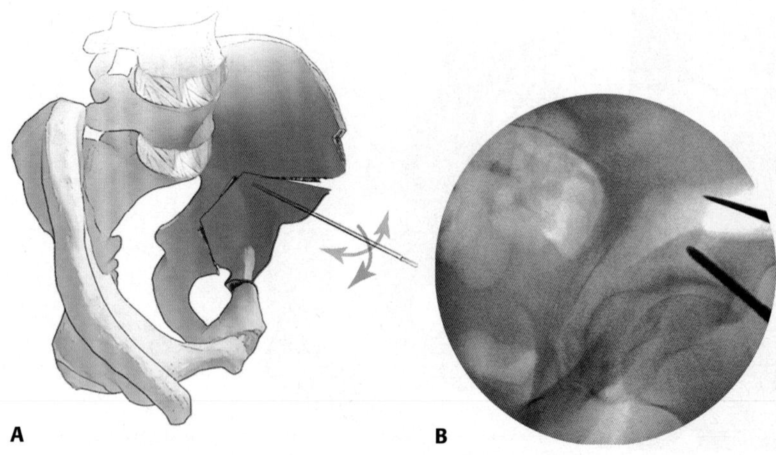

TECH FIG 5 • A. An illustration of the completed osteotomy and Schanz pin placement for assistance in mobilization of the fragment. **B.** Intraoperative fluoroscopic images at the beginning, showing the mobilized acetabular fragment.

  - The ideal final position can be confirmed using a nonsterile assistant to overlay a protractor on the image intensifier's screen.
- Once positioned, two small fragment screws are directed from the stable ilium into the superior portion of the osteotomy fragment and a single large fragment screw is directed from the supra-acetabular region of the mobile fragment into the stable ilium. Some surgeons prefer to place all screws antegrade from the stable ilium to the fragment. Final screw placement is checked with image intensification, and stability, along with range of motion, is assessed.
  - Kirschner wires can be used as needed for provisional fixation.
  - Flexion and internal rotation should be assessed to ensure repositioning has not caused iatrogenic FAI.
  - A Horsley bone cutter can be used to remove the excess bone from the superior aspect of the osteotomy fragment and the resected bone can be placed into the space between the ilium and PAO fragment and impacted into place (see **FIG 6** in the Postoperative Care section).
- At this point, the surgeon may opt to perform an open arthrotomy for any planned intracapsular work.

Closure

- The rectus femoris is reattached to the AIIS through a drill hole and augmented with another no. 1 nonabsorbable stitch.
- A final small fragment screw is used to fix the osteotomized ASIS back into position.
- The TFL, subcutaneous, and skin layers are closed with the surgeon's preference of suture.
  - A deep and superficial drain may be placed if the surgeon prefers.

PEARLS AND PITFALLS

Indications	■ Symptomatic acetabular dysplasia or retroversion ■ Anterior/lateral CEA: <15–20 degrees ■ Tönnis angle (acetabular index): >10–15 degrees ■ Kellgren-Lawrence grade: 0–2
Contraindications	■ Open triradiate cartilage ■ Asymptomatic dysplasia ■ Kellgren-Lawrence grade: 3–4 ■ Age 50 years or older (relative)
Preoperative	■ The patient and family must understand the risks of a highly complex procedure. ■ The surgeon must assess the amount of anticipated correction as well as proximal femoral morphology to avoid iatrogenic impingement.

Technique	▪ Newer rectus-sparing approaches may allow easier early ambulation, improve limb proprioception, and perhaps decrease pain. ▪ The LFCN should be identified and protected during the approach. ▪ The femoral and obturator neurovascular bundles are protected by flexion and adduction. The sciatic nerve is protected by extension and abduction. ▪ Free mobility of the fragment is essential and lack of mobility indicates a likely incomplete osteotomy. ▪ Final positioning of the osteotomy fragment is the most critical step and must be individualized for each patient, with the basic goal of producing a near-horizontal sourcil and an appropriately anteverted acetabulum. A nonsterile protractor may be placed on the fluoroscopy screen to assess positioning. ▪ Ideal patient positioning and imaging at the time of the procedure will help prevent suboptimal fragment positioning. ▪ Early training should involve assisting a surgeon experienced in performing PAO, cadaver-based dissection and osteotomy training, and a mentoring relationship with a senior surgeon who is willing to assist and monitor early cases.
Arthrotomy/ arthroscopy	▪ Arthrotomy at the time of PAO is considered conventional but is not always necessary, nor should it be considered the standard of care.[39] ▪ Pre-PAO hip arthroscopy by an experienced arthroscopist may allow better preoperative assessment of articular cartilage damage and allow staged treatment of labral pathology or abnormal femoral neck morphology prior to performance of a PAO, but it is not standard of care.

POSTOPERATIVE CARE

- Patients should anticipate a 4- to 5-day hospital stay, especially when an epidural is used for postoperative pain control for the first 48 hours.
- For anticoagulation, a single dose of low-molecular-weight heparin is given 24 hours postoperatively and then restarted 12 hours after epidural removal until discharge.
  - Unless stronger anticoagulation is indicated by a personal or direct family history of deep vein thrombosis or clotting disorder, patients who are ambulating well are discharged on a full-strength (325 mg) aspirin daily for 6 weeks.
- After removal of the epidural, patients begin ambulation with 50% weight bearing on the affected extremity for 6 weeks. After the 6-week follow-up appointment, patients may slowly transition to weight bearing as tolerated.
- At the 6-week point, patients are prescribed physical therapy for abductor and core strengthening.
  - Patients should expect a mild limp for around 3 months postoperatively.
- At both the 6-week and 3-month follow-up appointments, standard postoperative imaging is obtained to evaluate interim bony healing (**FIG 6**).

OUTCOMES

- In 2008, Steppacher et al[47] reported on a 20-year follow-up of the first 63 patients (75 cases) who underwent Bernese PAO by Ganz. They were able to contact 58 patients, accounting for 68 of the original 75 cases.
  - Forty-one hips (60%) were preserved at 20 years. Hips with Tönnis grade 0 or 1 preoperatively (n = 52) had a survivorship of 75%, whereas those with a preoperative grade 2 or 3 hips (n = 16) had a survivorship of 13%. In those hips that survived, the Tönnis grade increased, on average, 0.7 from baseline.
  - The average Merle d'Aubigné and Postel score decreased in comparison to the previously reported 10-year value (15.8 vs. 16.7), but it was still slightly higher than patients' preoperative scores (15.8 vs. 15.2). A score of 18 is excellent, 15 to 17 is good, 13 to 14 is fair, and below 13 is poor.[34]
- Several studies have reported on midterm follow-up after PAO (average follow-up, 6 to 12 years).
  - Matheney et al[32] described outcomes on 135 hips followed for 9 ± 2.2 years. At final follow-up, 102 hips (76%) remained preserved, with a Western Ontario and McMaster Universities Arthritis Index (WOMAC) pain score of lower than 10. Seventeen underwent THA at an average of 6.1 years after the PAO and 16 had a WOMAC pain score of 10 or higher. Kaplan-Meier analysis, with arthroplasty as the end point, revealed a survival rate of 96% (95% CI, 93% to 99%) at 5 years and 84% (95% CI, 77% to 90%) at 10 years.
  - Troelsen and colleagues[53] reported on 116 PAOs followed for an average of 6.8 years. Kaplan-Meier analysis showed a hip survival rate of 81.6% at 9.2 years. The median physical component score on the Short Form-36 at final follow-up was 48.31, whereas a nonaffected population has a mean score of 50 ± 10. The median pain score on the visual analog scale was 0 at rest and 1 after 15 minutes of normal walking.
  - Kralj et al[29] in 2005 described 26 patients (26 hips) with a mean follow-up of 12 years (range, 7 to 15 years). Four hips (15%) required conversion to THA at a mean of 4.5 years (range, 2 to 7 years). All four hips had preoperative Tönnis grade 2 or 3 osteoarthritis. Thirteen hips (50%) had no radiographic signs of arthritis, but the Tönnis grade increased, on average, 0.8 from preoperative values.

COMPLICATIONS

- A meta-analysis on complications after PAO revealed that 62% of the studies make note of the substantial learning curve and the potential for a higher complication rate during a surgeon's initial cases.
- Reported major complication rates range from 6% to 37%.[7]
  - The most commonly reported complications included the following:
    - Symptomatic heterotopic ossification
    - Wound hematomas
    - Major nerve (sciatic or femoral) palsies

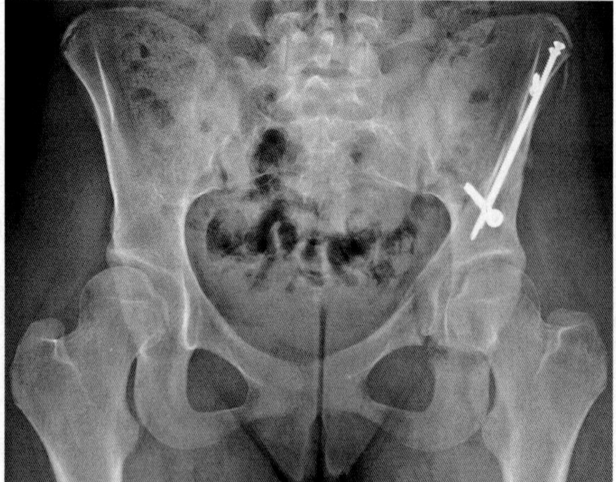
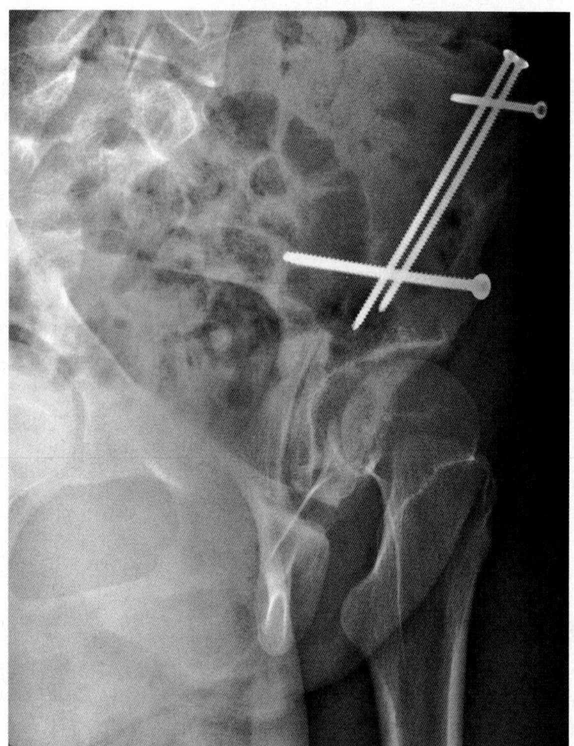
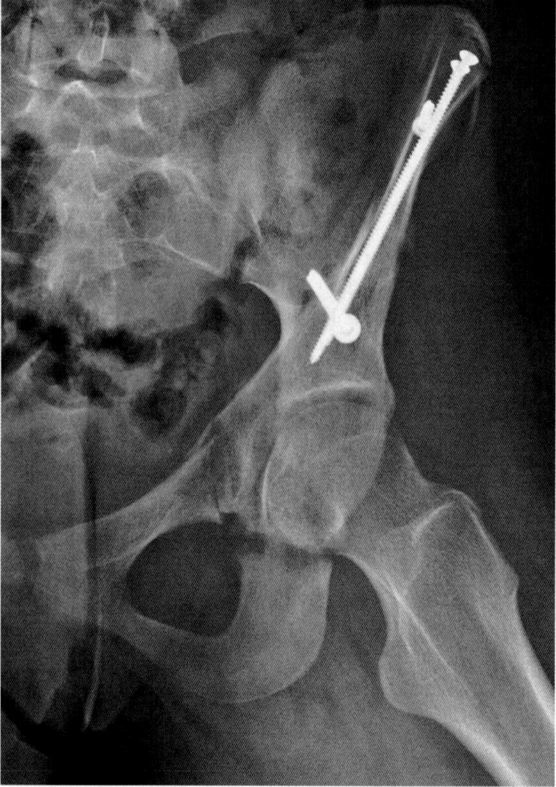

FIG 6 • Postoperative AP (**A**), false-profile (**B**), and Dunn lateral (**C**) radiographs showing final acetabular fragment position and screw fixation.

- Minor nerve (lateral femoral cutaneous) dysfunction
- Intra-articular osteotomies
- Loss of fixation
- Malreduction
- Symptomatic hardware
- Nonunion of at least one osteotomy

- Less common complications included the following:
  - Deep vein thrombosis
  - Pulmonary embolism
  - Arterial laceration or thrombosis
  - Intra-articular fracture
  - Infection
  - Major blood loss requiring transfusion
  - Femoral head or acetabular osteonecrosis
  - Posterior column discontinuity
  - Nonunion requiring revision surgery

- In 1999, Hussell et al[22] reported on the technical complications in his first 508 consecutive cases. Thirteen of the 508 patients (2.6%) required a salvage arthroplasty due to complications. Eighty-five percent of the complications occurred within the first 50 PAOs performed. Complications consisted of the following:
  - Intra-articular extension (n = 11, 2.2%)
  - Malreduction (n = 11, 2.2%)
  - Single osteotomy nonunions (n = 7, 1.4%)
  - Posterior column fractures (n = 6, 1.2%)
  - Fragment osteonecrosis (n = 5, 1.0%)
  - Brooker type IV heterotopic ossification (n = 5, 1.0%)
  - Sciatic nerve palsy (n = 5, 1.0%)
  - Failure of fixation (n = 4, 0.8%)
  - Postoperative subluxation of the femoral head (n = 4, 0.8%)
  - Femoral nerve palsy (n = 3, 0.6%)

REFERENCES

1. Anderson LA, Gililland J, Pelt C, et al. Center edge angle measurement for hip preservation surgery: technique and caveats. Orthopedics 2011;34(2):86.
2. Bardakos NV, Villar RN. The ligamentum teres of the adult hip. J Bone Joint Surg Br 2009;91(1):8–15.
3. Byrd JW. Evaluation of the hip: history and physical examination. N Am J Sports Phys Ther 2007;2(4):231–240.
4. Carlioz H, Khouri N, Hulin P. Triple juxtacotyloid osteotomy [in French]. Rev Chir Orthop Reparatrice Appar Mot 1982;68(7): 497–501.
5. Chan A, McCaul KA, Cundy PJ, et al. Perinatal risk factors for developmental dysplasia of the hip. Arch Dis Child Fetal Neonatal Ed 1997;76(2):F94–F100.
6. Clohisy JC, Barrett SE, Gordon JE, et al. Medial translation of the hip joint center associated with the Bernese periacetabular osteotomy. Iowa Orthop J 2004;24:43–48.
7. Clohisy JC, Schutz AL, St John L, et al. Periacetabular osteotomy: a systematic literature review. Clin Orthop Relat Res 2009;467(8): 2041–2052.
8. Cooperman DR, Wallensten R, Stulberg SD. Acetabular dysplasia in the adult. Clin Orthop Relat Res 1983;(175):79–85.
9. Darmanis S, Lewis A, Mansoor A, et al. Corona mortis: an anatomical study with clinical implications in approaches to the pelvis and acetabulum. Clin Anat 2007;20(4):433–439.
10. Dimeglio A. Growth in pediatric orthopaedics. J Pediatr Orthop 2001;21(4):549–555.
11. Dunn DM. Anteversion of the neck of the femur; a method of measurement. J Bone Joint Surg Br 1952;34(2):181–186.
12. Dunn PM. Perinatal observations on the etiology of congenital dislocation of the hip. Clin Orthop Relat Res 1976;(119):11–22.
13. Eppright R. Dial osteotomy of the acetabulum in the treatment of dysplasia of the hip. J Bone Joint Surg Am 1975;57:1172.
14. Furnes O, Lie SA, Espehaug B, et al. Hip disease and the prognosis of total hip replacements. A review of 53,698 primary total hip replacements reported to the Norwegian Arthroplasty Register 1987-99. J Bone Joint Surg Br 2001;83(4):579–586.
15. Ganz R, Klaue K, Vinh TS, et al. A new periacetabular osteotomy for the treatment of hip dysplasias. Technique and preliminary results. Clin Orthop Relat Res 1988;(232):26–36.
16. Garbuz DS, Awwad MA, Duncan CP. Periacetabular osteotomy and total hip arthroplasty in patients older than 40 years. J Arthroplasty 2008;23(7):960–963.
17. Ginnetti J, Erickson J, Peters C. Periacetabular osteotomy: intra-articular work. Instr Course Lect 2012;62:279–286.
18. Gosvig KK, Jacobsen S, Sonne-Holm S, et al. Prevalence of malformations of the hip joint and their relationship to sex, groin pain, and risk of osteoarthritis: a population-based survey. J Bone Joint Surg Am 2010;92(5):1162–1169.
19. Grothaus MC, Holt M, Mekhail AO, et al. Lateral femoral cutaneous nerve: an anatomic study. Clin Orthop Relat Res 2005;(437):164–168.
20. Guille JT, Pizzutillo PD, MacEwen GD. Development dysplasia of the hip from birth to six months. J Am Acad Orthop Surg 2000;8(4): 232–242.
21. Hussell JG, Mast JW, Mayo KA, et al. A comparison of different surgical approaches for the periacetabular osteotomy. Clin Orthop Relat Res 1999;(363):64–72.
22. Hussell JG, Rodriguez JA, Ganz R. Technical complications of the Bernese periacetabular osteotomy. Clin Orthop Relat Res 1999;(363):81–92.
23. Ito H, Song Y, Lindsey DP, et al. The proximal hip joint capsule and the zona orbicularis contribute to hip joint stability in distraction. J Orthop Res 2009;27(8):989–995.
24. Itokazu M, Takahashi K, Matsunaga T, et al. A study of the arterial supply of the human acetabulum using a corrosion casting method. Clin Anat 1997;10(2):77–81.
25. Jacobsen S, Sonne-Holm S, Soballe K, et al. Hip dysplasia and osteoarthrosis: a survey of 4151 subjects from the Osteoarthrosis Substudy of the Copenhagen City Heart Study. Acta Orthop 2005;76(2):149–158.
26. Kalhor M, Horowitz K, Beck M, et al. Vascular supply to the acetabular labrum. J Bone Joint Surg Am 2010;92(15):2570–2575.
27. Klaue K, Durnin CW, Ganz R. The acetabular rim syndrome. A clinical presentation of dysplasia of the hip. J Bone Joint Surg Br 1991;73(3):423–439.
28. Kohnlein W, Ganz R, Impellizzeri FM, et al. Acetabular morphology: implications for joint-preserving surgery. Clin Orthop Relat Res 2009;467(3):682–691.
29. Kralj M, Mavcic B, Antolic V, et al. The Bernese periacetabular osteotomy: clinical, radiographic and mechanical 7-15-year follow-up of 26 hips. Acta Orthop 2005;76(6):833–840.
30. Le Coeur P. Correction des défauts d'orientation de l'articulation coxofémorale par ostéotomie de l'isthme iliaque. Rev Chir Orthop 1965;51:211–212.
31. Lequesne M, de Seze S. False profile of the pelvis. A new radiographic incidence for the study of the hip. Its use in dysplasias and different coxopathies. Rev Rhum Mal Osteoartic 1961;28:643–652.
32. Matheney T, Kim YJ, Zurakowski D, et al. Intermediate to long-term results following the Bernese periacetabular osteotomy and predictors of clinical outcome. J Bone Joint Surg Am 2009;91(9):2113–2123. doi:10.2106/JBJS.G.00143.
33. Martin HD, Savage A, Braly BA, et al. The function of the hip capsular ligaments: a quantitative report. Arthroscopy 2008;24(2):188–195.
34. Matta JM. Fractures of the acetabulum: accuracy of reduction and clinical results in patients managed operatively within three weeks after the injury. J Bone Joint Surg Am 1996;78(11):1632–1645.
35. Murphy SB, Ganz R, Muller ME. The prognosis in untreated dysplasia of the hip. A study of radiographic factors that predict the outcome. J Bone Joint Surg Am 1995;77(7):985–989.
36. Myers SR, Eijer H, Ganz R. Anterior femoroacetabular impingement after periacetabular osteotomy. Clin Orthop Relat Res 1999;(363):93–99.
37. Nunley RM, Prather H, Hunt D, et al. Clinical presentation of symptomatic acetabular dysplasia in skeletally mature patients. J Bone Joint Surg Am 2011;93(suppl 2):17–21.
38. Peters CL, Erickson JA, Anderson L, et al. Hip-preserving surgery: understanding complex pathomorphology. J Bone Joint Surg Am 2009;91(suppl 6):42–58.
39. Peters CL, Sierra RJ. Report of breakout session: intraarticular work during periacetabular osteotomy—simultaneous arthrotomy or hip arthroscopy? Clin Orthop Relat Res 2012;470(12):3456–3458.
40. Philippon MJ. The role of arthroscopic thermal capsulorrhaphy in the hip. Clin Sports Med 2001;20(4):817–829.
41. Ponseti IV. Growth and development of the acetabulum in the normal child. Anatomical, histological, and roentgenographic studies. J Bone Joint Surg Am 1978;60(5):575–585.
42. Reynolds D, Lucas J, Klaue K. Retroversion of the acetabulum. A cause of hip pain. J Bone Joint Surg Br 1999;81(2):281–288.
43. Schramm M, Hohmann D, Radespiel-Troger M, et al. The Wagner spherical osteotomy of the acetabulum. Surgical technique. J Bone Joint Surg Am 2004;86(suppl 1):73–80.
44. Seldes RM, Tan V, Hunt J, et al. Anatomy, histologic features, and vascularity of the adult acetabular labrum. Clin Orthop Relat Res 2001;(382):232–240.
45. Smoll NR. Variations of the piriformis and sciatic nerve with clinical consequence: a review. Clin Anat 2010;23(1):8–17.
46. Steel HH. Triple osteotomy of the innominate bone. J Bone Joint Surg Am 1973;55(2):343–350.
47. Steppacher SD, Tannast M, Ganz R, et al. Mean 20-year followup of Bernese periacetabular osteotomy. Clin Orthop Relat Res 2008;466(7):1633–1644.
48. Svenningsen S, Terjesen T, Auflem M, et al. Hip motion related to age and sex. Acta Orthop Scand 1989;60(1):97–100.
49. Tan V, Seldes RM, Katz MA, et al. Contribution of acetabular labrum to articulating surface area and femoral head coverage in adult hip joints: an anatomic study in cadavera. Am J Orthop (Belle Mead NJ) 2001;30(11):809–812.
50. Tönnis D. Normal values of the hip joint for the evaluation of X-rays in children and adults. Clin Orthop Relat Res 1976;119:39–47.
51. Tönnis D, Behrens K, Tscharani F. A modified technique of the triple pelvic osteotomy: early results. J Pediatr Orthop 1981;1(3):241–249.

52. Tornetta P III, Hochwald N, Levine R. Corona mortis. Incidence and location. Clin Orthop Relat Res 1996;(329):97–101.
53. Troelsen A, Elmengaard B, Soballe K. Medium-term outcome of periacetabular osteotomy and predictors of conversion to total hip replacement. J Bone Joint Surg Am 2009;91(9):2169–2179.
54. Uzel M, Akkin SM, Tanyeli E, et al. Relationships of the lateral femoral cutaneous nerve to bony landmarks. Clin Orthop Relat Res 2011;469(9):2605–2611.
55. Wagner FV, Negrao JR, Campos J, et al. Capsular ligaments of the hip: anatomic, histologic, and positional study in cadaveric specimens with MR arthrography. Radiology 2012;263(1):189–198.
56. Watanabe RS. Embryology of the human hip. Clin Orthop Relat Res 1974;(98):8–26.
57. Wertheimer LG, Lopes Sde L. Arterial supply of the femoral head. A combined angiographic and histological study. J Bone Joint Surg Am 1971;53(3):545–556.
58. Wiberg G. Studies on dysplastic acetabula and congenital subluxation of the hip joint, with special reference to the complication of osteoarthritis. Acta Chir Scand 1939;83(suppl 58):1–135.
59. Wilkinson JA. A post-natal survey for congenital displacement of the hip. J Bone Joint Surg Br 1972;54(1):40–49.
60. Wynne-Davies R. Acetabular dysplasia and familial joint laxity: two etiological factors in congenital dislocation of the hip. A review of 589 patients and their families. J Bone Joint Surg Br 1970;52(4):704–716.
61. Yang ZG, Chen WP, Wu LD. Effectiveness and safety of tranexamic acid in reducing blood loss in total knee arthroplasty: a meta-analysis. J Bone Joint Surg Am 2012;94(13):1153–1159.

Surgical Dislocation of the Hip

Farshad Adib and Young-Jo Kim

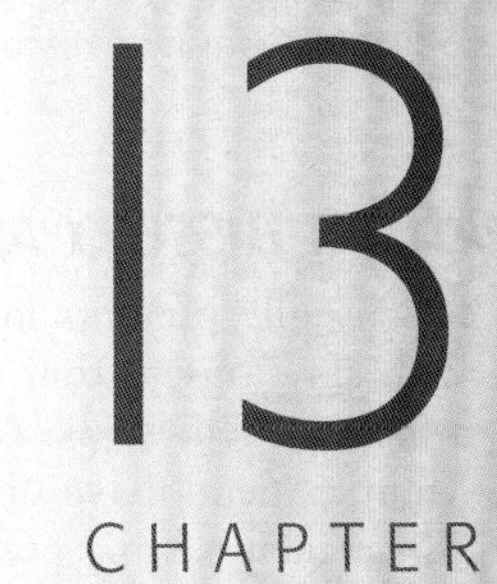

DEFINITION

- Surgical dislocation of the hip can be done safely to treat a number of conditions, including femoroacetabular impingement (FAI), labral tears, chondral injuries, reduction of femoral neck fractures, femoral head, acetabular fractures, excision of tumors, reduction of acute severe slipped capital femoral epiphysis (SCFE), or any condition that requires wide complete access to the hip joint.[14,15]
- There is little morbidity associated with this procedure, and avascular necrosis of the femoral head is a rare complication.[5]
- This technique allows functional assessment of motion intraoperatively which is the most critical step in the treatment of FAI. Majority of reoperations after FAI treatment is due to under- or overcorrection.[4]
- Also, surgical hip dislocation approach is comprehensive enough to assess and treat extra-articular impingement at the same time.[16]

ANATOMY

- The blood supply to the femoral head is mainly from the medial femoral circumflex artery (MFCA) (**FIG 1A**).[17]
- The intact external rotator muscles, most notably the obturator externus muscle, protect the MFCA during the dislocation (**FIG 1B**).[7]

PATHOGENESIS

- In FAI, anatomic deformity leads to abnormal contact between the proximal femur and the acetabular rim at the terminal extent of motion. This repetitive collision damages the soft tissue structures within the joint.[3]
- In cam impingement, an abnormal prominence on the femoral neck passes into the hip beneath the labrum and mechanically damages the labrum and cartilage of the acetabulum.
- Pincer impingement occurs with overcoverage of the acetabular rim impinging on the anterior femoral neck or head–neck junction with terminal flexion.
  - Both cam and pincer impingement can, and frequently do, coexist.
- The early chondral and labral lesions that occur in physically active adolescents and young adults can progress and result in degenerative joint disease of the hip.
- Causes of FAI can be idiopathic, secondary to an SCFE, anterior overcoverage of the hip with a retroverted acetabulum, residual deformity from Perthes disease, or posttraumatic changes.

NATURAL HISTORY

- A pistol grip deformity of the femoral head has been associated with early arthrosis of the hip.[9]
- End-stage osteoarthrosis of the hip, once thought to be mainly idiopathic, is now believed to be a result of mild deformities similar to those caused by childhood diseases of the hip such as developmental hip dysplasia, SCFE, and Legg-Calvé-Perthes.[1]

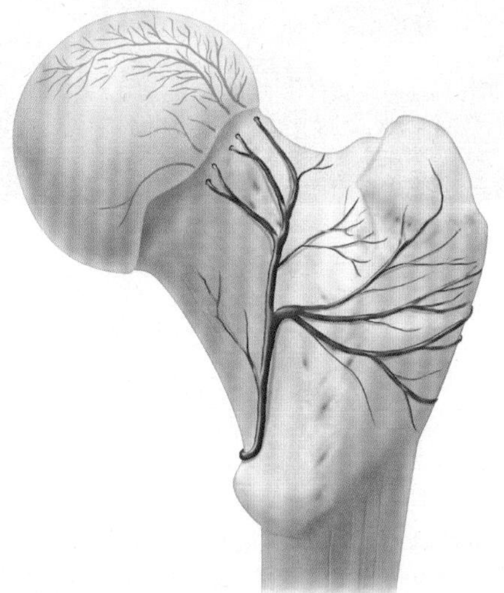

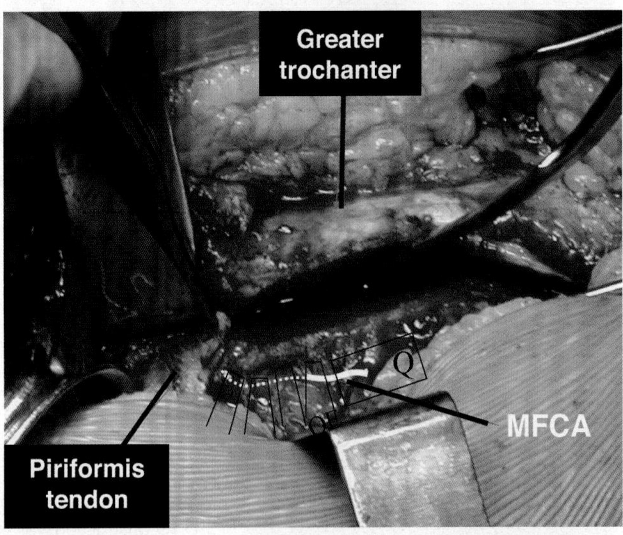

FIG 1 • **A.** Vascular anatomy of the femoral head. Note the proximity of the terminal branches of the MFCA to the insertion of the piriformis tendon. **B.** Intraoperative photograph showing the path of the MFCA over and behind the intact short external rotators, including the quadratus femoris (*Q*) and the obturator externus (*OE*).

PATIENT HISTORY AND PHYSICAL FINDINGS

- FAI usually presents in active adolescents or young adults with slow onset groin pain, which may be exacerbated by athletic activities.
- Many patients have difficulty sitting for long periods and adjust their seating posture to decrease lumbar lordosis to allow less flexion at the hips. Frequently, they complain of difficulty getting into or out of a car.
- There can be a family history of hip pain, early arthrosis, or hip arthroplasty.
- Patients may walk with an antalgic gait, favoring the side of impingement. A foot progression angle externally rotated may indicate a chronic SCFE or femoral retroversion.
- The impingement test, if positive, shows reproducible groin pain with internal rotation, which is relieved with external rotation.
- The physical examination should include both flexion and internal rotation range-of-motion tests.
  - Patients with impingement will have less than 90 degrees of true hip flexion.
  - Patients with impingement will have less internal rotation in flexion than extension and may have a compensatory external rotation of the hip as it is flexed.
- Radiographic findings of FAI are common in the normal, healthy population; therefore, it is paramount that good clinical–radiographic correlation be done. Additionally, other causes of hip pain such as osteoid osteoma, stress fracture, osteonecrosis are ruled out.

IMAGING AND OTHER DIAGNOSTIC STUDIES

- Plain radiographs should include an anteroposterior (AP) view of the pelvis and a lateral view of the hip (**FIG 2A,B**).

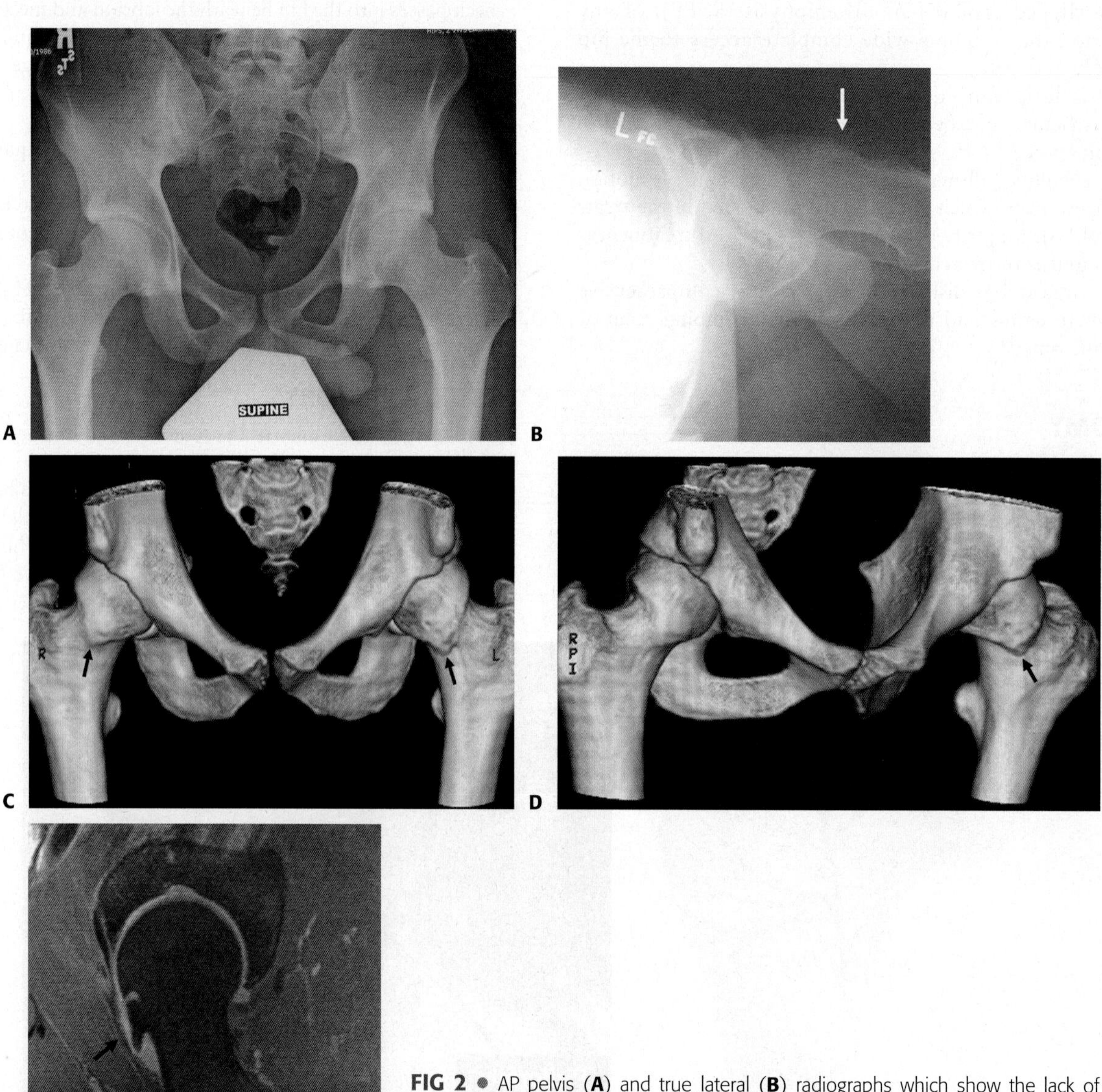

FIG 2 • AP pelvis (**A**) and true lateral (**B**) radiographs which show the lack of femoral head–neck offset anteriorly (*arrow* in **B**) that is causing cam impingement. 3-D reconstructions of the same pelvis from an AP (**C**) and a slightly left rotated (**D**) perspective. The large "bumps" (*arrows*) obscuring the anterior femoral head–neck junction account for the lack of offset appreciated in **B. E.** T1-weighted sagittal magnetic resonance imaging (MRI) showing a large anterior osteophyte (*arrow*).

The maximal deformity of the head–neck junction in FAI could be localized best by the 45-degree Dunn view.[10]

- Computed tomography (CT) scans with two- and three-dimensional (3-D) reconstructions are helpful for preoperative planning and detecting subtle femoral head–neck junction prominence (**FIG 2C,D**).
- Magnetic resonance imaging can further delineate the labral and cartilage pathology (**FIG 2E**). If the study is performed with gadolinium and high-resolution sagittal oblique or radial sequences, labral pathology can be detected.

DIFFERENTIAL DIAGNOSIS

- FAI
- Labral tear
- Hip dysplasia
- SCFE
- Acetabular retroversion

NONOPERATIVE MANAGEMENT

- Nonoperative management includes cessation of aggravating activities and symptomatic treatment using nonsteroidal anti-inflammatories.
- Physical therapy to strengthen the hip musculature does not address the mechanical impingement of FAI but may have a role in affecting pelvic inclination.

SURGICAL MANAGEMENT

- Hip pathology may be addressed through hip arthroscopy. However, it may be difficult to dynamically assess hip mechanics before and after débridement.
- Femoral head–neck osteoplasty may be performed through an anterior approach to the hip without a surgical dislocation. However, the articular cartilage of the acetabulum and most of the femoral head cannot be evaluated with this limited approach.

Preoperative Planning

- All imaging studies are reviewed.
- The lack of femoral head–neck offset is best appreciated on the 45-degree Dunn lateral view of the hip (see **FIG 2A,B**) or on the radial reformats of CT or magnetic resonance (MR) scans around the femoral neck axis or 3-D reconstruction of a CT scan.
- A CT scan that includes cuts through the distal femoral condyles may be used to accurately measure the amount of femoral version.[11]
- After general anesthesia is administered, the patient's hips are examined. The amount of true hip flexion and internal and external rotation with the hip extended and hip flexed are noted and compared to the preoperative assessment.

Positioning

- The patient is placed in the full lateral position, secured on a pegboard. A flat-top cushion (with a half-moon–shaped cutout for the down leg) placed beneath the operative side helps to stabilize the leg during the approach (**FIG 3A–C**).
- A hip drape with a sterile side bag is used, which will capture the leg during the dislocation maneuver (**FIG 3D**).

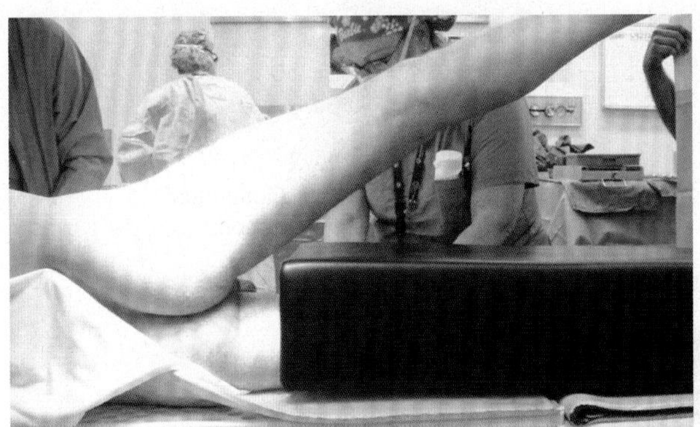
A

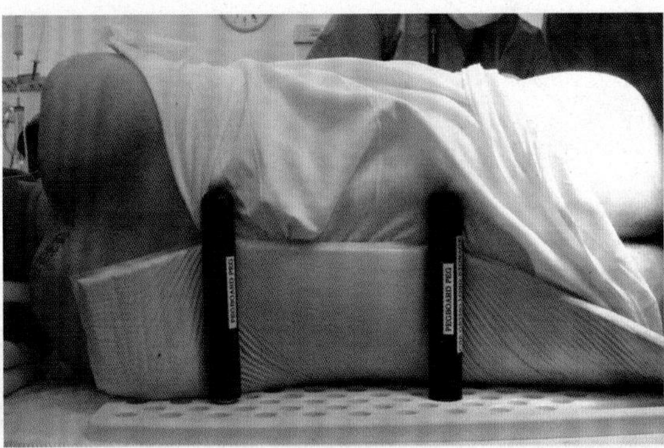
B

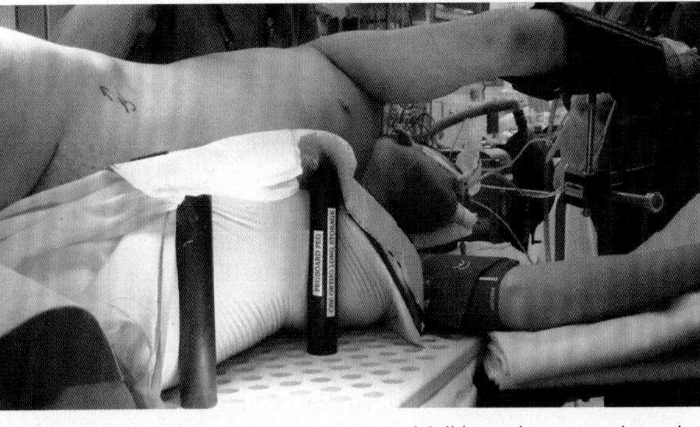
C

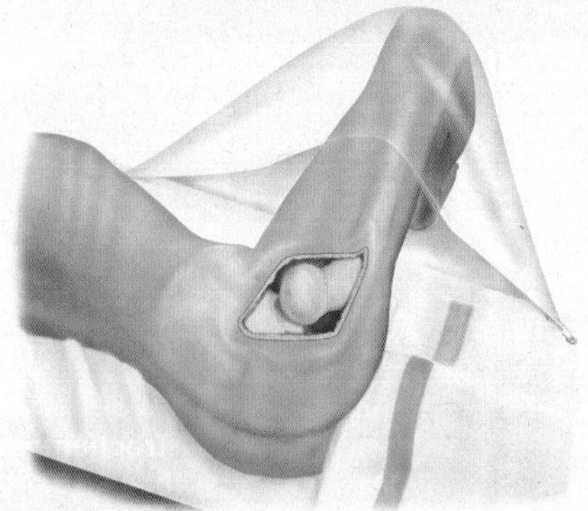
D

FIG 3 • **A–C.** The patient is positioned full lateral on a pegboard. Before patient preparation, the surgeon should ensure that the leg can be flexed and adducted fully and is not blocked by the anteroinferior peg. **D.** Position of the leg in the sterile leg holder after dislocation. The hip is flexed, adducted, and externally rotated.

Approach

- The approach consists of an anterior dislocation through a Kocher-Langenbeck or a Gibson approach with a trochanteric flip osteotomy (**FIG 4A,B**).
- A Kocher-Langenbeck incision is followed by splitting the gluteus maximus muscle.
- The abductors and gluteus maximus muscles can be spared by performing a Gibson approach, which proceeds between the gluteus medius and maximus (**FIG 4C,D**).[8]
  - The Gibson approach may result in less hip extensor dysfunction but may make anterior exposure more difficult.
- A Z-shaped capsulotomy is made to allow entry to the hip joint while protecting the deep branch of the MFCA (**FIG 4E**).[5]

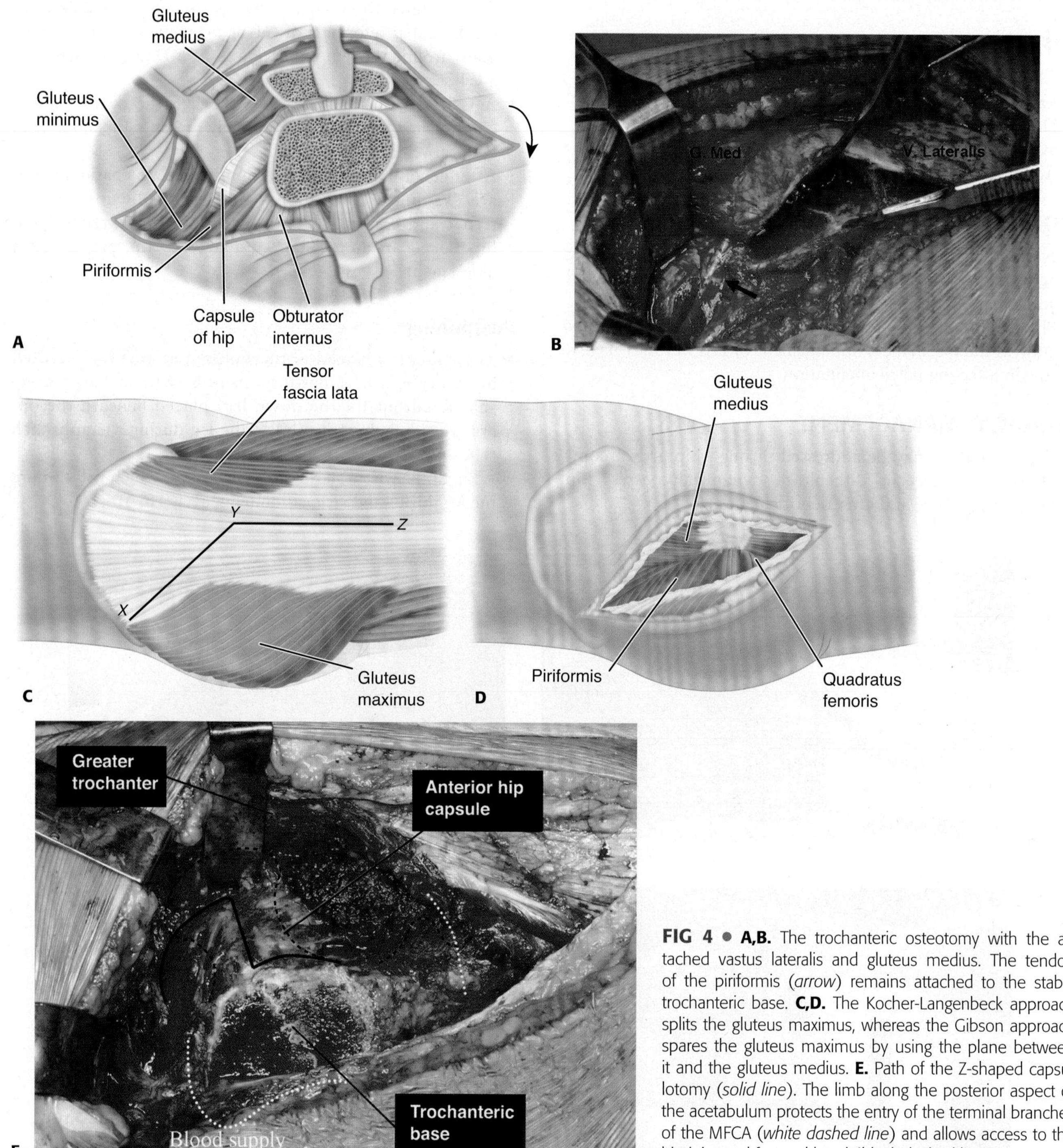

FIG 4 • **A,B.** The trochanteric osteotomy with the attached vastus lateralis and gluteus medius. The tendon of the piriformis (*arrow*) remains attached to the stable trochanteric base. **C,D.** The Kocher-Langenbeck approach splits the gluteus maximus, whereas the Gibson approach spares the gluteus maximus by using the plane between it and the gluteus medius. **E.** Path of the Z-shaped capsulotomy (*solid line*). The limb along the posterior aspect of the acetabulum protects the entry of the terminal branches of the MFCA (*white dashed line*) and allows access to the hip joint and femoral head (*black dashed line*).

Surgical Hip Dislocation by a Transtrochanteric Approach

Approach to Hip Capsule

- A longitudinal lateral incision is made, centered over the junction between the anterior and middle thirds of the greater trochanter (**TECH FIG 1A**).
- The fascia lata is split distally in line with the incision. The proximal dissection progresses through the interval between the anterior edge of the gluteus maximus and the tensor (**TECH FIG 1B**).
- The proximal 4 to 5 cm of fascia of the vastus lateralis is incised, and the vastus muscle fibers are reflected anteriorly.
- The gluteus maximus, along with the fascia of the gluteus medius, which is left on the undersurface of the gluteus

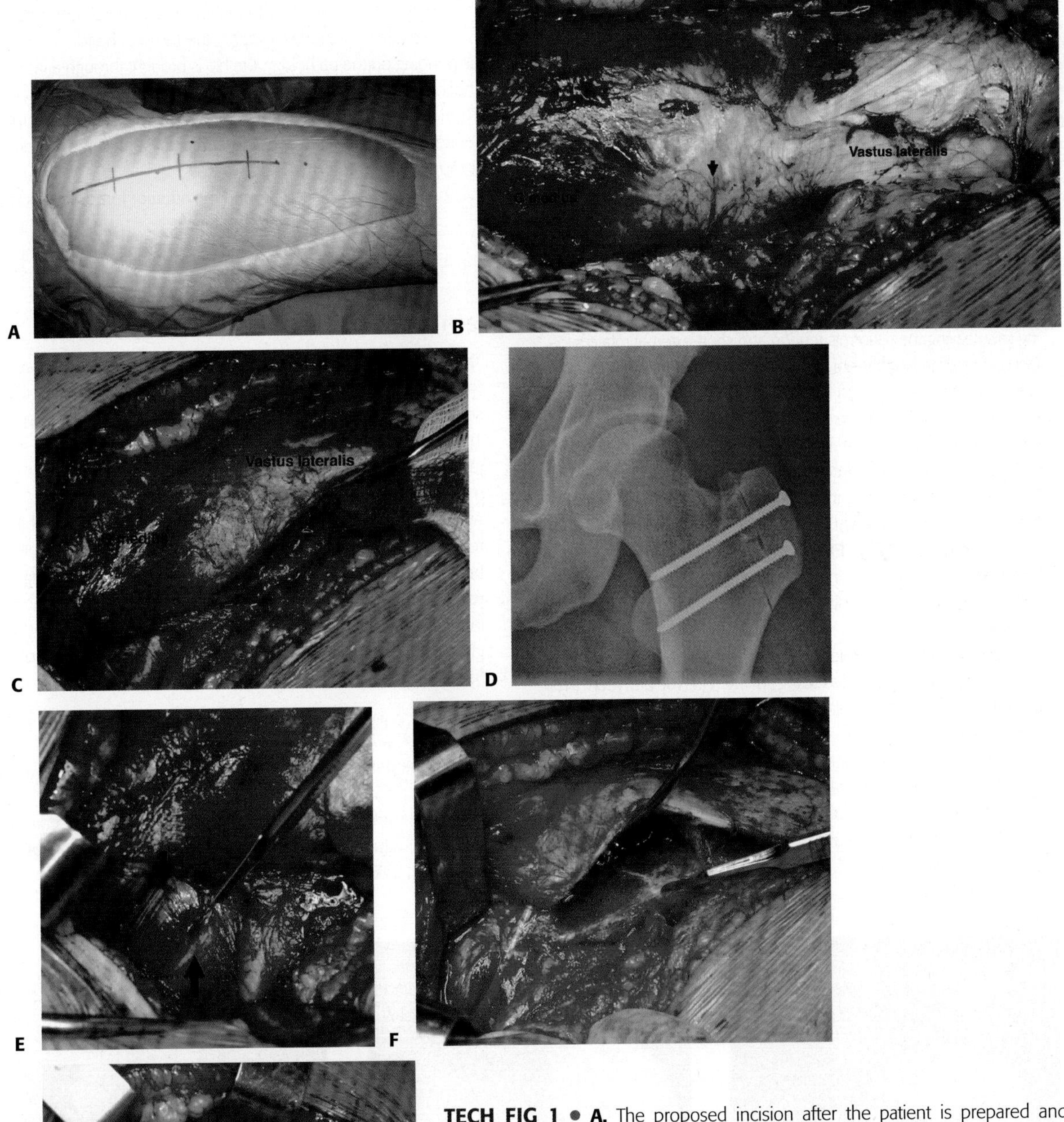

TECH FIG 1 • **A.** The proposed incision after the patient is prepared and draped. **B.** The Gibson approach is between the gluteus maximus and medius. Note the trochanteric branches of the MFCA on the greater trochanter (*black arrow*). **C.** The trochanteric osteotomy is made with an oscillating saw. **D.** A step cut osteotomy provides improved stability and healing of the trochanteric osteotomy. **E.** The fascia over the piriformis tendon (*bottom arrow*) is divided to develop the interval between it and the capsular minimus (*top arrow*). **F.** A 1- to 1.5-cm trochanteric wafer is lifted anteriorly with the gluteus medius and vastus lateralis left attached. **G.** The anterior capsule is completely exposed before the arthrotomy is made.

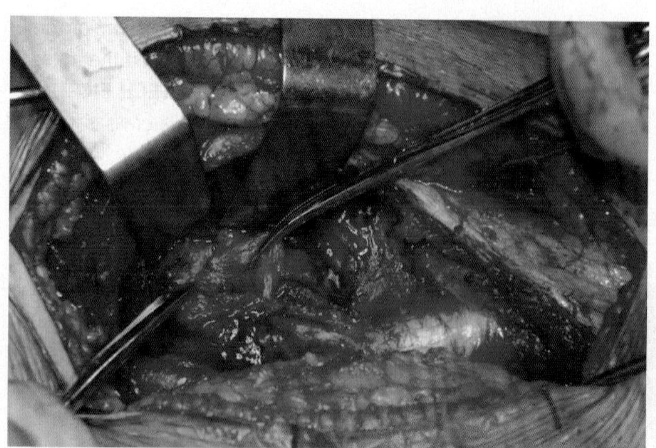

TECH FIG 2 • The longitudinal limb of the capsulotomy is first made. This will allow visualization and prevent inadvertent cutting of the labrum while the posterior limb of the capsulotomy is made.

maximus for protection, is reflected posteriorly to expose the gluteus medius and insertion.

- A 1- to 1.5-cm thick trochanteric osteotomy is made with an oscillating saw, leaving the piriformis tendon and short external rotators intact on the remaining base of the greater trochanter (**TECH FIG 1C**).
- A trochanteric step cut can be performed using two saw blades 6 mm apart if a relative neck lengthening is not planned. This provides excellent stability of the trochanteric osteotomy with lower rates of trochanteric delayed union (**TECH FIG 1D**).
- The fascia overlying the piriformis tendon is incised to identify the tendon and the interval between the piriformis and capsular minimus muscles (**TECH FIG 1E**).
- The trochanteric wafer is next reflected and flipped anteriorly with its attached sleeve of vastus lateralis and the gluteus medius (**TECH FIG 1F**).
- The capsular minimus is elevated in an anterior direction off the hip capsule by carefully dissecting in the interval between the posterior edge of the capsular minimus and the piriformis tendon (**TECH FIG 1G**).
  - An assistant may use a right angled retractor to assist with the exposure of the capsule.
  - Progressive hip flexion, external rotation, and adduction further aid the exposure.
- The hip capsule is exposed up to the rim of the acetabulum.

Hip Arthrotomy and Dislocation

- A Z-shaped capsulotomy is then performed, with the longitudinal arm of the Z in line with the anterior neck of the femur (**TECH FIG 2**).
  - The distal arm of the capsulotomy extends anteriorly well proximal to the lesser trochanter.
  - The proximal arm is extended posteriorly along the acetabular rim, just distal to the labrum and well proximal to the retinacular branches of the MFCA entering the capsule posteriorly to supply the femoral head.
- Depending on the pathology, the hip is brought through a range of motion to determine areas of impingement in a dynamic fashion.
- The leg is then placed in the sterile side bag, flexed, externally rotated, and adducted while the hip is subluxated anteriorly through the arthrotomy.
  - A bone hook placed around the anterior femoral neck may be needed to subluxate the hip.
  - The ligamentum teres is then divided using curved meniscus scissors to allow full dislocation of the hip.

Dynamic Assessment and Osteoplasty

- The entire femoral head and acetabulum can now be assessed for chondral flaps or labral tears, which can be repaired using suture anchors spaced about 7 to 10 mm apart or débrided.
- The aspherical segment of the femoral head at the head–neck junction can be resected using a quarter-inch osteotome and rongeur (**TECH FIG 3A,B**).
- After reestablishing sphericity of the femoral head, the hip is reduced and the results of the débridement are assessed by bringing the hip through a range of motion and confirming the relief of impingement and improvement in range of motion.
- Intraoperative fluoroscopy showing a lateral of the hip in 90 degrees of flexion will determine if the femoral head–neck offset has been reestablished (**TECH FIG 3C**).

Osteotomy Fixation

- The trochanteric wafer is reduced and held in position with a towel clip.
- Three 3.5-mm small fragment screws are placed to secure the trochanter. Fluoroscopy confirms reduction and fixation of the osteotomy (**TECH FIG 4**).

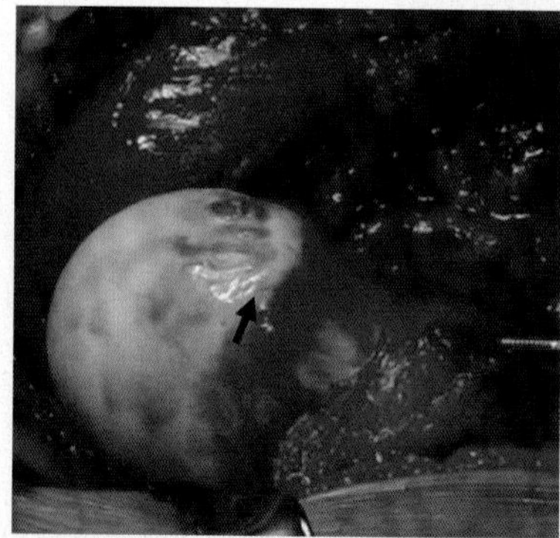
A

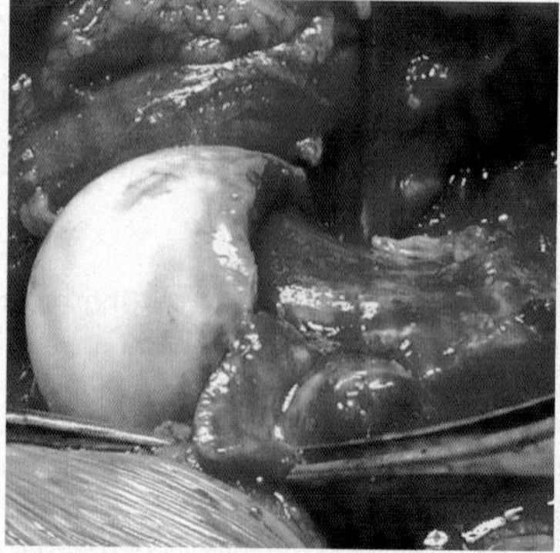
B

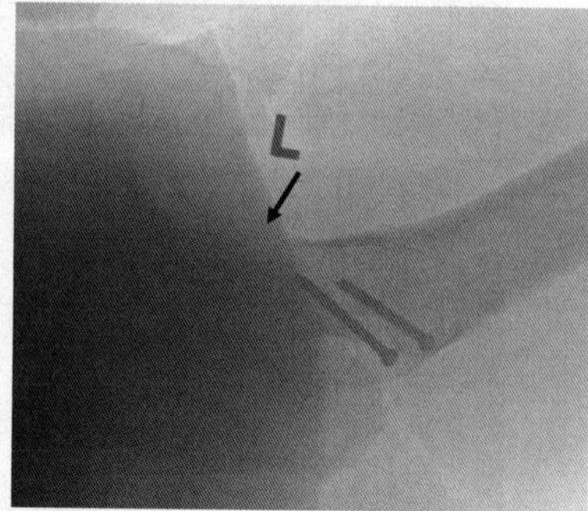

C

TECH FIG 3 • **A.** The hips have been dislocated, and the lack of femoral head–neck offset as well as the cartilage damage is readily apparent (*black arrow*). **B.** The femoral head–neck offset has been restored, eliminating the cam-type FAI. **C.** The *black arrow* shows the restoration of the femoral head–neck offset (compare with **FIG 2B**).

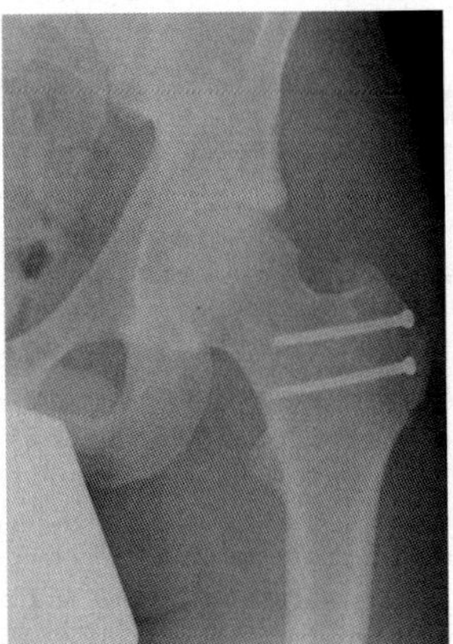

TECH FIG 4 • The trochanteric osteotomy is fixed with two or three 3.5-mm screws.

- Alternatively, 4.0-mm cannulated screws or 4.5-mm cortical screws may be used for trochanteric fixation.

Closure

- The Z-shaped capsulotomy is loosely repaired using absorbable 2-0 suture (**TECH FIG 5**).

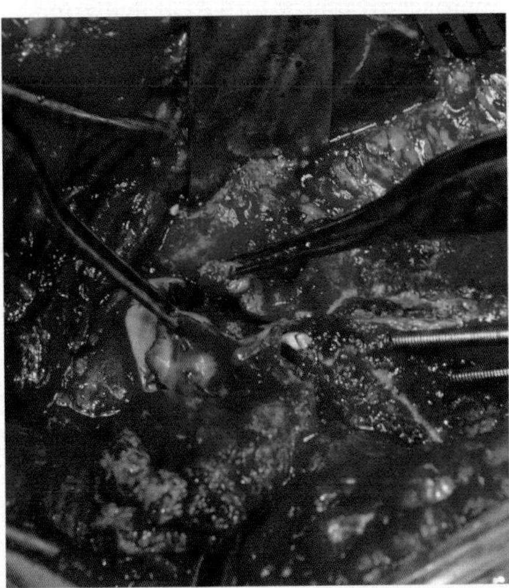

TECH FIG 5 • The Z-shaped capsulotomy is loosely reapproximated with absorbable suture.

- The fascia of the vastus lateralis is closed with a running absorbable suture. The fascia lata and the fascia between the tensor and gluteus maximus are reapproximated.
- Skin is closed in routine fashion.

PEARLS AND PITFALLS

Indications	▪ A complete history and physical examination should be performed. ▪ All associated pathology should be addressed.
Approach	▪ Exposure may be easier when the gluteus maximus is split as opposed to the Gibson approach.
Trochanteric osteotomy	▪ A small muscular cuff of gluteus medius may be left on the stable trochanteric base so the blood supply from the MFCA is not disrupted. ▪ After scoring the greater trochanter, the full thickness of the trochanter should first be cut anteriorly to safely assess the size of the wafer.
Heterotopic ossification	▪ If a large portion of capsular minimus is left on the capsule during the dissection, the patient may develop heterotopic ossification.
Femoral neck fracture	▪ Aggressive resection of the bone at the femoral head–neck junction can weaken the bone and theoretically cause a fracture during relocation or dislocation of the hip.

POSTOPERATIVE CARE

- The hip is held flexed and in neutral rotation by placing two pillows under the leg and one under the greater trochanter.
- The patient is placed in a continuous passive motion machine for 6 hours a day, set from 30 to 80 degrees of flexion.
- Prophylaxis for deep venous thrombosis is individualized; however, all patients should be started on mechanical compression devices immediately.
- After the epidural is removed (if used), out-of-bed ambulation is permitted with one-sixth body weight partial weight bearing.
- Range-of-motion exercises are started, but care is taken to protect the greater trochanter osteotomy by limiting adduction to midline and avoiding resisted abduction exercises for 6 weeks.
- Some patients may benefit from heterotopic ossification prophylaxis using indomethacin.
- AP view of the pelvis or hip and true lateral hip radiographs are obtained 6 weeks postoperatively. Weight bearing is increased to full, and hip strengthening exercises are prescribed.

OUTCOMES

- Ganz et al[6] has performed over 1200 surgical hip dislocations with no cases of osteonecrosis reported.
- Generally, outcomes are excellent if the correct pathology is addressed in a joint without significant preexisting arthrosis.
- In a clinical assessment in adults by Murphy et al[12] using the Merle d'Aubigné scale, hip scores improved significantly.

- Almost 80% of patients were satisfied with results of surgical dislocation approach treatment for FAI at midterm.[13]

COMPLICATIONS

- Avascular necrosis of the femoral head can occur if care is not taken to follow the technique and to preserve the retinacular vessels.
- Femoral neck fracture if the femoral head–neck junction is aggressively débrided.
- Sciatic or femoral nerve neurapraxia
- Greater trochanteric nonunion
- Heterotopic ossification
- Repeat labral tear
- Continued arthrosis of the joint
- Painful postoperative joint adhesions[2]

REFERENCES

1. Aronson J. Osteoarthritis of the young adult hip: etiology and treatment. Instruct Course Lect 1986;35:119–128.
2. Beck M. Groin pain after open FAI surgery: the role of intraarticular adhesions. Clin Orthop Relat Res 2009;467:769–774.
3. Clohisy JC, Kim YJ. Femoroacetabular impingement research symposium. J Am Acad Orthop Surg 2013;21(suppl 1):vi–viii.
4. Clohisy JC, Nepple JJ, Larson CM, et al. Persistent structural disease is the most common cause of repeat hip preservation surgery. Clin Orthop Relat Res 2013;471(12):3788–3794.
5. Ganz R, Gill T, Gautier E, et al. Surgical dislocation of the adult hip. J Bone Joint Surg Br 2001;83(8):1119–1124.
6. Ganz R, Parvizi J, Beck M, et al. Femoroacetabular impingement: a cause for osteoarthritis of the hip. Clin Orthop Relat Res 2003;(417):112–120.
7. Gautier E, Ganz K, Krügel N, et al. Anatomy of the medial femoral circumflex artery and its surgical implications. J Bone Joint Surg Br 2000;82(5):679–683.
8. Gibson A. Posterior exposure of the hip joint. J Bone Joint Surg Br 1950;32-B(2):183–186.
9. Goodman DA, Feighan JE, Smith AD, et al. Subclinical slipped capital femoral epiphysis. Relationship to osteoarthrosis of the hip. J Bone Joint Surg Am 1997;79(10):1489–1497.
10. Meyer DC, Beck M, Ellis T, et al. Comparison of six radiographic projections to assess femoral head/neck asphericity. Clin Orthop Relat Res 2006;445:181–185.
11. Murphy SB, Simon SR, Kijewski PK, et al. Femoral anteversion. J Bone Joint Surg Am 1987;69(8):1169–1176.
12. Murphy S, Tannast M, Kim YJ, et al. Debridement of the adult hip for femoroacetabular impingement: indications and preliminary clinical results. Clin Orthop Relat Res 2004;(429):178–181.
13. Naal FD, Miozzari HH, Schär M, et al. Midterm results of surgical hip dislocation for the treatment of femoroacetabular impingement. Am J Sports Med 2012;40:1501–1510.
14. Spencer S, Millis M, Kim YJ. Early results of treatment for hip impingement syndrome in slipped capital femoral epiphysis and pistol grip deformity of the femoral head–neck junction using the surgical dislocation technique. J Pediatr Orthop 2006;26:281–285.
15. Tannast M, Krüger A, Mack PW, et al. Surgical dislocation of the hip for the fixation of acetabular fractures. J Bone Joint Surg Br 2010;92(6):842–852.
16. Tibor LM, Sink EL. Pros and cons of surgical hip dislocation for the treatment of femoroacetabular impingement. J Pediatr Orthop 2013;33(suppl 1):S131–S136.
17. Trueta J, Harrison MH. The normal vascular anatomy of the femoral head in adult man. J Bone Joint Surg Br 1953;35-B(3):442–461.

Surgical Hip Dislocation (Femoroacetabular Impingement)

14 CHAPTER

Luis Pulido and Rafael J. Sierra

DEFINITION

- Femoroacetabular impingement (FAI) is a common cause of hip pain and hip osteoarthritis in the young adult.[5]
- FAI is a dynamic pathologic condition that occurs when an abnormally shaped femoral head–neck and/or an overcovered acetabulum abut each other under physiologic range of motion (ROM), causing damage to the acetabular labrum and articulating cartilage.[9]
- The Ganz technique of safe surgical hip dislocation (SHD) of the hip was the first method described for treatment of FAI and helped refine the concept of FAI.[1,4]
- The greatest advantage of the SHD technique is a 360-degree visualization and access to the acetabulum and femoral neck. Unobstructed visualization allows the hip surgeon to address FAI as well as other intra-articular and extra-articular hip disorders that may require correction at the time of surgery.

ANATOMY

The Deep Branch of the Medial Femoral Circumflex Artery

- Knowledge of the anatomy of the deep branch of the medial femoral circumflex artery (MFCA) allowed Ganz et al[6] to develop a safe approach to dislocate the hip without the risk of avascular necrosis of the femoral head.
- The MFCA branches from the deep femoral artery and has five constant branches: superficial, ascending, acetabular, descending, and deep. The deep branch of the MFCA supplies blood to the femoral head.[6]
- The deep branch of the MFCA lies at an average of 8.8 mm from the insertion of the obturator externus. It runs between the pectineus medially and iliopsoas tendon laterally along the inferior border of the obturator externus. It reaches the trochanter proximal to the quadratus femoris muscle, where it leads to the trochanteric branch. The trochanteric branch of the deep MFCA crosses over the trochanteric crest toward the lateral aspect of the greater trochanter.
- The main deep branch of the MFCA crosses the tendon of the obturator externus posteriorly and continues its course anteriorly to the tendons of the superior gemellus, obturator internus, and inferior gemellus. It is found at an average of 1.5 cm from the lesser trochanter. The deep branch perforates the capsule just proximal to the insertion of the tendon of the superior gemellus and distal to the tendon of the piriformis, where it commonly divides into two of four terminal branches. Covered by synovium, these branches continue their course and perforate the femoral head at 2 to 4 mm lateral to the bone–cartilage junction.
- The anastomosis between the inferior gluteal artery and the MFCA occurs at the inferior border of the piriformis. This constant anastomosis must be preserved.
- Surgical dislocation of the hip does not cause significant strain on the deep branch of the MFCA.

Trochanteric Trigastric (Flip) Osteotomy

- During the trochanteric flip osteotomy, the trochanter is cut from posterior to anterior. The flip osteotomy allows the hip to be exposed anteriorly and dislocated in the same direction without disrupting the short external rotators or the MFCA. The trochanteric osteotomy also minimizes injury to the superior gluteal neurovascular bundle by maintaining the abductors in continuity.

Acetabular Labrum

- The acetabular labrum is a triangular fibrocartilaginous structure that is attached to the bony acetabular rim. The labrum is a relatively avascular structure. The main blood supply is from the hip capsule to the periphery of the labrum.
- The labrum helps with the stability of the hip by lateralizing femoral head coverage as well as maintaining a suction seal of the hip joint.
- The labral innervation comes from a branch of the nerve to the quadratus femoris and from the obturator nerve. Sensory nerve organs as well as free nerve endings suggest that the injury to the labrum causes pain and is important in proprioception.

Femoral Head–Neck Osteopathy

- A precise knowledge of superior retinacular vessel anatomy is necessary for any procedures at the femoral neck. The femoral head–neck osteochondroplasty is performed in FAI surgery to increase the femoral head offset.
- The superior retinacular vessels are located over the posterosuperior neck. They are covered by synovial tissue and perforate 2 to 4 mm lateral to the articular margin. The retinacular vessels must be always visualized.

PATHOMECHANICS

- FAI is a dynamic process where there is abutment between the acetabular rim and the femoral neck under physiologic ROM of the hip. Repetitive trauma during impingement leads to labral pathology and cartilage degeneration.[5]
- The decreased femoral offset at the head–neck junction and the lack of sphericity of the femoral head is known as a *cam morphology* (also described as a pistol grip or head tilt deformity). Cam impingement is more common in young males.[3]

- Cam deformity causes damage mainly to the anterior superior acetabular cartilage during hip flexion, causing chondrolabral separation and shearing of the acetabular cartilage from subchondral bone.
- Pincer impingement is caused by excessive coverage of the acetabulum. This can be seen in patients with acetabular retroversion or coxa profunda. Pincer is more common in females and the pattern of labral injury is seen in the anterior superior acetabulum, globally or posteriorly (coup–contrecoup).
- The combination of cam and pincer is most commonly the mechanism in FAI.

NATURAL HISTORY

- FAI is a major etiologic factor in the development of early degenerative joint disease of the hip. Although the natural history of FAI needs further understanding, the pathophysiology and clinical data suggest that FAI plays an important role in early hip osteoarthritis in the young adult.[5]

PATIENT HISTORY AND PHYSICAL FINDINGS

- The main goal of performing a clinical history and physical examination in the young adult with hip pain is to establish a differential diagnosis and determine if the origin of pain is intra- or extra-articular.[10]
- FAI is one cause of intra-articular hip pain in the young adult.
- Most patients are active and pain is related to activities that flex, rotate, or load the joint. Pain is usually reproduced in positions of hip flexion such as prolonged sitting.
- The distribution of pain in FAI includes the groin (88%), lateral hip (67%), anterior thigh (35%), and buttocks (29%).[8]
- Associated symptoms include hip snapping, catching, locking, and weakness.
- The physical evaluation includes observation of gait pattern (foot progression angle and abductors' strength) and seating posture, passive hip ROM,[11] and provocative hip tests.
- Common provocative hip tests include the following:
  - The classic FAI impingement test (flexion, adduction, and internal rotation)
  - Flexion, abduction, and external rotation
  - Lateral rim impingement (abduction)
  - Posterior rim impingement (extension, abduction, and external rotation)
  - Stinchfield (hip flexion–straight-leg raise against resistance)
- A diagnostic image-guided intra-articular hip injection can help to determine if the pain is related to an intra-articular hip disorder.

IMAGING AND OTHER DIAGNOSTIC STUDIES

- Radiographs are the main diagnosis modality for FAI. Advanced cross-sectional studies, such as computed tomography (CT) and magnetic resonance arthrogram (MRA), are used to further characterize the acetabulum and femur's bony and soft tissue structures.
- Plain radiographs are used in the evaluation of subtle bony structural abnormalities such as hip dysplasia or FAI. The recommended views include a true standing anteroposterior pelvis, frog-leg lateral, cross-table lateral, and false-profile pelvis.
- The orthopaedic surgeon needs to assess the degree of hip osteoarthritis, amount of anterior and lateral acetabular coverage, acetabular version and depth, femoral head sphericity, and amount of femoral head–neck offset seen on plain radiographs.
- MRA is commonly used to detect the presence of labral and chondral damage associated with FAI. Additionally, MRA can help rule out other differential diagnosis of hip pain.

DIFFERENTIAL DIAGNOSIS

- See Table 1.

NONOPERATIVE MANAGEMENT

- Nonsurgical management should be the first line of treatment for FAI. This includes restriction of activities that place the hip in extreme ROM or high-impact activities.
- Nonsteroidal anti-inflammatory medications are recommended to alleviate symptoms.
- Physical therapy to maintain core and hip muscle strength is recommended.
- Physical therapy aiming to improve ROM is contraindicated.

SURGICAL MANAGEMENT

- The decision to proceed with open versus arthroscopic surgery for surgical treatment of FAI should be based on the patient's anatomy, surgeon's experience/preference, and potential rehabilitation.[7]

Indications for Surgical Hip Dislocation to Treat Femoroacetabular Impingement

- Patients younger than 40 years with preserved articular cartilage and the following:
  - Coxa profunda, defined as lateral center edge angle greater than 40 degree
  - Cam lesions extending over the retinacular vessels as seen on CT scan or radiographs
  - High-riding trochanter from old Perthes or slipped capital femoral epiphysis
    - Trochanteric advancement and relative lengthening can be performed.

Table 1 Differential Diagnosis of Intra-articular and Extra-articular Causes of Hip Pain

Intra-articular	Extra-articular

• Acetabular dysplasia
• Femoroacetabular impingement
• Labral tears
• Chondral injuries
• Avascular necrosis
• Ligamentum teres tears
• Synovitis
• Loose bodies
• Tumors
• Infection
	• Anterior inferior iliac spine impingement (subspinal)
	• Proximal hip muscular injuries
	  • Adductors
	  • Hamstrings
	  • Rectus femoris
	  • Abductors
	• Bursitis (trochanteric and iliopsoas bursitis)
	• Referred lumbosacral pain
	• Sports hernias
	• Intra-abdominal and intrapelvic disorders (hernia, diverticulosis, endometriosis)

- Combined procedures to address both intra-articular and extra-articular impingement
  - Combined periacetabular osteotomy and SHD
  - Combined derotational femoral osteotomy and SHD
- Anticipated labral reconstruction (fascia lata or round ligament autograft)

- Other non-FAI indications for SHD include the following:
  - Femoral head and/or acetabular fracture
  - Removal of intra-articular heterotopic bone
  - Benign tumors
    - Synovial chondromatosis
    - Pigmented villonodular synovitis
    - Proximal femur osteochondromas and enchondromas

Contraindications for Surgical Hip Dislocation to Treat Femoroacetabular Impingement

- Patients age 40 years old and older[2]
- Extensive cartilage damage
  - Anterior hip subluxation
  - Anterior and posterior cartilage damage (coup–contrecoup)
- No clearly defined pathology causing hip pain
- Pain out of proportion
- Smokers

Preoperative Planning

- Preoperative planning is based on clinical evaluation and radiographic assessment.
- The amount of acetabular bony resection should not exceed 25 degrees of lateral coverage.
- The cam deformity is resected until impingement-free ROM is obtained. Thirty percent of the head and neck diameter is considered the maximum amount of cam resection without affecting the load to failure, but the correction never extends to that amount.

Positioning

- The patient is placed in the lateral decubitus position.
- Hip ROM and impingement with internal rotation at 90 degrees is measured. This is used as future reference during the offset procedure.

Approach

- Posterior Kocher or Gibson approach with osteotomy of the greater trochanter
- Perform a straight lateral incision centered over the greater trochanter. The size of the incision averages 15 cm. Incise skin and subcutaneous tissue down to the fascia.
- Elevate the subcutaneous tissue from the anterior fascia until perforators are encountered.
- Leg position 1: straight lateral on the table (tensions fascia, allowing easy visualization of Gibson interval if the surgeon prefers)
- These vessels mark the plane that divides the anterior border of the gluteus maximus with the underlying muscles. Incise the fascia through this interval starting from distal to proximal, ensuring that the gluteus maximus fibers head posteriorly.
- Peel the gluteus maximus posteriorly off the gluteus medius, including its overlying shiny fascia, because the pedicle to the anterior half of the gluteus maximus muscle runs within this gluteus medius fascia. Dissect the interval proximally as far up as possible.

TECHNIQUES

Trochanteric Trigastric (Flip) Osteotomy

- The objective of the osteotomy is to leave the gluteus medius tendon, long tendon of the gluteus minimus tendon, and vastus lateralis tendon attached to the mobile trochanter. The stable trochanter is preserved with the piriformis and all other external rotators.
- Incise gliding tissue over the posterior border of the trochanter over the bursa in a straight line similar to fascia for closure over the trochanter and screws after surgery.
- Leg position 2: Internal rotation and extension of the hip allows better visualization of the posterior trochanter, short rotators, and sciatic nerve.
- A safe distance to mark the proximal starting point of the osteotomy is 5 mm anterior to the trochanteric overhang (**TECH FIG 1A,B**).
- Perform the osteotomy from the posterior trochanter toward the vastus ridge. The saw blade must be parallel to the long axis of the leg (tibia) with the hip internally rotated over the table (**TECH FIG 1C**). Stop the saw at the anterior cortex (**TECH FIG 1D**). Complete the osteotomy by levering the fragment with an osteotome. The anterior ridge created potentially increases rotational stability of the trochanter after fixation (**TECH FIG 1E**).
- Open the osteotomy using a Hohmann retractor. Beware of potential damage to the femoral head if the Hohmann retractor is placed too far anterior or left in place when exposing the anterior capsule (especially in a Perthes hip with a short neck).
- Use the knife to cut the remaining gluteus medius fibers and vastus lateralis intermedius fibers off the stable trochanter. Aim the knife blade parallel to the femur and stable trochanter.
- A shiny fat pad is visible anterior to the posterosuperior tip of the trochanter. Incise only through this gap to visualize the capsule. Occasionally, fibers of the piriformis tendon remain attached to the trochanteric fragment and must be cut to allow further mobilization of the trochanter. The anterior Hohmann retractor should be exchanged for a Meyerding or knee retractor.
- Incise the vastus fascia posteriorly, just anterior to the intramuscular septum. Using sharp dissection, elevate the vastus lateralis muscle subperiosteally in continuity with the trochanteric fragment. This dissection continues over the anterior border of the proximal femur by releasing proximal attachments of the vastus intermedius and lateralis up to the inferior medial aspect of the capsule. The mobile trochanter should become more and more retractable while the assistant flexes and externally rotates the hip.

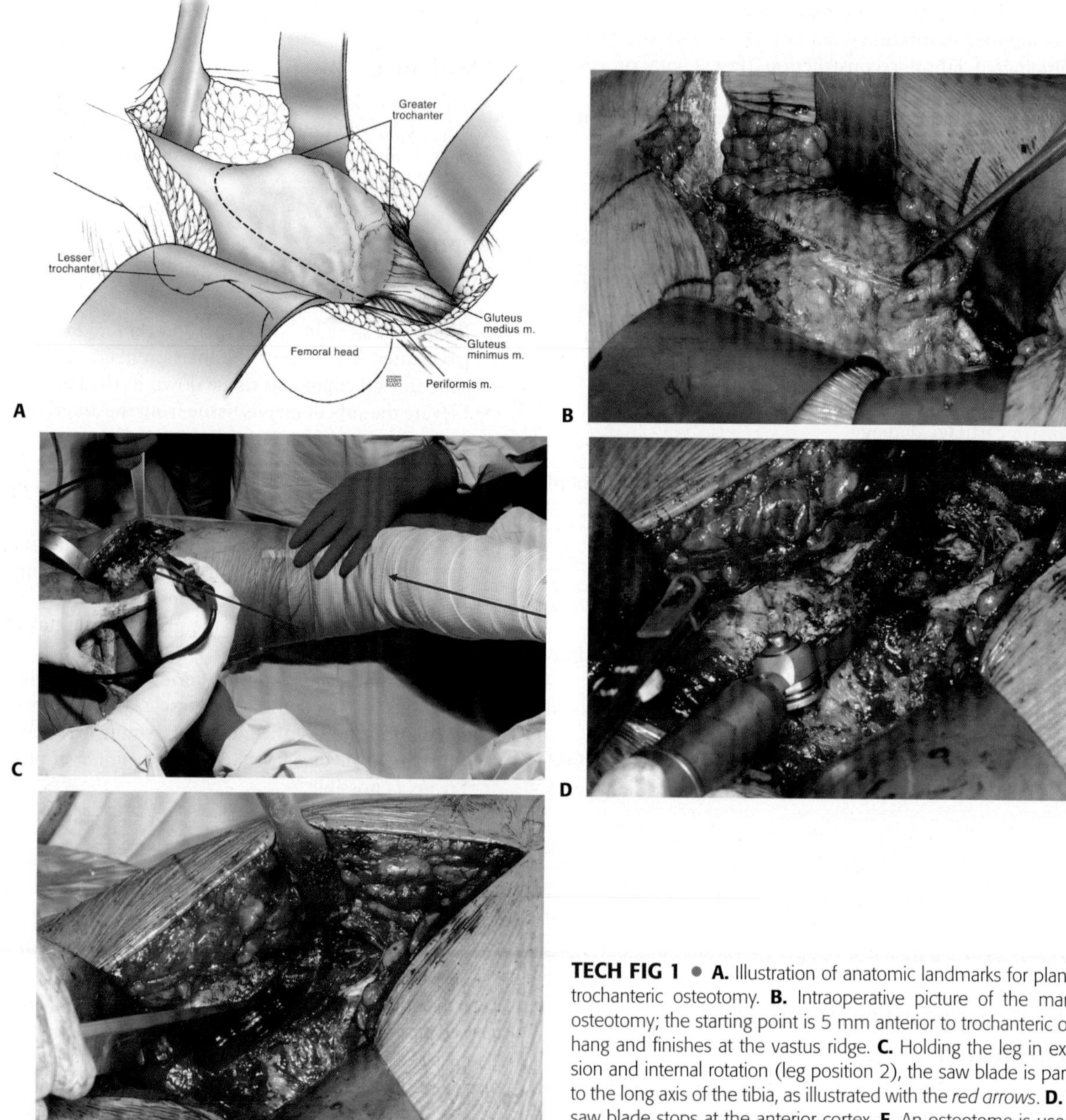

TECH FIG 1 • **A.** Illustration of anatomic landmarks for planned trochanteric osteotomy. **B.** Intraoperative picture of the marked osteotomy; the starting point is 5 mm anterior to trochanteric overhang and finishes at the vastus ridge. **C.** Holding the leg in extension and internal rotation (leg position 2), the saw blade is parallel to the long axis of the tibia, as illustrated with the *red arrows*. **D.** The saw blade stops at the anterior cortex. **E.** An osteotome is used to lever, leaving an anterior ridge to increase the rotational stability of the trochanter fixation.

Capsular Exposure

- Leg position 3: Flexion and external rotation of the hip decreases tension over the posterior interval between piriformis and gluteus minimus and trochanteric flip (**TECH FIG 2A**).
- The gluteus medius muscle is gently retracted in an anterosuperior direction using a narrow Deaver retractor. Mobilizing the gluteus medius provides exposure of the piriformis and gluteus minimus muscles.
- Find the interval between the piriformis and the gluteus minimus proximally (**TECH FIG 2B**). Stay proximal to the piriformis tendon because an anastomosis between the deep branch of the MFCA and inferior gluteal artery runs inferior to the piriformis.
- Elevate the gluteus minimus off the superior and posterior capsule down to the sciatic notch. Be careful because the nerve to the gluteus minimus runs anterior over the muscle and not far from the distal border. The gluteus minimus must be elevated enough to avoid damage at the time of femoral head dislocation.
- The superior dissection can be carried up anteriorly to the reflected head of the rectus, which becomes visible over the acetabular rim.

- Anteroinferiorly, the insertions of the short head of the minimus onto the capsule should be released. The remaining capsular thickening is known as a *Bigelow ligament*.
- The trochanteric fragment is retracted anteriorly throughout this exposure. Increasing flexion and abduction facilitates anterior retraction of the trochanteric fragment. A complete anterior, superior, and posterior capsular exposure should be obtained.
- The insertions of the short external rotator muscles and the piriformis muscle are left intact to protect the deep branch of the MFCA.

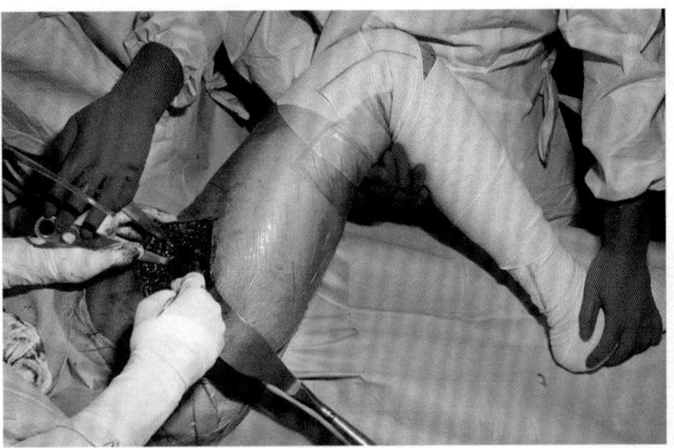

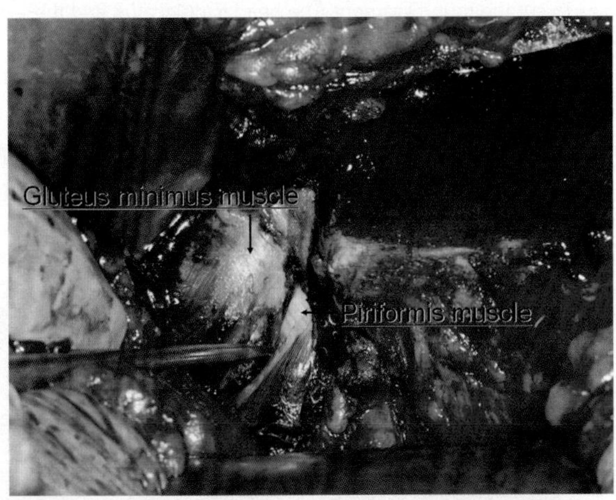

TECH FIG 2 • **A.** The capsular exposure begins by bringing the leg into position 3 with the hip flexed and externally rotated to decrease tension over posterior interval between piriformis, gluteus minimus, and the trochanteric mobile fragment. **B.** Intraoperative picture of the interval between the piriformis and the gluteus minimus.

Z-Shaped Capsulotomy

- A Z-shaped capsulotomy for the right hip and an inverse Z-shaped capsulotomy for the left hip are performed (**TECH FIG 3A**).
- Use the knife blade to perform the Z-shaped capsulotomy. Start at the anterosuperior edge of the stable trochanter toward the acetabular rim along the long axis of the neck from distal to proximal. Initially, start with 2 cm, then begin the perpendicular anterior limb (just 1 cm), enough to see the joint inside. Continue to carry the transverse limb of the capsulotomy with a knife from inside out, so that the labrum can be seen as the rim is approached. Use Vicryl 0 to tag each side of the transverse limb of the capsulotomy (**TECH FIG 3B**).
- Use an 8-mm Hohmann retractor in the anterior wall, taking care not to damage the anterior labrum or cartilage next to the rim. This places the anterior capsule at stretch.
- Complete the capsulotomy anteriorly inside-out until the iliacus muscle is visualized. Posteriorly carry the capsulotomy along the acetabular rim, taking care not to injure the labrum.
- Use a superior acetabular Hohmann or large Langenbeck retractor in the ilium.

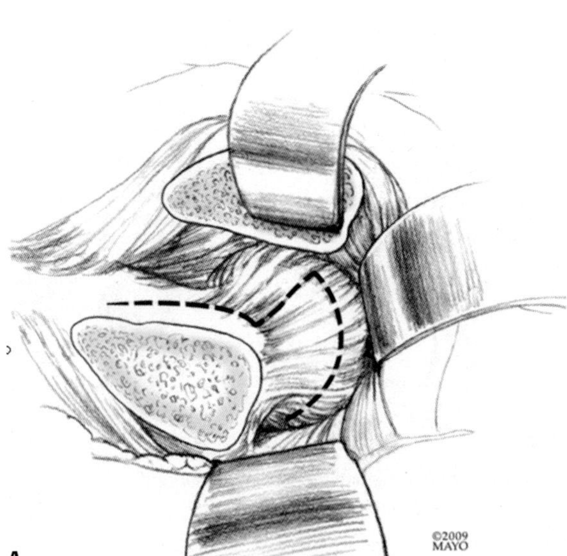

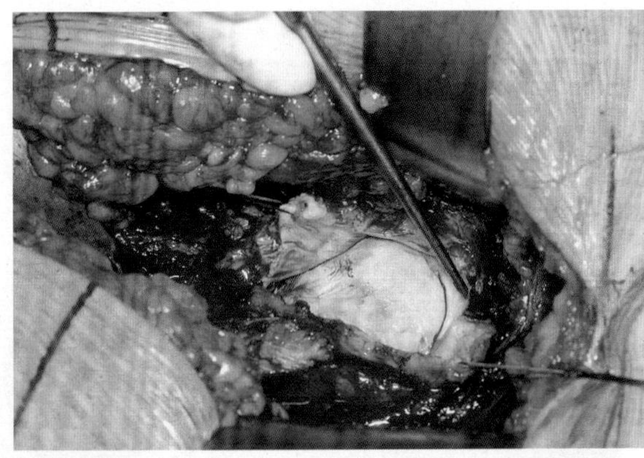

TECH FIG 3 • **A.** Illustration of the Z-shaped capsulotomy. **B.** Intraoperative picture of the Z capsulotomy showing the femoral head, neck, and acetabular labrum.

Femoral Head Dislocation

- Leg position 4: Hip is flexed and externally rotated, and foot is brought into sterile pocket.
- Use a bone hook on the neck to sublux the femoral head out of the acetabulum. Use large parametrium (90 degrees) scissors to cut the round ligament. The head is dislocated and the leg is flexed and externally rotated and placed inside the pocket.
- Leg position 5: leg in pocket. Elevate the knee higher than pelvis and toward the head of the patient (abduction, flexion, external rotation, and axial loading) with a gentle axial push at the knee to push the femoral head posteriorly, creating enough space to have 360-degree visualization of the acetabulum (**TECH FIG 4**).
- Place the inferior cobra retractor into the teardrop. This move assists posterior and inferior subluxation of the femoral head.

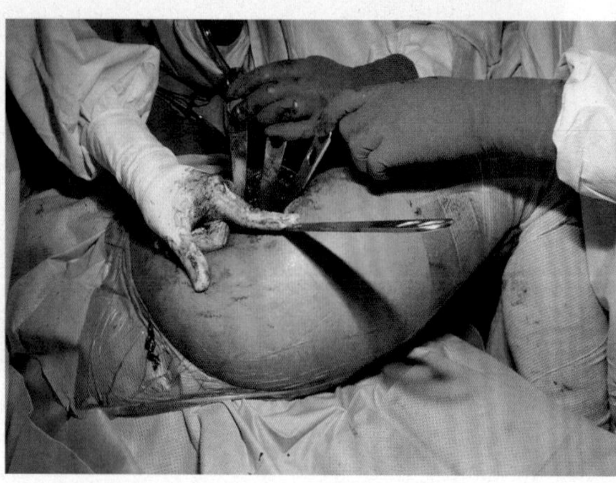

TECH FIG 4 • Intraoperative picture showing leg position 5 with the leg in pocket and the knee elevated higher than the pelvis (abduction, flexion, external rotation, and axial loading).

Acetabulum and Labrum

- Inspection, labral takedown, and rim trimming can be performed with a 360-degree direct visualization of the acetabulum (**TECH FIG 5A**).
- The rim trimming is performed at the site of acetabular impingement, most commonly located in the anterosuperior acetabulum at the 12 o'clock to 3 o'clock positions.
- Bone resection down to healthy rim cartilage can be performed with a high-speed burr or with a narrow curved osteotome (if roof is large enough). The amount of bone removed depends on the cartilage damage and the depth of the socket (**TECH FIG 5B–D**).
- Nonabsorbable anchored sutures (2-0 Ethibond) are used for labral refixation into the acetabular rim. The knots should be tied over the rim outside of the joint, taking care to pass the suture through the undersurface of the labrum so that it is not reattached in the inverted manner or too high. Three or four anchors are usually used.

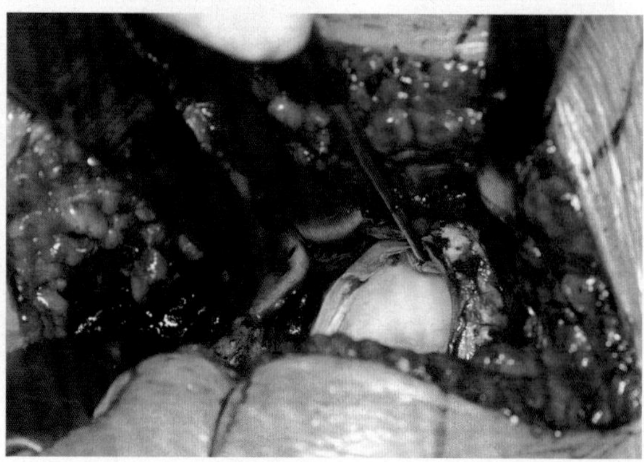

A

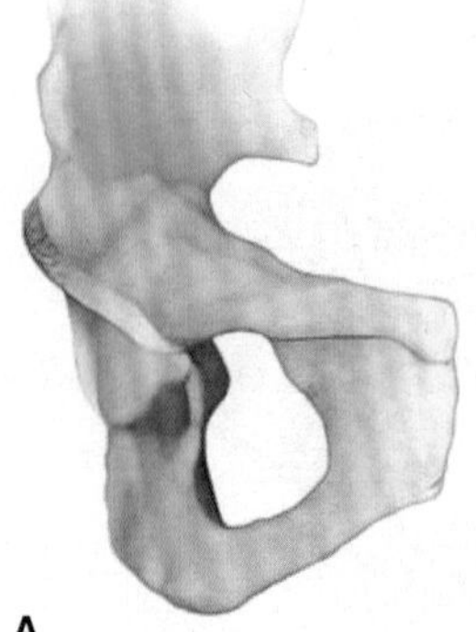

B A

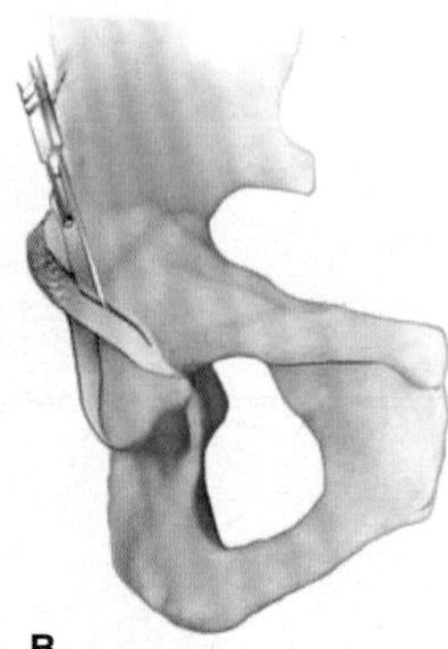

B

TECH FIG 5 • **A.** Acetabular exposure. **B.** Illustration of acetabular labral takedown, *(continued)*

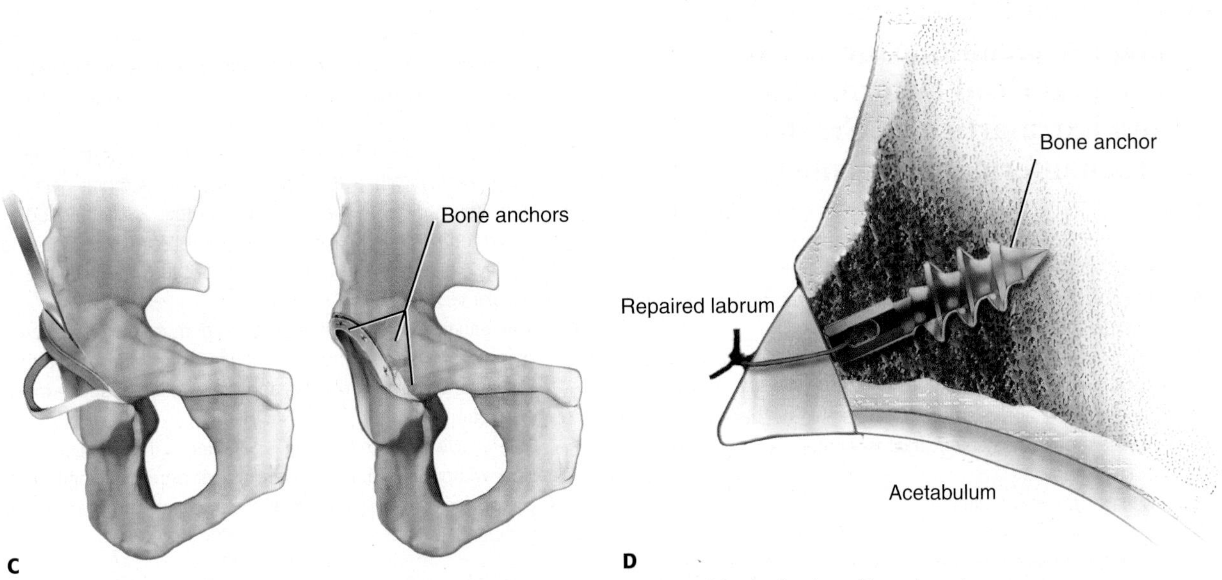

TECH FIG 5 • *(continued)* (**C**) bone trimming, and (**D**) labral refixation with anchored sutures.

Femoral Head and Neck Resection

- Leg position 6: Remove the inferior cobra retractor and bring the knee down (adduction), keeping the leg position within the sterile pocket for femoral head and neck exposure.
- Place two Eva retractors underneath the femoral neck.
- Remove the ligamentum teres at this time.
- Assess the femoral head offset and mark out the area to be removed.
- A change in cartilage color may be visible where the offset problem begins. Remove excess bone and recreate femoral neck waist (**TECH FIG 6A**).
- Always visualize the retinaculum. The retinacular vessels penetrate the femoral neck about 2 to 4 mm lateral to the cartilage bone junction posterosuperiorly. If an offset is present near the retinaculum, it is safer to bring the osteotome proximal to distal, not too deeply, because it may cross the intraosseous vessels. Stop at the superior border of retinaculum; break the piece of bone off and, using a knife in an inside-out maneuver, detach the piece from the soft tissues.
- After the femoral head–neck offset has been recreated, use femoral head templates to verify good neck clearance (**TECH FIG 6B**).
- Reduce hip and check ROM for impingement. Internal rotation of 45 degrees free of impingement should be obtained.
- Place bone wax into cancellous bone of the head–neck junction to prevent capsular adhesions.
- Loose capsular closure prevents hematoma formation and stretch of retinacular vessels, decreasing blood flow to the femoral head.
- Evaluate for extra-articular impingement (posterior trochanter on pelvis). If necessary, trim the posterior stable trochanter.

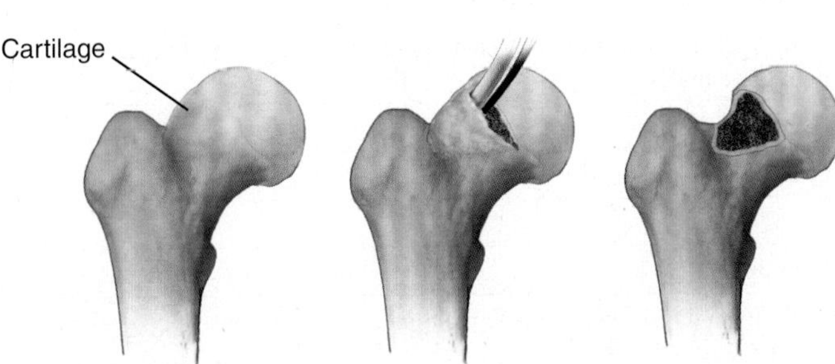

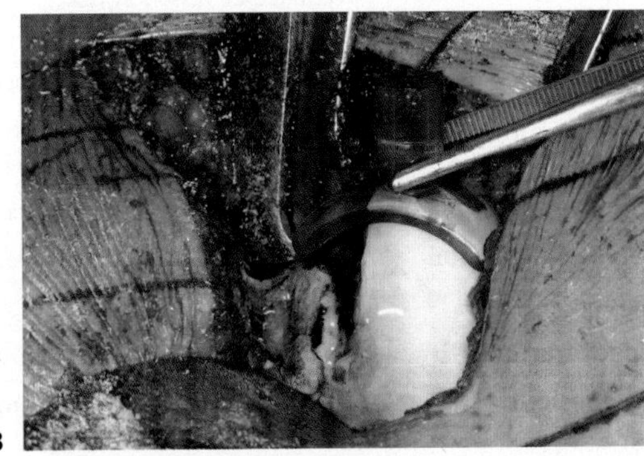

TECH FIG 6 • **A.** Illustration of the femoral head and neck osteochondroplasty. **B.** Intraoperative picture using the spherical guide and improved offset following femoral head–neck osteochondroplasty.

Extended Retinacular Soft Tissue Flap: A Technique for Severe Femoral Head Deformities and Extra-articular Greater Trochanteric Impingement

- The medial retinacular soft tissue flap as described by Ganz et al[6] allows extending the SHD approach to treat sequelae of slipped capital epiphysis or Perthes deformities.
- The soft tissue flap is developed by subperiosteal release of the external rotators.
- Leg position 1: straight lateral on the table. Femoral head is reduced into the acetabular socket.
- Expose the cancellous bone of the stable trochanter by retracting the mobile trochanteric fragment anteriorly with a Meyerding or knee retractor.
- Visualize the retinaculum.
- Using a small osteotome, the posterior stable trochanter is reduced in a piecemeal fashion. Avoid posterior penetration with the osteotome. The mobilized fragments are turned and subperiosteal elevation of the osteotomized pieces is performed under direct visualization with a knife. This is performed until the osteotomy surface levels the posterior and superior surface of the neck.
- The periosteum anterior to the retinacular vessels is incised longitudinally with a knife at the superior femoral neck. The periosteum distal to the quadratus femoris is also incised and mobilized posteriorly. The subperiosteal flap is developed posteriorly, containing the deep branch of the MFCA and the retinacular vessels.
- The retinacular soft tissue flap allows performing relative lengthening of the femoral neck to manage intra- and extra-articular impingement, improve ROM, and improve the abductor mechanism strength.
- The relative neck lengthening is obtained at the superior femoral neck without affecting the overall lower extremity length. This is performed by distally advancing the trochanter and trimming the posterior superior circumference of the trochanter.

Trochanteric Reattachment and Closure

- For trochanteric reattachment, use a bone hook to pull distally and internally rotate the fragment. The fragment is reduced in anatomic position with the bone hook or with a ball spike pusher (Picador) held by the assistant.
- Two or three 4.5-mm screws, commonly 65 to 70 mm in men and 55 to 60 mm in women, are used for fixation of the greater trochanter. Medial and lateral are the preferred location for screw fixation.
- The bursa is closed over the screws with a running 2-0 Vicryl suture for gliding tissue reconstruction.
- Layered closure including the fascia, subcutaneous tissues, and skin is performed.
- Subcutaneous tissue and skin closure is routine. Suction drainage is only occasionally needed.

PEARLS AND PITFALLS

Trochanteric osteotomy	▪ Avoid smaller trochanteric mobile fragments. Starting the cut 5 mm anterior to the trochanteric overhang will avoid cutting small trochanteric piece at risk for fracture. ▪ Starting the trochanteric osteotomy 5 mm anterior will prevent undercutting the trochanter and placing the retinacular vessels at risk. ▪ Use washers in soft bone.
Capsule exposure	▪ Avoid injury to the anastomosis to prevent damage to the blood supply of the femoral head.
HO	▪ Elevate the minimus in its entirety off the capsule. The more muscle damage, the higher risk of HO. ▪ Indomethacin is used postoperatively in large males.
Labral injury at exposure	▪ During capsulotomy, use the knife from inside out.
Sciatic nerve compression	▪ Limit time for posterior displacement of the femoral head.
Painful screws	▪ Close bursa over screws.
Femoral neck fractures	▪ Avoid overresection of cam greater than 30%.
Capsular adhesions	▪ Encourage passive ROM postoperatively from day 1 using a CPM machine.

POSTOPERATIVE CARE

- Patients undergoing surgery for FAI are mobilized the day following surgery.
- Passive- and active-assisted internal or external rotation is permitted to protect trochanteric fixation. Passive ROM is initiated immediately with the use of a continuous passive motion (CPM) machine 6 hours a day for 6 weeks. A stationary bike may begin at week 2.
- Hip flexion is limited to 90 degrees.
- The patients are touch weight bearing for the first 4 weeks after surgery.
- Weight bearing is advanced after 4 weeks.
- Active abductor strengthening begins at week 4.
- Our protocol is to see patients for follow-up 8 weeks after surgery. At that time, patients are typically on one crutch or using no support.
- Muscle weakness may persist for 3 months after surgery and abductor rehabilitation is continued throughout the ensuing months.
- A therapist who specializes in return to sports programs supervises the return to high-impact pivoting sports, which usually does not occur before 6 months.
- Screws are removed at 3 months in athletes.

OUTCOMES

- The current literature to assess the outcomes of SHD is level IV, evidence from small case series studies reporting early and midterm results.
- Good to excellent results have been seen in 70% to 90% of patients at 2 to 5 years follow-up.
- Patient selection is very important. Those older than 40 years or patients with degenerative changes have less favorable results.

COMPLICATIONS

- Heterotopic ossification (HO) (37%; most were Brooker type 1)
- Trochanter nonunion and failure of trochanteric fixation (1% to 2%)
- Sciatic nerve neurapraxia (<1%)

REFERENCES

1. Beck M, Leunig M, Parvizi J, et al. Anterior femoroacetabular impingement: part II. Midterm results of surgical treatment. Clin Orthop Relat Res 2004;(418):67–73.
2. Boone GR, Pagnotto MR, Walker JA, et al. Caution should be taken in performing surgical hip dislocation for the treatment of femoroacetabular impingement in patients over the age of 40. HSS J 2012;8:230–234.
3. Clohisy JC, Baca G, Beaule PE, et al. Descriptive epidemiology of femoroacetabular impingement: a North American cohort of patients undergoing surgery. Am J Sports Med 2013;41:1348–1356.
4. Espinosa N, Beck M, Rothenfluh DA, et al. Treatment of femoro-acetabular impingement: preliminary results of labral refixation. Surgical technique. J Bone Joint Surg Am 2007;89(suppl 2, pt 1):36–53.
5. Ganz R, Parvizi J, Beck M, et al. Femoroacetabular impingement: a cause for osteoarthritis of the hip. Clin Orthop Relat Res 2003;417:112–120.
6. Gautier E, Ganz K, Krugel N, et al. Anatomy of the medial femoral circumflex artery and its surgical implications. J Bone Joint Surg Br 2000;82:679–683.
7. Nepple JJ, Byrd JW, Siebenrock KA, et al. Overview of treatment options, clinical results, and controversies in the management of femoroacetabular impingement. J Am Acad Orthop Surg 2013;21(suppl 1):S53–S58.
8. Nepple JJ, Prather H, Trousdale RT, et al. Clinical diagnosis of femoroacetabular impingement. J Am Acad Orthop Surg 2013;21(suppl 1):S16–S19.
9. Parvizi J, Leunig M, Ganz R. Femoroacetabular impingement. J Am Acad Orthop Surg 2007;15:561–570.
10. Sierra RJ, Trousdale RT, Ganz R, et al. Hip disease in the young, active patient: evaluation and nonarthroplasty surgical options. J Am Acad Orthop Surg 2008;16:689–703.
11. Yuan BJ, Bartelt RB, Levy BA, et al. Decreased range of motion is associated with structural hip deformity in asymptomatic adolescent athletes. Am J Sports Med 2013;41:1519–1525.

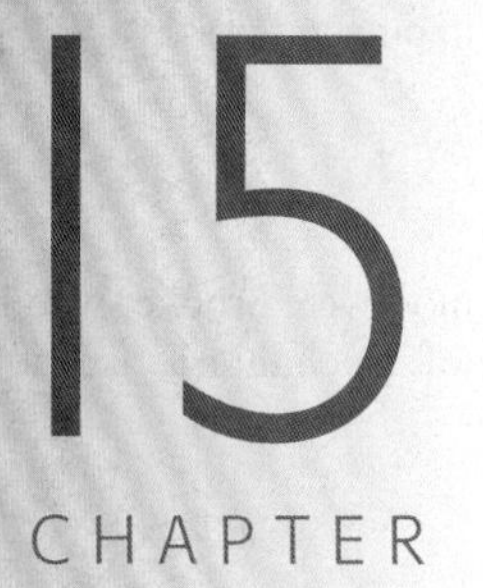

CHAPTER 15

Treatment of Anterior Femoroacetabular Impingement through the Mini-Open Anterior Approach

Diana Bitar and Javad Parvizi

DEFINITION

- Femoroacetabular impingement (FAI) is a mechanical hip disorder defined as abnormal abutment between the femoral head or the femoral head–neck junction and the acetabulum. It was initially described as a distinct physiologic entity by Myers et al,[28] who noted abnormal contact between the femoral neck and the acetabular rim in a cohort of patients undergoing periacetabular osteotomy (PAO) to correct hip dysplasia.
- One of the earlier descriptions of this condition was by Smith-Petersen[35] in 1936, when a case of malum coxae senilis was described. The case in that original article resembled what we now describe as FAI. Another description of this condition came in 1970s when the term *pistol grip deformity* was introduced. The latter was a description of aberrant morphologic features of the femoral head and neck on anteroposterior (AP) radiographs of patients with early idiopathic hip osteoarthritis (OA).[24]
- FAI can be anterior or posterior, with anterior abnormalities being more frequent. The estimated prevalence of FAI in the general population is 10% to 15%[38] and is increasingly being recognized as a cause of hip pain in young, active individuals. Repetitive anterolateral impingement produces acetabular articular cartilage delamination, labral disease, and eventually secondary OA. Establishment of a correlation between clinical picture, physical findings, suggestive radiographic structural abnormalities, and positive magnetic resonance angiogram (MRA) is crucial for diagnosis and appropriate treatment of this condition.

ANATOMY

- Establishing an accurate diagnosis and selecting the optimal surgical treatment strategy relies on a thorough understanding of the pathoanatomy of hip impingement disorders.
- Two different structural impingement types have been described:
  - Femoral-based abnormality (ie, cam impingement) is more common in the young, athletic male[16] (M:F ratio = 14:1).[38] Cam is a term applied to an eccentric prominence in a rotating mechanism which converts rotary motion into linear motion.[26]
  - Acetabular-based abnormality (ie, pincer impingement) is seen more commonly in athletic middle-aged women (M:F ratio = 1:3).[38] Pincer comes from the French word meaning "to pinch" (**FIG 1**).[1,13,23]
- It is important to note that most FAI cases are likely to be a combination of cam and pincer impingement. In this state, both the proximal femur and the acetabulum present with distorted structural characteristics. Isolated cam or pincer deformities are rare; in 86% of cases, a combined deformity is present.[38] In one study of 149 hips with FAI lesions, only 26 hips presented with an isolated cam lesion and 16 hips presented with an isolated pincer lesion.[1]
- Cam-type impingement syndrome can be primary (reduced femoral head–neck offset or an aspherical femoral head) with abnormal physeal development or secondary to previous pathologies (eg, slipped capital femoral epiphysis [SCFE], Perthes abnormalities, developmental dysplasia of the hip [DDH], or as a result of a prior trauma to the proximal femur and/or acetabulum).
- Morphologically, cam lesions can result from an osseous bump or from angular deformities of the proximal femur (eg, femoral retrotorsion or coxa vara). The osseous bump location further divides cam lesions into lateral-based prominence (pistol grip) or anterosuperior-based prominence, which is only detected on lateral radiographic views of the hip. Cam impingement owing to femoral angular deformities is uncommon.
- Pincer-type impingement syndrome consists of an overcoverage abnormality, which can be focal or global. Focal overcoverage can be anterior (acetabular retroversion with or without a deficient posterior wall) or posterior (prominent

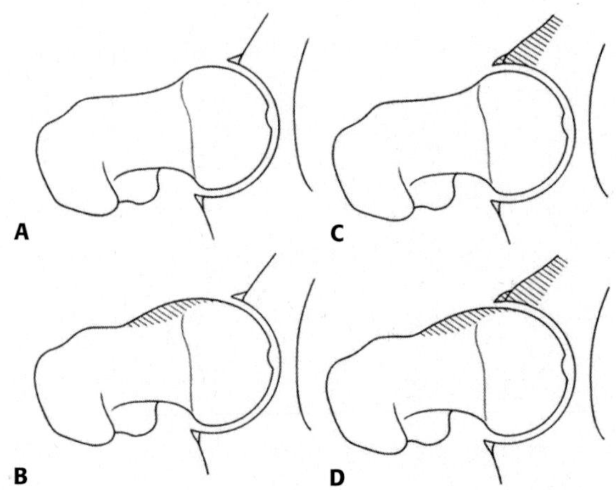

FIG 1 • The factors causing FAI are shown. Reduced clearance during joint motion leads to repetitive abutment between the proximal femur and the anterior acetabular rim. **A.** Normal clearance of the hip. **B.** Reduced femoral head and neck offset. **C.** Excessive overcoverage of the femoral head by the acetabulum. **D.** Combination of reduced head and neck offset and excessive anterior over coverage can be seen.

posterior wall). Global overcoverage consists of concentric deepening of the acetabulum (acetabular dome breaching the pelvic brim) which presents as coxa profunda or protrusio acetabuli, with the latter being the most severe form.

PATHOGENESIS

- If left untreated, the process of FAI is likely to lead to hip joint degeneration.[13,23,39] Mechanical impingement is most noticeable with hip flexion alone or hip flexion combined with internal rotation.
- In pincer impingement, a linear contact occurs between the acetabular overcovering rim with a labrum, which acts like a bumper.[1] The head–neck junction, with the maximal impact force tangential to the joint surface,[38] leads to a full tear of the labrum, which is the first structure to fail in this situation. Sustained mechanical abutment results in degeneration of the labrum with intrasubstance ganglion formation; ossification of the injured labrum leads to further deepening of the acetabulum and worsening of the overcoverage.[24]
- In cam impingement, a jamming of the aspherical head portion (shear stress) into the acetabulum occurs, with the maximal impact force perpendicular to the joint surface, leading to an undersurface tear of the labrum fibrocartilaginous separation,[38] which more accurately should be called *separation of the acetabular cartilage from the labrum.*[1]
- Based on this pathophysiology, the typical location of femoral cartilage damage is circumferential in pincer impingement with contrecoup lesion and is localized between 11 o'clock and 3 o'clock positions in cam impingement.[38] A contrecoup lesion is acetabular cartilaginous damage in the opposite part of the femoroacetabular abutment. It is seen in one-third of all cases of pincer impingement and is associated with slight joint subluxation.[38] Therefore, the cartilaginous lesions are more benign in pincer impingement than those seen in cam impingement with an average depth of 4 mm in the former and 11 mm in the latter.[1,38]

ETIOLOGY

Genetics

- Numerous studies conducted on family members, especially sets of twins, have demonstrated a genetic component to OA, which is mostly seen in Caucasians. Furthermore, it has been shown that genetic factors are largely responsible for variations in hip and acetabular morphology and cartilage thickness.[26]
- Based on one genetic study, cam deformity tends to be more prevalent in the family members of affected patients than pincer deformity. There is a relative risk of 2.8 and 2, respectively, that a sibling will have the same abnormal anatomy. Likewise, a positive family history increases the risk of bilateralism of the deformity.[18]

Geographical Variation

- FAI is more prevalent in the Western world where the majority of hip OA, previously labeled primary OA, is currently considered to be the consequence of abnormal hip joint anatomy.
- In contrast, in a retrospective study of 946 primary total hip arthroplasty (THA) conducted in Japan, Takeyama et al[37] identified FAI as an underlying pathology in only six hips.

Underlying Hip Pathologies

- In some cases, FAI is secondary to childhood hip disorders such as SCFE, DDH, Legg-Calvé-Perthes disease, or femoral neck fracture complicated by malunion.
  - In one study that followed patients for 15 years, those formerly treated for SCFE subsequently displayed signs of FAI.[18]
  - As reported by Eijer et al,[9] previous femoral neck fractures may result in secondary FAI, specially if the reduction is not completely anatomic.
  - Snow et al[36] reported four cases of anterior cam impingement which occurred after an asymptomatic period following reossification of the femoral head in Legg-Calvé-Perthes disease.

NATURAL HISTORY

- Because FAI is a newly identified condition, the natural history of its development has not been clearly defined in the literature. However, there is an association between morphologic deformities and secondary OA of the hip.
- Not all patients with FAI will progress to end-stage disease that requires intervention. It is estimated that one-third of patients with mild OA in the presence of FAI will take more than 10 years to develop end-stage OA, if at all.[26]
- Symptomatic impingement disorders most likely progress to secondary OA, making surgical treatment a rational option.
- Close observation and follow-up or prompt and timely conservative surgical treatment should be tailored to each case, taking into consideration clinical presentation, radiographic findings, family history, and especially, the rate of disease progression. Clinicians should be aware that delay of surgical correction may lead to chondral damage and disease progression to a stage where joint preservation procedures may be of little benefit.[26]

PATIENT HISTORY AND PHYSICAL FINDINGS

History

- FAI usually affects active young adults and begins with slow onset of activity-related anterior inguinal (groin) pain that is often preceded by a minor traumatic event.[24]
- Associated lateral (trochanteric) and posterior hip (gluteal) pain is common but the pain is most commonly felt in the groin (83% of cases).[26] The pain is often manifested after sitting for a prolonged period.[24]
- In the early stages of the disease, the pain or aching is intermittent and could be aggravated by excessive physical demands on the hip, such as prolonged walking or high-demand athletic activities, including running, cutting, pivoting, and repetitive hip flexion.
- Labral disease or unstable articular cartilage flaps[3] may cause mechanical symptoms of locking and catching. Anterior FAI is almost always associated with labral tears,[5] which are rarely isolated and most likely indicate underlying bony pathologies. Acetabular labral tears should be considered in active patients with a history of groin pain that is exacerbated by activity without radiologic evidence or other hip pathology.[3]
- Stiffness is common, with reductions in the range of hip flexion, adduction, and internal rotation in particular,[26] whereas overall hip function is almost unaffected.[24]

- After inquiring about the overall performance of the patient (including age, activity level, and comorbidities), a detailed hip-focused history should be conducted to determine any trauma, childhood hip disease, previous surgeries and treatments as well as the impact of hip pain on quality of life.

Physical Examination

- After assessment of overall health and body habitus, the hip clinical examination should be done with great care because it provides the most reliable diagnostic information. Physical findings will dictate further tests and necessary management.
- Observation of sitting posture, gait, palpation of the hip, abductor strength testing, careful hip range-of-motion (ROM) assessment, and specific provocative tests should be performed.
  - Anterior FAI commonly provokes discomfort/pain in an upright sitting position, which involves hip flexion greater than 90 degrees.
  - The gait pattern over short distances and abductor strength are usually normal in the early stages of the disease. A limp, secondary to mild abductor weakness, and positive Trendelenburg test may develop as labral disease and joint degeneration progress.
- Hip ROM testing should be performed carefully with stabilization of the pelvis to accurately define motion end points. Passive flexion is often limited to approximately 90 degrees and reduced compared with the contralateral hip. Internal rotation may be severely restricted to just a few degrees. Hip discomfort is often reproduced at the end points of passive motion.
- Surgical scars from any previous procedures are inspected to aid in planning of any subsequent surgery. When in doubt, infection should be ruled out.
- The anterior impingement test and Patrick test are sensitive maneuvers to detect intrinsic hip disease and usually reproduce hip symptoms in patients with anterior FAI.
  - The anterior impingement test, also known as the *flexion*, *adduction*, and *internal rotation test*, is performed by flexing the patient's hip to 90 degrees, adducting and internally rotating it simultaneously.
  - Patrick test, which is also known as the *flexion*, *abduction*, and *external rotation test*, is performed by crossing the examined limb on the other in a figure-of-four (the ipsilateral heel resting on the contralateral knee) and by applying downward pressure to the knee. If pain is elicited on the ipsilateral side anteriorly, it is suggestive of a hip joint disorder on the same side. If pain is elicited on the contralateral side posteriorly around the sacroiliac joint, it is suggestive of pain caused by dysfunction in that joint.
  - Moreover, the distance from the ipsilateral knee to the bed should be noted. The test is positive if this distance is greater than the corresponding measurement on the opposite side, if the contralateral hip is considered normal.[26]
- For posterior FAI, an impingement test (performed in the prone position) is considered positive if forced external rotation in full extension is reproducibly painful. Posterior impingement results from focal acetabular overcoverage (pincer); it is manifested radiographically by a posterior wall sign where the too prominent posterior acetabular wall runs lateral to the femoral head center (normally, the posterior rim runs approximately through the femoral head center).[38]
- A posterior impingement test can also be positive in anterior FAI when the disease progresses and posteroinferior traction osteophytes develop, producing clinical symptoms of posterior impingement in extension.
- The Drehman sign is positive if hip flexion produces unavoidable passive external rotation of the hip.[38]
- Logroll test is also a useful provocative test in patients with FAI. With the patient in supine position and with the hip and knee in full extension, the foot on the affected extremity is externally rotated. Positive sign is present if this maneuver results in pain in the anterior hip of the rotated extremity.

IMAGING AND OTHER DIAGNOSTIC STUDIES

- Investigation of FAI requires a combination of roentgenographic examination and more sophisticated cross-sectional studies, such as magnetic resonance imaging (MRI)/MRA and sometimes a computed tomography (CT) scan.

Roentgenography

- Is the first-line investigation and ideally may include five views: a supine AP view of the pelvis, an axial cross-table lateral view (surgical profile of Arcelin and Danelius-Miller view), a frog-leg lateral view, a false profile (Lequesne view), and a Dunn-Rippstein view in 45 or 90 degrees of flexion.[4,27,31]
- The AP and axial cross-table views are crucial and should be taken with the legs in 15 degrees of internal rotation to adjust for femoral antetorsion and fully expose the femoral neck length.
- Obtaining an AP view in the supine position allows for a direct comparison with intraoperative and immediate postoperative roentgenograms.[38] Standing AP views are important to accurately evaluate and follow joint space narrowing and to apply coxometric measurements.
- The AP view of the pelvis mainly detects pincer lesions and laterally based cam lesions (pistol grip). Anterosuperior cam lesion can be missed on AP views and should be investigated on at least one, if not all, of the three lateral views (**FIG 2**).
- Lequesne view (false profile) is not used for diagnosing FAI because it does not show the relationship between the anterior and posterior acetabular walls. However, it is more likely used for the diagnosis of early joint degeneration in the posteroinferior part of the acetabulum, which is a relative contraindication for joint-preserving surgery.[38] The Lequesne view should be included in a thorough radiologic evaluation to exclude associated mild hip dysplasia because it highlights anterior femoral head coverage (anterior center-edge angle of Lequesne) (**FIG 3**). Attention should be paid to radiographs where the pelvic tilt, rotation, and inclination are seen. X-ray beam centralization should be taken into consideration for correct interpretation of the radiologic hip parameters. The film-focus distance is different for each view: It should be 120 cm in AP and cross-table views but 102 cm in Dunn, frog-leg, and Lequesne views.[38]
- The structural parameters of the hip are assessed on all radiographic views (**FIGS 4** and **5**).

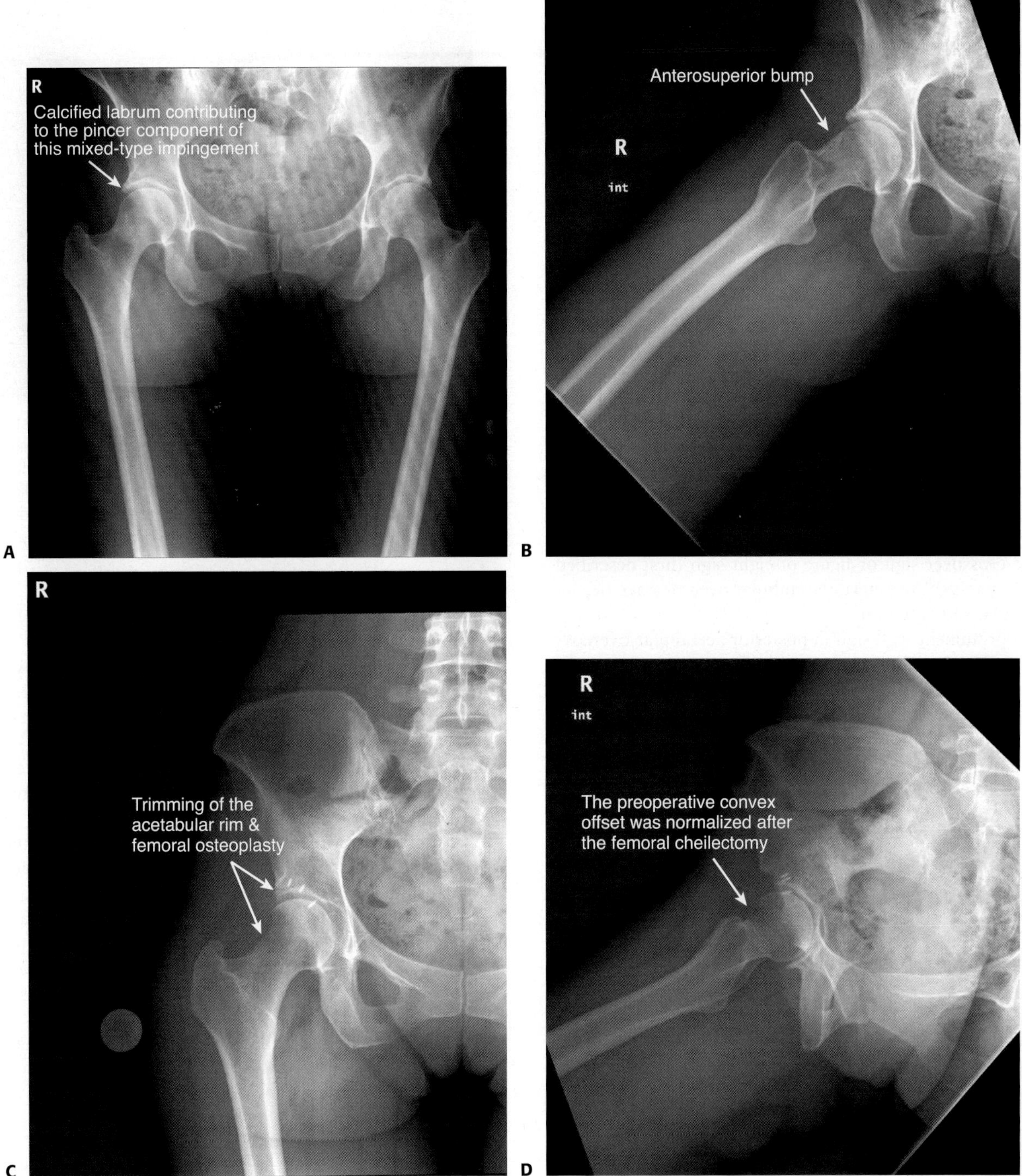

FIG 2 • **A.** AP pelvis view of 34-year-old female complaining of 1-year duration of right hip groin pain, noticed after a minor motor vehicle accident. This view shows a calcified labrum posteriorly and laterally, a finding that was confirmed on the MRA. Note the relatively normal head–neck junction on this view. **B.** Frog-leg lateral view of the right hip shows an anterosuperior prominence responsible for decreased offset, contributing to impingement during hip flexion and internal rotation. **C,D.** AP and lateral views of the right hip after femoroacetabular osteoplasty through mini-open direct anterior approach, showing the trimmed acetabular rim, reattached superolateral labrum, and femoral bump osteoplasty.

- AP view of the pelvis can identify the following:
  - Lateral cam lesion, which is a pistol grip deformity that has a prominent, convex head–neck junction with reduced head–neck offset[26] and an aspherical femoral head (alpha angle measurement)
  - Acetabular depth, where the acetabular fossa location is noted relative to the Kohler line to look for general acetabular overcoverage. Normally, the fossa is lateral to the Kohler line; coxa profunda is noted when the fossa is medial to this line and protrusio acetabuli when the medial aspect of the

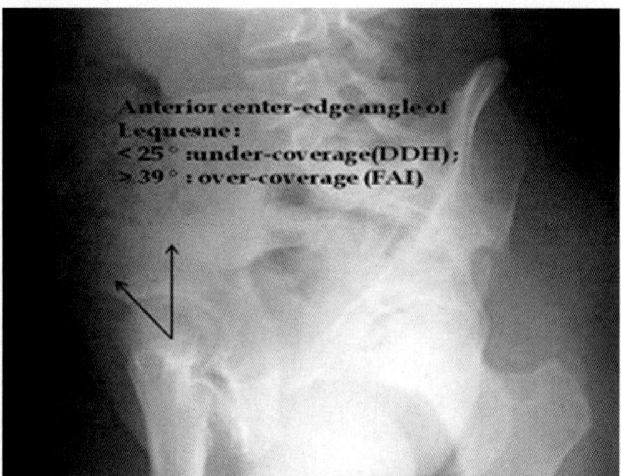

FIG 3 • False profile of the angle of Lequesne, which measures the anterior coverage of the femoral head. The anterior center-edge angle is measured between the vertical line passing through the femoral head center and the line connecting the femoral head center to the anterior sourcil edge.

femoral head is medial to this line. Acetabular version: look for the following:

- The crossover sign or figure-of-eight sign (first described by Reynolds)[26] in anterior acetabular overcoverage (ie, acetabular retroversion)
- The prominent wall sign in posterior acetabular overcoverage. Normally, the posterior wall passes approximately through the femoral head center.

- Often, with so-called acetabular retroversion, the ischial spine is abnormally prominent into the true pelvis medially.[38] Acetabular inclination is quantified by the Tönnis

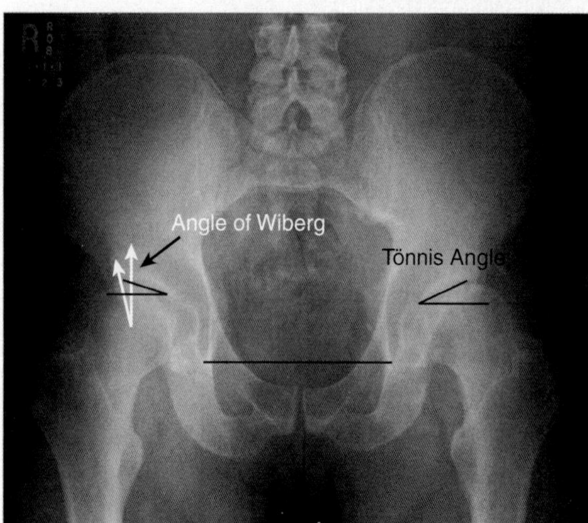

FIG 4 • Pelvis AP view of a 43-year-old gentleman complaining of bilateral groin pain. The *black lines* represent the Tönnis angle, which measures 25 degrees bilaterally in this case; it is the angle between the horizontal line (in reference to the bi-tear drop line) and the line joining the medial edge to the lateral edge of the acetabular sourcil. The *white arrows* depict the LCE angle of Wiberg, measured between the vertical line passing through the femoral head center and the line joining this center to the lateral sourcil edge; it measures 7 degrees on the left side and 10 degrees on the right. These values are consistent with bilateral hip dysplasia with coxa valga (femoral neck–shaft angle measuring 160 degrees on the right side and 152 degrees on the left).

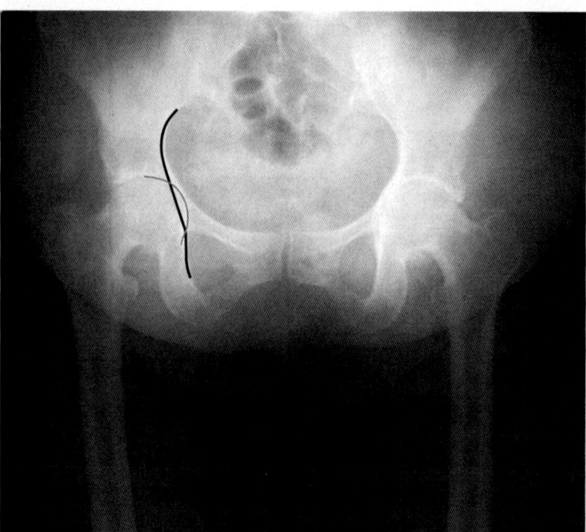

FIG 5 • AP pelvis view of 57-year-old lady complaining of long-standing left hip pain. It shows right hip coxa profunda where the acetabular fossa is medial to the Kohler line and left hip protrusio acetabuli where the femoral head is medial to this line. The *thick line* depicts the ilioischial line (Kohler line) and the *thin line* designs the acetabular fossa. Advanced bilateral OA is noted on this x-ray, making left THA option undisputable.

angle (acetabular index and acetabular roof angle), which is normally 10 degrees or slightly less.

- Other coxometric measurements noted on the AP view that quantify acetabular depth include the following:
  - The lateral center-edge (LCE) of Wiberg: normally varies between 25 and 39 degrees[38]
  - The femoral head extrusion index, where the uncovered horizontal portion of the femoral head is quantified, should not exceed 20% to 25%.
- The lateral views are examined to assess the following (**FIG 6**):
  - Femoral head sphericity: either by gross visual inspection or using the Mose template. Asphericity can be quantified by measuring the alpha angle of Nötzli (abnormal if >50 degrees in women and >68 degrees in men[38]). However, this angle measurement is subject to poor intraobserver reliability, with 30% of reliability based on an MRI study.[23]
    - The triangle index has better reproducibility than the alpha angle because it is constructed using clear geometric landmarks and is more independent from femoral rotation.[38]
  - Femoral head–neck offset is normally 11.6 ± 0.7 mm.[8] Generally, a value inferior to 10 mm is a strong indicator of cam impingement. The offset ratio (femoral offset divided by femoral head diameter) can also be deduced where a value inferior to 0.17 is considered abnormal.[21] Indentation sign on the femoral head in pincer impingement.[38]
- These projections best visualize the anterior and anterolateral femoral head–neck deformity that characterizes cam impingement disease.
- Joint space narrowing, periarticular cysts, and labral ossification are also noted on AP and lateral views.
- The alpha angle and head–neck offset can be measured on the AP view only in the case of pistol grip deformity. Both AP and lateral views should be scrutinized for abnormal morphologic features consistent with FAI.

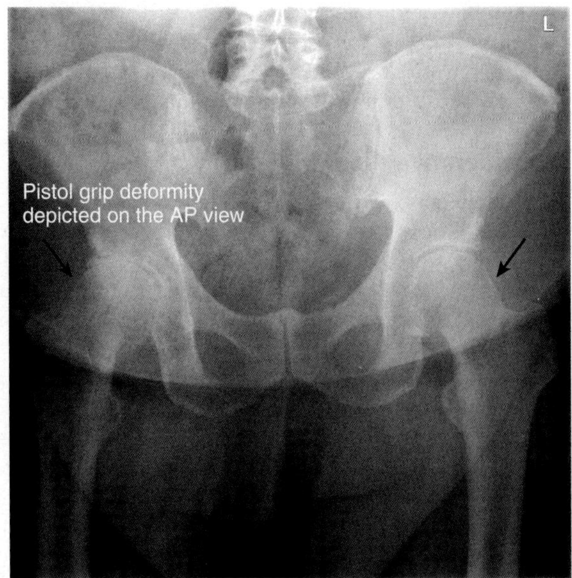

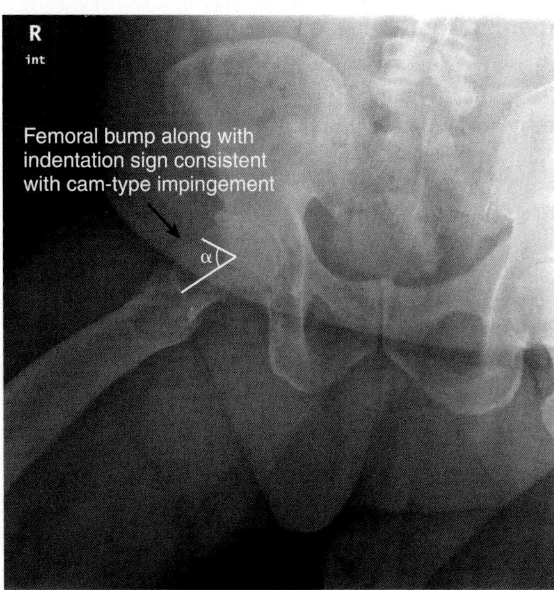

FIG 6 • AP and frog-leg lateral views of the hip of a 60-year-old man complaining of right hip pain. The roentgenograms shows advanced right hip OA with underlying etiology of a cam-type impingement. The anterolateral femoral osseous bump is noted on both hips, which is quantified by the alpha angle, calculated between the femoral neck axis and the line connecting the femoral head center to the point of beginning of the asphericity on the anterior femoral head contour. It measures 66 degrees on the right hip.

- Secondary changes in impingement can include labral ossification, acetabular stress fracture, and herniation pits (defined as radiolucencies surrounded by a sclerotic margin and located in the anterosuperior quadrant of the femoral neck).

Magnetic Resonance Angiogram

- MRA of the hip has been increasingly used in recent years for all patients with suspected impingement and associated intra-articular diseases.
  - The contour of the femoral head–neck junction,[19] labral disease,[7] and associated articular cartilage disease (especially in the posteroinferior joint) are better visualized on the MRA. The alpha angle and head–neck offset can be measured more accurately this way.
  - MRI also excludes other uncommon disorders such as stress fracture, osteonecrosis of the femoral head, neoplasm, infection, and synovial diseases.
- The sensitivity of an MRA is estimated to be 90% with a specificity of 91%.[11]
- Kassarjian et al[22] reported that in 88% of cases of symptomatic cam-type impingement, MRA detects a triad of abnormal head–neck morphology, anterosuperior cartilage abnormality, and anterosuperior labral abnormality.
- Using gadolinium-enhanced MRA, Nötzli et al[29] produced the first quantitative study of femoral head asphericity, describing the alpha angle and reporting that values of greater than 55 degrees on average are indicative of FAI.
- MRA is the most reliable technique to detect intra-articular lesions and should be performed in conjunction with x-rays whenever FAI is suspected.

Computed Tomography Scan

- It is the best investigation tool for bone characterization and can be useful in defining the extent of osseous impingement lesions. It shows in detail the contour of the femoral head–neck junction and the exact morphology of the femoral bump and complements other radiologic modalities.
- Alpha angles can be quantified using three-dimensional (3-D) reconstruction of CT scan. The beta angle (the angle at which the posterior aspect of the femoral head becomes aspherical) can also be measured.[26]
- All coxometric measurements (such as acetabular version) can be assessed thoroughly on CT images, confirming the roentgenographic findings.

DIFFERENTIAL DIAGNOSIS

- Differential diagnosis of FAI is mainly that of groin pain and other pathologies, including multiple hip disorders and pathologies of the adjacent bony and soft tissue structures.
- Mild hip dysplasia (joint instability) is the first and most important diagnosis to rule out. Usually, most dysplastic hips have excessive acetabular anteversion; however, as stated by Li and Ganz,[25] one in six dysplastic hips have some degree of retroversion. This finding should be noted preoperatively to avoid impingement worsening following routine anterior repositioning at the time of PAO.
- Isolated intra-articular hip disease (such as villonodular synovitis, chondrocalcinosis, isolated labral tear, chondral disease, and loose body) could explain hip pain in the absence of an impingement deformity.[3]
- Extra-articular hip disorders (such as sacroiliac joint disorders, tendinitis, and bursitis) or referred pain (lumbar spine diseases, inguinal hernia, and symptomatic femoral artery aneurysm) should not be overlooked.
- In cases where multiple disorders coexist or overlap, a diagnostic hip injection can be performed in order to confirm that the hip joint is the pain generator, with complete or near-complete pain relief indicating an intra-articular hip pathology.

Conservative Treatment

- Nonoperative measures to treat FAI have not been documented in the literature. However, this option should always be considered first. Conservative treatment may help and should be applied as a first-line treatment in symptomatic hips, especially those with mild and intermittent symptoms, before surgery is considered. Treatment may include activity restrictions, hydrotherapy, anti-inflammatory medicines, and intra-articular cortisone injections. The severity of the clinical picture will dictate the eventual therapeutic modalities.
- Physical therapy, emphasizing the improvement of passive hip ROM or stretching, is counterproductive and should be avoided because it will irritate the hip and subsequently worsen the pain by sustaining and evolving articular surface damage.
- Anti-inflammatory medicines may be appropriate to relieve acute-onset pain but may also mask the symptoms of an underlying destructive process.[23] These medications should be prescribed with caution and administered for a short period of time, given their side effects and taking into consideration symptoms necessitating an extended course of analgesics.
- Activity restriction or cessation may alleviate symptoms in some patients. Athletes involved in repetitive hip flexion activities may experience significant relief of discomfort if they refrain from their sport. Although conservative measures are likely to be temporarily successful in some patients, those with a high activity level and athletic ambitions usually have low compliance.[23]

SURGICAL MANAGEMENT

- Recognition of the detrimental effect of FAI has led to the development of novel joint-preserving techniques[24] aimed at restoring normal structural configurations of the proximal femur and/or acetabulum, interrupting the advancement of osseous morphology, and preventing the development of end-stage OA.
- Corrective surgery can be performed via several modalities, including a mini-open anterior approach, surgical dislocation of the hip,[12] combined hip arthroscopy and limited open decompression,[5] and arthroscopic decompression alone.[15]
- Selection of the adequate treatment option depends on multiple factors but is mainly dictated by the type and severity of the underlying abnormal anatomy.
- Open surgical dislocation of the hip with trochanteric flip osteotomy to perform osteochondroplasty, initially described by Ganz et al[12] in 2001, was the mainstay of early surgical management of FAI before the encouraging results of less invasive techniques were published.[26]
- Independently of the chosen technique, the primary goal of surgery is to address osseous structural impingement lesions and associated soft tissue intra-articular injuries (eg, labrum or articular cartilage). Many studies have demonstrated more favorable clinical, radiologic, and functional outcomes with labral repair compared to labral débridement in selected cases.[2,10,23,32]
- Surgical dislocation of the hip is reserved for less common cases with nonfocal (global) impingement problems or severe deformities such as advanced nonfocal femoral head deformity encountered in Legg-Calvé-Perthes disease or circumferential pincer impingement where the posterior acetabular rim cannot be exposed via the minimally invasive anterior approach or arthroscopy.
- For hips with focal cam-type FAI, the mini-open anterior surgical approach may provide excellent exposure, allowing appropriate correction of the osseous pathology on both sides of the joint while being a minimally invasive procedure.

Preoperative Planning

- The patient's history and physical examination findings should be reviewed shortly before proceeding with the surgery, with specific attention drawn to preoperative hip ROM, especially flexion and internal rotation, because these clinical parameters should improve after recontouring of the anterolateral femoral head–neck junction.
- Preoperative radiographic studies (x-rays, MRA, and CT scan if obtained) are reevaluated. The size and location of the impingement lesion or lesions are determined, as well as the status of the acetabular labrum and articular cartilage, and are correlated with intraoperative findings.
- It is of utmost importance to determine the type (cam, pincer, or a combined cam-pincer) and subtype of the impingement lesion (focal or global, femoral bump or angular deformity) because the characteristics of the specific deformity will dictate the surgical decision making:
  - On the acetabular side, the focal or global overcoverage can be corrected by resection osteoplasty of the excessive acetabular brim or by a reverse PAO to reorient a retroverted acetabulum.[24] The presence or absence of posterior overcoverage (as detected by the posterior wall sign) as well as the status of the acetabular articular cartilage determines which of these options is elected[24]; a reverse PAO is preferred if the posterior wall is deficient or the acetabular cartilage is injured.
  - On the femoral side, an osseous bump is nearly always the culprit lesion in reducing the clearance of the femoral neck during flexion; it can be corrected by resection osteoplasty.
- Although infrequent, proximal femur reorientation osteotomies can be done to address the FAI lesion such as femoral neck lengthening with trochanteric advancement or flexion-valgus intertrochanteric osteotomy (in case of decreased anteversion or varus position of the femoral neck).[24]
- In our practice, osteochondroplasty of the femoral head–neck junction and/or acetabular brim via mini-open anterior approach of the hip is used for the treatment of anterior cam-type impingement and associated intra-articular lesions.

Positioning

- Spinal or general anesthesia can be administered. However, regional anesthesia resulting in optimal muscle relaxation is preferred to facilitate joint distraction.
- The patient is positioned supine on a regular operating table. We prefer manual distraction of the joint while assessing the central compartment of the hip to minimize the risk of osteonecrosis of femoral head, which is correlated with the duration and force of traction applied through a fracture table.
- The hip region from the umbilicus to the upper thigh is scrubbed and draped. The whole leg is also scrubbed and draped free to allow unrestricted ROM of the hip during the procedure, a crucial surgical time for the assessment of the adequacy of the osteoplasty.

Techniques of Mini-Open Osteochondroplasty through the Direct Anterior Approach

Surgical Approach (Hueter Approach or Smith-Petersen Approach)

- A 3- to 4-cm incision is made extending from the lateral aspect of the anterior superior iliac spine heading distally toward the lateral side of the patella (**TECH FIG 1A**).
- This approach is a muscle-splitting approach, which dissects the interval between the sartorius (innervated by the femoral nerve) and the tensor fascia lata (TFL) (innervated by the superior gluteal nerve). We avoid developing this interval to protect the lateral femoral cutaneous nerve (LFCN) of the thigh.
- The dissection is carried through the subcutaneous tissue to the perimysium of the TFL muscle. The subcutaneous dissection is performed slightly lateral to the sartorius–tensor interval. The gap between the sartorius and the TFL can be easily identified and avoided by externally rotating the lower extremity to stretch the sartorius, making it more prominent.
- The fascia of the tensor muscle is incised over the muscle belly (**TECH FIG 1B**), and the TFL muscle is reflected downward and laterally. The medial soft tissue flap, including the tensor perimysium and the sartorius, is reflected upward and medially. The underlying rectus tendon is exposed.
- The original deep dissection of this approach involves an internervous passage between the rectus femoris (innervated by the femoral nerve) and the gluteus medius (innervated by the superior gluteal nerve). We do not dissect this interval; instead, we medially retract the rectus femoris without division of any of its insertions to avoid weakness of hip flexion.
- After medial retraction of the rectus, the soft tissue and iliocapsularis muscle fibers (iliacus minor, which originates from the

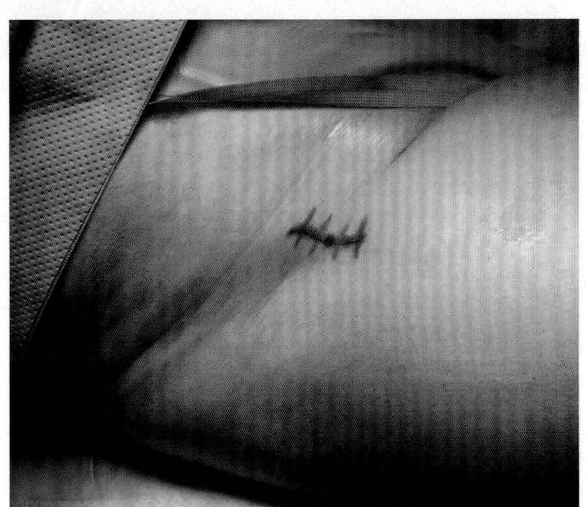

A

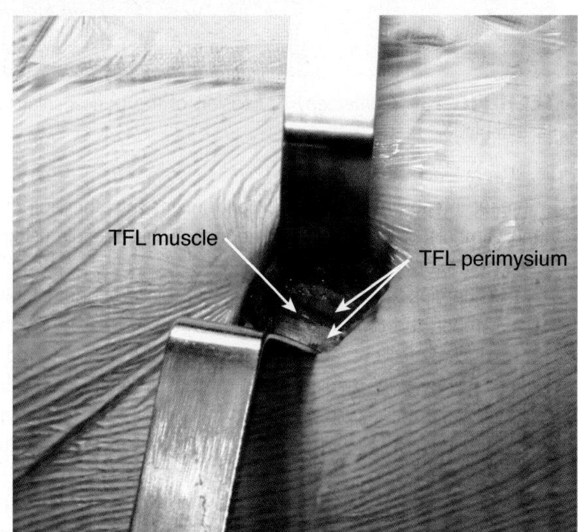

B

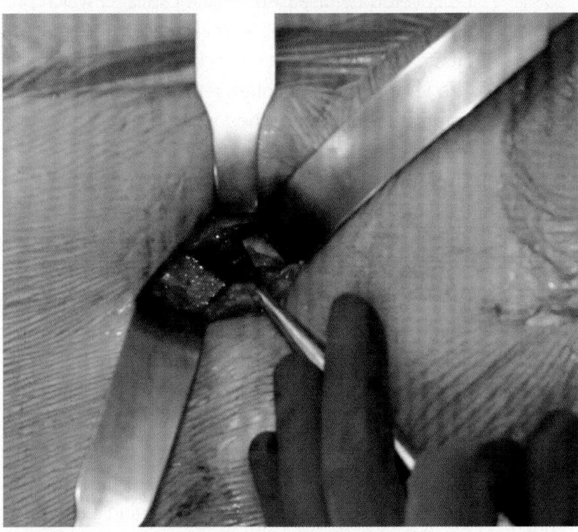

C

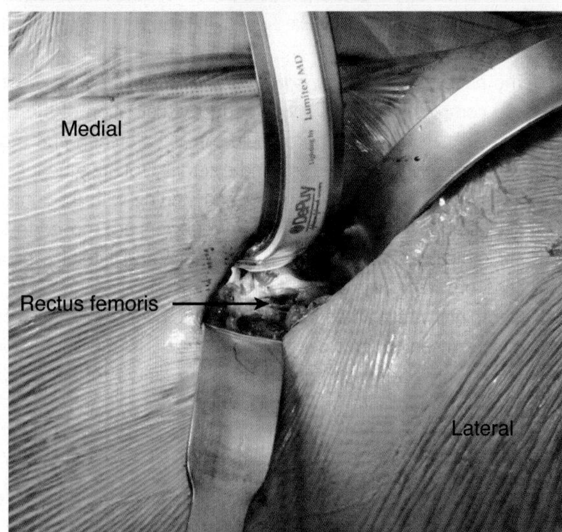

D

TECH FIG 1 • Mini-open anterior approach. **A.** Laterally to the ASIS, a 3-cm incision is drawn heading distally toward the lateral side of the patella. **B.** The TFL perimysium is opened, exposing the TFL muscle belly. **C.** Stripping of the pericapsular fat pad and the iliocapsularis muscle fibers using a Cobb elevator. **D.** Exposure of the rectus femoris after extra-articular placement of three curved retractors; the TFL and sartorius muscles are retracted laterally and medially, respectively, using two blunt-tipped retractors. A sharp-tipped retractor equipped with source light is placed proximally to the AIIS and medially to the origin of the rectus femoris. *(continued)*

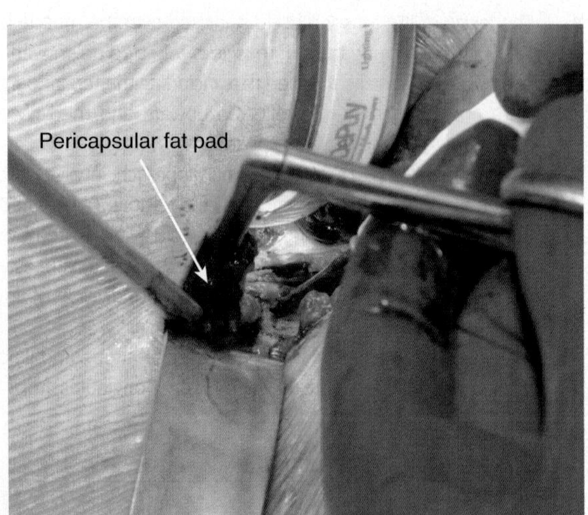

E

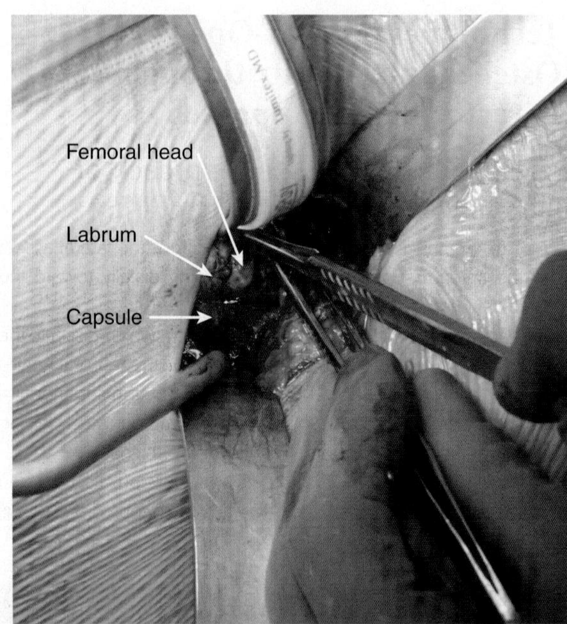

F

TECH FIG 1 • *(continued)* **E.** Excision of the pericapsular fat pad using Bovie cautery. **F.** I-shaped capsulotomy is performed with scalpel blade.

anterior inferior iliac spine [AIIS] and inserts into the iliofemoral ligament) are stripped from the anterior hip capsule using a Cobb elevator (**TECH FIG 1C**).

- Blunt-tipped curved retractors are placed, one laterally around the capsule overlying the neck of the femur and one medially retracting the sartorius and rectus muscles to expose the medial capsule of the femoral neck. At this point, the ascending branch of the lateral femoral circumflex artery is ligated or electrocoagulated if it crosses the surgical field.
- A third sharp-tipped retractor with a light source is placed at the upper part of the AIIS and under the rectus femoris; the hip should be flexed during placement of this retractor (**TECH FIG 1D**).

- The pericapsular fat pad is grasped with a pituitary instrument and completely excised, giving perfect visualization of the capsule (**TECH FIG 1E**). The capsule can be stretched and more easily identified by adducting and externally rotating the leg. An "I"-shaped capsulotomy is performed starting with the longitudinal limb (**TECH FIG 1F**), and the retractors are moved to the intra-articular space to reflect the medial and lateral capsular flaps, providing ample access to the femoral head and neck.
- Our mini-invasive anterior approach, which does not detach any muscle insertion, provides excellent access to the joint, which can be inspected with specific attention drawn to the femoral head–neck junction.

Femoral Head–Neck Reshaping Osteoplasty

- Based on the preoperative roentgenograms, after adequate exposure of the joint, a thorough assessment of the ROM is done to locate the FAI lesion. This step is crucial in the decision-making process for treatment of FAI.[23] The femoral head–neck junction should be inspected while the hip is brought into full and extreme motion. Although impingement in flexion and internal rotation is by far the most common, impingement also may occur in flexion–adduction, flexion–abduction, and rarely in extension and external rotation.[23]
- The lower extremity should be brought up into a figure-of-four position to provide adequate visualization of the posteromedial head–neck junction.
- The extent of the femoral bump, the presence of labral tear, and cartilaginous lesions are assessed and documented.
  - There is usually a clear delineation between the normal area of white femoral articular cartilage and the area of the femoral head afflicted with the impingement. The area of FAI (femoral bump) is convex shaped and may be covered by diseased hyaline cartilage, which presents as obvious wear and abnormal creases (indentation sign) created by repetitive contact with the acetabular rim. The femoral bump is often red or blue in appearance, in contrast to the untarnished white hyaline cartilage of the femoral head.[23]
  - The labrum should be carefully examined for evidence of tear and/or degeneration. A nerve hook is used to palpate the articular surface of the labrum[6] to reveal any tear concealed by the integrity of the capsular aspect of the labrum. Every effort should be made to repair an injured labrum[6,23]; resection should be reserved only for ossification, attrition, or extensive degeneration and scarring.
  - The central compartment of the hip is inspected and palpated by applying a manual traction to the extremity; with the arthrotomy done, minimal traction is sufficient to allow adequate subluxation of the hip and visualization of the weight-bearing dome region of the acetabulum.[6] To adequately palpate the cartilage using a hook, the joint subluxation can be maintained and optimized by inserting a smooth Cobb retractor into the joint. Any cartilaginous lesion should be noted and addressed either with conservative débridement, resection of the unstable

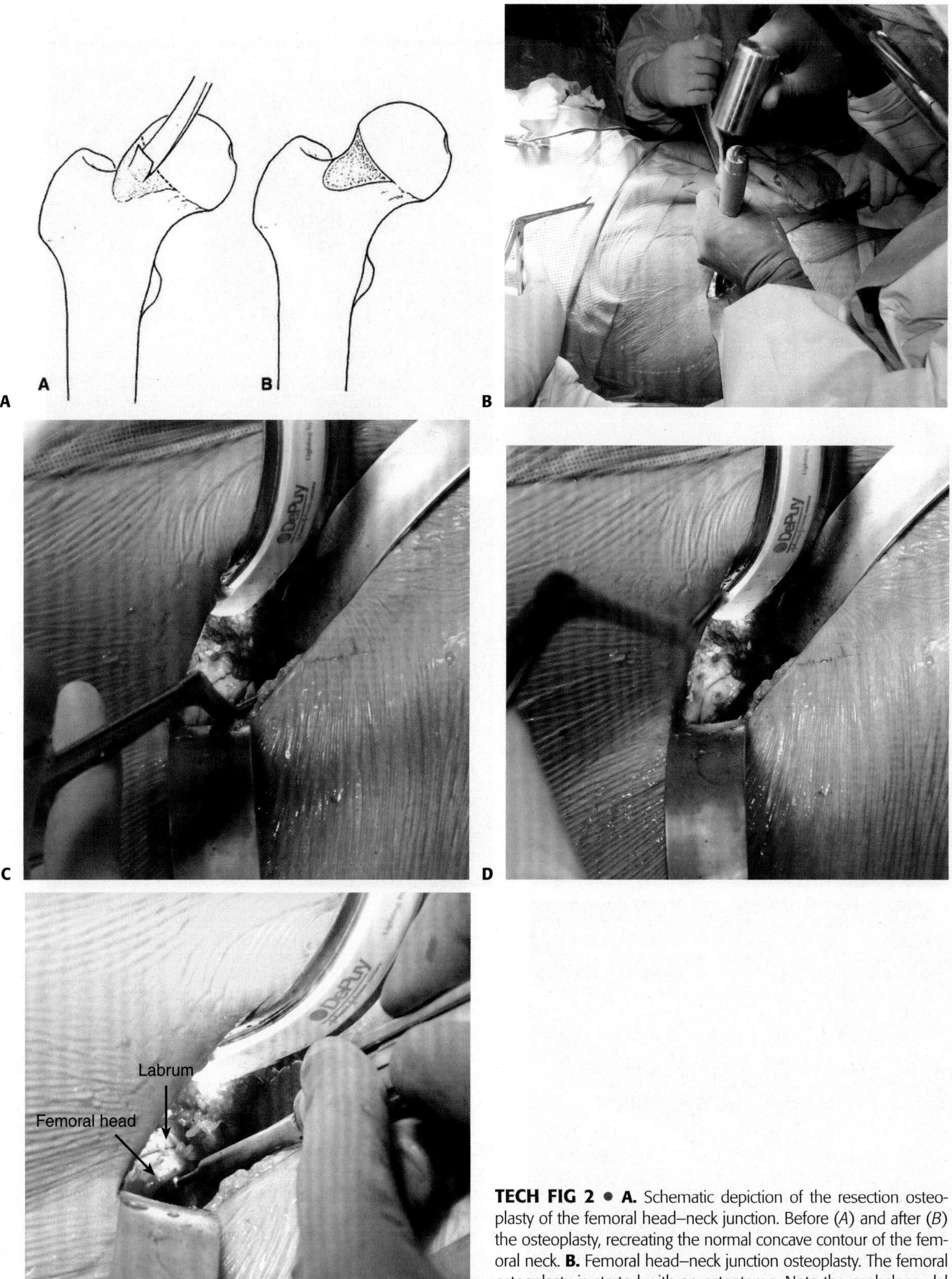

TECH FIG 2 • A. Schematic depiction of the resection osteoplasty of the femoral head–neck junction. Before (*A*) and after (*B*) the osteoplasty, recreating the normal concave contour of the femoral neck. **B.** Femoral head–neck junction osteoplasty. The femoral osteoplasty is started with an osteotome. Note the cephalocaudal orientation of the osteotome. **C,D.** Removal of the osteotomized bump. **E.** A high-speed pneumatic burr is used to fine-tune the femoral reshaping. *(continued)*

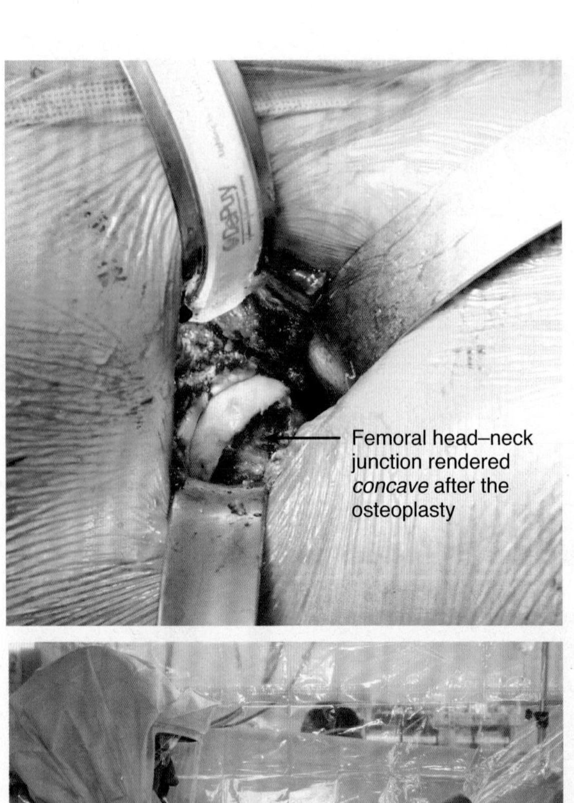

F

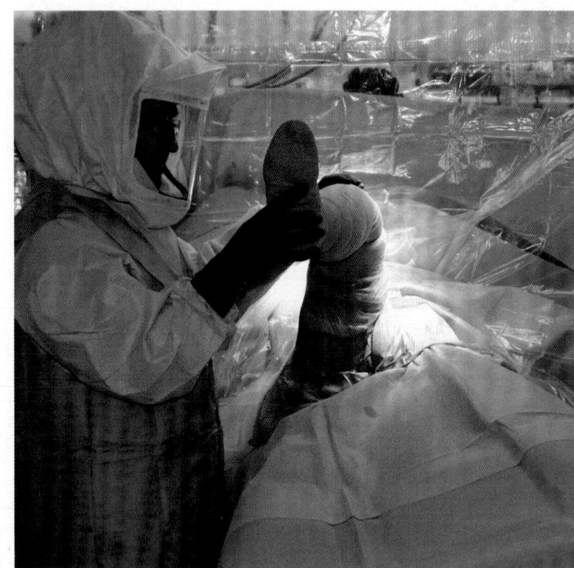

G

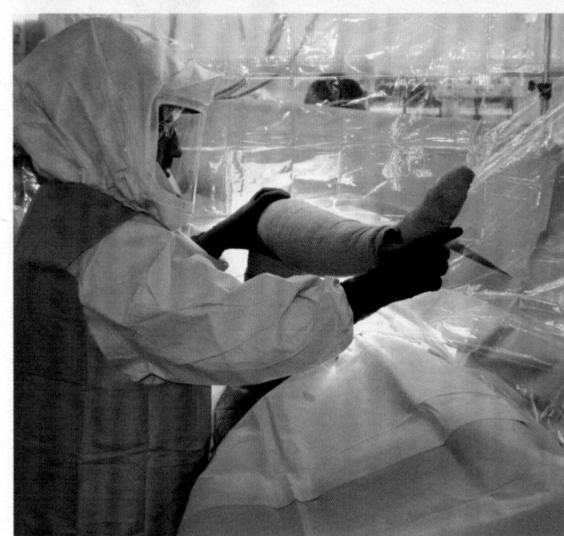

H

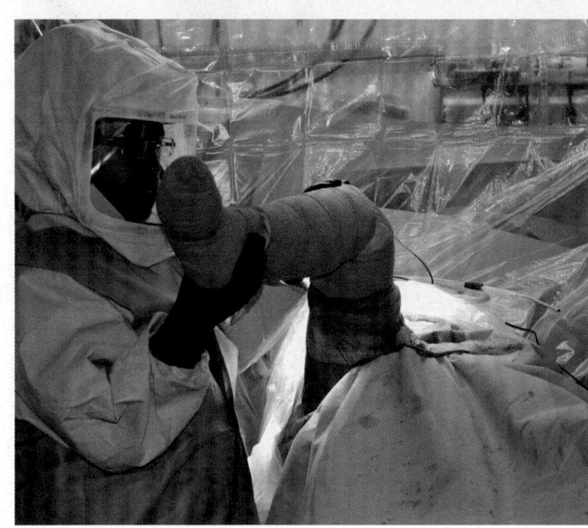

I

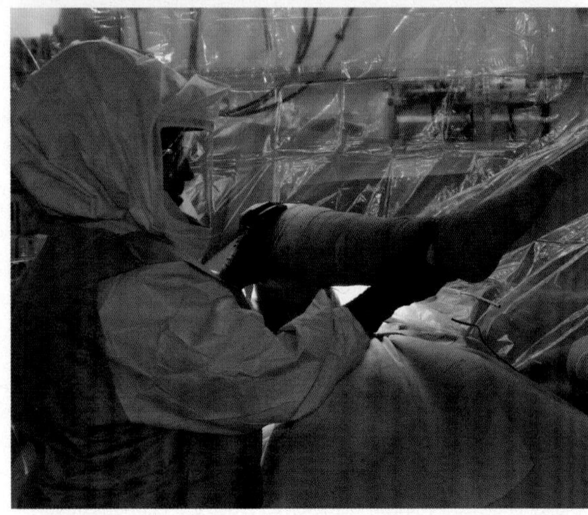

J

TECH FIG 2 • *(continued)* **F.** Note the restored normal concave shape of the head–neck junction after completion of the osteoplasty. **G.** ROM before and after the osteoplasty. Extremely limited internal rotation of the hip (<5 degrees) before the osteoplasty. **H.** Preoperative external rotation. **I,J.** Note the remarkable improvement of ROM after completion of the femoral osteoplasty, especially internal rotation, which increased about 30 degrees.

displaced cartilage flap (which can be responsible for clicking and catching), or microfracture of a full-thickness Outerbridge IV lesion, exposing the underlying subchondral bone.

- With the mini-open anterior approach, 60% to 70% of the acetabular cavity can be adequately visualized; the only portion that cannot be exposed is the posteroinferior part of the socket, which can be alternatively palpated by a blunt-tipped nerve hook.[6]
- The osteochondroplasty of the neck can be performed using a combination of osteotomes (**TECH FIG 2A**) (half- and quarter-inch curved osteotomes) and pneumatic burr (**TECH FIG 2B**). The femoral bump is located in the anterosuperior region and has a characteristic bluish-reddish discoloration. During this fundamental surgical step, the articular cartilage of the femoral head is protected by releasing the manual traction, allowing the head to re-sit inside the acetabulum.[6] If the socket contributes to the impingement lesions, it should be trimmed before proceeding with the femoral osteoplasty.
- The reshaping of the femoral head–neck junction should begin proximal to the impingement site (**TECH FIG 2B**) and tapered distally in a near circumferential manner, avoiding the superior portion of the neck where the posterosuperior retinacular vessels enter the bone[23]; these vessels are the terminal branches of the medial femoral circumflex artery.[14]
- The femoral cheilectomy should proceed in a stepwise manner, resecting at once a small bony sleeve. The adequacy of the resection is dynamically assessed perioperatively by bringing the hip into full ROM. The visualization of the lateral neck is maximized by internal rotation of the hip. The posteroinferior part of the neck is reached by placing the leg in a figure-of-four position.[6]
- If direct visualization and the palpation of the femoral head–neck junction detect residual impingement, the osteoplasty is incrementally refined until it is deemed to be adequate. Ultimately, it should be smoothly beveled inferiorly to prevent notching of the femoral neck.
- The extent of bone removal, as well as its depth (which ranges from 5 to 10 mm), is determined by the recreation of the normal smooth concave contour of the head–neck junction and achievement of impingement-free ROM.[6] In severe cases, the resection may expand to cover more than 180 degrees of the femoral head–neck circumference.
- After completion of the femoral head recontouring, the hip motion should improve at least 10 to 15 degrees in flexion and at least 15 to 20 degrees in internal rotation (**TECH FIG 2C**), with the concave femoral neck remaining free of abutment with the acetabular brim.[23]
- Fluoroscopic examination can be performed after completion of the cheilectomy, especially at the beginning of the procedure to confirm establishment of head sphericity and adequate osteochondral resection, with special attention paid to match the preoperative views based on the obturator foramen and the ischial tuberosity.
- AP and frog-leg lateral views should be obtained to better visualize the anterolateral head–neck junction. Varying degrees of flexion and internal–external rotation permit excellent assessment of the osteochondroplasty. In our practice, where FAI surgical correction is routine, we do not use perioperative fluoroscopic control.

Acetabular Rim Trimming by Resection Osteoplasty

- Whether to address the acetabular rim in the treatment of FAI is governed by two essential factors: the existence of anterior focal overcoverage and the condition of the acetabular articular cartilage and the labrum. Taking both factors into consideration will dictate the nature of treatment that should be done on the acetabular side: limited rim osteoplasty versus reverse PAO. If acetabular trimming is deemed necessary to restore normal hip morphology, it should be done before the femoral reshaping.
- Acetabular trimming necessitates full exposure of the bony acetabular ridge (**TECH FIG 3B**); for this purpose, the acetabular labrum must be carefully mobilized. As stated previously, resection of the labrum is done when it is ossified or when it is afflicted with attrition or excessive scarring. If required, the excision of the labrum should be as conservative as possible and limited to the injured area only. Otherwise, a healthy labrum with firm substance or minimally damaged (linear tears) should be preserved and repaired.
- If a focal anterior overcoverage contributes to FAI (acetabular retroversion with a positive crossover sign), a resection osteoplasty of the anterosuperior rim should be performed.
  - Before the osteoplasty of the rim is accomplished, the labrum, if not torn, is detached cautiously from the anterosuperior acetabular rim using a sharp blade[23] while preserving its continuity with the uninvolved normal segment.
- Once the bony lip of the acetabulum is adequately exposed, a 10-mm curved osteotome or 5-mm high-speed burr is used to trim the overhanging part of the brim (between 2 and 5 mm).[6,23] As for the femoral osteoplasty, the acetabular trimming should be carried out in a stepwise manner until the overcoverage has been entirely resected (**TECH FIG 3B**).
- The amount of rim resection is determined by the magnitude of the anterior overcoverage and extent of the chondral lesion as detected intraoperatively where the area of cartilage damage should be included in the trimming, but excessive (>1 cm) resection should be avoided at all costs to prevent any iatrogenic instability. Roughly 1 mm of resected acetabular edge corresponds to 2 to 3 degrees of correction of the Wiberg angle.
- After completion of the acetabular osteoplasty, the labrum is reattached with anchored sutures to the underlying cancellous acetabular rim, which is trimmed down to bleeding bone.[6] Three to four anchors are needed to reattach the labrum, and if the acetabular rim is analogous to a clock face, there should be an interval of 1 hour between the two anchors, with 6 hours located at the transverse ligament level.
- In cases where the acetabular retroversion is coexistent with a deficient posterior wall (running medial to the femoral head center) or at least lack of posterior overcoverage[23] (posterior wall passing through the head center), a reverse PAO should be done after confirming the integrity of the acetabular articular cartilage through MRA. Routine arthrotomy of the hip should always be done at the time of PAO to evaluate the labrum and the articular cartilage for the presence of lesions and to ensure impingement-free hip ROM. However, describing the PAO surgical technique is beyond the scope of this chapter.

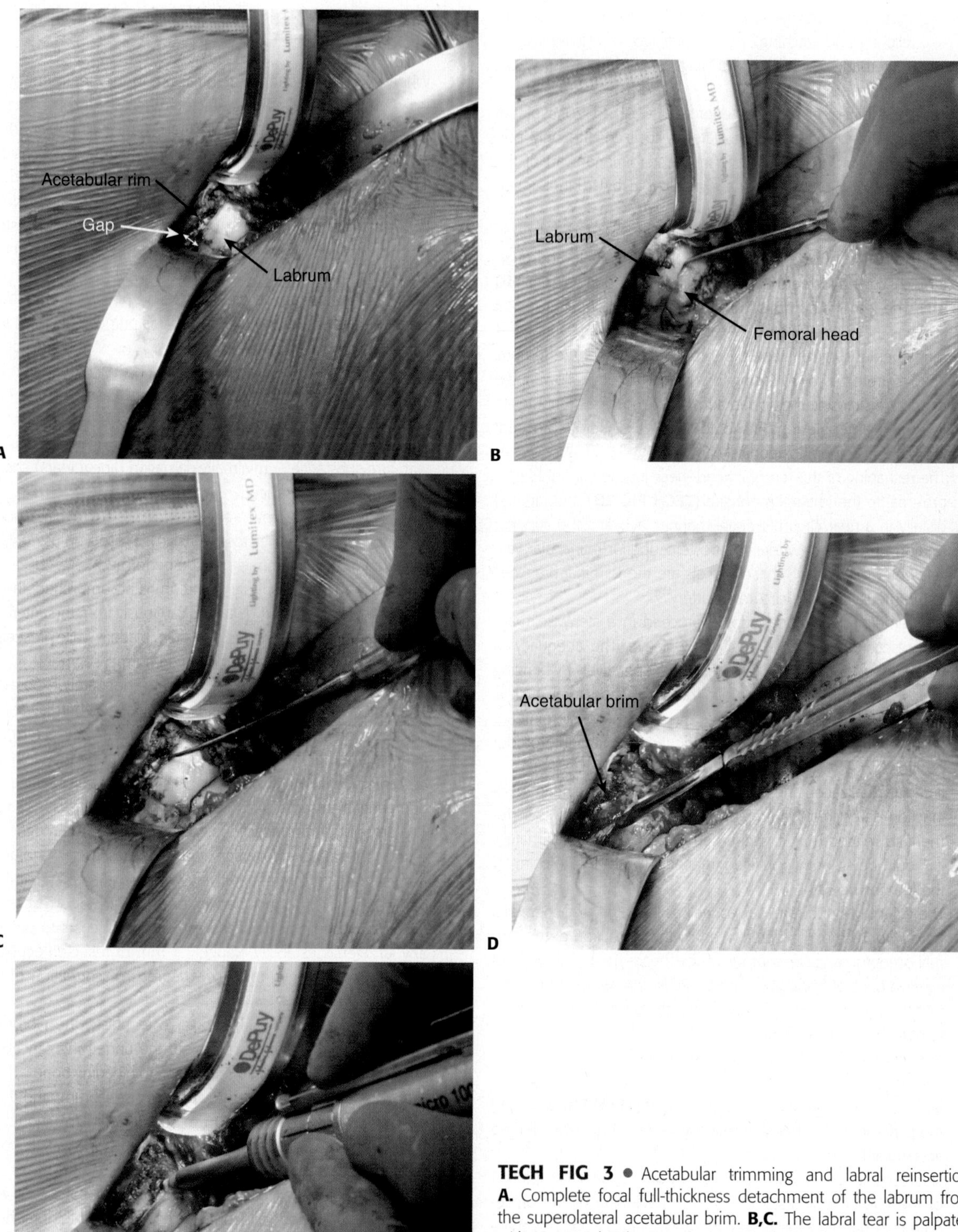

TECH FIG 3 • Acetabular trimming and labral reinsertion. **A.** Complete focal full-thickness detachment of the labrum from the superolateral acetabular brim. **B,C.** The labral tear is palpated with a nerve hook passed respectively on the articular and capsular surfaces of the labrum. **D.** The labral detachment is further extended with a blade, giving access to the anterolateral rim of the acetabulum. **E.** Trimming of the overhanging acetabular edge using a 5-mm high-speed burr. *(continued)*

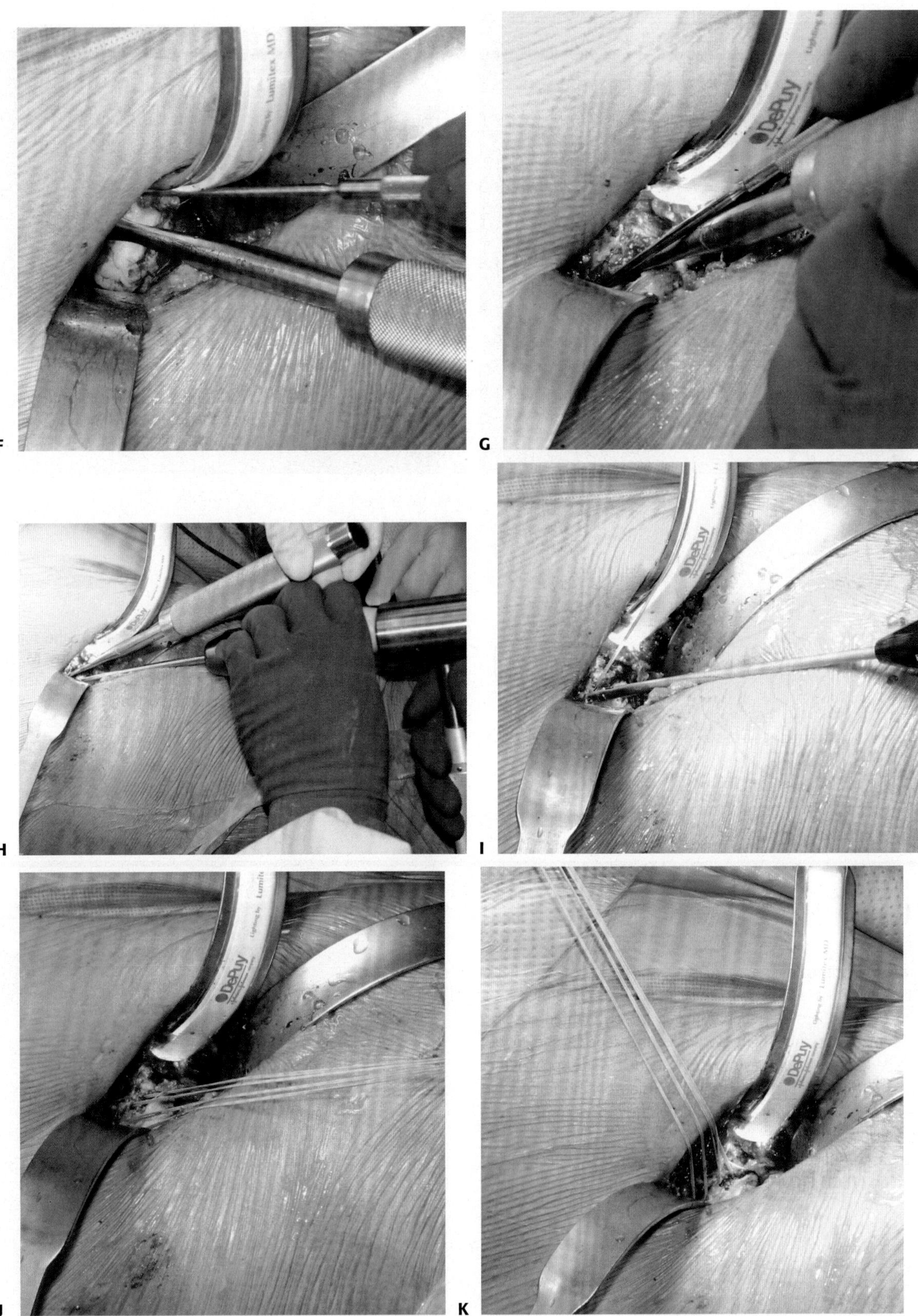

TECH FIG 3 • *(continued)* **F,G.** The cartilage of the central compartment is circumferentially palpated with the hook, whereas a Cobb retractor is placed inside the joint to maintain and enhance the femoroacetabular subluxation conferred by the manual traction. **H.** Microfracture is realized in the acetabular zone of full-thickness cartilaginous loss. **I–K.** Nonabsorbable suture anchors are inserted into the trimmed and revived acetabular rim; in this case, four anchors were used. *(continued)*

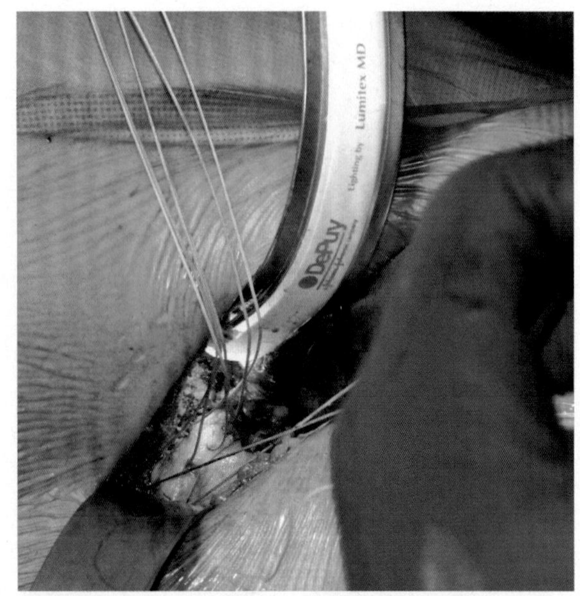

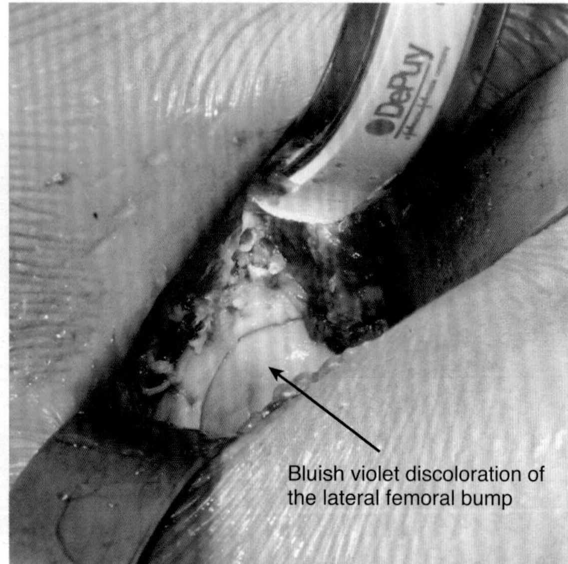

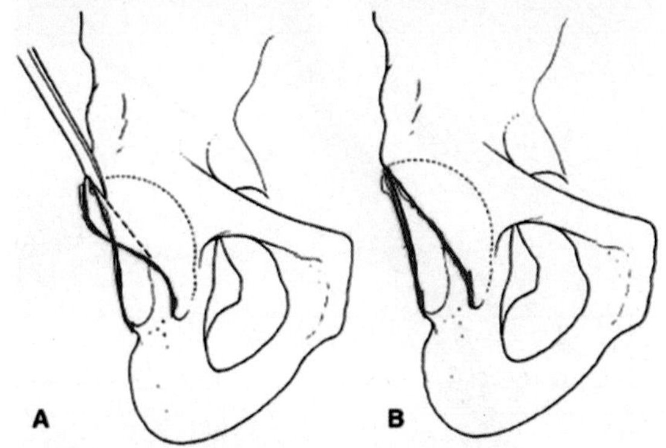

TECH FIG 3 • *(continued)* **L.** Equidistant passage of the sutures through the labral substance, taking good and stable bites. **M.** The sutures are tied, reattaching the labrum to its acetabular rim and reproducing its sealing effect. **N.** Resection osteoplasty of the excessive anterior rim of the acetabulum. Before (*A*) and after (*B*) the osteoplasty, removing the site of anterior impingement. Note the preoperative crossover sign, which disappeared after achievement of the trimming.

Closure

- After copious irrigation of the hip joint, bone wax is applied to the areas of bone resection on the femoral neck. After a final check of the hip ROM, a meticulous capsulorrhaphy is performed.[6]
- The capsular flaps are reapproximated loosely with an absorbable running suture. Tight closure of the capsule should be avoided because this may compromise the blood supply of the femoral head by placing excessive tension on the retinacular vessels.[23] Only the longitudinal limb of the capsulotomy needs to be closed.
- The fascia, subcutaneous tissue, and skin are closed in standard fashion (**TECH FIG 4**).

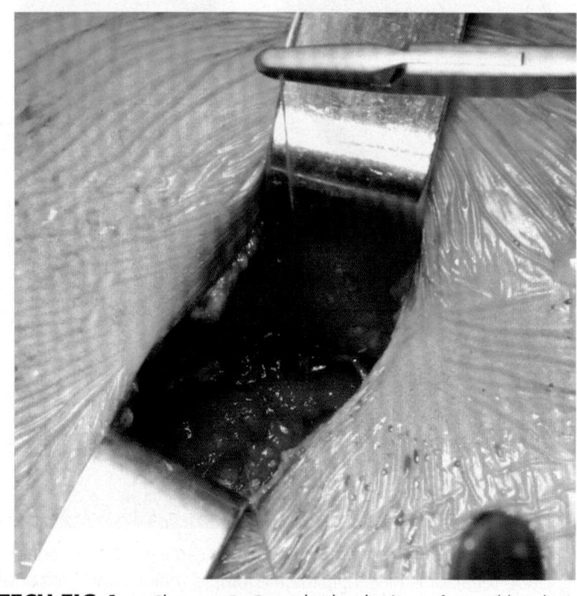

TECH FIG 4 • Closure. **A.** Capsulorrhaphy is performed by closing the longitudinal capsular limb. *(continued)*

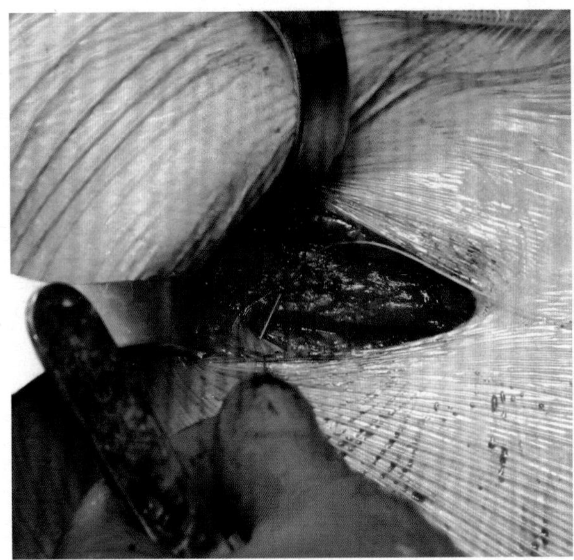
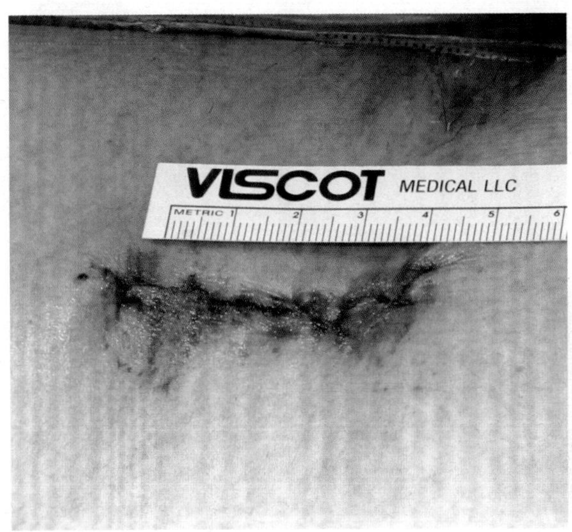

TECH FIG 4 • *(continued)* **B.** Closure of the TFL perimysium with absorbable running suture. **C.** Incision length of 4 cm.

PEARLS AND PITFALLS

Indications	■ Ideal surgical candidates are young (younger than 50 years old), have symptomatic FAI that has failed all conservative means, are well-conditioned, or have no or mild secondary cartilaginous damage. ■ Every aspect of the clinical picture should be taken into consideration to make a definitive diagnosis of anterior FAI. ■ The type of impingement disease should be accurately classified to exclude a coexistent hip dysplasia. ■ The surgical strategy presented here is primarily used for the treatment of anterior cam-type deformities. For severe and global deformities, hip dislocation is a valuable option and should be considered.
Articular cartilage and labrum	■ Cartilaginous lesions of the anterior and superolateral acetabular rim are common in both types of impingement.[23] ■ Articular flaps should be débrided back to stable articular cartilage. ■ Microfracture of the acetabular rim disease should be performed for full-thickness cartilage defects. ■ In rare cases where the labrum is revealed to be completely normal, it should not be detached from the acetabular rim.
Limited open osteochondroplasty	■ The sartorius–tensor muscle interval should not be developed in order to avoid damaging the LFCN. ■ None of the rectus femoris heads should be released. ■ For mixed FAI cases, the acetabular trimming and labral reinsertion should be performed first in order to accurately judge the adequacy of femoral recontouring back into a normalized acetabular socket. ■ The posteroinferior acetabular rim can be reached and, if needed, trimmed by placing the lower limb in a figure-of-four position (**FIG 7**). ■ A combination of curved osteotomes and pneumatic burr facilitates the osteoplasty through this surgical approach. ■ Perioperative dynamic examination of the hip and palpation through the arthrotomy ensures complete resection of the impinging structures.
Postoperative rehabilitation	■ Partial weight bearing should be continued for 6 weeks postoperatively to minimize the risk of iatrogenic femoral neck fracture. ■ Excessive therapy within the first 2 months after surgery should be avoided because it can hamper the rehabilitation process. ■ Emphasis should be on gentle ROM within the patient's comfort zone and gentle, progressive strengthening as tolerated by the patient.

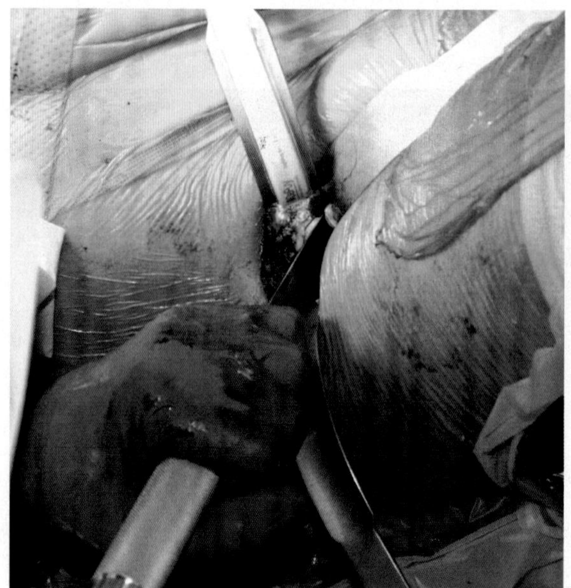

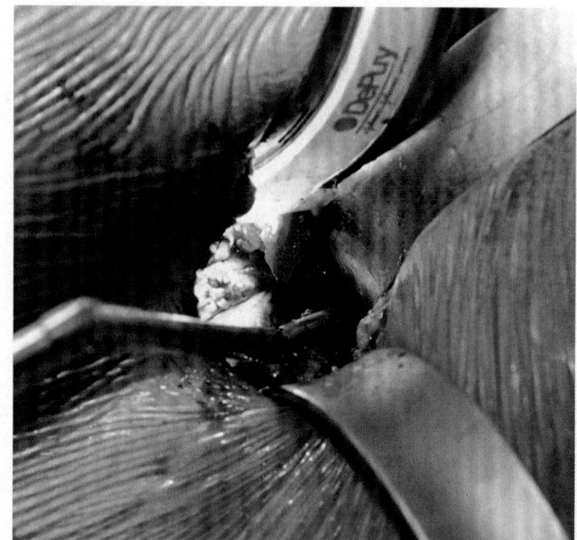

FIG 7 • Posteroinferior acetabular rim resection. **A,B.** By placing the lower limb in a figure-of-four position, the posteroinferior aspect of the medial acetabular brim can be reached and osteotomized.

POSTOPERATIVE CARE

- The patients are usually hospitalized for 24 hours and postoperative radiographs are obtained to verify the adequate recontouring of the femoral head–neck junction and to document the integrity of the femoral neck (see **FIG 2**). Postoperative films should be compared to the preoperative films, avoiding any pelvic tilt or malrotation.
- Pharmaceutical deep venous thrombosis prophylaxis is treated with aspirin, one tablet of 325 mg administered two times a day for 6 weeks.
- Heterotopic ossification (HO) risk can be minimized with prophylactic administration of anti-inflammatory medications for 6 weeks: celecoxib (400 mg/day) or indomethacin (75 mg/day). The mini-open anterior approach involves little surgical dissection and avoids any muscular detachment, decreasing the risk of HO with minimal blood loss. Copious irrigation of the joint also reduces the risk of HO development.
- The rehabilitation program consists of touchdown partial weight bearing using crutches for 6 weeks to decrease the risk of femoral neck stress fracture, and then progresses gradually to full weight bearing. During this period, hip flexion is limited to 70 degrees.
- To prevent adhesions between the capsule and the osteotomized zone of the femoral neck, continuous passive motion (no more than 70 degrees of hip flexion) can be used for 4 to 6 hours per day for 1 or 2 weeks postoperatively.[23]
- Formal physical therapy can be started 6 weeks after surgery. The rehabilitation should consist of a gentle ROM program and progressive strengthening within the patient's comfort zone. Because the surgical technique does not involve trochanteric osteotomy, abduction strengthening can be initiated early in the postoperative period.
- The patient may return to normal daily activities (such as walking, ascending or descending stairs, and riding a stationary bicycle) as tolerated 4 to 6 weeks after surgery and may return to full activity once ROM and strength are restored and pain reduced, typically 4 to 6 months postoperatively.

OUTCOMES

- Because FAI has gained significant interest only during the last decade, only a small number of studies have been published documenting the clinical outcome of conservative surgical treatment.[2,10,15,32] Good midterm results have been reported using various surgical approaches for treatment of FAI, including surgical dislocation, arthroscopy, combined arthroscopy, and limited open and direct anterior mini-open approaches.[30]
- As surgical dislocation of the hip was the mainstay of treatment for FAI, several studies evaluated this particular surgical option, providing early- to midterm clinical outcomes which are promising.[2,10,32,40] Despite its ease of performance and relatively good clinical outcome, dislocation carries a risk of developing complications, mainly HO[12] (37%) and greater trochanter malunion (up to 20%).[40]
- In addition, although there were no reported cases of avascular necrosis (AVN), in the initial description of the procedure, laser Doppler flowmetry showed transient changes in head perfusion during the procedure, which returned to baseline after reduction of the joint.[5] Dislocation also requires the rupture or division of the ligamentum teres with loss of its proprioceptive nerve fibers, the consequences of which are currently unknown.[5]
- Arthroscopic osteochondroplasty has certain potential disadvantages, including the risk of inadequate exposure of the anterolateral head–neck junction, entrapment of bony debris within the joint, increasing the risk of HO, and the possibility of inadequate osseous débridement, leading to failed procedure.
- The mini-open anterior approach combine the advantages of arthroscopic decompression and open surgical dislocation while avoiding the main drawbacks of these two techniques:
  - Similar to hip arthroscopy, no traction is required, and the mini-open procedure carries less risk of neural damage and scuffing of the femoral head cartilage.

- It is a minimally invasive approach that avoids hip dislocation and the need for trochanteric osteotomy, which is top on the list of complications (trochanteric malunion) associated with this surgical method.
- It provides a wide and comprehensive view of all the compartments of the hip, which can be suboptimal in the technically demanding arthroscopic-only procedure, allowing adequate care for chondral and labral lesions.

- Our experience with the mini-open anterior approach has been encouraging when applied to appropriately indicated impingement cases. Analysis of 293 consecutive cases performed in 265 patients between January 2006 and February 2011 revealed good to excellent clinical outcomes; 156 hips (149 patients) achieved a minimum of 2-year follow-up. Out of these, 11 hips underwent THA and 1 hip underwent resurfacing due to degenerative joint disease at an average of 1.4 years postoperatively.[30]
- Despite the auspicious outcome of this technique, it may not be advocated for more advanced disease with posterior impingement lesions or for hips that have circumferential lesions of the femoral head where surgical dislocation, as described by Ganz et al,[12] seems to be more accommodating.

COMPLICATIONS

General Complications

- As with any surgical procedure, this less invasive intervention carries a risk for general complications not directly related to the surgical technique; the most relevant are the following:
  - Infection
  - Deep venous thrombosis
- The relatively short operative time and young age of the patients, along with the fast recovery following the procedure, indicates that the likelihood of developing these complications is exceedingly small.

Specific Complications Related to the Surgical Technique

- The rate and nature of complications associated with the surgical treatment of FAI differ according to the type of surgical procedure performed. The mini-open approach nullifies the risk of trochanteric malunion observed with the surgical dislocation technique and reduces significantly the risk of articular cartilage scuffing, which can occur in hip arthroscopy, especially if the instruments are introduced before obtaining sufficient hip distraction of 8 to 10 mm.
- Neurovascular injury
  - The LFCN is at greatest risk of injury through the mini-open approach.[6] If the interval between the TFL and the sartorius is dissected, the fascia of the latter should be avoided because the LFCN runs over it. Dissection of this interval is not mandatory to provide wide access to the hip joint.
  - This approach does not carry the risk of neurologic damage associated with the arthroscopy where
    - Excessive hip flexion can injure the sciatic nerve.
    - An inadequately padded perineal post can compress the pudendal nerve.
  - Transient neurapraxia has been reported with the use of excessive traction applied during hip arthroscopy.
  - The femoral artery and nerve can be injured through both the arthroscopic and open approaches. Following anatomic landmarks carefully during the mini-open anterior approach spares these vital structures.
- HO
  - Copious irrigation of the joint after the cheilectomy is completed and before proceeding with the capsulorrhaphy decreases the risk of HO. This risk is higher with the purely arthroscopic technique where osteochondroplasty is performed with a high-speed burr, yielding osseous debris; in this case, high-flow hip irrigation along with continuous suction should be used all the time.
  - In addition to profuse irrigation, prophylactic use of indomethacin minimizes the risk of HO development.
- Femoral neck fracture
  - Removing more bone proximally than distally on the head–neck junction can create an apple-bite[20] defect instead of the normal concave-shape junction; this defect can get wedged into the acetabular dome during hip flexion, breaking the suction seal of the labrum and increasing the risk of postoperative femoral neck fracture.
  - In contrast, incomplete reshaping of the head–neck junction is probably more frequent with the purely arthroscopic technique, which has a long learning curve. Several publications have stated that the main reasons for hip arthroscopy revision are inadequate remodeling of FAI deformities.[17]
  - The technique described here provides an excellent visualization of the hip and is associated with lesser risk of failure due to inadequate osteoplasty. However, recurrence of the osseous bump can still occur with any technique used to treat FAI; applications of bone wax on the bleeding reshaped bony cuts reduce the risk of bump reappearance.
- AVN of the femoral head
  - The risk of AVN following hip arthroscopy was theoretical until the results of two cases were published in the literature.[33,34] It is believed that femoral head osteonecrosis may develop secondary to a combination of increased intra-articular pressure and traction.
  - A constant and reliable landmark to identify the hip blood supply arthroscopically is the lateral synovial fold.[17]
  - Because no traction is needed during the mini-open approach, it can be hypothesized that the risk of AVN is less with this procedure, but special care needs to be taken to avoid the zone of the femoral neck where the retinacular vessels run. Because FAI treatment through hip dislocation has not been shown to increase the risk of AVN,[12] this risk is small after cheilectomy through an anterior approach, sparing the need for hip dislocation.
  - In our large series of patients operated on using the mini-open anterior approach, postoperative complications included one neuroma (0.6%) that required excision, one subtrochanteric hip fracture (0.6%) that required open reduction and internal fixation, one repeat labral tear (0.6%) that underwent arthroscopic débridement, and one case of persistent trochanteric bursitis (0.6%) that required iliotibial band lengthening/greater trochanteric bursa excision.[30]

REFERENCES

1. Beck M, Kalhor M, Leunig M, et al. Hip morphology influences the pattern of damage to the acetabular cartilage: femoroacetabular impingement as a cause of early osteoarthritis of the hip. J Bone Joint Surg Br 2005;87:1012–1018.
2. Beck M, Leunig M, Parvizi J, et al. Anterior femoroacetabular impingement: part II. Midterm results of surgical treatment. Clin Orthop Relat Res 2004;(418):67–73.
3. Burnett RS, Della Rocca GJ, Prather H, et al. Clinical presentation of patients with tears of the acetabular labrum. J Bone Joint Surg Am 2006; 88:1448–1457.
4. Clohisy JC, Keeney JA, Schoenecker PL. Preliminary assessment and treatment guidelines for hip disorders in young adults. Clin Orthop Relat Res 2005;441:168–179.
5. Clohisy JC, McClure JT. Treatment of anterior femoroacetabular impingement with combined hip arthroscopy and limited anterior decompression. Iowa Orthop J 2005;25:164–171.
6. Cohen SB, Huang R, Ciccotti MG, et al. Treatment of femoroacetabular impingement in athletes using a mini-direct anterior approach. Am J Sports Med 2012;40:1620–1627.
7. Czerny C, Hofmann S, Neuhold A, et al. Lesions of the acetabular labrum: accuracy of MR imaging and MR arthrography in detection and staging. Radiology 1996;200:225–230.
8. Eijer H, Leunig M, Mohamed N, et al. Cross table lateral radiographs for screening of anterior femoral head neck offset in patients with femoro acetabular impingement. Hip Int 2001;11:37–41.
9. Eijer H, Myers SR, Ganz R. Anterior femoroacetabular impingement after femoral neck fractures. J Orthop Trauma 2001;15(7):475–481.
10. Espinosa N, Rothenfluh DA, Beck M, et al. Treatment of femoroacetabular impingement: preliminary results of labral fixation. J Bone Joint Surg Am 2006;88:925–935.
11. Ferguson TA, Matta J. Anterior femoroacetabular impingement: a clinical presentation. Sports Med Arthrosc 2002;10:134–140.
12. Ganz R, Gill TJ, Gautier E, et al. Surgical dislocation of the adult hip: a technique with full access to the femoral head and acetabulum without the risk of avascular necrosis. J Bone Joint Surg Br 2001;83: 1119–1124.
13. Ganz R, Parvizi J, Beck M, et al. Femoroacetabular impingement: a cause for osteoarthritis of the hip. Clin Orthop Relat Res 2003;417:112–120.
14. Gautier E, Ganz K, Krügel N, et al. Anatomy of the medial femoral circumflex artery and its surgical implications. J Bone Joint Surg Br 2000;82:679–683.
15. Guanche CA, Bare AA. Arthroscopic treatment of femoroacetabular impingement. Arthroscopy 2006;22:95–106.
16. Hack K, Di Primio GD, Rakhra K, et al. Prevalence of cam-type femoroacetabular impingement morphology in asymptomatic volunteers. J Bone Joint Surg Am 2010;92(14):2436–2444.
17. Ilizaliturri VM Jr. Complications of arthroscopic femoroacetabular impingement treatment: a review. Clin Orthop Relat Res 2009;467: 760–768.
18. Imam S, Khanduja V. Current concepts in the diagnosis and management of femoroacetabular impingement. Int Orthop 2011;35:1427–1435.
19. Ito K, Minka MA II, Leunig M, et al. Femoroacetabular impingement and the cam-effect. An MRI-based quantitative anatomical study of the femoral head-neck offset. J Bone Joint Surg Br 2001;83:171–176.
20. Jackson T, Stake CE, Trenga AP, et al. Arthroscopic technique for treatment of femoroacetabular impingement. Arthrosc Tech 2013;2(1): e55–e59.
21. Kappe T, Kocak T, Bieger R, et al. Radiographic risk factors for labral lesions in femoroacetabular impingement. Clin Orthop Relat Res 2011;469(11):3241–3247.
22. Kassarjian A, Yoon LS, Belzile E, et al. Triad of MR arthrographic findings in patients with cam-type femoroacetabular impingement. Radiology 2005;236:588–592.
23. Lavigne M, Parvizi J, Beck M, et al. Anterior femoroacetabular impingement: part I. Techniques of joint preserving surgery. Clin Orthop Relat Res 2004;418:61–66.
24. Leunig M, Parvizi J, Ganz R. Nonarthroplasty surgical treatment of hip osteoarthritis. Instr Course Lect 2006;55:159–166.
25. Li PL, Ganz R. Morphologic features of congenital acetabular dysplasia: one in six is retroverted. Clin Orthop Relat Res 2003;(416): 245–253.
26. Macfarlane RJ, Haddad FS. The diagnosis and management of femoro-acetabular impingement. Ann R Coll Surg Engl 2010;92: 363–367.
27. Meyer DC, Beck M, Ellis T, et al. Comparison of six radiographic projections to assess femoral head/neck asphericity. Clin Orthop Relat Res 2006;445:181–185.
28. Myers SR, Eijer H, Ganz R. Anterior femoroacetabular impingement after periacetabular osteotomy. Clin Orthop Relat Res 1999;(363): 93–99.
29. Nötzli HP, Wyss TF, Stoecklin CH, et al. The contour of the femoral head-neck junction as a predictor for the risk of anterior impingement. J Bone Joint Surg Br 2002;84(4):556–560.
30. Parvizi J, Huang R, Diaz-Ledezma C, et al. Mini-open femoroacetabular osteoplasty: how do these patients do? J Arthroplasty 2012;27 (8 suppl):122–125.
31. Peelle MW, Della Rocca GJ, Maloney WJ, et al. Acetabular and femoral radiographic abnormalities associated with labral tears. Clin Orthop Relat Res 2005;441:327–333.
32. Peters CL, Erickson JA. Treatment of femoroacetabular impingement with surgical dislocation and debridement in young adults. J Bone Joint Surg Am 2006;88:1735–1741.
33. Sampson TG. Complications of hip arthroscopy. Clin Sports Med 2001;20:831–835.
34. Scher DL, Belmont PJ Jr, Owens BD. Osteonecrosis of the femoral head after hip arthroscopy. Clin Orthop Relat Res 2010;468: 3121–3125.
35. Smith-Petersen MN. The classic: treatment of malum coxae senilis, old slipped upper femoral epiphysis, intrapelvic protrusion of the acetabulum, and coxa plana by means of acetabuloplasty. J Bone Joint Surg 1936;18:869–880.
36. Snow SW, Keret D, Scarangella S, et al. Anterior impingement of the femoral head: a late phenomenon of Legg-Calvé-Perthes' disease. J Pediatr Orthop 1993;13(3):286–289.
37. Takeyama A, Naito M, Shiramizu K, et al. Prevalence of femoroacetabular impingement in Asian patients with osteoarthritis of the hip. Int Orthop 2009;33(5):1229–1232.
38. Tannast M, Siebenrock K. Conventional radiographs to assess femoroacetabular impingement. Instr Course Lect 2009;58:203–212.
39. Tanzer M, Noiseux N. Osseous abnormalities and early osteoarthritis: the role of hip impingement. Clin Orthop Relat Res 2004;429: 170–177.
40. Yun HH, Shon WY, Yun JY. Treatment of femoroacetabular impingement with surgical dislocation. Clin Orthop Surg 2009;1:146–154.

Basics of Total Hip Arthroplasty: The Preoperative Patient Evaluation

16 CHAPTER

Scot Brown and William Hozack

DEFINITION

- Total hip arthroplasty (THA) is one of the most successful operations performed today.[3]
- This elective procedure provides significant pain relief and improved functional status to millions of patients globally every year.
- Due to its elective nature, careful preoperative screening, evaluation, and medical workup are important to continue to reproduce or improve on the historical success of this operation.

PATHOGENESIS

- There are many varied causes of hip pain or limited function that makes a patient a good candidate for THA (Table 1).

PATIENT HISTORY AND PHYSICAL FINDINGS

- A detailed history and examination is necessary to delineate the etiology of the pain and functional limitations.
- The history of the present illness should include, but is not limited to, the following:
  - Evaluation of pain severity, quality, location, and duration
    - Attention should be paid to mitigating and exacerbating factors.*
    - Hip-related pain typically is felt in the groin but may present atypically as anterior thigh or knee pain.
    - Functional limitations such as inability to engage in activities of daily living (ADLs), work, exercise, or have a problem with travel. Some of these patients may also be at risk of falls due to gait problems.*
  - Interventions attempted to date and their effectiveness
    - Modification of activities
    - Medications
    - Injections*
    - Use of assistive devices*
    - Physical therapy and associated modalities*
    - Weight loss*
  - Specific questions should be asked to differentiate true hip pain from lateral thigh pain or sciatica; for example, asking about the primary location of the pain (groin versus thigh or buttock) and associated symptoms such as radiation past the knee, distal weakness, or paresthesias.
- The past medical history should include the following:
  - Disease processes that require more extensive preoperative workup and clearance prior to surgery, such as coronary and pulmonary disorders, diabetes, and immune-related diseases, may affect surgery, anesthesia, recovery, and healing time.
  - Medications, especially blood thinners, disease-modifying antirheumatic drugs, and steroids, which may need to be stopped in the perioperative period
  - Allergies to medication, especially antibiotics and analgesics, as well as latex allergies. For example, a patient with a documented penicillin allergy will need to have either vancomycin or clindamycin administered pre- and postoperatively for prophylaxis.[4]
- A physical examination is important to document the preoperative status of the affected hip and ipsilateral lower extremity. It also helps identify other causes of symptoms that patients perceive as hip pain, such as back pain, where a significant number of patients have compounding pathologies.[6]
- A thorough neurovascular examination documents preoperative status and can indicate patients who may require more intensive preoperative testing. The examination should include the following:
  - Pedal pulses—if absent, ankle–brachial indices and a vascular surgery evaluation may be needed.
  - Distal motor strength, noting any grade of preexisting foot drop
  - Distal sensation
  - Notation of edema, skin changes, or hair loss that may indicate severe vascular dysfunction and increased risk for wound healing problems and infection
- Evaluate hip range of motion in the affected leg as well as the patient's gait.[10]
- Note any preexisting limb length inequality, which will need to be addressed in the preoperative planning for correction.
- Evaluate the planned surgical site for preexisting scars, rashes, or plaques that may affect the approach. For example, psoriatic plaques may need to be treated and resolved prior to surgery as they present greater potential for wounds and infectious complications.[1,2]

Table 1 Etiology of Symptoms That Necessitate Total Hip Arthroplasty

Osteoarthritis
Osteonecrosis
Posttraumatic arthritis
Inflammatory arthropathies (RA, JRA, psoriatic arthritis)
Developmental etiologies (DDH, LCP, SCFE, FAI)
Acute femoral neck fracture[12]

RA, rheumatoid arthritis; JRA, juvenile rheumatoid arthritis; DDH, developmental dysplasia of the hip; LCP, Legg-Calvé-Perthes disease; SCFE, slipped capital femoral epiphysis; FAI, femoroacetabular impingement.

* = Centers for Medicare & Medicaid Service requirements

IMAGING AND OTHER DIAGNOSTIC STUDIES

- Initial diagnostic investigation should begin with x-rays. A standard set that includes an anteroposterior (AP) pelvis, AP hip, and frog-leg lateral versus cross-table lateral should be obtained.
- In addition to evaluating the extent of arthritis, imaging studies are used for preoperative planning via digital or acetate templating. A standardized marker should be placed at the level of the joint to allow for correction of magnification. In the case of dysplasia, x-rays of the contralateral hip can be helpful in templating for the size of components.[13] If initial x-rays appear inconsistent with the extent of the patient's complaints, further investigation may be undertaken.[5]
  - Magnetic resonance imaging (MRI) can demonstrate preradiographic avascular necrosis, transient osteoporosis, labral pathology, and occult hip fractures.
  - Bone scan can be used when a patient is not able to undergo MRI.
  - Computed tomography scan can be used to evaluate bony morphology in cases of congenital or posttraumatic deformity.

NONOPERATIVE MANAGEMENT

- Healthy patients with functional limitations related to their pathology who have failed conservative management are good candidates for THA.
- Young, healthy patients with bilateral disease in which both hips are indicated for surgery may undergo a one-stage bilateral THA, a procedure that has been proven to have lower complication rates and significant cost savings compared to two-stage procedures.[7]
- Absolute contraindications for surgery
  - Patients with active infections
  - Patients not medically cleared should be managed with nonoperative measures until the underlying disease preventing operative candidacy is treated.
- Relative contraindications for surgery
  - Morbid obesity (body mass index [BMI] >40 kg/m^2)[9]
  - Uncontrolled diabetes[8]
  - Narcotic dependence
  - Active smokers[11]

SURGICAL MANAGEMENT

- Various approaches and techniques for fixation will be discussed in the following chapters.

Preoperative Planning

- Consent: After determining a patient is a satisfactory candidate for THA, a detailed discussion must be had that details the diagnosis and prognosis for the patient's condition. Risks, benefits, and alternatives to surgery (including their inherent risks and benefits) should be discussed with the patient at this time.
- The surgeon and patient should approach informed consent from a shared decision-making perspective. This leads to greater patient investment in and cooperation with the plan of care, improved outcomes, and decreased risk of medical malpractice claims.[14]
- Once a patient has elected to undergo surgery, there are several steps that must be completed prior to conducting the procedure. The protocol committee at our institution recommends the following as part of the preoperative assessment for primary joint replacement candidates:
  - Routine preoperative testing consists of a complete blood count (CBC) and chem-7 panel. In diabetic patients, hemoglobin A1c may be evaluated at the discretion of the surgeon.
  - Urinalysis should be considered for symptoms consistent with a urinary tract infection (UTI), a UTI in the past 6 months, a history of diabetes mellitus, a history of prostate disease, or a history of urologic surgery requiring instrumentation.
  - Preoperative clearance must be obtained from appropriate medical doctors as the patient's past medical history dictates.
  - Dental evaluation should be undertaken to ensure there are no active infections prior to surgery.
  - For patients with a BMI greater than 40, weight reduction should be attempted prior to surgery. For those who are unable to meet this goal, a discussion regarding the increased risk for perioperative complications should be conducted.
  - Patients on aspirin should not stop taking it prior to surgery due to increased cardiac risk.
  - Patients taking nonsteroidal anti-inflammatory drugs should not stop these medications prior to surgery as the increase in preoperative pain can make postoperative pain control more difficult. However, the surgeon must accept the potential for increased perioperative bleeding.
  - Plavix, Aggrenox, and Coumadin should all be stopped 1 week prior to the planned surgery and Pradaxa and Xarelto stopped at least 3 days before. If the patient is not an appropriate candidate for neuraxial anesthesia and general anesthesia is planned, the patient may continue these medications as indicated by his or her medical consultants.
  - Patient education programs are a valuable resource to help a patient prepare his or her expectations related to the surgery, hospitalization, and subsequent recovery.
  - Preoperative skin cleansing should begin at home prior to the day of surgery. The International Consensus on Periprosthetic Joint Infection (http://www.msis_na/international consensus) recommends the use of over-the-counter Hibiclens for 2 days preoperatively.

REFERENCES

1. Day MS, Nam D, Goodman S, et al. Psoriatic arthritis. J Am Acad Orthop Surg 2012;20:28–37.
2. Della Valle C, Parvizi J, Bauer T, et al. The diagnosis of periprosthetic joint infections of the hip and knee. Guideline and evidence report. American Academy of Orthopaedic Surgeons Web site. Available at: http://www.aaos.org/research/guidelines/PJIguideline.pdf. Accessed November 13, 2014.
3. Learmonth ID, Young C, Rorabeck C. The operation of the century: total hip replacement. Lancet 2007;370:1508–1519.
4. Matar WY, Jafari SM, Restrepo C, et al. Preventing infection in total joint arthroplasty. J Bone Joint Surg Am 2010;92:36–46.
5. Newberg AH, Newman JS. Imaging of painful hip. In: McCarthy JC, ed. Early Hip Disorders: Advances in Detection and Minimally Invasive Treatment. New York: Springer, 2003:17–43.
6. Parvizi J, Pour A, Hillibrand A, et al. Back pain and total hip arthroplasty. Clin Orthop Relat Res 2010;468:1325–1330.

7. Parvizi J, Tarity TD, Sheikh E, et al. Bilateral total hip arthroplasty: one-stage versus two-stage procedures. Clin Orthop Relat Res 2006; 453:137–141.
8. Pedersen AB, Mehnert F, Johnsen SP, et al. Risk of revision of a total hip replacement in patients with diabetes mellitus. J Bone Joint Surg Br 2010;92-B:929–934.
9. Rajopal R, Martin R, Howard JL, et al. Outcomes and complications of total hip replacement in super-obese patients. Bone Joint J 2013; 95-B:576–763
10. Roder C, Staub L, Eggli S, et al. Influence of preoperative functional status on outcome after total hip arthroplasty. J Bone Joint Surg Am 2007;89:11–17.
11. Singh J. Smoking and outcomes after knee and hip arthroplasty: a systematic review. J Rheumatol 2011;38:1824–1834.
12. Tidermark J, Ponzer S, Svensson O, et al. Internal fixation compared with total hip replacement for displaced femoral neck fractures in the elderly. J Bone Joint Surg Br 2003;85-B:380–388.
13. Unnanuntana A, Wagner D, Goodman S. The accuracy of preoperative templating in cementless total hip arthroplasty. J Arthroplasty 2009;24:180–186.
14. Youm J, Chenok KE, Belkora J, et al. The emerging case for shared decision making in orthopaedics. Instr Course Lect 2013;62: 587–594.

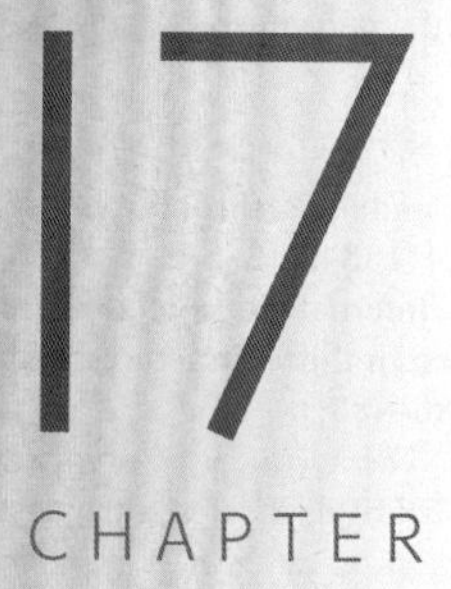

CHAPTER

Bearing Surface Options for Total Hip Arthroplasty

Eric A. Levicoff, Robert P. Good, and Peter F. Sharkey

DEFINITION

- The bearing surface in total hip arthroplasty (THA) is defined by the contacting materials that form the articulation between the reconstructed acetabulum and the replaced femoral head.

ANATOMY

- The native femoroacetabular joint is formed by a nearly frictionless articulation between the cartilage elements of the acetabulum and the femoral head. Upon reconstruction, all remaining cartilage is removed and a new articulation occurs between materials with various mechanical properties.
- The relevant anatomy of this articulation involves gravitational and musculotendinous elements that impart forces around the center of rotation (CoR) of the hip: (**FIG 1A**)
  - The sum of the forces about the hip is zero when rotational and axial stability is present.
  - The combination of these force vectors results in a joint reactive force (JRF), which is defined as the sum of forces acting on the hip CoR.
  - The major variables contributing to JRF include the following:
    - Body weight (BW)
    - Distance from the center of gravity (CoG) to the CoR (the lever arm [L])
  - It is easiest to consider two main forces acting on the CoR:
    - A downward force (D), consisting of the BW times the lever arm for the body weight (L)
    - An upward force (U), equal and opposite to D, made up by the pull of the abductor muscles (Ab) times the lever arm for this muscle (l)
    - The JRF is the absolute sum of these two forces or essentially force D multiplied by a factor of two.
    - This can be represented by the equation:

      $JRF = (BW \times L) + (Ab \times l)$ or
      $JRF = D + U$, and because D must equal U
      $JRF = 2D$

    - The greater the BW and the further the CoR is from the CoG (increasing lever arm [L]), the greater D becomes, therefore increasing the JRF.

PATHOGENESIS

- As degenerative arthritis develops in the hip, often an osteophyte forms along the medial wall of the acetabulum, causing lateral migration of the femoral head and the CoR.
  - This creates a vicious cycle whereby the lever arm increases, as does the JRF, causing further buildup of medial osteophyte and further lateralization of the femoral head (**FIG 1B**).
  - In addition, the contact area between the acetabulum and the femoral head is reduced, further increasing contact stresses on the articular surface.
- Increasing JRF can result in pain, decreased function, and an accelerated rate of cartilage degradation.
- In addition, patients will often reflexively lean over the affected hip, attempting to move their CoG toward the hip CoR, decreasing the lever arm, JRF, and pain.
  - This leads to an altered gait pattern called a *Trendelenburg gait.*
  - A Trendelenburg gait pattern also lessens the workload of the abductor by decreasing the amount of force needed to counteract downward force.
  - Over time, this can lead to significant atrophy of the abductor and persistent dysfunction, even following THA.
- The concept of JRF remains relevant during and following THA, as the JRF following THA equates to the force on the bearing surface.
  - The greater the JRF following THA, the greater the forces on the bearing surface and theoretically the higher the rate of wear and osteolysis.
  - Medialization of the socket during THA has the effect of decreasing the body weight lever arm, thereby decreasing JRF on the bearing surface and decreasing the rate of wear (**FIG 1C**).
- Following THA, increases in JRF can lead to accelerated production of wear particles, causing several potential problems:
  - Osteolysis
  - Increased risk of component loosening and failure
  - Increased risk of component fracture
  - Increased risk of modular junction issues (eg, taper corrosion)

NATURAL HISTORY

- Because cartilage has little restorative capacity, the natural history of arthritis is typically progressive dysfunction and gradually worsening pain over time.
- Progressive biomechanical and structural changes include the following:
  - Cartilage delamination
  - Osteophyte formation
  - Lateral migration of the femoral head and hip CoR
  - Abductor weakness
  - Ambulatory dysfunction
- Following THA, the bearing surface is subjected to the same principles determining JRF as the cartilage in the native joint.
  - Like any nonbiologic material, the materials used in THA break down over time via a process generically termed *wear.*

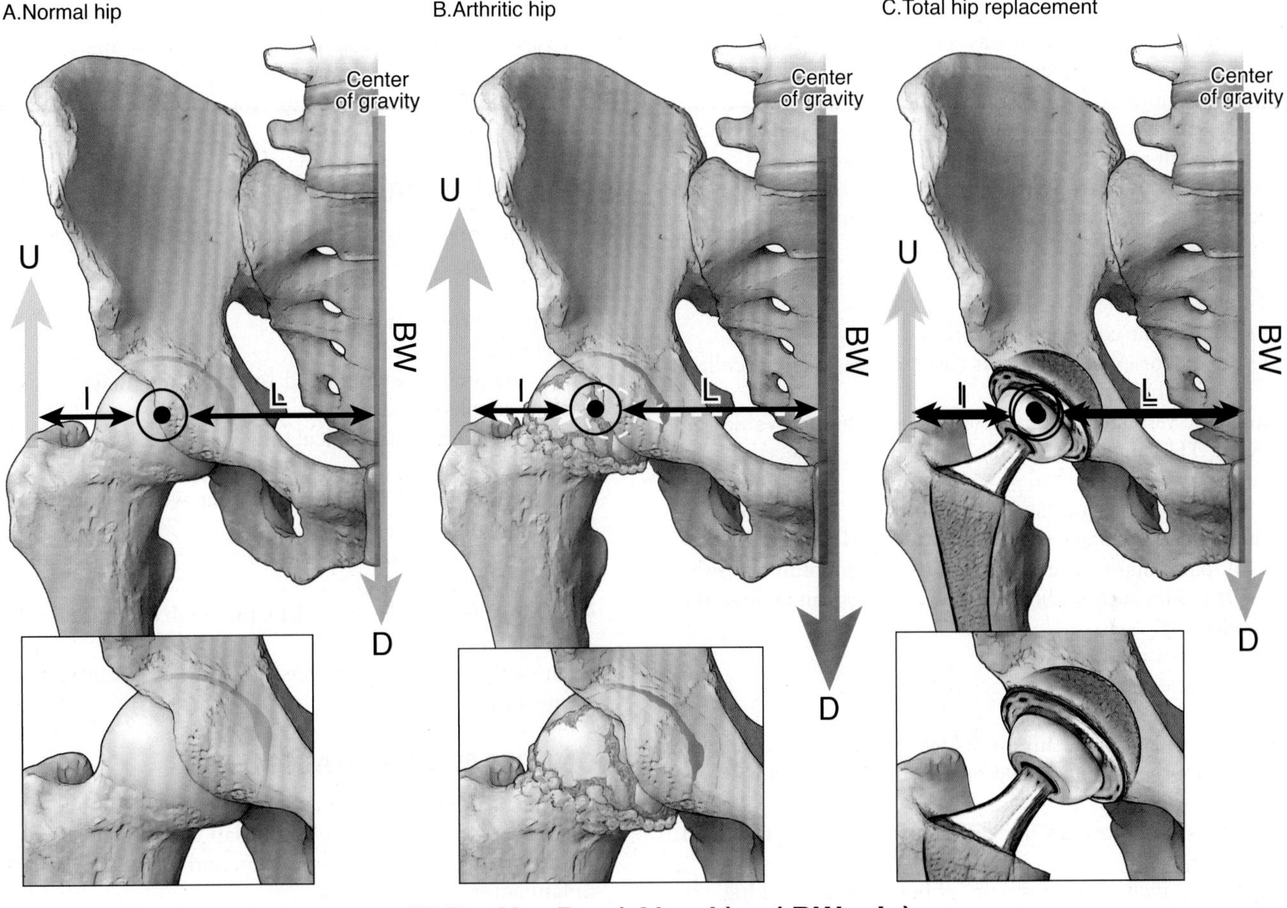

FIG 1 • **A.** A schematic demonstrating the forces that contribute to JRF around the hip CoR. "D" is the downward vector, consisting of the body weight (*BW*) times the lever arm (*L*). "U" is the upward vector, consisting of the pull of the abductors times the lever arm (*l*). **B.** A schematic demonstrating how these forces change in an arthritic hip. Note the increase in lever arm with progressive medial acetabular osteophyte moving the CoR laterally. The overall downward force becomes larger, as does the compensatory upward force, significantly increasing the total JRF. **C.** A schematic demonstrating how medialization of the acetabular socket moves the CoR back to its native state, decreasing JRF following THA.

- Regardless of bearing surface materials, over time, wear particles are released into the local tissues following THA and can cause:
  - Osteolysis
  - Synovitis and local tissue irritation
  - Metal ion-related pathology
  - Systemic side effects

PATIENT HISTORY AND PHYSICAL FINDINGS

- Frequently, osteolysis is asymptomatic and seen either incidentally on plain radiographs or noticed on routine, scheduled follow-up films.
- If osteolysis is severe, it can cause loosening of the prosthesis, which can manifest as:
  - Pain in the groin or thigh
    - Thigh pain typically correlates with stem loosening.
    - Groin pain typically correlates with cup loosening or synovitis.
    - Pain worsens over time.
  - "Start-up" pain
    - Pain that is significant at the beginning of ambulation but recedes with continued ambulation
    - Usually secondary to initial settling of a loose prosthesis
- Wear particles can produce synovitis in the hip that may manifest as:
  - Groin pain
  - Weakness
  - Joint swelling
- Physical examination findings consistent with advanced osteolysis and/or loosening include the following:
  - Pain with ambulation
  - Pain with active hip flexion, particularly active straight-leg raising
  - Swelling
  - Tenderness to palpation

IMAGING AND OTHER DIAGNOSTIC STUDIES

- As bearing surface wear and osteolysis are often asymptomatic, it is important to take serial plain radiographs at routine intervals following THA.
  - With the use of conventional highly cross-linked polyethylene (PE), routine follow-up films should be obtained 5 years postoperatively.[17,27]
    - Subsequent films should be taken every 2 to 3 years thereafter.

   - If an osteolytic lesion is noted, serial radiographs should be obtained at least every year and occasionally every 6 months, depending on the size and extent of the lesion.
  - The sensitivity of plain radiographs is quite low, particularly with respect to detecting smaller lesions.
- Computed tomography (CT) can be very useful for the detection and monitoring of osteolytic lesions about the pelvis[15] (**FIG 2**).
  - CT is often used to:
    - Detect smaller lytic lesions
    - Determine component position
    - Look for evidence of soft tissue masses or fluid collections about the hip
- Magnetic resonance imaging (MRI) is of limited value following THA due to the significant artifact produced by the metal components.
  - Newer MRI sequences that reduce the amount of artifact (metal artifact reduction [MAR] MRI) can be useful, particularly when evaluating for pseudotumor in the soft tissues surrounding a THA. Findings can include the following:
    - Solid or cystic masses
    - Muscle wasting
    - Soft tissue destruction
- Bone scans can be useful means for the detection or exclusion of loosening but should not be used as the primary diagnostic tool.
  - Bone scans often do not differentiate between lysis and loosening.
  - The specificity and sensitivity of bone scans is lacking.
- Laboratory studies are often used to distinguish between infection, wear, and aseptic loosening and should include the following:
  - Complete blood count (CBC) with differential, which is often normal but can be elevated with significant infection
  - Erythrocyte sedimentation rate (ESR), which is often normal in cases of aseptic loosening but elevated with infection
  - C-reactive protein (CRP), which is also often normal in cases of aseptic loosening but elevated with infection
  - Serum cobalt and chromium levels (in metal on metal articulations or to evaluate for corrosion at modular junctions)

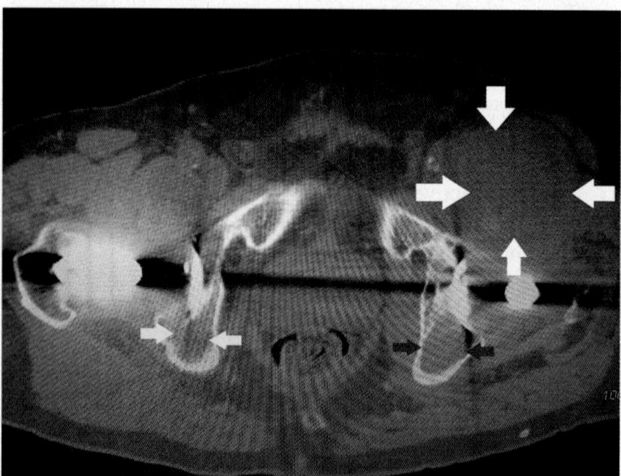

FIG 2 • A CT scan image demonstrating significant lysis in the ischium posterior to the left acetabular shell (*red arrows*) compared to a smaller osteolytic lesion on the opposite side (*yellow arrows*). Also, notice the large fluid collection anterior to the left hip joint representing significant particle-induced periarticular synovitis (*white arrows*).

DIFFERENTIAL DIAGNOSIS

- The major materials used for THA bearing surfaces include the following:
  - PE
  - Cobalt-chromium (CoCr)
  - Ceramic
- These materials are combined to form four major bearing surface couplets:
  - CoCr femoral heads articulating with PE acetabular liners (MoP)
  - Ceramic femoral heads articulating with PE acetabular liners (CoP)
  - CoCr femoral heads articulating with CoCr acetabular liners (MoM)
  - Ceramic femoral heads articulating with ceramic acetabular liners (CoC)
- Each of these bearing couplets has distinct advantages and disadvantages (Table 1).

NONOPERATIVE MANAGEMENT

- Management of asymptomatic, stable osteolysis and wear consists of serial radiographs and laboratory studies, regular follow-up, activity modification, and limited use of anti-inflammatory medications.
  - If asymptomatic osteolysis becomes progressive, surgery may be indicated to prevent further bone destruction and potentially more complicated revision surgery.

Table 1 Major Advantages and Disadvantages of the Four Main Bearing Surface Couplets

Bearing Couplet	Advantages	Disadvantages
CoCr on UHMWPE (MoP)	• Most studied • Longest follow-up • Biologically kind • Cost-effective	• Slightly higher wear rate relative to other couplets • Emerging risk of "trunnionosis"
Ceramic on UHMWPE (CoP)	• High wettability • Lower wear rate than MoP • Biologically kind	• Costly • Small risk of ceramic head fracture
CoCr on CoCr (MoM)	• Low risk of femoral head or liner fracture • Low wear rate	• Higher risk of early revision • Local and systemic reaction to metal debris and ion release
Ceramic on Ceramic (CoC)	• Highest wettability and lowest friction • Extremely low wear rate • Biologically kind	• Most costly couplet • Typically fewer liner and femoral neck length options • Risk of fracture • Risk of squeaking

CoCr, cobalt-chromium; UHMWPE, ultra-high-molecular-weight polyethylene.

- Symptomatic osteolysis is typically severe and often requires operative management.
  - Exceptions to this rule include the following:
    - Older patients with prohibitive medical comorbidities
    - Minimal or nonambulators
    - Extreme osteolysis that makes reconstruction impossible

SURGICAL MANAGEMENT

- The goal of THA is to restore as closely as possible the natural biomechanics of the hip joint, allowing for a return to normal gait and improved function, pain relief, and quality of life.
  - Restoration of the hip CoR, native femoral offset, and limb length is critical.
- Appropriate choice of bearing surface options is an important component to the overall success of THA.

Preoperative Planning

- Choice of bearing surface is usually determined preoperatively and depends on the following:
  - Patient characteristics that contribute to the expected overall lifetime wear of the prosthesis, including the following:
    - Age
    - Body weight
    - Life expectancy
    - Activity level
    - Generally speaking, the younger and more active the patient, the more consideration that should be given to alternative bearing surfaces (options other than MoP).
  - Technical considerations
    - Larger femoral heads offer enhanced stability but typically higher wear rates.
    - Larger femoral heads also impart greater shear force to the modular trunnion and potentially increase the risk of fretting corrosion at the modular interface.
    - Alternative bearing surfaces may not be available with as many options as MoP.
    - Some neck length options necessitate the need for skirts, decreasing the head–neck ratio and range of motion to impingement.
  - Cost
    - Ceramic components tend to be more expensive, whereas metal femoral heads and PE liners are usually the least expensive.
    - Cost will likely become increasingly important as health care systems attempt to address the growing need for THA with limited available funds and begin to consider demand matching when choosing devices.

Tribology

- Tribology is defined as the study of design, friction, wear, and lubrication of interacting surfaces in relative motion, which is critical for the understanding of bearing couplets in THA.
- Conceptually, friction can be thought of as the force resisting motion between two surfaces.
  - The coefficient of friction (CoF) is a value used to compare friction of different surface couplets (Table 2).
    - It is a ratio of the force needed to produce movement, divided by the normal force between the surfaces.
    - The lower the CoF, the less friction there is between two bodies.

Table 2 Relative Coefficients of Friction of Different Material Combinations

Material Combination	Coefficient of Friction (approximate)
Cartilage : cartilage	0.003
Ice : ice (wet)	0.02
Cobalt-chromium : UHMWPE	0.09
Ceramic : UHMWPE	0.1
Cobalt-chromium : Cobalt-chromium	0.1
Ceramic : ceramic	0.05

Note: The values given for the bearing surface materials take into account the surface lubrication found in vivo.

  - In THA, friction results in the delamination of material from the surface of the bearings, the major cause of wear, and subsequent osteolysis.
  - The CoF in THA bearings is influenced by several factors, including the following:
    - Contact area
    - Clearance
    - Surface roughness
    - Lubrication
- Contact area and clearance
  - Contact area is inversely proportional to clearance.
  - In general, lower clearance and higher contact area are preferred.
    - Higher contact area leads to lower contact stress.
    - Lower contact stress leads to lower rates of wear.
    - Lower clearance leads to more favorable lubrication dynamics.
  - However, clearance below a certain point can lead to extremely high friction.
    - No potential space for fluid leads to complete loss of lubrication.
    - Direct contact between the surfaces (equatorial contact)
- Surface roughness
  - Can be thought of as the smoothness of the bearing surface
  - At a microscopic level, the surface of any material is not completely uniform, with pits and projections into and out from the intended diameter.
  - The more uniform the diameter (ie, fewer pits and projections), the less the surface roughness and the less friction and wear that occurs.
  - Surface roughness can change over time.
    - As opposed to hard-on-soft bearing couplets (ie, MoP and CoP), hard-on-hard bearing couplets (ie, MoM and CoC) can have an initial run-in phase, during which surface roughness is reduced.
    - The harder the femoral head, the less susceptible it will be to scratching from third bodies (ie, bone debris within the articulation), which can negatively impact surface roughness after implantation.
- Lubrication occurs when a film of fluid is interposed between two surfaces.
  - Fluid film lubrication in THA can be full or mixed.
    - Mixed-fluid film lubrication results in variable degrees of surface contact, whereas full-fluid film lubrication completely separates the two surfaces and reduces wear.

- To a certain degree, fluid film lubrication permits small variations in surface roughness by slightly separating the bearing surfaces.
- Lubrication is influenced by several factors:
  - Fluid viscosity, with higher viscosity leading to a more favorable lubrication scheme
  - Clearance between the two articulating surfaces
  - Surface material and wettability
  - Wettability refers to the ability of fluid to interact with another material and improves lubrication by allowing a more uniform fluid layer.
  - CoC couplets tend toward full lubrication, whereas MoM, CoP, and MoP couplets tend toward mixed lubrication.[10]

Bearing Surface Options

Polyethylene

- PE has been in use for THA since the early 1960s.
- Traditional PE is made of ultra-high-molecular-weight polyethylene (UHMWPE).
  - UHMWPE is composed of ethylene polymer chains.
  - Contains two major structural regions:
    - Crystallites are regions of folded chains that confer the mechanical properties to the material.
    - Amorphous regions constitute the remainder of the material and do not contribute significantly to the mechanical properties.
- PE technology has evolved; today, most UHMWPE used for THA uses cross-linking technology to improve wear characteristics.
  - Cross-linking refers to a process by which adjacent ethylene polymers are covalently bonded together (**TECH FIG 1A**).
    - Cross-linking is usually achieved using either gamma or electron-beam irradiation.
    - Radiation causes the formation of free radicals that have the potential to join together in a covalent bond between polymers.
    - Cross-linking occurs predominantly in the amorphous regions.
    - The amount of cross-linking is proportional to the dose of radiation.
  - The advantages of cross-linking include the following:
    - Decreased wear
    - Decreased risk of osteolysis
    - Improved material longevity
  - The disadvantages of cross-linking include the following:
    - Alteration of mechanical properties, specifically decreased fatigue and fracture resistance, especially when subject to impingement following component malposition in THA[11]
    - Any residual free radicals can lead to oxidation of the PE and early failure.
- Oxidation is one of the main causes of PE failure.
  - Occurs when free radicals react with oxygen[18] (**TECH FIG 1B**)
    - Forms peroxy free radicals which steal hydrogen from other ethylene chains, forming unstable hydroperoxides
    - Hydroperoxides then react with ethylene polymers and degrade into products (ketones, acids, esters) associated with diminution of PE mechanical properties.
    - The hydrogen theft creates another free radical to start this process over again, leading to a vicious cycle of PE deterioration.
  - Any process that results in the creation of free radicals can lead to oxidative instability and the risk of PE failure.
    - Cross-linking
    - Gamma sterilization
  - Oxidation can occur during or after manufacturing, including *in vivo* following component implantation.
- Manufacturers take advantage of several technologies to reduce the risk of oxidation while improving the wear characteristics of PE:
  - Sterilization technique
    - Conventional PE historically was sterilized using gamma irradiation in air (high oxygen content) which led to high levels of early oxidation and failure.
    - Newer generation PE is often sterilized with gas to reduce free radical production.
    - Sterilization also now takes place in an inert environment (typically nitrogen) to eliminate early oxidation.
  - Thermal treatment
    - Heating of PE following irradiation converts the crystalline regions to amorphous matter, allowing free radicals to migrate and bond with each other.
    - Annealing is performed by heating the PE to just below its 137° C melting point, which allows the PE to retain its mechanical properties, but results in a lower degree of free radical reduction.
    - Melting heats the PE to above the melting point and permits the conversion of all crystalline matter to amorphous matter, resulting in a higher degree of free radical elimination, but some loss of crystallization and ultimate mechanical strength.
  - Vitamin E infusion
    - Vitamin E is a natural scavenger of free radicals and is present throughout the body to protect tissues from oxidative degradation.
    - Vitamin E can be added to PE in several different manners, leading to either a surface concentration of vitamin E or an even distribution of vitamin E throughout the PE structure.
    - "Diffusion" refers to the postmanufacturing addition of vitamin E, whereas "blending" refers to the addition of vitamin E to PE resin during the manufacturing process.
    - In UHMWPE, vitamin E lends hydrogen to peroxy free radicals eliminating the free radical, avoiding oxidation, and halting the cycle of free radical production (**TECH FIG 1C**).

Cobalt-Chromium

- CoCr is a group of alloys using different proportions of cobalt and chromium, in addition to other metals typically including nickel and molybdenum.
  - Cobalt provides the mechanical strength and hardness to the material, whereas the chromium is soluble in the cobalt and confers resistance to corrosion.
  - Different concentrations of metals results in varying degrees of strength and resistance to corrosion.

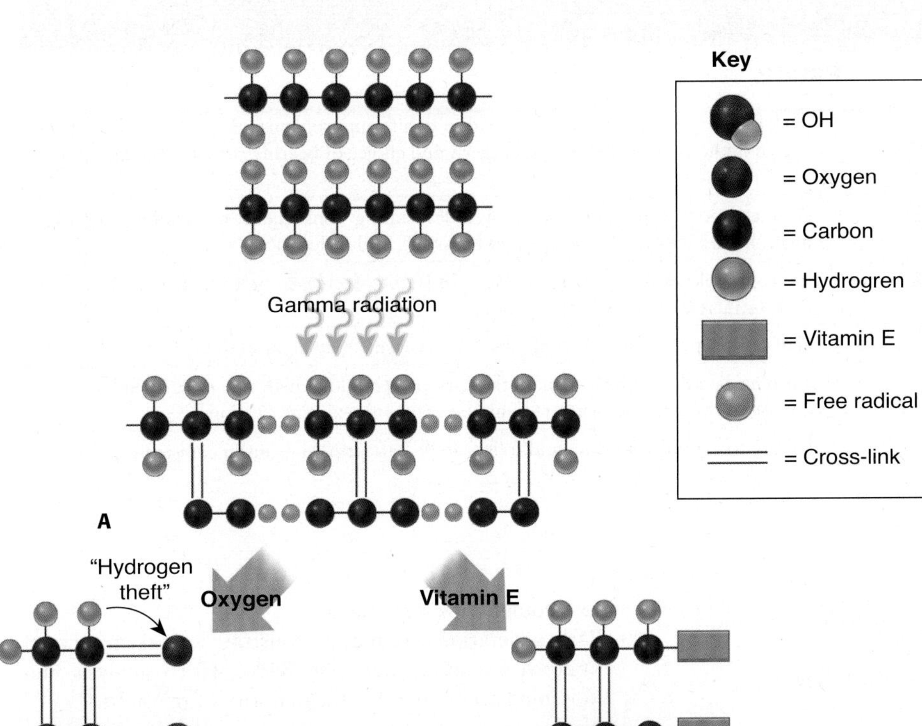

TECH FIG 1 • A schematic of cross-linking of PE. Radiation breaks the PE chains, producing free radicals that can react in several ways. **A.** Free radicals can react with each other, forming a cross-link. **B.** Free radicals can react with oxygen to form a peroxide and another unstable free radical. **C.** In the presence of vitamin E, the free radical can react with the hydrogen from vitamin E, avoiding production of peroxides. The vitamin E remains stable even after donating hydrogen.

- CoCr has been used to manufacture both femoral heads and acetabular components and can serve as the acetabular bearing surface.
  - CoCr is currently the material most commonly used for femoral heads.
    - It has better hardness compared to titanium and therefore is more resistant to in vivo conformational changes and third body damage that can increase wear.
  - The use of CoCr as an acetabular liner has rapidly decreased recently due concerns about local and systemic reactions to metal wear products.

Ceramics

- Bearing surface ceramics can be manufactured using both aluminum and zirconium oxide.
- Ceramics are made from crystalline powders that are sintered into their general shape.
  - The crystallites within the structure are referred to as *grains*.
  - Grain size is inversely proportional to material strength.
    - Higher grain size results in lower strength and decreased fracture resistance.
    - Reduced grain size results in higher strength and enhanced fracture resistance.
- Advantages of ceramics include the following:
  - Increased hardness, allowing for finer material polishing and enhanced scratch resistance
  - Increased wettability, improving lubrication characteristics
  - Decreased wear
- Disadvantages of ceramics include the following:
  - Currently, there are fewer neck length and liner options.
  - Decreased ductility and increased brittleness
  - Risk of possible fracture and catastrophic failure
  - Risk of bearing surface noise including squeaking
- There are two major types of ceramics used today for THA, both of which are made and distributed by one company (CeramTec, Plochingen, Germany).
  - Pure alumina oxide (Biolox forte), introduced in 1994
  - Aluminum oxide matrix (Biolox delta), approved in the United States in 2003
    - The most recent generation of ceramic bearing surfaces.
    - In addition to aluminum, this material contains yttria-stabilized zirconium and platelet-shaped strontium oxide particles which improve the mechanical properties of the ceramic by decreasing the risk of both fracture initiation and propagation.

PEARLS AND PITFALLS

Pearls	Pitfalls
Choice of bearing surface should be made preoperatively, with proper consideration of intraoperative backup plans.	■ Lack of preoperative planning can lead to significant problems, particularly when unexpected findings are noted during surgery, and choice of bearing surface is no exception.
Proper component orientation is imperative for all bearing surfaces.	■ Poor component placement can have devastating consequences, including impingement, higher wear rates, component breakage, and dislocation.
Choice of bearing surface is not a one size fits all proposition.	■ Improper selection of bearing surface can lead to decreased performance, unnecessary cost, or increased risk of early failure.
Routine follow-up is essential.	■ Without proper follow-up, early deleterious events may be missed.
MoM have been noted to demonstrate significantly higher rates of early failure.	■ Current data do not fully explain the reasons behind the high rate of early failure, and the use of this bearing couplet should be used with extreme caution.
Squeaking following CoC THA may be an indication of impending failure.	■ Failure to carefully workup and follow these patients can result in catastrophic failure.

POSTOPERATIVE CARE

- Postoperative care following THA should follow specific standards, regardless of bearing surface choice.
- Early postoperative visits should focus on the following:
  - Wound healing
  - Early radiographic stability of components
    - Lack of subsidence
    - Appropriate component position
  - Progression of activities, relief of pain, and improvement in quality of life
- Later postoperative visits should concentrate on detecting signs of component failure such as the following:
  - Osteolysis
  - Eccentric PE wear
  - Instability
  - Pain
  - Bearing noise
  - Biologic reactions to metal debris

OUTCOMES

- CoCr and CoP
  - Most commonly used bearing couplet
  - Excellent long-term outcomes for both cross-linked and traditional PE acetabular liners
  - Larger femoral heads (≥36 mm) in this cohort impart substantially improved stability but at a cost of higher volumetric wear rates than smaller head sizes.[20]
  - Cross-linked PE liners and ceramic femoral heads are more costly than their conventional counterparts, but midterm clinical data have demonstrated that they have distinct advantages.
  - Advantages of cross-linked PE over conventional PE liners are that[7,9,14,29]:
    - Wear rate is approximately 8- to 10-fold lower.
    - Lower incidence of osteolysis
    - Fewer revisions due to osteolysis
  - Advantages of ceramic femoral heads versus CoCr femoral heads may include the following:
    - Lower wear rates[22,28]
    - Elimination of chrome and cobalt leads to a lower risk of femoral neck taper corrosion (trunnionosis).[19]
- CoC
  - Exceedingly low wear rates
  - Early generation ceramics demonstrate long-term survival (>20 years) of greater than 84%, with osteolysis and loosening accounting for the majority of revisions.[25]
  - Newer generation ceramics show excellent midterm survival rates, demonstrating greater than 98% survival at 10 years.[5,32]
  - Reasons for aseptic THA failure include the following:
    - Osteolysis
    - Loosening
    - Squeaking
    - Component fracture
- MoM
  - Reported advantages include the following:
    - Decreased wear
    - Low risk of fracture
    - Low dislocation rates (secondary to increased femoral head diameter)
  - Use has dwindled in recent years out of concern for early failure and adverse local tissue reaction (ALTR) related to metal wear particles.
  - Demonstrates significantly lower survival rates compared to other bearing couplets.[23,30]
  - Most common reasons for failure include the following:
    - Early osteolysis
    - Early loosening
    - ALTR
  - Should be used with caution due to reports of higher early failure compared to other bearing couplets. It is not yet clear whether certain subsets of patients are more susceptible than others to early failure when MoM constructs are used.[4]

COMPLICATIONS

- Osteolysis is the progressive deterioration of periprosthetic bone following joint arthroplasty.
  - It is typically caused by the biologic response to small wear particles.[8]
    - Can occur with any bearing couplet
    - The degree of osteolysis depends on the biologic activity of wear particles.

- Particle material is an important characteristic in their biologic activity, with chrome and cobalt particles being particularly active.
- Size is also an important determinant of biologic activity and it is commonly thought that particles between 0.2 and 7 μm in diameter create the highest degree of biologic activity.

- Degradation of bone is a side effect of the body's attempt to eliminate small wear particles.
- Osteolysis is a primary cause of aseptic loosening and periprosthetic fracture (**FIG 3**).
- It is often asymptomatic until complications occur (ie, painful loosening).
- The development of osteolysis is closely associated with wear debris particles and their effect on cell differentiation, cell proliferation, and cytokine regulation.[12,24]
  - Increased proliferation of osteoclasts
  - Decreased proliferation of osteoblasts
  - Upregulation of interleukin-1(IL-1) and tumor necrosis factor alpha (TNF-α), amongst other proinflammatory cytokines
  - Downregulation of procollagen α-1
- Increased rates of wear and lysis is associated with the following:
  - Poor component position
  - Manufacturing techniques
  - Increased body weight and activity level[21]

- ALTR and pseudotumor
  - Thought to develop from release of local metal debris
  - Can occur in any type of hip replacement construct, but the risk is dramatically higher in cases involving:
    - MoM articulations, with a reported incidence as high as 6.5% in this population[33]
    - Increased modularity (ie, modular neck/stem constructs), particularly when dissimilar metals are mated at the modular junction
  - Significant local pathology resulting in the following:
    - Soft tissue compromise including muscle, tendon, and bone (**FIG 4**)
    - Mass effect from solid, cystic, or mixed tumors
    - Pain
    - Osteolysis
    - Loosening
  - Although definite risk factors are poorly understood, certain constructs should be considered hips at risk (**FIG 5**).
  - Patients can often present with pain and/or hip dysfunction but can be asymptomatic.
  - Clinical evaluation of these patients should include the following:
    - Thorough history and physical examination, specifically considering:
      - Pain
      - Ambulatory dysfunction
      - Abductor insufficiency

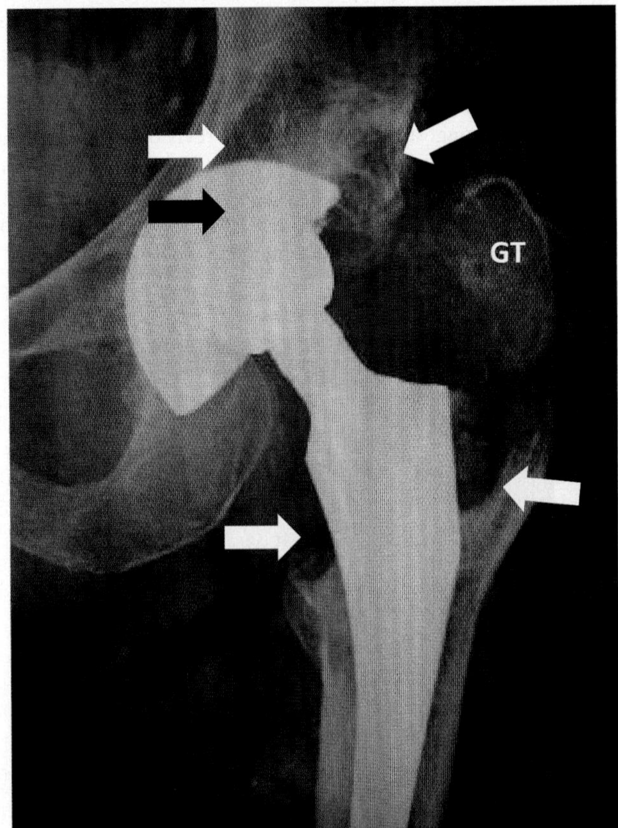

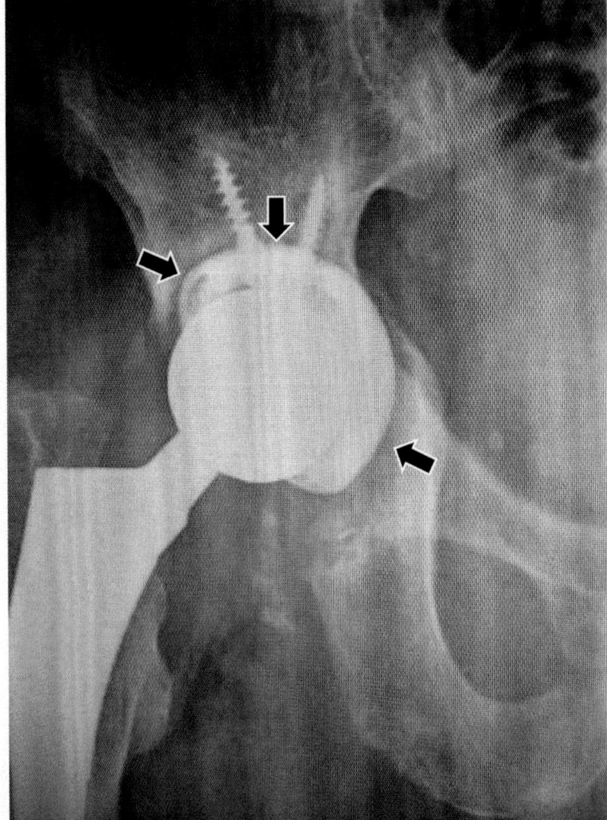

FIG 3 • **A.** A picture of severe osteolysis about a THA that caused a fracture of the greater trochanter (*GT*). Note the eccentric PE wear (*black arrow*) and the lysis about both the femoral and acetabular components (*white arrows*). **B.** A picture of periprosthetic osteolysis causing loosening of an acetabular socket. Note the radiolucent line surrounding the component (*black arrows*).

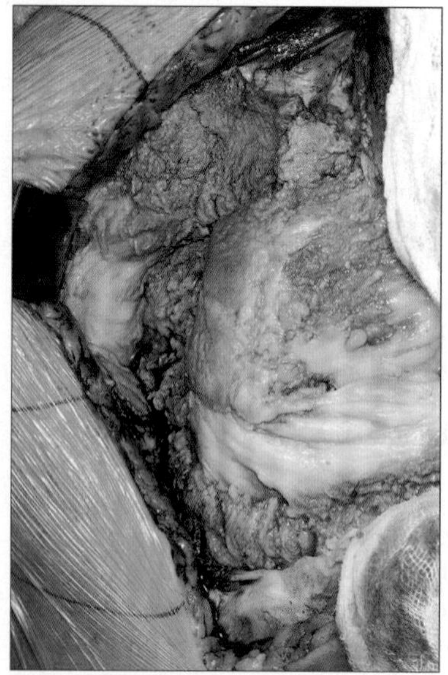

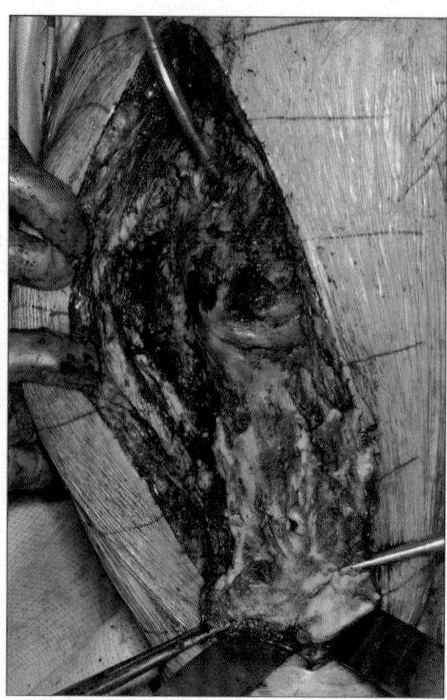

FIG 4 • **A.** An intraoperative photograph of a large pseudotumor surrounding a MoM THA. **B.** Another photograph of the same patient during removal of the pseudotumor demonstrating significant tissue loss and necrosis.

        - Soft tissue swelling
        - History of instability
    - Imaging, including the following:
        - Plain x-rays
        - CT scan
        - MRI using a metal artifact reduction series (MARS), looking for evidence of space-occupying lesion and periarticular tissue destruction (**FIG 6**)
    - Lab work should include the following:
        - ESR
        - CRP
        - Serial serum cobalt and chromium levels
        - Hip aspiration with cell count, differential, and gram stain/culture
  - Treatment typically requires revision surgery such as the following:
    - Exchange of metal components to either PE or ceramic when possible
    - Dèbridement of all necrotic tissue
    - The possibility of the need for full revision surgery, including the use of constrained components if necessary secondary to soft tissue compromise
- Bearing surface fracture
  - Occurs almost exclusively with ceramic components
  - Overall incidence of fracture is low.
    - Reported to be between 0% and 2.6% in clinical series[3,13,26]
    - More commonly involves the acetabular liner but can also involve the femoral head

Risk factors for the development of pseudotumor or ALTR

- MoM constructs
- Modular neck constructs
- Females
- Older than 65 years of age
- Larger femoral heads
- Cup inclination angles greater than 50°

FIG 5 • A list of the most common risk factors for the development of ALTR.

    - Increased risk with component malposition and resultant impingement
  - Newer generation ceramics are believed to have a reduced risk of fracture due to the following:
    - Smaller grain size
    - Stabilizing particles mixed into components to prevent fracture initiation and propagation.
  - Principles of treatment include the following:
    - Immediate joint immobilization and bed rest to prevent fragment dispersal and destruction of well-fixed components
    - Urgent revision
    - Total synovectomy with removal of ceramic debris
    - Profuse joint lavage
  - Studies suggest that outcomes for revision following fractured ceramic components may be improved with newer ceramics.[31]
  - Complete component revision may be necessary as opposed to simple head and liner revision in some cases.[2]

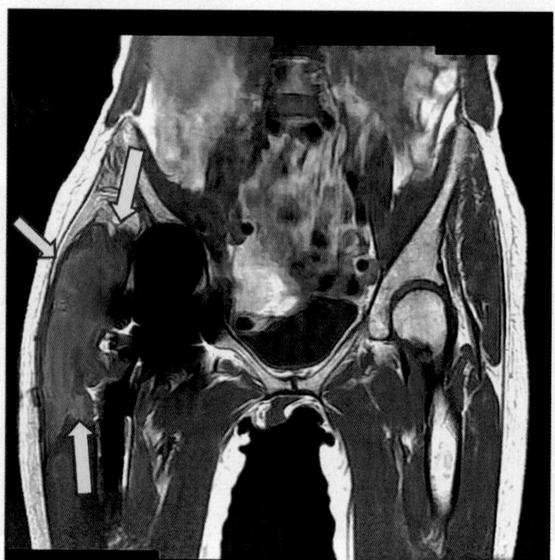

FIG 6 • An MRI (with MARS) of a large pseudotumor surrounding a MoM THA.

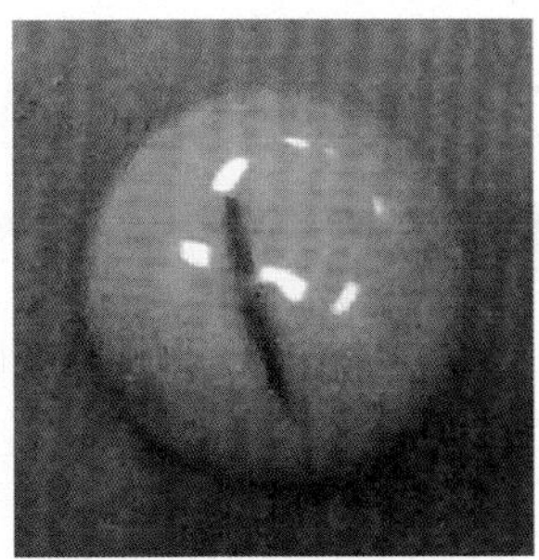

FIG 7 • A photograph demonstrating stripe wear found on a ceramic femoral head that was revised for squeaking.

- Squeaking and bearing surface noise
  - Highest incidence found with CoC constructs.
  - Risk factors and mechanism are poorly understood, but edge loading seems to be a critical factor.
  - Overall reported incidence varies between less than 1% and 10%, depending on study methodology (eg, definition of noise).[16] Higher rates are noted when patients are specifically asked about noises.
  - Squeaking is often associated with stripe wear found at the time of revision[6] (**FIG 7**). It is thought to be connected with lubrication that allows surface contact and metal transfer.
  - Squeaking can be an early indicator of impending liner fracture and should be worked up and followed carefully.[1]

REFERENCES

1. Abdel MP, Heyse TJ, Elpers ME, et al. Ceramic liner fractures presenting as squeaking after primary total hip arthroplasty. J Bone Joint Surg Am 2014;96(1):27–31.
2. Allain J, Roudot-Thoraval F, Delecrin J, et al. Revision total hip arthroplasty performed after fracture of a ceramic femoral head. A multicenter survivorship study. J Bone Joint Surg Am 2003;85-A(5):825–830.
3. Amanatullah DF, Landa J, Strauss EJ, et al. Comparison of surgical outcomes and implant wear between ceramic-ceramic and ceramic-polyethylene articulations in total hip arthroplasty. J Arthroplasty 2011;26(6 suppl):72–77.
4. Bozic KJ, Browne J, Dangles CJ, et al. Modern metal-on-metal hip implants. J Am Acad Orthop Surg 2012;20(6):402–406.
5. Brandt JM, Gascoyne TC, Guenther LE, et al. Clinical failure analysis of contemporary ceramic-on-ceramic total hip replacements. Proc Inst Mech Eng H 2013;227(8):833–846.
6. Chevillotte C, Trousdale RT, Chen Q, et al. The 2009 Frank Stinchfield Award: "hip squeaking": a biomechanical study of ceramic-on-ceramic bearing surfaces. Clin Orthop Relat Res 2010;468(2):345–350.
7. Digas G, Kärrholm J, Thanner J, et al. The Otto Aufranc Award. Highly cross-linked polyethylene in total hip arthroplasty: randomized evaluation of penetration rate in cemented and uncemented sockets using radiostereometric analysis. Clin Orthop Relat Res 2004;(429):6–16.
8. Dowd JE, Cha CW, Trakru S, et al. Failure of total hip arthroplasty with a precoated prosthesis. 4- to 11-year results. Clin Orthop Relat Res 1998;(355):123–136.
9. Engh CA, Hopper RH, Huynh C, et al. A prospective, randomized study of cross-linked and non-cross-linked polyethylene for total hip arthroplasty at 10-year follow-up. J Arthroplasty 2012;27(8 suppl):2–7.
10. Flanagan S, Jones E, Birkinshaw C. In vitro friction and lubrication of large bearing hip prostheses. Proc Inst Mech Eng H 2010;224(7):853–864.
11. Gencur SJ, Rimnac CM, Kurtz SM. Fatigue crack propagation of virgin and highly cross-linked, thermally treated ultra-high molecular weight polyethylene. Biomaterials 2006;27(8):1550–1557.
12. Goodman SB, Huie P, Song Y, et al. Cellular profile and cytokine production at prosthetic interfaces. Study of tissues retrieved from revised hip and knee replacements. J Bone Joint Surg Br 1998;80:531–539.
13. Hannouche D, Nich C, Bizot P, et al. Fractures of ceramic bearings: history and present status. Clin Orthop Relat Res 2003;(417):19–26.
14. Harsha AP, Joyce TJ. Comparative wear tests of ultra-high molecular weight polyethylene and cross-linked polyethylene. Proc Inst Mech Eng H 2010;227(5):600–608.
15. Howie DW, Neale SD, Martin W, et al. Progression of periacetabular osteolytic lesions. J Bone Joint Surg Am 2012;94(16):e1171–e1176.
16. Jarrett CA, Ranawat AS, Bruzzone M, et al. The squeaking hip: a phenomenon of ceramic-on-ceramic total hip arthroplasty. J Bone Joint Surg Am 2009;91(6):1344–1349.
17. Kitamura N, Sychterz-Terefenko CJ, Engh CA. The temporal progression of pelvic osteolysis after uncemented total hip arthroplasty. J Arthroplasty 2006;21(6):791–795.
18. Kurtz SM. The UHMWPE Biomaterials Handbook: Ultra High Molecular Weight Polyethylene in Total Joint Replacement and Medical Devices, ed 2. Burlington, MA: Academic Press, 2009.
19. Kurtz SM, Kocagöz SB, Hanzlik JA, et al. Do ceramic femoral heads reduce taper fretting corrosion in hip arthroplasty? A retrieval study. Clin Orthop Relat Res 2013;471(10):3270–3282.
20. Lachiewicz PF, Heckman DS, Soileau ES, et al. Femoral head size and wear of highly cross-linked polyethylene at 5 to 8 years. Clin Orthop Relat Res 2009;467(12):3290–3296.
21. McClung CD, Zahiri CA, Higa JK, et al. Relationship between body mass index and activity in hip or knee arthroplasty patients. J Orthop Res 2000;18(1):35–39.
22. Meftah M, Klingenstein GG, Yun RJ, et al. Long-term performance of ceramic and metal femoral heads on conventional polyethylene in young and active patients: a matched-pair analysis. J Bone Joint Surg Am 2013;95(13):1193–1197.
23. Milošev I, Kovac S, Trebse R, et al. Comparison of ten-year survivorship of hip prostheses with use of conventional polyethylene, metal-on-metal, or ceramic-on-ceramic bearings. J Bone Joint Surg Am 2012;94(19):1756–1763.
24. O'Neill SC, Queally JM, Devitt BM, et al. The role of osteoblasts in peri-prosthetic osteolysis. Bone Joint J 2013;95-B(8):1022–1026.
25. Petsatodis GE, Papadopoulos PP, Papavasiliou KA, et al. Primary cementless total hip arthroplasty with an alumina ceramic-on-ceramic bearing: results after a minimum of twenty years of follow-up. J Bone Joint Surg Am 2010;92(3):639–644.
26. Porat M, Parvizi J, Sharkey PF, et al. Causes of failure of ceramic-on-ceramic and metal-on-metal hip arthroplasties. Clin Orthop Relat Res 2012;470(2):382–387.
27. Ries MD, Link TM. Monitoring and risk of progression of osteolysis after total hip arthroplasty. Instr Course Lect 2013;62:207–214.
28. Roy ME, Whiteside LA, Magill ME, et al. Reduced wear of cross-linked UHMWPE using magnesia-stabilized zirconia femoral heads in a hip simulator. Clin Orthop Relat Res 2011;469(8):2337–2345.
29. Thomas GE, Simpson DJ, Mehmood S, et al. The seven-year wear of highly cross-linked polyethylene in total hip arthroplasty: a double-blind, randomized controlled trial using radiostereometric analysis. J Bone Joint Surg Am 2011;93(8):716–722.
30. Topolovec M, Milošev I. A comparative study of four bearing couples of the same acetabular and femoral component: a mean follow-up of 11.5 years. J Arthroplasty 2014;29(1):176–180.
31. Traina F, Tassinari E, De Fine M, et al. Revision of ceramic hip replacements for fracture of a ceramic component: AAOS exhibit selection. J Bone Joint Surg Am 2011;93(24):e147.
32. Yeung E, Bott PT, Chana R, et al. Mid-term results of third-generation alumina-on-alumina ceramic bearings in cementless total hip arthroplasty: a ten-year minimum follow-up. J Bone Joint Surg Am 2012;94(2):138–144.
33. Wiley KF, Ding K, Stoner JA, et al. Incidence of pseudotumor and acute lymphocytic vasculitis associated lesion (ALVAL) reactions in metal-on-metal hip articulations: a meta-analysis. J Arthroplasty 2013;28(7):1238–1245.

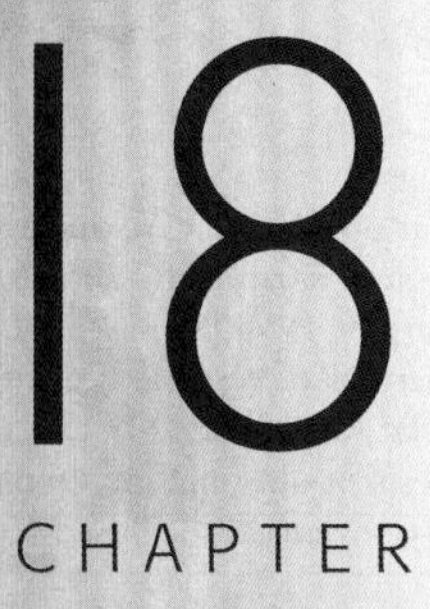

CHAPTER

Prevention of Complications in Total Hip Arthroplasty

Eric B. Smith

DEFINITION

- Total hip arthroplasty (THA) is successfully performed around the world for the treatment of arthritis, osteonecrosis, and femoral neck fracture, with predictably excellent results. The criteria for successful THA are no different today than they were 50 years ago: The procedure should be safe, effective, and durable. There is no doubt about the effectiveness of THA relieving pain and improving function. Additionally, there have been dramatic advances in bioengineering that have improved the durability of implants so that most THA patients will never need to be concerned that their hip implant will need to be revised. With appropriate preoperative planning and precise surgical techniques, THA is a very safe procedure. Despite this, complications can and do occur, and it is imperative that we minimize the risks of surgery.
- Intraoperative complications during THA can range from minor, such as a subtle crack seen during broaching of the femur that is easily remedied with a cerclage cable, to major, such as a catastrophic vascular injury that could lead to loss of life or limb. A thorough understanding of the bony structure of the pelvis and the surrounding neurovascular anatomy is necessary to minimize risks of injury. This knowledge allows for optimal surgical exposure with safe placement of retractors. Complications can be due to direct injury such as vascular injury, peripheral nerve injury, or intraoperative fracture. Additional complications can be due to poor technical technique that can lead to infection or instability and dislocation. It is important to note that the incidence of all these complications is higher in revision surgery and surgeons and patients should be appropriately prepared and counseled on the possibility of their occurrence.
- Although it is out of the scope of this chapter, perioperative complications after THA unrelated to surgical technique are often preventable. A thorough medical and surgical preoperative evaluation along with appropriate patient selection can dramatically impact the surgical outcomes of THA patients. Patients with significant comorbidities should be medically optimized prior to surgery. Those with diabetes or significant renal or liver disease are at increased risk for surgical site infection (SSI). Patients with morbid obesity need greater surgical complexity and have higher risks of wound complications, infections, and fractures. It is also imperative that the orthopaedic surgeon be actively involved in managing patients postoperatively to ensure the medical and physical well-being of their patients.
- Additionally, complications can develop from the implants and bearing surfaces themselves. Discussion regarding tribology and implant materials is found in other chapters. However, many of the complications we most commonly deal with as orthopaedic joint reconstruction surgeons are not typically due to technical mistakes but occur due to decisions we make. Using the latest breakthrough in THA is often a dangerous proposition and many intelligent surgeons have succumbed to this pressure only to find that they were faced with unexpected complications.
- This chapter consists of a review of the anatomy surrounding the hip and then discusses the following complications: vascular injury, peripheral nerve injury, periprosthetic fracture, periprosthetic joint infection (PJI), and dislocation.

ANATOMY

- The hip is a diarthrodial synovial joint consisting of articulation of the femoral head with the acetabulum. The acetabulum is a concave socket formed within the innominate bone of the pelvis. At puberty, the ilium, ischium, and pubis unite together to form the acetabulum. The acetabulum is surrounded by vital neurovascular structures, and their anatomic locations are critical to understand.
- Posteriorly, the sacrospinous ligament extends from lateral border sacrum to ischial spine. The sacrotuberous ligament is larger and extends from dorsum and lateral border sacrum and posterior surface ilium to the ischial tuberosity. The attachments of the sacrospinous and sacrotuberous ligaments enclose the lesser and greater sciatic notches, respectively, forming the greater and lesser foramina. Structures passing through the greater sciatic foramina are the piriformis muscle; sciatic nerve; superior and inferior gluteal nerve and artery; internal pudendal nerve, artery, and vein; nerve to the obturator internus muscle; nerve to the quadratus femoris; and the posterior cutaneous nerve of the thigh. Structures passing through the lesser sciatic foramina are the tendon of the obturator internus, nerve to the obturator internus, pudendal nerve, and the internal pudendal artery. The superior gluteal nerve and artery exit above the piriformis. The inferior gluteal nerve and artery as well as the sciatic nerve exit posterior to the hip joint, inferior to the piriformis, and superior to the superior gemellus muscle (**FIG 1**).
- The sciatic nerve is the largest nerve in the body. It arises from the sacral plexus (L4–S3) and exits through the greater sciatic foramen anterior and medial to the piriformis muscle. The sciatic nerve will split into the common peroneal and tibial nerves at the popliteal fossa. Proximally, the common peroneal portion of the sciatic nerve sits more laterally and has thinner connective tissue coverage. When the sciatic nerve is injured, it is typically the common peroneal branch that is affected.[44] There are anatomic variations of the sciatic nerve as it emerges from the greater sciatic notch.

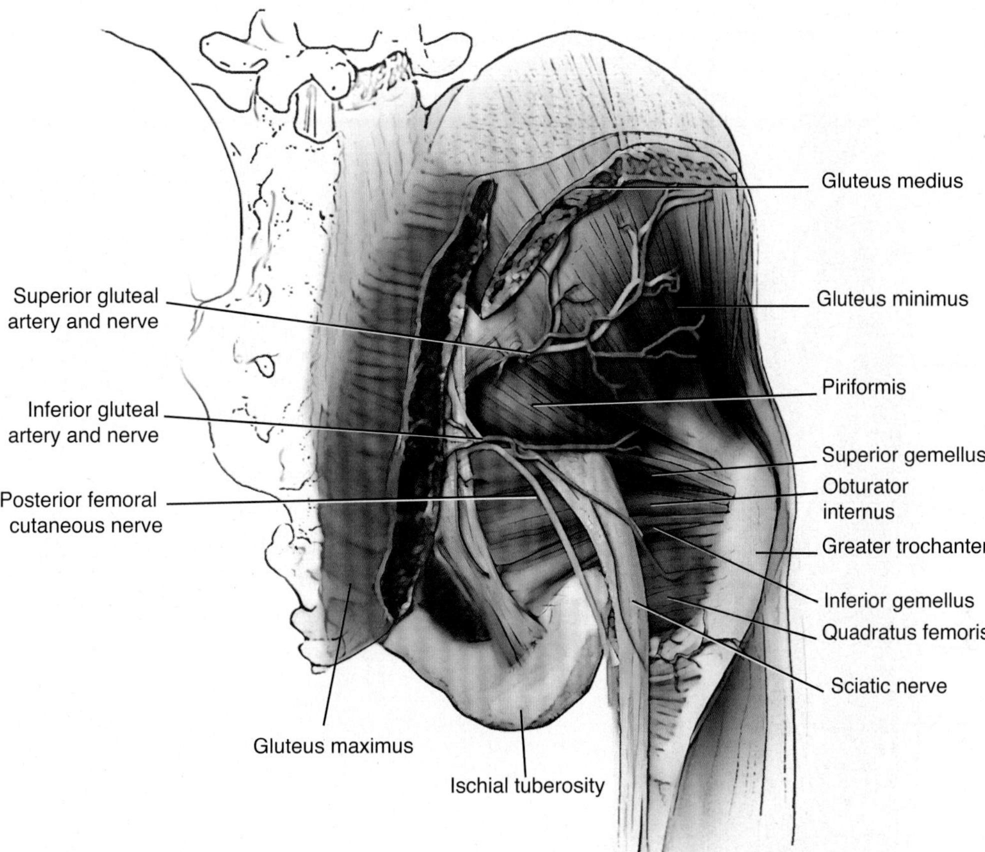

FIG 1 • Posterior aspect of the hip. The sciatic nerve is the main structure at risk posteriorly.

Eighty-four percent of the time, it exits as one nerve distal to the piriformis. Sixteen percent of the time, there can be a branch passing proximally, posteriorly, or through the muscle.

- Anteriorly, the neurovascular structures enter the thigh under the inguinal ligament within the femoral triangle. The borders of the triangle are the sartorius laterally, pectineus medially, and the inguinal ligament superiorly. Within the triangle, from lateral to medial, are the femoral nerve, artery, and vein and the lymphatic vessels. The muscles that make up the floor of the femoral triangle, from lateral to medial, are the iliacus, psoas, pectineus, and adductor longus muscles. The lateral femoral cutaneous nerve lies on the surface of the iliacus muscle and exits the pelvis under the lateral attachment of the inguinal ligament. It can be found medially and travels superficially to the sartorius muscle about 6 to 8 cm below the anterior superior iliac spine. The femoral artery lies on the surface of the iliopsoas and delivers the profunda femoris, which supplies the anteromedial portion of the thigh, perforators, and vastus lateralis. The lateral and medial femoral circumflex arteries arise from the profunda femoris. The lateral femoral circumflex artery gives off an ascending branch toward the greater trochanter that is at risk during anterolateral approaches. The medial femoral circumflex artery, which provides the majority of blood flow to the femoral head, proceeds posteriorly between the iliopsoas and pectineus and lies anteriorly to the quadratus femoris (**FIG 2**).
- The femoral nerve (L2–L4) lies on the psoas muscle belly and passes through the femoral triangle as the most lateral structure. It is at risk to injury during the approach to the hip with retractors rather than with reaming or drilling.
- Inferiorly, the obturator nerve and artery exit the pelvis via the obturator canal. The posterior branches run inferiorly to the transverse acetabular ligament.
- Superiorly, the superior gluteal nerve and artery run between the gluteus minimus and medius to the tensor fascia lata. Branches of the superior gluteal nerve can pass within 5 cm to the greater trochanter.
- Because it is common to place screws for cementless acetabular component fixation during THA, it is necessary to understand the anatomy deep to the acetabulum as well. Running along the inner cortical surface of the acetabulum are the external iliac, femoral and obturator vessels, and nerves. Wasielewski et al[49] described a four-quadrant system for safe placement of acetabular screws (**FIG 3**). The quadrants are formed by drawing a line from the anterior superior iliac spine through the center of the acetabulum to the posterior fovea, forming acetabular halves. A second line is drawn perpendicular to the first at the midpoint of the acetabulum, forming four quadrants. The posterior superior and posterior inferior quadrants contain the best bone stock and are considered safe for screw placement. The anterior superior and anterior inferior quadrants are considered dangerous and should be avoided due to risks to the external iliac and obturator vessels and nerves, respectively.

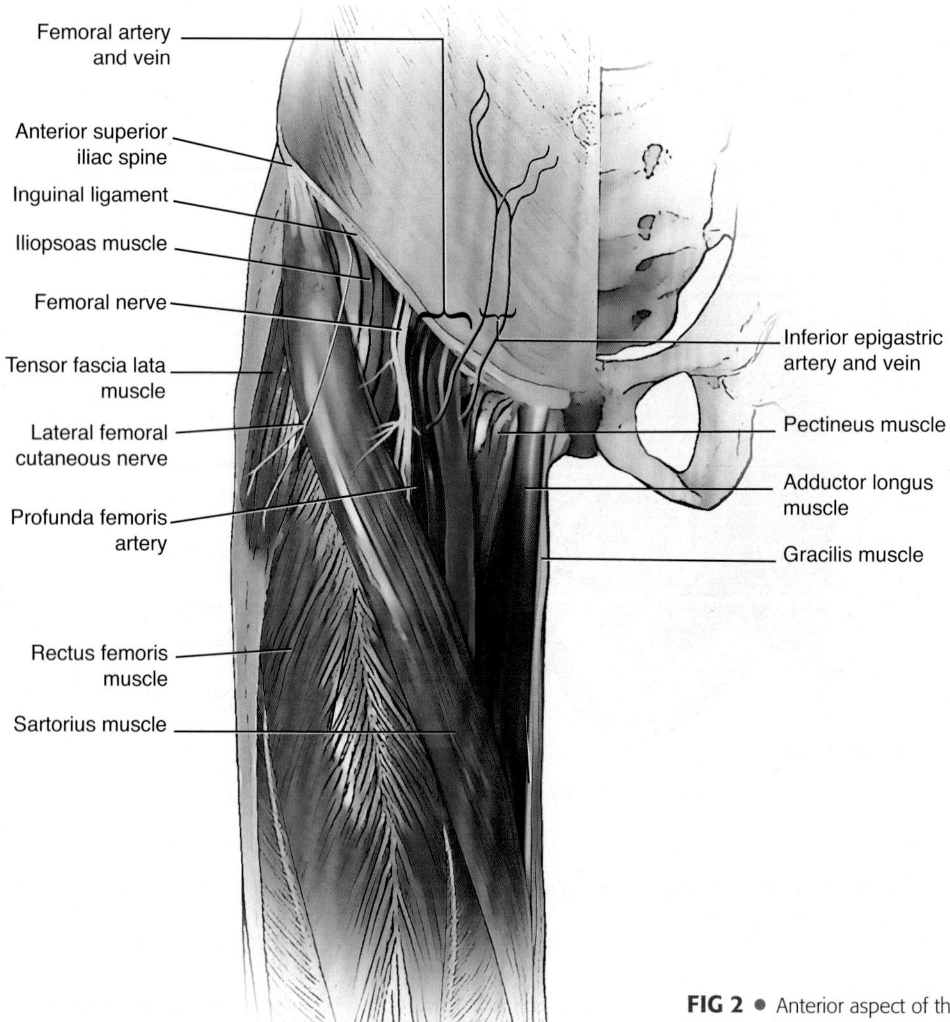

FIG 2 • Anterior aspect of the hip. Note the proximity of the neurovascular bundle just anterior and medial to the hip joint. In addition, note the lateral femoral cutaneous nerve on the anterior aspect of the sartorius muscle. It is at risk during the direct anterior approach to the hip.

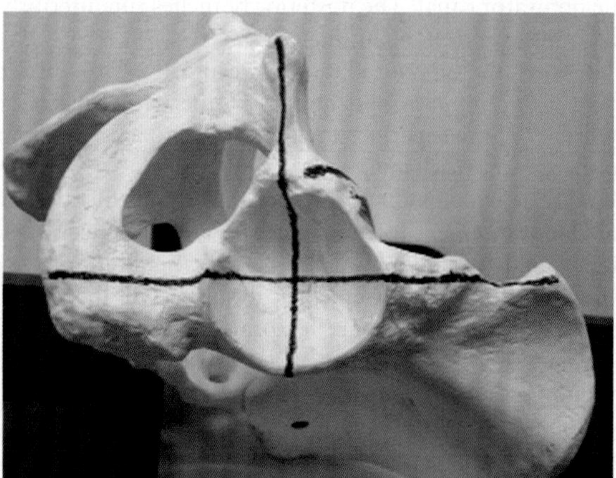

FIG 3 • Model of the pelvis in supine position. The quadrants described by Wasielewski et al[49] are formed by drawing a line from the anterior superior iliac spine through the center of the acetabulum to the posterior fovea. A second line is drawn perpendicular to the first at the midpoint of the acetabulum, forming four quadrants. The posterior superior and posterior inferior quadrants are considered safe for screw placement, whereas the anterior superior and anterior inferior quadrants are considered dangerous and should be avoided.

Vascular Injury

- Vascular injury is one of the most catastrophic complications in THA and can lead to loss of life or limb. The reported incidence of injury is between 0.08% and 0.25%.[8,16,33,35] Sharma et al[46] reported an overall mortality rate of 7% and a 15% incidence of limb loss in patients with vascular injury after THA. The most important treatment for vascular injury is prevention. Surgeons must be keenly aware of the surrounding anatomy and have a high index of suspicion if excessive bleeding is encountered or unexplained hypotension exists during the surgery or postoperatively. Besides the obvious monitoring for acute hypotension performed by the anesthesiologist, careful monitoring of patients for changes in vital signs in the recovery room postoperatively is paramount to prompt recognition of a vascular injury. Although direct injury to vessels can occur that would lead to hemorrhage, indirect injury can occur during routine manipulation of the limb as vessels can be stretched, torqued, and compressed. Strain on the vessels can cause intimal tears and flaps that can fully clot off arteries.
- Generally, the most common vessels at risk during THA are the external iliac artery and vein, femoral artery and vein,

profunda femoris artery and vein, and obturator artery and vein. All of these vessels can be at risk regardless of the approach to the hip joint as they come into play mainly during exposure of the acetabulum. The risk of vascular injury increases substantially during conversion and revision procedures. The need to remove implants and/or cement along with the presence of scar tissue, heterotopic ossification, and bony abnormalities all contribute to the higher risk. Additionally, patients with a history of trauma, previous radiation, congenital malformation, and existing peripheral vascular disease are at increased risk for vascular injury.

- Precise understanding of the anatomy surrounding the hip is critically important for a safe exposure. Protecting the vessels with appropriate retractors and avoidance of straying into the soft tissue can help avoid injury. Direct injury can occur from a variety of sources: scalpels, osteotomes, retractors, bone fragments, reamers, drills, screws, cement, and the implants themselves. Careful dissection and placement of retractors during exposure through a variety of approaches leads to a safe outcome. It is also the surgeon's responsibility to ensure retractors held by their assistants do not drift or migrate into unsafe positions.
- Anteriorly, the external iliac and femoral vessels are at risk. They pass anteriorly to the hip joint on the surface of the iliopsoas muscle. Cadaveric dissection has shown that the femoral vessels lie within an inch of the anterior capsule of the hip.[11] Therefore, it is critical that the anterior retractor be placed directly onto the anterior acetabular wall, superficial to any labral tissue but deep to the indirect head of the rectus femoris and the iliopsoas muscles (**FIG 4**). If it is noted that the retractor has pierced into the muscle, it should be carefully removed and visualized for blood extravasation. Inferiorly, the obturator vessels are at risk during dissection, retractor placement, or implant/cement removal. The profunda femoris vessels are at risk during instrumentation of the femur, especially when placing cerclage wires.[1] However, the major risk of vascular injury during THA comes from the use of acetabular screws. As indicated in the Anatomy section, the quadrant system described by Wasielewski et al[49] is crucial to avoiding injury to the external iliac and obturator vessels when drilling and inserting acetabular screws. Screws should only be placed in the posterior superior and posterior inferior quadrants (see **FIG 3**).

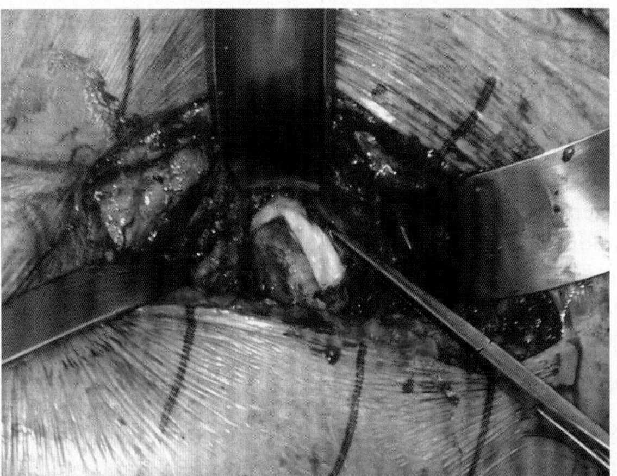

FIG 4 • Exposure of the acetabulum. Note that the anterior retractor (at the top of the photo) is placed directly superficial to the labrum and deep to the indirect head of the rectus femoris muscle. The Kocher is pointing at the space between these two structures.

- During revision surgery, safe component removal is also paramount. If implants or cement have migrated into the pelvis, vascular surgical support should be on hand during the procedure. Lewallen[24] has suggested that intrapelvic mobilization of vessels be performed prior to hip exposure. Another option is to place an intravascular balloon sheath in the common femoral artery prior to hip exposure. It could be inflated to tamponade the vessel if major bleeding is encountered on intrapelvic implant removal. Emergency vascular surgery intervention for repair could be performed in a somewhat managed fashion while the bleeding is controlled.
- The hallmark signs of vascular injury are sudden hemorrhage (pulsatile if arterial), hypotension, tachycardia, decreasing hemoglobin, low urine output, and/or thigh or abdominal distention. If massive bleeding occurs, apply direct pressure to the area and obtain immediate vascular assistance. The anesthesiologist should administer blood products immediately. If the patient is hemodynamically stable, angiography and transcatheter embolization can be performed. If the patient is unstable, immediate exploration must be performed.[3]
- Early recognition and prompt action is necessary (whether intraoperatively or in the postoperative period) to save the patient's life and/or limb in the case of vascular complications. These unfortunate outcomes are real and a high index of suspicion is critical in avoiding their occurrence.

Peripheral Nerve Injury

- The overall incidence of major nerve injury after primary THA is 0.6% to 2.9% regardless of approach.[12,20,38,44] The incidence has been reported from 3.2% to7.6% after revision THA, and nerve injury was found in 5.2% of patients undergoing primary THA for congenital dislocation or dysplasia of the hip.[22,41,44] Additionally, it is generally accepted that lengthening the lower extremity greater than 4 cm is a risk factor for neurapraxia[13]; however, other studies have shown that there is no relation between the amount of lengthening and nerve injury.[38]
- The two largest and most critical structures are the femoral and sciatic nerves (see **FIGS 1** and **2**). The superior gluteal and obturator nerves are also at risk, and, with the increasing use of the direct anterior approach, lateral femoral cutaneous neurapraxia is commonly seen. The most common motor nerve injury is to the sciatic nerve followed by the superior gluteal, obturator, and femoral nerves, respectively. The common peroneal portion of the sciatic nerve is more often injured due to its anatomic characteristics. As noted, the peroneal portion is more lateral and has thinner connective tissue coverage, which makes it more susceptible to injury.[44]
- Although nerve injuries can occur with any approach to the hip, certain nerves can be at higher risk depending on the dissection method. During acetabular exposure via the posterior approach, the sciatic nerve should be palpated and protected with a posterior Hohmann retractor. The position of the leg is important during exposure of the proximal femur. Increased tension on the sciatic nerve is seen with flexion, internal rotation, and adduction. Therefore, placing a soft roll under the thigh to avoid adduction during femoral preparation can decrease tension on the nerve. During the lateral, anterolateral, and direct anterior approaches, the

femoral nerve is at risk with the anterior acetabular retractor. As mentioned earlier, precise placement along the bone and deep to the indirect head of the rectus is important to protect the nerve. Specifically with the direct anterior approach, the lateral femoral cutaneous nerve is affected frequently. In one report, 81% of patients reported neurapraxia; however, this did not lead to any functional limitations.[17] The superior gluteal nerve is at risk during the direct lateral (Hardinge) approach. The nerve passes within 5 cm of the tip of the greater trochanter; therefore, avoidance of extending the split in the gluteus medius more than 5 cm should protect the nerve.

- Similar to vascular injuries, damage to peripheral nerves can occur from direct mechanical compression, distraction, or thermal injury. If deformity exists, or if excessive scar, heterotopic ossification, prior radiation, or previous hardware is present, the risk of injury is increased. Understanding of the surrounding anatomy is again critical to protecting these structures. During revision THA, entrapment of nerves with cerclage wires has been reported.[28] The femoral, sciatic, and obturator nerves can be adherent or encased in acetabular bone cement.[27] If there is posterior wall deficiency, the sciatic nerve can adhere to a porous-coated acetabular component and be at risk with removal of the implant. However, when a nerve injury is diagnosed postoperatively, it is frequently impossible to determine its origin. The cause of nerve injury after THA is still poorly understood and is likely multifactorial.
- Patients who have had damage to a peripheral nerve will present with motor and sensory deficits in the anatomic distribution and dermatome of that particular nerve. If a direct injury to the nerve has occurred, the nerve deficit will typically be evident immediately after surgery. However, nerve palsies can occur for up to 36 hours or more postoperatively. Neurovascular monitoring of all postoperative THA patients is vitally important for the first 2 days after surgery. Immediate evaluation in the recovery room is paramount. Early nerve palsy can be the first sign of a vascular injury and this should be ruled out immediately.
- Accurate serial physical examination results regarding neurovascular status as well as wound assessment for drainage or swelling should be recorded. Immediate postoperative radiographs should be evaluated to assess the location of implants, screws, cerclage wires, cement, or bone fragments. Computed tomography (CT) scans or magnetic resonance imaging (MRI) should be obtained for further clarification of hardware position or the presence of an expanding hematoma if there is any uncertainty. An MRI of the lumbar spine (if spinal anesthesia was performed) should be obtained if there is concern for an epidural hematoma. Urgent evacuation of the hematoma has been shown to improve outcomes.[7] If hardware is causing damage to a nerve, it should be removed.[24] To prevent nerve injuries, intraoperative monitoring with somatosensory evoked potentials has been recommended by some; however, it is time consuming and can give a significant number of false-positive results.[43] Additionally, in a study comparing THA cases using monitoring versus those that did not, the use of monitoring did not decrease the number of nerve injuries.[41]

Prognosis

- Neurologic recovery after injury is variable. Improvement may occur for 2 to 3 years and is unpredictable. Where some authors suggest that recovery is associated with the extent of injury, others found no correlation.[24,38] Direct injury to nerves tends to have a better outcome than stretch injuries. Femoral nerve palsy improves better than sciatic nerve palsies and isolated peroneal palsies tend to do better than complete sciatic nerve palsies.[13,50] If the nerve palsy involves only sensory and not motor, or if the motor function begins to return in the early postoperative period, then prognosis is good for recovery.[44]

Intraoperative Periprosthetic Fracture

- Periprosthetic fractures can be challenging for both inexperienced and seasoned orthopaedic surgeons. Intraoperative femur fractures occur in approximately 0.1% to 3.2% of primary cemented THA and 3% to 5.4% of primary uncemented THA. The rate of fracture during revision surgery is significantly higher with some reporting an incidence of 30%.[5,31] Intraoperative acetabular fractures are less common. Fractures can occur during bone preparation; when dislocating or relocating the hip, preparing the bone, inserting a new implant; or, if revision surgery, removal of preexisting implants.
- Patients with osteoporosis, deformity, osteolysis, bone defects, and small size are at increased risk for fracture. Sheth et al[47] reviewed over 5000 THA patients and found female gender, increasing age, and hip dysplasia to have an increased risk for fracture. Additional risk factors include a diagnosis of rheumatoid arthritis, Paget disease, and chronic steroid usage.[26] Surgical techniques and the design of implants can also increase the risk of intraoperative fracture. Minimally invasive surgical (MIS) approaches are associated with a higher risk of intraoperative fracture.[18,19] As with many complications, understanding the risk factors for fracture can help to prevent them from occurring.

Fractures of the Femur

- The most commonly used system that describes periprosthetic femur fracture patterns and can guide treatment is the Vancouver classification described by Masri et al.[29] This system is based on the location of the fracture and the fixation of the stem. Type A fractures are stable fractures involving only the greater trochanter (AG) or the lesser trochanter (AL). Type B fractures occur around the stem or just below its tip. Type B1 indicates a fracture involves the stem where the stem remains well fixed. Type B2 also involves the stem; however, the stem is loose. Type B3 fractures involve a loose stem with poor available bone stock. Type C fractures occur distally beyond the stem tip and therefore do not affect the fixation of the implant. The Vancouver system for intraoperative fractures keeps the same anatomic definitions (types A, B, C); however, additional subtypes were added to indicate the quality of the fracture. Subtype 1 refers to a simple cortical perforation; subtype 2 represents a nondisplaced, linear fracture; and subtype 3 indicates a displaced or unstable fracture.[10]

Surgical risks

- Surgical exposure is critical in performing a safe, well-functioning hip replacement. If exposure is compromised due to MIS, morbid obesity, or muscular body habitus, the risk of periprosthetic fracture increases.[18] Straining to access the femoral canal can cause perforation or fracture during reaming, broaching, or implantation. The use of cementless implants inherently increases the risk of fracture. In an effort to gain press-fit stability, the strength of the underlying bone can be overcome. Stem design has been shown to affect fracture rates. Revision of femoral components carries the highest risk of fracture. The weakened bone is at risk due to osteolysis or stress shielding. Fracture can occur due to implant or cement removal. The presence of an endosteal pedestal can lead to eccentric reaming or broaching that can cause perforation. Long straight reamers and implants inserted into the curved bow of the femur also increase the risk of perforation and fracture.

- During surgery, a high index of suspicion and thorough exposure and inspection of the surrounding bone are fundamental to immediate diagnosis and treatment of intraoperative fractures. Fractures can occur during impaction or removal of implants or during reaming, broaching, or dislocation of the hip. During impaction of the implants, any of the following subtleties can indicate that a fracture has occurred: sudden change in the position of the implant, sudden lack of resistance to impaction, or a change in the audible pitch made when impacting the implant. Wedge-tapered stems have been found to have the highest rate of fracture when compared with metaphyseal or diaphyseal engaging stems or cemented stems.[30] Cortical perforations can also occur during reaming, broaching, or implant insertion. The risk of perforation is significantly increased when exposure is not adequate (due to poor exposure by the surgeon and/or with morbidly obese or very muscular patients) and reaming or insertion is forced (**FIG 5**).

Treatment

- Appropriate treatment of recognized fractures can lead to very successful outcomes. Identifying the fracture, full exposure to determine its extent, and stable internal fixation are all imperative for appropriate treatment. If a fracture is suspected, remove the implant, broach, or reamer, and expose the fracture fully to obtain direct visualization. If there is any difficulty determining the full extent of propagation, fluoroscopy or radiographs should be used.
- Greater trochanteric fractures can be treated with trochanteric claws and/or cerclage cables. Nondisplaced linear fractures around the metaphysis can be stabilized with a cerclage cable and reinsertion of the stem. Excellent results have been shown with this technique, with 100% femoral component survival up to 16 years.[4] A displaced fracture can be reduced and fixed with cerclage cables; however, a diaphyseal stem should be used. A diaphyseal fracture can be treated with standard reduction and internal fixation with a plate, screws, and cables if the stem is stable. However, if the stem is unstable, a long-stemmed implant and fixation is necessary. If the bone stock is poor, cortical allograft can be used as supplemental fixation.
- Cortical perforations can be identified with curettes, curved hemostats, or intraoperative fluoroscopy/radiographs. If a perforation is noted, full exposure of the defect is necessary to ensure no fracture line has propagated distally beyond the defect. A long-stem implant should be used to bypass the perforation by a distance of two cortical diameters. A cerclage cable can be placed around the bone distal to the perforation to ensure no propagation while reaming, broaching, and inserting the implant. If the perforation is substantial, consider augmenting the repair with a cortical strut graft placed over the defect.
- Fractures can be missed intraoperatively. Therefore, all patients should receive postoperative radiographs in the

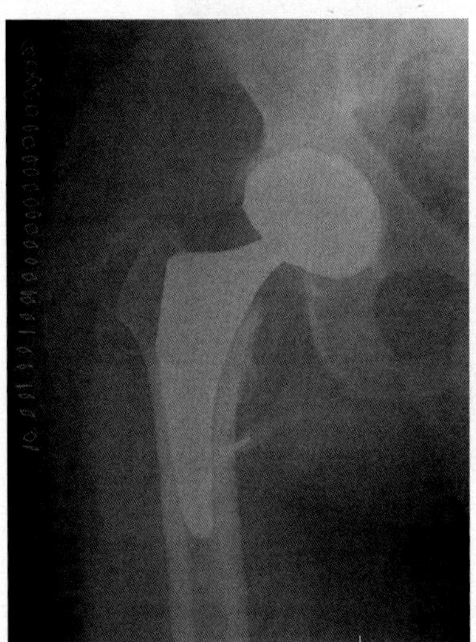
A

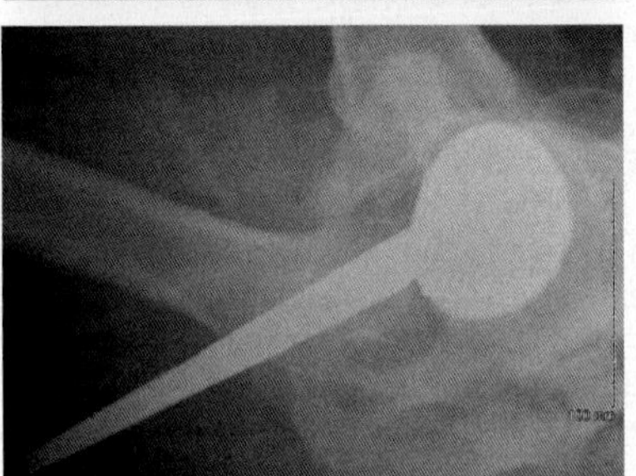
B

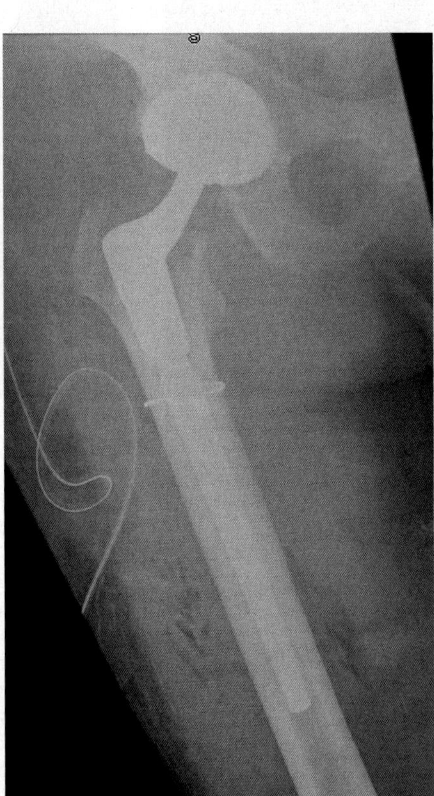
C

FIG 5 • **A.** Immediate anterior posterior (AP) postoperative radiograph showing apparent appropriate position of the femoral implant after THA via an anterior approach. **B.** Follow-up lateral radiograph was obtained showing stem that was placed through a perforation in the posterior metaphyseal femur, likely due to a difficult exposure. **C.** AP radiograph after femoral stem revision to a diaphyseal engaging stem.

recovery room. Besides evaluation of the implant for positioning, sizing, etc., these radiographs should be carefully scrutinized for the presence of a periprosthetic fracture. If a fracture line is seen on the postoperative radiograph, the fracture and stem are evaluated for stability. If both appear stable, protected weight bearing can be ordered. Close radiographic follow-up is necessary to monitor for displacement. If the fracture or implant are initially unstable or become unstable during follow-up, revision surgery should be performed.

Fractures of the Acetabulum

- Intraoperative periprosthetic acetabular fractures are uncommon; however, with increased use of press-fit cups, the incidence is increasing. To achieve adequate fixation and stability, acetabular components are designed to create plastic deformation of the host bone when impacted. Commonly, the components are slightly larger than the amount that is reamed (ie, under-reaming) and this can lead to fracture when impacting. Peterson and Lewallen[39] classified periprosthetic acetabular fractures into two types: implant stable (type 1) and implant unstable (type 2).

Surgical risks

- Screws are often used to augment fixation of cementless acetabular components. Due to concerns regarding fretting and osteolysis with screws, the use of oversized components that are press-fit into an under-reamed acetabulum can be used. This can lead to fracture during component insertion, especially in osteoporotic bone. Curtis et al[9] found a significant risk of fracture when under-reaming a hemispherical, uncemented cup by 4 mm. Sharkey et al[45] reported on 13 cases with acetabular fracture and found osteoporosis and component oversizing to be risk factors for fracture. The authors recommended line-to-line reaming in patients with osteoporosis. As with the femur, the risk of fracture is increased during revision surgery. Removal of a well-fixed cup can lead to damage of the surrounding bone stock. Also, impacting implants into bone that is significantly weakened by osteolysis can lead to fracture and loss of fixation.

Treatment

- The treatment of an intraoperative acetabular fracture is dependent on fixation of the implant. If a fracture is identified while impacting the component and the component is well fixed, the implant can remain in place and the fracture can be treated with protected weight bearing. If there are screw holes, screws can be added to augment fixation (**FIG 6**). If the implant is unstable, it must be removed and the surrounding bone stock assessed. Bone grafting of defects and impacting a multihole revision shell can achieve fixation in most fractures, but plate fixation prior to cup insertion may be

A
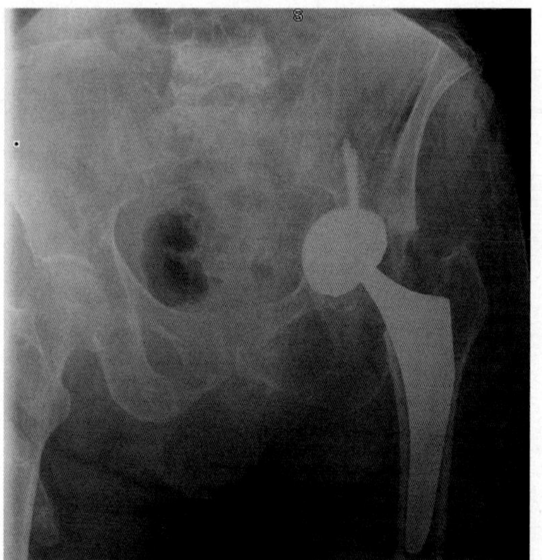

B
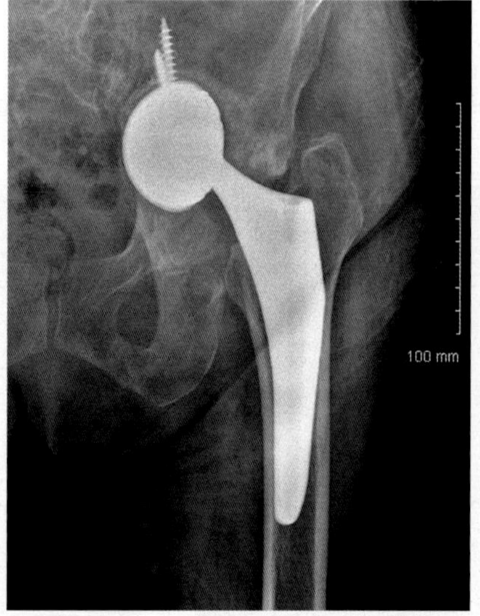

C
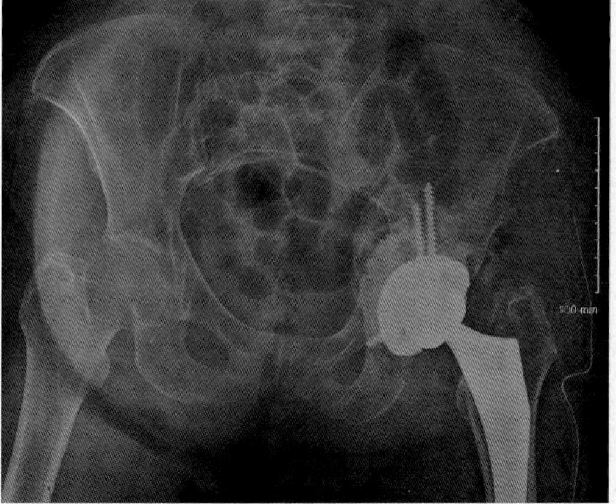

FIG 6 • **A.** Immediate anterior posterior (AP) postoperative radiograph showing protrusion of the acetabular component after THA. The surgeon realized there was weakness of the medial wall but felt the component was secure with acetabular screws. **B.** Follow-up AP radiograph showing intrapelvic migration of the acetabular component through the medial wall. **C.** AP radiograph after successful acetabular component revision. The posterior column, superior dome, and a portion of the pubic root allowed for rim fit fixation with screw augmentation and bone grafting.

necessary. Despite these recommendations, these patients need to be followed carefully. Peterson and Lewallen[39] noted that even when the fracture heals, 80% of the cases in their series eventually required revision.

Preventing Intraoperative Fractures

- As always, preventing intraoperative fractures from happening is the best course. Preoperative preparations, including patient evaluation for risk factors, templating of sizes, and determining the type of implant, will help avoid periprosthetic fracture. When faced with a high-risk patient with osteoporotic bone, cementing the femoral and/or acetabular components is a reliable alternative that has a much lower risk of fracture. If press-fit implants are used, performing line-to-line reaming of the acetabular component and avoiding under-reaming can lessen the risk of fracture.[45] It is helpful to use multiple senses when inserting press-fit femoral implants. The use of auditory, visual, and tactile senses can ensure appropriate broaching and implantation of the implants. The force of impacting press-fit femoral stems and frequency analysis of hammering sound data have been studied. Finite element analysis has shown that a decrease in hammering sound frequency indicates adequate hammering has occurred and any further hammering risks fracture.[42] Therefore, when the broach stops moving and a change in pitch is heard when impacting, no further impaction should occur.
- During revision THA, removal of well-fixed cemented or cementless implants requires special preparation to avoid fracture. A review of these techniques is found in Chapter 24. Specialized instruments can be used such as cup-out systems that use a precisely curved blade to remove fixed, cementless acetabular components (**FIG 7**). On the femoral side, burrs, flexible osteotomes, and ultrasonic cement removal systems can help remove fixed stems. However, if a stem is well fixed, an extended trochanteric osteotomy should be performed. This allows for controlled removal of implants and cement and lessens the risk of a comminuted, unstable fracture.
- Recognition of fractures intraoperatively is paramount. During surgery, if a fracture is recognized, appropriate treatment can be taken to ensure the components are stable, whether it is on the femoral or acetabular side. A treated small, nondisplaced fracture will likely go on to heal without issue, but an unrecognized fracture could lead to unnecessary morbidity and additional surgery. If there is any suspicion for fracture, intraoperative fluoroscopy should be used, especially in high-risk patients.

Periprosthetic Joint Infection

- PJI, an often-studied and dreaded complication of total joint arthroplasty (TJA), is addressed in Chapters 33 and 34. In conjunction with the Musculoskeletal Infection Society, an International Consensus Meeting was held in Philadelphia, Pennsylvania in 2013.[34] The recommendations from this meeting were not level 5 expert advice; however, thousands of articles were studied, discussed, and agreed on by hundreds of experts from all over the world. The following is a list of the recommendations from this historical meeting that pertain specifically to preventing PJI.

Consensus Recommendations for Prevention of Periprosthetic Joint Infection[34]

- Avoid performing TJA in patients with an active infection. Active infection of the arthritic joint (septic arthritis); presence of septicemia; and/or presence of active local cutaneous, subcutaneous, or deep tissue infection are all significant risk factors predisposing patients to SSI or PJI and are contraindications to undertaking elective TJA.
- Dental hygiene is important. All patients undergoing elective arthroplasty should be screened for evidence of active oral/dental infection. This may be performed by administration of a questionnaire or dental examination.
- Consensus does not exist for routine screening for methicillin-resistant *Staphylococcus aureus* (MRSA) and methicillin-sensitive *Staphylococcus aureus* (MSSA) other than for high-risk patients. For those colonized, short-term nasal application of mupirocin is the most accepted current method of decolonization for MRSA and/or MSSA.
- Routine urine screening is *not* warranted for patients undergoing elective arthroplasty. Urine screening prior to elective

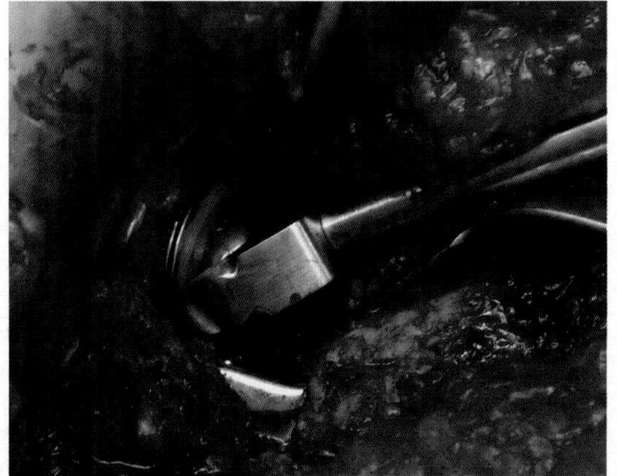

A

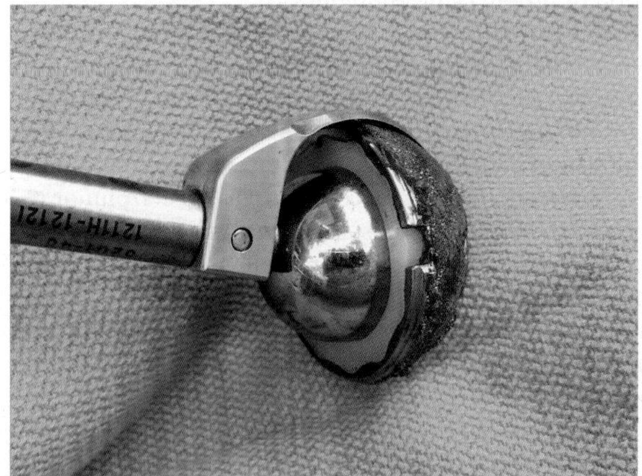

B

FIG 7 • **A.** Removal of a well-fixed, retroverted, uncemented acetabular implant using a cup removal device. This device is centered in the socket using an appropriately sized femoral head. The blades are sized to match the diameter of the component to allow for precise removal without bone loss. **B.** The cutting blades can break through bone ingrowth surrounding the cup. The component shown here was removed successfully without any bone adherent to the implant.

arthroplasty should be reserved for patients with a present history or symptoms of a urinary tract infection.

- Disease-modifying agents (ie, antirheumatologic medications or immunosuppressants) should be stopped prior to elective TJA. The timing of drug discontinuation should be based on the specific medication and the individual patient. The cessation of immunosuppressant medications should be performed in consultation and under the direction of the treating physician.
- *All* patients with prior septic arthritis should undergo evaluation by serology and aspiration of the joint whenever possible, prior to arthroplasty.

Skin Preparation

- Preoperative cleansing of the skin with chlorhexidine gluconate (CHG) should be implemented. In the presence of sensitivity to CHG, or when it is unavailable, it is our consensus that antiseptic soap is appropriate.
- We recommend that whole body skin cleansing should start at least the night prior to elective arthroplasty. It is a consensus that after bathing, patients are advised to sleep in clean garments and bedding without the application of any topical products.
- Clipping, as opposed to shaving, is the preferred method for hair removal at the surgical site. If necessary, hair removal should be performed as close to the time of the surgical procedure as possible.
- Elective arthroplasty should *not* be performed in patients with active ulceration of the skin in the vicinity of the surgical site. It is our consensus that incisions should not be placed through active skin lesions. For certain lesions such as those due to eczema and psoriasis, surgery should be delayed in these patients until their lesions have been optimized.
- The surgeon and operating room personnel should mechanically wash their hands with an antiseptic agent for a minimum of 2 minutes for the first case. A shorter period may be appropriate for subsequent cases. There is no clear difference among various antiseptic agents for hand washing.

Perioperative Antibiotics

- We support the surgical checklist protocol as beneficial to patient safety and specifically as it applies to correct administration of prophylactic antibiotics.
- The preoperative dose of antibiotics should be administered within 1 hour of surgical incision; this can be extended to 2 hours for vancomycin and fluoroquinolones. Postoperative antibiotics should not be administered for greater than 24 hours after surgery.
- A first- or second-generation cephalosporin (cefazolin or cefuroxime) should be administered for routine perioperative surgical prophylaxis. Isoxazolyl penicillin is used as an appropriate alternative.
- Currently, teicoplanin and vancomycin are reasonable alternatives when routine antibiotic prophylaxis cannot be administered.
- In a patient with a known anaphylactic reaction to penicillin, vancomycin or clindamycin should be administered as prophylaxis. Teicoplanin is an option in countries where it is available.
- Preoperative antibiotics have different pharmacokinetics based on patient weight and should be weight-adjusted.
- For current MRSA carriers, vancomycin or teicoplanin is the recommended perioperative antibiotic prophylaxis.
- Patients with prior history of MRSA should be rescreened preoperatively. If patients are found to be negative for MRSA, we recommend routine perioperative antibiotic prophylaxis.
- The type of preoperative antibiotic administered to a patient with prior septic arthritis or PJI should cover the previous infecting organism of the same joint.
- An additional dose of antibiotic should be administered intraoperatively after two half-lives of the prophylactic agent. The general guidelines for frequency of intraoperative antibiotic administration are cefazolin every 2 to 5 hours,[4] cefuroxime every 3 to 4 hours, clindamycin every 3 to 6 hours, isoxazolyl penicillin every 3 hours, and vancomycin every 6 to 12 hours.
- We recommend that redosing of antibiotics be considered in cases of large blood volume loss (>2000 mL) and fluid resuscitation (>2000 mL). As these are independent variables, redosing should be considered as soon as the first of these parameters are met.

Operating Environment

- We believe that arthroplasty surgery may be performed in operating theaters without laminar flow. Laminar flow rooms and other strategies that may reduce particulates in operating rooms would be expected to reduce particulate load. Studies have not shown lower SSI in laminar flow rooms, and some cases are associated with increased rates of SSI.
- We recommend that operating room traffic should be kept to a minimum.
- We agree that ultraviolent light environments can lower infection rates but recognize that this can pose a risk to operating room personnel.
- We recommend that all personnel wear clean theater attire, including disposable head covering, when entering an operating room. Garments worn outside of the hospital should not be worn during TJA.
- We recommend that a coordinated effort be made to minimize the duration of surgery without technical compromise of the procedure. Increased surgical time is a risk factor for PJI.
- We recognize the significance of patient normothermia and the data from nonorthopaedic procedures. We support general recommendations from the general surgery literature and identify this as a field that requires further research.
- We recommend double gloving and recognize the theoretical advantage of triple gloving.
- We recognize the advantage of glove changes at least every 90 minutes or more frequently and the necessity of changing perforated gloves.
- We recommend that the timing of opening trays should occur as close to the start of the surgical procedure as possible with the avoidance of any delays between tray opening and the start of surgery.
- We recognize high contamination rates in studies of scalpel blades that have been used for the skin incision and recommend changes after skin incision.
- We recommend changing suction tips every 60 minutes based on studies showing higher rates of contamination.
- We recommend against the use of fluid-filled basins that sit open during the surgery.
- We recognize the theoretical basis for irrigation to dilute contamination and nonviable tissue and that a greater

volume of irrigation would be expected to achieve greater dilution. We recognize advantages and disadvantages of different methods of delivering fluid but make no recommendations of one method over another.

- We recognize the mechanical advantage of irrigation but that conflicting evidence exists supporting the use of one agent over the other and make no recommendation regarding type of solution.
- Antibiotic-impregnated polymethylmethacrylate cement reduces the incidence of PJI following TJA and should be used in patients at high risk for PJI following elective arthroplasty.
- In a patient with prior septic arthritis or PJI, we recommend the use of antibiotic-impregnated cement if a cemented component is used.
- Antibiotic should be added to cement in all patients undergoing cemented or hybrid fixation as part of revision arthroplasty.
- If possible, avoid allogeneic blood transfusions as they are associated with an increased risk of SSI/PJI.
- Compared to general anesthesia, neuraxial anesthesia reduces the amount of blood loss during THA.
- Avoid metal-on-metal bearing surfaces as observational data suggest that these bearings may be associated with a higher risk of PJI.

Dislocation

- Although dislocation is not considered an intraoperative complication during THA, it deserves special consideration as it can have a devastating impact on the outcome of patients. The incidence of dislocation is approximately 1% to 10% after primary THA and as high as 27% after revision THA.[2,15,21] An epidemiologic study found that dislocation was the number one cause for THA revision.[6] The purpose of this section is to focus on preventing dislocation through appropriate patient selection and surgical technique.

Risk Factors

- There are many factors that increase the risk of dislocation including patient characteristics, implant design, and surgical-related factors. Patient characteristics that may lead to higher rates of dislocation are female, age older than 80 years, previous surgery, rheumatoid arthritis, hip trauma, developmental dysplasia of the hip, neuromuscular disorders, dementia, alcoholism, and psychosis. These factors are not adjustable. Surgeon experience has a positive impact on reducing dislocation, and an inexperienced low-volume surgeon should consider obtaining assistance when treating the high-risk patient.
- From a surgical standpoint, it is imperative to use appropriate implants, position them appropriately, and ensure the soft tissues are tensioned properly.[14] It has been shown that implants designed to maximize the head–neck ratio (ie, larger head with smaller neck) provide a greater impingement-free range of motion. Larger diameter heads also increase the jump distance necessary for the femoral head to disengage from the liner. Avoiding skirts on the femoral head will minimize the neck size and the chance for impingement. A larger head–neck ratio, combined with an increased jump distance, gives greater range of motion without impingement, therefore reducing dislocation rates.[23] However, very large heads (>36 mm) have shown no increased benefits for stability versus their smaller counterparts and can cause iliopsoas impingement, leading to postoperative groin pain. Additional stability can be obtained with dual mobility bearing surfaces, especially in challenging revision THA procedures.[40]
- Exposure to the hip is an important factor for hip stability. Visualizing all areas of the surgical field is critically important to place the implants appropriately. It is well known that dislocation rates differ for the various approached to the hip; however, surgeons must be comfortable that the joint can be exposed properly to ensure appropriate implant positioning. Morrey's classic meta-analysis revealed the following dislocation rates based on the approach: 3.2% posterior, 0.55% direct lateral, 2.2% anterolateral, and 1.3% transtrochanteric.[32] Repairing the posterior capsule reduces the incidence of dislocations performed via the posterior approach.[48]
- Once the hip is exposed, appropriate implant orientation and positioning are crucial. A safe zone for the acetabulum has been defined as 40 ± 10 degrees of cup inclination or abduction and 15 ± 10 degrees of anteversion.[25] Excessive anteversion can lead to anterior dislocations, whereas retroversion can lead to posterior dislocations. Excessive abduction can lead to dislocation when the hip is adducted, whereas a horizontal cup lacking abduction can cause an impingement-related dislocation. Also, acetabular osteophytes can lead to impingement and should be removed.
- Normal femoral version is 10 to 15 degrees and restoration of this is important in achieving hip stability. Rarely is femoral version in itself an issue with stability during primary THA but careful attention to version is necessary during revision THA and patients with dysplasia. Characteristics of the femur have more to do with soft tissue tensioning (ie, offset and length are important elements to restore for hip stability). Increased lateral offset tensions the abductor muscles. Conversely, the lack of offset results in abductor weakness, possible impingement, and loss of soft tissue tension, resulting in increased risk of dislocation. Offset and length need to be checked carefully so as to not overlengthen the limb. Also, excessive lateral offset can lead to lateral hip pain. Tensioning can be assessed by distracting the limb distally and ensuring the femoral head does not disengage from the acetabular liner (Shuck test).

Preventing Hip Dislocation

- Appropriate implant positioning and soft tissue balancing are the key surgical principles of performing a stable THA. A systematic approach should start with preoperative planning. Start by templating the size, position, and offset of the components, restoring leg lengths and femoral offset. Choose an implant that is unlikely to impinge and sizes that give a high head–neck ratio. In challenging cases, be prepared to use modular components and dual mobility bearings. Choose the surgical approach to the hip that gives you the best exposure and comfort with dissection. If a posterior approach is used, repair of the posterior capsule is imperative.
- Careful positioning of the implants is crucial. Place the acetabular component at 40 ± 10 degrees of cup inclination or abduction and 15 ± 10 degrees of anteversion. Maintain the femoral anteversion of 15 degrees. Combined anteversion of the acetabulum and femur should be approximately 35 to 45 degrees in females and 25 to 35 degrees in males. Ensure that there is no Shuck. Take the limb through a full range of motion while

monitoring the implants for impingement or frank dislocation. If these occur, build offset or length (ie, tension the soft tissues) and reevaluate. Verify that the leg has not been inappropriately lengthened. If the leg is long, carefully reevaluate the position and orientation of the acetabulum. Frequently, the leg can be lengthened indirectly in an attempt to tighten the soft tissues when the acetabulum version is incorrect.[36] Reposition and reorient the acetabulum if this is the case. High wall liners can be placed to assist in stability; however, these will reduce the available range of motion and can lead to impingement. If necessary, intraoperative radiographs could be obtained to evaluate positioning of the implants. Postoperatively, hip precautions can be ordered, especially if there is any concern for instability. However, it has been shown that hip precautions are not necessary when a THA has been performed in a stable fashion via the direct lateral approach.[37]

PEARLS AND PITFALLS

Vascular injury

- The acetabulum is surrounded by vital neurovascular structures and their anatomic locations are critical to understand.
- Place screws only in the posterior superior and posterior inferior quadrants of the acetabulum.
- Place anterior retractors directly onto the anterior acetabulum wall. Straying into the soft tissue can damage the femoral vessels.
- Have a high index of suspicion for vascular injury if excessive bleeding is encountered or unexplained hypotension exists during the surgery or postoperatively.
- In the event of a vascular injury, act fast to save the life and/or limb of the patient. Communicate with your anesthesiologist to administer blood products expeditiously.
- In high-risk revision cases, have a vascular surgeon available for immediate action.

Peripheral nerve injury

- The femoral nerve is at risk with the anterior acetabular retractor. Precise placement of the retractor along the bone and deep to the indirect head of the rectus femoris muscle is important to protect the nerve.
- The superior gluteal nerve is at risk during the direct lateral (Hardinge) approach. Avoid extending the gluteus medius split more than 5 cm proximal to the greater trochanter.
- During acetabular exposure via the posterior approach, the sciatic nerve should be palpated and protected with a posterior retractor.
- Preoperatively, inform high-risk patients that they are at increased risk of nerve injury if they have a deformity of the hip, excessive scar tissue, heterotopic ossification, existing hardware, or had prior radiation.
- Nerve deficits are typically evident immediately after surgery but may develop for up to 36 hours or more postoperatively so careful monitoring is imperative.
- CT scan or MRI should be obtained for further clarification of hardware position or the presence of an expanding hematoma if there is any suspicion of neurologic injury. Remove any hardware causing damage to a nerve and evacuate any causative hematoma.

Intraoperative periprosthetic fracture

- Use caution when preparing for and inserting implants in high-risk patients—those with osteoporosis, deformity/dysplasia, osteolysis, bone defects, small size, rheumatoid arthritis, Paget disease, or chronic steroid use.
- Consider cementing implants in high-risk patients.
- Use an appropriate exposure to allow for unimpeded access to the hip. Straining to access the joint can lead to perforation or fracture during reaming, broaching, or implantation.
- When placing a hemispherical, uncemented acetabular cup, avoid under-reaming by 4 mm. Ream line-to-line when dealing with significant osteoporosis.
- During acetabular revisions, cup-out systems can be used to remove fixed, cementless components.
- During femoral revisions, do not hesitate to use an extended trochanteric osteotomy if the implant is not easily removable.
- Obtain postoperative radiographs in the recovery room and carefully scrutinize for the presence of a periprosthetic fracture.

Periprosthetic joint infection

- Avoid performing TJA in patients with an active infection.
- Disease-modifying agents (antirheumatologic medications, immunosuppressants) should be stopped prior to elective TJA.
- The preoperative dose of antibiotics should be administered within 1 hour of surgical incision.
- Use vancomycin or teicoplanin as the perioperative antibiotic for current MRSA carriers.
- An additional dose of antibiotic should be administered intraoperatively after two half-lives of the prophylactic agent and/or for cases with a large blood loss.
- Minimize operating room traffic.
- Minimize the duration of surgery without technical compromise of the procedure.
- Antibiotic-impregnated cement should be used in patients at high risk for PJI and in revision procedures.

Dislocation

- Start with a systematic approach of preoperative planning. Template the size, position, and offset of the components.
- Use appropriate implants, position them appropriately, and ensure the soft tissues are tensioned properly.
- Maximize the head–neck ratio (36-mm head maximum).
- Place the acetabular component in 40 ± 10 degrees of cup inclination and 15 ± 10 degrees of anteversion.
- Place the femoral component in 10–15 degrees of anteversion.
- Repair the posterior capsule if the posterior approach to the hip is used.
- In challenging cases, be prepared with modular components, dual mobility, or constrained bearings.

CONCLUSION

- THA has revolutionized the management of patients crippled with arthritis, providing excellent long-term results. The effectiveness of the procedure and the durability of implants have been superb. Despite the evolution in techniques for THA, complications can still occur. These complications can range from minor inconveniences to extremely serious, life- and/or limb-threatening injuries.
- Complications after THA can have a profound effect on patients' lives. Similar to all complications, it is best to prevent them from happening rather than treat them after they have occurred. Understanding the anatomy surrounding the hip, diligent preoperative planning, and meticulous surgical technique are required to avoid these potentially tragic complications. Prompt recognition of neurovascular injuries and swift action can be the difference between life and death. Recognition and stabilization of intraoperative fractures can ensure an excellent outcome and avoid the need for further surgery. Proper preparation and precaution can help to prevent PJI. Precise technique can avoid an unstable THA.

REFERENCES

1. Aleto T, Ritter MA, Berend ME. Case report: superficial femoral artery injury resulting from cerclage wiring during revision THA. Clin Orthop Relat Res 2008;466(3):749–753.
2. Ali Khan MA, Brakenbury PH, Reynolds IS. Dislocation following total hip replacement. J Bone Joint Surg Br 1981;63(2):214–218.
3. Barrack RL. Neurovascular injury: avoiding catastrophe. J Arthroplasty 2004;19(4 suppl 1):104–107.
4. Berend KR, Lombardi AV Jr, Mallory TH, et al. Cerclage wires or cables for the management of intraoperative fracture associated with a cementless, tapered femoral prosthesis: results at 2 to 16 years. J Arthroplasty 2004;19(7 suppl 2):17–21.
5. Berry DJ, Lewallen DG, Hanssen AD, et al. Pelvic discontinuity in revision total hip arthroplasty. J Bone Joint Surg Am 1999;81(12): 1692–1702.
6. Bozic KJ, Kurtz SM, Lau E, et al. The epidemiology of revision total hip arthroplasty in the United States. J Bone Joint Surg Am 2009;91:128–133.
7. Butt AJ, McCarthy T, Kelly IP, et al. Sciatic nerve palsy secondary to postoperative haematoma in primary total hip replacement. J Bone Joint Surg Br 2005;87(11):1465–1467.
8. Calligaro KD, Dougherty MJ, Ryan S, et al. Acute arterial complications associated with total hip and knee arthroplasty. J Vasc Surg 2003;38:1170–1177.
9. Curtis MJ, Jinnah RH, Wilson VD, et al. The initial stability of uncemented acetabular components. J Bone Joint Surg Br 1992;74(3): 372–376.
10. Davidson D, Pike J, Garbuz D, et al. Intraoperative periprosthetic fractures during total hip arthroplasty. Evaluation and management. J Bone Joint Surg Am 2008;90:2000–2012.
11. Davis ET, Gallie PA, James SL, et al. Proximity of the femoral neurovascular bundle during hip resurfacing. J Arthroplasty 2010;25(3): 471–474.
12. Dehart MM, Riley LH Jr. Nerve injuries in total hip arthroplasty. J Am Acad Orthop Surg 1999;7:101–107.
13. Edwards BN, Tullos HS, Noble PC. Contributory factors and etiology of sciatic nerve palsy in total hip arthroplasty. Clin Orthop Relat Res 1987;(218):136–141.
14. Eftekhar NS. Dislocation and instability complicating low friction arthroplasty of the hip joint. Clin Orthop Relat Res 1976;(121):120–125.
15. Ekelund A, Rydell N, Nilsson OS. Total hip arthroplasty in patients 80 years and older. Clin Orthop Relat Res 1992;(281):101–106.
16. Feugier P, Fessy MH, Carret JP, et al. Total hip arthroplasty. Risk factors and prevention of iatrogenic complications [in French]. Ann Chir 1999;53:127–135.
17. Goulding K, Beaulé PE, Kim PR, et al. Incidence of lateral femoral cutaneous nerve neurapraxia after anterior approach hip arthroplasty. Clin Orthop Relat Res 2010;468:2397–2404.
18. Graf R, Azizbaig-Mohajer M. Minimally invasive total hip replacement with the patient in the supine position and the contralateral leg elevated. Oper Orthop Traumatol 2006;18:317–329.
19. Graw BP, Woolson ST, Huddleston HG, et al. Minimal incision surgery as a risk factor for early failure of total hip arthroplasty. Clin Orthop Relat Res 2010;468(9):2372–2376.
20. Johanson NA, Pellicci PM, Tsairis P, et al. Nerve injury in total hip arthroplasty. Clin Orthop Relat Res 1983;(179):214–222.
21. Kavanagh BF, Fitzgerald RH Jr. Multiple revisions for failed total hip arthroplasty not associated with infection. J Bone Joint Surg Am 1987;69(8):1144–1149.
22. Kennedy WF, Byrne TF, Majid HA, et al. Sciatic nerve monitoring during revision total hip arthroplasty. Clin Orthop Relat Res 1991;264:223–227.
23. Krushell RJ, Burke DW, Harris WH. Range of motion in contemporary total hip arthroplasty. The impact of modular head-neck components. J Arthroplasty 1991;6(2):97–101.
24. Lewallen DG. Neurovascular injury associated with hip arthroplasty. Instr Course Lect 1998;47:275–283.
25. Lewinnek GE, Lewis JL, Tarr R, et al. Dislocations after total hip replacement arthroplasties. J Bone Joint Surg Am 1978;60(2):217–220.
26. Lindahl H. Epidemiology of periprosthetic femur fracture around a total hip arthroplasty. Injury 2007;38:651–654.
27. Mahadevan D, Challand C, Keenan J. Cement extrusion during hip arthroplasty causing pain and obturator nerve impingement. J Arthroplasty 2009;24(1):158.
28. Mallory TH. Sciatic nerve entrapment secondary to trochanteric wiring following total hip arthroplasty. A case report. Clin Orthop Relat Res 1983;(180):198–200.
29. Masri BA, Meek RM, Duncan CP. Periprosthetic fractures evaluation and treatment. Clin Orthop Relat Res 2004;(420):80–95.
30. Mayle RE, Della Valle CJ. Intra-operative fractures during THA: see it before it sees us. J Bone Joint Surg Br 2012;94(11 suppl A):26–31.
31. Meek RM, Garbuz DS, Masri BA, et al. Intraoperative fracture of the femur in revision total hip arthroplasty with a diaphyseal fitting stem. J Bone Joint Surg Am 2004;86(3):480–485.
32. Morrey BF. Instability after total hip arthroplasty. Orthop Clin North Am 1992;23(2):237–248.
33. Nachbur B, Meyer RP, Verkkala K, et al. The mechanisms of severe arterial injury in surgery of the hip joint. Clin Orthop Relat Res 1979;141:122–133.
34. Parvizi J, Gehrke T, et al. Proceedings of the International Consensus Meeting on Periprosthetic Joint Infection. Brooklandville, MD: Data Trace Publishing, 2013:1–140.
35. Parvizi J, Pulido L, Slenker N, et al. Vascular injuries after total joint arthroplasty. J Arthroplasty 2008;23(8):1115–1121.
36. Parvizi J, Sharkey PF, Bissett GA, et al. Surgical treatment of limb-length discrepancy following total hip arthroplasty. J Bone Joint Surg Am 2003;85(12):2310–2317.
37. Peak EL, Parvizi J, Ciminiello M, et al. The role of patient restriction in reducing the prevalence of early dislocation following total hip arthroplasty. A randomized, prospective study. J Bone Joint Surg Am 2005;87(2):247–253.
38. Pekkarinen J, Alho A, Puusa A, et al. Recovery of sciatic nerve injuries in association with total hip arthroplasty in 27 patients. J Arthroplasty 1999;14(3):305–311.
39. Peterson CA, Lewallen DG. Periprosthetic fracture of the acetabulum after total hip arthroplasty. J Bone Joint Surg Am 1996;78(8): 1206–1213.
40. Philippot R, Adam P, Reckhaus M, et al. Prevention of dislocation in total hip revision surgery using a dual mobility design. Orthop Traumatol Surg Res 2009;95(6):407–413.
41. Porter SS, Black DL, Reckling FW, et al. Intraoperative cortical somatosensory evoked potentials for detection of sciatic neuropathy during total hip arthroplasty. J Clin Anesth 1989;1:170–173.
42. Sakai R, Kikuchi A, Morita T, et al. Hammering sound frequency analysis and prevention of intraoperative periprosthetic fractures during total hip arthroplasty. Hip Int 2011;21(6):718–723.

43. Satcher RL, Noss RS, Yingling CD, et al. The use of motor-evoked potentials to monitor sciatic nerve status during revision total hip arthroplasty. J Arthroplasty 2003;18:329–332.
44. Schmalzreid TP, Amstutz HC, Dorey FJ. Nerve palsy associated with total hip replacement. J Bone Joint Surg Am 1991;73:1074–1080.
45. Sharkey PF, Hozack WJ, Callaghan JJ, et al. Acetabular fractures associated with cementless acetabular component insertion: a report of 13 cases. J Arthroplasty 1999;14(4):426–431.
46. Sharma DK, Kumar N, Mishra V, et al. Vascular injuries in total hip replacement arthroplasty: a review of the problem. Am J Orthop 2003;32:487–491.
47. Sheth NP, Brown NM, Moric M, et al. Operative treatment of early peri-prosthetic femur fractures following primary total hip arthroplasty. J Arthroplasty 2013;28(2):286–291.
48. Suh KT, Park BG, Choi YJ. A posterior approach to primary total hip arthroplasty with soft tissue repair. Clin Orthop Relat Res 2004;418:162–167.
49. Wasielewski RC, Cooperstein LA, Kruger MP, et al. Acetabular anatomy and the transacetabular fixation of screws in total hip arthroplasty. J Bone Joint Surg Am 1990;72:501–508.
50. Yacoubian SV, Sah AP, Estok DM II. Incidence of sciatic nerve palsy after revision hip arthroplasty through a posterior approach. J Arthroplasty 2010;25:31–34.

Cemented Total Hip Arthroplasty

Matthew S. Hepinstall and José A. Rodriguez

19

CHAPTER

DEFINITION

- For the past 50 years, cemented total hip arthroplasty (THA) has been a highly successful surgical solution for end-stage hip disease.
- Although cementless fixation has grown in popularity and now dominates North American practice, cemented THA remains an evidence-based and appropriate treatment of hip pathology caused by a variety of degenerative, inflammatory, traumatic, vascular, developmental, and metabolic disorders.

ANATOMY

- The hip is a diarthrodial synovial joint consisting of the articulation of the femoral head with the acetabulum. It functions as a ball-and-socket joint, with inherent bony constraints that define the range of motion. The laxity or tightness of the associated soft tissue also affects kinematics and function.
- The acetabulum develops at the junction between three embryologically distinct bones—the ilium, ischium, and pubis—which fuse at the triradiate cartilage during adolescence.
- The acetabulum typically demonstrates 15 to 20 degrees of anteversion, as does the femoral neck. Normal combined anteversion is therefore 30 to 40 degrees, although the degree of anteversion varies considerably between individuals.

PATHOGENESIS

- Degenerative joint disease (DJD) is a final common pathway for various hip disorders of distinct etiologies.
  - Developmental abnormalities of the hip can lead to impingement and/or subluxation, abnormal joint reaction and articular shear forces, and consequent mechanical joint degeneration. These abnormalities include the following:
    - Developmental dysplasia
    - Coxa profunda
    - Protrusio acetabuli
    - Acetabular retroversion or pincer deformity of the acetabulum
    - Pistol grip or cam deformity of the proximal femur
    - Legg-Calvé-Perthes disease
    - Slipped capital femoral epiphysis
  - Posttraumatic arthritis can develop after fractures of the femoral head, femoral neck, or acetabulum.
  - Osteoarthritis may also be idiopathic.
- Rheumatologic conditions such as rheumatoid arthritis and the seronegative spondyloarthropathies are caused by autoimmunity.
- Osteonecrosis of the femoral head can result from many etiologic factors:
  - Alcoholism
  - Corticosteroid use
  - Chemotherapy
  - Sickle cell disease
  - Systemic lupus erythematosus
  - Vasculitis
  - HIV infection
  - Coagulopathy
- Osteonecrosis may also be idiopathic.
- Less commonly, metabolic disorders such as hemochromatosis and ochronosis, as well as hematologic abnormalities such as hemophilia and sickle cell disease, can cause advanced degeneration of the hip, as can rare congenital disorders, including epiphyseal and spondyloepiphyseal dysplasias.

NATURAL HISTORY

- The natural history of DJD is progression of disease. Although clinical symptoms may wax and wane, they generally become more severe, frequent, and debilitating over time.
  - Although medications can help control the progression of rheumatoid arthritis and other inflammatory conditions, no medical therapies currently have been proven to act as disease-modifying agents in DJD.
- When osteoarthritis is a consequence of anatomic abnormalities, there is hope that surgical correction of these abnormalities may unload the joint, halt progression of the disease, and even allow for biologic repair.
  - Periacetabular osteotomy may positively impact the natural history of joint degeneration in acetabular dysplasia,[25] but the long-term effect of osteotomy on hip function and progression of arthrosis is unknown. In the presence of moderate DJD, progression of the disease commonly occurs in spite of a well-performed osteotomy.
  - Similarly, osteochondroplasty of the femoral neck and acetabular rim may relieve symptoms associated with femoroacetabular impingement, but it is not known whether these procedures will reduce the progression of arthrosis.

PATIENT HISTORY AND PHYSICAL FINDINGS

- Initial evaluation should focus on identifying the extent to which hip pain can be attributed to intra-articular hip pathology. Hip pain may be localized to the groin, peritrochanteric region, thigh, knee, or, occasionally, below the knee. Lumbar spine disease may also cause pain in these regions.
  - Although the source of the pain can usually be identified on the basis of physical examination, occasionally, selective anesthetic injection is helpful to elucidate the relative

contributions of overlapping pathologies to a patient's symptoms.
- Palpation is performed to assess for areas of tenderness, warmth, fluctuance, or mass.
  - Trochanteric bursitis is a common cause of hip area pain that can be ruled out by identifying a nontender bursa.
  - An inguinal mass may suggest that groin pain is related to a hernia.
- Active and passive range of motion should be assessed.
  - Flexion contracture commonly is encountered, as are limited internal rotation and abduction.
  - Limited external rotation, if present, impairs activities of daily living.
- Motor power of the abductors, adductors, flexors, and extensors is assessed and documented using a 5-point scale.
  - Abductor weakness diminishes the likelihood of achieving a limp-free hip after arthroplasty.
- Gait should be assessed with the patient's legs exposed and with and without use of walking aids.
  - Trendelenburg gait suggests abductor weakness or hip discomfort.
  - Coxalgic gait suggests hip pain of any etiology.
  - Stiff hip gait may be present with hypertrophic osteoarthritis.
  - Short limb gait may be present with developmental dysplasia of the hip.
- Legs should be observed for leg length discrepancy (LLD). Some shortening is usually present in DJD. Severe shortening may be present in developmental dysplasia of the hip. Adduction contracture may cause apparent shortening, whereas abduction contracture may cause apparent lengthening. Pelvic tilt from spinal deformity may contribute to functional LLD. Pelvic tilt should be assessed in the standing and seated positions to determine whether it arises from LLD or spinal deformity.
- Examination of the spine should include inspection for deformity, palpation for tenderness, evaluation for pain with passive straight-leg raise, and a neurologic examination.
- Examination of distal pulses and capillary refill may reveal peripheral vascular disease that could be associated with vascular claudication.
- Tests of the hip include the following:
  - *Thomas test:* Inability to maintain extension of the ipsilateral hip reveals flexion contracture.
  - *Patrick test:* Discomfort with flexion, abduction, and external rotation of the hip suggests intra-articular hip pathology; however, this test may also provoke sacroiliac pain.
  - *Ober test:* Persistent abduction of the hip reveals tightness of the iliotibial band. This finding is important to note preoperatively so that it is not misinterpreted intraoperatively as overlengthening.
  - *Impingement test:* Hip pain with passive flexion, adduction, and internal rotation suggests intra-articular pathology but is not specific for femoroacetabular impingement.
  - *Stinchfield test:* Hip pain with resisted straight-leg raise suggests intra-articular pathology, typically affecting the central joint rather than the labrum.
  - *Passive straight-leg raise:* Radicular pain suggests lumbar pathology.
- Once pain has been localized to the hip, an assessment of pain, limp, extent of disability, and desired level of activity is warranted. This information allows the practitioner to give the patient a realistic assessment of the potential benefits of various therapeutic modalities.
- Skin over the affected hip should be assessed for mobility and the presence and location of scars from any prior surgical procedures, which may influence surgical approach.

IMAGING AND OTHER DIAGNOSTIC STUDIES

- Plain radiographs should be obtained, weight bearing if possible.
  - Low anteroposterior (AP) view of the pelvis centered over the pubic symphysis and including the proximal third of the femora. Slight internal rotation of the hips allows accurate assessment of the neck–shaft angle. The coccyx should be pointing directly to the symphysis pubis and located about 3 cm above the symphysis pubis if pelvic rotation is neutral.
  - AP and false-profile views of the involved hip
  - AP and lateral lumbar spine
  - Computed tomography, magnetic resonance imaging, and other supplemental studies are indicated if the cause of pain is not evident on plain radiographs.

DIFFERENTIAL DIAGNOSIS

- Lumbar spine pathology
  - Spinal stenosis and neurogenic claudication
  - Herniated nucleus pulposus
  - Degenerative disc disease or spondylitis
- Sacroiliac joint pathology
- Trochanteric bursitis
- Tendinopathy of the gluteus medius or minimus
- Iliopsoas bursitis
- Inguinal hernia
- Vascular claudication
- Femoroacetabular impingement without advanced arthritis

NONOPERATIVE MANAGEMENT

- Nonoperative options include weight loss, activity modification, physical therapy, injections, pain management, and the use of walking aids. These interventions do not alter the underlying disease process, but they may substantially diminish pain and disability.

SURGICAL MANAGEMENT

- Cemented THA has been a highly successful operation. Significant early complications are uncommon, and patient outcomes are outstanding in the short and intermediate term. Long-term outcomes beyond 10 to 15 years are limited by component wear, fixation failure, and biologic reaction to wear debris.
- In most reported series,[1,5–8,17] fixation has been the limiting factor for the survival of hip implants in patients with long life expectancies.
- The durability of cement fixation is highly dependent on meticulous surgical technique. Bone cement is vulnerable to failure under tension and shear, which can be caused by gaps in the cement mantle. Stress risers increase the risk of cement fracture.

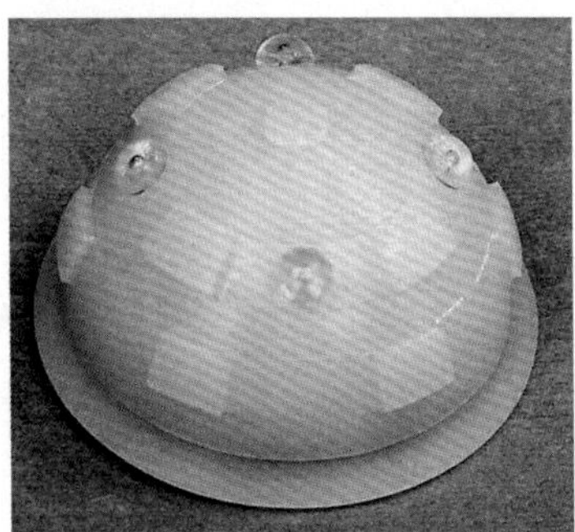

FIG 1 • Polyethylene acetabular components are the accepted standard for cemented acetabular fixation.

- Improvements in cement technique have resulted in a reduction in the rates of aseptic loosening of femoral components.[13,17]
- Acetabular cement fixation remains challenging for many surgeons, with variable results over the long term.[3,6,7,9,22] Appearance of the bone–cement interface on the immediate postoperative radiograph predicts the durability of cemented acetabular fixation.[22]
  - Surgeons who consistently achieve good cement technique can expect reproducible long-term results.

Preoperative Planning

Indications

- Reproducible, durable, long-term outcomes using cement fixation have been achieved in older, lighter weight patients, particularly women, with low to moderate activity levels and relatively normal anatomy of the pelvis and proximal femur. If THA is indicated for such a patient, cement fixation remains an excellent option for both components.
- When distorted femoral anatomy interferes with the use of standard press-fit prostheses, cement fixation may be the best and simplest option.
- Cement fixation may also be the best option in pathologic bone associated with tumor or radiation or in any other situation in which bone in- or ongrowth cannot be anticipated.
- Cement fixation of the femoral component increases the quantity of fat and marrow embolization that occurs with THA. We therefore prefer to avoid cement fixation in patients with significant cardiopulmonary disease.

Implant Selection

- Choice of prosthesis should be based on critical review of the published outcomes and the surgeon's familiarity with the implant. This includes design features and rationale, instrumentation, and potential technical pitfalls.
- It is generally agreed that the optimal cemented acetabular component is all polyethylene (**FIG 1**), with multiple pegs to ensure concentric insertion within a cement mantle of appropriate thickness and a peripheral flange to optimize pressurization of cement during component insertion. Recent data challenge the value of polyethylene pegs, demonstrating an association with radiographic evidence of loosening.[11]
- On the femoral side, there has been debate whether the optimal prosthesis is roughened to allow interdigitation of cement and rigid fixation at the cement–prosthesis interface or polished and tapered to allow slight subsidence into a stable position without generating wear particles.
  - Both design philosophies have resulted in good to excellent long-term results when properly employed.[13,17]
  - Conversely, simply roughening the surface of a successful smooth stem has led to a surprising number of early failures of fixation.[13]
  - Polished and tapered femoral stems have emerged as the most commonly used cemented stems worldwide.

Templating

- Once the implant system has been chosen, templates can be compared to patient radiographs to predict implant size and determine the implant placement that will best reconstruct the patient's center of rotation, offset, and leg length.
- A horizontal reference line is drawn between the inferior tips of the acetabular teardrops (**FIG 2A**). Both lesser trochanters are marked at their medial points (the medial tip of the lesser trochanter is the most reproducible landmark on the proximal femur radiographically). The perpendicular distance between the interteardrop line and the medial point of the

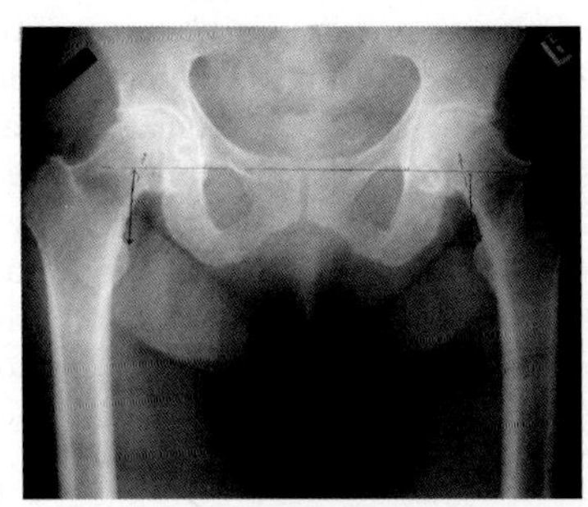

A

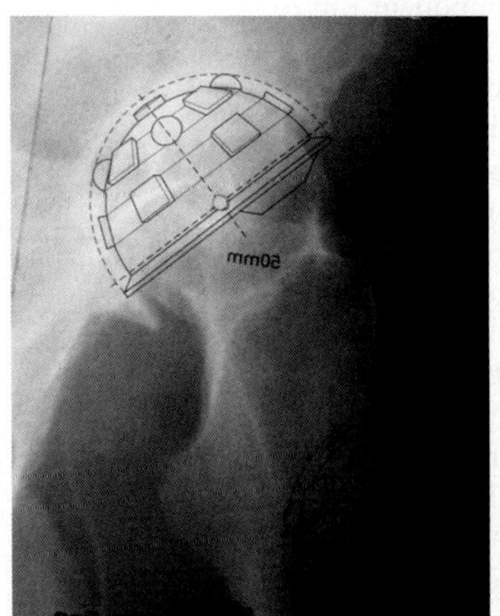

B

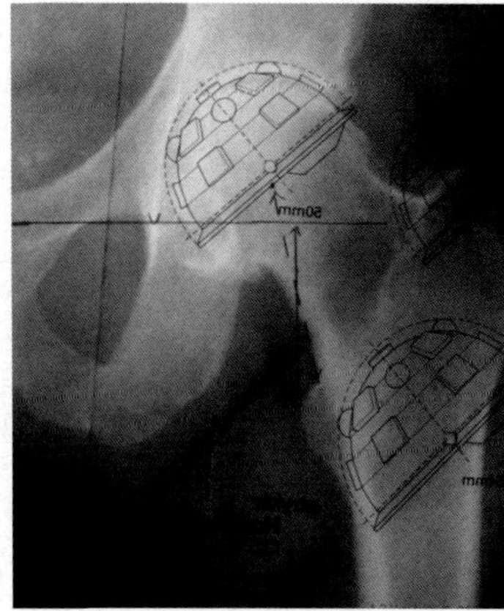

C

FIG 2 • Templating. **A.** The LLD and LTC are measured on the low AP pelvis radiograph. **B.** The false-profile view of Lequesne provides a lateral view of the proximal femur and an oblique view of the pelvis. It is the most reliable view for templating acetabular size. **C.** The selected acetabular template is positioned on the AP radiograph. *(continued)*

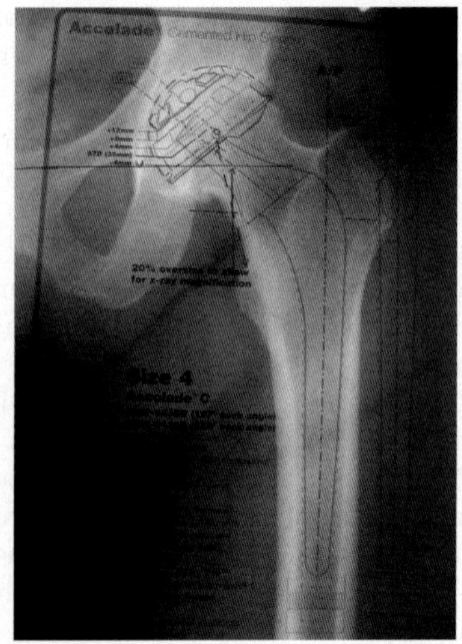

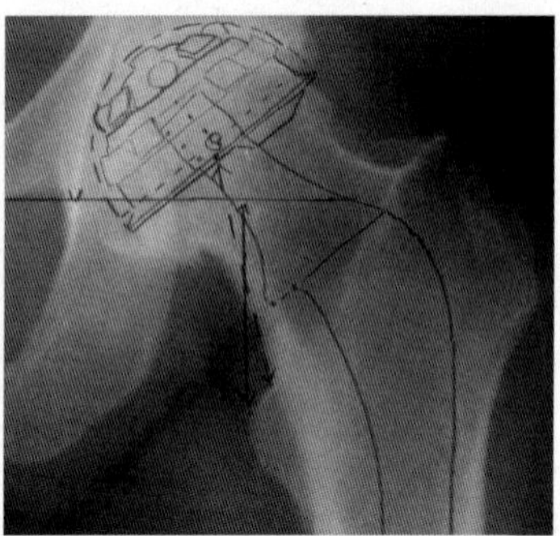

FIG 2 • *(continued)* **D.** Femoral component templating to restore leg length and offset. **E.** The vertical distance between the center of the acetabular component and the center of the prosthetic head represents the anticipated change in leg length—we seek an increase in leg length of 2 to 5 mm in most cases.

lesser trochanter is measured for each hip (represented by the solid vertical lines in **FIG 2A**).

- The LLD is calculated by subtracting the value measured for the nonoperative hip from the value obtained for the operative hip.

- The centers of the femoral heads are marked. These are the preoperative centers of rotation of the hip joints. A mark is also placed on the superior aspect of the lesser trochanter on the operative hip (this can be identified intraoperatively). The distance between the superior aspect of the lesser trochanter and the center of the femoral head (LTC) (represented by the dashed lines in **FIG 2A**) is measured and recorded for each hip.
- Selection of the appropriate acetabular component requires a measurement of the acetabular size. Cemented socket templating accounts for a 2-mm cement mantle in approximating the reamed hemispherical cavity. Implant size is estimated most accurately on the false-profile radiograph (**FIG 2B**).
- The acetabular template is positioned on the AP radiograph in 40 to 45 degrees of abduction,[18,25] with its inferomedial border placed approximately 10 mm lateral to the teardrop (**FIG 2C**). The prosthesis should remain at or lateral to the medial floor of the acetabulum, and the superolateral corner of the component should fall near the superolateral border of the acetabulum.
  - Incomplete coverage of the acetabular component (up to 20%) may be acceptable.
- Once the desired position of the acetabular component is selected, the new center of rotation of the hip is determined using the template. In most cases, the goal is to recreate the normal anatomic center of rotation. Changing the center of rotation up to 10 mm may be acceptable to optimize bone stock for component fixation. Such a change may be necessary in cases of dysplasia with a high hip center.
- Attention then is turned to templating the femoral component. The goal is to choose an implant that permits an adequate cement mantle without excessive removal of cancellous bone and restores anatomic leg length and offset.
- The template is placed in neutral position in the femoral canal. Its proximal–distal position should be selected on the basis of the bony constraints, the desire for a circumferential 2-mm cement mantle, and the goal of restoring leg length (**FIG 2D**).
  - Most implant systems are available with standard or enhanced offset necks; the implant that optimizes the patient's offset in relation to the new center of rotation of the socket is chosen.
  - Modular femoral heads with the option of plus and minus sizes allow the surgeon to lengthen or shorten the femoral neck, affecting both leg length and offset.
- Once the optimal component position is selected, the level of the femoral neck osteotomy is marked, and the distance from the lesser trochanter is recorded.
- After marking socket and femoral component positions on the radiograph, the vertical distance between the center of the acetabular component and the center of the femoral head will approximate the leg length correction (**FIG 2E**).
  - The goals of leg length equality and optimal stability should be balanced. In most cases, optimal stability can be achieved with 0 to 5 mm of lengthening compared to the prearthritic state.[23]

Positioning

- Positioning of the patient depends on the choice of surgical exposure.
- For the posterolateral approach to the hip, we use the lateral decubitus position with the pelvis secured to prevent rotation.
  - An axillary roll is used to prevent injury to the brachial plexus, and all bony prominences are carefully padded to avoid pressure-related complications.
  - Many surgeons attempt to establish a fixed relationship between the pelvis and the floor to allow positioning of the acetabular component in reference to the plane of the floor. The use of internal landmarks is more reproducible and permits the surgeon more freedom in positioning.
  - We tilt the table toward the surgeon during acetabular preparation and component insertion, optimizing visualization. A backrest is used to stabilize the patient during this maneuver.
- For the direct anterior approach to the hip, we place the patient in the supine position on a radiolucent table with a table attachment used to facilitate femoral elevation. Custom traction tables and table attachments are also available but increase reliance on nonsterile personnel.

Approach

- Multiple surgical approaches can adequately expose the hip joint for THA.

- The posterolateral approach is desirable for its excellent extensile exposure and avoidance of trauma to the abductor mechanism. With modern techniques of posterior soft tissue repair and implant positioning that restore the center of rotation, offset, leg length, and combined anteversion,[2] dislocation rates are comparable to those observed with other approaches.[21]
- The direct anterior approach is gaining popularity for its preservation of the gluteus maximus and minimal disruption of the short external rotators as well as improved ability to use intraoperative fluoroscopy and directly assess LLD. There is an associated rate of lateral femoral cutaneous nerve injury. We have used this approach successfully for cementless and cemented femoral applications but have not routinely cemented the acetabulum with this approach.
- Anterolateral, direct lateral Hardinge, and transtrochanteric approaches have all been used with success for the performance of THA. As each of these approaches can compromise the abductor attachment, they have not been used routinely in our practice.

TECHNIQUES

Exposure (Posterior Approach)

- A gently curved skin incision is made starting posterior and slightly proximal to the tip of the greater trochanter, passing about 1 cm posterior to the most prominent point of the greater trochanter on the lateral aspect of the femur and distally along the shaft of the femur to approximately the level of the gluteus maximus insertion.
- The iliotibial band is incised slightly anterior to the line of the skin incision so that the fascial incision extends distally from the most prominent point of the trochanter and remains 5 to 10 mm anterior to the insertion of the gluteus maximus tendon into the proximal femur.
- The proximal portion of the fascial incision is performed in line with the fibers of the underlying gluteus maximus. The muscle fibers of the gluteus maximus are split bluntly.
- Partial or complete release of the gluteus maximus insertion into the linea aspera can be performed at this time. This is seldom necessary for exposure but may reduce the small risk of postoperative sciatic nerve palsy.[15]
- The hip is internally rotated and release of the quadratus femoris off the posterior femur is performed with the electrocautery. This step is complete when the lesser trochanter is exposed.
  - The first perforator off the profunda femoris artery is often encountered during this step. This vessel is easily cauterized before it is transected, but hemostasis can be more difficult if it is transected before it is recognized.
  - Leaving a small cuff of quadratus and attached to the femur laterally facilitates repair, but medial dissection is best carried out close to bone so as to minimize bleeding.
- The gluteus medius is retracted anteriorly and proximally so the superior border of the piriformis tendon is clearly visualized.
- The piriformis tendon, the conjoint tendon of the obturator internus and gemelli, the obturator externus tendon, and the posterior capsule are released as a single flap from the greater trochanter and the lateral portion of the femoral neck.
- Superior and inferior capsulotomies create a quadrangular flap of capsule, tendon, and muscle for repair at the end of the case.
  - The superior capsulotomy is performed along the inferior edge of the gluteus minimus.
  - The inferior capsulotomy is performed at approximately the 7:30 position for a right hip, separating the posterior capsule from the inferior capsule. The obturator externus muscle is adjacent to the capsule but is not visible until the lateral portion of the inferior capsulotomy is performed. After initiating the inferior capsulotomy, a retractor placed between the capsule and the underlying obturator externus will protect the muscle and minimize bleeding associated with the capsulotomy.

Intraoperative Assessment of Leg Length

- Prior to dislocation of the hip, a Steinmann pin is placed into the obturator foramen at the level of the infracotyloid groove.[23] This landmark can be reproducibly identified by passing the pin just distal to the ischium at the level of the acetabulum.
  - The surgeon should experience a pop as the pin pierces the obturator membrane; the pin should be inserted no further.
- The femur is placed in a neutral and reproducible position on the operating table and the position of the vertical Steinmann pin is marked on the femur using the electrocautery and a marking pen (**TECH FIG 1**).
  - The Steinmann pin can be replaced later in the case and the mark on the femur provides a reference for assessment of change in leg length.

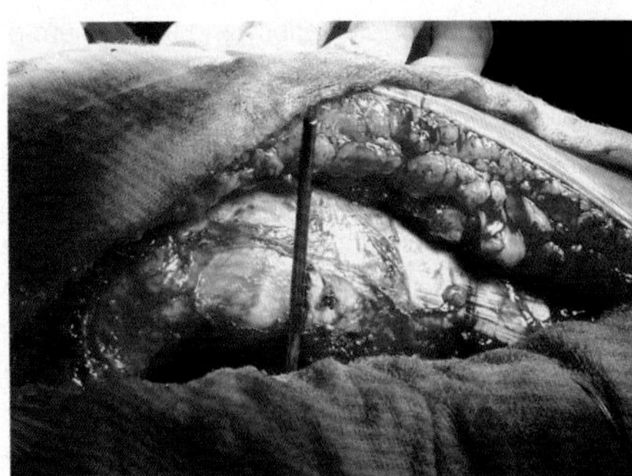

TECH FIG 1 • A Steinmann pin placed in the obturator foramen at the level of the infracotyloid groove provides a fixed pelvic reference point for assessment of changes in leg length.

Dislocation of Hip and Osteotomy of Femoral Neck

- The hip is dislocated posteriorly using gentle flexion, adduction, and internal rotation.
- The center of the femoral head is then estimated and marked, and the LTC is measured and recorded (**TECH FIG 2**).
  - Reconstruction of the anatomic geometry of the hip, including leg length and offset, is aided by approximate reproduction of this distance.
  - A slight (<5 mm) increase in the LTC can optimize hip stability without excessive lengthening of the leg or stretching the iliotibial band.
- The femoral neck osteotomy is performed at the templated level, aiming at the junction of the femoral neck with the greater trochanter.
  - The femoral neck can be left a few millimeters longer than templated, allowing for measurement error. Additional bone can easily be removed during femoral preparation using the sagittal saw or the calcar planar.

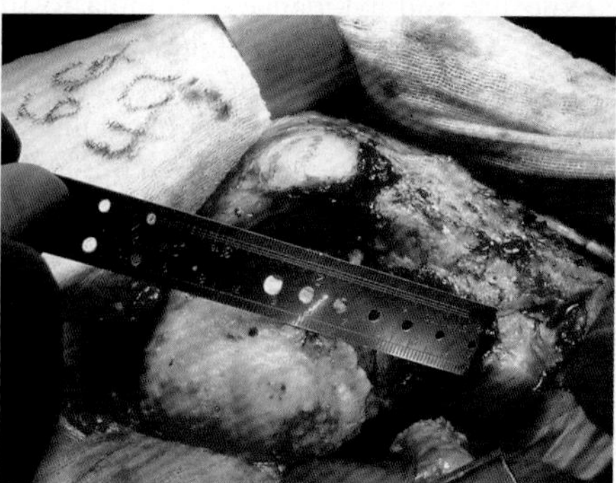

TECH FIG 2 • The LTC is measured intraoperatively prior to osteotomy of the femoral neck.

Acetabular Exposure

- Wide exposure of the acetabulum is achieved by translating the femur anteriorly.
  - This typically requires release of the superior capsule, which should be divided at its acetabular insertion with care to avoid trauma to the overlying gluteus minimus.
  - In stiff hips, further mobility can be achieved by releasing the reflected head of the rectus femoris muscle, which becomes evident after the anterior portion of the superior capsular release is performed.
  - Release of the tendinous insertion of the gluteus maximus into the linea aspera allows further anterior translation, if necessary.
- The labrum should be resected, but the transverse acetabular ligament should be preserved to provide a landmark for the placement of the inferior portion of the acetabular component and a restraint to the extrusion of cement inferiorly during cement pressurization and component insertion.
- The pulvinar should be removed from the fovea using electrocautery to allow visualization of the medial wall of the acetabulum.

Acetabular Preparation

- A slightly undersized reamer is used initially to ensure appropriate medialization without penetrating the medial wall, followed by sequential concentric reaming until the blush of cancellous bone is seen in the pubis anteriorly and the ischium posteriorly.
  - Historically, the first reamer chosen was several sizes smaller than the templated size.
  - Starting with a reamer the size of the removed femoral head saves time and minimizes eccentric reaming.
- Most of the strong subchondral bone of the ilium in the superior aspect of the acetabulum is typically preserved to provide support for the prosthesis. However, sclerotic bone must be penetrated sufficiently to permit cement interdigitation using multiple holes with a high-speed burr.
  - A randomized controlled clinical trial demonstrated the significantly improved radiographic appearance of the cement mantle with careful removal of most of the subchondral bone to allow cement interdigitation into cancellous bone of the roof of the acetabulum.[12]
- The appropriate position for the acetabular component is selected using a trial prosthesis. Insertion of the trial component should be easy and free of bone or soft tissue obstruction to allow for unencumbered insertion of the actual component. If the margins of the acetabular cavity remain tight, it can be reamed an additional 1 mm at the periphery.
  - Internal landmarks used for positioning the acetabular cup include the anterior wall and pubic ramus, posterior wall, transverse acetabular ligament, and superior acetabular rim.
  - With normal acetabular morphology, positioning the prosthesis just within the confines of the acetabulum with a small amount of implant exposed posterosuperiorly and the inferior aspect tucked inside and parallel to the transverse acetabular ligament ensures appropriate component abduction of 40 to 45 degrees and anteversion of 10 to 20 degrees.
  - In cases with large anterior osteophytes or preoperative acetabular retroversion as noted by a positive crossover sign, the posterior wall and the transverse acetabular ligament are used preferentially to gauge proper anteversion. Anterior osteophytes should be debulked using a burr or an osteotome; this reduces the risk of anterior bony impingement with hip flexion and internal rotation.

- Once the appropriate component position is selected using the trial, it can be marked on the bone using methylene blue, and the relationship of the component to the aforementioned landmarks can be noted visually to assist in placement of the final component (**TECH FIG 3A**).
- A high-speed burr is then used to create holes in the pubis, ischium, and ilium for cement intrusion and "macrolock" to complement the "microlock" achieved by interdigitation in bony trabeculae of cancellous bone.
- If acetabular cysts are present, these are débrided and the sclerotic margins are removed using the burr.
- A dry operative field free of debris is necessary for maximal cement interdigitation into cancellous bone (**TECH FIG 3B**).
  - This is achieved by the use of hypotensive regional anesthesia with arterial pressure in the range of 45 to 70 mm Hg and pulse irrigation to remove fat and blood followed by drying with a sponge, with or without local use of epinephrine.
  - Although it is not our practice, others have demonstrated improved cement intrusion when suction aspiration of the ilium was performed at the time of cementing to help maintain a dry bone surface.[14]

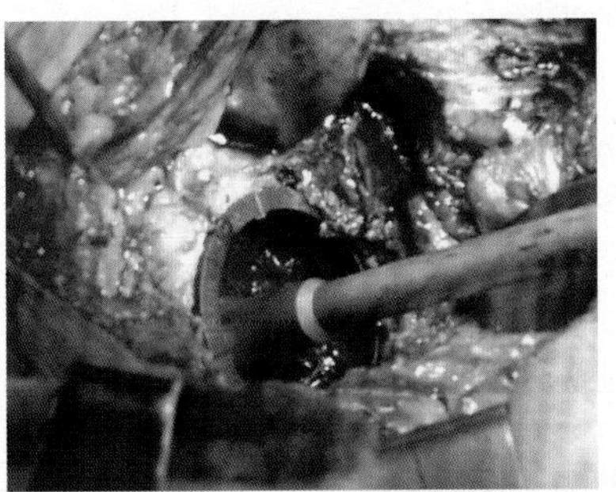

A

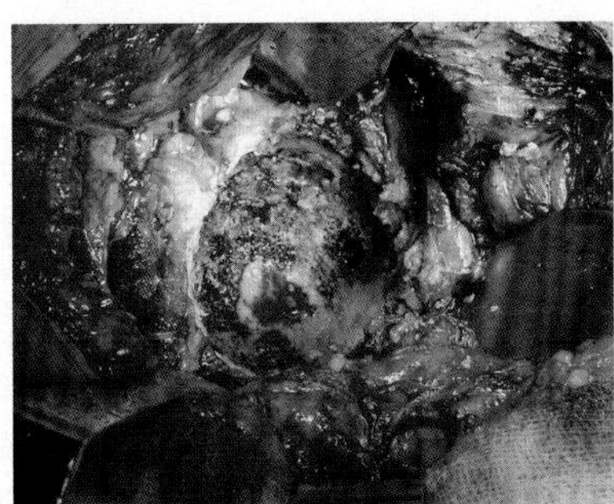

B

TECH FIG 3 • Acetabular preparation. **A.** Once the optimal position of the acetabular trial has been achieved, the position should be marked on the surrounding bone. **B.** A dry surgical field after preparation of the acetabulum is essential for optimal cement interdigitation. This is best achieved with the use of hypotensive anesthetic techniques.

Cementing the Acetabular Component

- Cement should be doughy but still relatively low in viscosity when it is placed in the acetabulum. Uniform simultaneous cement pressurization is then achieved using a rubber balloon that is pressed into the acetabulum (**TECH FIG 4A**).
- After pressurization has been maintained for 30 to 60 seconds, the balloon is removed, and the transverse acetabular ligament is cleared of cement (**TECH FIG 4B**). This minimizes intrapelvic extrusion and allows visualization of the floor of the acetabulum to guide placement of the acetabular component.
- The acetabular component is then inserted, with care to match the abduction and anteversion selected at the time the trial prosthesis was inserted. The component should have an outer diameter 2 mm smaller than that of the final reamer, allowing for an adequate cement mantle.
- Extra cement is removed while pressure is maintained on the acetabular component using a Charnley pusher centrally to minimize angular forces on the cement mantle until the cement has hardened.

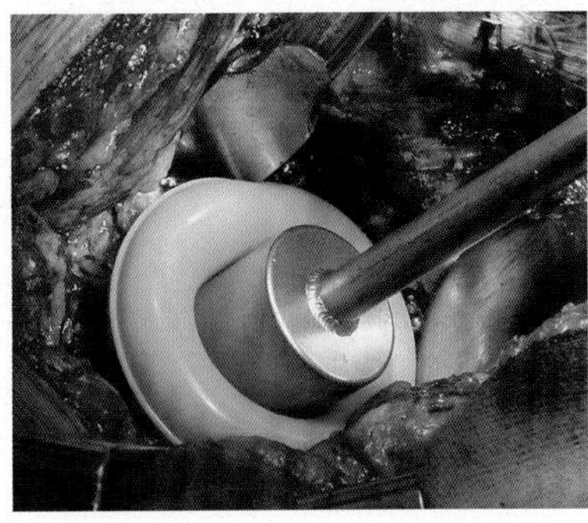

A

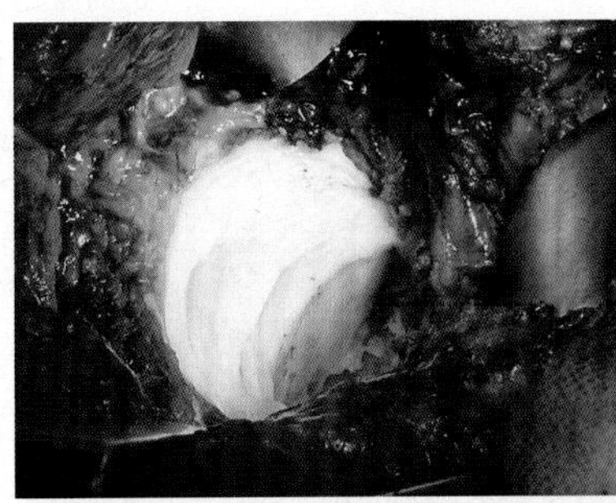

B

TECH FIG 4 • Cementing the acetabular component. **A.** Pressurization of acetabular cement is maintained for 30 to 60 seconds. **B.** Cement is removed from the region of the transverse acetabular ligament to minimize intrapelvic extrusion.

Femoral Preparation

- Exposure requires proper delivery of the proximal femur out of the wound by flexion, adduction, and internal rotation. Difficulty achieving this position can be remedied by release of the gluteus maximus tendon.
- The starting point for entry into the femoral canal is in the posterolateral femoral neck. This allows cylindrical reamers and straight broaches to be inserted along the anatomic axis of the proximal femoral diaphysis while maintaining a uniform cement mantle despite the proximal femoral bow.
  - To achieve the appropriate starting point, all residual soft tissue must be removed from the posterolateral femoral neck and remaining bone must be removed using a high-speed burr or other tool.

- Many surgeons successfully use a box osteotome to achieve this goal, although it does not have the precision of the burr (**TECH FIG 5**).
- Once the starting point has been prepared, a conical canal-finding reamer is introduced to aid in the identification of the anatomic axis of the femur. The entry point into the femur is opened, while reaming of the diaphyseal endosteum is minimized. Broach preparation of the canal without extensive reaming preserves cancellous bone to permit optimal cement interdigitation.
  - Sequential broaching is then performed, with care to insert the broaches in appropriate anteversion (typically 10 to 15 degrees). This is achieved by following the patient's native version, unless the patient has significant deformity of the proximal femur or the acetabular component is known to be in excessive anteversion or retroversion.
  - The degree of anteversion is best assessed visually if the assistant holds the tibia perpendicular to the plane of the floor.
- Sequential broaching is continued until torsional stability is achieved at a depth of broach insertion that brings the proximal surface of the broach into the plane of the neck cut.
  - If careful preoperative templating was performed, this should result in restoration of leg length and offset with the implant system being used. This can be confirmed following the attachment of trial necks and heads.

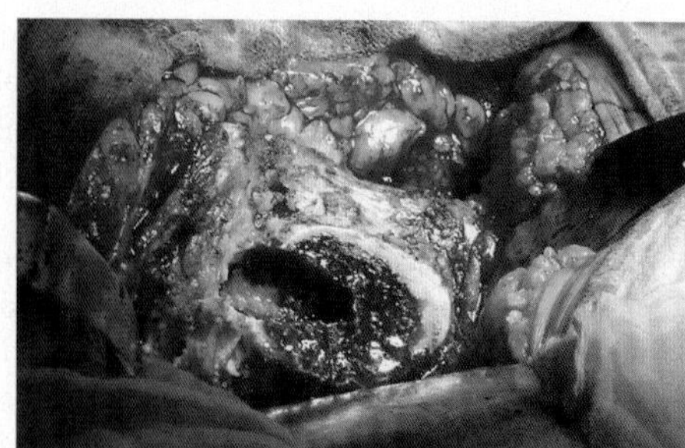

TECH FIG 5 • Residual bone of the posterolateral femoral neck must be removed to access the optimal starting point for femoral preparation and component insertion.

- Many hip systems have options for standard or extended offset necks; these can be defined by the amount of offset or by the neck–shaft angle.
  - In general, the neck that best recreates the anatomic geometry on preoperative templating should be selected.
  - However, be aware that radiographs may underestimate offset if the hip is not internally rotated to bring the femoral neck perpendicular to the x-ray beam.
- A trial femoral head is selected using the preoperative plan and attempting to recreate or minimally increase the LTC.

Assessment of the Reconstruction and Soft Tissue Balance Using Trial Components

- A trial reduction is performed and the adequacy of the reconstruction is assessed using four principal maneuvers:
  - First, the hip is internally rotated until the femoral head trial and acetabular component are coplanar (**TECH FIG 6A,B**) and the knee is bent 90 degrees.
    - If the coronal plane of the pelvis is perpendicular to the floor, the angle between the tibia and the floor is the combined anteversion of the femoral and acetabular components.[16]
    - Combined anteversion of 35 to 40 degrees is optimal in women, whereas somewhat less anteversion is desirable in men, who usually have less lumbar lordosis.
  - Second, the hip is externally rotated with the hip and knee in extension. The anterior capsule should be loose enough to allow external rotation of the femur so that the greater trochanter approaches one fingerbreadth away from the ischium but not so loose as to allow impingement of the trochanter against the ischium or of the prosthetic neck against the posterior socket.
  - Third, the Steinmann pin is replaced in the obturator foramen at the level of the infracotyloid groove and the relative lengthening or shortening of the leg is measured and noted.
    - In general, the goal is to increase the leg length sufficiently to eliminate any preoperative LLD. An additional

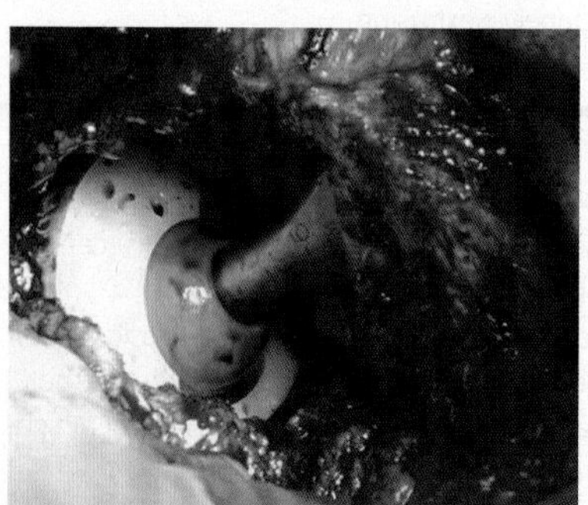

A

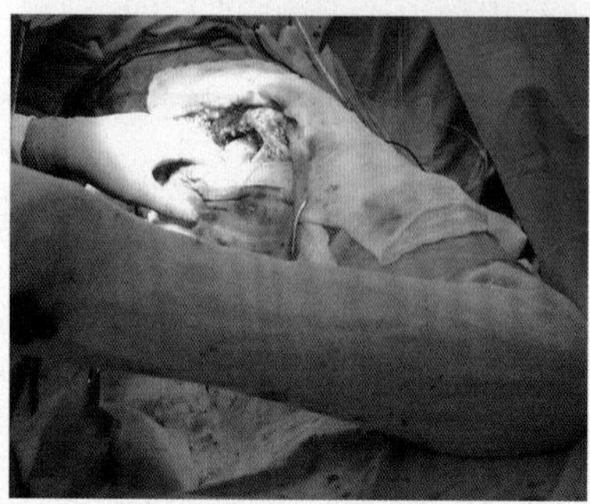

B

TECH FIG 6 • The coplanar test. **A.** The hip is internally rotated until the femoral head trial is coplanar with the rim of the acetabular component. **B.** The position of the leg then allows the surgeon to estimate combined anteversion.

2 or 3 mm of lengthening can optimize the perceived stability of the hip, but additional lengthening beyond 5 mm can generate a clinically meaningful LLD. This may vary with preoperative clinical LLD and other factors.

- Fourth, the hip is flexed and internally rotated and stability is assessed. The surgeon should feel a clear soft tissue resistance prior to dislocation rather than a smooth unimpeded motion.

- Additional information may be gained from the Ober test, in which the knee is flexed 90 degrees and the hip is extended to neutral and abducted. The knee is then released while the examiner continues to support the foot.
  - If the offset has been substantially increased, the knee will remain elevated (ie, the hip will remain abducted), indicating tightness of the iliotibial band.
  - Results of this test are meaningless unless they are compared to preoperative findings, as the iliotibial band may be tight preoperatively.
- A commonly used test that provides more limited information is the shuck or push–pull test, in which an assistant applies traction on the femur with the hip reduced but internally rotated and the surgeon subjectively assesses the extent to which the femoral head can be distracted from the acetabulum.
  - There should be some give with push–pull, but the assistant should be unable to completely dislocate the hip with simple traction.
  - Used in isolation, this test may lead the surgeon to overlengthen the leg.
- If the hip is found to be too loose, several options exist:
  - The size of the femoral stem can be increased. Larger stems may also have longer necks, depending on the implant system.
  - If leg length is appropriate but offset is insufficient, the surgeon can switch from a standard to an extended-offset stem.
  - A plus-sized modular head can be used. We recommend against use of skirted heads, but modern implant systems typically provide femoral heads of several lengths without the need for a skirt. We recommend against using the longest femoral head without a skirt. If the final reconstruction varies from the trial reconstruction, the surgeon is left without the option of further increasing leg length and offset.
- If the anterior capsule is found to be tight in a hip with an otherwise acceptable reconstruction, we advocate anterior capsulotomy to balance the hip.
- If the hip is too tight, with excessive anterior capsular tightness, a positive Ober test, and excessive lengthening, several options exist:
  - The femoral trial can be downsized or implanted deeper into the femur.
  - A minus-sized femoral head can be selected. We recommend against using the shortest femoral head. If the final reconstruction varies from the trial reconstruction, the surgeon is left without the option of further decreasing leg length and offset.

Cementing the Femoral Component

- The femoral trials are removed and the femur is prepared for cement fixation. A distal cement restrictor (**TECH FIG 7**) is placed approximately 1 cm past the anticipated depth of stem insertion.
  - This helps avoid unnecessarily long cement mantles that are difficult to remove at revision and enhances cement pressurization.
- The femoral canal is irrigated using pulse lavage, dried using suction, and packed with vaginal packing or a surgical sponge.
- Cement for the femoral side should be prepared under vacuum or using centrifugation, both of which increase cement strength by reducing cement porosity. Cement is then poured into a cement gun. The cement is ready to be injected when it has reached an intermediate viscosity low enough to be inserted with the cement gun and to easily interdigitate in cancellous bone but high enough to allow pressurization.

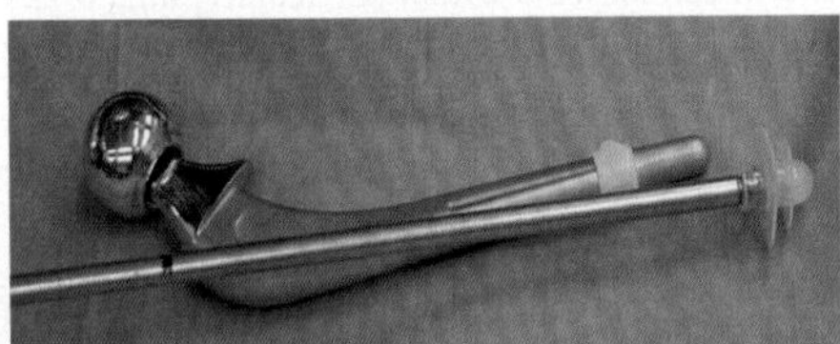

TECH FIG 7 • A cement restrictor placed distal to the tip of the stem allows for cement pressurization. The appropriate depth of insertion is marked on the insertion device.

- After ensuring that there is no air in the tip of the cement gun, cement is injected in a retrograde fashion from distal to proximal, allowing the cement to push the cement gun out of the canal.
- Once the canal is filled to the level of the neck cut, the tip is removed from the cement gun and replaced with a cement-pressurizing device that occludes the proximal femoral canal.
  - Any holes in the femoral shaft should be occluded prior to cement pressurization.
  - As pressurization is performed, cement, fat, and marrow contents should be seen extruding from small vascular foramina in the femoral neck. When the pressurizer is removed from the femur, the void should be filled with more cement.
- The surface of the cement is dried with a sponge, and cement is used to coat the femoral stem, concentrating on the metaphyseal region. These measures diminish the amount of blood, fluid, and other debris present in the cement and at the cement–prosthesis interface. Such impurities have been shown to have significant effects on cement strength.
- If the femur has a relatively wide diaphysis, addition of a distal centralizer is advised to reduce the risk of varus malpositioning of the stem.
- The stem is best inserted when the cement is in the medium dough phase. The amount of time required for the cement to reach this state varies with room temperature and rate of mixing.
  - Preheating the stem will further reduce cement porosity and accelerate cement polymerization.[18]

TECHNIQUES

- To avoid the creation of voids in the cement mantle, the stem should be inserted in one continuous smooth motion, without adjusting varus/valgus or rotational alignment. Insertion is started by hand, impacting the insertion device with a mallet as needed.
- Once the position of the trial stem has been reproduced, gentle pressure is maintained on the stem while excess cement is removed and cement around the stem is pressurized by finger.
- When the cement has polymerized, the previously selected trial head is placed on the stem, and the LTC, leg length and soft tissue balance, and combined anteversion are reassessed.
  - Once the appropriate head is selected, the trunnion of the stem is carefully cleaned and dried, and the implant is gently impacted in place.
- The acetabulum is cleared of debris using irrigation and suction, and reduction is performed.

Soft Tissue Repair and Wound Closure

- Injection of the deep soft tissues (ie, hip capsule, gluteus medius tendon, vastus lateralis, and iliotibial band) with a combination of local anesthetic, narcotic, and either corticosteroid or nonsteroidal anti-inflammatory medication results in decreased postoperative pain and narcotic requirements.[19]
- After copious irrigation of all exposed tissues, an extended posterior soft tissue repair is performed (**TECH FIG 8**).
- The quadratus femoris is repaired to its insertion, along with repair of the gluteus maximus insertion if this tendon was released.

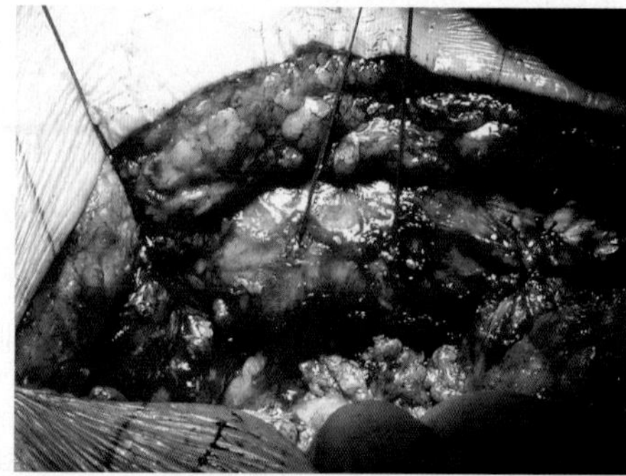

TECH FIG 8 • A meticulous posterior soft tissue repair should include the posterior capsule as well as the piriformis and obturator tendons. Inspection of the repair is essential prior to closure of the fascia.

- A figure-8 suture is placed approximating the superior aspect of the piriformis to the superior capsule and/or gluteus minimus tendon; this suture is not tied initially.
- Transosseous repair of the short external rotators and posterior capsule to the posteromedial aspect of the greater trochanter is performed.
  - A nonabsorbable suture is passed through the superolateral portion of the posterior capsular flap and the piriformis tendon in a single pass, with a second pass through the capsule and the conjoint tendon.
  - A second nonabsorbable suture is passed through the inferolateral portion of the capsular flap and the obturator externus tendon and then again through the capsule.
  - The two sutures are passed through drill holes in the greater trochanter and tied to each other. Prior to tying the sutures, the leg is abducted and externally rotated, minimizing tension on the posterior soft tissue flap.
- The suture connecting the piriformis to the superior capsule and/or abductors is tied last.
- The repair should be inspected carefully to make sure that the posterior flap is in intimate contact with the femur before the fascia is closed.
  - An inadequate repair can easily be revised. If the soft tissues cannot reach the bone, a significant increase in length and/or offset is implied. If this was not planned, femoral modularity can be used to shorten the limb and avoid severe LLD.
- The wound is once again copiously irrigated and routine closure of the fascia, subcutaneous tissue, and skin is performed.

PEARLS AND PITFALLS

Leg length and offset	▪ Optimal function requires restoration of leg length and offset. Patients with a particularly high offset should be warned that mild lengthening of the leg may be necessary to achieve appropriate soft tissue tension.
Indications	▪ Concomitant spine pathology can lead to persistent symptoms after otherwise successful THA. ▪ Older, lighter weight, less active women with osteoporosis generally have excellent outcomes after cemented THA and may be spared the thigh pain that remains common after noncemented femoral fixation.
Exposure	▪ Effort should be made to minimize soft tissue trauma. However, small skin incisions that limit exposure may place important deeper structures at risk for increased trauma.
Hypotensive anesthesia	▪ Optimal cement fixation of the acetabular component is difficult to achieve without a dry surgical field, making hypotensive anesthesia a crucial aspect of cement technique.

POSTOPERATIVE CARE

- Blood management
  - Preoperative medical management of anemia is the best approach to minimizing transfusions.
  - Preoperative autologous blood donation is not routinely required but can be used to reduce postoperative exposure to allogenic blood in patients with mild preoperative anemia.
  - Preoperative recombinant human erythropoietin may be considered in patients unable to donate blood.
  - Allogenic transfusion may be used as indicated for symptomatic anemia related to surgical blood loss.
- Pain control
  - Patient satisfaction is improved by the use of multimodal analgesia protocols,[19] combining soft tissue injections at the time of surgery, acetaminophen, nonsteroidal anti-inflammatory medications, and both long- and short-acting narcotics.
  - These regimens reduce both pain and narcotic requirements, thereby reducing perioperative nausea, emesis, sedation, and confusion and enabling more rapid rehabilitation.
- Intravenous antibiotics
  - Antibiotics are given within 1 hour before surgery and continued postoperatively for 24 hours.
  - Cefazolin is the preferred antibiotic.
  - Vancomycin or clindamycin are typically used in the patient allergic to penicillin or cephalosporins. Vancomycin may be preferable, as *Staphylococcus epidermidis* isolates are often resistant to clindamycin.
- Prophylaxis against venous thromboembolic disease
  - Intermittent pneumatic compression devices provide mechanical prophylaxis, which has been proven to reduce the risk of venous thromboembolism (VTE), both as the sole mode of prophylaxis and as an adjunct to pharmacologic prophylaxis.
  - The optimal pharmacologic prophylaxis remains a matter of debate, but some form of prophylaxis should be started inthe hospital and continued after discharge in the vast majority of patients. We typically use aspirin for patients at low or standard risk of VTE and low or standard risk of surgical site bleeding. Patients with a history of VTE or who are otherwise deemed to be at high risk for thrombosis, as well as those with a prior indication for anticoagulation, are typically kept on extended warfarin prophylaxis after discharge. Patients at high risk of bleeding require an individualized approach. In some such cases, withholding pharmacologic prophylaxis may be appropriate during the period when bleeding is most likely. Mechanical prophylaxis may play a particularly important role in these patients.
  - Accelerated rehabilitation protocols further reduce the risk of thromboembolic disease and are an important part of most multimodal prophylaxis regimens.
  - Screening Doppler ultrasounds are no longer recommended.
- Physical therapy
  - Posterior hip dislocation precautions are recommended for patients undergoing THA through a posterior approach. Our standard physical therapy regimen is 6 weeks, although precautions can be relaxed earlier in patients who are stiff at their first follow-up visit. Precautions may not be required with other surgical approaches.[20] A recent study in which limited posterior precautions (avoiding flexion greater than 100 degrees or marked internal rotation of the hip) were used showed a very low dislocation rate with a modified posterior soft tissue repair.[4]
  - Weight bearing is permitted as tolerated with a walker or two crutches starting within 24 hours of surgery.
  - Patients are weaned off walking aids as tolerated.
- Discharge
  - Most patients can be discharged home 2 to 3 days after surgery.
  - Patients with other severely affected joints, difficult home environments, or poor social support may require a brief period of inpatient rehabilitation.

OUTCOMES

- Relief of hip pain and restoration of function are remarkable after THA. Thigh pain is rare after cemented THA, whereas it is relatively common after noncemented femoral fixation.
- The clinical success of cemented THA has been documented at long-term follow-up (**FIG 3**). Although function may decline with age and comorbidities, 94% of patients followed for 30 years were free from hip pain or reported minimal discomfort.[27]
- Minimum 25-year follow-up data after cemented THA using first-generation cement techniques are available.[1,6,7] Each center reported a single-surgeon series consisting of consecutive cases performed in the late 1960s and early 1970s.
  - Implant survivorship was 94% at 10 years, 90% at 15 years, 84% to 85% at 20 years, 77% to 81% at 25 years, and 68% at 30 years.
  - Revision with removal of at least one component was required in 12% of hips at 30-year follow-up,[7] with the remainder of the original implants either still functioning well in vivo (7%) or in place at the time of patient death (81%).
- Minimum 20-year follow-up data after cemented THA using improved cement technique in the 1970s and early 1980s are also available.[3,5,24,26]
  - Revision with removal of at least one component has been required in 3% to 10% of patients at 10 to 15 years and in 5% to 12% of patients at 20 to 25 years.
- Reasons for revision
  - Aseptic loosening accounts for most revision procedures after cemented THA, with rates ranging from 62% to 100%.[1,3,17,26]
  - Deep infection, recurrent dislocation, and periprosthetic fracture account for most other revisions.

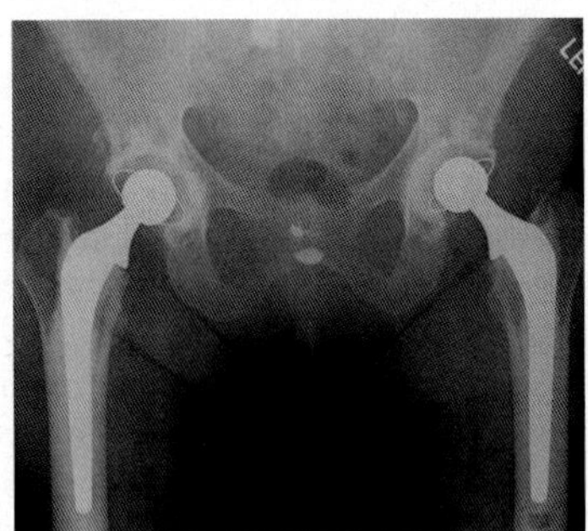

FIG 3 • Radiograph of cemented THA.

- Less common reasons for revision after cemented THA include osteolysis, isolated polyethylene wear, and technical errors such as LLD.
- Component fracture, a major cause of revision with early implant systems, is very uncommon with modern implants.

COMPLICATIONS

- Embolism of fat and bone marrow occurs whenever the marrow space of a long bone is instrumented but seldom results in fat embolism syndrome. Cement fixation of the femoral component may increase the quantity of fat displaced, the consequent pulmonary shunt, and the risk of fat embolism syndrome.[24] For this reason, we avoid cement fixation in patients with significant cardiopulmonary disease.
- VTE is common in THA if prophylaxis is not used. Most prophylactic regimens are associated with low rates of symptomatic deep vein thrombosis (DVT) and pulmonary embolism, with fatal pulmonary embolism occurring in fewer than 0.5% of patients. Aggressive pharmacologic anticoagulation has been proven to reduce the rate of asymptomatic DVT, but no regimen has been found to decrease the low rate of fatal pulmonary embolism.
- Cardiopulmonary complications are uncommon with appropriate preoperative medical optimization and conservative surgical indications, but at-risk patients should be monitored carefully in the perioperative period.
- Clinically meaningful LLD is an avoidable complication in most patients. In a prospective study,[23] the methods for equalizing leg lengths described in this chapter resulted in postoperative LLD that averaged +2.6 mm (range, −7 to +9 mm), with 87% having inequality of 6 mm or less. None of the patients reported symptoms of LLD or required the use of a shoe lift.
- Infection can be a devastating complication after THA.
  - Perioperative intravenous antibiotics and antibiotic-laden bone cement[10] have both been associated with decreased risk of deep infection.
  - Laminar flow and body exhaust suits have been demonstrated to decrease the risk of infection in the setting of inconsistent antibiotic use, but additive benefit in the setting of consistent use of prophylactic antibiotics is unproven.
  - The use of iodine-impregnated adhesive plastic drapes and the minimization of operating room traffic may also reduce bacteria counts in the surgical wound.
- Dislocation after THA is one of the more common causes of early revision surgery. Dislocation risk is minimized when the reconstruction restores leg length, offset, and center of rotation, with appropriate femoral and acetabular anteversion. Improving the head–neck ratio with the use of large-diameter heads can reduce dislocation risk, but polyethylene thickness should not be compromised in cemented THA, as thin polyethylene implants transfer load to the cement mantle less uniformly.
- Periprosthetic fracture can occur intra- or postoperatively. The key to management is intraoperative recognition, as most fractures can be managed expediently at the time of surgery. If an appropriate starting point is used for femoral preparation, intraoperative fractures in primary cemented THA are uncommon. Postoperative fractures typically are associated with trauma, often in the setting of osteolysis, and their management is beyond the scope of this chapter.
- Aseptic loosening is the most common cause of failure after cemented THA. The risk of aseptic loosening can be decreased by the use of well-designed implants and modern cement techniques. Nevertheless, several patient factors influence the rates of aseptic loosening after cemented THA.
  - Male gender is strongly associated with increased risk of revision for aseptic loosening.[1]
  - The severity of acetabular dysplasia is also a risk factor for aseptic loosening, with increased rates of revision associated with Crowe types III and IV hip dysplasia compared with those with less or no dysplasia.[8]
  - Inflammatory arthritis is associated with decreased risk of revision for aseptic loosening.[1]
  - Patient age at time of surgery is inversely correlated with risk of revision for aseptic loosening. Twenty-five-year survivorship free of revision for aseptic loosening was 68.7% in patients who were younger than 40 years of age at the time of primary arthroplasty and 100% in patients older than 80 years of age, with incremental increases in survival observed for each decade of increased age between 40 and 80 years.[1]
- Osteolysis, a common cause of failure in uncemented implants, is less common after cemented THA and possibly related to decreased polyethylene wear in cemented THA. Although ballooning osteolysis is uncommon when cement is used, fixation failure in cemented THA is related to the biologic reaction to wear debris.
- Sciatic nerve palsy is an uncommon complication after cemented THA. It most commonly occurs when the operated extremity is lengthened substantially after a long-standing (especially congenital) shortening of the limb, resulting in traction-related nerve ischemia. We routinely palpate the sciatic nerve before the hip is dislocated and again after the arthroplasty is performed to assess whether the tension in the nerve has been excessively increased.
  - The sciatic nerve may also be compressed under the tendon of the gluteus maximus during surgery if the hip is maintained in severe flexion and internal rotation. For this reason, Hurd et al[15] recommended routine release of the gluteus maximus tendon during THA.

REFERENCES

1. Berry DJ, Harmsen WS, Cabanela ME, et al. Twenty-five-year survivorship of two thousand consecutive primary Charnley total hip replacements: factors affecting survivorship of acetabular and femoral components. J Bone Joint Surg Am 2002;84:171–177.
2. Biedermann R, Tonin A, Krismer M, et al. Reducing the risk of dislocation after total hip arthroplasty: the effect of orientation of the acetabular component. J Bone Joint Surg Br 2005;87:762–769.
3. Bourne RB, Rorabeck CH, Skutek M, et al. The Harris design-2 total hip replacement fixed with so-called second-generation cementing techniques: a ten to fifteen-year follow-up. J Bone Joint Surg Am 1998;80:1775–1780.
4. Brown JA, Pagnano MW. Surgical technique: a simple soft-tissue-only repair of the capsule and external rotators in posterior-approach THA. Clin Orthop Relat Res 2012;470:511–515.
5. Buckwalter AE, Callaghan JJ, Liu SS, et al. Results of Charnley total hip arthroplasty with use of improved femoral cementing techniques: a concise follow-up, at a minimum of twenty-five years, of a previous report. J Bone Joint Surg Am 2006;88:1481–1485.

6. Callaghan JJ, Albright JC, Goetz DD, et al. Charnley total hip arthroplasty with cement: minimum twenty-five-year follow-up. J Bone Joint Surg Am 2000;82:487–497.
7. Callaghan JJ, Templeton JE, Liu SS, et al. Results of Charnley total hip arthroplasty at a minimum of thirty years: a concise follow-up of a previous report. J Bone Joint Surg Am 2004;86:690–695.
8. Chougle A, Hemmady MV, Hodgkinson JP. Severity of hip dysplasia and loosening of the socket in cemented total hip replacement: a long-term follow-up. J Bone Joint Surg Br 2005;87:16–20.
9. Crites BM, Berend ME, Ritter MA. Technical considerations of cemented acetabular components: a 30-year evaluation. Clin Orthop Relat Res 2000;381:114–119.
10. Engesaeter LB, Lie SA, Espehaug B, et al. Antibiotic prophylaxis in total hip arthroplasty: effects of antibiotic prophylaxis systemically and in bone cement on the revision rate of 22,170 primary hip replacements followed 0–14 years in the Norwegian Arthroplasty Register. Acta Orthop Scand 2003;74:644–651.
11. Faris PM, Ritter MA, Keating EM, et al. The cemented all-polyethylene acetabular cup: factors affecting survival with emphasis on the integrated polyethylene spacer: an analysis of the effect of cement spacers, cement mantle thickness, and acetabular angle on the survival of total hip arthroplasty. J Arthroplasty 2006;21:191–198.
12. Flivik G, Kristiansson I, Kesteris U, et al. Is removal of subchondral bone plate advantageous in cemented cup fixation? A randomized RSA study. Clin Orthop Relat Res 2006;448:164–172.
13. Herberts P, Malchau H. How outcome studies have changed total hip arthroplasty practices in Sweden. Clin Orthop Relat Res 1997;344:44–60.
14. Hogan N, Azhar A, Brady O. An improved acetabular cementing technique in total hip arthroplasty: aspiration of the iliac wing. J Bone Joint Surg Br 2005;87:1216–1219.
15. Hurd JL, Potter HG, Dua V, et al. Sciatic nerve palsy after primary total hip arthroplasty: a new perspective. J Arthroplasty 2006;21:796–802.
16. Lucas DH, Scott RB. Coplanar test: the Ranawat sig. A specific maneuver to assess component position in total hip arthroplasty. J Orthop Tech 1994;2:59.
17. Malchau H, Herberts P, Eisler T, et al. The Swedish Total Hip Replacement Register. J Bone Joint Surg Am 2002;84(suppl 2):2–20.
18. Parks ML, Walsh HA, Salvati EA, et al. Effect of increasing temperature on the properties of four bone cements. Clin Orthop Relat Res 1998;355:238–248.
19. Parvataneni HK, Shah VP, Howard H, et al. Controlling pain after total hip and knee arthroplasty using a multimodal protocol with local periarticular injections: a prospective, randomized study. J Arthroplasty 2007;22(6):33–38.
20. Peak EL, Parvizi J, Ciminiello M, et al. The role of patient restrictions in reducing the prevalence of early dislocation following total hip arthroplasty. A randomized, prospective study. J Bone Joint Surg Am 2005;87:247–253.
21. Pellicci PM, Bostrom M, Poss R. Posterior approach to total hip replacement using enhanced posterior soft tissue repair. Clin Orthop Relat Res 1998;355:224–228.
22. Ranawat CS, Deshmukh RG, Peters LE, et al. Prediction of the long-term durability of all-polyethylene cemented sockets. Clin Orthop Relat Res 1995;317:89–105.
23. Ranawat CS, Rao RR, Rodriguez JA, et al. Correction of limb-length inequality during total hip arthroplasty. J Arthroplasty 2001;16:715–720.
24. Ries MD, Lynch F, Rauscher LA, et al. Pulmonary function during and after total hip replacement: findings in patients who have insertion of a femoral component with and without cement. J Bone Joint Surg Am 1993;75:581–587.
25. Siebenrock KA, Leunig M, Ganz R. Periacetabular osteotomy: the Bernese experience. J Bone Joint Surg Am 2001;83:449.
26. Skutek M, Bourne RB, Rorabeck CH, et al. The twenty to twenty-five-year outcomes of the Harris design-2 matte-finished cemented total hip replacement: a concise follow-up of a previous report. J Bone Joint Surg Am 2007;89:814–818.
27. Wroblewski BM, Fleming PA, Siney PD. Charnley low-frictional torque arthroplasty of the hip: 20-to-30 year results. J Bone Joint Surg Br 1999;81:427–430.

CHAPTER 20

Uncemented Total Hip Arthroplasty

Matthew S. Austin, Brian A. Klatt, and Paul B. McKenna

DEFINITION

- Total hip arthroplasty (THA) is the standard of care for symptomatic degenerative joint disease (DJD) of the hip that is unresponsive to nonoperative treatment.
- Cementless THA has demonstrated excellent mid- to long-term results.
- The acetabular component obtains initial fixation through a press-fit and has a surface that allows for in- or ongrowth of bone.
- The femoral component obtains initial fixation through a press-fit in either the metaphysis or diaphysis and has a surface that allows for in- or ongrowth of bone. The metaphyseal-fit prosthesis may be either wedge-shaped or fit-and-fill.

ANATOMY

- The acetabulum must be exposed so that the anterior and posterior walls, superior dome and rim, and teardrop are visualized.
- The proximal femur must be exposed so that the periphery of the proximal femoral neck cut is visualized.

PATHOGENESIS

- DJD of the hip is the end point of many hip disorders, including osteoarthritis, inflammatory arthritis, dysplasia, osteonecrosis, trauma, and sepsis.

NATURAL HISTORY

- DJD of the hip often follows a variable symptomatic course. It is unknown why it progresses more rapidly in some patients than others and why some patients are more symptomatic than others.

PATIENT HISTORY AND PHYSICAL FINDINGS

- The history should be directed to determine whether the patient's pain is extrinsic or intrinsic.
- The patient's pain may be extrinsic (eg, lumbar radiculopathy or intrapelvic pathology) and THA may fail to relieve the patient's pain completely, even in the face of severe degenerative changes of the hip.
- Pain usually is located in the groin but may be located in the medial thigh, buttock, or the medial knee.
- Range of motion (ROM) should be observed. Normal ROM of the hip is an arc of motion of 120 to 140 degrees of flexion–extension, 60 to 80 degrees of abduction–adduction, and external–internal rotation of 60 to 90 degrees. Loss of motion may be due to pain, contracture, or abnormal biomechanics.
- Nonoperative treatment must be optimized before consideration is given to surgery.
- Leg lengths should be measured and recorded preoperatively and the patient should be counseled about reasonable postoperative expectations.
- Examinations to perform include the following:
  - *Trendelenburg test.* The test is positive if the contralateral hip drops inferiorly; this may indicate that the hip abductors are compromised.
  - *Hip flexion–internal rotation.* The test is positive if the patient's pain is recreated. Pain that is not recreated with this examination may be from an extrinsic source.

IMAGING AND OTHER DIAGNOSTIC STUDIES

- Plain radiographs, including anteroposterior (AP) views of the pelvis and AP and true lateral views of the hip, should be obtained to evaluate the anatomy, assess for deformity, and devise an adequate plan preoperatively (**FIG 1**).

DIFFERENTIAL DIAGNOSIS

- Lumbar radiculopathy
- Spinal stenosis
- Sacroiliac DJD
- Intra-abdominal pathology
- Intrapelvic pathology
- Neuropathy

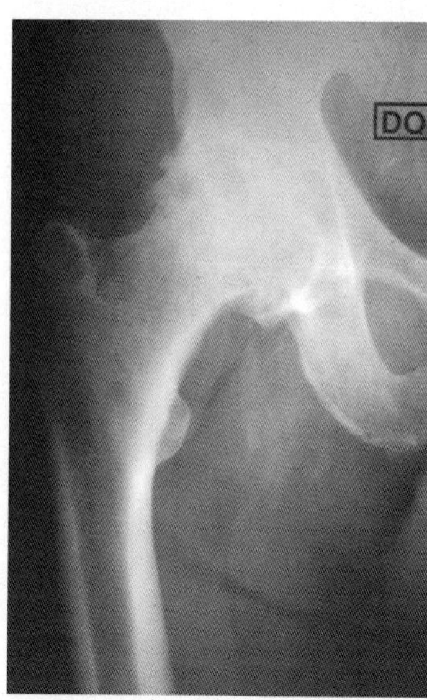

FIG 1 • AP radiograph of the hip demonstrates advanced degenerative changes of osteophytes and joint space obliteration.

- Meralgia paresthetica
- Complex regional pain syndrome
- Vascular claudication
- Primary bone tumors
- Metastasis
- Infection

NONOPERATIVE MANAGEMENT

- Acetaminophen
- Nonsteroidal anti-inflammatory drugs
- Glucosamine
- Chondroitin sulfate
- Physical therapy

SURGICAL MANAGEMENT

- The primary indication for cementless THA is painful, severe DJD of the hip that has been nonresponsive to appropriate nonoperative treatment modalities.

Preoperative Planning

- Preoperative planning for routine cementless primary THA can be accomplished with plain radiographs at standard magnifications.
  - Standard templates are available for the components and many are available for digital templating.
- The acetabular component is placed so that the inferomedial edge of the cup is at the radiographic teardrop. The inclination is 35 to 45 degrees and the cup should contact the superolateral rim of the acetabulum.
- The femoral component is placed so that the center of rotation is at the level of the greater trochanter. The femoral offset should be reproduced. However, the femur must be internally rotated 10 to 15 degrees on the radiograph to bring the femoral neck into the plane of the radiograph. Externally rotated femora will appear to be in coxa valga.
- Proximal-fit femoral prostheses are designed to obtain fit in the metadiaphyseal region.
- Diaphyseal-fit femoral prostheses are designed to obtain fit in the diaphysis.

Modular Femoral Stems

- Despite good results with fully monoblock stems introduced in the 1960s, surgeons had difficulty fine-tuning leg length and soft tissue tensioning during THA. Meticulous attention to preoperative planning, neck resection levels, and cementation technique along with adjustment of soft tissue tension via repair of trochanteric osteotomy were used to restore appropriate hip biomechanics.
- The primary benefit of modularity is the relative ease with which surgeons can optimize hip biomechanics, and it is for this reason that the vast majority of surgeons today use femoral implants with at least one modular junction.
- Other benefits include the following:
  - Aids in exposure at the time of revision by removing the modular parts and retaining the osseointegrated portion of the implant
  - Alterations to modular parts can be easily adjusted at revision, especially in the presence of instability. This has led to clinically apparent reductions in the dislocation rates in hip revisions.[8,32]
  - Replacement of worn or damaged parts without requiring removal of the osseointegrated portion of the implant

Femoral Modularity: The Basics

- Femoral modularity can exist at one or more junctions.
  - Head–neck: Nearly all modern femoral stems have modularity at this junction. It allows adjustment of head size and neck length.
  - Metaphyseal: Metadiaphyseal modular junction of the femur, distal to the femoral neck osteotomy (S-ROM [DePuy, Warsaw, IN], Emperion [Smith & Nephew, Memphis, TN], Restoration [Stryker Orthopaedics, Kalamazoo, MI]). This allows for multiple neck options for offset, version, neck–shaft angle, and neck length in addition to femoral head–neck options.
  - Dual neck: Double modularity of the neck with a head–neck junction and a junction proximal to the femoral neck osteotomy, unsupported by host bone (ProFemur [Wright Medical Technology, Arlington, TN]; M-L Taper with Kinectiv Technology [Zimmer, Warsaw, IN]; Anatomic Benoist Girard [ABG] [Stryker Orthopaedics], Rejuvenate [Stryker Orthopaedics]). These stems also allow for multiple neck options for offset, version, neck–shaft angle, and neck length in addition to femoral head–neck options. However, the latter two stems have been recalled.
- Modularity of femoral stems occurs at a Morse style tapered junction. The trunnion compresses into the bore as it expands, creating an interference fit. In this way, it provides both axial and rotational stability.
- Tapers exist in proprietary geometries, depending on the component design. It is important to know the taper type, particularly in revision situations, in order to have the proper instruments and implants available.

Potential Advantages of Modular Stems

- Biomechanical goals of THA
  - Restore the normal hip center.
  - Recreate the bony anatomy.
  - Optimize soft tissue tension.
- The use of modular femoral components may allow for optimal restoration of hip biomechanics.
- Most nonmodular (monolithic) femoral stems are based on a range of normal femoral morphology. This may not allow for accurate restoration of individual biomechanics.
  - Noble et al[39] analyzed 200 cadaveric femurs and found that there is no specific relationship between the size and shape of the metaphysis and diaphysis.
  - Anthropologic literature has demonstrated the effect of aging on femoral morphology. Endosteal changes occur primarily in the diaphysis, with cortical thinning and medullary expansion beginning in the fourth decade. A practical consequence of the effect of age on the size of the endosteal surface is the possible need for femoral components of varying neck length and offset for a given canal size.
- Adequate soft tissue tension is created through the offset and neck length. Insufficient soft tissue tension may lead to a decreased abductor lever arm and weakness and/or instability. Excessive soft tissue tension may result in pelvic tilt, leg length inequality, and/or greater trochanteric pain syndrome.

- Certain anatomic variants such as the increased femoral neck anteversion seen in developmental dysplasia of the hip, retroversion in slipped capital femoral epiphysis, coxa vara, and malunions from previous fractures can increase the difficulty in restoring proper hip biomechanics. In a study of 1000 primary THAs using the S-ROM prosthesis, Kindsfater et al[29] found that the anteversion needed adjustment to enhance stability in over 47% of the cases.
- Modular systems can provide up to 10,398 combinations of sizes and shapes. This enables the surgeon to adjust the prosthesis to the patient and not the patient to the prosthesis.[5]
- Therefore, the establishment of immediate rigidity, including resistance to torsional forces, is imperative for the long-term survivorship of the prosthesis.
- Ohl et al[40] and Otani and Whiteside[41] determined biomechanically that both proximal and distal fixation of the prosthesis resisted torsional loads better than either proximal fixation or distal fixation.
- The difficulty with a nonmodular stem is that the proximal metaphyseal and proximal diaphyseal areas of human femur tend not to correlate in terms of size and geometry.[33,39]
- Midstem modular prostheses and some proximal stem systems (S-ROM) allow the surgeon to achieve a tight fit both proximally and distally. The surgeon can independently size components that tightly fit in both anatomic areas.

Concerns

- The major concern with modular femoral components is the addition of another junction. The major problems associated with these additional articulations are as follows:
  - Fretting/corrosion
  - Fracture
  - Dissociation
  - More recent concerns include the generation of metal debris and soft tissue reaction to the debris.
- Fretting and corrosion are often linked, synergistic processes that can lead to poor outcomes for two reasons[26]:
  - The degradation process can lead to a decrease in the structural integrity of the metal.
  - The release of degradation products may elicit an adverse biologic reaction in the host.
- Fretting
  - Results from micromotion between two surfaces. The movement required for disruption of the passive oxidation layer on metal can be as little as 3 to 4 nm and depends on the frequency of motion and the amount of load on the construct.
  - Motion leading to reduction of the oxide layer on the surface can expose the base alloy to an aqueous solution.
  - Exposure to the aqueous solution oxidizes the alloy into ionic form (dissolution) or reacts with oxygen to reform the oxide film (repassivation).
  - When this repassivation occurs in a crevice, such as that associated with a modular neck–stem interface, it depletes the local oxygen supply, creating a more acidic environment. This situation creates accelerated corrosion, pitting, and cracks.
  - Metals that are repeatedly stressed in a corrosive environment can experience catastrophic failure.
  - Fretting at the neck–stem junction in proximal modular stems occurs more frequently and to a greater extent than that of the head–neck taper.
    - A retrieval of 16 dual modular stem were analyzed, 6 of which demonstrated significant fretting and crevice corrosion at the neck–stem junction. This contrasted with only 3 of the stems having any sign of corrosion at the head–neck junction.[30]
    - Another retrieval analysis of a proximal dual modular stem found evidence of abrasion and corrosion, indicating that initiation and propagation of the fatigue crack could have been corrosion assisted. The neck in question was the largest size neck available for this implant.[13]
- Femoral stem fractures are rare events. However, there have been several case reports of proximal modular stem fractures.[3,13,22,49]
  - Huot Carlson et al[25] examined 78 retrieved modular stems and found 7 with fractures. They correlated the presence of stem fracture with the combination of small stem; large femoral neck offset; and active, heavy patients.
  - Atwood et al[3] analyzed a retrieved proximal modular femoral stem (ProFemur Z) that experienced catastrophic failure at the modular neck less than 2 years after implantation. Analysis of the fractured stem revealed large (200 μm) crevices and areas of burnishing, which indicated that fretting occurred. There was also an absence of evidence to support simple cyclic fatigue failure.
  - Skendzel et al[49] reported two dual modular stem failures. Both occurred in men weighing over 220 pounds whose index procedure was less than 4 years before the time of failure.
- Dissociation of the modular components is another concern.
  - The majority of reported cases are those of femoral head–neck dissociation. These usually occur after a hip dislocation and the subsequent reduction attempt.[9,47,56]
  - Others have reported dissociation at other levels of modularity.[1,50,51] Microscopic examination of the retrieved prostheses have also shown the presence of fretting at the neck–stem interface, suggesting that there may be micromotion present, leading to corrosion, dissolution of the metal, and eventual dissociation of the taper.[50]
- Adverse reaction to metal debris (ARMD)
  - Collier examined the extent of corrosion at modular junctions in two studies. In one study, they found corrosion present in more than 30% of retrievals when mixed alloy head–stem combinations were used. When all cobalt–chrome and all-titanium combinations were used, corrosion was present in less than 6% and 10%, respectively.[10,11]
  - It is now well established that metallic particulate debris can initiate ARMD, a cell-mediated hypersensitivity reaction.[23] ARMD may lead to destructive lesions. This was recently reported initially with metal-on-metal articulations in resurfacings and THA, but concern has been growing regarding the junctions associated with modular hip stems.[19]
  - There have been increasing reports of adverse soft tissue reactions (pseudotumor) in THAs with a metal-polyethylene articulation. Crevice corrosion at the head–neck taper (trunnionosis) is thought to be the source.[12,34,35,37,52] Others have reported the presence of a pseudotumor in dual modular stems where retrieval analysis shows large degrees of fretting and corrosion at the neck–stem interface but pristine trunnions at the head–neck junction.[55]

- The material makeup of the head–neck junction has a large effect on the degree of corrosion seen in retrieval studies. There is a higher incidence of corrosion in the presence of mixed alloy combinations. This is due to the mechanical and tribologic properties of the metals.[18] When two dissimilar metals are in contact in an electrolyte solution, there is an electrical potential difference between them, resulting in a flow of electrons creating galvanic corrosion.
- Ceramic heads appear to reduce the amount of taper corrosion, but they do not eliminate it. Taper corrosion occurs with a similar frequency with ceramic heads on metal tapers, but not to the same extent. The mechanism of the development of corrosion is similar, but in the presence of a ceramic head, it only occurs on the metal taper.[31]

Conclusions

- Modularity may have a role in THA in select cases.
- Such cases may include deformity, abnormal femoral morphology, or inability to achieve stability with nonmodular implants.
- Risks of modularity include ARMD, failure of the modular junction, and/or subsequent need for reoperation.
- The two materials used at the modular junction may be important in terms of adverse reactions.
- Therefore, modularity should be used selectively and after careful consideration.

Positioning

- The patient is positioned according to surgeon preference and in accordance with the surgical approach.
  - The hip should be draped to allow a wide surgical exposure should an extensile approach be required in the event of a complication.
- The pelvis must be stabilized in a secure fashion to avoid pelvic tilt, which may affect the surgeon's perception of the acetabular position.

Approach

- The hip can be exposed for primary routine arthroplasty via a variety of approaches:
  - Anterior
  - Anterolateral
  - Direct lateral
  - Posterior
  - Two-incision
  - Small-incision variants of these approaches

TECHNIQUES

Acetabular Exposure

- The approach to the hip is chosen according to the surgeon's preference. The approach illustrated here is the direct lateral (modified Hardinge) approach in the supine position.
- Retractors are placed in the anterior, superior, and inferior positions, thereby exposing the entire periphery of the acetabulum (**TECH FIG 1**).
- The labrum is resected.
- The soft tissue in the cotyloid fossa is removed, allowing exposure of the medial wall and teardrop.

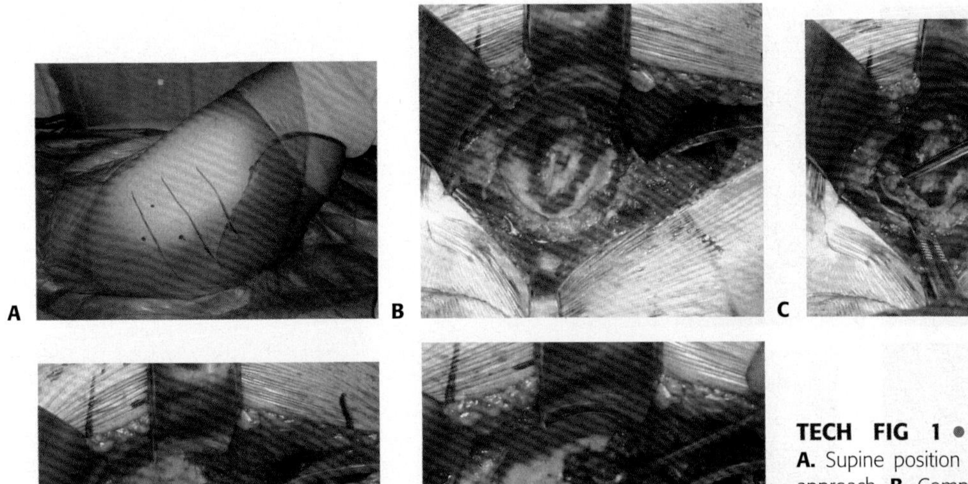

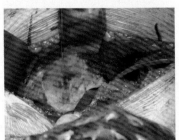

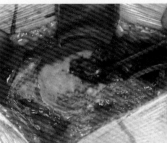

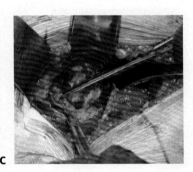

TECH FIG 1 • Acetabular exposure. **A.** Supine position for modified Hardinge approach. **B.** Completed acetabular exposure. The medial wall and native acetabular anatomy are easily visualized. **C.** Labrum is resected. **D.** Osteotome removes osteophytes from cotyloid fossa. **E.** Curette removes remaining tissue to expose teardrop.

Acetabular Preparation

- Before reaming, the entire periphery of the acetabulum, medial wall, and teardrop must be directly visualized (**TECH FIG 2**).
- The initial reaming must be done with moderate pressure until the quality of bone is assessed.
  - The goal of the initial reaming is to medialize the reamer fully. The cotyloid fossa should be eliminated without penetrating the medial wall.
- Reaming then proceeds sequentially. The goal is to recreate the center of rotation by placing the inferomedial aspect of the socket at the level of the teardrop with the component inclined at 35 to 45 degrees, with 10 to 20 degrees of anteversion and good initial fixation obtained through a press-fit.
- The templated size should be used as a guide; intraoperatively, an increase or decrease in cup diameter may be found to be appropriate.
  - Failure to recognize the need for a different cup diameter may lead to iatrogenic fracture or a failure to achieve initial fixation.
- The bony bed should be bleeding but not devoid of sclerotic bone.
- The pelvis must remain in a stable position to avoid malpositioning of the acetabular component.

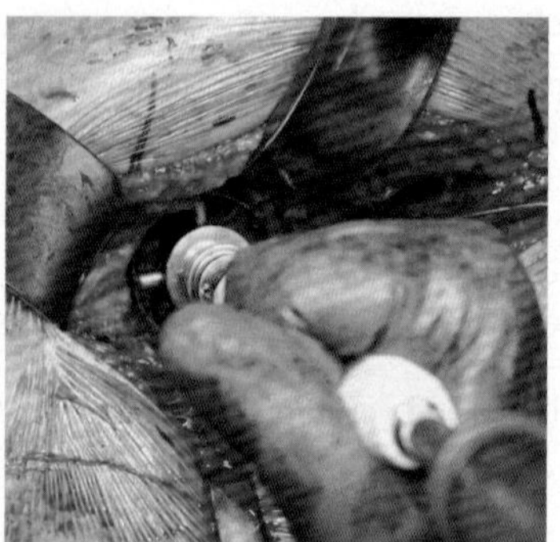
A
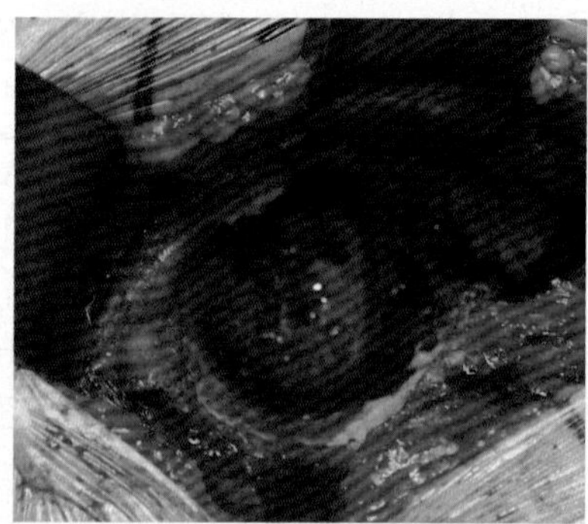
B
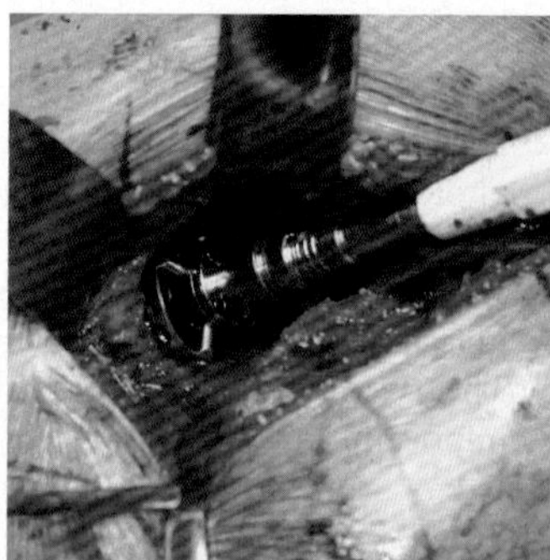
C

TECH FIG 2 • Acetabular preparation. **A.** Initial reaming to medialize acetabulum fully. **B.** Reaming completed to medial wall. **C.** Reaming proceeds sequentially at 35 to 45 degrees of abduction and 10 to 20 degrees of anteversion.

Acetabular Component Implantation

- The position of the pelvis is reassessed. Any tilt is corrected.
- The trial component or reamer is used to assess bone coverage of the component and position (**TECH FIG 3**). If the trial or reamer is not seated properly, then further reaming may be necessary. If deemed appropriate, implantation of the actual component may proceed.

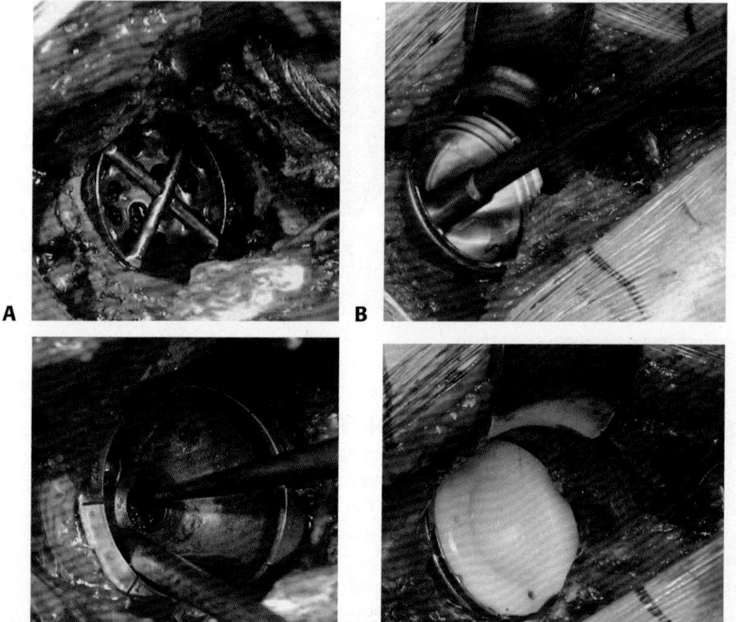

TECH FIG 3 • Acetabular component implantation. **A.** Final reamer is used to assess component position, bony coverage, and seating. **B.** Acetabular component is implanted. **C.** Central hole is used to verify that the cup is fully seated. **D.** Actual liner is inserted into the cup.

- The actual implant should be 1 to 2 mm larger than the last reamer. The surgeon must know the actual diameter of the implant, taking into account any rim or coating.
  - Implants that are larger than the size of the last reamer by 4 mm or more are associated with risk of fracture.
- The acetabular component is then implanted, with care taken to medialize the implant. The inferomedial aspect of the cup should be at the level of the teardrop in 35 to 45 degrees of abduction and 10 to 20 degrees of anteversion.
- A trial liner or the actual liner is then inserted.

Femoral Exposure

- The femur is exposed by elevating it out of the wound with a retractor (Bennett or double-footed).
- The periphery of the femur is exposed with another retractor (**TECH FIG 4**).
- The soft tissues must be protected so that iatrogenic damage by reamers or broaches is avoided.

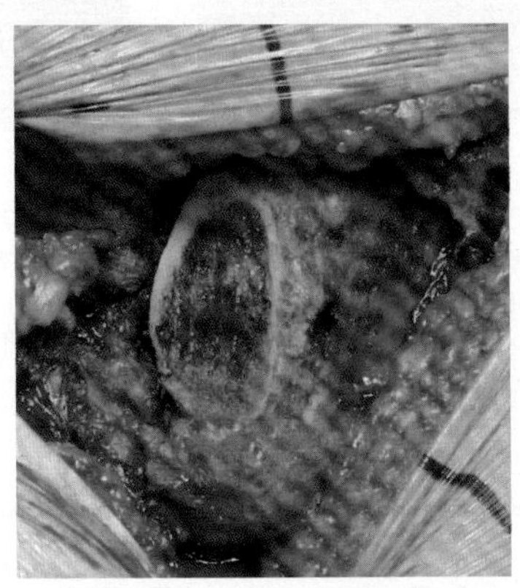

TECH FIG 4 • Femoral exposure. The femur is elevated and exposed with two double-footed retractors to allow atraumatic broaching.

Femoral Preparation (Proximal-Fit Prosthesis)

- The femur is prepared as delineated by the surgical protocol for each prosthesis (**TECH FIG 5**). The surgeon should be familiar with the prosthesis and all of the available options and idiosyncrasies.
- The proximal-fit prosthesis usually requires a starter reamer, which is used as a canal finder. In addition, the reamer should be lateralized to avoid broaching and subsequent varus positioning of the implant.
- The femur then is broached sequentially, with care taken to lateralize the broach. Broaching is complete when the broach ceases to advance, the pitch of impaction increases, and good cortical contact is obtained.
  - Improper broaching can lead to fracture, malposition, or undersizing.

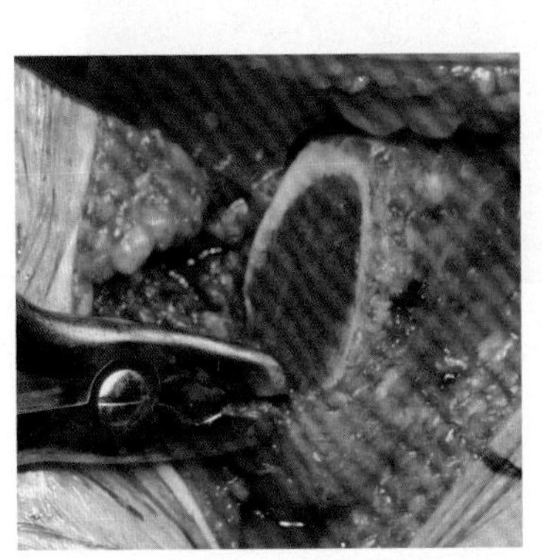

A

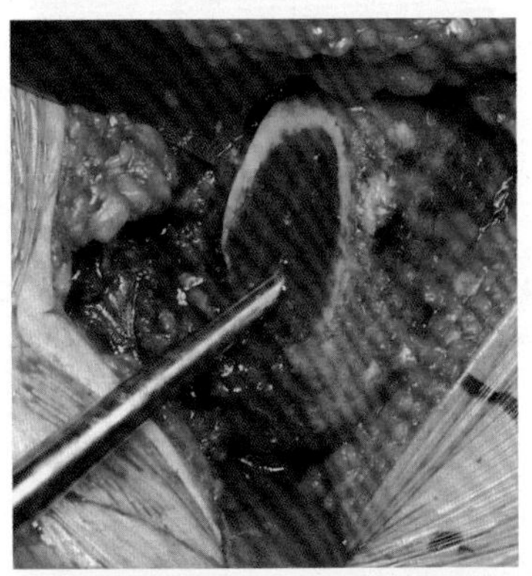

B

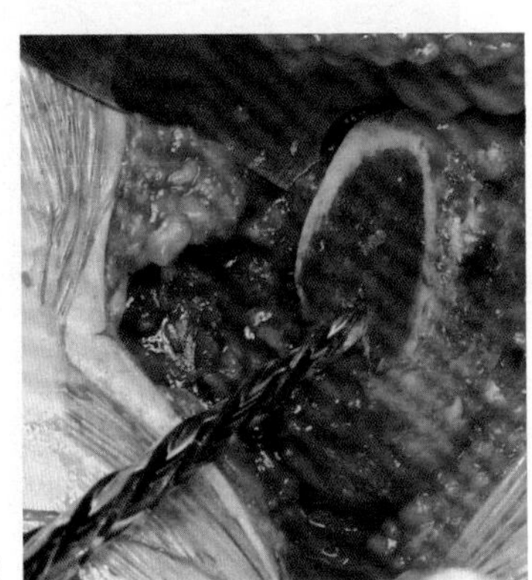

C

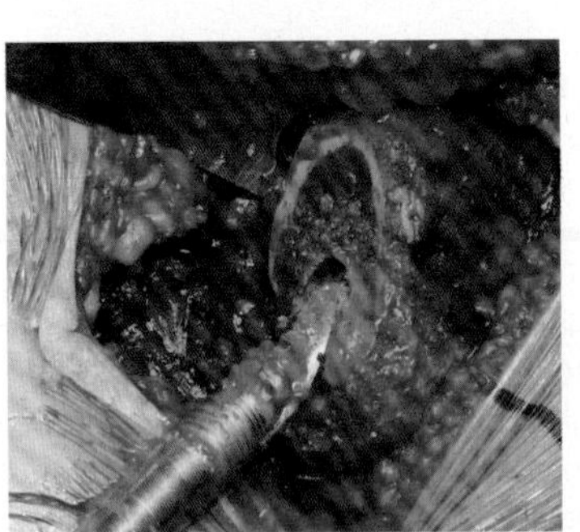

D

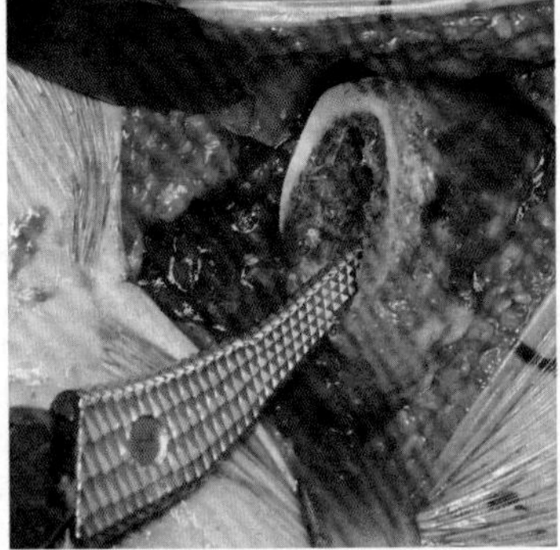

E

TECH FIG 5 • Femoral preparation. **A.** Rongeur is used to clear tissues and lateral cortical bone. **B.** Curette is used to find canal. **C,D.** Canal is reamed to open canal and care is taken to lateralize. **E.** Broaching proceeds. *(continued)*

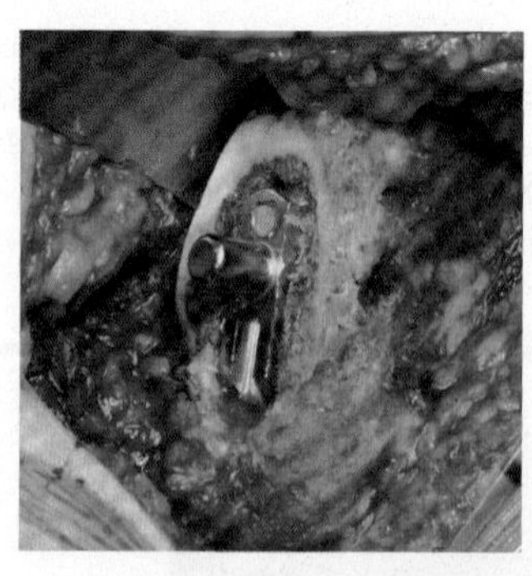

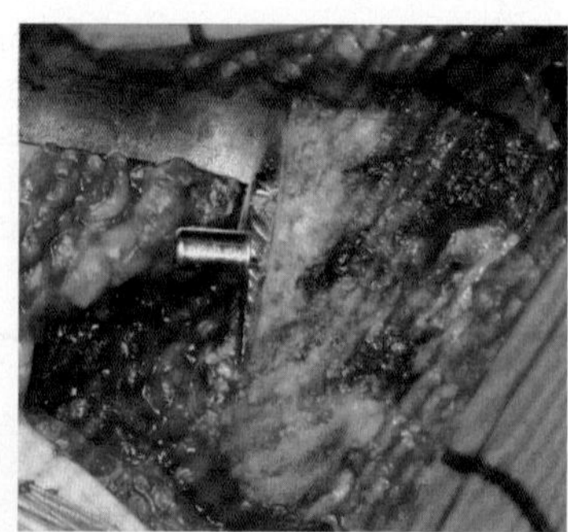

TECH FIG 5 • *(continued)* **F,G.** Final broach is seated.

- The component should be anteverted 10 to 15 degrees.
- The greater trochanter can be used as a reference to recreate the center of rotation.
- It may be necessary to adjust the neck cut to allow for further seating of the prosthesis.
- The templated size should be used as a guide and an increase or decrease in stem size intraoperatively may be appropriate.
  - Failure to recognize the need for a different size may lead to iatrogenic fracture or failure to achieve initial fixation.
- A standard or varus neck is selected based on the soft tissue tension and the patient's anatomy.

Femoral Component Implantation (Proximal-Fit Prosthesis)

- The implant chosen usually matches the size of the last broach.
- The proximal-fit femoral component is inserted, with care taken to avoid varus positioning (**TECH FIG 6**).
- The implant is impacted until it ceases to advance, the pitch of impaction increases, there is good cortical contact, and the implant has reached the level of the last broach.

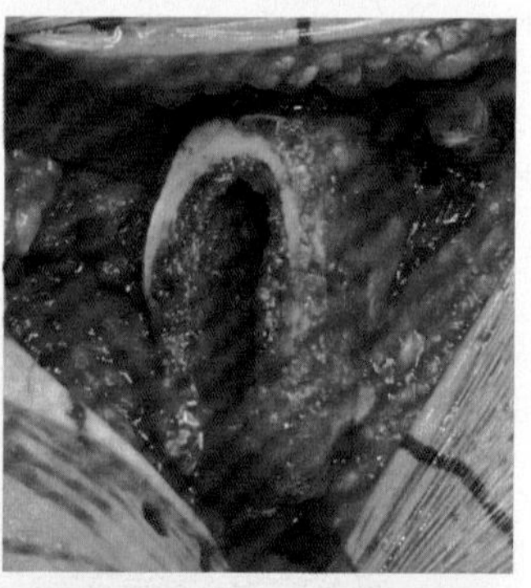

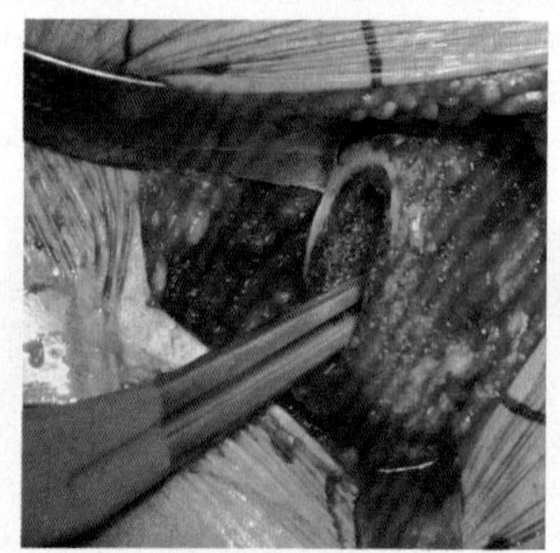

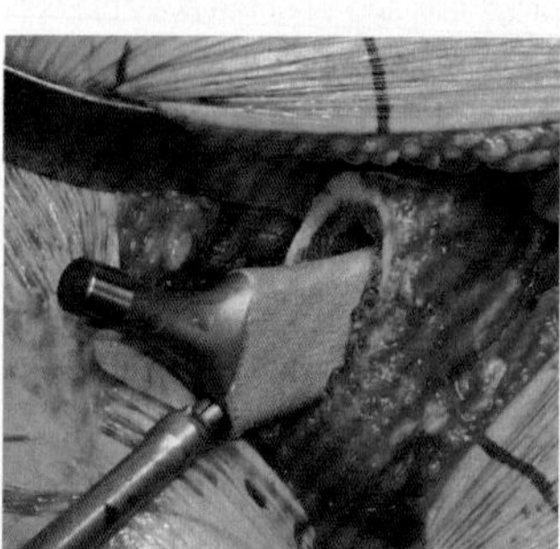

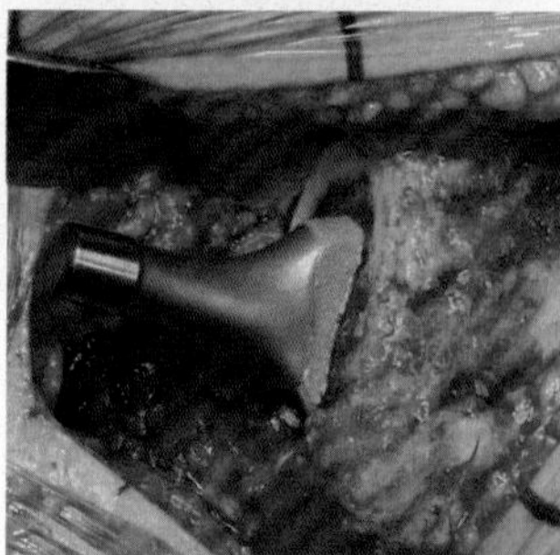

TECH FIG 6 • Femoral component implantation (proximal-fit prosthesis). **A.** Canal appearance before implantation. **B,C.** Component is introduced in proper orientation until resistance is met. **D.** Component fully seated.

Soft Tissue Tension/Leg Length Determination

- The hip is trial reduced and assessed for soft tissue tension, stability, ROM, impingement, and leg length.
- The soft tissue tension should allow for no more than 1 to 2 mm of toggle (**TECH FIG 7**).
- The hip should be stable within the patient's physiologic ROM. If instability exists, the position of the components must be reassessed.
- The ROM should be physiologic for the patient.

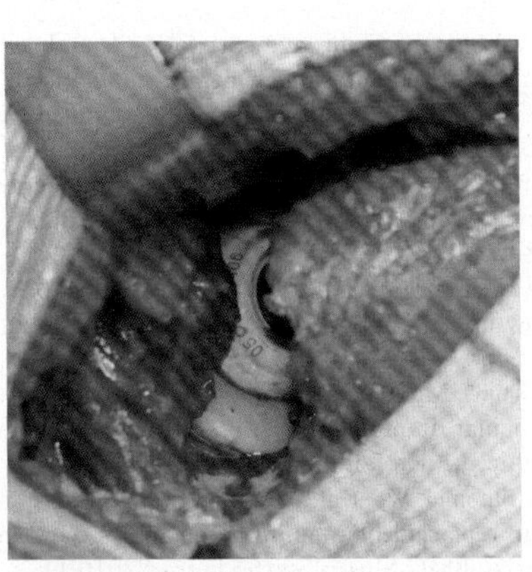

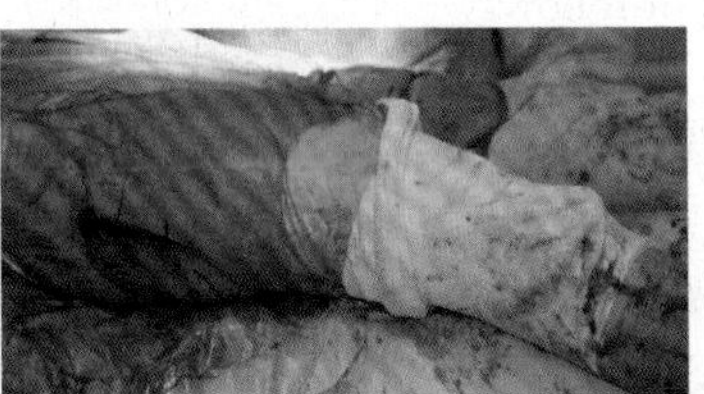

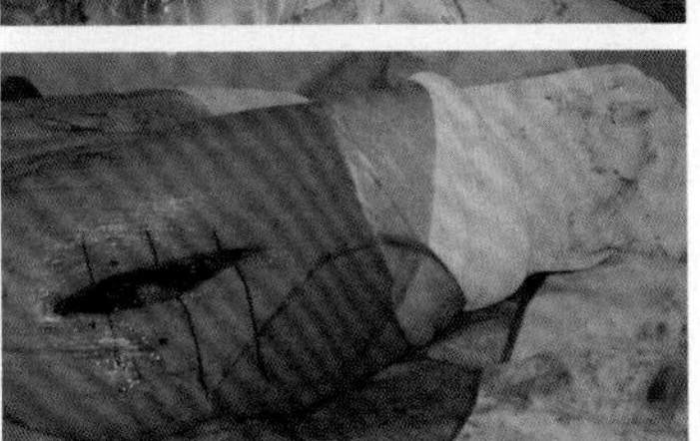

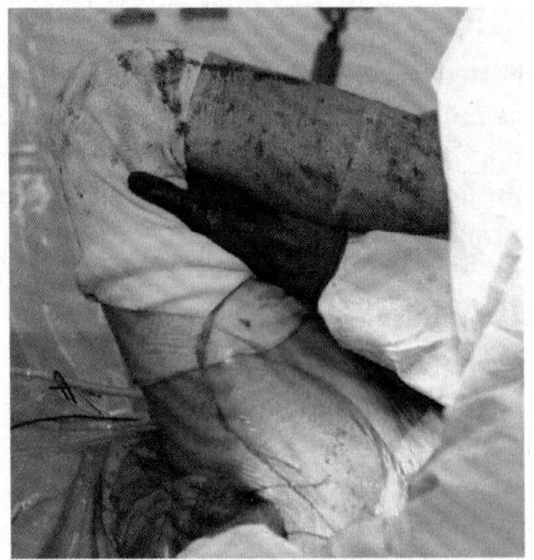

TECH FIG 7 • Soft tissue tension and leg length determination. **A.** Hip is reduced. Soft tissue tension is evaluated. **B.** Abduction/external rotation. **C.** Adduction/internal rotation. **D.** Flexion/adduction/internal rotation.

- Impingement must be assessed and rectified with removal of any remaining osteophytes.
  - Increased offset may aid in decreasing impingement.
  - Proper component position must be verified to exclude positioning as a source of impingement.
- The patient's leg length is assessed either directly through palpation of the heels or malleoli or indirectly through the use of a pin placed in the ilium and a marker placed on the femur.
  - One must be careful to position the limb accurately to avoid inducing error during the measurement process.

Closure

- The wound is thoroughly irrigated.
- Drains are placed at the discretion of the surgeon.
- The capsule is closed meticulously, especially if a posterior approach is used.
- The soft tissues are closed with absorbable suture.
- The skin is closed according to surgeon preference.

PEARLS AND PITFALLS

Preoperative planning	▪ Preoperative radiographs must be evaluated for any unusual findings (eg, dysplasia) that may require techniques or implants not routinely performed or available.
Intraoperative decision making	▪ The templated component size must be used as a guide. Proper implant sizing must be guided by visual, auditory, and tactile feedback.
Implantation	▪ The components must be implanted properly. Failure to achieve soft tissue tension, physiologic ROM, stability, and reasonable leg lengths must be followed by reevaluation of the component positioning.
Soft tissues	▪ Care must be taken to perform gentle dissection and thorough closure of the capsule and soft tissue to minimize pain, instability, and limp.

POSTOPERATIVE CARE

- Weight bearing after cementless THA is controversial. Some surgeons routinely restrict weight bearing for 6 weeks, whereas others allow weight bearing as tolerated.
- Hip precautions are prescribed according to the approach.
  - Posterior approaches avoid flexion, internal rotation, and adduction, whereas anterior approaches avoid extension, external rotation, and adduction.
  - The hip precautions are discontinued at 6 weeks.
  - Some surgeons who perform the anterior approach have discontinued the use of traditional hip precautions.[46]
- The patient ambulates with the aid of crutches or a walker for several weeks and progresses to use of a cane. Generally, the cane is discontinued at 6 weeks.

OUTCOMES

- The survivorship of cementless THA components generally has been excellent, although isolated reports of high failure rates exist for certain designs, which have subsequently been abandoned. Most modern, uncemented acetabular and femoral components have a reported survivorship of 95% to 100% at mid- to long-term follow-up.[2,4,6,7,14–17,20,21,24,27,28,36,38,42–45,48,53]

- Overall survival of cementless acetabular components has ranged from 83% to 99.1% at 8.5 to 16.3 years of follow-up.[2,6,14,16,21,24,28,38,48,54]
- The reported survivorship of cementless femoral components has ranged from 82% to 100% at 6.6 to 17.5 years of follow-up.[2,4,15,17,20,27,28,36,42–45,53]
- The main limitation to long-term clinical success has been wear and subsequent osteolysis.

COMPLICATIONS

- Iatrogenic fracture
- Stress shielding of proximal bone
- Blood loss
- Infection
- Neurovascular injury
- Anesthetic and medical complications
- Loosening
- Osteolysis

REFERENCES

1. Abdel-Aal AM. Dissociation of modular total hip arthroplasty at different levels due to subsidence of cementless stems. A report of three cases. Orthopedics 2008;31:82.
2. Archibeck MJ, Berger RA, Jacobs JJ, et al. Second-generation cementless total hip arthroplasty: eight to eleven-year results. J Bone Joint Surg Am 2001;83:1666–1673.
3. Atwood SA, Patten EW, Bozic KJ, et al. Corrosion-induced fracture of a double-modular hip prosthesis: a case report. J Bone Joint Surg Am 2010;92(6):1522–1525.
4. Bojescul JA, Xenos JS, Callaghan JJ, et al. Results of porous-coated anatomic total hip arthroplasty without cement at fifteen years: a concise follow-up of a previous report. J Bone Joint Surg Am 2003;85:1079–1083.
5. Buly R. The S-ROM stem: versatility of stem/sleeve combinations and head options. Orthopedics 2005;28(9 suppl):S1025–S1032.
6. Callaghan JJ, Savory CG, O'Rourke MR, et al. Are all cementless acetabular components created equal? J Arthroplasty 2004;19(4 suppl 1):95–98.
7. Capello WN, D'Antonio JA, Feinberg JR, et al. Ten-year results with hydroxyapatite-coated total hip femoral components in patients less than fifty years old: a concise follow-up of a previous report. J Bone Joint Surg Am 2003;85:885–889.
8. Carter A, Mortazavi SMJ, Sheehan E, et al. Revision for instability: what are the predictors of failure? In: 78th Annual Meeting Proceedings. Rosemont, IL: American Academy of Orthopedic Surgeons, 2011:500–501.
9. Chu CM, Wang SJ, Lin LC. Dissociation of modular total hip arthroplasty at the femoral head-neck interface after loosening of the acetabular shell following hip dislocation. J Arthroplasty 2001;16:806–809.
10. Collier JP, Mayor MB, Jensen RE, et al. Mechanisms of failure of modular prostheses. Clin Orthop Relat Res 1992;285:129–139.
11. Collier JP, Mayor MB, Williams IR, et al. The tradeoffs associated with modular hip prostheses. Clin Orthop Relat Res 1995;311:91–101.
12. Cooper HJ, Della Valle CJ, Berger RA, et al. Corrosion at the head-neck taper as a cause for adverse local tissue reactions after total hip arthroplasty. J Bone Joint Surg Am 2012;94(18):1655–1661.
13. Dangles CJ, Altstetter CJ. Failure of the modular neck in a total hip arthroplasty. J Arthroplasty 2010;25(7):1169.e5–1169.e7.
14. Della Valle CJ, Berger RA, Shott S, et al. Primary total hip arthroplasty with a porous-coated acetabular component. A concise follow-up of a previous report. J Bone Joint Surg Am 2004;86:1217–1222.
15. Della Valle CJ, Paprosky WG. The middle-aged patient with hip arthritis: the case for extensively coated stems. Clin Orthop Relat Res 2002;(405):101–107.
16. Duffy GP, Prpa B, Rowland CM, et al. Primary uncemented Harris-Galante acetabular components in patients 50 years old or younger: results at 10 to 12 years. Clin Orthop Relat Res 2004;427:157–161.
17. Engh CA Jr, Claus AM, Hopper RH Jr, et al. Long-term results using the anatomic medullary locking hip prosthesis. Clin Orthop Relat Res 2001;393:137–146.
18. Gilbert JL, Buckley CA, Jacobs JJ. In vivo corrosion of modular hip prosthesis components in mixed and similar metal combinations. The effect of crevice, stress, motion, and alloy coupling. J Biomed Mater Res 1993;27(12):1533–1544.
19. Gill IP, Webb J, Sloan K, et al. Corrosion at the neck-stem junction as a cause of metal ion release and pseudotumour formation. J Bone Joint Surg Br 2012;94:895–900.
20. Grant P, Nordsletten L. Total hip arthroplasty with the Lord prosthesis. A long-term follow-up study. J Bone Joint Surg Am 2004;86:2636–2641.
21. Grubl A, Chiari C, Gruber M, et al. Cementless total hip arthroplasty with a tapered, rectangular titanium stem and a threaded cup: a minimum ten-year follow-up. J Bone Joint Surg Am 2002;84:425–431.
22. Grupp TM, Weik T, Bloemer W, et al. Modular titanium alloy neck adapter failures in hip replacement—failure mode analysis and influence of implant material. BMC Musculoskelet Disord 2010;11:3.
23. Hallab NJ, Anderson S, Caicedo M, et al. Immune responses correlate with serum-metal in metal-on-metal hip arthroplasty. J Arthroplasty 2004;19(8):88–93.
24. Herrera A, Canales V, Anderson J, et al. Seven to 10 years followup of an anatomic hip prosthesis: an international study. Clin Orthop Relat Res 2004;423:129–137.
25. Huot Carlson J, Citters D, Currier J, et al. Femoral stem fracture and in vivo corrosion of retrieved modular femoral hips. J Arthroplasty 2012;27(7):1389–1396.
26. Jacobs JJ, Gilbert JL, Urban RM. Corrosion of metal orthopaedic implants. J Bone Joint Surg Am 1998;80:268–282.
27. Kim YH, Kim JS, Oh SH, et al. Comparison of porous-coated titanium femoral stems with and without hydroxyapatite coating. J Bone Joint Surg Am 2003;85:1682–1688.
28. Kim YH, Oh SH, Kim JS. Primary total hip arthroplasty with a second-generation cementless total hip prosthesis in patients younger than fifty years of age. J Bone Joint Surg Am 2003;85:109–114.
29. Kindsfater KA, Politi JR, Dennis DA, et al. The incidence of femoral component version change in primary THA using the S-ROM femoral component. Orthopedics 2011;11:34–38.
30. Kop AM, Swarts ES. Corrosion of a hip stem with a modular neck taper junction. J Arthroplasty 2009;24(7):1019–1023.
31. Kurtz M, Kocagöz BS, Hanzlik MS, et al. Do ceramic femoral heads reduce taper fretting corrosion in hip arthroplasty? A retrieval study. Clin Orthop Relat Res 2013;471:3270–3282.
32. Lachiewicz PF, Soileau E, Ellis J. Modular revision for recurrent dislocation for primary or revision total hip arthroplasty. J Arthroplasty 2004;19(4):424–429.
33. Laine HJ, Lehto MUK, Moilanen T. Diversity of the proximal femoral medullary canal. JA Arthroplasty 2000;15:86–92.
34. Leigh W, O'Grady P, Lawson E, et al. Pelvic pseudotumor: an unusual presentation of an extra-articular granuloma in a well-fixed total hip arthroplasty. J Arthroplasty 2008;23:934–938.
35. Mao X, Tay GH, Godbolt DB, et al. Pseudotumor in a well-fixed metal-on-metal polyethylene uncemented hip arthroplasty. J Arthroplasty 2012;27(3):493–938.
36. Marshall AD, Mokris JG, Reitman RD, et al. Cementless titanium tapered-wedge femoral stem: 10- to 15-year follow-up. J Arthroplasty 2004;19:546–552.
37. Meftah M, Nicolaou N, Rodriguez JA. Metal allergy response to femoral head-neck corrosion after total hip replacement. Curr Orthop Pract 2010;21:530.
38. Moskal JT, Jordan L, Brown TE. The porous-coated anatomic total hip prosthesis: 11- to 13-year results. J Arthroplasty 2004;19:837–844.
39. Noble PC, Alexander JW, Lindahl LJ, et al. The anatomic basis of femoral component design. Clin Orthop Rel Res 1988;235:148–165.
40. Ohl MD, Whiteside LA, McCarthy DS, et al. Torsional fixation of a modular femoral hip component. Clin Orthop Relat Res 1993;287:135–141.
41. Otani T, Whiteside LA. Failure of cementless fixation of the femoral component in total hip arthroplasty. Orthop Clin North Am 1992;23:335–346.

42. Park MS, Choi BW, Kim SJ, et al. Plasma spray-coated Ti femoral component for cementless total hip arthroplasty. J Arthroplasty 2003;18:626–630.
43. Parvizi J, Keisu KS, Hozack WJ, et al. Primary total hip arthroplasty with an uncemented femoral component: a long-term study of the Taperloc stem. J Arthroplasty 2004;19:151–156.
44. Parvizi J, Sharkey PF, Hozack WJ, et al. Prospective matched-pair analysis of hydroxyapatite-coated and uncoated femoral stems in total hip arthroplasty: a concise follow-up of a previous report. J Bone Joint Surg Am 2004;86:783–786.
45. Parvizi J, Sullivan T, Duffy G, et al. Fifteen-year clinical survivorship of Harris-Galante total hip arthroplasty. J Arthroplasty 2004;19:672–677.
46. Peak EL, Parvizi J, Ciminiello M, et al. The role of patient restrictions in reducing the prevalence of early dislocation following total hip arthroplasty. A randomized, prospective study. J Bone Joint Surg Am 2005;87:247–253.
47. Pellicci PM, Hass SB. Disassembly of a modular femoral component during closed reduction of the dislocated femoral component. A case report. J Bone Joint Surg Am 1990;72:619–620.
48. Robertson A, Lavalette D, Morgan S, et al. The hydroxyapatite-coated JRI-furlong hip. Outcome in patients under the age of 55 years. J Bone Joint Surg Br 2005;87:12–15.
49. Skendzel JG, Blaha JD, Urquhart AG. Total hip arthroplasty modular neck failure. J Arthroplasty 2011;26(2):338.e1–338.e4.
50. Sporer SM, DellaValle C, Jacobs J, et al. A case of disassociation of a modular femoral neck trunion after total hip arthroplasty. J Arthroplasty 2006;21(6):918–921.
51. Star MJ, Colwell CW Jr, Donaldson WF, et al. Dissociation of modular hip arthroplasty components after dislocation: a report of three cases at differing dissociation levels. Clin Orthop Relat Res 1992;278:111–115.
52. Svensson O, Mathiesen EB, Reinholt FP, et al. Formation of a fulminant soft-tissue pseudotumor after uncemented hip arthroplasty. A case report. J Bone Joint Surg Am 1988;70:1238–1242.
53. Teloken MA, Bissett G, Hozack WJ, et al. Ten to fifteen-year follow-up after total hip arthroplasty with a tapered cobalt-chromium femoral component (trilock) inserted without cement. J Bone Joint Surg Am 2002;84:2140–2144.
54. Udomkiat P, Dorr LD, Wan Z. Cementless hemispheric porous-coated sockets implanted with press-fit technique without screws: average ten-year follow-up. J Bone Joint Surg Am 2002;84:1195–2000.
55. Werner SD, Bono JV, Nandi S, et al. Adverse tissue reactions in modular exchangeable neck implants: a report of two cases. J Arthroplasty 2013;28:543.e13–543.e15.
56. Woolson ST, Potteroff GT. Disassembly of a modular femoral prosthesis after dislocation of the femoral component. A case report. J Bone Joint Surg Am 1990;72:624–625.

CHAPTER 21

Total Hip Arthroplasty in Severe Deformity

Chloe E.H. Scott, Frazer A. Wade, and Colin R. Howie

DEFINITION

- Severe deformity is a congenital (acquired or iatrogenic) abnormality in the size and shape of the native acetabulum or proximal femur, and special techniques or implants must be employed by the surgeon to perform a primary total hip arthroplasty (THA).

ANATOMY

- Severe deformities around the hip typically result from pediatric hip disease, skeletal dysplasia, infection, metabolic bone disease, or trauma; or are the consequences of the treatment.
- The American Academy of Orthopaedic Surgeons' classification can be used to describe both acetabular-sided[11] and femoral-sided[12] deformity:
  - Acetabular deficiencies in deformity are frequently segmental (type I), cavitary (type II), or combined (type III).
  - Femoral abnormalities are typically malalignment (type IV) or stenosis (type V). The Paprosky classification does not include these deformities. However, occasionally, the proximal femur is completely absent.
- Although we focus on bony abnormality because of technical problems with fit and fix, deformed anatomy around the hip also alters local hip biomechanics with subsequent overloading and secondary osteoarthritis (OA) because of changes in the insertion and lever arm of muscles around the hip, particularly the abductors.
- Deformed anatomy at the hip affects the mechanical alignment of the entire lower limb and alters the biomechanics of the knee, ankle, and foot, and can lead to degenerative joint disease at these locations.
- Abnormal anatomy creates difficulties in approach (identifying true anatomy), implant selection (because of problems with endosteal anatomy), size, and the challenges of restoring lower limb biomechanics.
- The most common cause of hip deformity in adults is developmental dysplasia of the hip (DDH), where a small dysplastic acetabulum is coupled with an anteverted femur with a narrow canal which may have been treated with previous proximal femoral osteotomy, further complicating the deformity. DDH itself can be caused by congenital dysplasia (most commonly dislocation), the consequences of infantile infection, neuromuscular disease, or inflammatory joint disease.
- There are several classifications of deformity severity in DDH: Crowe and Hartofilakidis[25] are widely used classification systems and are composite for both sides of the hip. The Edinburgh system[17] uses similar criteria but divides the problems into femur and acetabulum to allow a detailed plan for each bone to be formulated (Table 1).

PATHOGENESIS

- Specific conditions and their treatment cause specific deformities and ultimately specific patterns of secondary OA and symptomatology.

Table 1 Classification System for Developmental Dysplasia of the Hip

Crowe

Grade	**I**	**II**	**III**	**IV**
Percent subluxation of femoral head	<50%	50%–74%	75%–100%	>100%
Proximal displacement of femur (% of pelvic height)	<10%	10%–15%	16%–20%	>20%

Hartofilakidis[25]

A	Dysplasia	Head in acetabulum
B	Low dislocation	Head in false acetabulum which contacts the true acetabulum
C	High dislocation	Head superiorly migrated and not in any contact with true acetabulum

Edinburgh[17]

Acetabulum			**Femur**		
AI	Dysplastic		**FI**	Dysplastic	
AII	Low dislocation		**FII**	Low dislocation	
AIIIa	Postsurgical	Retained metalwork	**FIIIa**	Postsurgical	Retained metalwork
AIIIb		No metalwork	**FIIIb**		No metalwork

Table 2 Congenital and Acquired Hip Conditions with Corresponding Characteristic Deformities

Etiology	Femoral Deformity	Acetabular Deformity
Pediatric hip disease		
DDH	Anteverted neck, short offset, diaphyseal canal stenosis, coxa valga	Small triangular shaped, deficient anterolateral cover with superior segmental defect, and large medial osteophyte in the true acetabulum
Perthes (other AVN)	Coxa magna, coxa plana, coxa breva +/− trochanteric overgrowth	Secondary acetabular dysplasia (congruent to deformed femoral head)
SCFE	Pistol grip deformity with external rotation	
Septic arthritis	Depends on age of onset 1. Similar to DDH with high dislocation 2. Similar to Perthes/AVN with coxa magna, plana, breva with GT overgrowth 3. Hip ankylosis	
Skeletal dysplasias		
MED/SED	Coxa magna, coxa plana, coxa breva	Similar to DDH when coxa magna and subluxation present (superior segmental defect) or protrusio when small head
Osteogenesis imperfecta	Fracture malunions, hyperplastic callus, anterior bowing	Protrusio
Diastrophic dysplasia	Narrow canal, anterior bow	Reduced bone stock
Congenital coxa vara	Varus with trochanteric overgrowth	
PFFD	Short femur, hypoplastic head	Dysplastic small head usually in dysplastic acetabulum
Metabolic bone disease		
Fibrous dysplasia	Shepherd crook femur	
Paget disease	Coxa vara, femoral bowing, wide canal	Protrusio
Trauma		
Fractures	Malalignment, canal stenosis	Heterotopic ossification

DDH, developmental dysplasia of the hip; AVN, avascular necrosis; SCFE, slipped capital femoral epiphysis; GT, greater trochanter; MED, multiple epiphyseal dysplasia; SED, spondyloepiphyseal dysplasia; PFFD, proximal femoral focal deficiency.

- Congenital and acquired causes of deformity around the hip joint are listed in Table 2.
- Osteotomies performed as realignment or conservative joint-sparing procedures to treat these conditions create new iatrogenic deformities and technical difficulties when hip reconstruction is considered:
  - Perthes—valgising proximal femoral osteotomy +/− trochanteric advancement
  - DDH—varising proximal femoral osteotomy, +/− derotation, +/− extension
  - Slipped capital femoral epiphysis (SCFE)—valgising proximal femoral osteotomy, +/− derotation, +/− flexion
  - Coxa vara—valgising proximal femoral osteotomy, +/− derotation
- Retained metalwork may be overgrown, broken, or obsolete. Careful planning is required to decide whether metalwork should be removed or retained and consideration given to the consequences of its removal.
- Deformity of the acetabulum and proximal femur disrupts hip kinematics and generates pain via the following:
  - Increased joint reaction force—secondary to abductor dysfunction and coupled with reduced joint contact area leads to high load per unit area and early failure with secondary OA.
  - Impingement of the following:
    - Large, abnormal nonconcentric femoral head on the acetabulum (**FIG 1**)
    - Overgrown greater trochanter (GT) on the ilium during hinged abduction
    - Highly dislocated femoral head with the false acetabulum or ilium
  - Leg length discrepancy (LLD) and altered gait kinematics, causing abnormal loading of the lumbar spine and lower limbs.
  - Lower limb mechanical axis disruption with overloading and subsequent OA of the knee and lumbar spine
- Deformities at different levels create different problems as outlined in Table 3.

NATURAL HISTORY

- Patients with deformity develop OA at an earlier age than those without deformity. The mean age at the time THA is performed in patients with deformity is 45 to 50 years old.[7,20,23]

PATIENT HISTORY AND PHYSICAL FINDINGS

- Patients with degenerative joint disease resulting from deformity around the hip present with exertional groin pain,

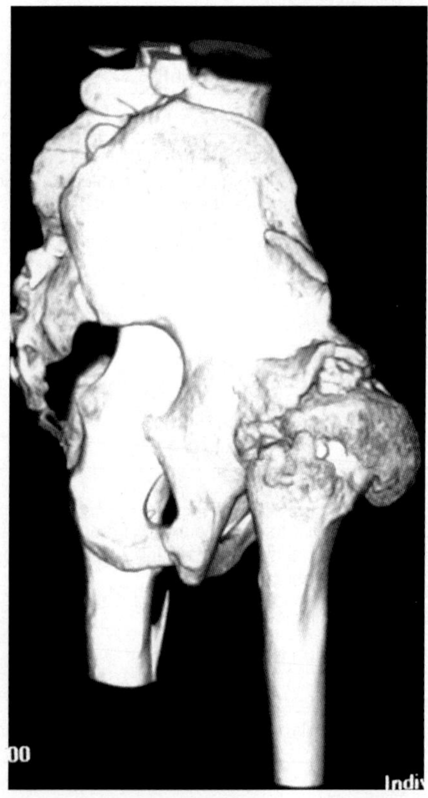

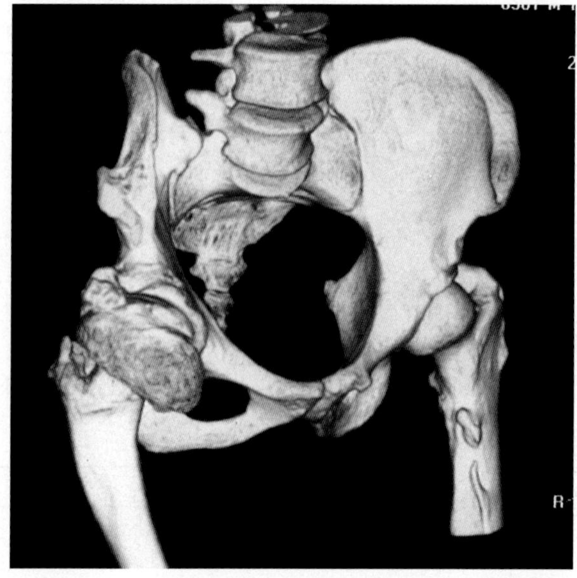

FIG 1 • 3-D reconstruction images of a low dislocation type (Hartofilakidis: B, Edinburgh AIIIb FII) dysplastic hip with a "mega-head" coxa magna, a large impinging anterior osteophyte, and an external rotation deformity of the proximal femur with posteriorly located GT. Accessing the hip joint through a posterior approach alone would not be possible.

knee pain (either referred or secondary long-leg arthritis), or lower back pain in addition to what may be a long-standing deformity, with or without LLD.

- Symptoms may have been present chronically with recent progression of functional limitations.
- Patients with underlying DDH may present with iliopsoas tendon snapping over an anteverted, uncovered, sometimes large, femoral head or secondary acetabular osteophyte (see **FIG 1**).
- Patients with congenital deformities may have associated conditions which must be considered; for example, fixed scoliosis (congenital, idiopathic, or acquired) or complex medical problems.
- Short stature/dwarfism will affect implant sizes.
- LLD may not be obvious in bilateral disease.
- Following fracture with or without fixation, degenerative joint disease with pain, stiffness, and functional limitation may have developed rapidly following the acute development of deformity and mechanical malalignment.
- Examination must include the following:
  - Observation of *gait* and Trendelenburg test with Medical Research Council (MRC) Scale for Muscle Strength grading of hip abductor power
  - Observation of surgical scars to indicate previous hip approaches
  - Hip range of motion—increased internal rotation and decreased external rotation is indicative of excessive femoral anteversion prior to the stiffness of advanced OA.
  - Anterior impingement test
  - Accurate documentation of true and apparent leg lengths
  - Neurologic assessment and documentation of lower limb vascular status
  - Examination of ipsilateral knee, lumbar spine, and contralateral hip
  - Examination of the spine and sitting posture to determine if any spinal curvature secondary to leg length problems is correctable. This is important in older patients in whom correcting an LLD may create an unstable spinal deformity.

IMAGING AND OTHER DIAGNOSTIC STUDIES

- Sufficient imaging should be performed to gain an understanding of the three-dimensional (3-D) anatomy of the deformity and facilitate planning of its correction and the implantation of THA components.
- In many cases for the experienced surgeon, this requires plain radiographs only:
  - Weight-bearing anteroposterior (AP) pelvis plus lateral of hip
  - Full-length femur AP and lateral to assess femoral deformity and anterior femoral bow
  - Judet views to assess anterior and posterior columns in acetabular deformity
  - Standing hip-knee-ankle x-rays to assess leg lengths and knee joint level. Some patients who have undergone surgery around the hip in childhood may experience overgrowth distally.
- Computed tomography (CT) scan with or without 3-D reconstruction (see **FIG 1**) enables visualization of multiplanar deformities in addition to assessment of acetabular bone stock, femoral canal diameter, GT position, and femoral neck version relative to the condylar axis of the knee (**FIG 2**). This allows detailed planning to be carried out.

DIFFERENTIAL DIAGNOSIS

- See Pathogenesis section.

Table 3 The Effects of Deformity at Different Femoral Levels with Proposed Surgical Solutions

Deformity	Problem	Solution
Femoral neck		
Angular varus	Abductor defunctioning ↑ JRF LLD if unilateral	↑ neck length and valgise Bilateral—maintain length Unilateral—lengthen to normal side
Torsional version	↑ anteversion (DDH) "normal" acetabulum Anteversion with matching retroversion acetabulum	Cemented stem or cementless EPC stem +/− derotation ST osteotomy Consider altering acetabular version to match femoral anteversion (particularly important if considering surface replacement when femoral anteversion cannot be corrected)
Greater trochanter		
Overgrowth	Exposure and femoral canal access GT fracture	
High riding	Impingement and levering instability Abductor defunctioning ↑ JRF	Trochanteric osteotomy and advancement
Posterior	Nonphysiologic abductor orientation with relative defunctioning and ↑JRF Persisting Trendelenburg gait	Derotation ST osteotomy or trochanteric transfer both bringing trochanter into same plane as the transverse axis of knee
Metaphyseal		
Many geometries	Poor metaphyseal fit for proximally coated cementless stems Difficult diaphyseal access for stem in metaphyseal–diaphyseal offset Deviated lower limb mechanical axis	Custom-designed femoral component With diaphyseal fixation—cemented or cementless EPC or fluted tapered +/− ST osteotomy
Diaphyseal		
Torsion Angulation Translation Stenosis	Stem alignment Mechanical axis restoration	Diaphyseal fixation stem to bypass multiplanar ST osteotomy

JRF, joint reaction force; LLD, leg length discrepancy; DDH, developmental dysplasia of the hip; EPC, endoprosthetic replacement component; ST, subtrochanteric; GT, greater trochanter.
From Berry DJ. Total hip arthroplasty in patients with proximal femoral deformity. Clin Orthop Relat Res 1999;(369):262–272.

NONOPERATIVE MANAGEMENT

- As for primary hip OA, nonoperative management consists of simple analgesia, weight loss, activity modification, physical therapy, and orthotics to address LLD.

SURGICAL MANAGEMENT

- Surgical management is indicated when conservative management has failed. The goals of surgical management are as follows:
  - Restoration of hip kinetics and kinematics, including hip center, acetabular and femoral version, abductor length, and GT position
  - Correction of lower limb mechanical alignment
  - Reconstruction of femoral and acetabular integrity to provide prosthesis containment
  - Joint stability
- Achieving these goals may require adding acetabular bone stock and correcting deformities with multiplanar osteotomies.
- Subtrochanteric osteotomy should be performed if
  - Restoring the hip center will lengthen the limb by greater than 4 cm, producing sciatic nerve traction
  - Significant angular/rotational/translational deformity prohibits stem access down the diaphysis or disrupts the mechanical axis of the lower limb.
  - Removal of awkward metalwork under direct vision
- Use implants with which you are familiar for these difficult cases, make the hip look normal, and conduct the procedure as usual. Both cemented[23] and cementless stems with diaphyseal engagement[31] have been used successfully in deformity cases in combination with subtrochanteric osteotomy. Our practice is to use a cemented, collarless, polished tapered stem routinely or a cementless, modular, fluted tapered stem if required. Custom-made implants may be necessary in rare cases, particularly if the endosteal anatomy is abnormal.
- Cemented stems provide immediate stability in osteopenic bone with a narrow canal. They also provided proximal metaphyseal stability if osteotomy is required. Cemented stems do not depend on metaphyseal fit and fill to obtain stability, as proximally coated cementless stems do, and can be difficult in these cases.
- Modular cementless femoral reconstruction systems with metaphyseal sleeves and long stems can correct femoral version independently of metaphyseal fit and fill,[3,41] but they do

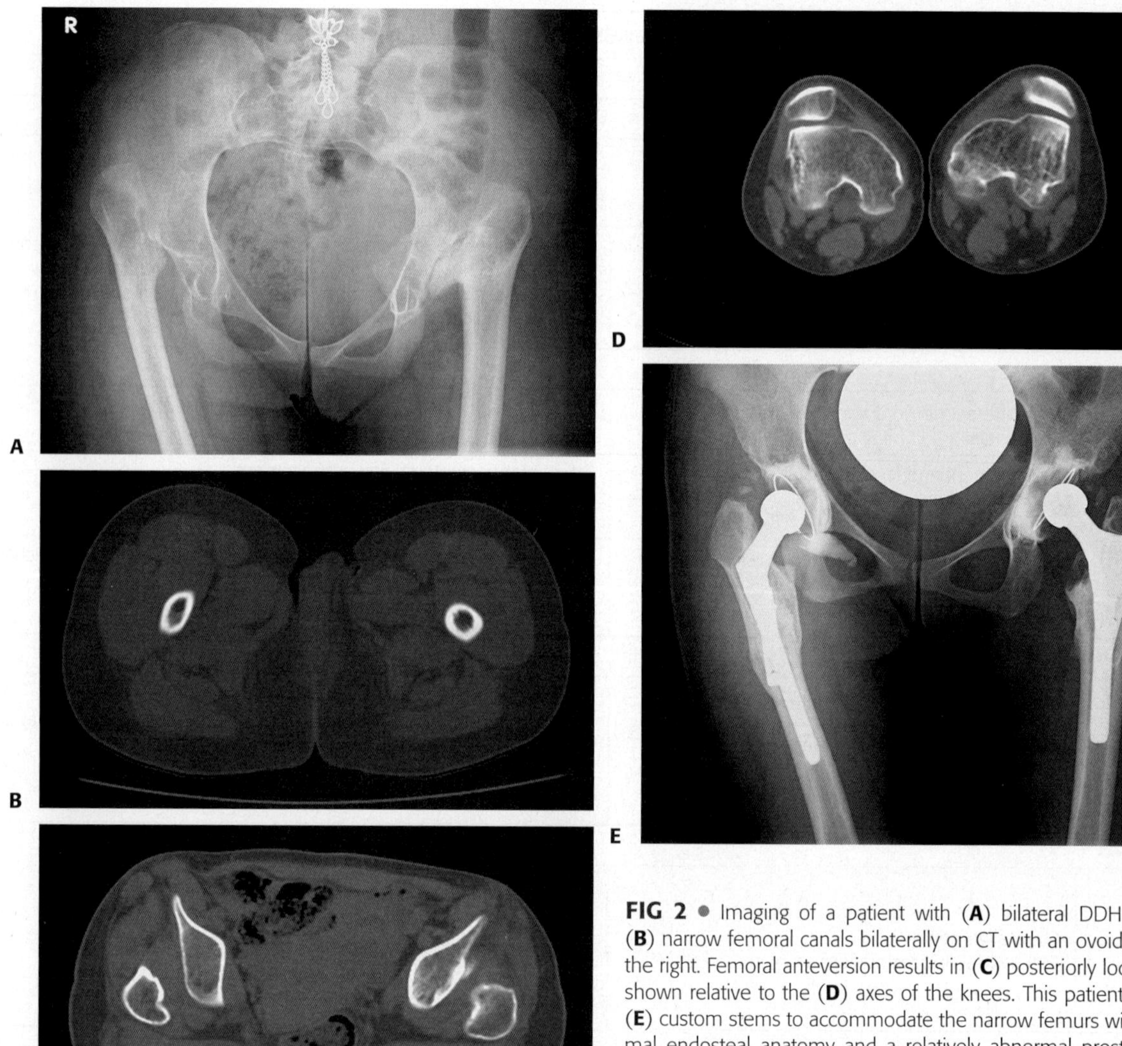

FIG 2 • Imaging of a patient with (**A**) bilateral DDH showing (**B**) narrow femoral canals bilaterally on CT with an ovoid canal on the right. Femoral anteversion results in (**C**) posteriorly located GTs shown relative to the (**D**) axes of the knees. This patient required (**E**) custom stems to accommodate the narrow femurs with abnormal endosteal anatomy and a relatively abnormal prosthetic anteversion angle required. Subtrochanteric shortening osteotomies were performed to avoid overlengthening soft tissues, with derotation to correct alignment of the hips with the knees and improve the abductor function.

not alter the position of the GT relative to the distal femoral condyles and thus do not restore physiologic abductor orientation or the mechanical alignment of the lower limb unless coupled with a trochanteric or subtrochanteric osteotomy (**FIG 3**). The diaphyseal stem provides relative stability in comparison to an osteotomy, but rotational stability depends on the diaphyseal cortical engagement of polished flutes only, with no ongrowth/ingrowth potential. Metaphyseal capture following a subtrochanteric osteotomy can be difficult with an incidence of nonunion that can be reduced by plating the osteotomy.

- Short-stem cementless components require a long, intact neck for rotational support and good-quality metaphyseal bone stock.[38] This is often absent in femoral deformity. These implants cannot correct for version or leg length and are not recommended when femoral deformity is present, although their short stem may seem attractive.
- Custom-made stems accommodate rather than correct deformity. They can be essential in very narrow femoral canals (see **FIG 2**) but are often also used in metaphyseal level deformity. When they are used to accommodate rather than correct metaphyseal level deformity, they do not restore mechanical alignment and are therefore exposed to high-bending moments with associated risks of aseptic loosening and cantilever bending. Failure to restore the mechanical axis of the lower limb can hasten ipsilateral knee OA development.
- Resurfacing does not correct deformity, particularly the often extreme femoral anteversion in DDH. In less severe cases, the acetabular version can be altered to accommodate excessive version of the femoral neck, but this must be planned if the acetabulum is inserted before the femoral head.
- Scarring from previous surgery can compromise ideal skin incision location and make exposure difficult with increased need for trochanteric osteotomy to obtain access to the diaphysis and difficulty reaming the femoral canal in up to 35% of cases.[6,16]
- Removal of retained metalwork adds to surgical time. Fresh screw holes act as stress risers and allow cement extrusion.

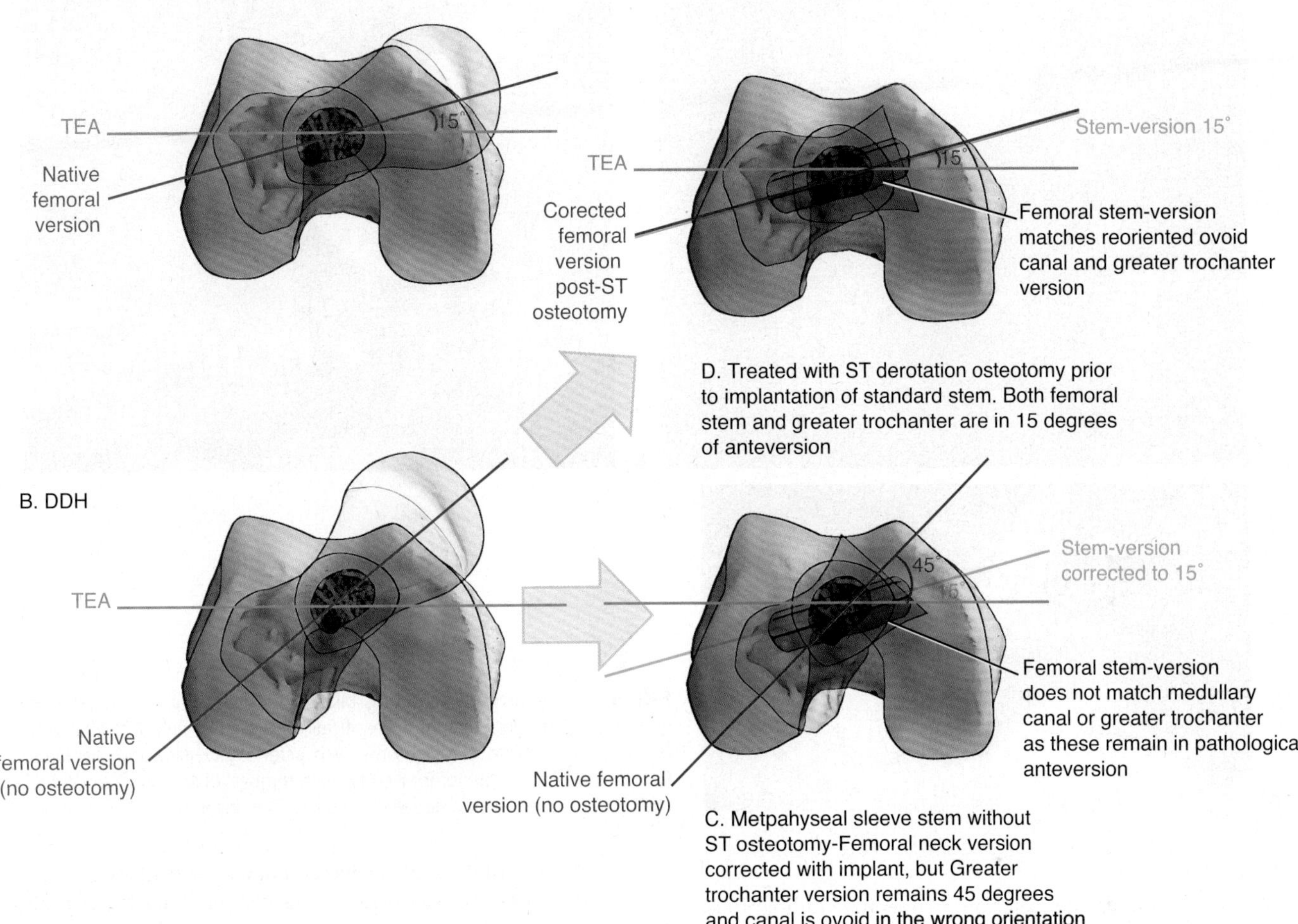
A. Normal
TEA
15°
Native
femoral
version
TEA
Corected
femoral
version
post-ST
osteotomy
15°
Stem-version 15°
Femoral stem-version
matches reoriented ovoid
canal and greater trochanter
version
D. Treated with ST derotation osteotomy prior
to implantation of standard stem. Both femoral
stem and greater trochanter are in 15 degrees
of anteversion
B. DDH
TEA
Native
femoral version
(no osteotomy)
45°
15°
Stem-version
corrected to 15°
Femoral stem-version
does not match medullary
canal or greater trochanter
as these remain in pathological
anteversion
Native femoral
version (no osteotomy)
C. Metpahyseal sleeve stem without
ST osteotomy-Femoral neck version
corrected with implant, but Greater
trochanter version remains 45 degrees
and canal is ovoid in the wrong orientation

FIG 3 • Diagrams to show the orientation in the transverse plane of proximal, distal, and diaphyseal femur in (**A**) normal anatomy and (**B**) DDH. Hip replacement using a modular metaphyseal sleeve (**C**) corrects femoral neck version, but the GT remains excessively anteverted relative to the transepicondylar axis (TEA) of the distal femur and the narrow ovoid canal is similarly maloriented. **D.** Subtrochanteric derotation osteotomy prior to standard femoral stem insertion restores GT alignment in addition to neck version and diaphyseal rotation.

They also act as stress risers for uncemented prosthesis, which rely on high initial hoop stresses. Although consideration should be given on removing metalwork as a separate earlier procedure, the implants are often overgrown with bone, and any defect created by removal rarely heals (**FIG 4**). Plate removal in particular can leave a gutter in the cortex, which is difficult to manage. Leaving the plate but removing the screws either in the usual manner or cutting endosteally under direct vision at the time of THA is recommended. Overdrilling leaves large defects in what is usually a small femur.

Approach Planning

- Previous surgery may determine skin incision.
- Trochanteric osteotomy (standard, extended, or subtrochanteric) may be required for access to the femur.
- Excessive anteversion and severe arthritis leading to stiffness or a megahead can lead to difficulties on dislocation of the hip (see **FIG 1**). A combined anterior and posterior approach should be used to release tight structures and identify bone anatomy before cutting bone.

Bone Quantity and Quality

- Acetabular defects may require bone stock restoration—is adequate autograft available or will trabecular metal or allograft be required?
- Medialization of the acetabulum is well reported with good results.[18]
- Cemented implants may be more appropriate in osteopenic bone.

Implant Type

- Templating is essential to decide whether standard, revision, or custom-made implants are necessary. A knowledge of the range of implants available is essential (eg, implants for the Asia Pacific market are often much smaller than for Western implants).
- Nonprimary implants have been required in up to 40% of femoral deformity cases[31]; however, this is not our experience with cemented prostheses.

Implant Size

- The acetabulum is often small anteroposteriorly and the femoral canal is narrow.

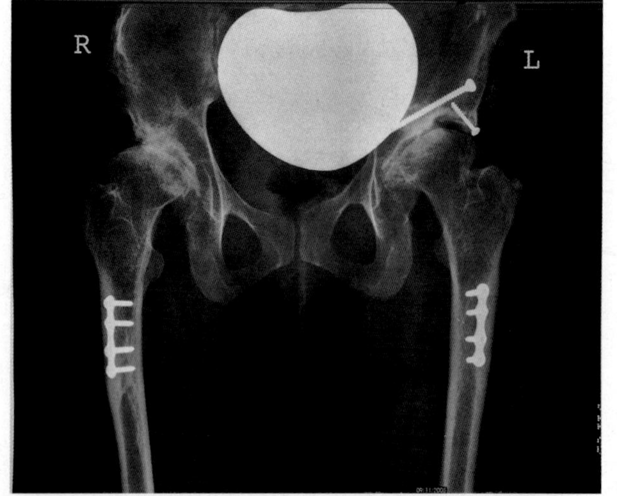

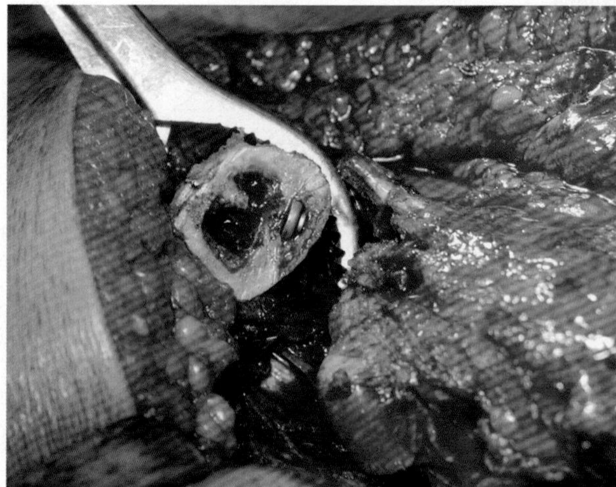

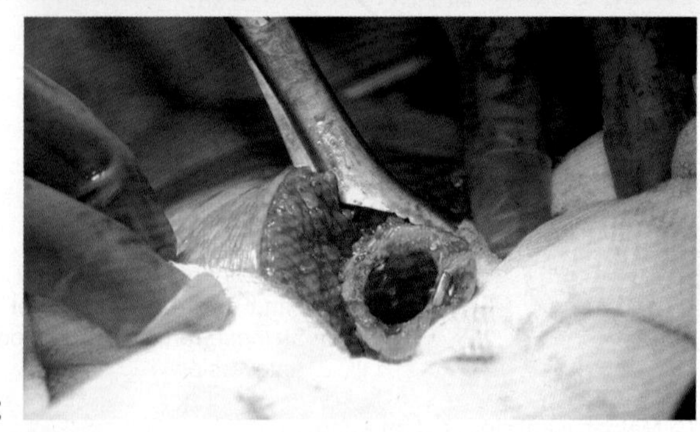

FIG 4 • A. Radiograph showing bilateral dysplastic hips with retained metalwork (Left hip, Edinburgh classification FIIIa, AIIIa; right hip, FIIIa, AII). **B.** Incarcerated plate at osteotomy with screws traversing the diaphysis. **C.** Plate left in situ in the femoral cortex with removal of screws via endosteal cutting to restore the intramedullary canal for THA insertion.

Acetabulum

- Measure acetabular diameter on preoperative radiographs.
- Ensure that small enough implants are available.
- This will also determine head size and may affect bearing selection.
- Use cemented for extremely small acetabula, and remove polyethylene from the anterior and posterior surface with a knife to fit.

Femur

- Measure canal diameter on preoperative radiographs/CT.
- Organize custom stems if endosteum is very narrow or abnormally shaped.
- Ensure that smaller stems are available to accommodate small, narrow femurs.
- Longer stems should be available if subtrochanteric osteotomy is planned, fracture/perforation is a significant risk, or screw holes will be present in removed metalwork.
- Long stems must be slim to accommodate narrow femurs but long enough to bypass the osteotomy site, screw holes, and fracture site by two cortical diameters.
- Usually, there is considerable anterior femoral bowing and stem entry, and length must be planned to avoid anterior perforation.

Other Hardware

- Retained metalwork
  - Metalwork is often still in situ from previous realignment, joint-sparing procedures, or fracture fixation.
  - Identify manufacturers and ensure that appropriate removal instrumentation is present.
  - Ensure that metal cutting equipment is available.
  - If plates are overgrown, consider retaining the plate but removing screws (see **FIG 4**).
  - Consider subtrochanteric femoral osteotomy to remove retained screws under direct vision.
- Wiring systems
  - Required for diaphyseal fracture prophylaxis if using cementless stem
  - Need to be available due to the high rate of intraoperative fracture (particularly when using cementless stems)
- Osteotomy stabilization
  - Plate and unicortical screws for subtrochanteric osteotomy stabilization
  - Temporary double plating to allow insertion may be necessary

Heterotopic Ossification Prophylaxis

- Consider if previous heterotropic ossification (HO), previous fracture surgery, or if trochanteric osteotomy is planned.

Consent

- Consent is to discuss with the patient the increased risk of complications (leg length, neurovascular complication, implant loosening, and fracture) and patient expectations need to be managed accordingly.

Bilateral Deformity

- In many cases, bilateral deformity exists, especially in DDH. Performing one THA may worsen LLD, and plans to schedule the second THA should be made early (see **FIG 4**) or acceptance of a shoe raise agreed (**FIG 5**).

Positioning

- The patient is placed in the lateral position with a posterior lumbosacral support and an anterior support placed on to the anterior superior iliac spine to stabilize the pelvis.

Approach

- Skin incisions from previous surgery are used with scar excision where possible to improve cosmesis.
- A posterior approach maintains abductor integrity, provides a circumferential view of the acetabulum, and is extensile to facilitate femoral osteotomy. Performing trochanteric osteotomy may defunction abductors in these extreme cases (reattachment is difficult), and subtrochanteric osteotomy, although sometimes necessary prior to dislocation, creates multiple fragments which can be difficult to manage while preparing the acetabulum.

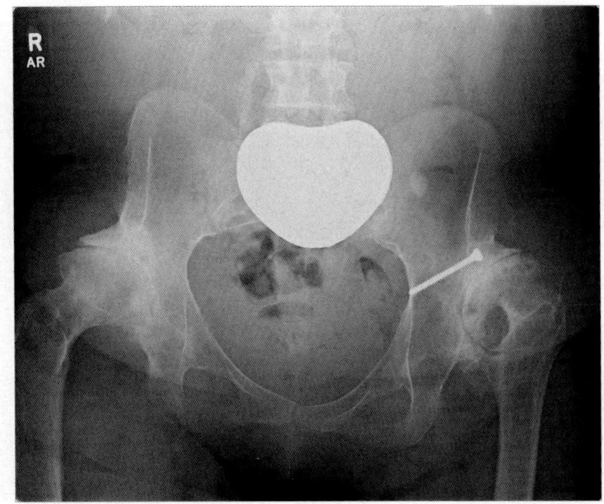

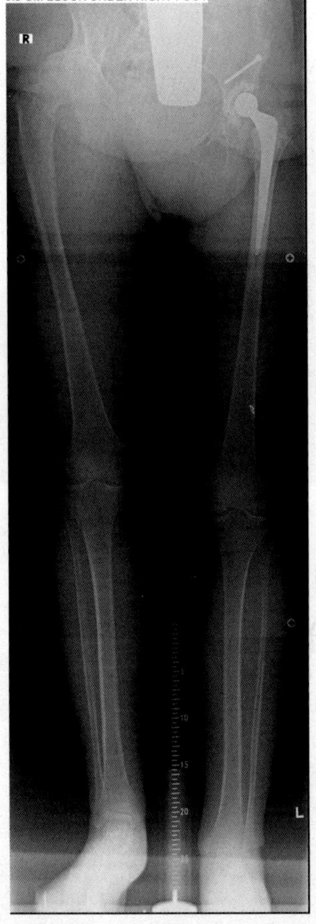

FIG 5 • Bilateral DDH with (**A**) low complete dislocation on the right with previous shelf osteotomy, coxa magna, and varising rotational flexion femoral osteotomy leaving the GT posteriorly (Hartofilakidis B; Edinburgh AIIIb, FIIIb). On the left, a previous pelvic osteotomy with a complete dislocation but a normal, small acetabulum (Hartofilakidis B; Edinburgh AIIIa, FII). **B.** Left THA with shortening derotation femoral osteotomy exacerbates LLD, pending right THA.

TECHNIQUES

Exposure

- A posterior approach, with the option of a direct anterior through the same incision, gives a circumferential view of the true acetabulum, preserves the abductors facilitating the soft tissue tension method for judging resection length in femoral osteotomy, and is extensile.
- Combining the posterior and true anterior approaches allows accurate neck resection in situ (or debulking of the often anteriorly subluxed femoral head) under direct vision prior to dislocation. This is particularly important in the stiff, fixed, externally rotated hip, which cannot be accessed from the back alone (see **FIG 1**).
- Occasionally, the head can be almost subcutaneous and removal of the anterior acetabular osteophyte is necessary to avoid impingement in flexion.
- Iliopsoas release from lesser trochanter allows proximal femoral descent.
- Total capsulectomy allows the proximal femur to be brought distally for hip center restoration.
- The sciatic nerve is usually found running over the ischium and can be traced back to the sciatic notch. It need not be mobilized unless a previous pelvic osteotomy has caused scarring and adhesions.
- The femoral bundle is rarely identified even when a direct anterior approach is added.

TECHNIQUES

Acetabular Reconstruction—Identifying the True Acetabulum in Severe DDH

- Indication: DDH or proximal femoral focal deficiency (PFFD) is where the femoral head does not articulate with the true acetabulum (**TECH FIG 1**).
- The femoral head may be articulating with a false acetabulum or may even be trapped in the abductor musculature in high dislocations.
- In these circumstances, the true acetabulum is often small and triangular with a narrow entry. Overhanging osteophytes close down the entry, but the transverse ligament is a constant indicator of the true acetabulum location.
- Medial osteophyte must be removed to identify the true floor.

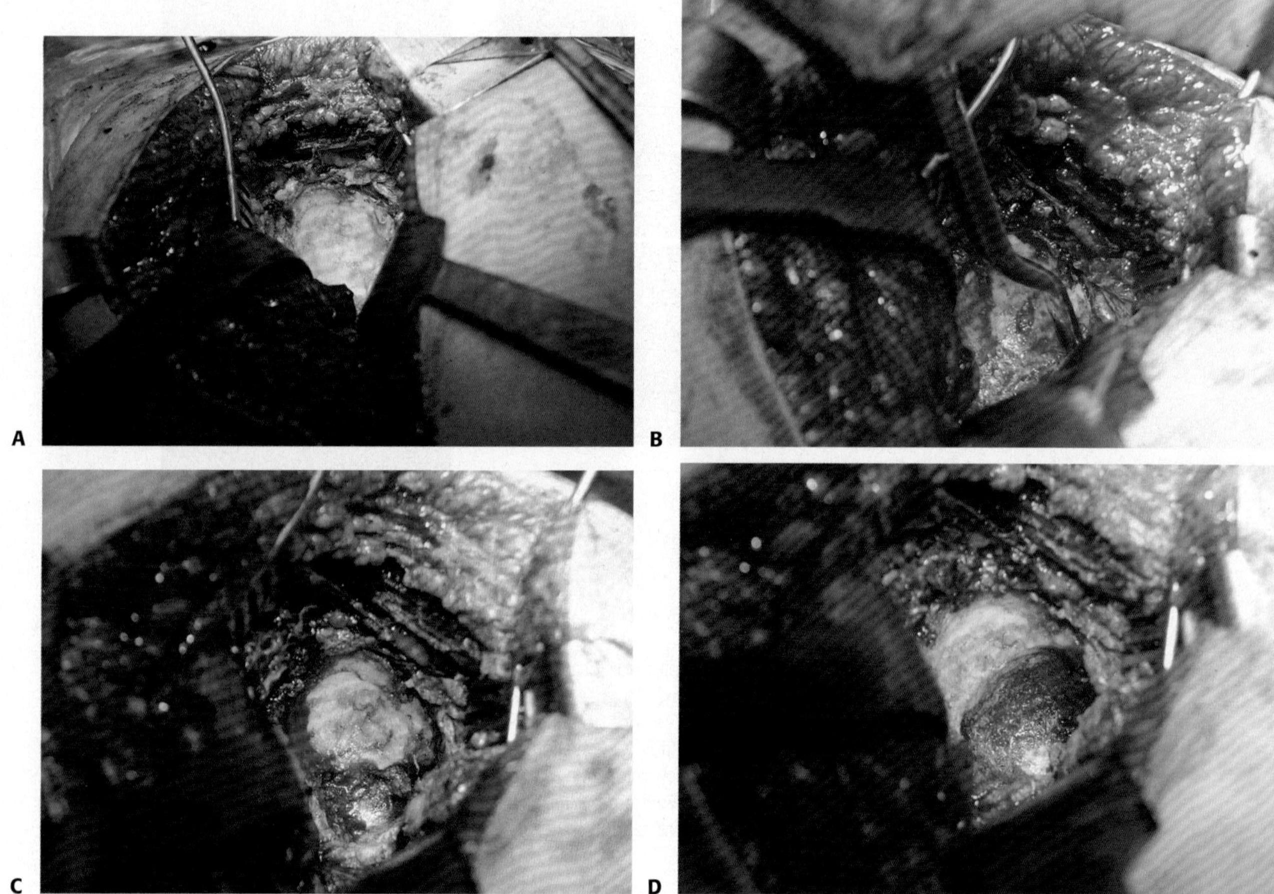

TECH FIG 1 • **A.** Uncontained superior acetabular defect in DDH with low dislocation. **B.** Gouge to remove medial wall osteophyte and identify the true floor. **C.** True floor and quadrilateral plate exposed after removal of osteophyte. **D.** Sequential reaming of true acetabulum delineates the extent of the superior defect.

Acetabular Reconstruction—Femoral Head Autograft

- Indication: Recreating an anatomic hip center when the resulting position is associated with anterosuperior roof deficiency of greater than 20%.
- The true acetabulum is prepared as for a standard cemented acetabular component (see **TECH FIG 1**). The final acetabular reamings are kept as graft for the procedure later.
- The superior segmental defect is delineated by inserting a trial cup (**TECH FIG 2A,B**). The defect is prepared using gouges to remove fibrocartilage. The femoral head is similarly prepared by removing fibrocartilage.
- A generous wedge of the resected femoral head, which came from the defect, is cut (**TECH FIG 2C,D**) and placed with its sclerotic convexity against the prepared concave defect with the reamings from the true acetabulum placed in the bed to improve contact. This is held temporarily with a K-wire (**TECH FIG 2E**) and fixed with two superiorly placed partially threaded cancellous screws.
- Any autograft overhanging the true acetabulum is then reamed away (**TECH FIG 2F**), leaving an acetabular bulk autograft supported by host bone and a contained socket into which a standard acetabular component can be cemented using third-generation cementing techniques (**TECH FIG 2G,H**).

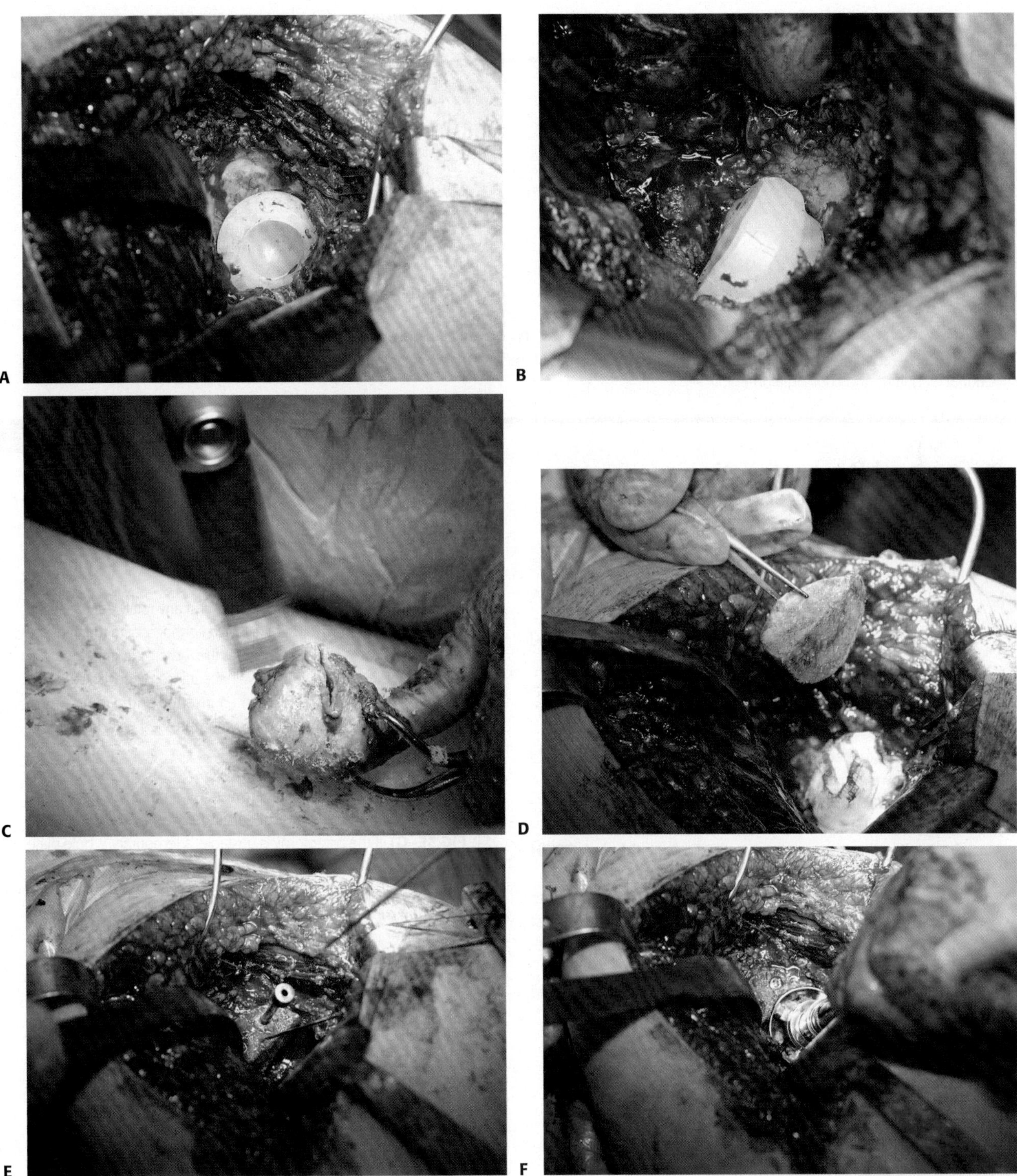

TECH FIG 2 • **A.** After preparing and reaming the true acetabulum, a trial cup is inserted to delineate the superior defect. **B.** Orthogonal view of acetabular deficiency. **C.** An appropriately sized wedge is cut from the resected femoral head. **D.** Wedge autograft. **E.** K-wire stabilization of wedge and drilling for partially threaded cancellous screw fixation. **F.** Reaming of overhanging graft edge. *(continued)*

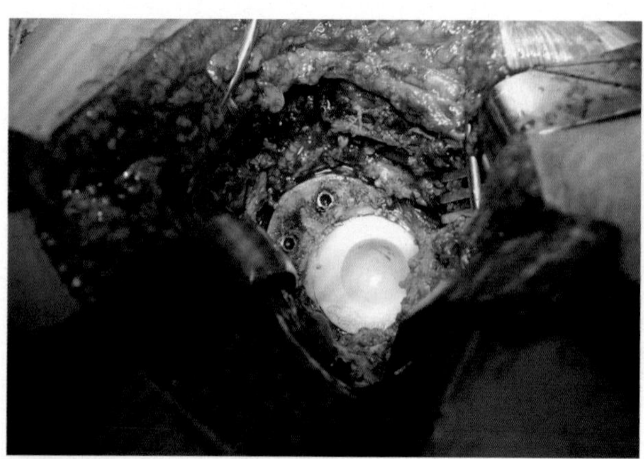
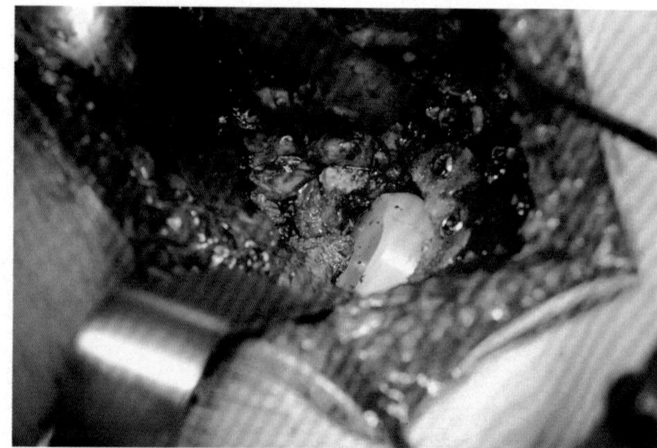

TECH FIG 2 • *(continued)* **G.** Final position of cemented cup with femoral head autograft. **H.** Orthogonal view showing reconstruction of the superior acetabulum and cup containment.

Femoral Reconstruction—Subtrochanteric Shortening Osteotomy

- Indication: When recreating an anatomic hip center, subtrochanteric shortening osteotomy will lengthen the lower limb by greater than 3 cm with risk of sciatic nerve palsy.
- Femoral length, angulation, and GT position can be addressed concurrently using this technique.
- It reduces the need for custom implants (although small sizes may be required) and restores lower limb mechanical alignment.
- Single-plane osteotomy is easier for correction of complex deformity than a stepped osteotomy and requires a shorter stem to bypass it by a minimum of two shaft diameters.
- Perform acetabular implantation first.
- Identify the level for osteotomy distal to the lesser trochanter.
- Create a transverse osteotomy perpendicular to the shaft (**TECH FIG 3A**).
- The proximal femoral fragment is prepared with serial rasps to accept the femoral component which best fits with the largest offset. A burr can be used in a retrograde manner at the osteotomy site to aid this.
- The proximal fragment with rasp and trial head in situ is reduced into the acetabulum (**TECH FIG 3B**).
- Longitudinal traction is applied to the distal fragment and the amount of overlap of proximal and distal fragments is noted and marked. This length is resected perpendicular to the diaphysis (**TECH FIG 3C**). The burr can then be used in an antegrade fashion on the distal fragment if needed to remove any sclerotic or stenotic bone under direct vision.
- The resultant bone ends are opposed, and any rotational correction is made to align the GT 15 degrees from orthogonal to the transepicondylar axis of the knee. This restores the anatomic alignment of the direction of pull of the abductors with the transepicondylar knee axis.
- The appropriate femoral trial is then inserted and passed across the osteotomy and the osteotomy compressed with fracture reduction forceps (**TECH FIG 3D**).
- A 5- or 6-hole, one-third tubular plate or dynamic compression plate (DCP) is applied posteriorly with a combination of unicortical and bicortical screws as the in situ femoral trial allows (**TECH FIG 3E–G**). If the osteotomy is unstable, a temporary 2-hole plate can be applied at right angles to stabilize the construct temporarily.
- The stem is then cemented using third-generation techniques while the assistant's fingers wrap around the femur anteriorly at the osteotomy site to prevent cement extrusion and provide tension against the plate and thus anterior compression at the osteotomy (**TECH FIG 3H,I**).
- After curing, morselized autologous graft is packed around the osteotomy site and the plate is left in situ.

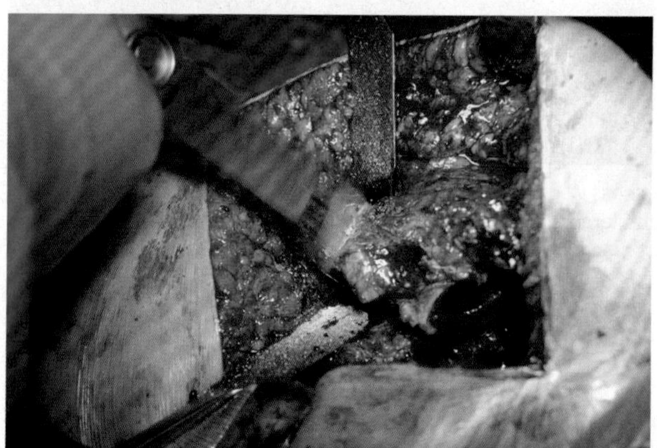
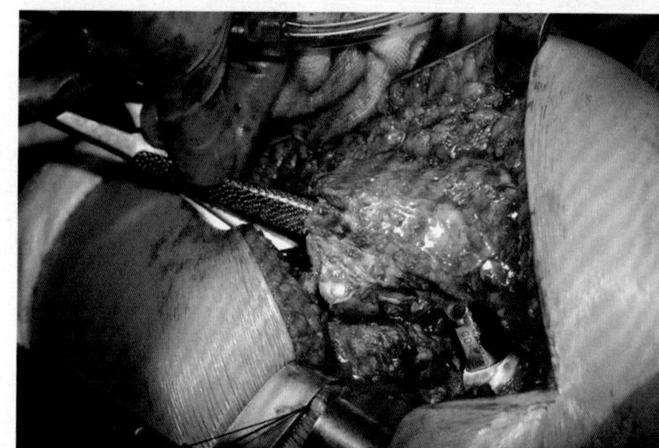

TECH FIG 3 • **A.** Perpendicular subtrochanteric osteotomy. **B.** Hip reduced to judge resection level on femur. *(continued)*

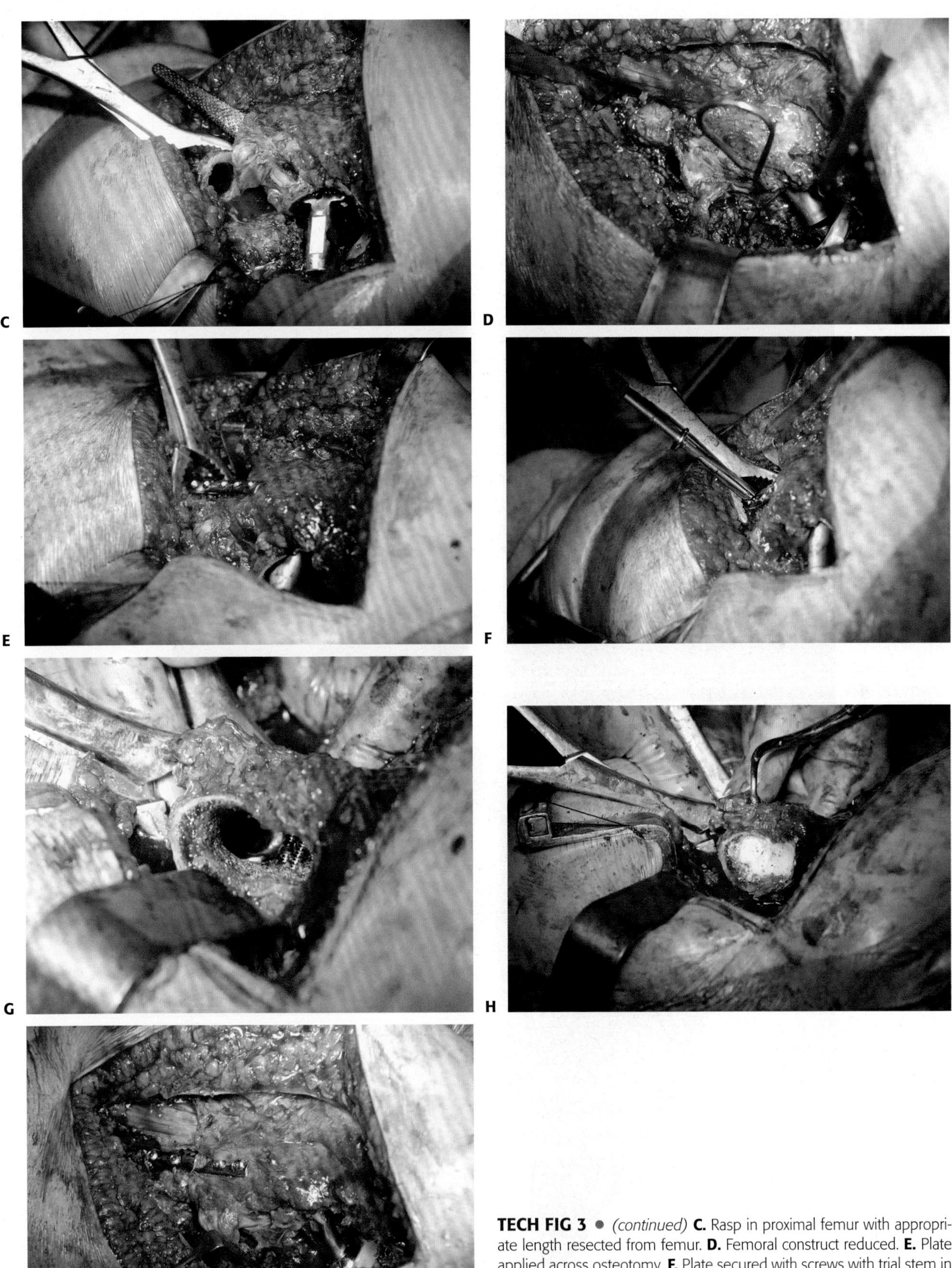

TECH FIG 3 • *(continued)* **C.** Rasp in proximal femur with appropriate length resected from femur. **D.** Femoral construct reduced. **E.** Plate applied across osteotomy. **F.** Plate secured with screws with trial stem in situ. **G.** Uni- and bicortical screws in situ with patent canal. **H.** Cementing with finger pressure around osteotomy. **I.** Final reduced construct—cemented THA.

TECHNIQUES

Femoral Reconstruction—Subtrochanteric Osteotomy with Derotation and angulation

- Indication: Angular deformity of femur requiring correction in order to implant stem and correct mechanical axis
- It is similar to shortening osteotomy, except the osteotomy made in the distal fragment should be oblique to correct angulation (**TECH FIG 4B**).
- The distal part has longitudinal traction applied, and the GT proximally is placed in the transepicondylar plane as before (**TECH FIG 4C**). The obliquity of the required osteotomy is determined by the overlap of the proximal osteotomy with the distal fragment (**TECH FIG 4D**). This is marked and the bone is resected accordingly.
- The distal fragment is prepared as before and the osteotomy is stabilized with a plate as before (**TECH FIG 4E–G**).

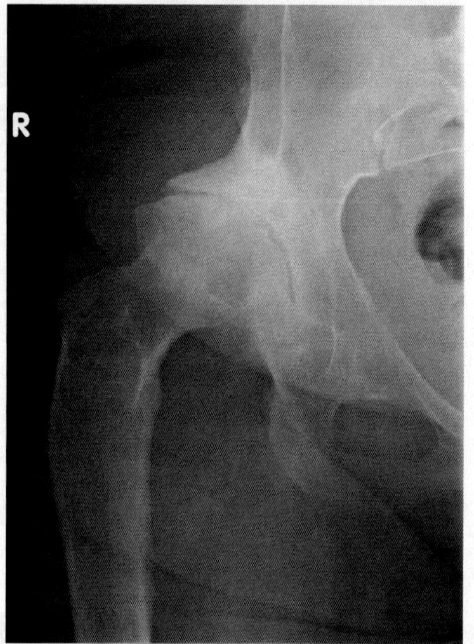

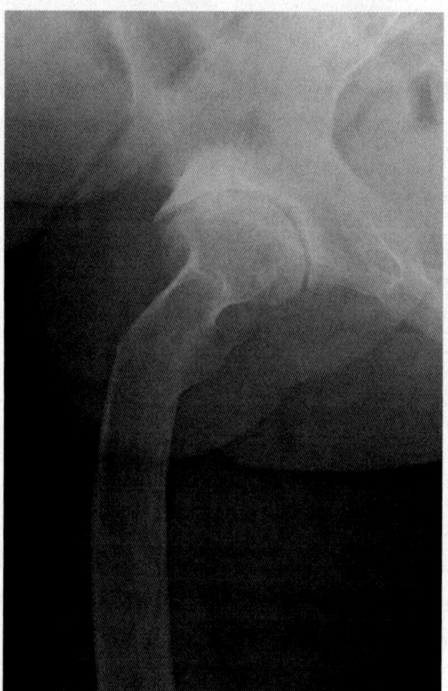

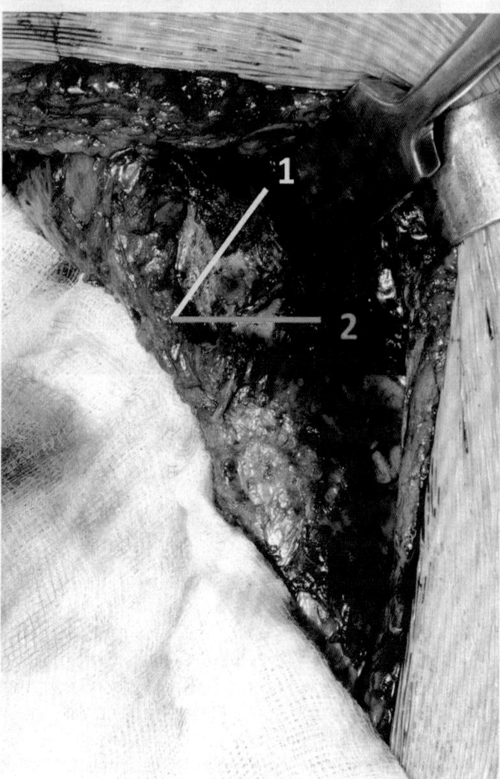

TECH FIG 4 • **A.** AP right hip (Edinburgh AIIIb, FIIIb). **B.** Lateral view showing complex proximal femoral deformity resultant of a varising rotational flexion femoral osteotomy. **C.** Proximal femur at posterior approach with marked bowing deformity. Planned osteotomies are marked. *(continued)*

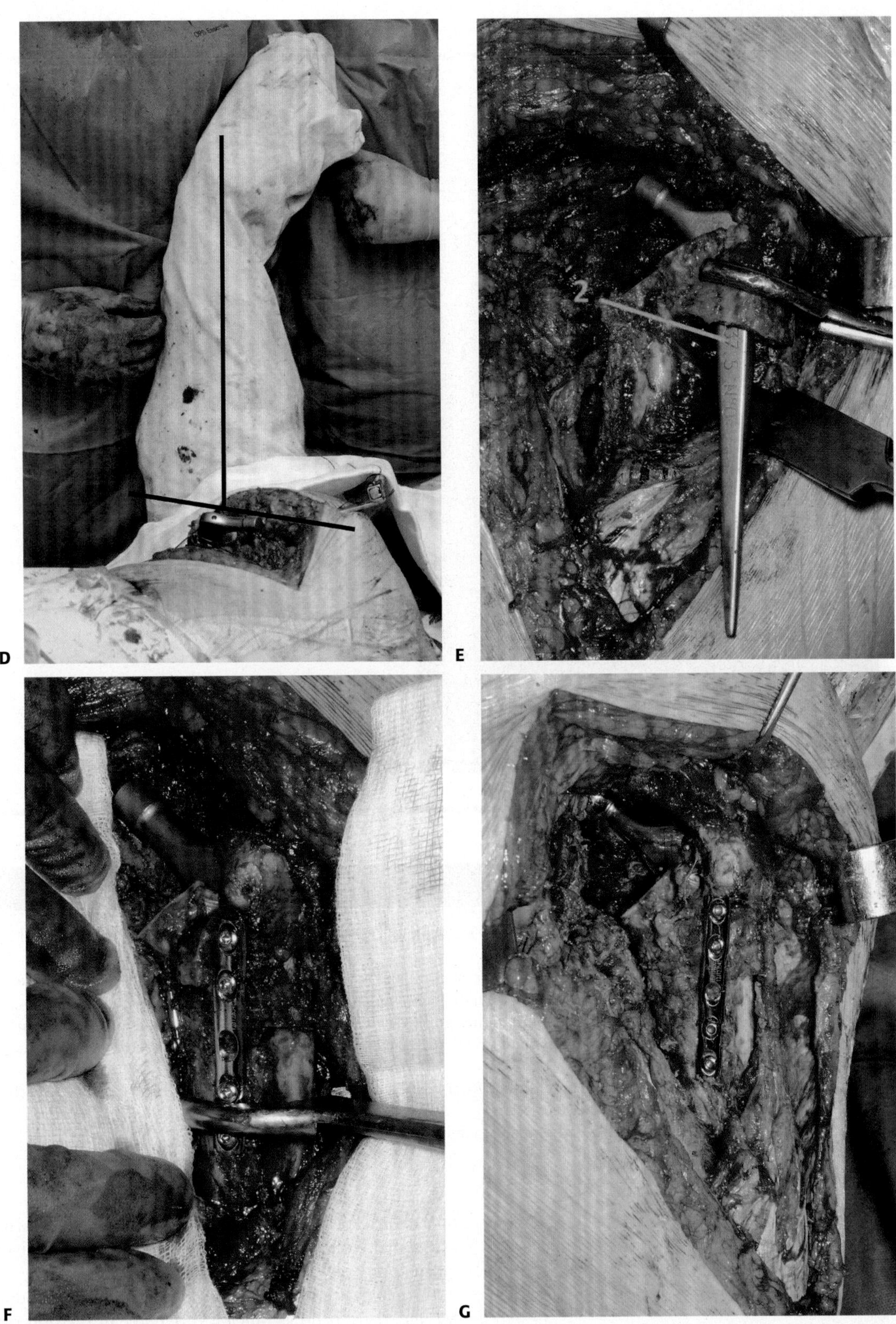

TECH FIG 4 • *(continued)* **D.** Following osteotomy 1 and proximal femoral preparation to accept a trial stem, femoral derotation and stem version are referenced from the long axis of the tibia and the knee TEA. **E.** With the desired version and length, the proximal femur with trial in situ is overlapped on the distal femur to clarify the angle of osteotomy 2 and amount of shortening required. **F.** Osteotomy 2 is made, the trial passed across into the distal fragment, and, after confirmation of version (using the TEA), the osteotomy is secured with plate and cortical screws as before with the trial in situ. **G.** Final femoral construct with cemented stem. *(continued)*

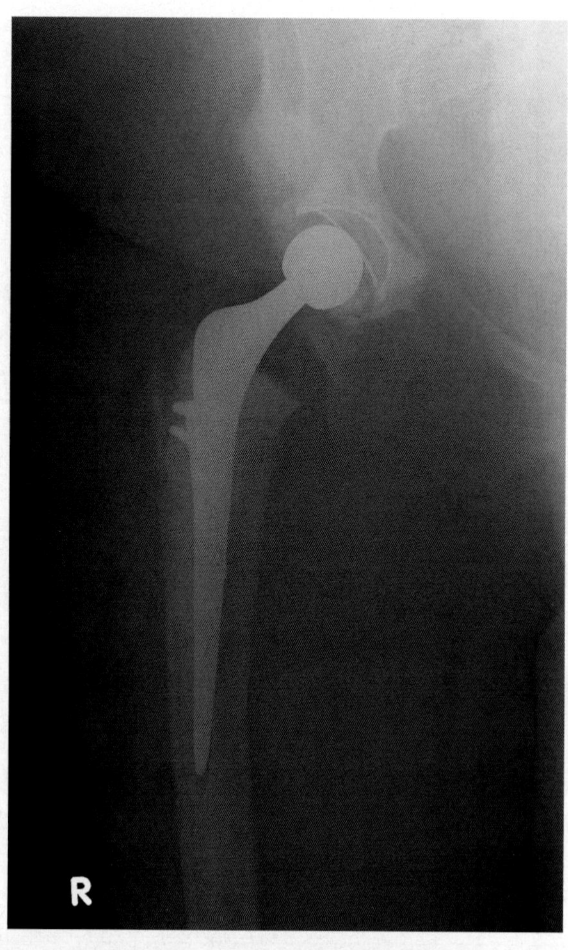

H

TECH FIG 4 • *(continued)* **H.** Radiograph.

PEARLS AND PITFALLS

- Bone is often osteopenic and soft in deformity—avoid overreaming the acetabulum, especially medially, and use prophylactic femoral cables if using cementless implants.
- THA stability depends on the relative relationship in space between the femoral and acetabular components, not only their absolute alignment. Attention should be paid to recreating this coupling not only on individual implant alignment.
- Femoral canals are often oval in shape and thus may be narrower than they appear on a single-plane radiograph. Obtain CT scans to measure this and ensure that narrow enough stems are available. Bear in mind that derotation osteotomy will change the orientation of an ovoid canal and custom-made implants may be necessary.
- All-polyethylene cups and cement allow on-table AP diameter customization if required by removing polyethylene from the outside of the cup with a knife. This is not possible with cementless metal-backed systems.
- Manage patient expectations particularly regarding LLD and outcome, which may take 2 years to plateau.

POSTOPERATIVE CARE

- Where structural autograft or femoral osteotomy has been used, patients should be partial weight bearing for 6 weeks with standard posterior approach dislocation precautions.

OUTCOMES

- In addition to being technically difficult cases, patients with deformity are young and active and often have multiple operations. As such, THA performed for severe deformity is associated with more complications and worse survivorship when compared to standard primary THA.
- Arthroplasty register data have suggested that after adjusting for age, there is no significant difference in revision risk for THA performed for sequelae of pediatric hip disease compared to THA performed for OA, with a 10-year survival rate of 93.6% compared to 93.8%.[14] However, more revisions were performed within 6 months in the pediatric hip

disease group, with significantly more revisions for dislocation.[14] These data do not consider the severity of deformity, which individual series have shown to be a key determinant of outcome.

- In DDH, mild deformity (eg, dysplasia without dislocation) rarely requires special techniques for deformity correction and is associated with THA survival comparable to that without deformity, with a 90% 15-year survival rate.[19] Worse deformity with dislocation (low or high) is associated with higher rates of failure and the 15-year survival rate reduces to 75%.[21]
- Using the technique of structural roof allograft to treat severe acetabular dysplasia, 10-year survivorship for aseptic loosening is reported as 80% to 100% when combined with cemented cups[5,23,32,40] and 91% to 100% with cementless.[22,26,39] Longer term, 12- to 15-year survival of 65% to 96% is reported with cemented cups.[1,13,24,29,37]
- When a subtrochanteric osteotomy is used, studies with mean follow-up of greater than 5 years have shown femoral stem survival of 90% to 100% when a cementless stem is used[8,15,30,33,35] and 80% to 91% with a cemented stem.[9,23,30] Osteotomy union of 93% to 100% is reported with cementless stems[8,15,30,33,35] and 90% to 97% with cemented stems.[23,30]
- Registry data have confirmed that there is no difference in the revision rate of short, cemented, collarless tapered stems (n = 1898; 7-year survival rate of 96.6%) compared to that of standard length stems (n = 39,956; 7-year survival of 96.5%) despite their use in a greater proportion of difficult DDH cases.[10] Concerns regarding the biomechanical strength and stability of these slighter stems have not been confirmed, with no documented cases of stem fracture and no increase in aseptic loosening.
- Using a variety of cementless stems in the management of proximal femoral deformity, Mortazavi et al[31] reported a mechanical failure rate (loose or revised) of 9% at 4 years. Twenty-one out of 58 (36%) required an osteotomy for exposure or deformity correction.
- Failure to restore the true hip center by positioning the acetabular component proximally and laterally increases the joint reaction force[4] and shearing forces on the cup[25] and does not restore the abductor moment arm. Cups placed 15 mm superiorly have significantly higher rates of aseptic loosening and revision of both acetabular and femoral components when compared to implants where the center of rotation has been anatomically restored.[36]
- Data on custom-made implants are difficult to interpret and long-term data are lacking. Medium-term follow-up of 48 cementless custom stems showed a survival rate of 96% at 4 years with failures due to early aseptic loosening.[27] Follow-up of 70 different custom-made cementless stems reports a 99% (95% confidence interval, 90 to 100) 12-year survival rate with no femoral loosening up to 16 years.
- Previous proximal femoral osteotomy adversely affects THA outcomes with an intraoperative complication rate of 11% to 23%,[6,16] increased risk of infection and septic THA failure rate of 8% at 5 to 10 years,[14] and an overall failure rate of 21% at 10 years in 215 patients.[16]

COMPLICATIONS

- Compared to THA for primary OA, there is a greater risk of complications when THA is performed in the presence of deformity:
  - The intraoperative fracture or femoral perforation rate is 5% to 22%.
  - The dislocation rate is 6% to 7%.[23,28]
  - The osteotomy nonunion rate is 3% to 7%.[9,23,28]
  - The nerve palsy rate is 1% to 5%.[3,6,16,23,27,36]
  - Residual LLD may still be present.[34]

REFERENCES

1. Akiyama H, Kawanabe K, Iida H, et al. Long-term results of cemented total hip arthroplasty in developmental dysplasia with acetabular bulk bone grafts after improving operative techniques. J Arthroplasty 2010;25(5):716–720.
2. Berry DJ. Total hip arthroplasty in patients with proximal femoral deformity. Clin Orthop Relat Res 1999;(369):262–272.
3. Biant LC, Bruce WJ, Assini JB, et al. The anatomically difficult primary total hip replacement: medium- to long-term results using a cementless odular stem. J Bone Joint Surg Br 2008;90(4):430–435.
4. Bicanic G, Delimar D, Delimar M, et al. Influence of the acetabular cup position on hip load during arthroplasty in hip dysplasia. Int Orthop 2009;33(2):397–402.
5. Bobak P, Wroblewski BM, Siney PD, et al. Charnley low-friction arthroplasty with an autograft of the femoral head for developmental dysplasia of the hip. The 10- to 15-year results. J Bone Joint Surg Br 2000;82(4):508–511.
6. Boos N, Krushell R, Ganz R, et al. Total hip arthroplasty after previous proximal femoral osteotomy. J Bone Joint Surg Br 1997;79(2): 247–253.
7. Busch VJ, Clement ND, Mayer PF, et al. High survivorship of cemented sockets with roof graft for severe acetabular dysplasia. Clin Orthop Relat Res 2012;470(11)3032–3040.
8. Chareancholvanich K, Becker DA, Gustilo RB. Treatment of congenital dislocated hip by arthroplasty with femoral shortening. Clin Orthop Relat Res 1999;(360):127–135.
9. Charity JA, Tsiridis E, Sheeraz A, et al. Treatment of Crowe IV high hip dysplasia with total hip replacement using the Exeter stem and shortening derotational subtrochanteric osteotomy. J Bone Joint Surg Br 2011;93:34–38.
10. Choy GG, Roe JA, Whitehouse SL, et al. Exeter short stems compared with standard length Exeter stems: experience from the Australian Orthopaedic Association National Joint Replacement Registry. J Arthroplasty 2013;28:103–109.
11. D'Antonio JA, Capello WN, Borden LS, et al. Classification and management of acetabular abnormalities in total hip arthroplasty. Clin Orthop Relat Res 1989;(243):126–137.
12. D'Antonio J, McCarthy JC, Bargar WL, et al. Classification of femoral abnormalities in total hip arthroplasty. Clin Orthop Relat Res 1993;(296):133–139.
13. de Jong PT, Haverkamp D, van der Vis HM, et al. Total hip replacement with a superolateral bone graft for osteoarthritis secondary to dysplasia: a long-term follow-up. J Bone Joint Surg Br 2006;88(2):173–178.
14. Engesaeter LB, Engesaeter IO, Fenstad AM, et al. Low revision rate after total hip arthroplasty in patients with pediatric hip diseases. Acta Orthop 2012;83(5):436–441.
15. Eskelinen A, Helenius I, Remes V, et al. Cementless total hip arthroplasty in patients with high congenital hip dislocation. J Bone Joint Surg Am 2006;88:80–91.
16. Ferguson GM, Cabanela ME, Ilstrup DM. Total hip arthroplasty after failed intertrochanteric osteotomy. J Bone Joint Surg Br 1994; 76(2):252–257.
17. Gaston MS, Gaston P, Donaldson P, et al. A new classification system for the adult dysplastic hip requiring total hip arthroplasty: a reliability study. Hip Int 2009;19(2):96–101.

18. Hartofilakidis G, Babis GC, Lampropoulou-Adamidou K, et al. Results of total hip arthroplasty differ in subtypes of high dislocation. Clin Orthop Relat Res 2013;471(9):2972–2979.
19. Hartofilakidis G, Karachalios T. Total hip arthroplasty for congenital hip disease. J Bone Joint Surg Am 2004:86(2):242–250.
20. Hartofilakidis G, Karachalios T, Georgiades G. Total hip arthroplasty in patients with high dislocation: a concise follow-up, at a minimum of fifteen years, of previous reports. J Bone Joint Surg Am 2011;93(17):1614–1618.
21. Hartofilakidis G, Stamos K, Karachalios T. Treatment of high dislocation of the hip in adults with total hip arthroplasty. Operative technique and long-term clinical results. J Bone Joint Surg Am 1998;80(4):510–517.
22. Hendrich C, Mehling I, Sauer U, et al. Cementless acetabular reconstruction and structural bone-grafting in dysplastic hips. J Bone Joint Surg Am 2006;88(2):387–394.
23. Howie CR, Ohly NE, Miller B. Cemented total hip arthroplasty with subtrochanteric osteotomy in dysplastic hips. Clin Orthop Relat Res 2010;468(12):3240–3247.
24. Iida H, Matsusue Y, Kawanabe K, et al. Cemented total hip arthroplasty with acetabular bone graft for developmental dysplasia. Long-term results and survivorship analysis. J Bone Joint Surg Br 2000;82(2):176–184.
25. Karachalios T, Hartofilakidis G. Congenital hip disease in adults: terminology, classification, pre-operative planning and management. J Bone Joint Surg Br 2010;92(7):914–921.
26. Kim M, Kadowaki T. High long-term survival of bulk femoral head autograft for acetabular reconstruction in cementless THA for developmental hip dysplasia. Clin Orthop Relat Res 2010;468(6):1611–1620.
27. Koulouvaris P, Stafylas K, Sculco T, et al. Custom-design implants for severe distorted proximal anatomy of the femur in young adults followed for 4-8 years. Acta Orthop 2008;79(2):203–210.
28. Krych AJ, Howard JL, Trousdale RT, et al. Total hip arthroplasty with shortening subtrochanteric osteotomy in Crowe type-IV developmental dysplasia: surgical technique. J Bone Joint Surg Am 2010;92 (suppl 1):176–187.
29. Lee BP, Cabanela ME, Wallrichs SL, et al. Bone-graft augmentation for acetabular deficiencies in total hip arthroplasty. Results of long-term follow-up evaluation. J Arthroplasty 1997;12(5):503–510.
30. Masonis JL, Patel JV, Miu A, et al. Subtrochanteric shortening and derotational osteotomy in primary total hip arthroplasty for patients with severe hip dysplasia: 5-year follow-up. J Arthroplasty 2003;18 (3 suppl 1):68–73.
31. Mortazavi SM, Restrepo C, Kim PJ, et al. Cementless femoral reconstruction in patients with proximal femoral deformity. J Arthroplasty 2011;26(3):354–359.
32. Mulroy RD Jr, Harris WH. Failure of acetabular autogenous grafts in total hip arthroplasty. Increasing incidence: a follow-up note. J Bone Joint Surg Am 1990;72(10):1536–1540.
33. Nagoya S, Kaya M, Sasaki M, et al. Cementless total hip replacement with subtrochanteric femoral shortening for severe developmental dysplasia of the hip. J Bone Joint Surg Br 2009;91(9):1142–1147.
34. Oe K, Iida H, Nakamura T, et al. Subtrochanteric shortening osteotomy combined with cemented total hip arthroplasty for Crowe group IV hips. Arch Orthop Trauma Surg 2013;133(12):1763–1770.
35. Onodera S, Majima T, Ito H, et al. Cementless total hip arthroplasty using the modular S-ROM prosthesis combined with corrective proximal femoral osteotomy. J Arthroplasty 2006;21(5):664–669.
36. Pagnano W, Hanssen AD, Lewallen DG, et al. The effect of superior placement of the acetabular component on the rate of loosening after total hip arthroplasty. J Bone Joint Surg Am 1996;78(7); 1004–1014.
37. Rodriguez JA, Huk OL, Pellicci PM, et al. Autogenous bone grafts from the femoral head for the treatment of acetabular deficiency in primary total hip arthroplasty with cement. Long-term results. J Bone Joint Surg Am 1995;77(8):1227–1233.
38. Schmidutz F, Bierer M, Weber P, et al. Biomechanical reconstruction of the hip: comparison between modular short-stem hip arthroplasty and conventional total hip arthroplasty. Int Orthop 2012;36(7):1341–1347.
39. Shetty AA, Sharma P, Singh S, et al. Bulk femoral-head autografting in uncemented total hip arthroplasty for acetabular dysplasia: results at 8 to 11 years follow-up. J Arthroplasty 2004;19(6):706–713.
40. Stringa G, Pitto RP, Di Muria GV, et al. Total hip replacement with bone grafting using the removed femoral head in severe acetabular dysplasia. Int Orthop 1995;19(2):72–76.
41. Tamegai H, Otani T, Fujii H, et al. A modified S-ROM stem in primary total hip arthroplasty for developmental dysplasia of the hip. J Arthroplasty 2013;28(10):1741–1745.

Hip Resurfacing

Kang-Il Kim and Young Soo Chun

22

CHAPTER

DEFINITION

- Hip resurfacing is a surgical procedure whereby the femoral head is preserved and a component (mostly metal) is placed like a cap on the femoral head. The acetabular component is also a monolithic piece made of metal.
- Hip resurfacing offers the advantage that femoral bone can be preserved, and the femoral canal is not violated for fixation of the femoral component.
- The current hip resurfacing technique has a hybrid fixation. The femoral head is resurfaced through insertion of a cemented component. The cup is press-fit.[18]

Resurfacing Systems

- Resurfacing total hip arthroplasty (THA) with metal-on-metal bearing and hybrid fixation (a cementless acetabular component and a cemented femoral component) has been performed for many decades. In recent years, and with the issue of metal-on-metal bearing surface failure, the popularity of this procedure has waned.
- Several hip resurfacing devices of various designs are available, but the most critical factor affecting the outcome of resurfacing is the surgeon's level of expertise.
- Several manufacturers now produce metal-on-metal surface replacement components with a cementless acetabular component, a cemented femoral component, and a cobalt-chromium articulation. These various devices differ in terms of material, surface treatments, cup design, manufacturing process, carbide content, component thickness, clearance, possibility of including a cement mantle under the femoral component, fixation methods, and size ranges offered (Table 1).

SURGICAL MANAGEMENT

Indications

- Hip resurfacing is used optimally in younger, active patients with good bone quality.
- This procedure is indicated for a degenerative hip joint with pain and decreased range of motion.
- When joint-preserving procedures such as femoral osteotomy, acetabular osteotomy, or vascularized bone grafting are not ideal for an early stage of unambiguous coxarthrosis, hip resurfacing can be considered.
- Osteoarthritis of the hip joint is a good indication for resurfacing arthroplasty. Selective cases of osteonecrosis of the femoral head could be an indication for the need for resurfacing arthroplasty.
- Resurfacing is usually reserved for patients with good bone stock, high activity level, and a need for a high degree of motion.
- Hemiresurfacing, in which only the femoral head is resurfaced, has largely been abandoned because it provided suboptimal results.
- Resurfacing has been approved by the U.S. Food and Drug Administration.
- General indications for hip resurfacing are as follows:
  - Primary osteoarthritis
  - Secondary osteoarthritis as sequela of childhood disease, including hip dysplasia or infection
  - Osteonecrosis of the femoral head
  - Posttraumatic arthritis
  - Ankylosing spondylitis
  - Rheumatoid arthritis

Contraindications

- Abnormal anatomy of the femoral head or neck
- Severe limb length discrepancy that may require some correction during arthroplasty
- Severe bone deficiency
- Large and cystic lesions of the femoral head
- Large necrotic area of the femoral head
- Severe dysplasia because screw fixation for the acetabulum cannot be performed with resurfacing
- Fertile female patient
- The patient with renal disease
- Patients who have a metal hypersensitivity

Special Considerations

Osteonecrosis of the Femoral Head

- Osteonecrosis of the femoral head presents a special problem for hip resurfacing.
- The presence of a necrotic lesion of the femoral head can compromise fixation of the component.
- In general, survival of hip resurfacing is lower for avascular necrosis than for osteoarthritis in the counterpart hip. However, resurfacing arthroplasty for selective cases of osteonecrosis of the femoral head has comparative results with other etiology.[2,19,31]

Use of a Computer-Assisted Navigation System

- A computer-assisted navigation system is an intraoperative image-guided localization system used to enable proper cutting of bone and exact location of the implants in total knee arthroplasty or THA and in minimally invasive surgery.
- Although hip resurfacing arthroplasty has been used for a long time with acceptable results without any navigation system, one of the main concerns following resurfacing arthroplasty is femoral neck fracture.
  - In general, slight valgus positioning of the implant is recommended to reduce the tension and shear stresses across

Table 1 Comparative Table for Representative Hip Resurfacing Systems Currently Available

Resurfacing System	Material	Acetabular Fixation	Femoral Fixation	Available Femoral Size (mm)	Available Acetabular Size (mm)	Cups for Dysplastic Hip	Surface Finish	Clearance (Diametral)	Cup Design	Cup Thickness
Cormet (Corin, Cirencester, United Kingdom)	Cast and heat-treated high-carbon CoCr	Uncemented TiVPS with HA	Cemented press-fit equatorially or uncemented Ti+HA internal coating	5 sizes, from 40 to 56 in 4-mm increments Available in cemented and uncemented versions	10 cup sizes, from 46 to 62 in 6-mm increments, with 2 cup sizes for every head size	Pegged and unpegged acetabular cups	10 nm	150–400	Full-hemisphere OD with 2-mm equatorial expansion with 3.5-mm offset bore	3–4 mm
Birmingham Hip Resurfacing (BHR; Smith & Nephew, Memphis, TN)	As cast high-carbon CoCR	Cast in CoCr beads with HA	Cemented, press-fit equatorially	6 sizes, from 38 to 58 in 4-mm increments	12 sizes, from 44 to 66 in 2-mm increments Two cups for every femoral size	Acetabular cups in congenital hip dysplasia and bridging range	20 nm	250–400	Full-hemisphere OD with 3.5-mm offset bore	3–4 mm
Conserve Plus (Wright Medical Technology, Memphis, TN)	Cast and heat-treated high-carbon CoCr	Uncemented sintered CoCr beads with HA	Cemented, full mantle	11 heads, from 36 to 56 in 2-mm increments	12 components, from 42 to 64 in 6-mm increments Two cups for every femoral size	Does not offer dysplasia and bridging cups	10 nm	200–350 (est)	170-degree truncated hemisphere	3- or 3.5-mm (new); 5-mm (old)

CoCr, Cobalt-Chromium; TiVPS, Vacuum plasma–sprayed pure titanium; HA, hydroxyapatite; OD, Outer diameter.

the head–neck junction, but intraoperative neck notching during femoral cutting often is a consequence of extreme valgus position.
  - Many mechanical femoral alignment guides have been developed to help surgeons achieve optimal positioning of the femoral implant.
- As for THA, early loosening or dislocation resulting from impingement due to the malposition of both components should be prevented.[18]
  - In hip resurfacing arthroplasty, avoidance of femoral notching by the femoral component and the position of the stem of the femoral component are critical. This may be technically difficult, even for an experienced surgeon, and it adds time to the procedure.
- Computer-assisted navigation systems have been developed to surmount the limitations of manual techniques.
  - Intraoperative navigation can demonstrate real-time positioning of instrumentation by imaging, thereby improving the accuracy of component positioning in hip resurfacing arthroplasty.
  - However, specific surface landmarks may be difficult to make out, and registration procedures are often the most time-consuming and accuracy-related segment of the procedure.
  - Irregular soft tissue distribution around the femoral neck also can affect navigation precision.
- Surgical navigation may be especially helpful during femoral procedures.
  - To reduce the potential risk of femoral neck fracture, we perform total hip resurfacing arthroplasty using computer-assisted navigation.
  - We have used the hip resurfacing systems from Vectorvision (BrainLAB, Munich, Germany) since 2005 (**FIG 1**).[14]
  - When using an image-free hip navigation system, the surgeon must digitize the pelvic and femoral planes of the patient to determine the individual pelvic and femoral coordinate system for prosthesis positioning.

Preoperative Planning

- Templates are used to determine approximate component sizes. Standard-sized conventional radiographs must be used rather than digital films, and the magnification factor must be taken into account.

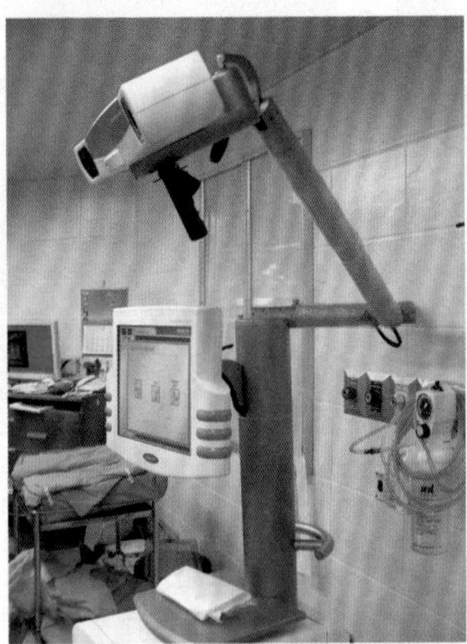

FIG 1 ● Image-free hip navigation system for hip resurfacing.

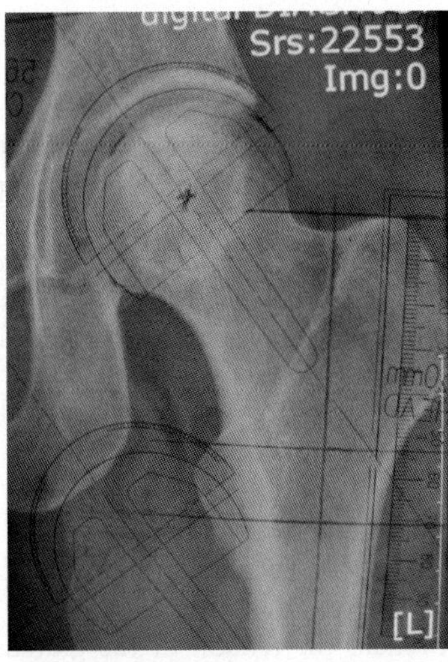

FIG 2 ● Templating. A slight valgus position without notching the femoral neck should be the goal. The distance (60 mm) between the tip of the greater trochanter and the lateral pin that is inserted to the lateral cortex of the proximal femur should be measured for conventional resurfacing procedures. The level of lateral pin insertion usually is similar to the level of the lesser trochanter.

- The femoral component must be sized so that there is no overreaming of the femur or risk of notching of the neck. Oversizing also should be avoided to preserve acetabular bone stock.
- Femoral component alignment is the most important preoperative consideration. Varus positioning must be avoided—neutral or slight valgus alignment is preferred (**FIG 2**). The authors recommend a femoral component axis shaft angle of 130 to 140 degrees.
- When optimum femoral template positioning has been achieved, the distance from the tip of the greater trochanter to the pin insertion point on the lateral femoral cortex is measured with the ruler printed on the template.
- The relation between the exit point of the guidewire on the template relative to the lesser trochanter should be noted and reproduced during surgery.
- An acetabular component should be selected to fill the acetabular fossa and accommodate the selected femoral component.

Approach

- All of the standard exposures of the hip have been successfully used to perform surface replacement.
- Hip resurfacing is technically demanding, and the surgical approach should allow adequate exposure of the acetabulum and proximal femur without compromising postoperative muscle function.
- The posterior approach is the most popular approach for total hip resurfacing.
- The anterior approach, advocated by Wagner,[28] is not popular.
- The anterolateral approach was described by Hardinge[11] and modified by Learmonth.
  - Exposure of the femoral head is achieved by flexion, adduction, and external rotation of the lower extremity. Exposure of the acetabulum is accomplished by depressing the femoral head into a posterior and inferior position.
  - This approach has the advantage of preserving the posterior retinacular vessels, which reduces the possibility that

an iatrogenic avascular state will develop postoperatively in the remaining femoral head.[13]
- Critics of this approach believe that the exposure offered is inadequate, leading to a greater risk of complications and improper component positioning of both implants in total hip resurfacing. There may be a higher incidence of heterotopic new bone formation, and decreasing abductor muscle function often is compromised following this approach.[21]

- The transtrochanteric approach for hip resurfacing was popularized by Amstutz and Le Duff.[2]
  - This approach provides excellent exposure, but it is rarely used for this operation primarily because of problems associated with trochanteric osteotomy and a higher incidence of heterotopic ossification.
- The posterior or posterolateral approach is the standard approach used for total hip resurfacing.
  - In this approach, the tendon of the gluteus maximus is released to allow easy anterior displacement of the femur.
  - The capsule and synovium around the femoral neck are preserved as much as possible to prevent further vascular damage to the femoral neck and head. The femoral head is then dislocated (**FIG 3**).

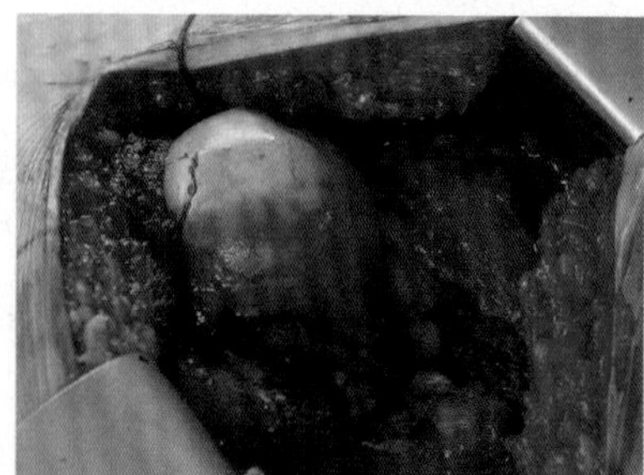

FIG 3 • Unlike conventional THA, the joint capsule and synovial membrane around the femoral neck should be preserved as much as possible to reduce vascular damage to the femoral head in hip resurfacing.

  - The femoral neck is sized using neck gauges. Sizing also gives an idea about the minimum acetabular size required.
  - Usually, the acetabular preparation is done first, unless the femoral head is especially large, which results in inadequate acetabular preparation. In such cases, the femoral head is prepared at one or two sizes larger than the targeted femoral component size.

TECHNIQUES

Posterolateral Approach

Exposure

- The patient is placed in the lateral position.
- The hip is flexed to 45 degrees and a straight incision is made, centered on the posterior edge of the greater trochanter.
  - Alternatively, the hip is extended and a conventional incision, curved posteriorly, is made (**TECH FIG 1A**).
- The fascia lata is incised, the fibers of the gluteus maximus are split, and a Charnley retractor is inserted (**TECH FIG 1B**).
- The tendon of insertion of the gluteus maximus is usually released to allow subsequent easy anterior displacement of the femur; the underlying perforator vessels may require coagulation (**TECH FIG 1C**).
- The trochanteric bursa is divided and swept posteriorly, after which the sciatic nerve may be easily seen or palpated.

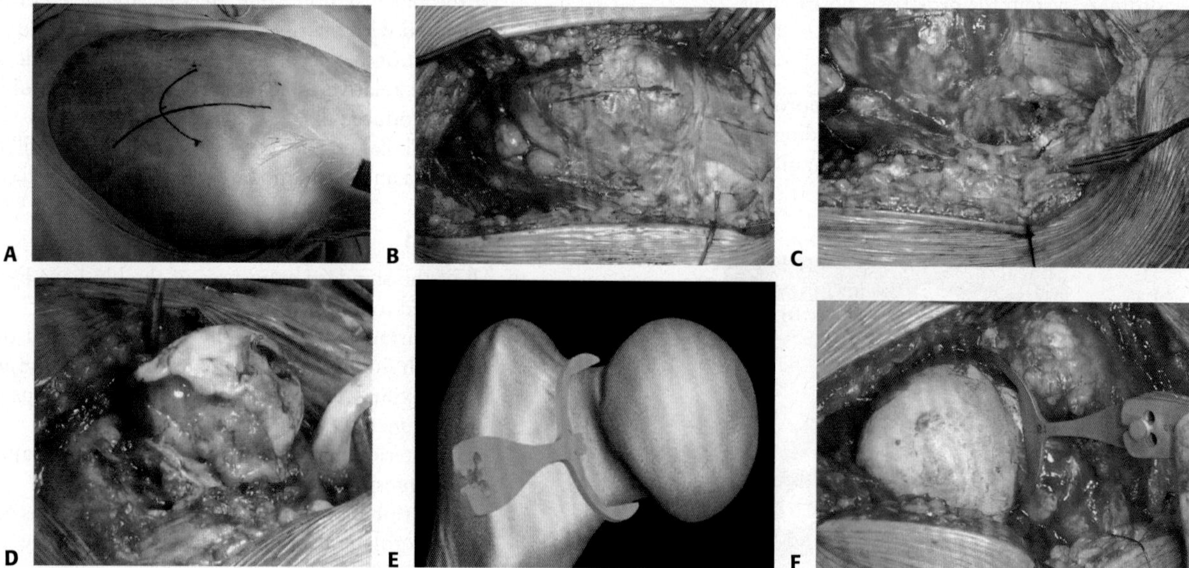

TECH FIG 1 • **A.** Posterolateral approach. The patient is in the lateral position with the affected hip flexed 45 degrees. A straight incision is made at the posterior border of the greater trochanter. **B.** The gluteus maximus fibers are split proximally and the iliotibial band is incised distally. **C.** A diathermy is used to release the insertion of the gluteus maximus tendon, leaving behind a small fringe for later suturing. Perforator vessels in this area may cause copious bleeding, requiring ligation or cauterization. **D.** Circumferential capsulotomy. With the hip fully extended and in maximal internal rotation, the anteroinferior capsule is divided inferiorly. The hip is then flexed to 45 degrees in maximum internal rotation and the anterosuperior hip capsule is divided superiorly. The capsulotomy is extended down to meet the previous inferior cut, giving a full circumferential capsulotomy. **E,F.** Diagram illustrating sizing of the femoral neck. The neck is sized in its maximum diameter.

- The posterior edge of the gluteus medius is retracted anteriorly to reveal the piriformis tendon.
- The fibers of the gluteus minimus are separated from the superior border of the piriformis tendon.
- The interval between the gluteus minimus and the superior acetabulum and superior hip capsule is developed with electrocautery.
- The hip is held in internal rotation and the piriformis tendon is divided as close as possible to its insertion, along with the hip capsule.
- The other external rotators and the hip capsule are divided with electrocautery, leaving a cuff of quadratus femoris for later suturing.
- The joint capsule is incised along the line formed by the superior margin of the piriformis muscle. The posterior capsule is detached cautiously, along with the base of the femur neck, to save intracapsular blood vessels around the femoral neck.
- The femoral head is dislocated, the hip is fully extended (by bringing the knee to the midline), and maximum internal rotation of the leg is performed (**TECH FIG 1D**).
- The anteroinferior hip capsule is divided, beginning inferiorly, just in front of the psoas tendon, using Muller capsular scissors or electrocautery.
- The femoral neck is sized using neck gauges or templates (**TECH FIG 1E,F**); this also gives an idea about the minimum acetabular size required.
- An anterolateral soft tissue pocket is created using a curved periosteal elevator or a Cobb elevator.
- A Hohmann retractor is placed over the anterosuperior acetabulum and impacted into the anterior inferior iliac spine, and the leg is externally rotated to allow the femoral head to prolapse under the abductors into the pocket.

Acetabular Preparation

- A pin retractor (Judd pin) is inserted into the ischium, retracting the posterior capsule and external rotators.
- Two Hohmann retractors are placed from inferior to the teardrop, directed antero- and posteroinferiorly (**TECH FIG 2A**).
- The labrum, transverse acetabular ligament, and other soft tissue in the cotyloid fossa are excised, giving a complete view of the bony acetabulum.
  - Sequential reaming is performed (**TECH FIG 2B**), with under-reaming by 1 to 2 mm.
- An acetabular component that provides the best possible fit without reaming excess acetabular bone is preferred; this choice determines the size of the femoral component.
  - A trial cup is inserted and tested for stability (**TECH FIG 2C**).
- The true acetabular component is then inserted in "native" version, usually 20 degrees and at a 45-degree angle (**TECH FIG 2D**).
- Any protruding acetabular osteophytes should be removed.
- The Hohmann retractors and pin retractor are removed.

Inserting the Guide Pin

- The limb is then internally hyperrotated to expose the femoral head.
- Lines are drawn on the center of the femoral head and neck in both anteroposterior (135 to 140 degrees of neck–shaft angle) and lateral planes (normal anteversion) and are extended up into the femoral head where they intersect (**TECH FIG 3A,B**).
  - The intersection point should be the entry point for the guide pin.
- A guide pin is drilled into the femoral head and neck using a guide instrument (**TECH FIG 3C**).
- A stylus is placed over the guide pin. This should pass around the femoral neck without impingement (**TECH FIG 3D**) to avoid notching of the femoral neck.
- The guide pin is normally inserted from the superior part of the femoral head about 1 to 2 cm above the fovea.
  - In the coronal plane, 5 to 10 degrees of valgus is desirable; a 135- to 140-degree angle must be maintained with the long axis of the femoral neck (**TECH FIG 3E**).
  - Because a deformed femoral head or osteophytes around the femoral head and neck may make it difficult to recognize the actual state and relation of the femoral head and neck junction, excessive osteophytes should be removed carefully before femoral pinning.

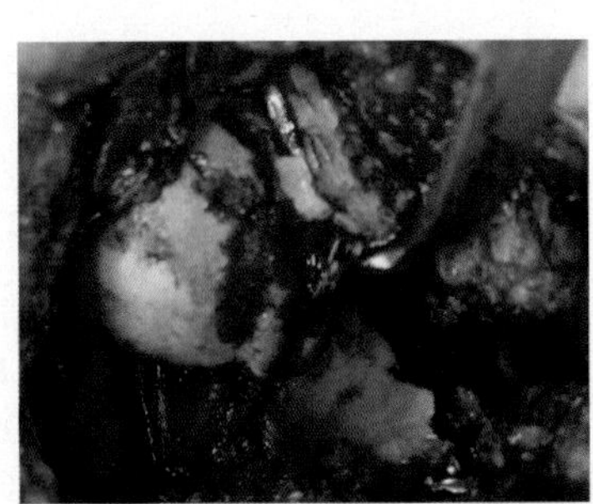
A

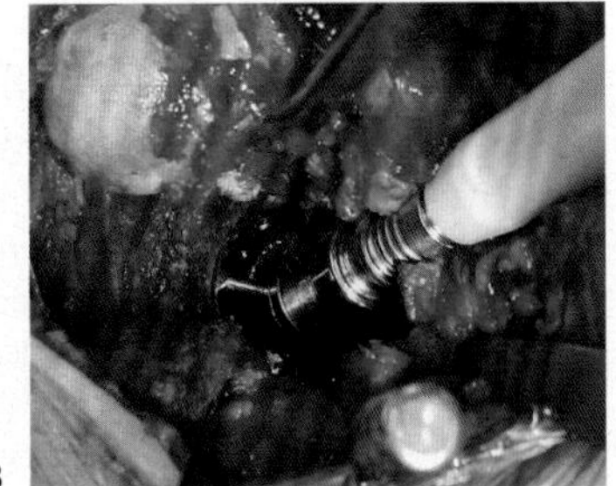
B

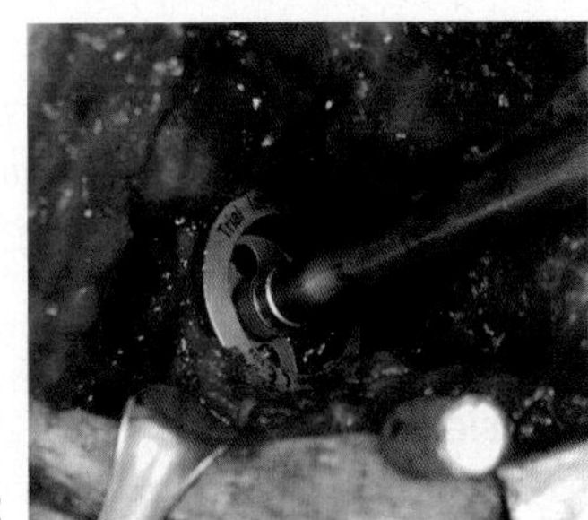
C

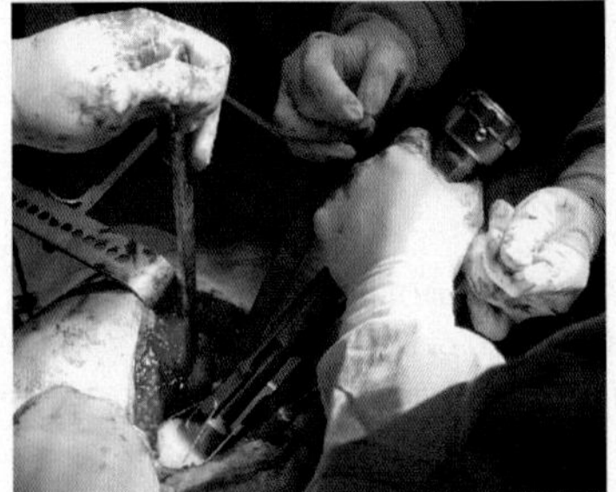
D

TECH FIG 2 • **A.** An anterosuperolateral acetabular pocket is created and the femoral head delivered into it with the hip in external rotation. **B.** The acetabulum is reamed in 2-mm increments, with 1-mm increments used in dense bone. The reamer handle is kept at 45 degrees inclination and native anteversion. **C.** Trial cup insertion after complete acetabular reaming. The trial's stability and the relation between the peripheral margin of the acetabulum and the trial after it is fully seated must be checked. **D.** Acetabular resurfacing with cup impaction in the desired position. The transverse ligament is a useful landmark for determining cup inclination.

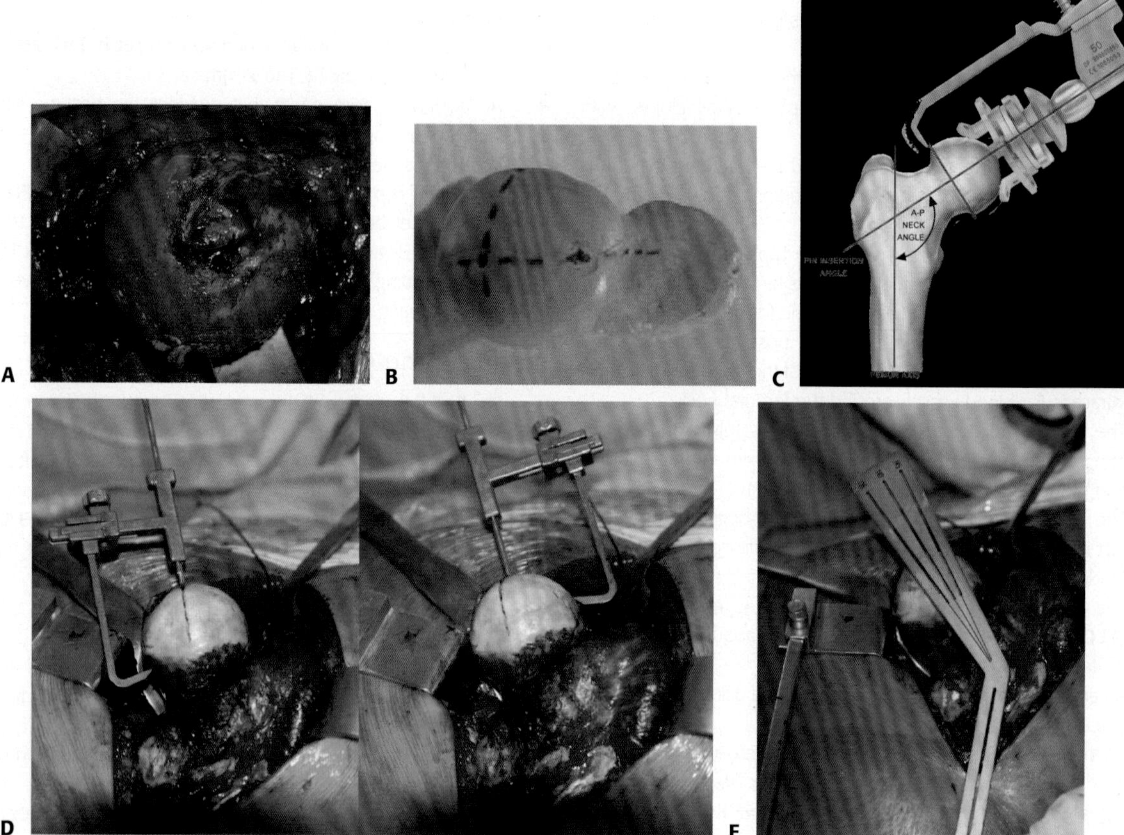

TECH FIG 3 • A,B. Planning the guidewire entry point in the anteroposterior (AP) plane. A line is drawn in the midlateral plane of the femoral neck. A second line is drawn in the center of the femoral neck so that it is parallel to the calcar femorale. This gives the guide pin a valgus orientation of about 5 to 10 degrees. The point where the two lines intersect, usually 1 to 1.5 cm superior to the fovea, should be the entry point for the guidewire. **C.** Planning the guidewire entry point in the superoinferior plane using guide instruments from various companies. **D.** Planning for slightly valgus placement for the femoral guide pin and checking for notching in the femoral neck. The stylus on the guide pin should move freely around the femoral neck at the head–neck junction without impingement. Moreover, the surgeon can confirm the head size through this procedure. **E.** The angle in the coronal plane is checked intraoperatively using a goniometer.

Femoral Head Resurfacing

- In most systems, femoral head preparation is done using cannulated reamers that pass over the previously inserted femoral guide pin (**TECH FIG 4A**).
- Consecutive reaming or milling using specialized instrumentation forms the femoral head into a chamfer-cut cylindrical shape (**TECH FIG 4B–D**).
- Nonimpinging osteophytes present on the femoral neck are best left untouched.
- Any necrotic bone in cases of osteonecrosis should be removed.
- The femoral head is then pulse lavaged, and a suction vent is placed into the lesser trochanter to keep the femoral head dry and to prevent embolism (**TECH FIG 4E**).
- A number of cement keyholes are drilled into the femoral head (**TECH FIG 4F**).
- A final check is made to confirm that there has been no notching from the trial component (**TECH FIG 4G**).

Cementing

- Bone cement is placed into the femoral component, which is then impacted onto the resurfaced femoral head (**TECH FIG 5A,B**).
  - Alternatively, in case of femoral head defect after curettage of necrotic bone, cement is applied to give a uniform 2-mm cement mantle around the femoral head (**TECH FIG 5C**), and the femoral component is placed over the head and lightly tapped into place (**TECH FIG 5D**).
- Check cement leakage; excess cement should be removed and pulse lavage used.
- The joint is then reduced and tested for stability and range of motion.

Wound Closure

- Good closure of the capsule and the external rotators is important.
- The tendinous insertion of the gluteus maximus also is repaired, and the fascia lata, subcutaneous fat, and skin are closed.

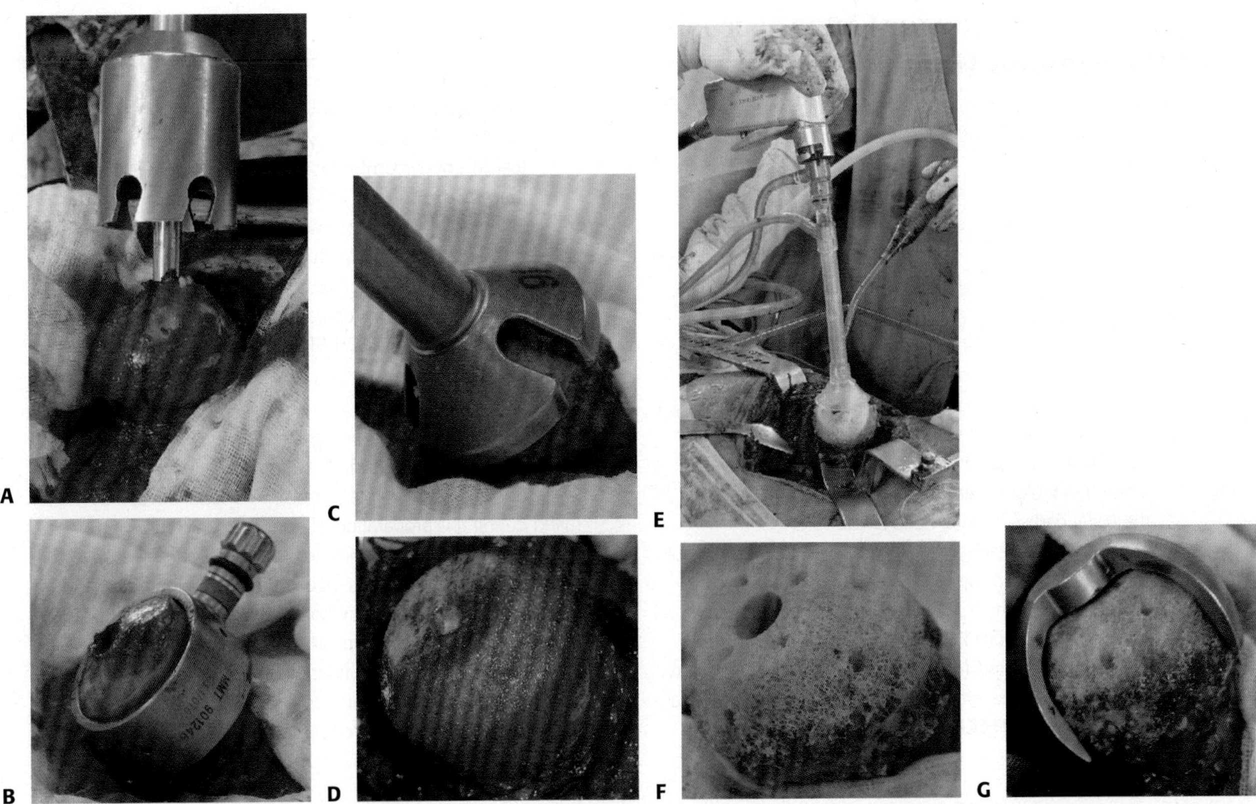

TECH FIG 4 • A. The guide rod is inserted after drilling over the guide pin and the head cutter is advanced through the guide rod. During this procedure, the surgeon should check for and avoid femoral notching at the head–neck junction. A head cutter one size larger may be used initially. **B.** After safe cutting has been accomplished, all instruments are removed, and the top of the head guide is placed through the prepared femoral head. The inferior margin of the guide is placed next to the superior margin of the head–neck junction. The locking lever is securely fixed, and the top area is resected using a saw. **C.** The chamfer cutter for the femoral head then is used on the reinserted guide rod. **D.** The final shape of the chamfer-cut femoral head. **E.** The prepared femoral head is irrigated using a motorized pulsatile lavage instrument. **F.** Multiple cement keyholes are made, being sure to keep the femoral head dry. **G.** A head trial is used to recheck the possibility of femoral notching and to determine the point between inferior margin of the trial and femoral head–neck junction.

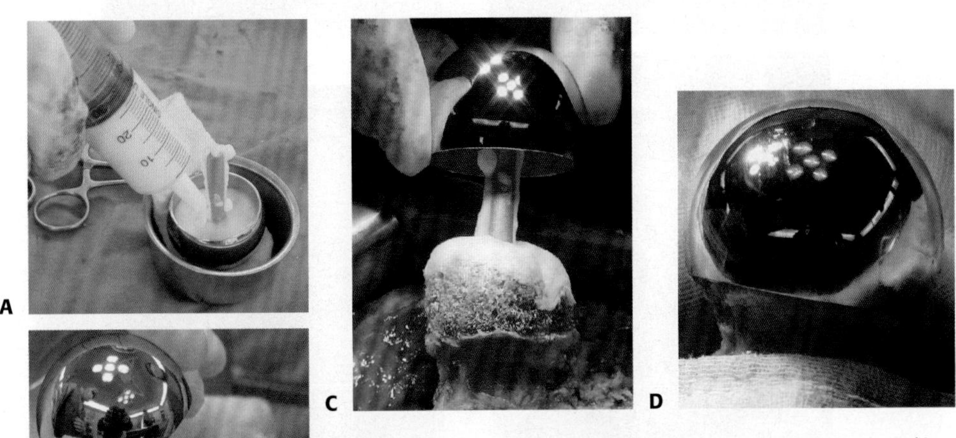

TECH FIG 5 • A. Low- or intermediate-viscosity cement is injected into the femoral component using a cement syringe. High-viscosity cement may alter full positioning of the component to the femoral head. **B.** The femoral component is advanced to the femoral head. **C.** In cases of femoral head defects, such as osteonecrosis, cement can be applied to the defect area of the femoral head and then the head component can be inserted. **D.** Femoral implant in place.

Special Technique for Osteonecrosis of the Femoral Head

- Because the surgical approach and acetabular preparation are almost the same, only the technique for the femoral side is described.

Femoral Preparation

- Accurate placement of the guide pin can be accomplished using pin alignment guides or a navigation system (**TECH FIG 6A,B**).
- In most systems, femoral head reaming is performed by cannulated reamers that pass over the central guide pin.
  - A series of reaming or milling devices form the femoral neck into a cylindrical shape (**TECH FIG 6C**).
  - To reduce the stress resulting from femoral notching, reaming should be stopped before the peripheral rim of the distal part of femoral head is cut.
  - The remaining distal rim of the femoral head is carefully removed using a rongeur (**TECH FIG 6D**).
- After chamfer cutting, the remaining necrotic area of the femoral head can be seen clearly (**TECH FIG 6E**).
- Using a small curette and rongeur, the remaining necrotic area is removed and irrigated with aseptic saline to remove tiny fragments of bone debris (**TECH FIG 6F**).
- The trial femoral head is inserted and the percentage of volume loss after removal of necrotic bone in the trial is measured (**TECH FIG 6G**).
  - In our experience, if the volume loss is less than 50% and the necrosis does not extend to the lower margin of the trial in any circumference of the femoral head and neck junction, resurfacing can be accomplished.
  - Otherwise, we recommend either metal-on-metal THA with a large diameter femoral head in cases where acetabular preparation has already been completed or conventional THA if preparation has not yet begun on the acetabular side (**TECH FIG 6H–J**).

Cementing

- Using pulsatile lavage, thorough saline irrigation is repeated, taking care to keep the femoral head dry. The carbon dioxide (CO_2) blow dry is useful for this purpose. A special suction system is used during the preparation of bone cement (**TECH FIG 7A**).
- The bone defect is filled with bone cement and pressurized.
- The femoral component is placed on the femoral head and impacted gently, with the cement inside the femoral component removed as a volume half using a cement syringe (**TECH FIG 7B–D**).
- The femoral component is applied to the femoral head with an impactor and extruding cement is removed with a curette, continuing until the bone cement hardens (**TECH FIG 7E–H**).

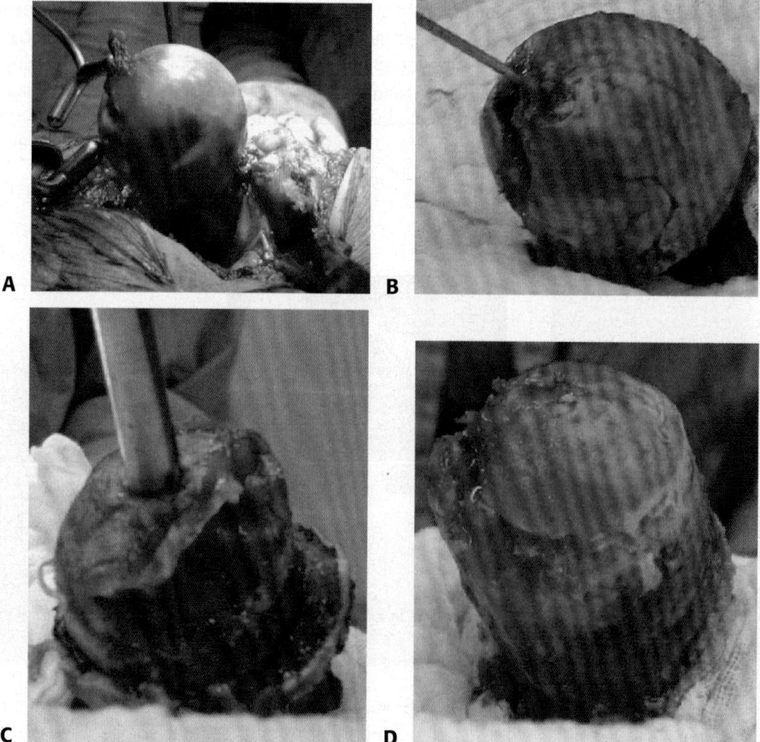

TECH FIG 6 • The centering jig is located over the guide pin (**A**), and the pin is then drilled through the centering jig (**B**). **C.** Femoral head reaming is performed by cannulated reamer through the central guide rod. The reaming should be stopped before the peripheral rim of the distal part of the femoral head is cut to reduce stress resulting from femoral notching. **D.** The final shape of femoral head reaming with distal peripheral cut using a rongeur. *(continued)*

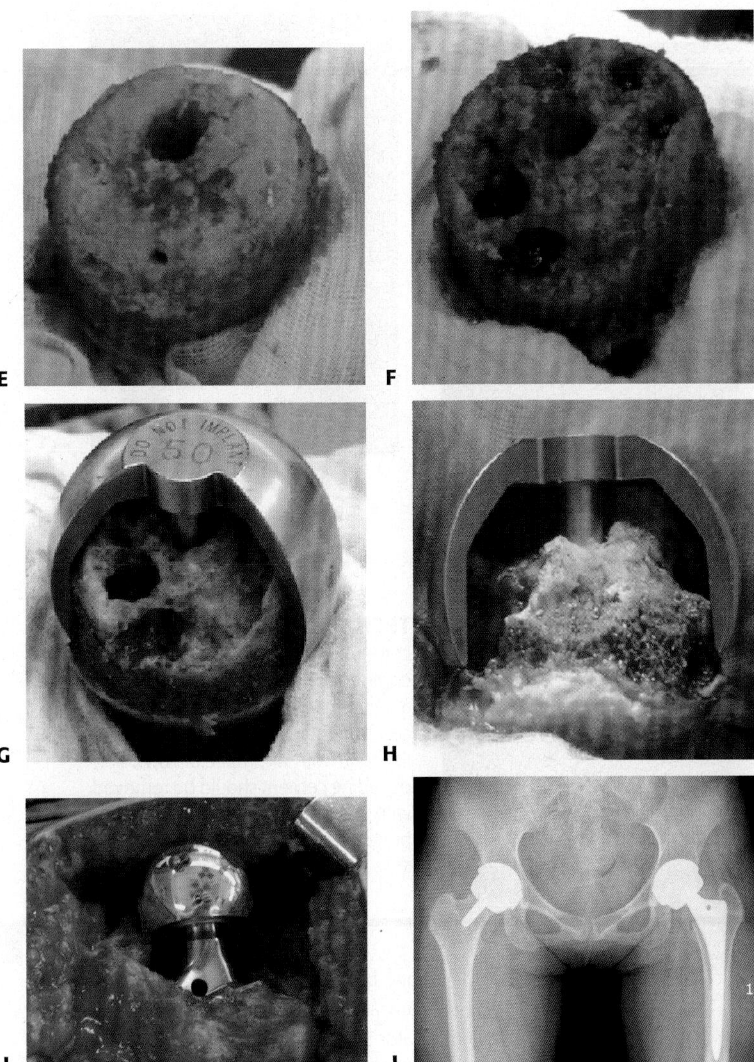

TECH FIG 6 • *(continued)* **E.** After chamfer cutting, the remaining necrotic area of the femoral head can be clearly recognized. Necrotic bone usually is yellowish because it does not bleed, so the margin between necrotic bone and living bone is well recognized. **F.** The necrotic part of the femoral head should be completely removed, and the remaining femoral head well bled. **G.** The percentage of volume loss of the inner femoral head after removal of necrotic bone can be measured using a size-matched femoral head trial. It has been our experience that resurfacing procedures can be continued if the volume loss is less than 50%. **H,I.** If the necrosis extends to the distal peripheral margin of the femoral head so that any circumference of the femoral head and neck junction is not covered by the lower margin of the head trial, we recommend a metal-on-metal, modular THA with large diameter femoral head or the conventional THA if the acetabular side is not yet finished for hip resurfacing. **J.** Postoperative radiograph shows both hip resurfacing and large head, metal-on-metal THA.

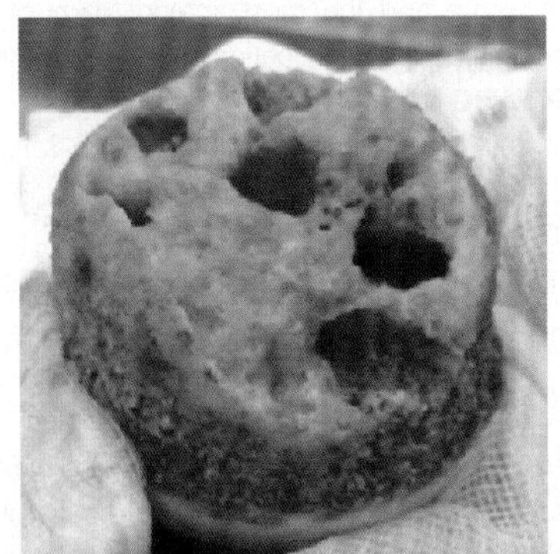
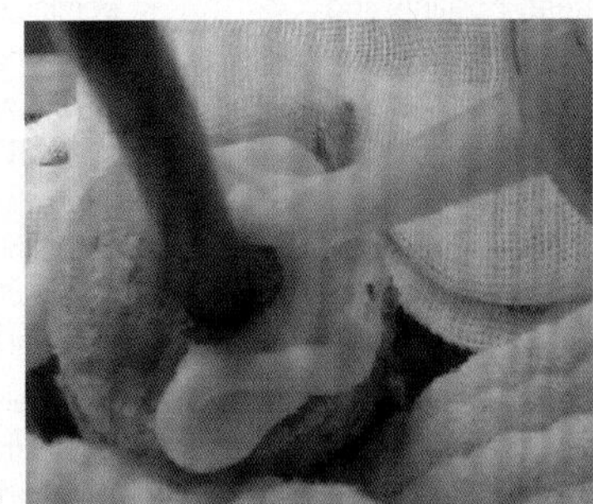
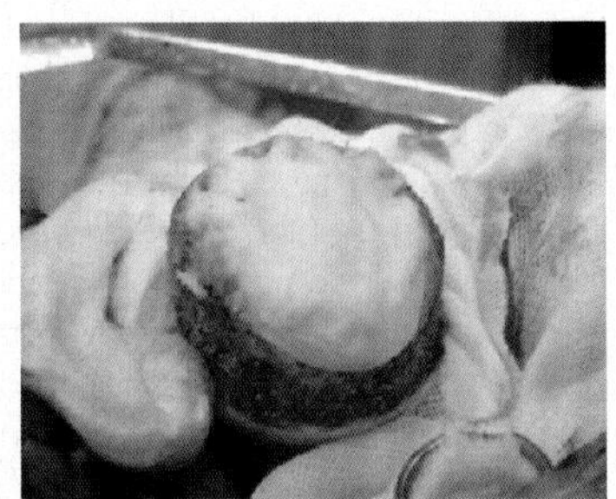

TECH FIG 7 • **A.** After thorough pulsatile saline irrigation, the femoral head is kept dry for implantation with cement. **B.** During cement filling of the defect area of the femoral head, a continuous suction drain is inserted into the central lumen for guide rod. **C.** The cement is applied onto the defect area of the femoral head with a bone cement syringe and finger pressure. *(continued)*

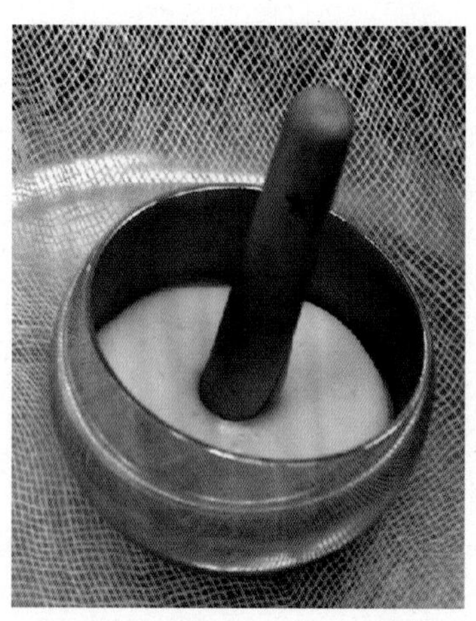
D

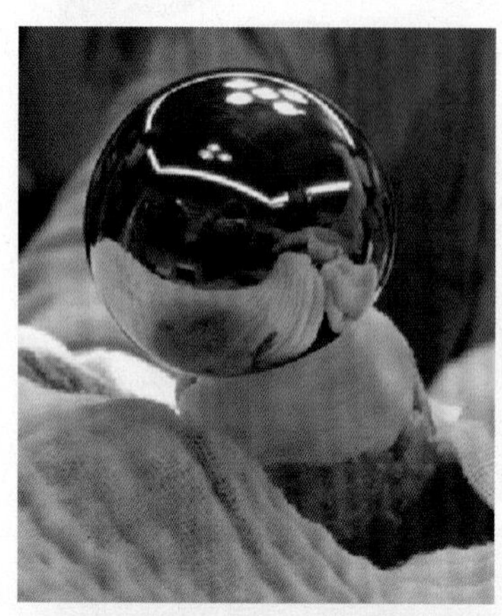
E

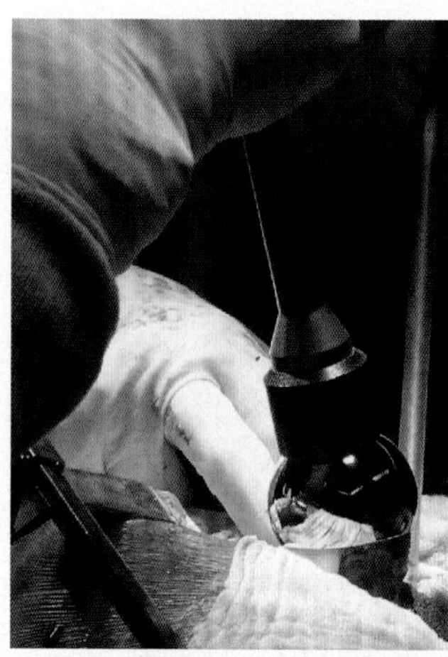
F

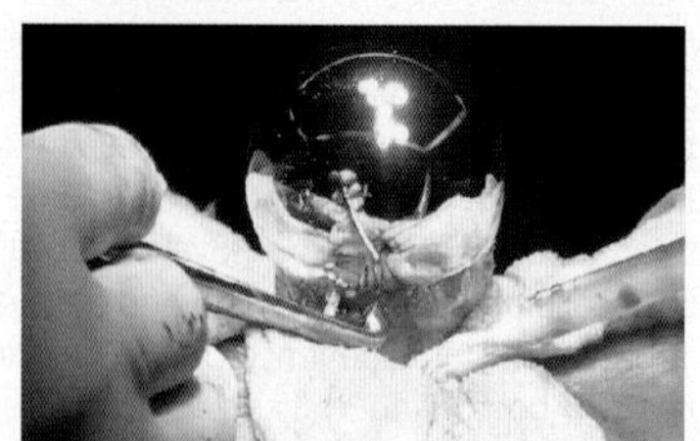
G

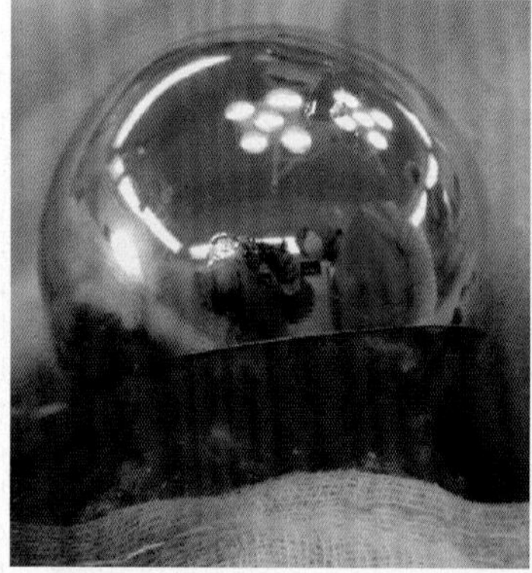
H

TECH FIG 7 • *(continued)* **D.** The cement is filled inside the femoral component as a volume half using a cement syringe. **E,F.** The femoral component is applied to the femoral head with an impactor. **G,H.** Any extruding cement should be removed with a curette, continuing until the bone cement becomes solid.

Hip Resurfacing Using a Navigation System

Patient Positioning

- At our institution, we use a posterolateral approach for hip resurfacing arthroplasty. When we use the hip resurfacing systems with image-free navigation for an acetabular procedure, certain initial maneuvers must be done with the patient in the supine position before moving the patient to the lateral position and undertaking the posterolateral approach because pelvis registration cannot be performed conveniently in the lateral position.
  - Once the pelvis registration has been completed, the patient can be moved to the lateral position.
- If the surgeon uses the navigation system only on the femoral side, the supine position for acetabular registration is not needed, and femoral registration is performed during surgery with the patient in the lateral position.
- Precise location of the registration points is a key factor in ensuring proper matching at every step.

Pelvis Registration

- A small-step incision is made on the iliac crest of the operative side and the fixation pin is inserted for the reference array, using an automatic drill at low speed (**TECH FIG 8A,B**).
  - The second pin is inserted in the same manner using a drill template (**TECH FIG 8C**).
- Once two pins have been inserted, the bone fixator and the pelvis reference array are attached (**TECH FIG 8D**).
  - The bone fixator should remain attached until the end of the entire navigation procedure.
- The plane of the pelvis is defined by entering points on the pelvis according to the navigation software (**TECH FIG 8E,F**).
  - Bony landmarks of interest are the left and right anterior superior iliac spine and the most anterior parts of both pubic bones, which, in most patients, are the pelvic tubercles (**TECH FIG 8G,H**).
- Once registration has been completed, the pelvis reference array is removed without dislodging the fixation pins and bone fixator (**TECH FIG 8I**).
  - The reference array is stored in a sterile location until it is reattached.

Repositioning the Patient

- When the pelvis registration procedure is finished, the patient is moved into the lateral decubitus position, and the surgical area is sterilized and draped thoroughly (**TECH FIG 9**).
- During draping, the surgical team should pay attention to the acetabular fixator and pins to protect against contamination or loosening.

Acquiring Acetabular Landmarks

- The skin is incised in a routine manner and the acetabulum is exposed.

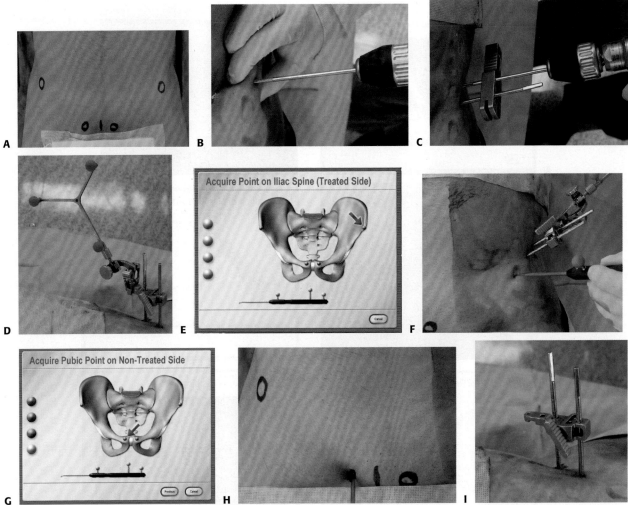

TECH FIG 8 • A. The anterior pelvic plane is defined using four points: the operated and contralateral sides of the anterior superior iliac spine and the most prominent pubic points on both the operated and the contralateral sides. **B.** After local sterilization, a small stab incision is made on the operated iliac crest and the fixation pin is inserted with a low-speed automated drill. The fixation pins should not be inserted near the anterior superior iliac spine point because this point is required for pelvic registration. **C.** The second pin is inserted in the same manner using a drill template. **D.** Once the second fixation pin has been inserted correctly, the bone fixator is attached, and the pelvic reference array is corrected to it. The reference array should be detected by the cameras both in the supine and lateral positions during the operation. **E.** The pelvic plane is defined by entering points on the pelvis as prompted by the software. **F.** The pointer is put in the left anterior superior iliac spine. **G,H.** The pointer is placed on the right pubic point according to the navigation system. **I.** Once registration has been completed, the pelvis reference array is removed without dislodging the fixation pins and bone fixator.

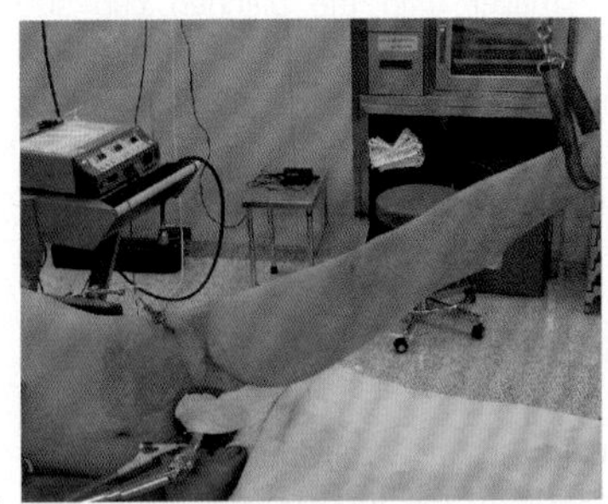

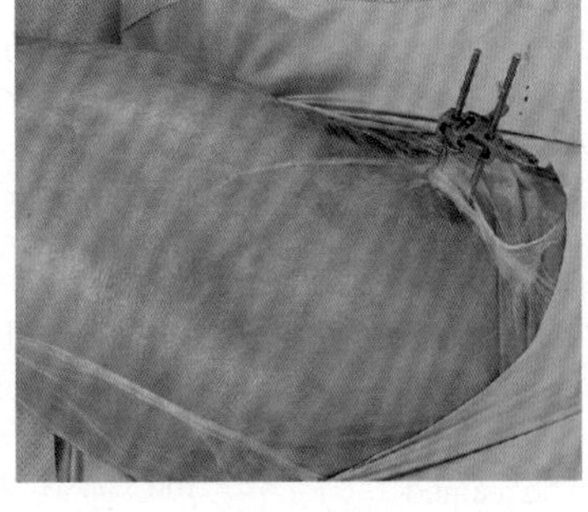

TECH FIG 9 • A. When the pelvis registration procedure is finished, the patient is moved into the lateral decubitus position. During this change in the patient's position and draping, the surgical team should pay attention to the acetabular fixator and pins to protect them from contamination or loosening. **B.** With the patient repositioned and secured, the surgical area is sterilized, and the patient is draped.

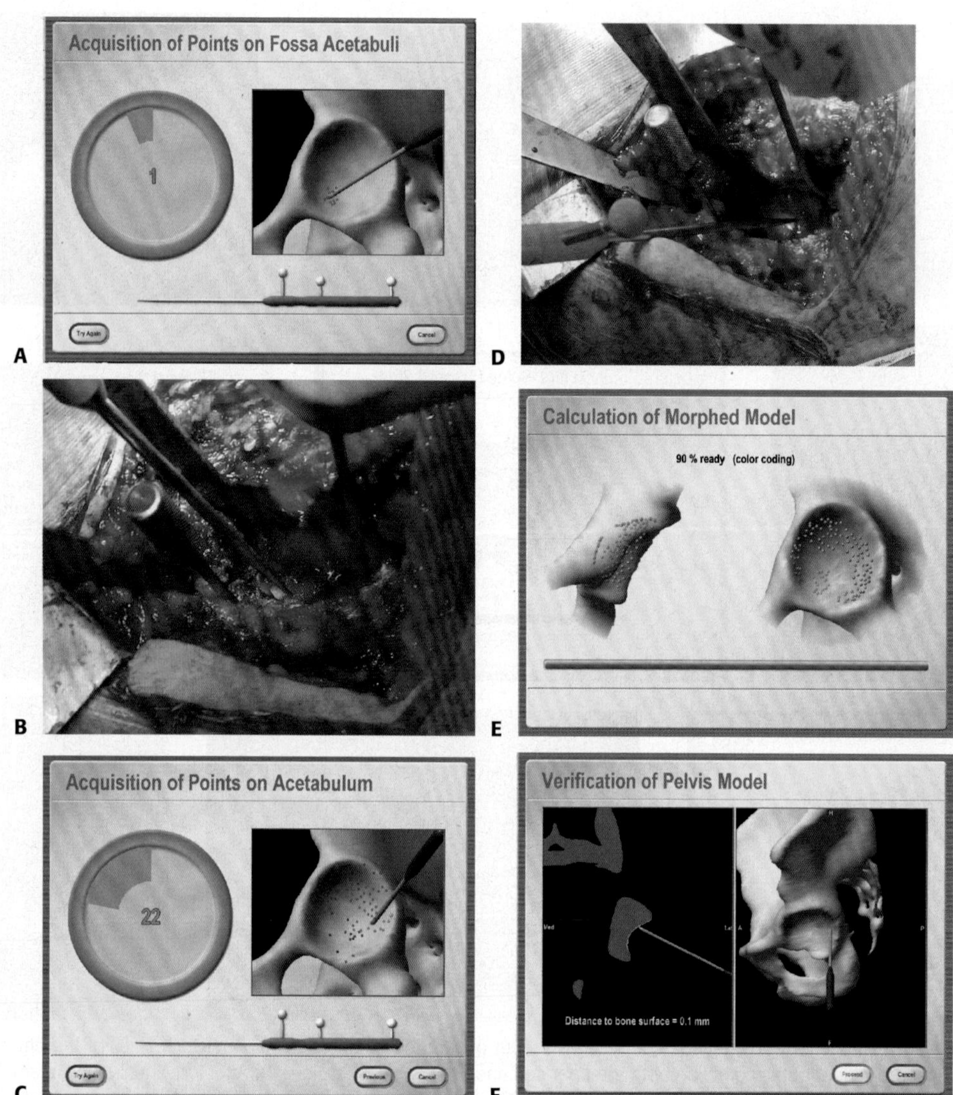

TECH FIG 10 • A,B. Multiple-point acquisition on the cotyloid fossa, the deeper part of the acetabulum, is used to register bony areas. Points acquired in this way are used to calculate the three-dimensional model. The number of points to be acquired is shown in the center of an acquisition clock. **C,D.** Acquiring points on the acetabular wall. **E,F.** Once the bone model has been calculated, pelvis registration is verified.

- Multiple landmark acquisition is used to register the cotyloid fossa and acetabular surface, including margins (**TECH FIG 10A–D**).
- To begin multiple landmark acquisition, the tip of the pointer is touched to the required structure and pivoted slightly.
  - Points are acquired by sliding the pointer tip along the defined structure.
  - Once the bone model has been calculated in the navigation monitor, pelvis registration should be verified immediately (**TECH FIG 10E,F**).

Inserting the Acetabular Cup

- To insert the cup at the desired angle, the bone must be reamed at the same angle as the planned cup (**TECH FIG 11A**).
- The acetabulum is initially reamed with an 8-mm diameter reamer, which is smaller than the planned cup size (**TECH FIG 11B,C**).
  - Subsequent reaming can then continue in increments of 2 mm.
- The planned inclination and version values for the implant are shown during reaming, and the values are updated dynamically (**TECH FIG 11D**).
- Once the reamer has been navigated to the planned position and reaming has been completed, a trial cup generally is used to confirm that the selected cup size is correct (**TECH FIG 11E**).
  - The cup is calibrated with the trial cup or cup inserted (**TECH FIG 11F,G**).

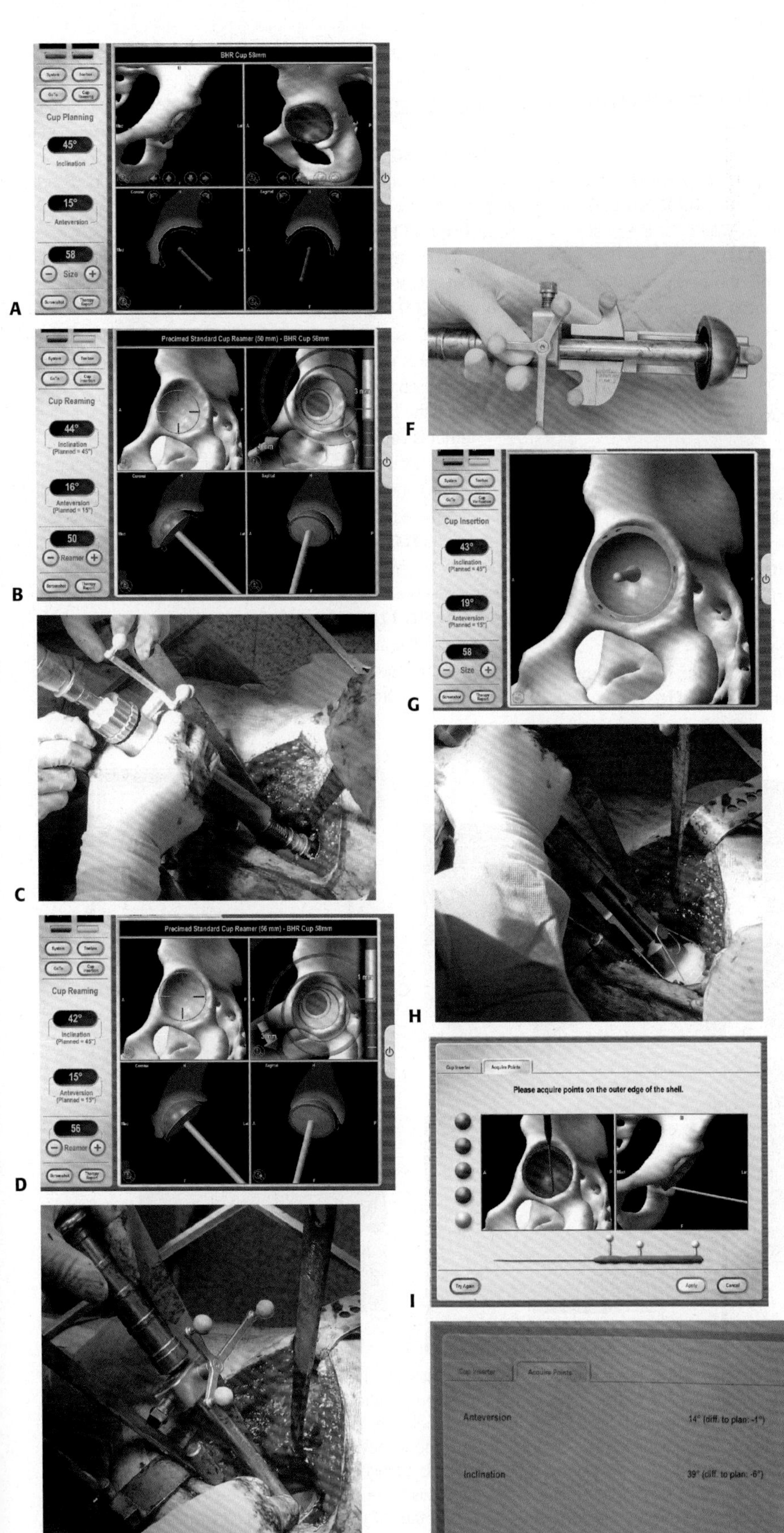

TECH FIG 11 • **A.** The size of the acetabular cup is calculated automatically, with the position of the cup planned per the surgeon's request. **B,C.** During acetabular reaming, these angles are updated dynamically, indicating how far they are inclined, anteverted, or retroverted. Ideally, the cup reamer should be directed according to the planned angles. **D.** Subsequent reaming can then continue in increments of 2 mm, with under-reaming by 2 mm less than the acetabular component to be inserted. Finally, the planned inclination and version values for the implant are shown. **E.** Before the actual acetabular cup is inserted, a trial cup generally is used to verify that the selected cup size and angle are correct. **F.** Calibrating the trial cup inserter with adapter. **G.** The angle of the acetabular cup is shown dynamically during insertion of the component. **H.** The cup inserter is used to place the acetabular cup in alignment with the bone. **I.** Cup placement is verified by acquiring five points along the peripheral margin of the acetabular cup. **J.** The tab page shows both inclination and version of the acetabular cup and compares the difference between real and planned angles.

- The cup inserter is navigated to the planned position, and the cup is inserted according to the manufacturer's recommendations until correct cup placement has been achieved (**TECH FIG 11H**).
  - The cup should be positioned using the anatomy as a reference and aligned with the bone.
  - To verify cup position, the pointer is used to acquire four or five points along the margin of the cup (**TECH FIG 11I**).
  - The navigation screen shows various values for the position of the cup implant (**TECH FIG 11J**).
- Once cup verification has been finished, the pelvic reference array, bone fixator, and two pins are removed, and femoral preparation proceeds.

Acquiring Femoral Landmarks

- For femoral pin insertion, two pins are inserted to the lesser trochanteric area (**TECH FIG 12A**).
- The location of the pins varies. They can be inserted into the proximal diaphyseal area, but the lesser trochanteric area is more comfortable and requires a smaller incision.
- Once two pins have been inserted, the bone fixator and femoral reference array are attached (**TECH FIG 12B**).
  - Before starting registration, as many osteophytes are removed as possible because the presence of osteophytes will affect the femoral notching calculation.
- The first step in femur registration is marking of the medial and lateral epicondyles using a sterile pointer (**TECH FIG 12C,D**). The pointer then is held to the piriformis fossa and head–neck junction (**TECH FIG 12E,F**).
- To acquire femoral head points, the pointer is slid across the surface of the bone following the navigator's direction (**TECH FIG 12G,H**).
- Once the femoral head points have been acquired, points are acquired on the anterior, superior, posterior, and inferior neck in sequence (**TECH FIG 12I,J**).
- Finally, it is necessary to ensure that there are sufficient points in the most critical area of the bone where notching is more likely to occur (**TECH FIG 12K,L**).
- Once registration has been accomplished, a three-dimensional bone model is made on the navigation monitor based on the points acquired (**TECH FIG 12M**).
  - Once the bone model has been made, registration of the femur is verified (**TECH FIG 12N,O**).
- The current neck–shaft angle (ie, varus or valgus, anteversion or retroversion) and calculated inner diameter of the head implant (head size) are shown automatically with images on the navigation screen (**TECH FIG 12P**).
- The software selects the implant size and angle to determine the smallest possible implant that will not cause femoral notching (**TECH FIG 12Q**).
- If necessary, the surgeon adjusts the implant size manually according to the preoperative planning and matches the size with the acetabular component.

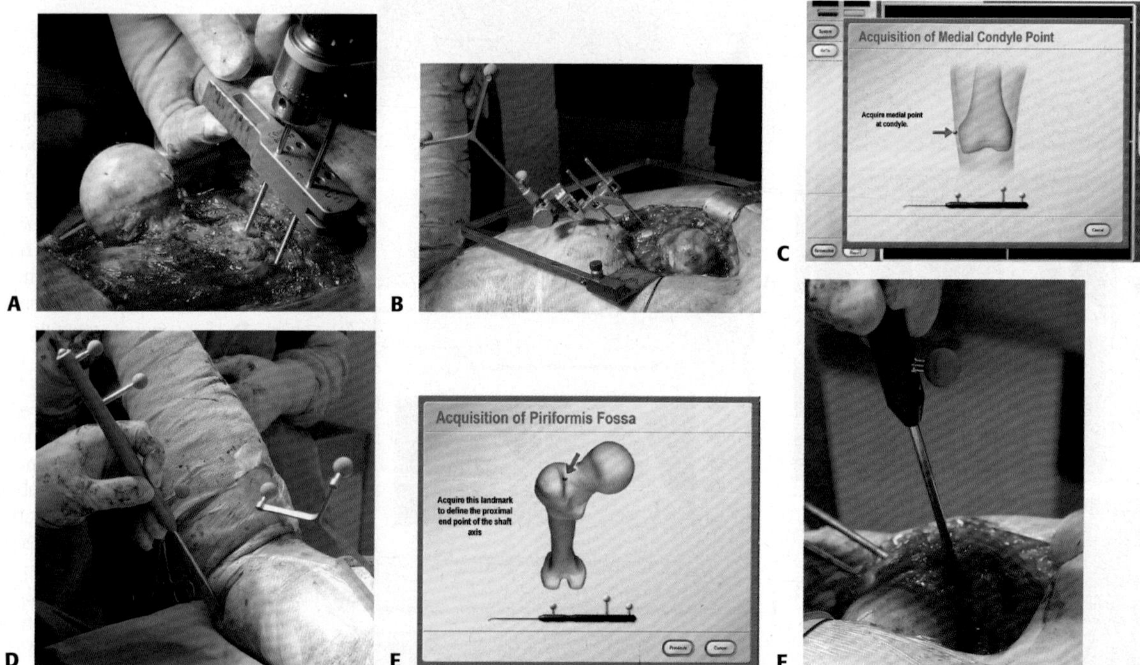

TECH FIG 12 • **A.** The fixation pin is inserted to the lesser trochanter using an automated drill at low speed. The second pin is inserted in the same manner using a drill template. The fixation pins should be placed bicortically for stability. **B.** Once the second fixation pin has been inserted correctly, the bone fixator is attached and the femoral reference array connected to it. Sufficient space should be available to facilitate drilling, reaming, and implant positioning without moving the reference array. **C,D.** Medial and lateral condyle points are acquired using single landmark acquisition. Each point is acquired by holding the tip of the pointer to the surface of the skin at the required location. **E,F.** Acquiring a point on the piriformis fossa. This point is essential for navigation to define the proximal end point of the shaft axis. If this point is not defined correctly, the calculated neck axis and implant position may not be accurate. *(continued)*

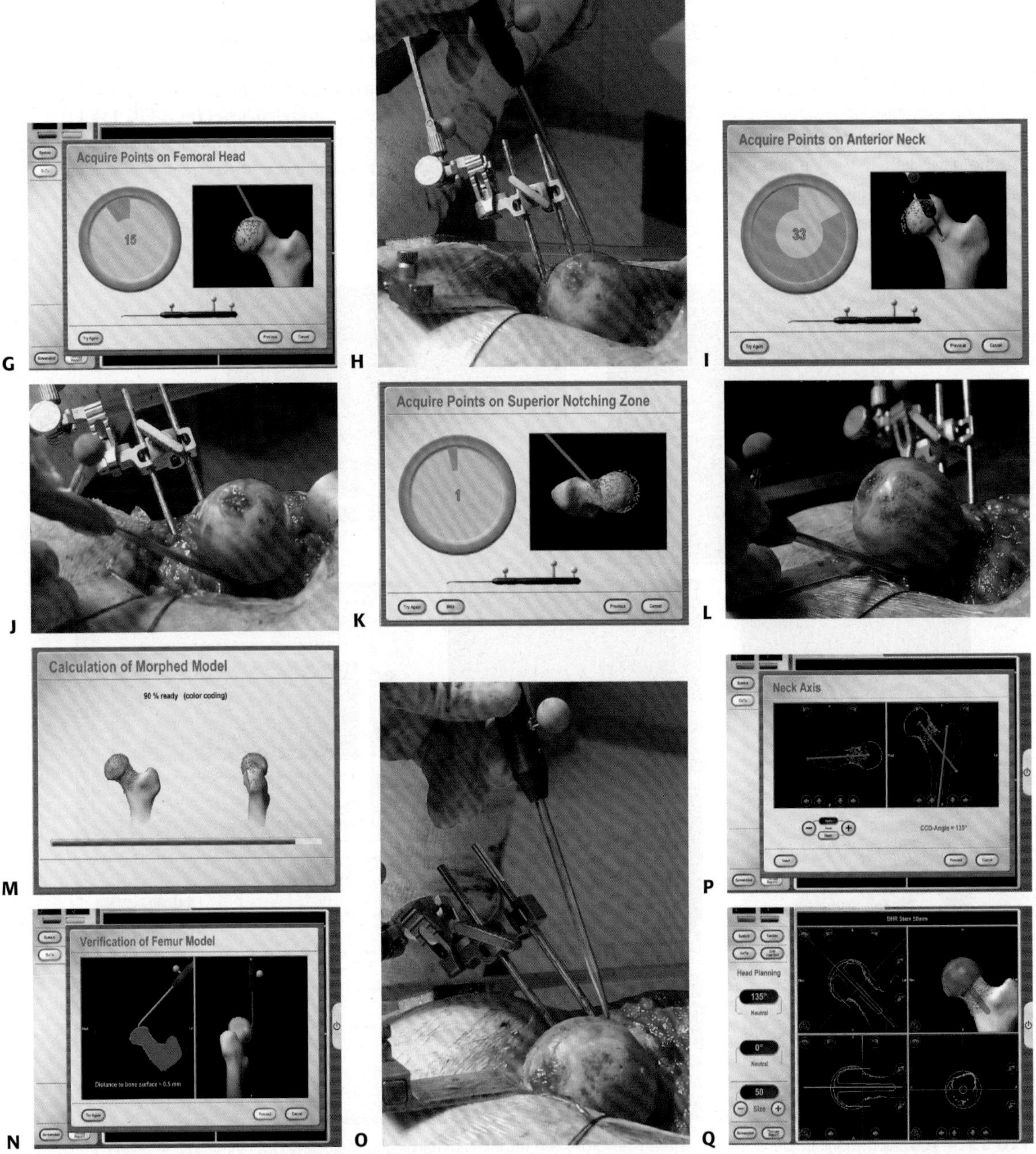

TECH FIG 12 • *(continued)* **G,H.** Acquiring points on the femoral head. To acquire points, the pointer is simply slid across the surface of the bone. This step is important for precise morphologic estimation and for determining the center of rotation and the required implant size. **I,J.** Acquiring points on the anterior, superior, posterior, and inferior neck. These points are used for estimating the neck axis and required implant size and for generating the femoral bony model. **K,L.** Acquiring points in the superior notching zone. This step is used to ensure that sufficient points have been acquired in the most critical area of the femur, where notching is most likely to occur. **M–O.** Once the bone model has been calculated, the femoral registration is verified. **P.** After verification of the femoral model, the current neck–shaft angle is shown automatically, and the surgeon can adjust the angle if necessary. **Q.** The size of the femoral component is calculated automatically, and the position of the component is planned per the surgeon's request.

Femoral Preparation Using Navigation

- Once navigation planning for head implantation has been finished, the drill guide pin is inserted into the femoral head using navigation.
  - The guide pin is moved along the varus–valgus axis and along the antegrade–retrograde axis. The drill guide pin is then relocated to the entry point selected following the navigation system so that it will not result in femoral notching (**TECH FIG 13A,B**).
  - Once the final adjustment has been made, drilling begins via the centering guide pin and femoral notching is rechecked using a stylus (**TECH FIG 13C,D**).
- Once the hole is successfully drilled and the implant positioned, femoral verification is undertaken (**TECH FIG 13E,F**).
- The remaining procedures for femoral component are done in the same manner as those for conventional resurfacing procedures described earlier.

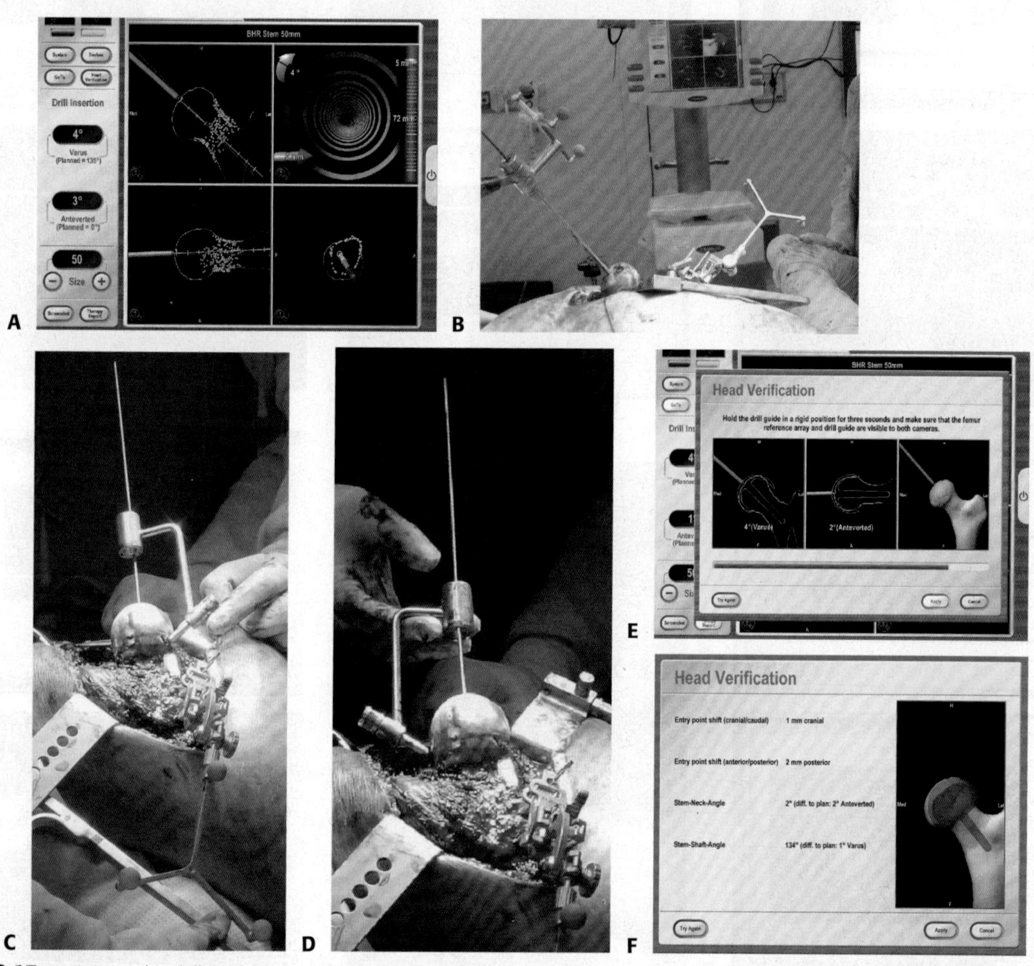

TECH FIG 13 • **A,B.** As the drill guide is moved, the angle values are updated dynamically, indicating how far varus or valgus, anteverted, or retroverted the implant is compared to the planned values. **C,D.** A stylus is used through the guide pin to estimate anterior, posterior, superior, and inferior femoral cutting lines and the possibility of femoral notching. **E,F.** The drill guide is placed over the pin and slid onto the surface of the femoral head to verify the position of the guide pin. The navigation system calculates the position of the implant according to the position of the drill guide. This is the last step in navigation for hip resurfacing. Once the verification process has been finished, the surgeon proceeds to the next step without navigation.

PEARLS AND PITFALLS

Acetabular position	■ Retract the femoral head sufficiently anterior to the acetabulum to provide a better view and to prevent unequal acetabular reaming or malposition of the component when the impactor handle meets the protruded anterior Hohmann retractor and femur. ■ Because the acetabular component has no screw holes and the inner surface consists entirely of polished area, the surgeon cannot see the inner acetabular surface during insertion of the acetabular component. ■ Furthermore, when acetabular osteoporosis is present, the surgeon should be careful to obtain a secure fit of the acetabular component because additional screw fixation is impossible. ■ To prevent under-seating of the acetabular cup, put the trial cup into the fully reamed acetabulum first and check the relation between the peripheral rim of the trial and the acetabulum. Then, when the cup is fully seated in the acetabulum, insert a real cup seated at the same depth as the trial.
Prevent femoral notching	■ Thorough preoperative templating to determine the ideal inlet point for the femoral guide pin is mandatory. ■ Avoid extreme valgus position of the femoral component. ■ Do not ream the entire femoral head all the way to the distal rim of the femoral head. ■ Use a rongeur to carefully remove any remaining distal rim of the femoral head to prevent further damage to the cervical blood supply and possible notching by a motorized reamer. ■ Check notching with the stylus several times during femoral preparation, especially in the anterior and superior portion of the femoral head, which is the most vulnerable for notching. ■ The patient must use crutches and then a cane to support weight bearing for 2 months to resist mechanical stress and permit femoral neck remodeling.
Femoral component seating	■ Use a custom-made femoral trial before insertion of the real component and check the level of the femoral component and relation (gap) between the lower peripheral margin of the trial and the distal rim of the femoral head when the trial is fully seated. Then insert a real femoral component of the same depth as the trial. ■ Insert the femoral component before the "dough" stage of cement is finished; cement that is too hard may prevent the femoral component from being seated.
Femoral side first	■ *Pros:* Retracting the femoral head for acetabular preparation is relatively easy because the femoral head is smaller after femoral preparation. ■ If the femoral head is not fit for resurfacing after preparation, conventional THA can be used. ■ *Cons:* A mismatch between the acetabular and femoral components can develop after femoral preparation. ■ An already prepared, mainly cancellous, femoral head may be damaged during retraction.
Acetabular side first	■ *Pros:* Avoid mismatch between acetabular and femoral components. Acetabular cup size dictates the femoral component size. ■ *Cons:* It is not easy to obtain sufficient anterior retraction of the whole femoral head during acetabular preparation. ■ If, after preparation, the femoral head is not suitable for resurfacing, large-head, metal-on-metal THA should be performed regardless of the surgeon's preference.

POSTOPERATIVE CARE

- The patient receives a second-generation cephalosporin 1 hour before the operation starts and for 36 to 48 hours postsurgery.
- An antithromboembolic stocking and pneumatic pump is applied immediately after the operation to prevent deep vein thrombosis (DVT) and permit mobilization on the first day after the operation.
- Low-molecular-weight heparin or indirect factor Xa inhibitor can be administered for medical prevention of DVT and pulmonary embolism (depends on DVT prevalence in each country).
- Various protocols for rehabilitation may be followed:
  - We continue partial weight bearing with crutches for 4 to 6 weeks to allow initial bony ingrowth on the acetabular side and to allow the patient to regain normal gait and balance.
  - To allow femoral remodeling around the neck area, we usually recommend that the patient use a cane until the end of the second month after the operation, after which full weight bearing is permitted. Light sports activity may begin no sooner than 3 months after the operation, after which the patient may even squat on the floor.
  - Patients are allowed to ride in a car as a passenger, drive a car, sleep on their side, or engage in any activities if able and so desired.
  - Regular sports activities are allowed after 6 months.

OUTCOMES

- Many authors have reported long-term results of metal-on-metal hip resurfacing arthroplasty. Treacy et al[26] reported a 95.5% survival rate at 10 years postoperatively in 144 consecutive patients, using the Birmingham hip resurfacing system (Smith & Nephew, Memphis, TN). Amstutz et al.[3] reported a survival rate of 93.9% at 5 years and 88.5% at 10 years postoperatively in 100 patients, using the Conserve Plus system (Wright Medical Technology, Memphis, TN). They also reported that the 10-year survival rates were 95.6% for those with a femoral component size of greater than 46 mm, 83.8% for 44 mm and 46 mm, and 78.9% for 42 mm or smaller. Gross et al[9] reported an 11-year survivorship rate of 93% using the hybrid Corin Cormet 2000 system (Corin Medical, Cirencester, United Kingdom).
- Mont et al[19] reported the results of metal-on-metal hip resurfacing for treatment of osteonecrosis of the femoral head in 42 hips with mean of 41 months follow-up. At the time of the final follow-up, the survival rate was 94.5% for patients with osteonecrosis and 95.2% for patients with osteoarthritis.
- Amstutz and Le Duff[2] reported no difference in survivorship between the osteonecrosis group and the control group after adjusting for head size, body mass index, and defect size.

The 8-year survival rate for the osteonecrosis group was 93.9% and the control group 93.4%.

- Daniel et al[6] reported on the results of metal-on-metal resurfacing in patients younger than 55 years with hip osteoarthritis.
  - Four hundred forty-six resurfacings were performed in 384 patients, with a maximum follow-up of 8.2 years (mean 3.3 years).
  - Out of 440 hips, there was only one failure (0.02%), giving a survival rate of 99.8%.
  - Thirty-one percent of the men with unilateral resurfacings and 28% with bilateral resurfacings could do heavy or moderately heavy jobs; 92% of men with unilateral resurfacings and 87% of the whole group could participate in leisure-time sports activity.
- Yoo et al[30] prospectively investigated the effect of resurfacing arthroplasty on the bone mineral density (BMD) of the femur by comparing 50 patients with hip resurfacing to 50 patients with uncemented THA.
  - The resurfacing patients demonstrated BMD loss of 2.6% in Gruen zone 1 and 0.6% in zone 7, whereas the THA patients had BMD loss of 7.8% in Gruen zone 1 and 7.7% in zone 7 at 1 year after surgery.
  - On the acetabular side, the resurfacing patients demonstrated BMD loss of 8% in Delee and Charnley zone 1 and 17.5% in zone 2, whereas the THA patients had BMD loss of 9.8% in zone 1 and 22.3% in zone 2.
- Hip resurfacing system transfers load to the proximal femur in a more physiologic manner than long-stem devices, and it may prevent stress shielding and preserves the bone stock of the proximal femur.[24]
- Cooke et al[5] reported that bone density of the femoral neck following hip resurfacing appears to decrease at 6 weeks and 3 months, returned to preoperative levels at 1 year, and was maintained at 3 years.
- Technetium 99m (Tc 99m) bone scan/single photon-emission computed tomography, microangiography with microcomputer tomography revealed that the intraosseous vascular network blood supply to the femoral head is maintained after hip resurfacing even if division of the deep branch of the medial femoral circumflex artery occurs during a posterior approach.[25] Forrest et al[8] suggested that femoral head viability after hip resurfacing can be evaluated with fluoride positron emission tomography. Nasser and Beaulé[20] recommended directing the reamer superolaterally and staying as close as possible to the inferomedial neck because damage to the retinacular vessels can occur without penetrating the femoral neck.
- Shimmin and Back[23] carried out a national review of fractures associated with hip resurfacing systems implanted between 1999 and 2003 in Australia.
  - Eighty-nine surgeons inserted the Birmingham hip resurfacing system in 3497 cases.
  - Fracture of the neck of the femur occurred in 50 patients with an incidence rate of 1.46%.
    - The relative risk of fracture was higher for women than for men.
    - The mean time to fracture was 15.4 weeks and it was often preceded by a prodromal phase of pain and limping.
    - Significant varus placement of the femoral component, intraoperative notching of the femoral component, and technical problems were the common risk factors in 85% of cases.
- McBryde et al[17] reported that although female patients may initially appear to have a greater risk for the need for revision, this increased risk is related to differences in the femoral component size and thus indirectly relates to sex.
- Amstutz et al[1] presented their experience with femoral neck fractures that occurred after metal-on-metal hybrid surface arthroplasty.
  - In a series of 600 resurfacings, five femoral neck fractures occurred (incidence 0.83%).
    - Four of the fractures occurred within the first 5 months after surgery.
    - All five fractures were associated with structural or technical risk factors, which may have weakened the femoral neck.
- Low bone density increases the risk of femoral neck fracture following resurfacing.[1]
- Schmalzried et al[22] reported that the outcomes of resurfacing are dependent on the preoperative characteristics of the proximal femur; patients with higher grade hips (those with earlier stage disease) have better outcomes.
- In cases of failed joint-preserving procedures such as core decompression or vascularized fibular grafting for osteonecrosis of the femoral head, hip resurfacing arthroplasty may play a role as a salvage operation.[4]
- Impingement between the acetabular cup and the femoral neck after hip resurfacing occurred mainly at the superior aspect of the femoral neck with an incidence rate between 6.3% and 22%.[10,29] However, most patients did not have symptoms affecting implant stability.
- de Steiger et al[7] reported that articular surface replacement (ASR, DePuy, Warsaw, IN) prostheses used in conventional hip arthroplasty and in hip resurfacing exhibited a greater revision rate compared with other prostheses. The cumulative revision rate of arthroplasties involving the ASR system at 5 years postoperatively was 10.9% compared with 4.0% for arthroplasties involving all other types of resurfacing prostheses.
- Kwon et al[15] reported that asymptomatic pseudotumor after metal-on-metal hip resurfacing arthroplasty was associated with significantly higher cobalt and chromium levels and inferior functional scores in 4% of the cases they studied.
- Langton et al[16] reported that in a multicenter study involving 4226 hips, the median chromium and cobalt concentrations in the failed group were significantly higher than in the control group. Survival analysis showed a failure rate in the patients with ASR of 9.8% at 5 years compared with less than 1% at 5 years for the Conserve Plus and 1.5% at 10 years for the Birmingham Hip Resurfacing systems.
- In 2008, there was a voluntary recall of the Durom acetabular component (Durom Cup, Zimmer, IN) because the instructions for use/surgical technique instructions were inadequate.
- In 2010, the Medicines and Healthcare Products Regulatory Agency in the United Kingdom recalled the ASR total hip system because of new unpublished data from the United Kingdom joint registry indicating that revision rates within 5 years were approximately 13%.[27]

COMPLICATIONS

- Femoral neck fracture
- Neck notching
- Neck narrowing (over 10% of normal width)
- Impingement between acetabular component and the femoral neck
- Femoral loosening[12]
- Femoral head collapse due to osteonecrosis
- Acetabular loosening
- Stem tip condensation
- Soft tissue reactions to metal ion
  - Adverse local tissue reaction/aseptic lymphocytic vasculitis–associated lesions
  - Metal hypersensitivity
  - Pseudotumor
- Metal ion release into the bloodstream
- Infection
- Femoral/sciatic nerve palsy
- DVT
- Dislocation
- Heterotopic ossification
- Spur formation

REFERENCES

1. Amstutz HC, Campbell PA, Le Duff MJ. Fracture of the neck of the femur after surface arthroplasty of the hip. J Bone Joint Surg Am 2004;86A:1874–1877.
2. Amstutz HC, Le Duff MJ. Hip resurfacing results for osteonecrosis are as good as for other etiologies at 2 to 12 years. Clin Orthop Relat Res 2010;468(2):375–381.
3. Amstutz HC, Le Duff MJ, Campbell PA, et al. Clinical and radiographic results of metal-on-metal hip resurfacing with a minimum ten-year follow-up. J Bone Joint Surg Am 2010;92(16):2663–2671.
4. Chun YS, Yoo MC, Kim KI, et al. Total Resurfacing arthroplasty after failed hip preserving procedures for osteonecrosis of the femoral head [abstract]. Abstract book of the 21st Annual Congress of the International Society for Technology in Arthroplasty (ISTA). Seoul, Korea, 2008.
5. Cooke NJ, Rodgers L, Rawlings D, et al. Bone density of the femoral neck following Birmingham hip resurfacing. Acta Orthop 2009;80(6):660–665.
6. Daniel J, Pysent PB, McMinn DJW. Metal-on-metal resurfacing of the hip in patients under the age of 55 years with osteoarthritis. J Bone Joint Surg Br 2004;86B:177–184.
7. de Steiger RN, Hang JR, Miller LN, et al. Five-year results of the ASR XL Acetabular System and the ASR Hip Resurfacing System: an analysis from the Australian Orthopaedic Association National Joint Replacement Registry. J Bone Joint Surg Am 2011;93(24):2287–2293.
8. Forrest N, Welch A, Murray AD, et al. Femoral head viability after Birmingham resurfacing hip arthroplasty: assessment with use of [18F] fluoride positron emission tomography. J Bone Joint Surg Am 2006;88(suppl 3):84–89.
9. Gross TP, Liu F, Webb LA. Clinical outcome of the metal-on-metal hybrid Corin Cormet 2000 hip resurfacing system: an up to 11-year follow-up study. J Arthroplasty 2012;27(4):533–538.
10. Gruen TA, Le Duff MJ, Wisk LE, et al. Prevalence and clinical relevance of radiographic signs of impingement in metal-on-metal hybrid hip resurfacing. J Bone Joint Surg Am 2011;93(16):1519–1526.
11. Hardinge K. The direct lateral approach to the hip. J Bone Joint Surg Br 1982;64B:17–18.
12. Howie DW, Cornish BC, Vernon-Roberts B. Resurfacing hip arthroplasty. Classification of loosening and the role of prosthetic wear particles. Clin Orthop Relat Res 1990;255:144–159.
13. Howie DW, Cornish BC, Vernon-Roberts B. The viability of the femoral head after resurfacing hip arthroplasty in humans. Clin Orthop Relat Res 1993;291:171–184.
14. Kim KI, Yoo MC, Cho YJ, et al. Comparison of results of resurfacing arthroplasty performed using a navigation system and conventional technique. Abstract book of the 21st Annual Congress of the International Society for Technology in Arthroplasty (ISTA). Seoul, Korea, 2008.
15. Kwon YM, Ostlere SJ, McLardy-Smith P, et al. "Asymptomatic" pseudotumors after metal-on-metal hip resurfacing arthroplasty: prevalence and metal ion study. J Arthroplasty 2011;26(4):511–518.
16. Langton DJ, Joyce TJ, Jameson SS, et al. Adverse reaction to metal debris following hip resurfacing: the influence of component type, orientation and volumetric wear. J Bone Joint Surg Br 2011;93(2):164–171.
17. McBryde CW, Theivendran K, Thomas AM, et al. The influence of head size and sex on the outcome of Birmingham hip resurfacing. J Bone Joint Surg Am 2010;92(1):105–112.
18. McMinn D, Treacy R, Lin K, et al. Metal on metal surface replacement of the hip: experience of the McMinn prosthesis. Clin Orthop Relat Res 1996;329(suppl):S89–S98.
19. Mont MA, Seyler TM, Marker DR, et al. Use of mental-on-metal total hip resurfacing for the treatment of osteonecrosis of the femoral head. J Bone Joint Surg Am 2006;88:90–97.
20. Nasser AB, Beaulé PE. Femoral head vascularity and hip resurfacing. In: Amstutz HC, ed. Hip Resurfacing Principles, Indications, Technique and Results. Philadelphia: Saunders Elsevier, 2008:17–22.
21. Ramesh M, O'Byrne JM, McCarthy N, et al. Damage to the superior gluteal nerve after the Hardinge approach to the hip. J Bone Joint Surg Br 1996;78B:903–906.
22. Schmalzried TP, Silva M, de la Rosa M, et al. Optimizing patient selection and outcomes with total hip resurfacing. Clin Orthop Relat Res 2005;441:200–204.
23. Shimmin AJ, Back D. Femoral neck fractures following Birmingham hip resurfacing. A national review of 50 cases. J Bone Joint Surg Br 2005;87B:463–464.
24. Sugano N. Femoral DEXA studies in hip arthroplasty. In: McMinn DJW, Modern Hip Resurfacing. London: Springer-Verlag, 2009:131–133.
25. Sugano N, Nishii T, Hananouchi T. Femoral head blood supply studies. In: McMinn DJW, Modern Hip Resurfacing. London: Springer-Verlag, 2009:125–127.
26. Treacy RB, McBryde CW, Shears E, et al. Birmingham hip resurfacing: a minimum follow-up of ten years. J Bone Joint Surg Br, 2011; 93(1):27–33.
27. U.S. Food and Drug Administration. Recalls. Available at: http://www.fda.gov/medicaldevices /productsandmedicalprocedures/implantsandprosthetics/metalonmetalhipimplants/ucm241770.htm. Accessed July 2, 2014.
28. Wagner H. Surface replacement arthroplasty of the hip. Clin Orthop Relat Res 1978;134: 102–130.
29. Yoo MC, Cho YJ, Chun YS, et al. Impingement between the acetabular cup and the femoral neck after hip resurfacing arthroplasty. J Bone Joint Surg Am 2011;93(suppl 2):99–106.
30. Yoo MC, Cho YJ, Kim KI, et al. Changes in BMD in the proximal femur after cementless total hip arthroplasty and resurfacing arthroplasty. Prospective, longitudinal, comparative study. J Korean Orthop Assoc 2006;41:212–219.
31. Yoo MC, Cho YJ, Kim KI, et al. Resurfacing arthroplasty in osteonecrosis of the femoral head [abstract]. Abstract book of the 23rd World Congress of the SICOT/SIROT. Istanbul, Turkey, 2005.

Total Hip Arthroplasty for Malignant Lesions

R. Lor Randall and Lisa A. Kafchinski

DEFINITION

- Metastatic bone disease (MBD) afflicts more than half of the 1.2 million patients newly diagnosed with cancer annually.[4,8]
- Bony involvement can be a major source of morbidity and mortality if not treated appropriately.
- The femur is the long bone most commonly affected, with 25% of cases involving the proximal third of the femur.[4,16,17]
- The pelvis is the third most common site for metastasis.[7]
- Seventy-five percent of all surgery for cancer that has metastasized to bone is performed in the hip area.[17]

ANATOMY

- Metastatic foci to any part of the areas around the hip substantially compromise the mechanical integrity of the bone, placing the patient at high risk for fracture and subsequent nonunion.
- The bony structure of the acetabulum consists of the anterior and posterior columns and their respective walls, which jut over laterally to cover the femoral head.
- The anterior column is defined as the bone that extends from the iliac crest to the pubic symphysis.
- The posterior column starts from the articulation of the superior gluteal notch with the sacrum and extends through the acetabulum and ischium to the inferior pubic ramus.
- The acetabular dome, the superior weight-bearing region, consists of both the anterior and posterior columns and is contributed to by both walls.
- The femoral head is not truly spherical; it is congruent only along the weight-bearing portion.
- The principal and secondary bony trabeculations of the head, neck, and intertrochanteric area enable the head and neck arcade to withstand tremendous compressive and tensile forces.

PATHOGENESIS

- The mechanism by which metastases occur is accounted for in a modified "seed/soil" theorem. Fewer than 1 in 10,000 neoplastic cells that escape into the circulation from the primary site are able to set up a metastatic focus. Metastasis, a complex, multistep process in which the cell first must break free, is a function of degradative enzymes such as collagenases, hydrolases, cathepsin D, and proteases. Once the cell invades the vascular channel, it circulates through the body.
- It is theorized that the cell is protected by a fibrin platelet clot. Clinical trials with heparin have not shown a significant change in metastatic outcome, however. Local factors such as integrins are instrumental in attracting the circulating metastatic cell to a particular remote tissue site. Once within the new tissue, the metastatic cell releases mediators such as tumor angiogenesis factor, inducing neovascularization, which in turn facilitates growth of the metastatic focus.
- Patients with advanced metastatic disease often experience dysfunction of hematopoietic and calcium homeostasis. They may develop a normochromic, normocytic anemia with leukocytosis. The increased number of immature cells, produced in response to the anemia and noted on the peripheral blood smear, is termed a *leukoerythroblastic reaction*.
  - Hypercalcemia may be seen in up to 30% of patients with extensive metastases, most commonly in myeloma, breast cancer, and non–small cell lung cancer.
- Blastic metastases are often painless and are associated with a lower incidence of pathologic fracture because the bone is not as severely weakened. Not all tumors that metastasize from the prostate to bone are blastic in nature, however. The lytic variants are painful and can cause pathologic fractures.
- Most tumors that metastasize from the breast to bone are blastic, but some demonstrate mixtures of blastic and lytic areas in the same bone. By taking serial radiographs and noting the appearance of bone metastases, it is possible to follow the progress of treatment with systemic hormone therapy or chemotherapy agents plus local radiation therapy. A favorable response may show a gradual conversion from a lytic to a blastic appearance as the pain decreases.
- Bone destruction in lytic lesions occurs as a result of the biologic response by native osteoclasts to the tumor. Neovascularization is common. Among the tumors that are characteristic for this hemorrhagic response are thyroid carcinomas, renal cell carcinomas, and multiple myelomas.
- Before surgical intervention is undertaken for these tumor types, it may be beneficial to perform a prophylactic embolization of the area to reduce perioperative bleeding. If a lesion is unexpectedly found to be aneurysmal at the time of surgical exploration, the friable tumor mass should be debulked rapidly down to normal bone, and the area should be packed until it can be stabilized with bone cement.

NATURAL HISTORY

- Metastatic involvement of the musculoskeletal system is one of the most significant clinical issues facing orthopaedic oncologists. The number of patients with metastasis to the skeletal system from a carcinoma is 15 times greater than the number of patients with primary bone tumors of all types. About one-third of all diagnosed adenocarcinomas include skeletal metastases, resulting in about 300,000 cases per year. Furthermore, 70% of patients with advanced, terminal carcinoma demonstrate bone metastases at autopsy.

- The carcinomas that commonly metastasize to bone are those of the prostate, breast, kidney, thyroid, and lung. One study showed that nearly 90% of patients with these types of carcinoma had bone metastases.
  - Among the carcinomas that less commonly metastasize to bone are cancers of the skin, oral cavity, esophagus, cervix, stomach, and colon.
- Because patients with MBD are surviving longer, surgeons must strive to perform an optimal reconstruction that can provide functional outcome for many years. However, once a pathologic fracture has occurred, a patient's life expectancy is considerably shorter. Therefore, stringent surveillance by medical oncologists for bony metastases must be encouraged, with early referral to the orthopaedic surgeon before pathologic fractures occur.
  - When patient survival is greater than 1 year after operative fixation for MBD, reoperation rates range from 3.1% to 42%.[3]

PATIENT HISTORY AND PHYSICAL FINDINGS

- In any patient with a history of cancer, especially those cancers that are well documented to metastasize to bone, any bone pain should raise suspicion for a metastatic focus.
- Pain at rest or at night that is or is not exacerbated with activity should heighten this suspicion.
- The hip examination may or may not be abnormal.

IMAGING AND OTHER DIAGNOSTIC STUDIES

- A methodical approach is mandatory in the workup of a patient with presumed metastatic disease to bone to locate the primary tumor.
  - A thorough history and physical examination must be completed before laboratory and radiographic analyses are done. The primary carcinoma may be detected on physical examination in as many as 8% of patients.
  - Laboratory analysis should include a complete blood count, erythrocyte sedimentation rate, renal and liver panels, alkaline phosphate, and serum protein electrophoresis.
- A plain chest radiograph and radiographs of known involved bones should follow.
  - For metastases to the hip, an anteroposterior (AP) radiograph of the pelvis and full AP and lateral radiographs of the entire femur should be obtained.
  - About 45% of all primary tumors will be detected in the lung on the chest radiograph.
- The workup also should include a staging bone scan.
  - If this scan is negative, myeloma should be suspected.
  - If the scan is positive, a lesion may be found at a more convenient biopsy site.
  - Bone scanning is more sensitive than plain radiographs in detecting early lesions.
- Computed tomography (CT) scans of the chest, abdomen, and pelvis should be performed.
  - CT of the lung can detect up to 15% of primary tumors missed on the plain radiograph.
- The use of positron emission tomography scanning, either in isolation or in conjunction with CT, is becoming more common in the workup of patients with possible metastatic cancer.
- These studies, in combination with a well-planned biopsy, will reveal the primary cancer for most patients.
  - Routine radiographic screening studies in search of early metastatic disease are not very helpful. Lytic changes become evident on routine radiographs only when cortical destruction approaches 30% to 50%.
- If a lesion is detected about the hip in the anatomic areas as described earlier, and a detailed pelvic and hip CT scan has not been performed within the past 6 to 8 weeks, one should be ordered.
  - Intravenous contrast medium is not necessary.
  - A recent CT scan is particularly important in the preoperative planning for an acetabular reconstruction.

DIFFERENTIAL DIAGNOSIS

- Prostate cancer
- Breast cancer
- Kidney carcinoma
- Thyroid carcinoma
- Lung carcinoma
- Myeloma
- Lymphoma of bone, although less common, can mimic these diagnoses.
- For a patient older than the age of 40 years, with no known history of metastatic carcinoma to bone, the osteophilic malignancies mentioned earlier must be considered and evaluated as described.

NONOPERATIVE MANAGEMENT

- Nonsurgical management of metastatic carcinoma to bone includes observation, radiation treatment, and hormonal or cytotoxic chemotherapy.
- Radiation is reserved for palliative intervention. Each patient's suitability for radiation therapy must be carefully determined. The histologic type of disease, extent of disease, prognosis, marrow reserve, and overall constitution must be assessed.
- Impending lesions about the proximal femur and acetabulum should dissuade the orthopedist from nonoperative management, particularly in renal cell and thyroid carcinoma, where bony destruction is likely to progress despite the best nonsurgical modalities.
- For a patient who has sustained a pathologic fracture secondary to metastatic carcinoma, the average survival time is 19 months.
  - Each histologic type has varying lengths of survival: prostate, 29 months; breast, 23 months; renal, 12 months; and lung, 4 months.
  - Moreover, each type of carcinoma exhibits varying radiosensitivity: prostate and lymphoreticular carcinomas, excellent; breast carcinoma, intermediate; and renal and gastrointestinal carcinomas, poor.
- When radiation therapy is used appropriately, 90% of patients gain at least minimal relief, with up to two-thirds obtaining complete relief. Seventy percent of patients who are ambulatory retain their ability to ambulate after radiation therapy to the lower extremities.
  - Systemic radioisotopes also may be used. Strontium 89 mimics calcium distribution in the body and has shown promise in clinical applications.

- When a patient has sustained a true pathologic fracture (rather than an impending lesion), surgical stabilization usually is indicated, with subsequent radiation therapy.
  - Because of poor bone quality, bone cement often must be used to augment the fixation.
- Hormonal therapy has an important role in the management of metastatic breast and prostate cancer. Fortunately, these agents are easy to administer and have few side effects.
- For breast cancer, medical hormonal manipulation can be done by use of antiestrogens, progestins, luteinizing hormone–releasing hormone, or adrenal-suppressing agents.
  - Tamoxifen is effective in 30% of all breast cancer cases; its effectiveness increases to 50% to 75% of cases in which the tumor is known to be estrogen receptor– and progesterone receptor–positive.
  - Surgical ablation (oophorectomy) also may have a role in certain cases.
- In some cases of prostate cancer, reduction in testosterone levels via bilateral orchiectomy or administration of estrogens or antiandrogens may produce dramatic results.
  - Estrogens are no longer used as a first-line agent because of the risk of cardiovascular complications.
- Cytotoxic chemotherapy is used extensively in the treatment of adenocarcinoma. However, in older patients with advanced disease, the side effects of the drugs may be too severe.

SURGICAL MANAGEMENT

- For cases involving the periacetabular area, femoral head, neck, and intertrochanteric area, cemented femoral arthroplasty components are an important surgical option for impending and realized fracture management.
- The goals for surgical intervention in the patient with metastatic carcinoma to bone are relief of pain; prevention of impending pathologic fracture; stabilization of true fractures; enhancement of mobility, function, and quality of life; and, for some, improved survival.
- It is generally agreed that a patient must have a life expectancy of at least 6 weeks to warrant operative intervention.
- Cancer patients, regardless of their age, may have increased difficulty protecting their fixation device or prosthesis secondary to systemic debilitation. Accordingly, rigid fixation, with polymethylmethacrylate (PMMA) augmentation as needed, is mandatory.

Preoperative Planning

- In many cases, the diagnosis of metastasis to the proximal femur will be made before a fracture occurs. In these cases, it is the responsibility of the orthopaedic surgeon to decide whether the patient should receive some form of internal stabilization before radiation therapy is begun. A CT scan of the involved area will help make this decision.
- Criteria for the performance of a prophylactic stabilization procedure include the following:
  - Fifty percent cortical lysis
  - A femoral lesion greater than 2.5 cm in diameter
  - An avulsion fracture of the lesser trochanter
  - Persistent pain in the hip area 4 weeks following the completion of radiation therapy

Table 1 Mirels Scoring System

Variable	1 Point	2 Points	3 Points
Site	Upper limb	Lower limb	Peritrochanteric
Pain	Mild	Moderate	Functional
Lesion	Blastic	Mixed	Lytic
Extent	Less than one-third	One to two-thirds	Greater than-two thirds

A mean score of 7 or below indicates a low risk of fracture; radiation therapy should be considered. A score of 8 or above suggests a substantial risk and surgical intervention is recommended.

- A Mirels score (Table 1) also may help in treatment decision making for hip and femoral lesions.
  - As elucidated in the Mirels score, the peritrochanteric area in general is at high risk for fracturing.
  - These criteria are not perfect, and large errors arise in estimation of the load-bearing capacity of the bone. For example, no system takes into account the histologic subtype, preexisting osteoporosis, and functional demands. Objective quantification of pain in the Mirels score is controversial as well.

Periacetabular Lesions and Impending and Realized Fractures

- Class I (minor): Lateral cortices, superior wall, and medial wall are intact (**FIG 1**). Treat with conventional cemented acetabular component with or without rebar (anchorage with large fragment screws) as needed (Table 2).
- Class II (major): Deficient medial wall (**FIG 2**) requires an antiprotrusio device, medial mesh, or rebar (Table 2).
- Class III (massive): Deficient lateral cortices and dome (**FIG 3**) mandate rebar augmentation of the posterior and sometimes the anterior columns; 6.5-mm cancellous screws or 5/16-inch Steinman pins are recommended (Table 2).

Table 2 Harrington Classification of Periacetabular Lesions

	Radiographic Findings	Treatment Options
Class I (minor)	Intact lateral cortices, superior and medial walls	Conventional cemented THA +/− rebar augmentation
Class II (major)	Deficient medial wall	Antiprotrusio device Medial mesh Rebar augmentation
Class III (massive)	Deficient lateral cortices and dome	Rebar augmentation of posterior (+/− anterior) column
Class IV (extensive)	Hemipelvic involvement	En bloc resection

From Harrington KD. The management of acetabular insufficiency secondary to metastatic malignant disease. J Bone Joint Surg Am 1981;63(4):653–664.

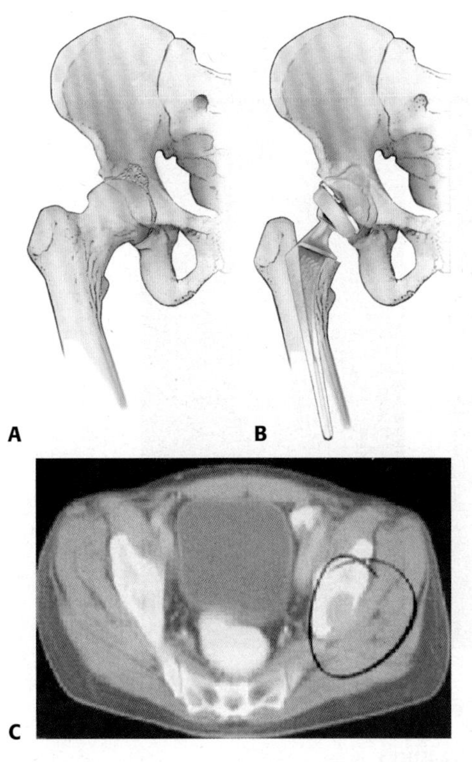

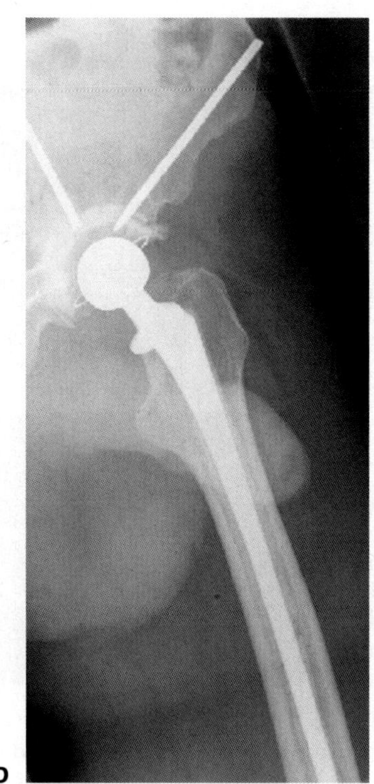

FIG 1 • Periacetabular lesions, class I (minor). Depiction of lesion (**A**) and repair (**B**). **C.** Left supracetabular lesion as seen on CT scan. **D.** Postoperative radiograph demonstrating reconstruction. Steinmann pin augmentation of the anterior and posterior columns was performed.

- Class IV: Resection is mandatory for attempted cure. Such cases should be referred to an orthopaedic oncologist and are beyond the scope of this chapter.

Femoral Head and Neck

- Impending fractures
  - Femoral head involvement is a reason to perform arthroplasty (**FIG 4**).
  - Modest femoral neck lesions may be stabilized with a reconstruction nail, with the exception of renal cell and thyroid carcinomas, in which cases arthroplasty is recommended.
- Realized fractures
  - Rarely heal
  - Internal fixation device failure is common.
- Procedure of choice: replacement arthroplasty
  - The decision to perform bipolar versus total hip arthroplasty is a result of acetabular involvement, preexisting arthritis, and life expectancy.
  - Acetabular disease may go unrecognized on plain radiographs in up to 83% of cases. Pelvic CT is imperative.

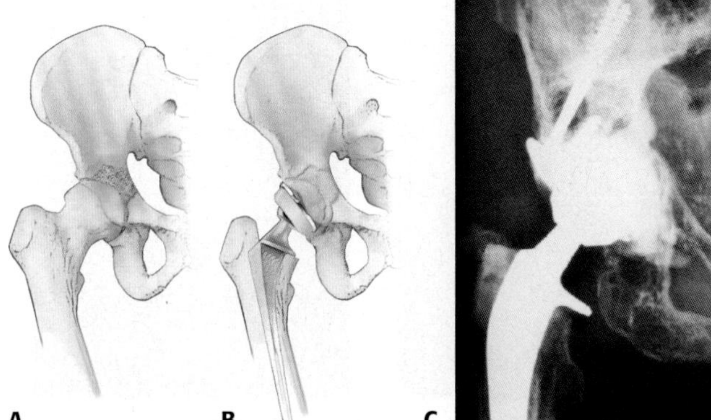

FIG 2 • Periacetabular lesions, class II (deficient medial wall). The lesion creates a deficient medial wall (**A**), requiring an antiprotrusio device (**B**). **C.** AP radiograph of a typical reconstruction.

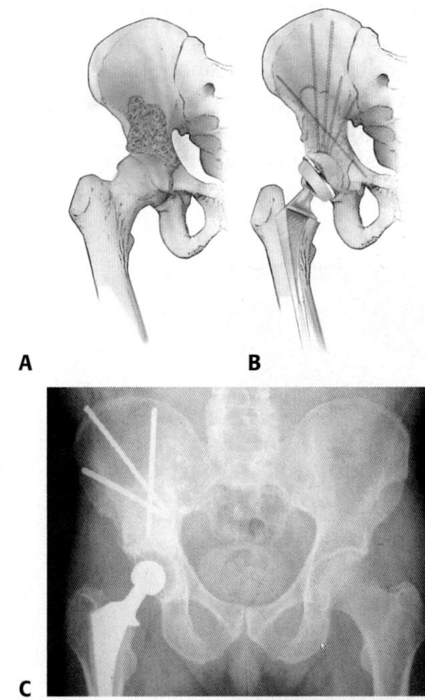

FIG 3 • Periacetabular lesions, class III (massive). Such lesions have deficient lateral cortices (columns) and dome (**A**) and necessitate the use of rebar to reconstruct the posterior or anterior columns with either 6.5-mm cancellous screws or 5/16-inch threaded Steinmann pins (**B**). **C.** AP radiograph of a typical reconstruction.

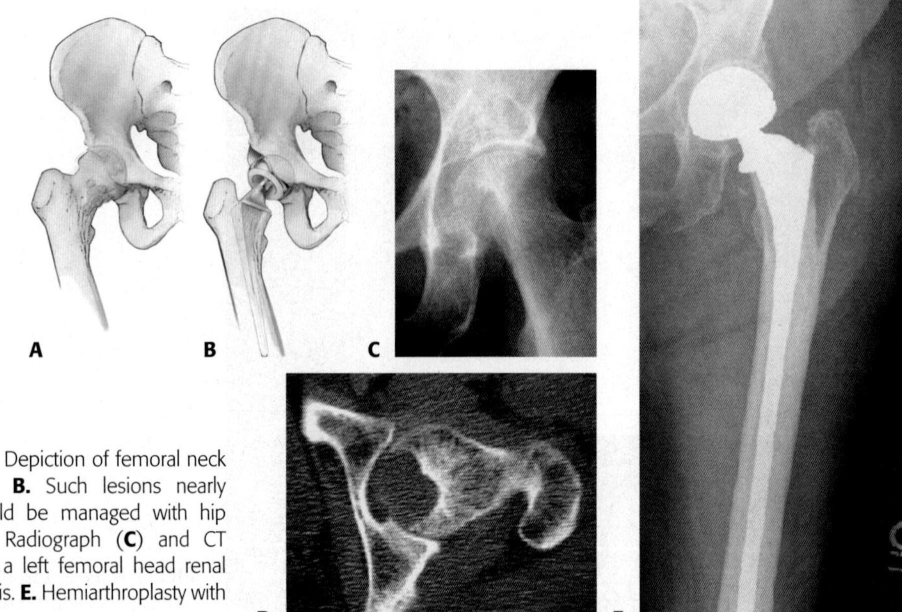

FIG 4 • **A.** Depiction of femoral neck involvement. **B.** Such lesions nearly always should be managed with hip arthroplasty. Radiograph (**C**) and CT scan (**D**) of a left femoral head renal cell metastasis. **E.** Hemiarthroplasty with long stem.

- Long-stem prostheses may be used for extensive femoral involvement, but attention must be paid to cement deployment during the early cure stage, use of a long laparoscopic sucker, or venting.

Peritrochanteric Neck

- Impending fractures
  - An intramedullary (IM) reconstruction-type device is strongly recommended. Screw and side plate constructs have a high failure rate (**FIG 5A**).
  - Long-stem stabilization and protection of the entire bone should be considered.[1]
  - For renal cell and thyroid cancer, the surgeon should proceed with cemented calcar-replacing arthroplasty.
- Realized fractures
  - Cemented calcar-replacing arthroplasty is the only appropriate option (**FIG 5B–E**).

Subtrochanteric

- Impending fractures
  - With the exception of renal cell and thyroid carcinoma, a cephalomedullary nail reconstruction is appropriate when bone loss is not extensive (**FIG 6A–E**).
  - Otherwise, proximal femoral replacement is necessary.
- Realized fractures
  - Cemented proximal femoral replacement is the only viable option to restore the patient to ambulatory status (**FIG 6F,G**).
  - Long-stem cemented femoral arthroplasty use in patients with MBD remains controversial. Some surgeons are cautious in the general use of cemented long-stem femoral arthroplasties in patients with MBD because of the risk of cardiopulmonary insult and collapse.

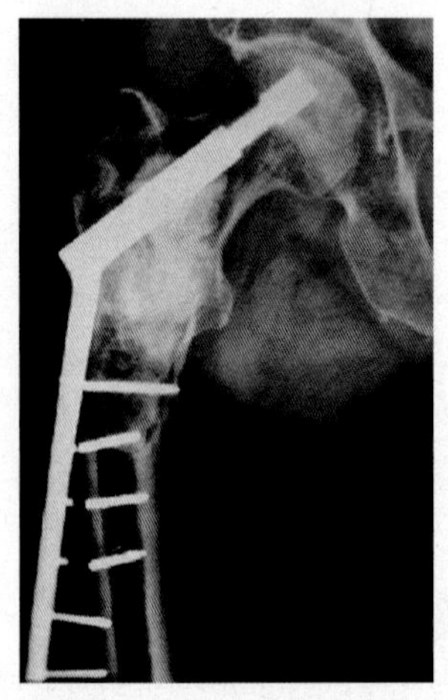

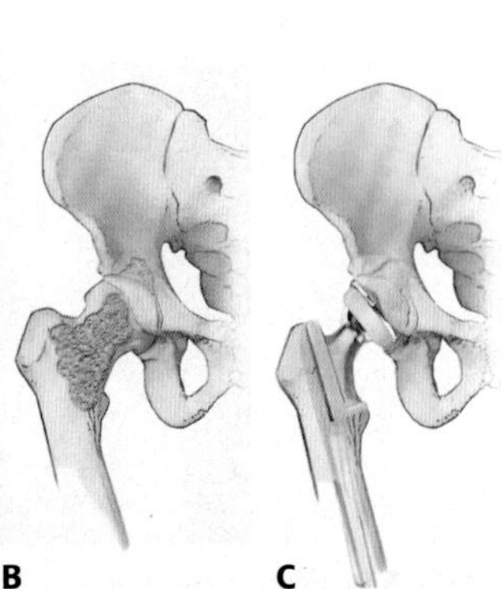

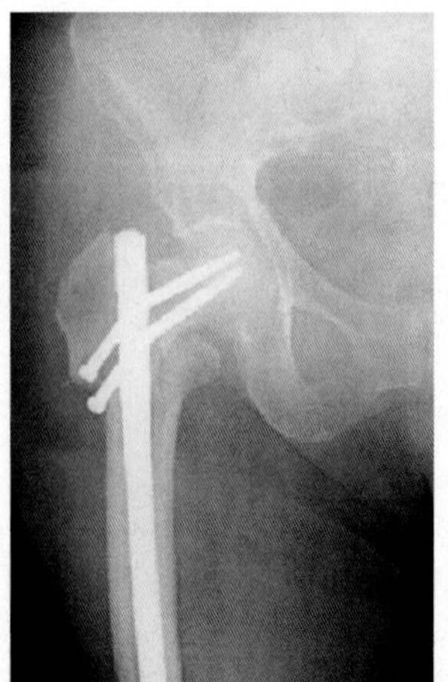

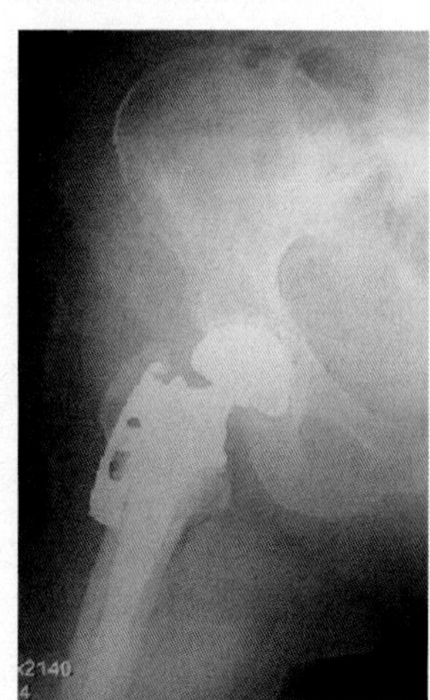

FIG 5 • **A.** Peritrochanteric metastatic lung cancer treated with screw and side-plate construct that failed within 4 months. For realized and large impending peritrochanteric lesions (**B**), the surgeon should have a low threshold for replacement arthroplasty (**C**). **D.** A realized intertrochanteric pathologic fracture from metastatic breast cancer was inappropriately treated with a reconstruction nail that went on to hardware failure within 3 months. **E.** The case shown in **D** was converted to a calcar-replacing hemiarthroplasty.

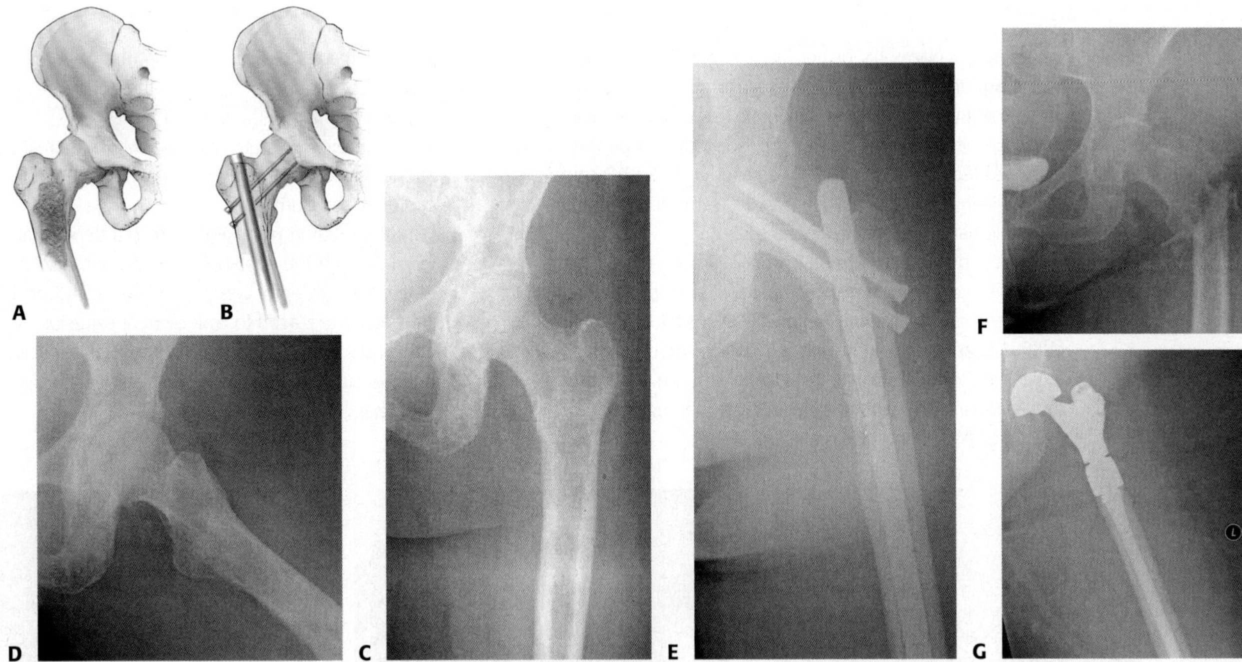

FIG 6 • Subtrochanteric femoral lesion (**A**) and cephalomedullary nail reconstruction (**B**). AP (**C**) and lateral (**D**) radiographs of an impending peri-subtrochanteric metastasis of breast carcinoma to bone treated with prophylactic stabilization (**E**). **F.** A patient with documented metastatic breast cancer to bone presented with a several-week history of progressive aching in the upper thigh. She was walking when she felt a snapping sensation and immense pain and was no longer able to ambulate. **G.** Treatment was with a proximal femoral replacement.

- Combining the use of bone cement with a long-stem femoral component further increases the possibility of complications, especially in a patient with MBD who has poor-quality bone and severe preexisting medical conditions. Deciding whether femoral stability from a cemented long-stem arthroplasty is worth the increased risk of a life-threatening cardiopulmonary embolic event is difficult. Certain steps listed in the following sections have been shown to minimize this risk, warranting long-stem use in cases of extensive femoral disease.[14]

Positioning

- Hip arthroplasty can be performed in either the supine or lateral decubitus position, but it is strongly recommended that the patient be placed in the decubitus position for anything other than a routine arthroplasty. This enables the surgeon to perform arthroplasty as well as extensive instrumentation of the posterior column when necessary.
- Reconstruction of impending proximal femoral lesions can be performed with the patient placed in the supine position on a fracture table that allows insertion of a cephalomedullary device and interlocking screws.

Approach

- Standard, but sometimes expanded, anterior, anterolateral, and posterior approaches may be used to access the acetabulum.
- For posterior column instrumentation, an extensile posterior approach is recommended.

TECHNIQUES

Periacetabular Reconstruction

- Rigid fixation of the acetabular component is critical to success. The preoperative CT and plain radiographs must be evaluated carefully before surgery (**TECH FIG 1A,B**).
- Class I defects can be managed with a conventional cemented acetabular component, with or without augmentation of fixation with large fragment screws (**TECH FIG 1C–E**).
- Class II defects
  - An antiprotrusio cage or a similar device must be used.
  - Any flanges or screws must be attached to healthy bone.
  - A posterior approach without a trochanteric osteotomy is usually adequate.
  - Nonunion of a trochanteric osteotomy is a major concern in patients with cancer and should be avoided unless absolutely necessary.
  - However, visualization of the posterior column is critical to confirm its mechanical integrity; therefore, an incision of adequate size must be used.
- Class III defects
  - An extensive posterolateral or lateral approach usually is chosen to deploy 6.5-mm cancellous screws or Steinmann pins under direct visualization with palpation of the sciatic notch and its contents.
  - Trochanteric osteotomy is operator dependent, but the surgeon must factor in the higher nonunion at this site given the patient's underlying condition and possible adjuvant radiation therapy.
  - If the disease is locally advanced, an extensile iliofemoral approach may be necessary to visualize the inner as well as the outer pelvis.

- The surgeon places his or her index finger into the sciatic notch and then aims the rebar screw or pin parallel to the notch into the posterior column of bone toward the sacral ala.
- Because threaded pins do not give adequate proprioceptive feedback, the surgeon is encouraged to use a 3.2-mm drill bit with a subsequent depth gauge to confirm that the drill hole has adequate wall integrity.
- At least two—preferably three or more—screws or pins are necessary to anchor the reconstruction. Intraoperative radiographs can be taken as needed (**TECH FIG 1F**).
- Although anterior column fixation is less important than posterior column fixation, if the anterior column is compromised, Steinmann pins may be deployed antegrade from the anterior crest into the acetabular defect.
- Some surgeons use targeting jigs, but we prefer to use a careful freehand technique with the nondominant hand in the defect to target the pin.
- These anterior pins are cut flush with the crest after they are deployed to the appropriate depth in the defect, ideally capturing the ilium.
- With the rebar in place and sunk to a depth that does not interfere with the acetabular component also being sunk to the correct depth, version, and verticality, mesh or similar material is placed to limit cement extrusion.
- The acetabular component is then cemented into place, making sure to get the PMMA fully interdigitated with the rebar.

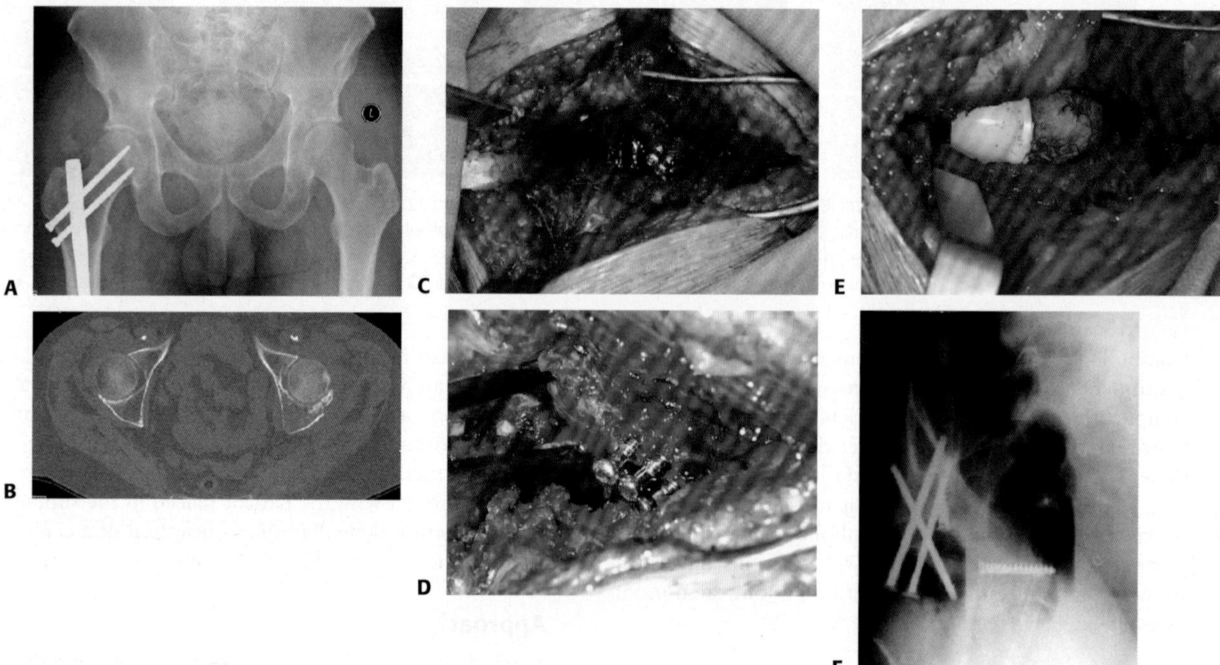

TECH FIG 1 • **A.** AP pelvic radiograph demonstrates a periacetabular metastatic focus. **B.** CT scan reveals the extent of posterior wall involvement of this class I defect. **C,D.** Posterior wall/column screws are used to augment the reconstruction. **E.** The screws are then incorporated in the cement mantle of the acetabular component. **F.** Intraoperative photos demonstrating adequate positioning of a combination of pins and screws to augment the cement fixation.

Long-Stem Cemented Femoral Components

- We prefer to use long-stem femoral components during hip arthroplasty for MBD, with a minimum stem length of 300 mm (**TECH FIG 2A**).
- Various surgical techniques have been proposed to reduce perioperative canal debris or IM pressurization.
  - Low-viscosity cement, IM venting, retrograde injection, thorough IM lavage, and intraoperative canal suctioning during cementing may decrease embolic events and decrease perioperative complications.
- Femoral preparation and component placement are performed in a similar systematic fashion.
  - After the femoral neck cut is completed with an oscillating saw, the canal is prepared with flexible reaming and broaching.
- The canal is suctioned between subsequent reamers with a long laparoscopic suction device (Sigmoidoscopic Suction device, Ref # 0033050; ConMed Corp., Utica, NY; **TECH FIG 2B,C**). The canal is then thoroughly brush-lavaged using the Pulsavac (Zimmer, Warsaw, IN) system.
- Three batches of Surgical Simplex P bone cement (Stryker, Mahwah, NJ) are mixed with 3.6 g of tobramycin for femoral cementation because of the patient's immunocompromised condition. We prefer Simplex P bone cement because of its low viscous qualities on immediate mixing. Once the cement is mixed (<1 minute), it is immediately injected into the femur in its early, liquefied cure state using a long cement gun.
- The long laparoscopic suction device (ConMed Corp.) is used to aspirate the canal immediately before and during insertion of the PMMA.

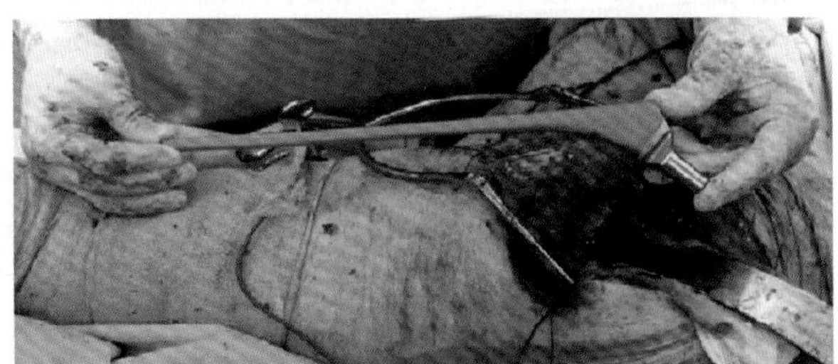

A

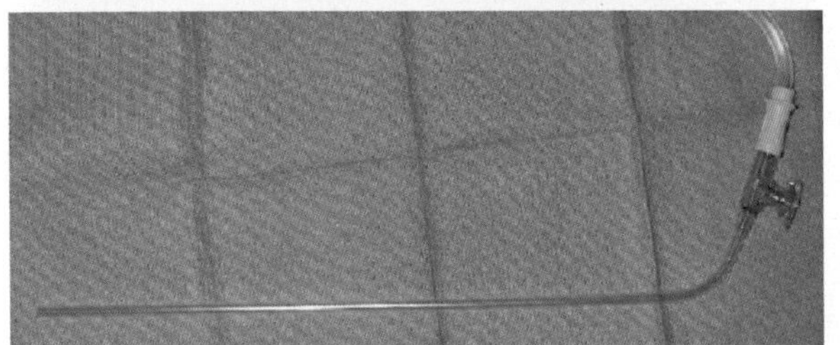

B

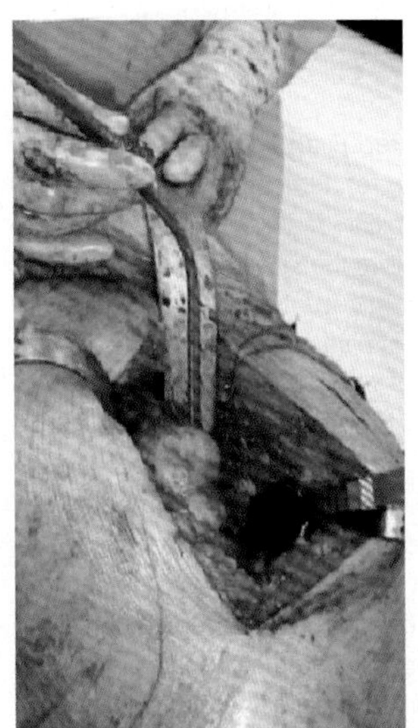

C

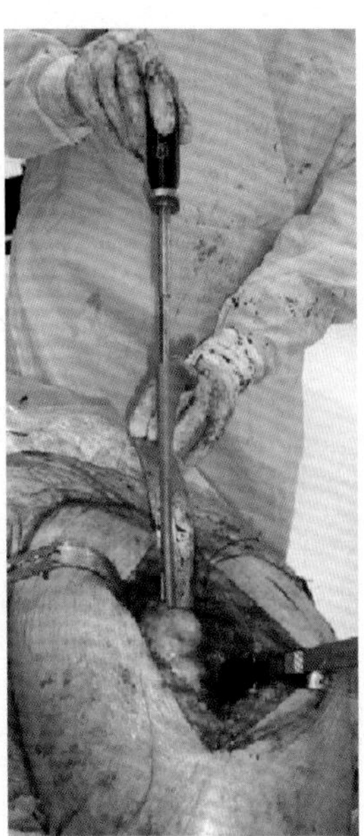

D

TECH FIG 2 • **A.** Typical long-stem femoral component used routinely in metastatic cases. **B,C.** During long-stem femoral component implantation, a long laparoscopic suction device is used to aspirate the medullary contents before and concurrent with cementation of early-cure state PMMA. **D.** The long-stem component is introduced slowly but early during the cement cure state, before the viscosity of the cement has increased.

- The femoral prosthesis is then slowly inserted into the femoral canal and allowed to settle with minimal manual force to avoid high-peak pressurization (**TECH FIG 2D**).
- All excess cement is removed and the implant is held in position until the PMMA has hardened.
- No distal venting is performed to avoid potential distal stress risers and minimize operative time. No cement restrictors are used.

Calcar-Replacing Hip Arthroplasty

- In the presence of peritrochanteric bone loss without subtrochanteric extension, a cemented calcar-replacing implant may be used.
- The surgeon may still consider using a longer cemented stem if the appropriate precautionary steps, as outlined earlier, are taken.

Proximal Femur Replacement

- For proximal femoral replacement, a long posterolateral incision is made to expose the proximal fourth to third of the femur.
- The iliotibial band is incised longitudinally to permit anterior and posterior exposure.
- The gluteus maximus is carefully split, with concurrent meticulous ligation of perforating arterioles.
- Time is taken to localize and protect the sciatic nerve in the retrogluteal area, where it lies immediately behind the external rotators.
- The abductors are defined, and the greater trochanter is osteotomized and preserved if it is not extensively involved with tumor.
- If the greater trochanter is too compromised, the abductors are transected at their tendinous attachment.
- The vastus lateralis muscle is reflected anteriorly, ligating the perforators serially. The main blood supply enters anteriorly.
- The external rotators are taken down using the surgeon's preferred technique.
- However, the hip capsule should be preserved as carefully as possible because it is instrumental in stabilizing the endoprosthetic reconstruction. It is recommended that the capsule be incised longitudinally, with the incision extending anteriorly over the neck, and detached circumferentially.
- It is strongly recommended that the entire limb, including the foot, be prepped in sterile fashion so that a distal pulse examination may be performed intraoperatively.
- The hip is dislocated anterolaterally.
- The acetabulum is inspected and assessed for possible reconstruction.
- Femoral resection level is determined by the lesion or fracture (**TECH FIG 3A,B**).
  - If the fracture under management is a realized fracture, a fresh transverse osteotomy should be performed at the level of healthy, uninvolved bone.
  - A malleable retractor is placed medially after the soft tissues have been emancipated with a Cobb or similar elevator.

- The psoas and adductors will be more easily tagged and released after the osteotomy, with retraction of the proximal femur segment laterally.
- Care must be taken to avoid injury to the profundus femoral vessels.

- The modular endoprosthetic reconstruction length is determined by the planned length of femoral resection (**TECH FIG 3C**). Careful preoperative planning and familiarity with the incremental reconstruction levels of the selected implant are important to facilitate efficient reconstruction.
- If no acetabular reconstruction is planned, a trial head is tested for size as usual.
- Although a large stem diameter is preferable, overzealous reaming in this patient population is discouraged. Continual lavage and irrigation of the medullary contents is of critical importance.
  - A cement mantle of at least 1 mm is preferred; therefore, the stem diameter should be at least 2 mm smaller than the last reamed size for ease of introduction at cementation and to avoid monomer introduction into the circulatory system.
  - Taper and face-reaming of the proximal femur as described by the implant manufacturer may be necessary.
- For cases of MBD, we prefer a longer, bowed stem. Cement precautions are mandatory.
- Neck length is determined by preoperative planning and trial reduction.
- After reduction of the trial, the capsule is pulled tight by stay sutures, and stability and length are assessed.
  - Anterior, posterior, and lateral stability should be evaluated. The sciatic nerve is evaluated.
  - Pulses should also be checked at this point. If they are diminished, that may indicate that the prosthesis is too long.
  - Orientation of the prosthesis is very important, with anteversion based on the sagittal plane created by the linea aspera. The prosthetic neck should be angled anteriorly 95 to 100 degrees off this plane.
- The prosthesis is assembled as described by the manufacturer.
- We strongly recommend against using cement that is too viscous.
- A long laparoscopic-type suction device should be used continually throughout instrumentation of the femoral canal, and consideration should be given to venting if a long stem is to be deployed.
  - The canal should be brushed as well.
  - As the cement matures after prosthetic deployment, the surgeon must immediately and carefully confirm the selected version.
- Soft tissue reconstruction is of paramount importance for a sound functional result.
- The hip capsule should be purse-stringed about the prosthetic neck using a no. 5 polyfilament, nondissolving stitch.
  - Once repaired, it should not be possible to dislocate the hip anteriorly, posteriorly, or laterally.
  - The tagged psoas tendon may be sewn to the anterior capsule. Likewise, the external rotators may be sewn to the posterior capsule.
  - At this point, the sciatic nerve is again checked to make sure it is not compromised.
- Numerous techniques have been described for reattaching the abductor mechanism to the implant. Manufacturers also describe various capture mechanisms. The surgeon must pay close attention to the reattachment mechanism because this is the limit of the functional reconstruction.
  - We prefer to use a soft tissue washer specific to the implant that can either be drilled through the residual trochanteric bone or harness the tendon itself (**TECH FIG 3D**).
- The vastus lateralis muscle is repaired, as are the gluteus maximus and iliotibial band.
- For metastatic cases, a drain is not mandatory unless the lesion is highly vascular (eg, renal cell and thyroid).

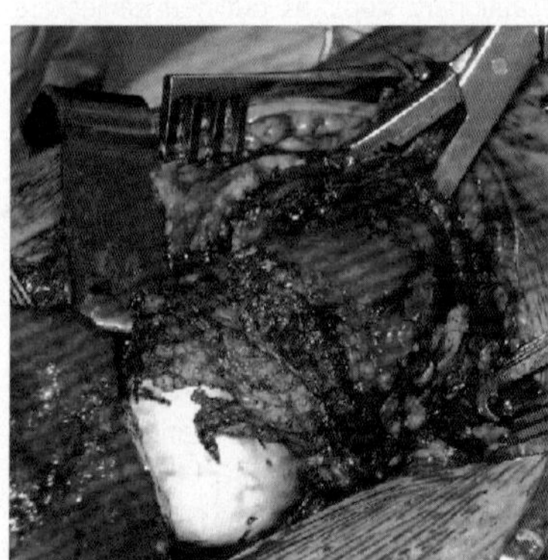
A

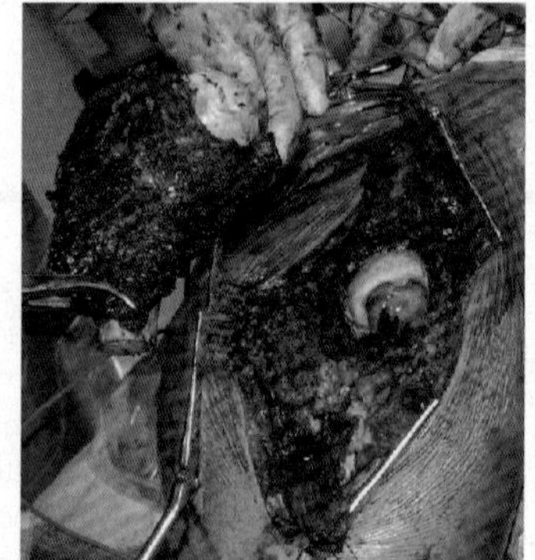
B

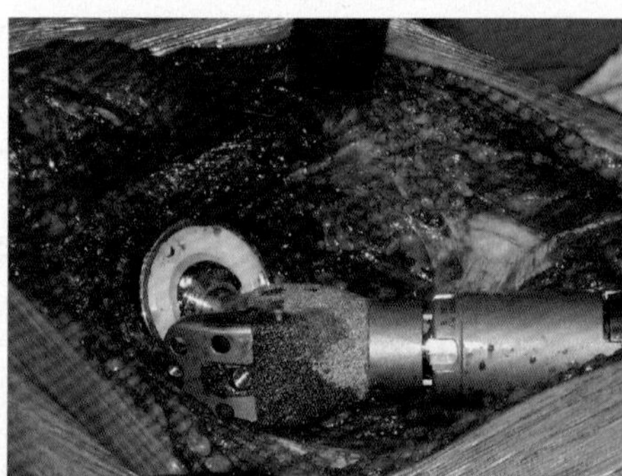
C

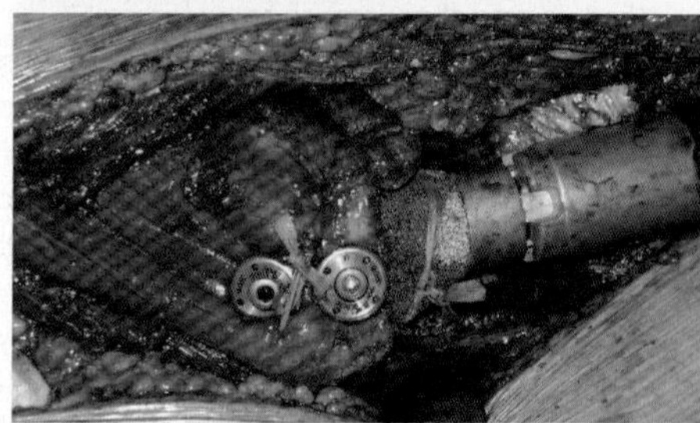
D

TECH FIG 3 • **A.** Resection of isolated renal cell carcinoma metastasis to the proximal femur. **B.** The femoral osteotomy is just below the lesion to provide disease-free bone stock for fixation of the proximal femur replacement. The size of the modular bodies available per the manufacturer is taken into account. **C.** The modular prosthesis in situ, corresponding to the length of the resected specimen. **D.** Durable abductor mechanism is critical to functional restoration. We prefer to use a soft tissue washer drilled through any residual greater trochanter that might be available.

PEARLS AND PITFALLS

Potential cardiopulmonary collapse secondary to cementation of femoral components	■ Low-viscosity cement, IM venting, retrograde injection, thorough IM lavage, and intraoperative canal suctioning during cementing are intended to decrease embolic events and decrease perioperative complications.
Extensive periacetabular bone loss	■ Rebar augmentation in the form of long, 6.5-mm cancellous screws or Steinmann pins should provide purchase for any posterior column bone and the sacral ala to gain fixation for cementation. Anterior augmentation may also be performed. The construct must be anchored in relatively healthy, noncontiguous bone so that if there is any local progression (such as that which may occur in thyroid and renal cancer), the reconstruction does not fail.
Instability of proximal femoral replacements	■ Intraoperatively, the surgeon must carefully determine the appropriate version, which is about 95–100 degrees off the midsagittal plane as determined by the linea aspera. Meticulous capsule repair with no. 5 nondissolving polyfilament suture is imperative. Overall length and offset also must be assessed carefully.
Abductor weakness in calcar- and proximal femoral–replacing reconstructions	■ Fixation of the residual abductor mechanism must be as rigid as possible. These patients will not be able to protect this reconstruction effectively. We prefer to use two smaller diameter soft tissue washers to screw down the mechanism. Larger bore bolts tend to destroy any residual greater trochanter in this compromised patient population.

POSTOPERATIVE CARE

- In this patient population, all reconstruction must permit weight bearing as tolerated, with an assistive device as needed.
- If a drain has been placed for metastatic cases, it should be discontinued within 72 hours.
- Depending on the approach and the extent of the dissection, hip precautions should be implemented for 6 to 12 weeks.

OUTCOMES

- Patients with periacetabular lesions have 70% to 75% satisfactory pain relief and return to at least partial mobility.
- Cemented total or hemiarthroplasty for femoral head, neck, and peritrochanteric lesions remains, in general, the procedure of choice in this patient population, with good to excellent outcomes relative to the omnipresent comorbidities.

COMPLICATIONS

- Periacetabular reconstructions are associated with complication rates of 20% to 30%.
- Cemented femoral arthroplasty is not without inherent risk.
  - Perioperative cardiopulmonary complications associated with cementing hip arthroplasty components are well described.[12,14–16]
  - Cement-associated desaturation and hypotension, pulmonary hypertension, cardiogenic shock, cardiac arrest, and intraoperative death are complications during femoral cementation and component placement secondary to canal pressurization.[2,6,10]
  - Cemented arthroplasty has been shown to be associated with more embolic events than noncemented arthroplasty, with higher IM pressures noted with cementation.[12,13]
  - Any factor that increases extrusion of femoral IM contents has been suggested to elevate the risk of cardiopulmonary embolic complications. In addition to cementation, this includes porous bone and the use of long-stem femoral implants. Long-stem components have been proposed to increase pressurization of the canal, producing more embolic events, with the rate of cardiopulmonary complications reported to be as high as 62%.[6,11]
  - Metastatic bone allows greater extrusion of emboli because of its permeative qualities and increased vascular supply. Thus, patients with MBD undergoing long-stem cemented femoral arthroplasty are at particularly high risk for cardiopulmonary compromise.
- Proximal femoral replacement is associated with complication rates as high as 28%.[9]
  - Most experienced surgeons believe that proximal femoral replacement remains the best option for subtrochanteric involvement in proximal femur pathologic fractures secondary to MBD.
  - No better alternatives with lower risks than proximal femoral replacement exist for this difficult patient population.

REFERENCES

1. Alvi HM, Damron TA. Prophylactic stabilization for bone metastases, myeloma, or lymphoma: do we need to protect the entire bone? Clin Orthop Relat Res 2013;471(3):706–714.
2. Fallon KM, Fuller JG, Morley-Forster P. Fat embolization and fatal cardiac arrest during hip arthroplasty with methylmethacrylate. Can J Anesth 2001;48:626–629.
3. Forsberg HA, Wedin R, Bauer H. Which implant is best after failed treatment for pathologic femur fractures? Clin Orthop Relat Res 2013;471(3):735–740.
4. Hage WD, Aboulafia AJ, Aboulafia DM. Incidence, location and diagnostic evaluation of metastatic bone disease. Orthop Clin North Am 2000;31:515–528.
5. Harrington KD. The management of acetabular insufficiency secondary to metastatic malignant disease. J Bone Joint Surg Am 1981;63(4):653–664.
6. Herrenbruck T, Erickson EW, Damron TA, et al. Adverse clinical events during cemented long-stem femoral arthroplasty. Clin Orthop Relat Res 2002;395:154–163.
7. Jansen JA, van de Sande MA, Dijkstra PD. Poor long-term clinical results of saddle prosthesis after resection of periacetabular tumors. Clin Orthop Relat Res 2013;471(1):324–331.
8. Landis SH, Murray T, Bolden S, et al. Cancer statistics, 1998. CA Cancer J Clin 1998;48:6–29.

9. Papagelopoulos PJ, Galanis EC, Greipp PR, et al. Prosthetic hip replacement for pathologic or impending pathologic fractures in myeloma. Clin Orthop Relat Res 1997;341:192–205.
10. Parvizi J, Holiday AD, Ereth MH, et al. Sudden death during primary hip arthroplasty. Clin Orthop Relat Res 1999;369:39–48.
11. Patterson BM, Healey JH, Cornell CN, et al. Cardiac arrest during hip arthroplasty with a cemented long-stem component. J Bone Joint Surg Am 1991;73A:271–277.
12. Pitto RP, Koessler M, Draenert K. Prophylaxis of fat and bone marrow embolism in cemented total hip arthroplasty. Clin Orthop Relat Res 1998;355:23–34.
13. Pitto RP, Koessler M, Kuehle JW. Comparison of fixation of the femoral component without cement and fixation with use of a bone-vacuum cementing technique for the prevention of fat embolism during total hip arthroplasty. J Bone Joint Surg Am 1999;81A:831–843.
14. Randall RL, Aoki SK, Olson PR, et al. Complications of cemented long-stem hip arthroplasties in metastatic bone disease. Clin Orthop Relat Res 2006;443:287–295.
15. Randall RL, Hoang BH. Musculoskeletal oncology. In: Skinner HB, ed. Current Diagnosis and Treatment in Orthopedics, ed 4. New York: McGraw-Hill, 2006.
16. Ward WG, Spang J, Howe D. Metastatic disease of the femur: surgical management. Orthop Clin North Am 2000;31:633–645.
17. Weber KL, Lewis VO, Randall RL, et al. An approach to the management of the patient with metastatic bone disease. Instr Course Lect 2004;53:663–676.

Revision Total Hip Arthroplasty with Well-Fixed Components

24

CHAPTER

Derek F. Amanatullah and Mark W. Pagnano

DEFINITION

- Well-fixed femoral and acetabular components often must be removed during revision total hip arthroplasty (THA).
- Determine which well-fixed components should be removed and which should be left in place at the time of revision THA.

ANATOMY

- Anatomic considerations during revision THA and the removal of well-fixed implants include pelvic landmarks as well as proximal femoral and diaphyseal landmarks.
  - The pelvic landmarks include the ischium, pubis, anterior and posterior acetabular columns, anterior inferior iliac spines, transverse acetabular ligament, sciatic notch, and acetabular walls.
  - The proximal femoral landmarks include the greater and lesser trochanters as well as the vastus ridge. These can be areas of relatively weak bone as a result of osteolysis, stress shielding, or previous surgery.
  - The femoral diaphyseal landmarks include the vastus ridge and linea aspera. These attachments for the vastus musculature must be reflected during an extended trochanteric osteotomy (ETO).
- The neurovascular structures at risk during revision THA and the removal of well-fixed implants include the sciatic, superior gluteal, and femoral nerves as well as the femoral vasculature.
- The sciatic nerve is at risk with the extensile posterior approach. The sciatic nerve can be identified in three distinct anatomic locations:
  - Exiting the sciatic notch deep to the piriformis muscle and superficial to the short external rotators (ie, superior gemellus, obturator internus, and inferior gemellus muscles)
  - Superficial to the ischium posterior and inferior to the posterior acetabular column superficial to the quadratus femoris muscle
  - Deep to the femoral insertion of the gluteus maximus tendon on the posterior femur
- The superior gluteal nerve is at risk during a transtrochanteric or extensile anterolateral approach. The superior gluteal nerve travels deep to the gluteus medius anteriorly along the ilium, approximately 4 to 5 cm proximal to the tip of the greater trochanter.
- The femoral nerve is at risk with excessive anterior dissection and retraction as well as approaches to the hip that are medial to the anterior superior iliac spine (eg, extended iliofemoral).
- The femoral vasculature is well anterior and usually protected by the iliopsoas muscle.

PATHOGENESIS

- Conditions that necessitate the removal of well-fixed femoral or acetabular components include the following:
  - Infection
  - Recurrent dislocation (eg, malpositioned components)
  - Limb length discrepancy
  - Severe osteolysis
  - Polyethylene damage or wear
  - Acetabular locking mechanism failure
  - Component failure (eg, femoral stem fracture)
- Component removal with attention to bone preservation for subsequent reconstruction is critical.

NATURAL HISTORY

- Retention of well-fixed acetabular or femoral components has acceptable long-term performance during isolated component revision THA.[2,16]

PHYSICAL FINDINGS

- The physical examination of the patient undergoing revision THA includes the following:
  - Gait pattern
  - Leg length discrepancy
  - Skin over the hip for previous scars
  - Muscle strength about the hip and leg
  - Distal neurovascular examination

IMAGING AND DIAGNOSTIC STUDIES

- Imaging studies identify which components are well fixed and evaluate the bone stock available for revision THA.
  - Biplanar radiographs of the entire implant as well as the joint above and below the components are essential. These should include the entire cement mantle if a cemented femoral implant is being evaluated.
  - Oblique, or Judet, views of the pelvis may be useful to evaluate the anterior and posterior columns. Some acetabular defects cannot be recognized using routine anteroposterior (AP) pelvis radiograph.
  - Plain radiographs greatly underestimate the extent of osteolysis and available bone stock for revision THA. Some surgeons find computed tomographic (CT) scanning as a useful asset to guide the bone grafting of osteolytic lesions and to identify remaining bone stock for fixation.

- Radiographic indicators of component stability include the following:

Stable	Unstable
No movement over time	Migration/subsidence
Streaming trabeculae	Circumferential lucency
Proximal stress shielding	Cortical thickening
Intact cement mantle	Pedestal formation
	Bead shedding
	Cement mantle fracture

- Scintillography (ie, bone scan) is sensitive to implant loosening that may not be viewed on plain radiographs or at the time of surgery and may help the surgeon decide whether to retain or remove implants that appear well fixed. Scintillography is not specific for loosening and detects other metabolic, oncologic, and infectious processes.

- Serum diagnostic studies evaluate infection prior to revision THA.
  - The combination of a normal erythrocyte sedimentation rate (ESR) and C-reactive protein (CRP) has a very high negative predictive value and indicate a very low (<1%) likelihood of infection.
  - Elevation of the ESR or CRP does not necessarily indicate infection but warrants an aspiration of the articulation with a manual cell count and differential as well as culture.

SURGICAL MANAGEMENT

Preoperative Planning

- The appropriate removal instruments and surgical approach are important considerations before revision THA with well-fixed implants.
- When performing revision THA with well-fixed implants, multiple options for the revision implant must be available to match the femoral and acetabular defect after extraction or discovered intraoperatively.

Positioning

- Patients can be positioned supine for the anterior or anterolateral approaches.
- Patients can be positioned in the lateral decubitus position for the anterolateral or posterior approaches.

TECHNIQUES

Surgical Approach

Posterior (Also Known as Moore or Southern)

- The patient is positioned in the lateral decubitus position, and the hip is exposed by splitting the iliotibial band and gluteus maximus muscle during the superficial dissection and reflecting the short external rotators and underlying hip capsule during the deep dissection. Deliberate repair of the posterior capsule and external rotators is required to reduce the incidence of dislocation after revision THA.

Anterolateral (Also Known as Watson-Jones or Hardinge)

- The patient is positioned in the supine or lateral decubitus position, and the hip is exposed by splitting the iliotibial band and gluteus maximus muscle during the superficial dissection and reflecting the anterior third of the gluteus medius and minimus muscles with or without a portion of the vastus lateralis muscle during the deep dissection. This approach maintains the posterior attachments of the hip, which reduces the incidence of dislocation after revision THA.

Anterior (Also Known as Modified Smith-Petersen)

- The patient is positioned in the supine position and the hip is exposed through the internervous plane between femoral and superior gluteal nerves, using the interval between the tensor fascia lata and the sartorius muscles during superficial dissection and the gluteus medius and rectus femoris muscles during deep dissection. This approach maintains the posterior attachments of the hip, which reduces the incidence of dislocation after revision THA.

Osteotomy

Extended Greater Trochanteric Osteotomy

- The ETO is determined by the amount of prosthesis that is well fixed or the distal extent of the cement column that needs to be removed. This is rarely less than 12 cm from the tip of the greater trochanter. Approximately one-third of the lateral portion of the femoral cortical circumference is included in the ETO (**TECH FIG 1A**).
- The vastus lateralis muscle remains attached to the lateral portion of the osteotomy at the vastus ridge, but distally, the vastus lateralis muscle is elevated off the linea aspera and retracted anteriorly to allow visualization of the lateral and posterior femoral cortex (**TECH FIG 1B**).
- An oscillating saw is used to perform the posterior portion of the osteotomy just superior to the linea aspera (see **TECH FIG 1B**).
- The distal extent of the osteotomy is beveled in the distal and AP direction. This portion of the osteotomy can be performed with a pencil-tipped high-speed burr (see **TECH FIG 1B**).
- The distal extent of the anterior portion of the osteotomy is made with an oscillating saw or small half-inch osteotome.
- The proximal extent of the anterior portion of the osteotomy is made with a small quarter-inch osteotome perforated through the vastus musculature. Multiple perforations are made in the same plane to complete the osteotomy (**TECH FIG 1C**). Alternatively, the proximal extent of the anterior portion of the osteotomy can be completed with a controlled fracture of the remaining cortex.
- The entire extended trochanteric fragment with the gluteus medius muscle remains attached to the greater trochanter, and the vastus lateralis muscle that remains attached to the vastus ridge is reflected anteriorly, with extreme care not to fracture the tip of the greater trochanteric fragment (**TECH FIG 1D**). The greater

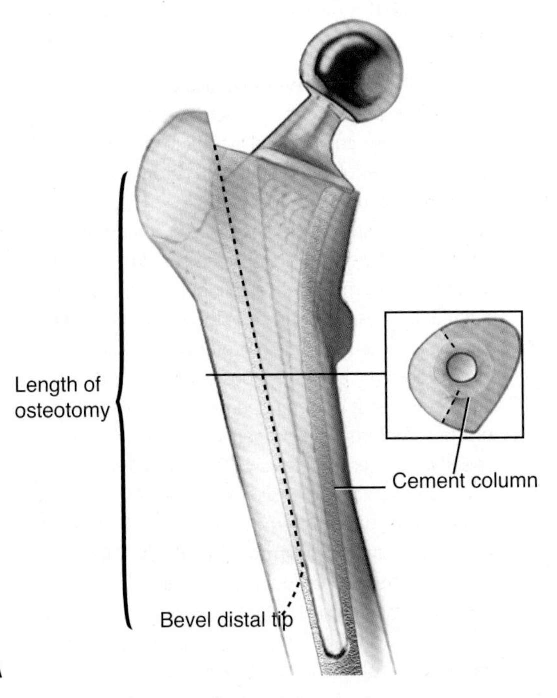

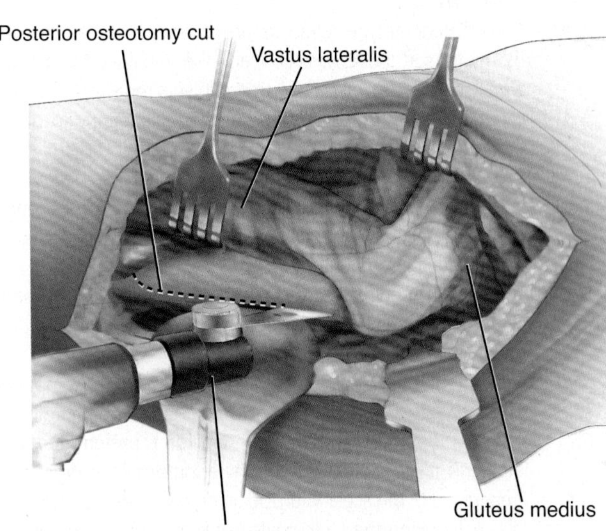

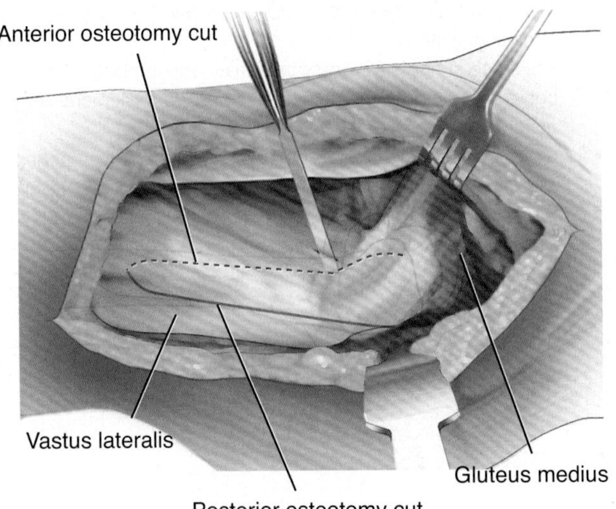

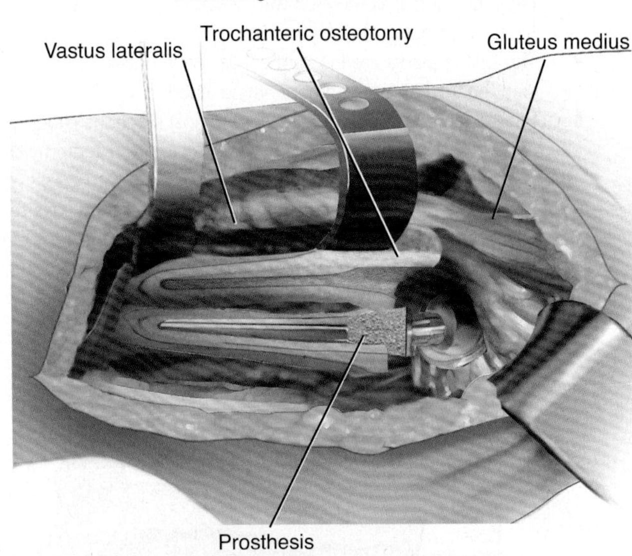

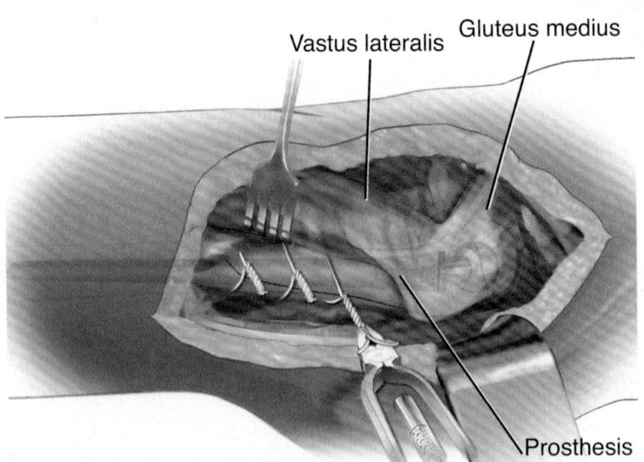

TECH FIG 1 • **A.** AP view of the planned femoral osteotomy demonstrating the length of the osteotomy needed to remove the prosthesis and/or cement mantle. About one-third of the lateral portion of the femoral circumference is part of the osteotomy. **B.** The vastus lateralis that remains attached to the lateral portion of the osteotomy is reflected anteriorly to allow visualization of the lateral and posterior femoral cortex. An oscillating saw is used to perform the posterior portion of the osteotomy just superior to the linea aspera. The distal extent of the osteotomy is beveled in the distal and AP direction. **C.** The anterior portion of the osteotomy is made with a quarter-inch osteotome perforated through the vastus musculature. The entire extended trochanteric fragment is reflected anteriorly, with care not to fracture the tip of the trochanteric fragment, which is the weakest point in the osteotomized fragment. **D.** Retract soft tissue and the trochanteric fragment to visualize the femoral prosthesis. All tissue lateral to the psoas tendon can be removed if necessary. The cement–implant and cement–bone interfaces or the ingrowth interface is now accessible. **E.** The trial implants are inserted and a trial reduction performed before the trochanteric fragment is reattached. The osteotomy is reduced and secured with looped Luque wires.

trochanter is the weakest point in the extended trochanteric fragment.

- The capsule surrounding the prosthesis below the greater trochanter is released or excised and the "shoulder" of the prosthesis exposed.
- Curved Bennett-type retractors are inserted distal to the osteotomy for soft tissue retraction, and the anterior arm Charnley-type hip retractor or curved Bennett-type retractor is used to carefully retract the trochanteric fragment anteriorly to expose the femoral prosthesis.
- Anterior and medial capsular attachments are taken down to the level of the psoas tendon. All tissue lateral to the psoas tendon can be removed at this point if needed to allow visualization of the femoral component.
- The surgeon now has access to the cement–implant, cement–bone, or bone–implant interfaces as needed for femoral component removal.
- Access to the acetabulum is obtained after femoral component extraction or with anterior dislocation of the hip. Anterior dislocation prior to femoral component extraction is preferred to avoid iatrogenic fracture of the osteotomy or proximal femur.
- Preparation of the acetabulum, if necessary, as well as the femoral canal for long-stem fully coated or fluted-tapered femoral implant insertion, is completed with flexible reamers and proximal tapered reamers.
- The trial implants are inserted and a trial reduction performed with the trochanteric fragment not attached.
- Prior to femoral component insertion, most surgeons choose to place a cable around the femur just distal to the osteotomy site to prevent iatrogenic femoral shaft fracture.
- ETO fixation is performed after the final implant is inserted. Often, small amounts of trochanteric bone must be removed to facilitate appropriate osteotomy reduction and fixation with looped Luque wires or cables (**TECH FIG 1E**).

Transfemoral (Also Known as Wagner) Osteotomy

- The length of the transfemoral osteotomy (TFO) is determined by the amount of prosthesis that is well fixed or the distal extent of the cement column that needs to be removed. The TFO is particularly useful in the setting of coronal fracture fragments or extensive proximal bone loss.
- The femur is split at the level of the greater trochanter using a large osteotome. The gluteus medius and minimus as well as vastus lateralis muscles are split but remain attached to the anterior and posterior portions of the osteotomy (**TECH FIG 2A**).
- The distal extent of the osteotomy is completed by beveling the osteotomy anteriorly, posteriorly, or making a complete transfemoral cut booking open the proximal femur. This portion of the osteotomy can be performed with a pencil-tipped high-speed burr or oscillating saw (**TECH FIG 2B**).
- The entire transtrochanteric fragment is reflected anteriorly and/or posteriorly with extreme care not to fracture the tip of the greater trochanteric fragment (**TECH FIG 2C**). The greater trochanter is the weakest point in the transtrochanteric fragment.
- The capsule surrounding the prosthesis is divided superiorly and inferiorly, leaving the anterior and posterior sleeves intact and the shoulder of the prosthesis exposed.
- A cerebellar-type or Charnley-type hip retractor is used to carefully retract the transtrochanteric fragment(s) to expose the femoral prosthesis.
- The surgeon now has access to the cement–implant, cement–bone, or bone–implant interfaces as needed for femoral component removal.
- Access to the acetabulum is obtained after femoral component extraction or with anterior or posterior dislocation of the hip. Dislocation prior to femoral component extraction is preferred to avoid iatrogenic fracture of the osteotomy or distal femur.

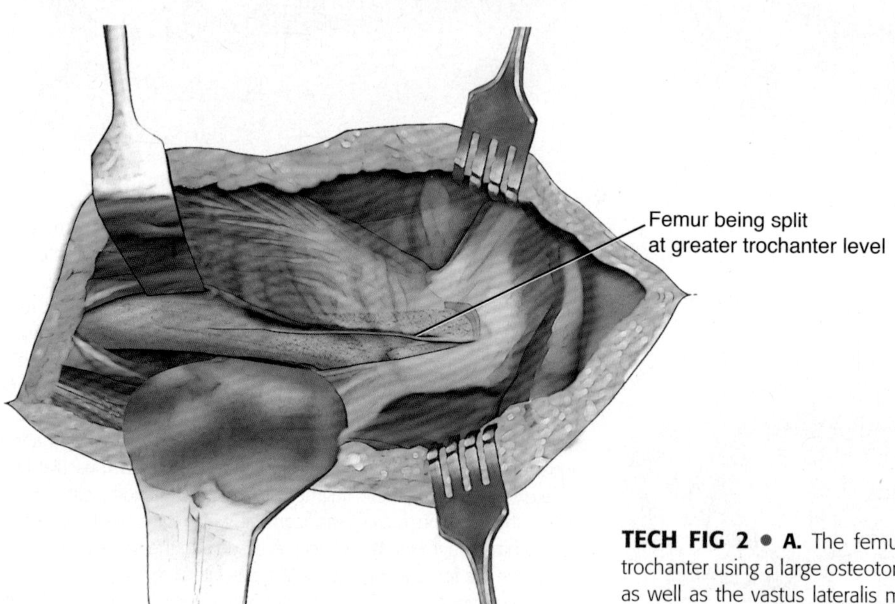

TECH FIG 2 • **A.** The femur is split at the level of the greater trochanter using a large osteotome. The gluteus medius and minimus as well as the vastus lateralis muscles are split but remain attached to the anterior and posterior portions of the osteotomy. *(continued)*

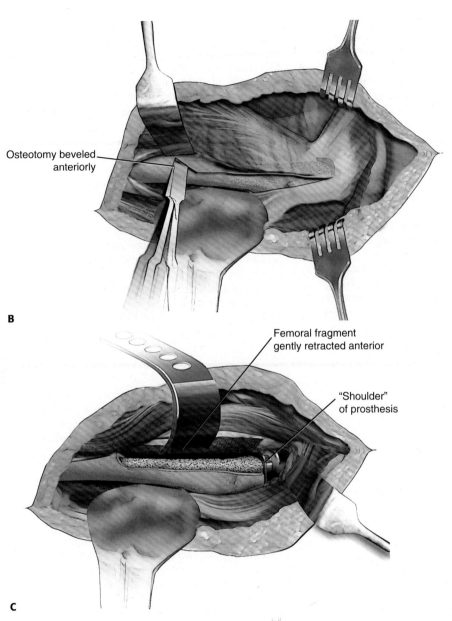

Osteotomy beveled anteriorly

B

Femoral fragment gently retracted anterior

"Shoulder" of prosthesis

C

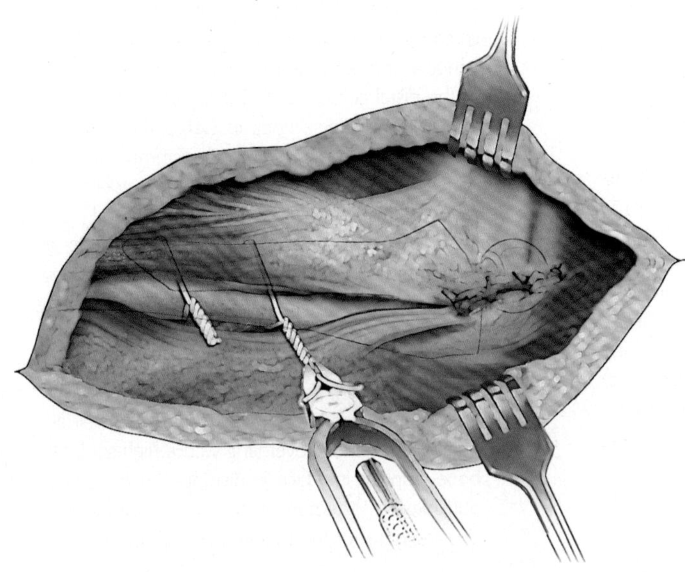

D

TECH FIG 2 • *(continued)* **B.** The distal extent of the osteotomy is completed by beveling the osteotomy anteriorly or posteriorly or making a complete transfemoral cut booking open the proximal femur. **C.** The entire transtrochanteric fragment is reflected anteriorly and/or posteriorly with care not to fracture the tip of the greater trochanteric fragment. The capsule surrounding the prosthesis is divided superiorly and inferiorly, leaving the anterior and posterior sleeves intact, and the shoulder of the prosthesis exposed. A cerebellar-type or Charnley-type hip retractor is used to carefully retract the transtrochanteric fragment(s), providing access to the cement–implant, cement–bone, or bone–implant interfaces as needed for femoral component removal and femoral instrumentation. **D.** Fixation is performed after the final implant is inserted. Often, small amounts of trochanteric bone must be removed to facilitate appropriate osteotomy reduction and fixation with heavy suture, looped Luque wires, or cables.

- Preparation of the acetabulum, if necessary, as well as the femoral canal for long-stem fully coated or fluted-tapered femoral implant insertion, is completed with flexible reamers and proximal tapered reamers.
- The trial implants are inserted and a trial reduction performed with the transtrochanteric fragment(s) not attached.
- Prior to femoral component insertion, most surgeons choose to place a cable around the femur just distal to the osteotomy site to prevent iatrogenic femoral shaft fracture.
- TFO fixation is performed after the final implant is inserted. Often, small amounts of trochanteric bone must be removed to facilitate appropriate osteotomy reduction and fixation with heavy suture, looped Luque wires, or cables (**TECH FIG 2D**).

Cortical Window

- The length of the cortical window is determined by the amount of prosthesis that is well fixed or the distal extent of the cement column that needs to be removed. Up to one-third of the lateral portion of the femoral cortical circumference may be included in a cortical window.
- As in the ETO, the vastus lateralis muscle remains attached to the lateral portion of the osteotomy at the vastus ridge, but distally, the vastus lateralis muscle is elevated off the linea aspera and retracted anteriorly to allow visualization of the lateral and posterior femoral cortex.
- Drill holes are made at the corner of the window to reduce any potential stress-risers that could lead to iatrogenic femur fracture.
- The drill holes are connected via osteotome or oscillating saw.
- The surgeon may remove the cortical window with an osteotomy and gain limited access to the cement–implant, cement–bone, or bone–implant interfaces as needed for femoral component removal. A carbide punch can be used to extract components in a retrograde fashion.
- The cortical window is temporarily held into position with Farabeuf clamps during trialing and final component placement.
- Fixation is performed after the final implant is inserted with looped Luque wires.

Implant Removal

Femoral Extraction

- Most well-fixed femoral components require a femoral osteotomy for safe extraction. A femoral osteotomy offers several advantages during the removal of a well-fixed femoral component:
  - Preservation of bone stock and soft tissue attachments
  - Exposure of the femoral canal for reconstruction
  - Deformity correction
  - Soft tissue balance
  - Bone grafting
  - Increased union rate when compared to an iatrogenic fracture
  - Decreased operating time
  - Distal cement removal
- Fracture planes may be used to gain access to well-fixed or loose femoral components in lieu of a femoral osteotomy or cortical window.
- To make the subsequent reconstruction straightforward, care should be taken to prevent femoral cortical penetration and preserve as much bone stock as possible during femoral component extraction. Intraoperative fluoroscopy may be useful to prevent a cortical breach.
  - Cemented femoral stems are disimpacted from their cement mantle after clearing the medial collar and lateral shoulder of the prosthesis as well as medial greater trochanteric overhang with a high-speed burr. The use of osteotomes should be avoided at this phase. Osteotomes increase hoop stresses and may heighten the risk of iatrogenic greater trochanter fracture. An implant-specific or universal extractor is applied to the neck of the cemented stem. The stem is disimpacted from its cement mantle with three to five firm but controlled blows with a slap hammer. If the femoral component does not have a lipped taper, it may be necessary to notch the inferior aspect with a diamond-cutting wheel to allow proper grasping of the femoral prosthesis for extraction. If the cemented stem is not easily disimpacted, consider performing an ETO and removal similar to an uncemented femoral stem (see in the following text) or free up the proximal cement mantle with a pencil-tipped high-speed burr or flexible osteotomes. If the cement mantle is to be removed, this may be accomplished with a combination of manual cement removal instruments (eg, splitter, V osteotome, T osteotome, reverse hook, or pituitary rongeur), motorized osteotomes, pencil-tipped high-speed burr to create fault lines and control cement fracture, round high-speed burr for metaphyseal cement, drill, and orthopaedic ultrasonic cement removal system (eg, OSCAR, Orthosonics, Chatham, NJ). The distal cement plug may be removed in a retrograde fashion, especially if loose, through a cortical window or in antegrade fashion by making a central hole in the distal cement with a drill, burr, or ultrasonic device and using a reverse hook to extract the distal cement. If the distal cement is distal to the isthmus of the femur, a cortical window or ETO should be considered. If the cement mantle is to be retained, the well-fixed, noninfected cement mantle can be contoured and texturized with a burr or ultrasonic device to create space for a new femoral component that is cemented into the existing cement mantel (ie, cement-in-cement technique).[12]
  - Proximally, porous-coated uncemented femoral stems are disimpacted from the bone after clearing the medial collar and lateral shoulder of the prosthesis as well as medial greater trochanteric overhang with a high-speed burr. The bone–implant interface is disrupted with a pencil-tipped burr, flexible osteotomes, motorized osteotomes, and a U osteotome for the medial calcar. If the medial calcar is

blocked by a collar, a metal-cutting burr is used to remove the collar and gain access to the calcar. Care should be taken, as osteotomes increase hoop stresses and may increase the risk of iatrogenic greater trochanter fracture. An implant-specific or universal extractor is applied to the neck of the cemented stem. The stem is disimpacted from its cement mantle with three to five firm but controlled blows with a slap hammer. If the femoral component does not have a lipped taper, it may be necessary to notch the inferior aspect of the femoral neck with a diamond-cutting wheel to allow proper grasping of the femoral prosthesis for extraction. If the proximally porous uncemented stem is not easily disimpacted, consider performing an ETO.

- Fully porous-coated uncemented femoral stems require a femoral osteotomy for extraction (**TECH FIG 3A**). After the femoral osteotomy, if the implant is not fractured, the implant can be cut with a metal-cutting high-speed burr at the distal extent of the femoral osteotomy (**TECH FIG 3B**). The distal portion of the remaining implant should be cylindrical. A Gigli saw is passed along the proximal portion of the implant along the calcar, removing any proximal medial fixation (**TECH FIG 3C**). An appropriately sized trephine is used in conjunction with copious irrigation to remove the remaining distal portion of the well-fixed, fully porous-coated femoral implant (**TECH FIG 3D**). Multiple trephines, a minimum of four to six that are one size above and one size below the expected implant size, should be available, as trephines dull quickly and implant sizes are dictated incorrectly. Flexible osteotomes and a pencil-tipped high-speed burr should also be available.

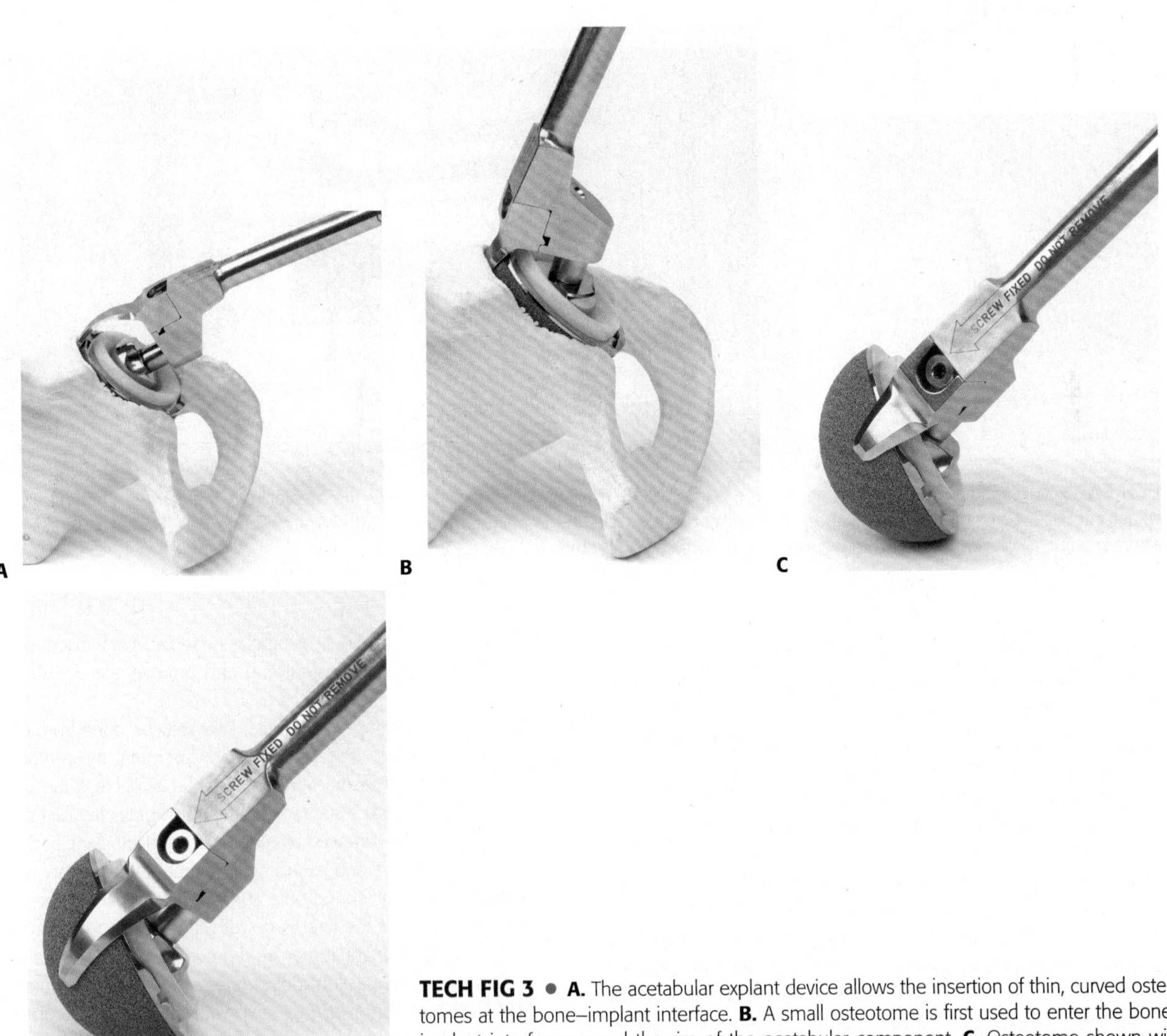

TECH FIG 3 • A. The acetabular explant device allows the insertion of thin, curved osteotomes at the bone–implant interface. **B.** A small osteotome is first used to enter the bone–implant interface around the rim of the acetabular component. **C.** Osteotome shown with the implant removed. **D.** A longer acetabular osteotome is used after the small osteotome. *(continued)*

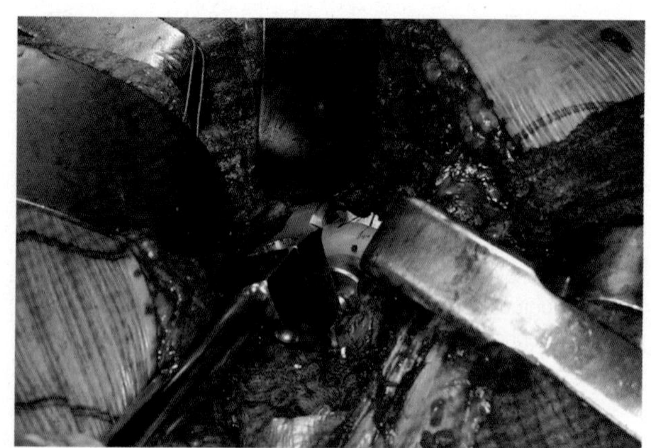
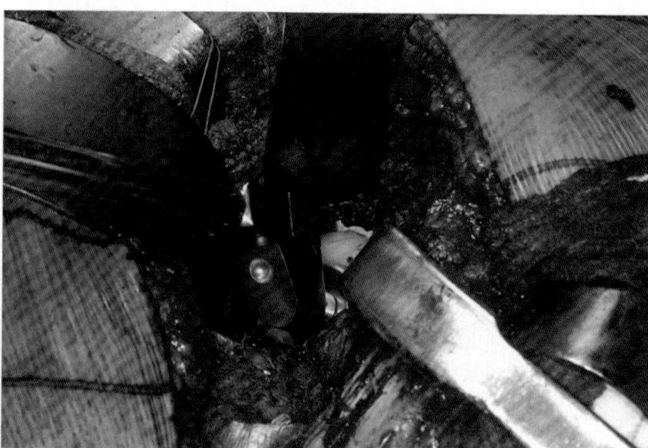
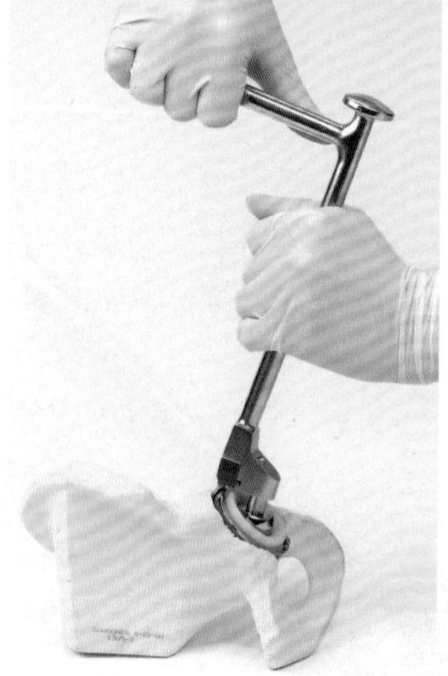
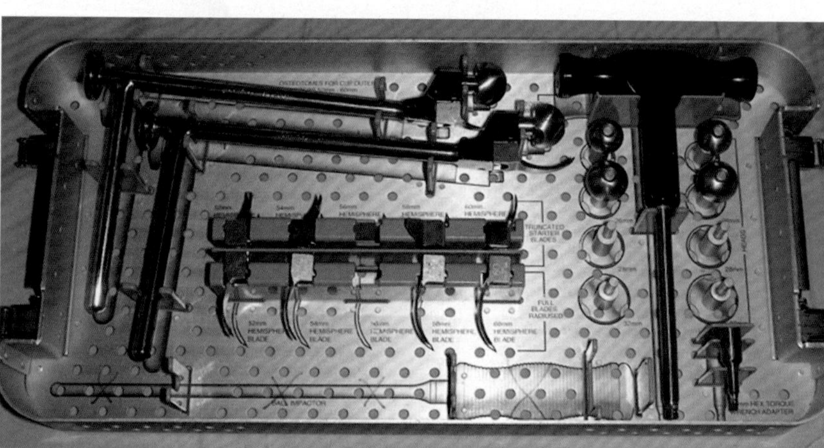

TECH FIG 3 • *(continued)* **E.** The large osteotome is inserted. **F.** The large osteotome removes the medial ingrown interfaces of the bone–implant interface. **G.** Using the acetabular explant chisel on a handle, the implant is removed with minimal bone loss. **H.** Tray with explant instrumentation. (Portions of this figure were provided Courtesy of Zimmer, Inc., Warsaw, IN.)

Acetabular Extraction

- Removal of a well-fixed acetabular component may be done from any approach to the hip.
- Care should be taken to preserve as much acetabular bone stock as possible during acetabular component extraction for subsequent reconstruction. Aggressively twisting or pulling a well-fixed component is seldom required and can lead to unintended major bone loss.
- An acetabular osteotome (Explant Acetabular Removal System, Zimmer Inc, Warsaw, IN) is designed to rotate short- and long-curved chisels at a fixed radius, corresponding to the size of the acetabular component, and disrupt the bone–implant interface to facilitate acetabular component removal (**TECH FIG 4A–D**). All screws should be removed with the appropriate driver or screw removal system prior to using the explant osteotome. The original liner, a trial liner, or bipolar head can be reinserted to center the acetabular osteotome and remove the acetabular component.
- Removal of a well-fixed acetabular liner may be done from any approach to the hip. If the liner is ceramic or metal, the appropriate implant-specific extraction tool must be available. If the liner is polyethylene and cemented into the pelvis or acetabular component, it may be removed by reaming the polyethylene back to the cement mantle and extracting the cement if necessary with osteotomes, a high-speed burr, and/or an orthopaedic cement removal system. If the liner is polyethylene and locked into an acetabular component, it may be removed with the appropriate implant-specific extraction tool, a one- or two-screw technique (**TECH FIG 4E,F**), or in fragments with reamers, osteotomes, and/or high-speed burr.

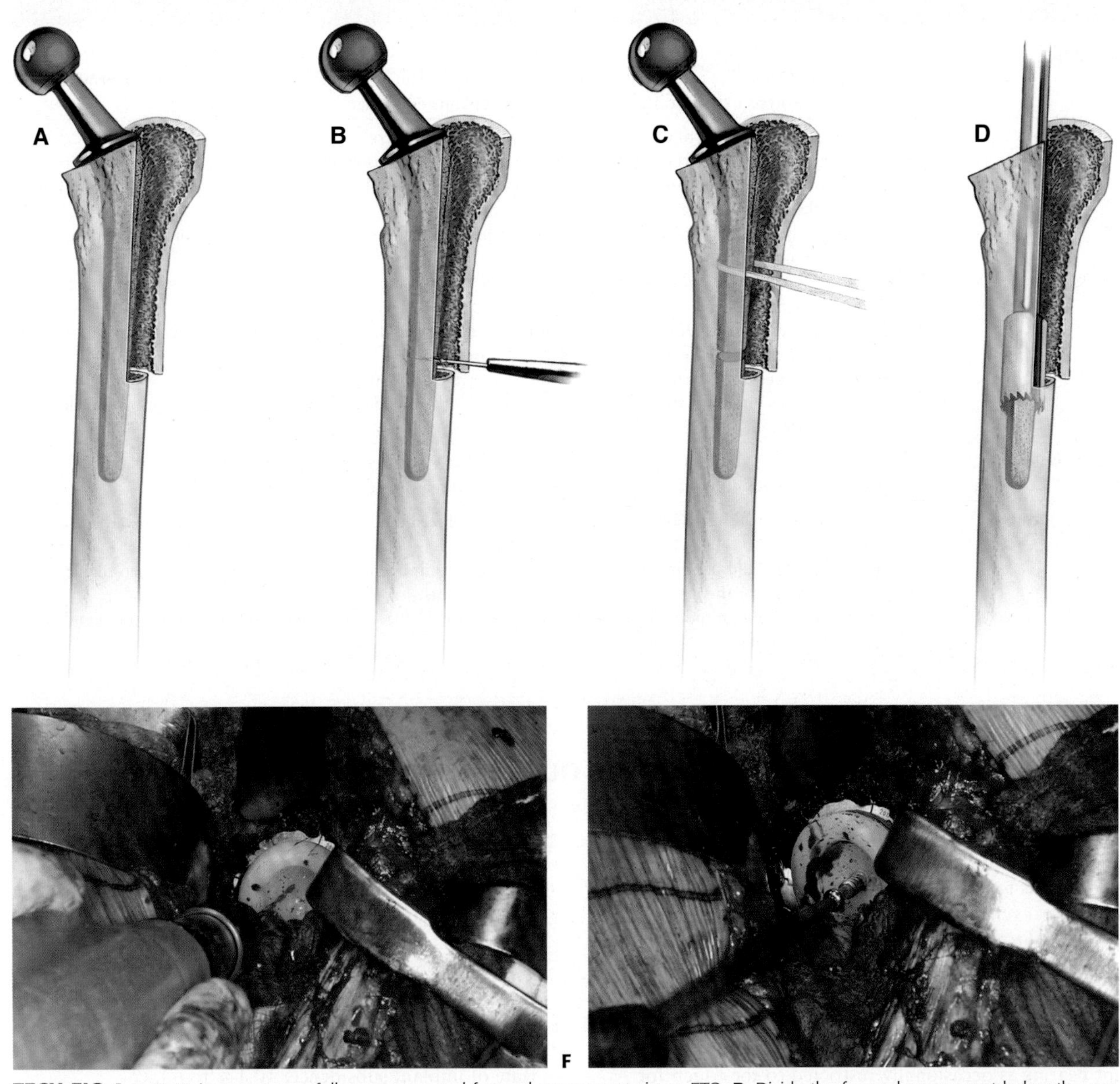

TECH FIG 4 • A. Gain access to a fully porous-coated femoral component via an ETO. **B.** Divide the femoral component below the metaphyseal flare with a metal-cutting high-speed burr if the implant has not already fractured. **C.** Use a Gigli saw medially to release the proximal and medial ingrowth surface. **D.** Trephine over the distal cylindrical portion of the femoral component to gain access to the remaining diaphysis. **E.** A drill bit is used to pierce the polyethylene. **F.** A cancellous screw is used to engage the polyethylene and back the polyethylene out of the acetabular cup once it strikes the metal shell. A second screw can be used as well. Care should be taken to avoid stripping the polyethylene when using this technique.

PEARLS AND PITFALLS

Acetabular deficiencies	■ Osteolysis and bone loss behind well-fixed acetabular components is often underestimated on plain radiographs. A simple polyethylene liner exchange may progress to complete acetabular revision if the socket proves to be loose or the osteolysis extensive and a surgical plan/implants/equipment must be available.
ETO	■ Bevel the distal transverse arm of the osteotomy to prevent distal fracture propagation. ■ Pass a cerclage wire distal to the osteotomy before femoral preparation and trial and final implant insertion. ■ Pay careful attention to trochanteric osteolysis and fracture risk at the vastus ridge at the junction of the vastus lateralis and the abductor attachment into the trochanter. ■ Have adequate bone graft available, including morselized cancellous graft and cortical struts for contained and uncontained defects. ■ With distally fixed stems combined with an ETO, a tight distal diaphyseal fit must be obtained, achieving three-point fixation. ■ Intraoperative and/or postoperative radiographs with the final implants in place are needed because intraoperative fracture rates are higher for revision THA and ETO cases. ■ An ETO can be combined with a proximal reduction or angular osteotomy. ■ Leave vastus muscle attached to the trochanteric fragment to provide adequate blood supply for osseous healing and implant stability.
Femoral component removal	■ Multiple trephines, a minimum of four to six, one size above and one size below the dictated implant, should be available, as trephines dull quickly and implant sizes are often dictated incorrectly.
Acetabular component removal	■ Thin curved osteotomes based on the cup and head size reduce bone loss during removal of well-fixed acetabular components. ■ The polyethylene should be removed from the acetabular component to allow screw removal, then replaced for a guide or reference for the curved-blade removal instruments. ■ Cementing an acetabular polyethylene shell is an option if the locking mechanism is not functional after polyethylene liner removal.

POSTOPERATIVE CARE

- Weight-bearing status is determined by a combination of bone quality, initial implant stability against that bone, and whether an osteotomy was used for exposure.
- Weight bearing as tolerated can typically begin after isolated head and liner exchange with the retention of osseointegrated components.
- Weight bearing is often restricted to 50% for 8 weeks with the use of a two-handed ambulatory assistive device if an extended osteotomy was done, if an implant was reinserted into relatively poor bone, and/or bone graft was used.
  - Weight bearing is occasionally restricted to toe-touch for 8 weeks or more after major reconstructive procedures in which the bone loss was extensive or the fixation obtained is judged to be at risk.
- When an implant is removed for infection and an antibiotic-impregnated articulated or static spacer is inserted, weight-bearing status is again based on the bone quality, implant stability, and need for an osteotomy and is often, but not always, restricted with an ambulatory assistive device used until replantation.

COMPLICATIONS

- Femoral fractures are common near the trochanteric region and in the femoral diaphysis during removal of well-fixed femoral implants.
- Nonunion can occur in the setting of ETO and TFO.
- Revision THA has a higher dislocation rate than primary THA.
- A tight diaphyseal fit is essential to prevent implant subsidence.
- Acetabular deficiencies may be extensive in the face of polyethylene wear and osteolysis.

OUTCOMES

- Short-term follow-up after ETO for revision THA[1,5,9,13–15,17]:
  - Osteotomy union rate: 97.8% to 100%
  - Greater trochanter fracture rate: 2.4% to 23.1%
  - Diaphyseal femoral fracture rate: 0.0% to 20.0%
  - Rate of implant subsidence: 1.4% to 23.0%
  - Dislocation rate: 7.1% to 30.8%
- Short-term follow-up after TFO for revision THA[3,4,6–8,10,11,18–20]:
  - Osteotomy union rate: 83.3% to 98.5%
  - Greater trochanter fracture rate: 60%
  - Diaphyseal femoral fracture rate: 0.0% to 17.6%
  - Rate of implant subsidence: 10.1% to 64.7%
  - Dislocation rate: 2.9% to 21.4%

REFERENCES

1. Aribindi R, Paprosky W, Nourbash P, et al. Extended proximal femoral osteotomy. Instr Course Lect 1999;48:19–26.
2. Berger RA, Quigley LR, Jacobs JJ, et al. The fate of stable cemented acetabular components retained during revision of a femoral component of a total hip arthroplasty. J Bone Joint Surg Am 1999;81:1682–1691.
3. Böhm P, Bischel O. Femoral revision with the Wagner SL revision stem: evaluation of one hundred and twenty-nine revisions followed for a mean of 4.8 years. J Bone Joint Surg Am 2001;83-A(7):1023–1031.
4. Böhm P, Bischel O. The use of tapered stems for femoral revision surgery. Clin Orthop Relat Res 2004;(420):148–159.
5. Chen WM, McAuley JP, Engh CA Jr, et al. Extended slide trochanteric osteotomy for revision total hip arthroplasty. J Bone Joint Surg Am 2000;82:1215–1219.
6. Fink B, Grossmann A, Schubring S, et al. A modified transfemoral approach using modular cementless revision stems. Clin Orthop Relat Res 2007;462:105–114.
7. Grunig R, Morscher E, Ochsner PE. Three-to 7-year results with the uncemented SL femoral revision prosthesis. Arch Orthop Trauma Surg 1997;116:187–197.

8. Hartwig CH, Böhm P, Czech U, et al. The Wagner revision stem in alloarthroplasty of the hip. Arch Orthop Trauma Surg 1996;115:5–9.
9. Huffman GR, Ries MD. Combined vertical and horizontal cable fixation of an extended trochanteric osteotomy site. J Bone Joint Surg Am 2003;85-A(2):273–277.
10. Isacson J, Stark A, Wallensten R. The Wagner revision prosthesis consistently restores femoral bone structure. Int Orthop 2000;24:139–142.
11. Kolstad K, Adalberth G, Mallmin H, et al. The Wagner revision stem for severe osteolysis. 31 hips followed for 1.5-5 years. Acta Orthop Scand 1996;67:541–544.
12. Lieberman JR, Moeckel BH, Evans BG, et al. Cement-within-cement revision hip arthroplasty. J Bone Joint Surg Br 1993;75:869–871.
13. Mardones R, Gonzalez C, Cabanela ME, et al. Extended femoral osteotomy for revision of hip arthroplasty: results and complications. J Arthroplasty 2005;20:79–83.
14. Miner TM, Momberger NG, Chong D, et al. The extended trochanteric osteotomy in revision hip arthroplasty: a critical review of 166 cases at mean 3-year, 9-month follow-up. J Arthroplasty 2001;16:188–194.
15. Morshed S, Huffman GR, Ries MD. Extended trochanteric osteotomy for 2-stage revision of infected total hip arthroplasty. J Arthroplasty 2005;20:294–301.
16. Moskal JT, Shen FH, Brown TE. The fate of stable femoral components retained during isolated acetabular revision: a six-to-twelve-year follow-up study. J Bone Joint Surg Am 2002;84-A(2):250–255.
17. Peters PC Jr, Head WC, Emerson RH Jr. An extended trochanteric osteotomy for revision total hip replacement. J Bone Joint Surg Br 1993;75:158–159.
18. Wagner M, Wagner H. The transfemoral approach for revision of total hip replacement [in German]. Oper Orthop Traumatol 1999;11:278–295.
19. Warren PJ, Thompson P, Fletcher MD. Transfemoral implantation of the Wagner SL stem. The abolition of subsidence and enhancement of osteotomy union rate using Dall-Miles cables. Arch Orthop Trauma Surg 2002;122:557–560.
20. Wilkes RA, Birch J, Pearse MF, et al. The Wagner technique for revision arthroplasty of the hip: a review of 24 cases. J Orthop Rheumatol 1994;7:196–198.

Fixation of Periprosthetic Fractures About/Below Total Hip Arthroplasty

Aaron Nauth, Iain Stevenson, Matthew D. Smith, and Emil H. Schemitsch

DEFINITION

- Periprosthetic fractures about a total hip arthroplasty are fractures which occur in the femur or acetabulum adjacent to either the femoral or acetabular component, respectively. These fractures can occur intraoperatively or postoperatively. The focus of this chapter will be postoperative fractures of the femur which occur adjacent to the femoral component of a total hip arthroplasty.

ANATOMY

- Fractures of the femur adjacent to the femoral component of a total hip arthroplasty are most commonly described using the Vancouver classification system which categorizes the fracture on the basis of anatomic location, stability of the femoral component, and surrounding bone stock (Table 1; **FIG 1**).[5] This classification system is simple, reliable, and serves to guide treatment.
- Type A fractures occur in the trochanteric region and involve either the greater trochanter (A_G) or the lesser trochanter (A_L).
- Type B fractures occur around or just distal to the stem of the femoral component and are subclassified based on the stability of the implant and the surrounding bone stock. Type B1 fractures occur around a stable implant. Type B2 fractures occur around a loose implant with adequate bone stock. Type B3 fractures occur around a loose implant with poor bone stock.
- Type C fractures occur well distal to a stable femoral component.

Table 1 Vancouver Classification of Periprosthetic Fractures of the Femur about a Total Hip Arthroplasty

Type	Fracture Description
A	Fracture around the trochanters
A_G	Greater trochanter
A_L	Lesser trochanter
B	Fracture about the stem or just distal to the stem
B_1	Stable implant
B_2	Loose implant with good bone stock
B_3	Loose implant with poor bone stock
C	Fracture well below the implant

PATHOGENESIS

- Postoperative periprosthetic fractures can occur in a variety of settings; however, major trauma accounts for a very small proportion.

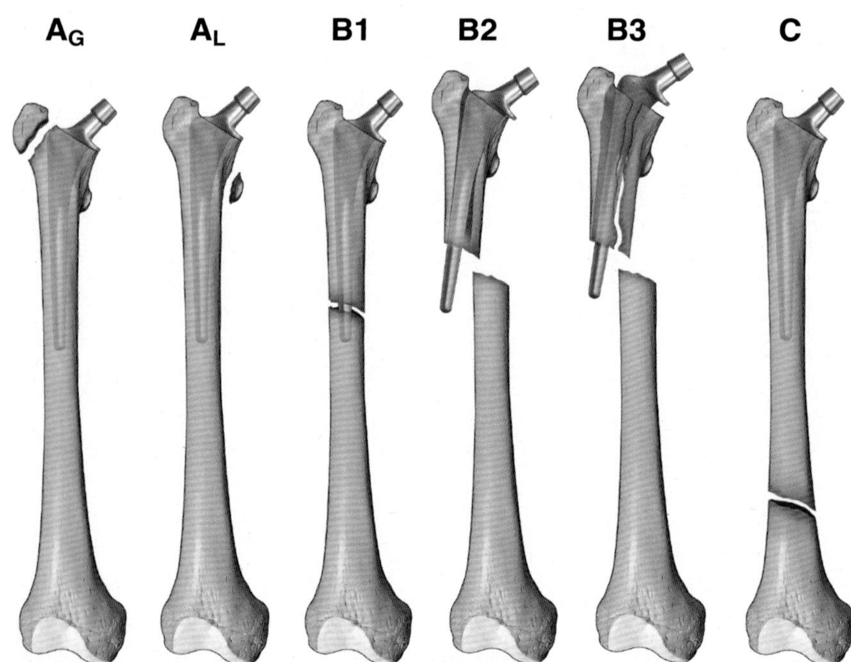

FIG 1 • The Vancouver classification of periprosthetic fractures of the femur about a total hip arthroplasty.

- The majority of these fractures occur with a low-energy fall and up to 25% occur without any significant trauma.
- A large proportion of these patients have pathologic and osteopenic bone due to a combination of factors including localized osteopenia of the proximal femur due to stress shielding and osteolysis as well as a high prevalence of osteoporosis in this patient population.

NATURAL HISTORY

- The vast majority of these fractures require surgical management for effective fracture healing and return of function.
- Retrospective literature has demonstrated a 1-year mortality of 11% and morbidity/mortality very similar to hip fracture patients.[1] This is an important consideration as these patients should be managed in a similar fashion to hip fracture patients by incorporating a multidisciplinary team approach (geriatrics assessment, delirium prevention etc.), carrying out early surgical intervention (<48 hours from injury), and using a surgical strategy that allows early weight bearing and mobilization.

PATIENT HISTORY AND PHYSICAL FINDINGS

- It is important to obtain information regarding the mechanism of injury and level of energy imparted as well as the cause of the fall.
- Information regarding prodromal symptoms such as thigh pain with weight-bearing or start-up pain should be obtained and may indicate a preexisting loose femoral stem prior to fracture.
- A history of past infections, wound healing complications, or constitutional symptoms may indicate a periprosthetic infection.
- A social history including the patient's prior ambulatory status, use of walking aids, level of independence, and overall functionality is helpful for setting reasonable treatment goals.
- Physical examination may indicate gross deformity of the limb in a displaced fracture or the findings may be more subtle in minimally displaced fractures such as pain with range of motion or rotation of the hip, difficulty weight bearing, or weakness of the limb. Physical examination should also focus on ruling out open wounds, neurovascular injury, and associated injuries.

IMAGING AND OTHER DIAGNOSTIC STUDIES

- Investigation begins with anteroposterior (AP) and lateral radiographs of the affected femur and an AP pelvis. Radiographs should be carefully inspected for the location of fracture lines, fragment displacement, implant loosening, and quality of bone stock.
- It is *critical* to identify any evidence of implant loosening as the surgical management of a periprosthetic fracture with a loose femoral component (Vancouver type B2) requires revision to a long-stem component in addition to fracture fixation, whereas a fracture with a stable component (Vancouver type B1) can be readily treated with fracture fixation alone. Lindahl et al[4] reported that the most common reason for treatment failure in the fixation of Vancouver type B1 fractures was loosening of the implant, presumably due to failure to recognize that the implant was loose at the time of fracture.
- Definite signs of radiographic loosening include progressive periprosthetic or cement mantle lucency, change in position of the stem, and component or cement mantle fracture (**FIG 2**). Radiographic signs of probable loosening include

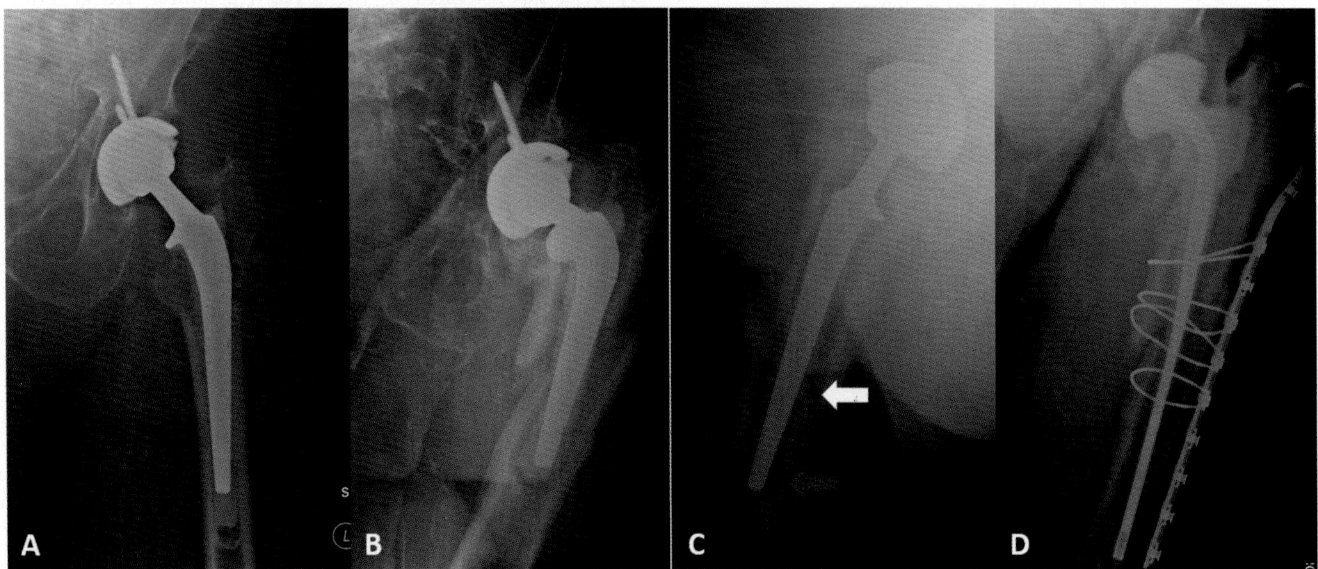

FIG 2 • Radiographs of a 91-year-old male patient with a Vancouver type B2 periprosthetic femur fracture 1 year following total hip arthroplasty. Comparison with immediate postoperative radiographs (**A**) shows definite signs of loosening including progressive radiolucency of the cement–bone interface, subsidence of the implant, fracture of the cement mantle (*white arrow*), and debonding of the cement mantle around the implant (*red arrow*) (**B,C**). The patient reported a 3-month history of prodromal thigh pain and his erythrocyte sedimentation rate (ESR) and C-reactive protein (CRP) were elevated significantly. The total hip arthroplasty was presumed to be infected, and revision to an antibiotic cement spacer combined with fixation of the fracture was performed (**D**) after infection was confirmed intraoperatively. (Reproduced with permission from Nauth A, Henry P, Schemitsch EH. Periprosthetic fractures of the femur after total hip arthroplasty: cable plate and allograft strut fixation of Vancouver B1 fractures. In: Sarwark JF, ed. Knowledge Online Journal. Rosemont, IL: American Academy of Orthopaedic Surgeons, 2014.)

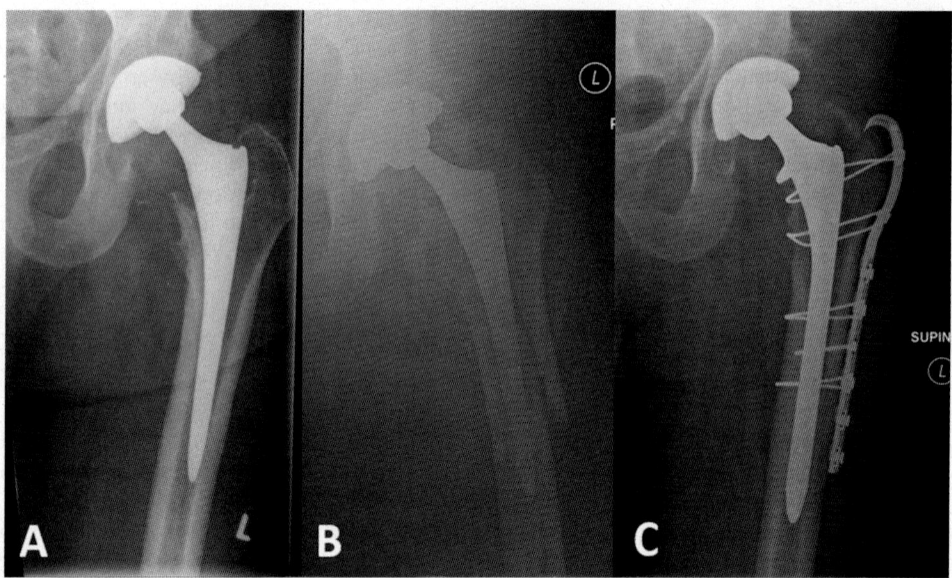

FIG 3 • Vancouver type B2 periprosthetic fracture in a 75-year-old male. Comparison with preinjury radiographs (**A**) shows noticeable subsidence and change of prosthesis position confirming loosening (**B**). Revision to a long-stemmed prosthesis combined with fracture fixation was performed (**C**).

greater than 2 mm of periprosthetic or cement mantle lucency, bead shedding, endosteal scalloping, and endosteal bone bridging at the tip of the stem.

- Whenever possible, preinjury radiographs should be obtained to assess for change in component position, as this is the best indication of a loose stem. Careful comparison of implant position on injury and preinjury radiographs is required, as the findings of implant subsidence can range from noticeable to relatively subtle (**FIGS 3** and **4**).
- Efforts should be made to obtain original operative reports in case revision of the implant is required.
- Inflammatory markers such as white cell count, erythrocyte sedimentation rate (ESR), and C-reactive protein (CRP) are often elevated in the setting of trauma, and therefore can be difficult to interpret in the setting of a fracture unless they are significantly elevated. If concern for infection exists on the basis of preinjury symptoms, a preoperative hip aspiration can be obtained or the surgeon should be prepared to proceed with a two-stage revision should infection be encountered at the time of surgery (see **FIG 2**).

DIFFERENTIAL DIAGNOSIS

- Periprosthetic infection
- Aseptic loosening
- Pathologic fracture

NONOPERATIVE MANAGEMENT

- Operative intervention is indicated for the vast majority of periprosthetic fractures of the femur with the exception of stable fractures of the lesser trochanter without shaft extension, minimally displaced fractures of the greater trochanter, and completely undisplaced fractures around the stem of a stable implant. In addition, minimally displaced fractures about the femoral stem in patients who are poor surgical candidates can be considered for a trial of conservative management.

SURGICAL MANAGEMENT

- The surgical management of periprosthetic femur fractures about a total hip arthroplasty is guided by the Vancouver classification.
- Type A_L fractures of the lesser trochanter are generally managed nonsurgically as are minimally displaced type A_G fractures of the greater trochanter. Displaced type A_G fractures are generally managed with open reduction and internal fixation (ORIF) +/− bone grafting and polyethylene liner exchange if they are associated with osteolysis and liner wear.
- Type B1 fractures have a stable implant and are managed with fracture fixation. The focus of this techniques chapter is on the fixation of these fracture types and techniques for type B1 fracture fixation are described below in detail. There is relative controversy in the literature regarding the optimal technique for fixation of Vancouver type B1 fractures, with the main controversy centered around the use of cable plating combined with allograft strut versus isolated lateral locked plating. The biomechanical literature suggests that the use of a lateral cable plate and screws combined with the use of an anterior allograft strut (90–90 fixation) is the optimal biomechanical construct.[7] Buttaro et al[2] retrospectively reviewed a 14 patient series of type B1 fractures treated with lateral locked plating +/− the use of a cortical strut. The authors reported a high rate of failure when isolated lateral locked plating was used (five of nine constructs) versus when lateral plating was combined with the use of a cortical strut (one of five constructs). In contrast, other authors have reported a very high rate of success when isolated lateral plating is combined with indirect reduction and biologically friendly techniques.[6] High-level prospective evidence comparing the

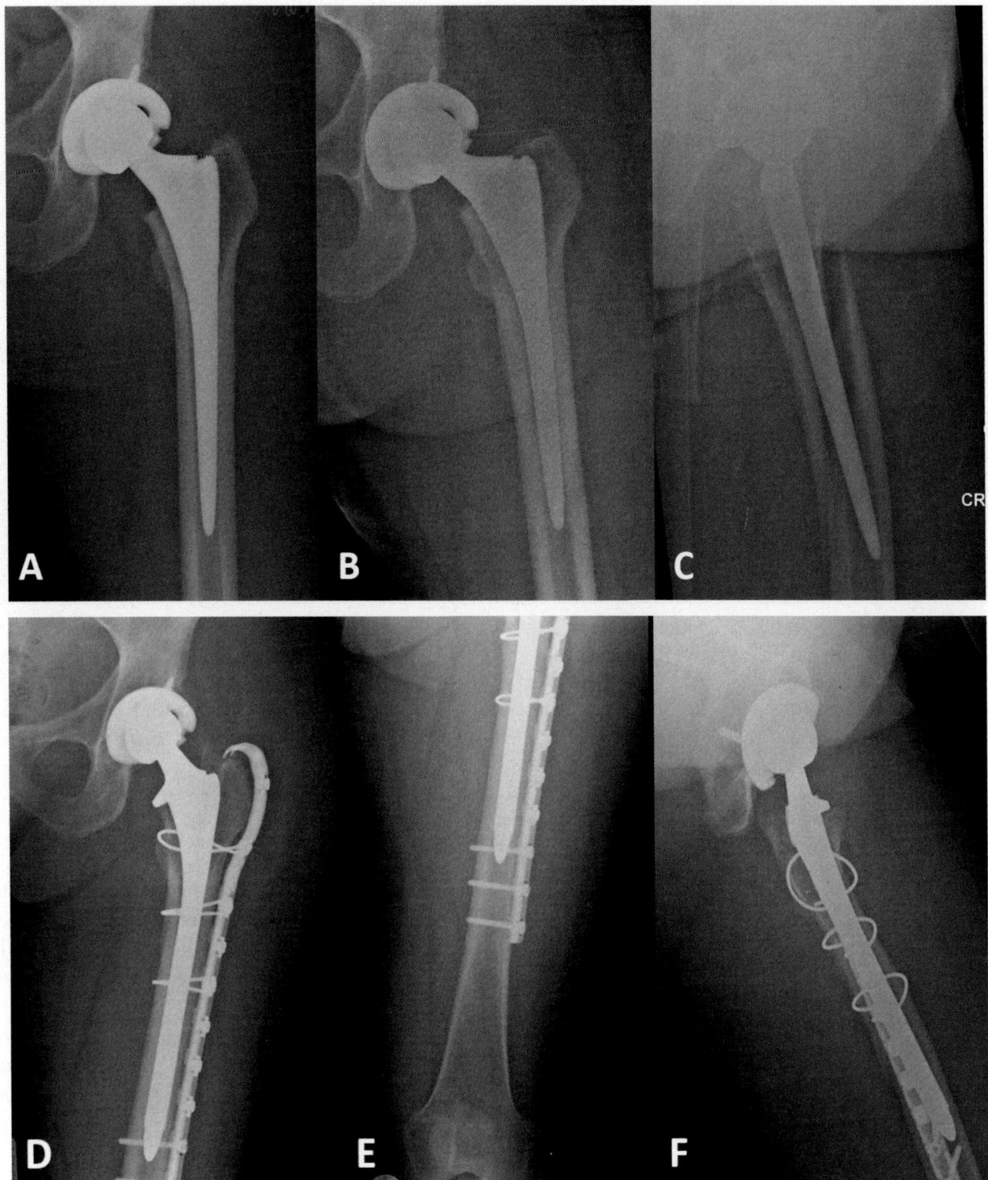

FIG 4 • Radiographs of a Vancouver type B2 periprosthetic femur fracture in 52-year-old female who suffered a fall at 3 weeks postoperatively. Comparison with immediate postoperative radiographs (**A**) shows subtle subsidence of the implant (**B,C**). The patient was brought to the operating room with plans for fixation of her fracture and revision to a long-stemmed implant. Implant loosening was confirmed at the time of the operation. Six-month postoperative radiographs in the same patient showing revision to a long-stemmed implant with cable plate and screw fixation of the fracture (**D–F**). (Reproduced with permission from Nauth A, Henry P, Schemitsch EH. Periprosthetic fractures of the femur after total hip arthroplasty: cable plate and allograft strut fixation of Vancouver B1 fractures. In: Sarwark JF, ed. Orthopaedic Knowledge Online Journal. Rosemont, IL: American Academy of Orthopaedic Surgeons, 2014.)

two techniques is lacking. Irrespective of the fixation strategy used, several biomechanical and surgical principles must be adhered to when treating these fractures. First, it is critical that the fracture is fixed without the stem in varus, as increased rates of fixation failure have been reported with varus positioning of the stem. Second, proximal fixation around the stem is best achieved with a combination of wires/cables and screws, and it is critical that sufficient overlap of the femoral prosthesis is obtained to avoid mechanical failure (**FIG 5**). This generally requires fixation to the level of the greater trochanter. Third, it is important to remember that these fractures commonly occur in pathologic/osteopenic bone, and the use of a plate of sufficient length to stabilize the entire length of the femur is recommended to avoid future peri-implant fracture. Finally, it is important to adhere to the principles of absolute versus relative stability depending on the type of fracture healing desired. In the setting of a simple transverse or spiral fracture, absolute stability and compression at the fracture site should be achieved using compression plating or lag screw fixation. This is in contrast to comminuted fractures which require relative stability and spaced fixation to allow for fracture healing indirectly by callus formation.

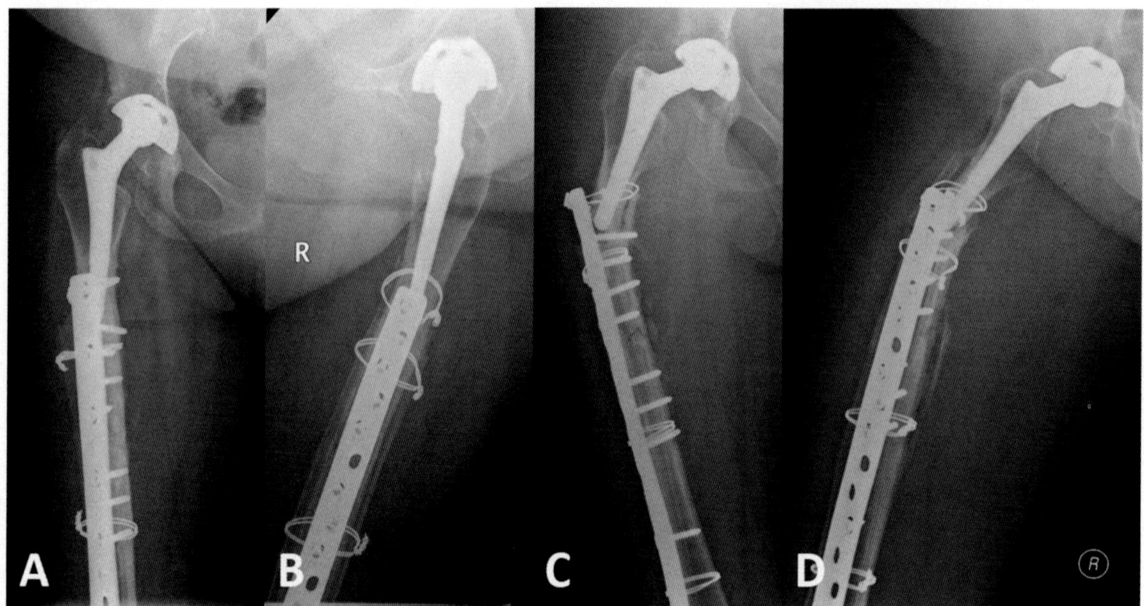

FIG 5 • Radiographs of a 41-year-old female patient with a Vancouver type B1 periprosthetic fracture that was fixed with lateral locked plating and fibular strut allograft (**A,B**). Radiographs show that insufficient overlap of the femoral component was obtained with the plate and predictable failure occurred (**C,D**). (Reproduced with permission from Nauth A, Henry P, Schemitsch EH. Periprosthetic fractures of the femur after total hip arthroplasty: cable plate and allograft strut fixation of Vancouver B1 fractures. In: Sarwark JF, ed. Orthopaedic Knowledge Online Journal. Rosemont, IL: American Academy of Orthopaedic Surgeons, 2014.)

- Vancouver type B2 fractures are treated with revision to a long-stemmed prosthesis and fixation of the fracture (see **FIGS 3** and **4**). The stem should bypass the fracture by at least two cortical diameters.
- Type B3 fractures require revision, ORIF, and possible structural allograft to restore bone stock.
- Vancouver type C fractures occur well below the stem and can be generally treated with isolated ORIF.

Preoperative Planning

- As indicated previously, multidisciplinary assessment is recommended to manage patient comorbidities and perioperative medical issues.
- At all times when managing periprosthetic fractures of the femur about a total hip arthroplasty, the surgeon should be prepared for the possible need for revision. This requires careful review of the initial operative report to ensure that revision implants of the appropriate type are available for possible revision of the femoral stem. Corten et al[3] reported that 20% of implants judged to be stable based on preoperative radiographs were found to be loose at the time of surgery. If any doubt exists regarding the stability of the femoral component, an arthrotomy of the hip with dislocation and stressing of the implant should be performed to rule out a loose femoral component.

Positioning

- The patient is positioned supine on a radiolucent (Jackson) table with a bump or inflated beanbag under the affected side to elevate the fractured limb (**FIG 6**). The limb is free-draped, and intraoperative fluoroscopy is placed on the contralateral side to the fracture.
- Alternatively, the patient can be positioned in the lateral decubitus position with the affected limb facing up and free-draped. This is the position of choice, if revision of the femoral component is planned.

Approach

- The approach involves a lateral incision using the distal aspect of the previous total hip arthroplasty incision extended distally toward the knee.
- If an arthrotomy is required for dislocation of the hip and evaluation of femoral component stability or for femoral component revision, the proximal aspect of the total hip incision can be used as well.
- If a minimally invasive approach and indirect reduction is being employed, then the distal aspect of the total hip incision is used to access the femur proximal to the fracture and a separate distal incision is made at the lateral aspect of the distal femur for distal plate placement.

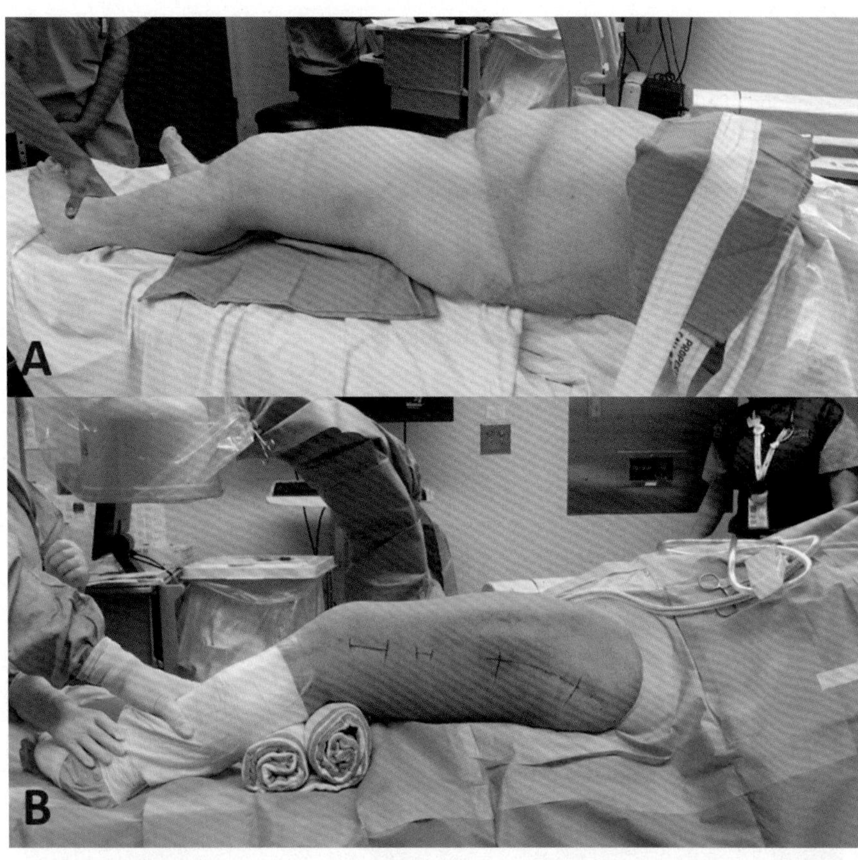

FIG 6 ● Intraoperative photographs showing patient positioning in the supine position with a beanbag used to elevate the operative hip and positioning of the C-arm on the patients contralateral side.

Cable Plating and Allograft Strut Fixation

- Surgical exposure: A lateral exposure is carried out to expose the entire femur extending from the distal aspect of the previous total hip arthroplasty incision to the level of the distal femur. For deep dissection, the fascia lata is split in line with the skin incision and the vastus lateralis is elevated anteriorly with dissection carried out along the posterior fibers (**TECH FIG 1C**). Perforating vessels are identified and coagulated. The entire lateral aspect of the femur, including the fracture, is exposed from the level just below the greater trochanter to the level of the metaphyseal flair. The lateral and anterior aspects of the femur are exposed. Although the exposure is extensile, care is taken to avoid stripping the soft tissues on the posterior and medial aspects of the femur (**TECH FIG 1D**).
- Fracture reduction and plate application: If doubt exists regarding the stability of the implant, the bone implant interface is carefully examined through the fracture site for any evidence of loosening. If loosening is suspected, proximal extension of the incision is carried out with an arthrotomy to evaluate implant stability at the level of the hip. Once implant stability is confirmed, fracture reduction is achieved with the use of reduction clamps (**TECH FIG 1E**). A plate of appropriate length is chosen to span the entire femur from the distal femur to the level just below the greater trochanter (it is critical to ensure adequate overlap of the plate with the femoral stem to avoid mechanical failure). Plate contouring is performed as necessary depending on the plate chosen to allow application of the plate to the lateral aspect of the femur. Newer generation precontoured locking plates have a contour to accommodate the anterior bow of the native femur. Provisional screw fixation is obtained through the plate both proximal and distal to the fracture. If the fracture pattern is amenable to absolute stability, then compression at the fracture site is obtained at this stage using the compression holes in the plate, lag screws, or an articulated tensioning device. Fluoroscopy is then used to confirm anatomic reduction and alignment as well as satisfactory positioning of the plate (**TECH FIG 1F**).
- Allograft preparation: Allograft preparation is begun as soon as the approach to the femur is complete and both infection and implant loosening have been definitively ruled out. The authors' preference is to use the anterior cortex of a distal femoral allograft as this provides a graft which accommodates the anterior bow of the femur and also allows for cancellous allograft to be obtained from the distal femur (**TECH FIG 1G**). Tibial or humeral strut allografts are acceptable alternatives. A strut allograft of appropriate length to allow adequate graft overlap with the femoral prosthesis and passage of two cables on either side of the fracture is necessary (generally, a minimum length of 25 to 30 cm is required). In addition, it is advisable to avoid ending the allograft at the same level distally as the plate and creating a stress riser. The anterior cortex of the distal femoral allograft is prepared using an oscillating saw and burr. Appropriate sizing and contouring of the graft is confirmed with provisional placement on the anterior cortex of the femur (**TECH FIG 1H**).

- Cable passage and allograft placement: Prior to definitive allograft placement, cables are passed around the femur using a cable passer, as these are more easily passed prior to graft placement. It is critical that these cables are passed directly on the bone to avoid entrapment of neurovascular structures (**TECH FIG 1I**). The authors typically use two cables proximal to the fracture and two cables distal to the fracture. The graft is then placed on the anterior aspect of the femur creating a 90–90 construct. The cables are then sequentially tightened, locked, and trimmed (**TECH FIG 1J**). At this stage, supplemental screw fixation is placed proximal and distal to the fracture. Proximally, this involves placing nonlocked screws or polyaxial locking screws around the well-fixed femoral stem or the use of unicortical locking screws. Intraoperative fluoroscopy is then used to confirm anatomic reduction and alignment of the fracture and satisfactory positioning of the plate, screws, cables, and allograft strut. At this point, the wound is irrigated copiously with normal saline. Cancellous allograft harvested from the distal femoral allograft is then placed at the fracture site and at the graft–host interface. A standard closure is then performed in layers.

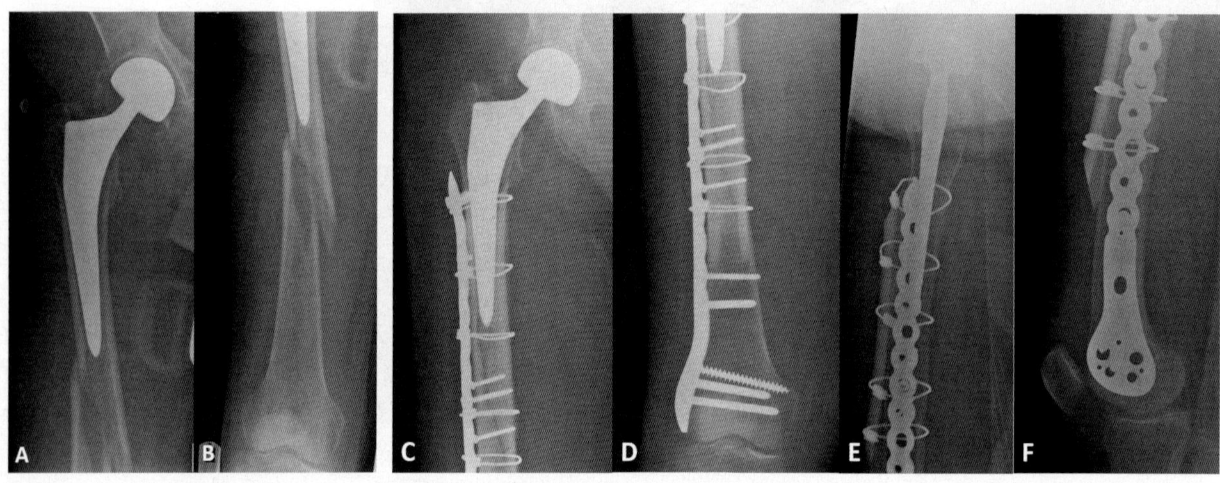

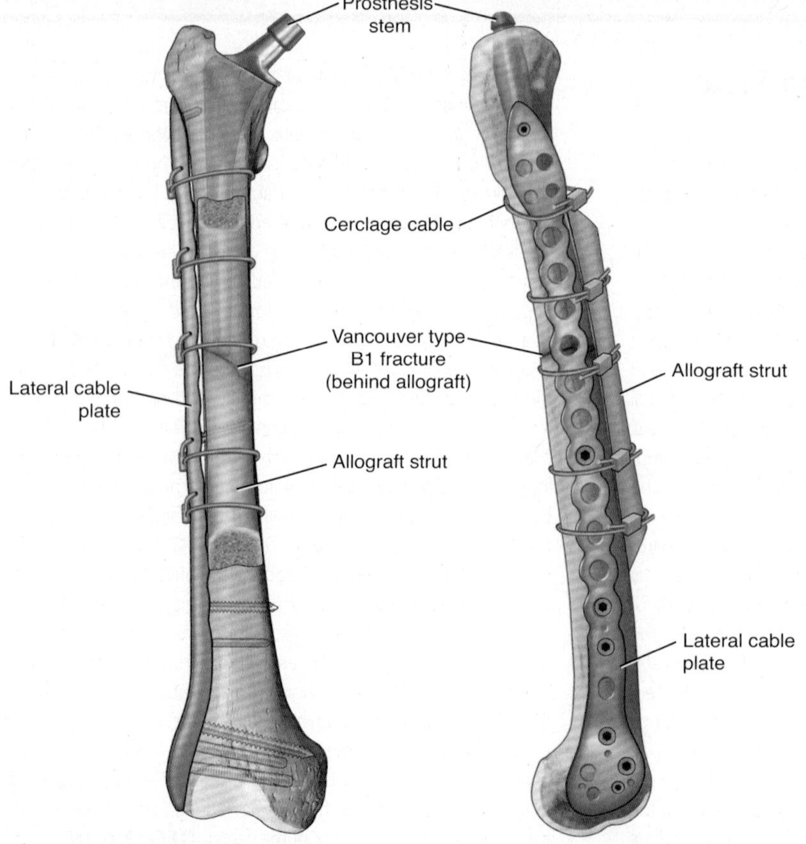

TECH FIG 1 • **A.** Radiographs of an 82-year-old female patient with a Vancouver type B1 periprosthetic fracture at the tip of a well-fixed stem that had been functioning well prior to a fall (*A,B*). Postoperative radiographs showing fixation of the fracture with a lateral distal femoral locking plate combined with an anterior allograft strut (90–90 fixation) and cables (*C–F*). **B.** Illustration depicting the construct of a lateral cable plate and anterior allograft strut (90–90 fixation) used for fixation of a Vancouver type B1 fracture. *(continued)*

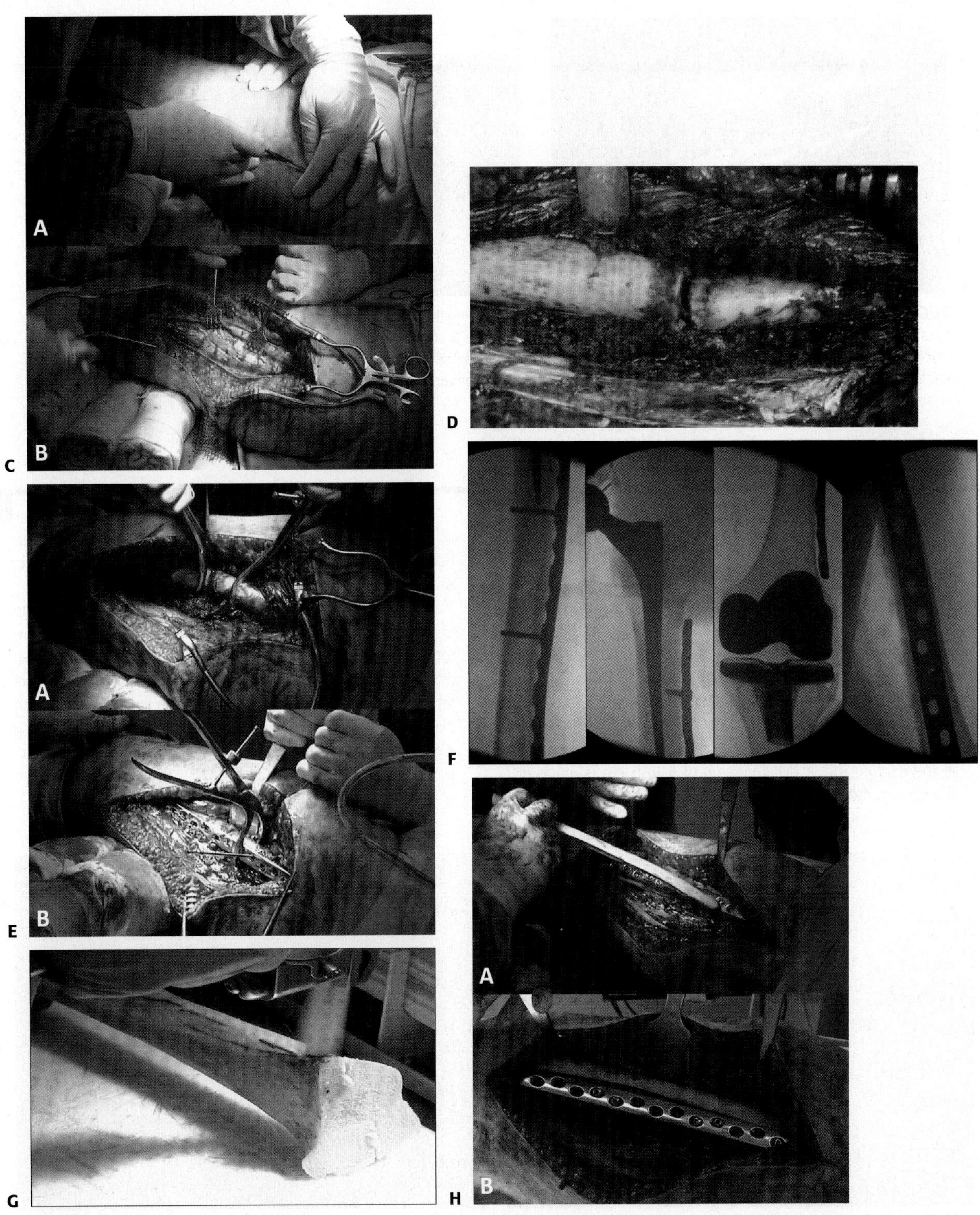

TECH FIG 1 • *(continued)* **C.** Intraoperative photographs showing the lateral incision and approach to the femur for fixation of a Vancouver type B1 fracture with a cable plate and anterior allograft strut. **D.** Intraoperative photograph of the fracture site of a Vancouver type B1 fracture demonstrating the avoidance of soft tissue dissection and stripping of the posterior and medial soft tissues. **E.** Intraoperative photographs of a Vancouver type B1 fracture demonstrating provisional reduction and lateral plate placement. **F.** Intraoperative fluoroscopy pictures demonstrating provisional reduction and plate fixation of the fracture. Note that the entire femur is spanned with the plate from just below the greater trochanter to the distal femur. **G.** Intraoperative photograph demonstrating preparation of the allograft strut from a distal femoral allograft. **H.** Intraoperative photograph demonstrating final allograft strut preparation and sizing. *(continued)*

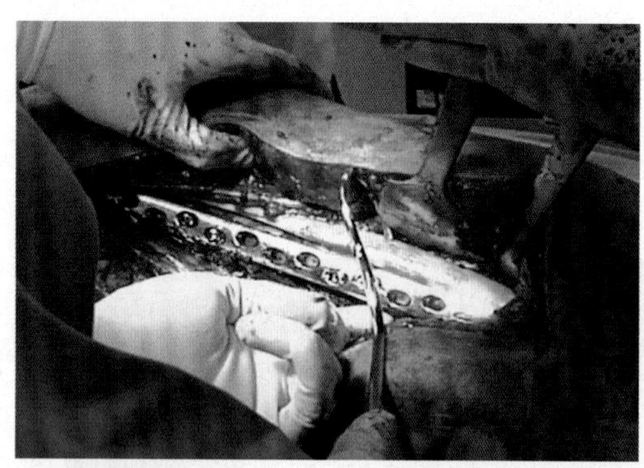

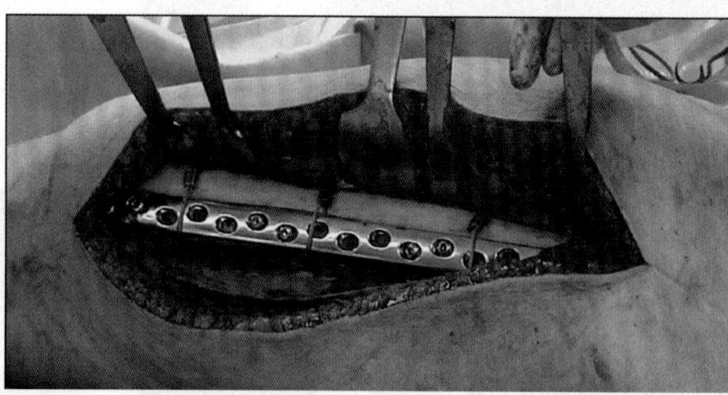

TECH FIG 1 • *(continued)* **I.** Intraoperative photograph demonstrating the technique for safe cable passage around the allograft strut and lateral plate. **J.** Intraoperative photograph demonstrating the final allograft strut and cable plate construct. (**C–J:** Reproduced with permission from Nauth A, Henry P, Schemitsch EH. Periprosthetic fractures of the femur after total hip arthroplasty: cable plate and allograft strut fixation of Vancouver B1 fractures. In: Sarwark JF, ed. Orthopaedic Knowledge Online Journal. Rosemont, IL: American Academy of Orthopaedic Surgeons, 2014.)

Minimally Invasive Isolated Lateral Locking Plate Fixation

- Surgical approach: A lateral exposure of the proximal femur is made using the distal aspect of the total hip arthroplasty incision with extension just proximal to the fracture. Deep dissection is carried out through fascia lata and posterior to vastus lateralis to expose the proximal femur from the level of the greater trochanter to just proximal to the fracture site. Care is taken to preserve the soft tissues and vascular supply at the fracture site. A distal incision of 4 to 5 cm is made at the level of the metaphyseal flare to expose the lateral aspect of the distal femur (**TECH FIG 2C**). A cobb elevator is then used to create a submuscular plane along the lateral aspect of the femur.
- Plate placement and indirect reduction: A lateral locking plate of appropriate length to span the entire femur is selected, contoured, and tunneled in the submuscular plane from the proximal incision to the distal incision (**TECH FIG 2D**). An indirect reduction is performed with traction of the limb and use of the plate as a reduction aid. The plate is reduced to the femur using a nonlocking screw distally and with the use of a cable or reduction clamp proximally (**TECH FIG 2E**). Fluoroscopy is used to confirm reduction in the coronal and sagittal planes.

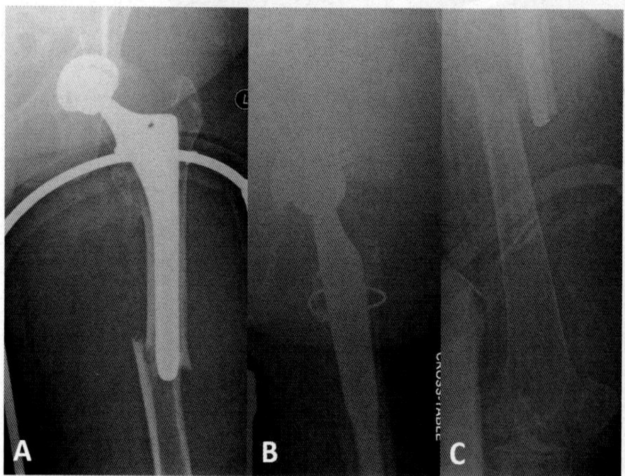

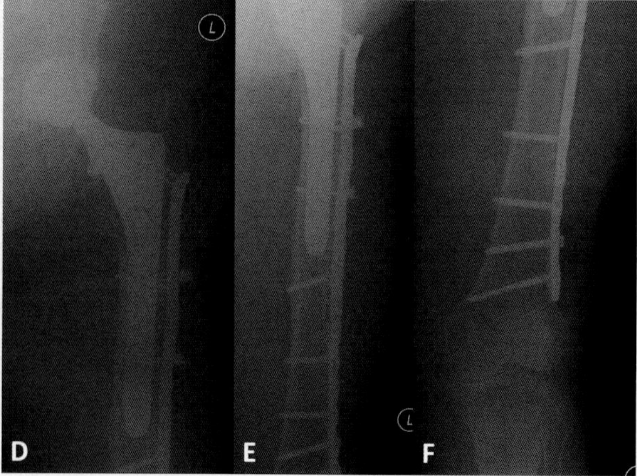

TECH FIG 2 • **A.** Radiographs of a 78-year-old female patient with a Vancouver type B1 periprosthetic fracture at the tip of a well-fixed stem that had been functioning well prior to a fall (*A–C*). Postoperative radiographs showing fixation of the fracture with isolated lateral locked plating using a minimally invasive approach (*D–F*). *(continued)*

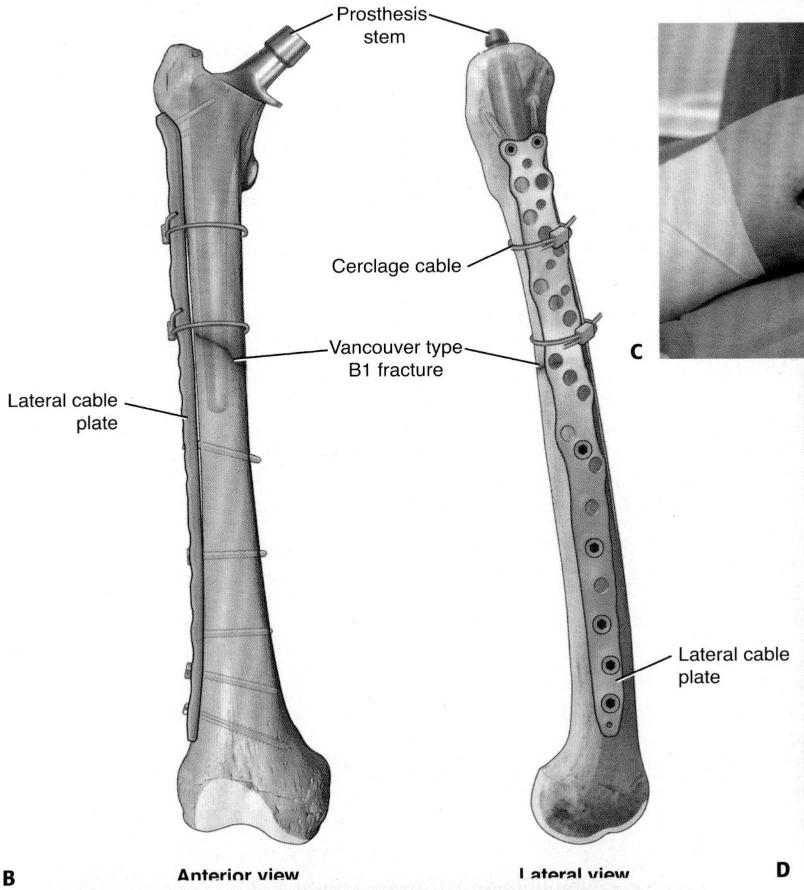

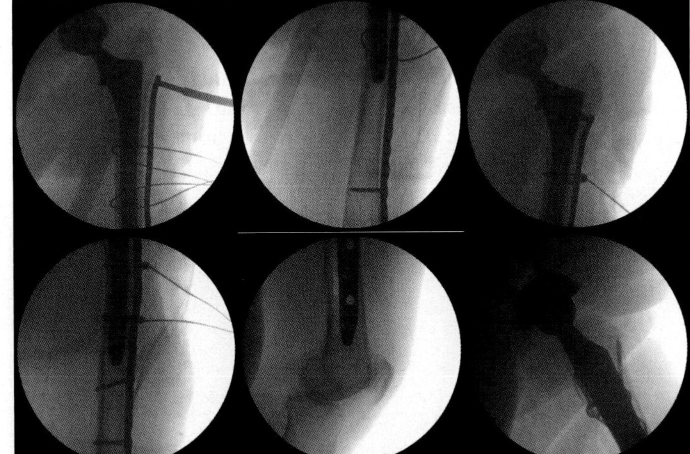
E

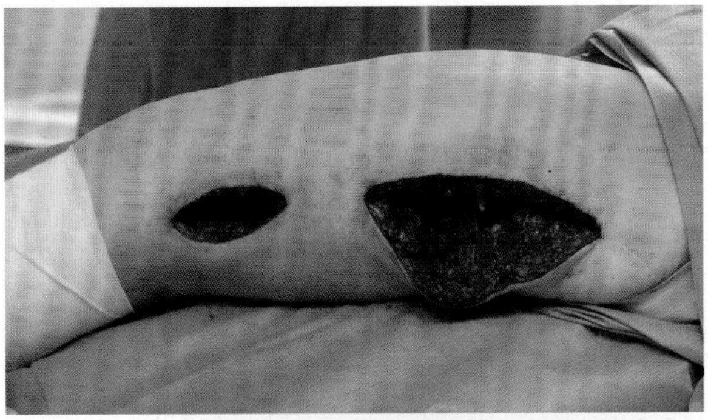

TECH FIG 2 • *(continued)* **B.** Illustration depicting isolated lateral locking plate fixation of a Vancouver type B1 fracture with the use of a combination of screws and cables for proximal fixation. **C.** Intraoperative photograph depicting the incisions for minimally invasive lateral locked plating of a Vancouver type B1 periprosthetic fracture. The skin, soft tissues, and vascular supply are left intact at the level of the fracture to preserve fracture healing biology as best as possible. **D.** Intraoperative photographs demonstrating plate selection and submuscular tunneling of the plate along the lateral aspect of the femur. **E.** Intraoperative and sequential fluoroscopic images demonstrating provisional plate placement and reduction followed by definitive fixation.

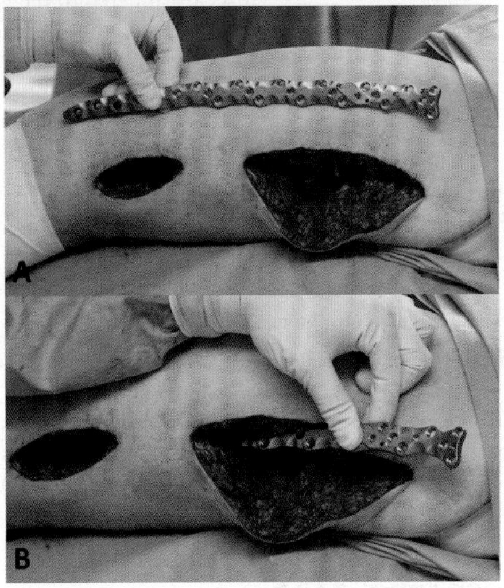

- Cable placement and definitive fixation: Once reduction is confirmed fluoroscopically, definitive fixation is carried out with a combination of locking and nonlocking screws distally and the use of cables and locking screws placed around the femoral component proximally. Newer generation periprosthetic locking plates allow for the placement of polyaxial locking screws around the prosthesis. Both cables and screws should be used to optimize proximal fixation, with the use of two to four cables combined with two to four screws based on bone quality. Distal fixation is obtained with a combination of locking and nonlocking screws, again based on bone quality. Spaced fixation and a screw density of 50% (ie, half of the distal screw holes should be left empty) should be used to prevent a large concentration of stress over a small length of plate at the fracture site (see **TECH FIG 2A**). Final fluoroscopic images (see **TECH FIG 2E**) are obtained and a standard layered closure is performed.

PEARLS AND PITFALLS

Periprosthetic fracture patient management	■ These patients should be managed in a similar fashion to hip fracture patients with the following: ■ Multidisciplinary assessment ■ Expedited surgery (within 48 hours) ■ Surgical goals of early weight bearing and mobilization
Implant loosening	■ It is critical that loosening of the femoral implant is ruled out prior to proceeding with fracture fixation by careful history and radiograph review (including preinjury films if available). If doubt exists regarding implant loosening, then the stability of the implant should be assessed intraoperatively (either with visualization of the implant–bone interface at the fracture site or with a formal arthrotomy and dislocation of the hip with stressing of the femoral component) and the surgeon should be prepared to proceed with revision to a long-stemmed component if it is determined that the implant is loose.
Fracture fixation	■ There is controversy with regard to the use of isolated locked plating versus cable plating and allograft strut and either strategy is acceptable. Irrespective of the strategy employed, it is critical that the following fixation principles are adhered to the following: ■ Avoid varus positioning of the femoral component. ■ Proximal fixation should be obtained with a combination of both cables and screws. ■ Sufficient overlap of the femoral component should be obtained with fracture fixation. ■ The entire length of the femur should be stabilized if possible. ■ Spaced fixation with a screw density of approximately 50% should be used distally.
Cable plating and allograft strut	■ If this strategy is selected, the following tips should be kept in mind: ■ Allograft strut can be obtained from the femur, tibia, or humerus. ■ Graft length should be a minimum of 25–30 cm. ■ Cable fixation around both the plate and allograft should be obtained with two cables, both proximal and distal to the fracture.
Isolated lateral locked plating	■ If this strategy is selected, the following tips should be kept in mind: ■ A biologically friendly surgical approach should be used to minimize disruption of soft tissues and vascular supply at the fracture site. ■ Proximal fixation should be obtained with a combination of cables and locking screws. ■ Distal fixation should be obtained with spaced fixation and a screw density of 50%.

POSTOPERATIVE CARE

- Postoperatively, the patient is typically kept touch weight bearing for a period of 6 weeks with range of motion of the knee and hip as tolerated. At 6 weeks, the patient is progressed to weight bearing as tolerated. The authors will allow patients treated with cable plating and strut allograft to weight bear as tolerated immediately after surgery, which is one of the advantages of using this construct as if facilitates more rapid mobilization and rehabilitation of the patient.

OUTCOMES

- As discussed before, Bhattacharyya et al[1] have demonstrated that patients presenting with a periprosthetic fracture about a total hip arthroplasty have similar rates of morbidity and mortality to that of the hip fracture population, with a 1-year mortality rate of approximately 11%.
- One-year mortality has been shown to be increased with delays to surgery of greater than 48 hours and it is vital that these patients receive surgery as soon as possible.[1]

COMPLICATIONS

- Variable outcomes have been reported in the literature with regard to complication and reoperation rates. Pooled assessment of the literature on outcomes following fixation of Vancouver type B1 fractures (based on a sample size of 333 patients) suggests the following rates:
  - Overall complication rate = 15%
  - Reoperation rate = 9%
  - Nonunion or hardware failure = 9%
  - Malunion = 6%
  - Infection = 5%
- Nonunion or hardware failure is reliably treated with revision ORIF using cable plating, strut allograft, and bone grafting (or use of an osteoinductive bone graft substitute) of the nonunion site (**FIG 7**).

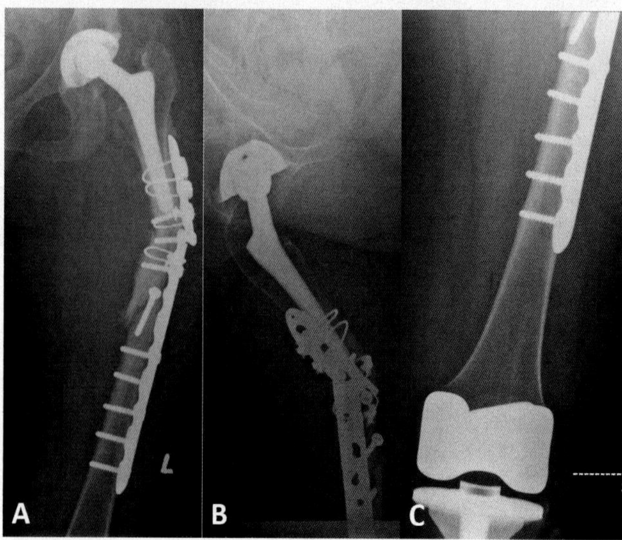

FIG 7 • Preoperative radiographs of a 47-year-old female patient showing nonunion and plate failure following lateral plate fixation of a Vancouver type B1 fracture (**A–C**). *(continued)*

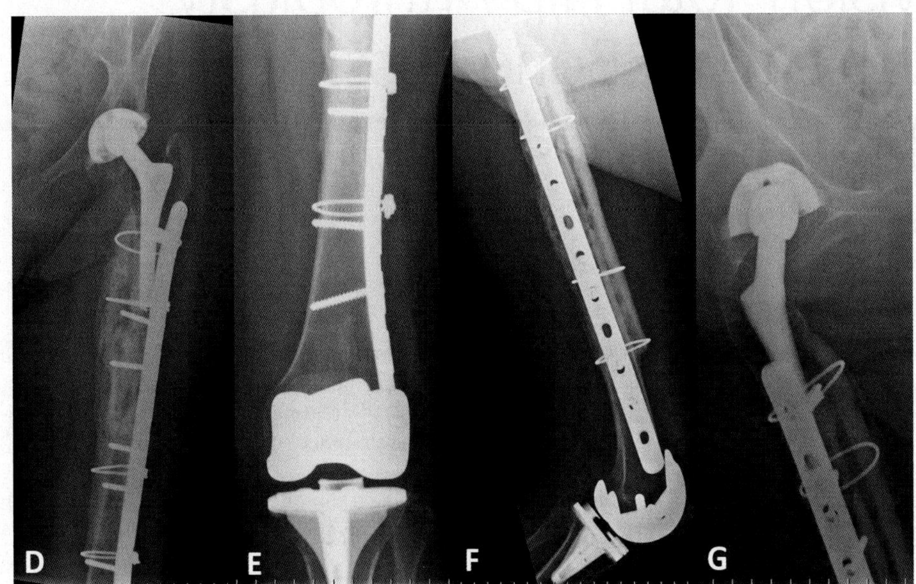

FIG 7 • *(continued)* One-year postoperative radiographs following revision fixation with a cable plate and anterior allograft strut combined with bone grafting of the nonunion and graft–host junction with allograft and bone morphogenetic protein (BMP) (**D–G**). Note: This represents an *off-label* use of BMP.

REFERENCES

1. Bhattacharyya T, Chang D, Meigs JB, et al. Mortality after periprosthetic fracture of the femur. J Bone Joint Surg 2007;89(12):2658–2662.
2. Buttaro MA, Farfalli G, Paredes Nunez M, et al. Locking compression plate fixation of Vancouver type-B1 periprosthetic femoral fractures. J Bone Joint Surg Am 2007;89(9):1964–1969.
3. Corten K, Vanrykel F, Bellemans J, et al. An algorithm for the surgical treatment of periprosthetic fractures of the femur around a well-fixed femoral component. J Bone Joint Surg Br 2009;91(11):1424–1430.
4. Lindahl H, Malchau H, Odén A, et al. Risk factors for failure after treatment of a periprosthetic fracture of the femur. J Bone Joint Surg Br 2006;88(1):26–30.
5. Masri BA, Meek RM, Duncan CP. Periprosthetic fractures evaluation and treatment. Clin Orthop Relat Res 2004;(420):80–95.
6. Ricci WM, Bolhofner BR, Loftus T, et al. Indirect reduction and plate fixation, without grafting, for periprosthetic femoral shaft fractures about a stable intramedullary implant. J Bone Joint Surg Am 2005;87(10):2240–2245.
7. Zdero R, Walker R, Waddell JP, et al. Biomechanical evaluation of periprosthetic femoral fracture fixation. J Bone Joint Surg Am 2008;90(5):1068–1077.

26 CHAPTER

Revision Total Hip Arthroplasty with Femoral Bone Loss: Impaction Allografting

Vishnu Prasad, Bas Weerts, and Michael Dunbar

DEFINITION

- One of the significant challenges in hip revision surgery is the absence of satisfactory proximal femoral bone stock.
- Restoration of the structural integrity of the proximal femur is paramount to the success of any revision surgery.
- Impaction allografting of bone has been used successfully as a technique to repair bone loss in the proximal femur; this procedure involves retrograde filling of the femoral canal with impacted particulate graft, thereby creating a neomedullary canal into which a cemented femoral stem can be placed.

ANATOMY

- Important anatomic considerations include the proximal femoral and diaphyseal anatomy and the assessment of the loss of proximal femoral bone stock.
- The proximal femoral anatomy includes the greater and lesser trochanters and the vastus ridge, which could be a point of relatively weak bone in revisions due to osteolysis, previous trochanteric osteotomies, or previous surgery in this area.
- The femoral diaphyseal anatomy includes the attachments of the vastus musculature at the vastus ridge and posteriorly at the linea aspera.
- The femur can be accessed through an anterior, posterior, transtrochanteric, or straight lateral Hardinge approach.

PATHOGENESIS

- In revision total hip replacements, the most common causes of bony deficiencies are aseptic loosening with debris-induced periprosthetic osteolysis, implant migration, infection, and iatrogenic bone loss during implant extraction.
- There is a higher risk of creating a false passage with cortical penetration in the presence of a pedestal and "egg-shell" bone in the elderly.
- Impaction bone grafting techniques are useful when faced with a large, ectatic femoral metaphysis or diaphysis (**FIG 1A–D**).

NATURAL HISTORY

- The impaction grafting technique allows the surgeon to achieve a stable construct while offering the potential to restore bone stock around the arthroplasty, which is appealing especially in young patients, and would be beneficial for future reconstructions, should they be required.
- When applied properly, it can provide sufficient support for an implant that otherwise would be inadequately supported by host bone.[4,10]
- The graft behaves as a friable aggregate and its resistance to complex forces depends on grading, normal load, and compaction.
- Histologic studies looking at graft incorporation have been carried out by several authors.[5] Ullmark and Obrant[15] have described a healing process that mimics fracture healing.
- Ultimately, the quality of the impacted bone and its remodeling potency determine prosthetic stability.

PATIENT HISTORY AND PHYSICAL FINDINGS

- A detailed history of the symptomatology of a failing arthroplasty includes the nature and quality of pain, instability, decrease in mobility, and quality of life.

A
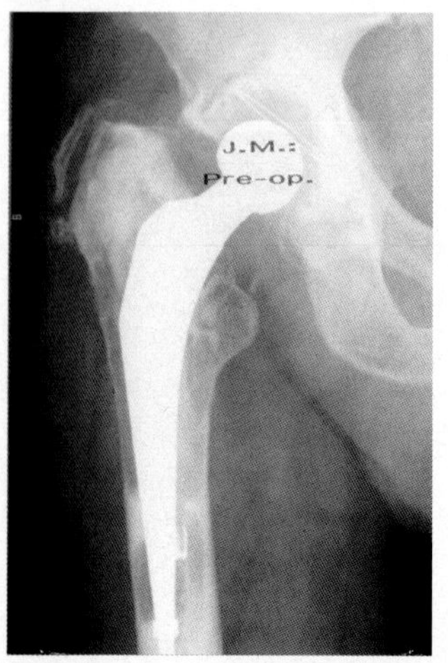

B
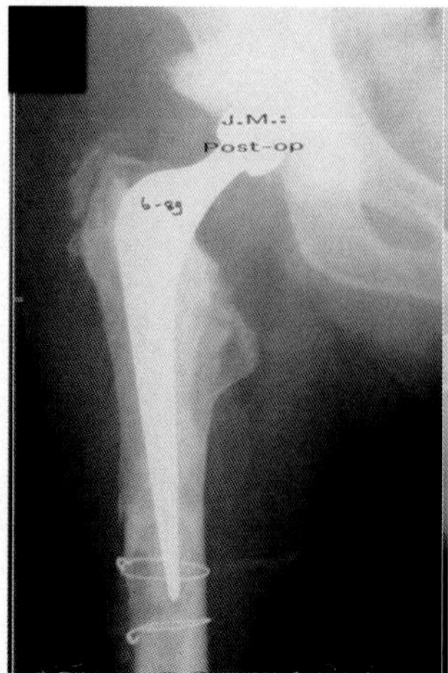

C
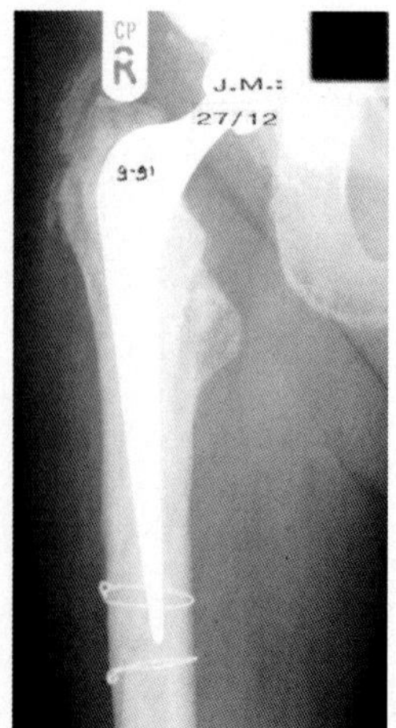

D
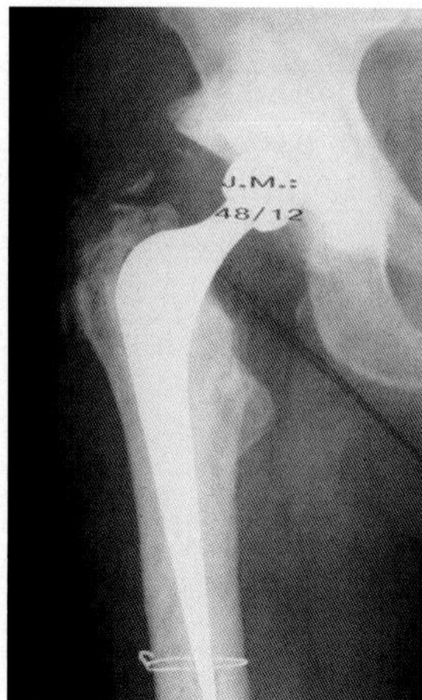

FIG 1 • Loose matt stem with endosteal lysis (**A**), immediate postoperative (**B**), 27 months postoperative. Note cortical healing (**C**) and 48 months postoperative (**D**) with good bone quality maintained. (Images reproduced with the kind permission of The Exeter Hip Unit publishers.)

- Detailed history of the index arthroplasty, postoperative course, and adverse complications such as delayed wound healing or infection
- Detailed history of any significant comorbidities, medications, and allergies
- Physical examination includes assessment of gait, leg lengths, skin and scars over the hip, and muscle strength of the hip and lower extremity, particularly assessment of abductor muscle integrity and distal neurovascular examination.

IMAGING AND OTHER DIAGNOSTIC STUDIES

- The goal of diagnostic imaging studies is to confirm the presence of a failing arthroplasty, exclude the presence of any infection, and ascertain what bone stock is available for the revision reconstruction.
- Confirmation of the presence of a failing arthroplasty and evaluation of the existing bone stock is accomplished by biplanar radiographs of the entire implant and the joint above and below the prosthesis, computed tomography scanning with possible three-dimensional (3-D) reconstruction, and scintigraphy (bone scans).
- Confirmation of a noninfected arthroplasty is vital prior to any revision arthroplasty.
  - This is best accomplished by laboratory evaluation, including erythrocyte sedimentation rate (ESR) and C-reactive protein (CRP). A combination of a normal ESR and CRP shows that the arthroplasty has a very low (<1%) likelihood of being infected.[12]
  - If ESR and CRP are elevated, an aspiration of the hip under image intensifier is warranted, with examination of the cell count with differential and culture of the fluid.
- Deficiency of proximal femoral bone stock can be assessed using the Endo-Klinik classification of femoral defects (**FIG 2**).

DIFFERENTIAL DIAGNOSIS

- Aseptic loosening
- Septic loosening
- Iatrogenic bone loss during implant extraction

NONOPERATIVE MANAGEMENT

- Nonoperative management of a failing hip arthroplasty with significant proximal femoral bone loss is only reserved for the patient with significant comorbidities where a complex revision procedure poses an extreme risk to limb or life.
- Nonoperative measures include optimization of analgesia and protected weight bearing with assistive walking devices or a wheel chair, as tolerated.

SURGICAL MANAGEMENT

- Femoral impaction grafting has been popularized by Gie et al[2,3] and Slooff et al.[11]
- The primary objective for the surgeon in using impacted allografts and cement is to achieve implant stability with preservation or restoration of bone stock.
- Implant stability in impaction grafting depends on constraint for the graft, impaction of the graft, and the injection of cement into the graft surface.
- Constraint is normally provided by the surrounding bone, but where this is defective, some form of artificial constraint must be created by the surgeon before the impaction is performed.
- The most effective way found so far to create this constraint is to use a perforated mesh, fixed appropriately to the bone so as to close off the bony defect or deficiency.[1,2] In simple cases, cerclage wires may suffice.
- The main purpose of the mesh is to provide constraint for the graft. Mesh has a limited effect on reinforcement of the

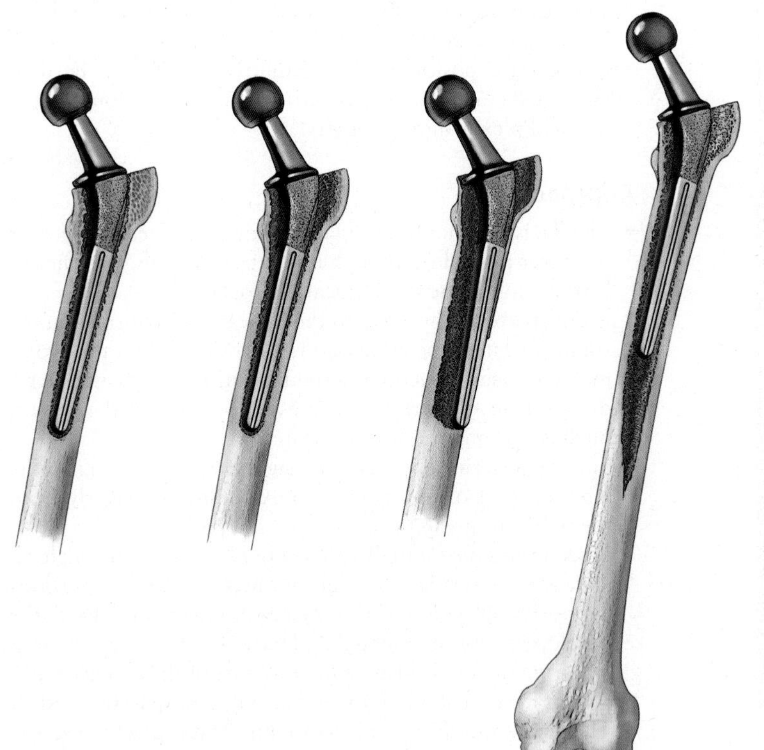

FIG 2 • Endo-Klinik classification of femoral defects. Grade 1—radiolucent zone confined to the upper half of the cement mantle with clinical signs of loosening. Grade 2—radiolucent zone around the cement mantle and endosteal erosion of the upper femur leading to widening of the medullary cavity. Grade 3—widening of the medullary cavity by expansion of the upper femur with proximal bone loss and perforation. Grade 4—gross destruction of the upper and middle thirds of the femur with damage to the distal third and loss of support, precluding the insertion of even a long stemmed prosthesis.

femoral diaphysis, and if used alone to make up circumferential deficits in the femoral diaphysis, mechanical failure is more likely to occur.

- Where replacement or reinforcement of the femoral diaphysis is needed, the mesh should be supplemented by the use of strut grafts, a plate, or a combination of the two. The struts and plate must extend a sufficient distance above and below the defect to be effective mechanically (**FIG 3**).
- Where femoral deficiencies are sited near the tip of a standard length stem, the mesh, strut graft, and/or plate may have to be reinforced by the use of a longer stem.

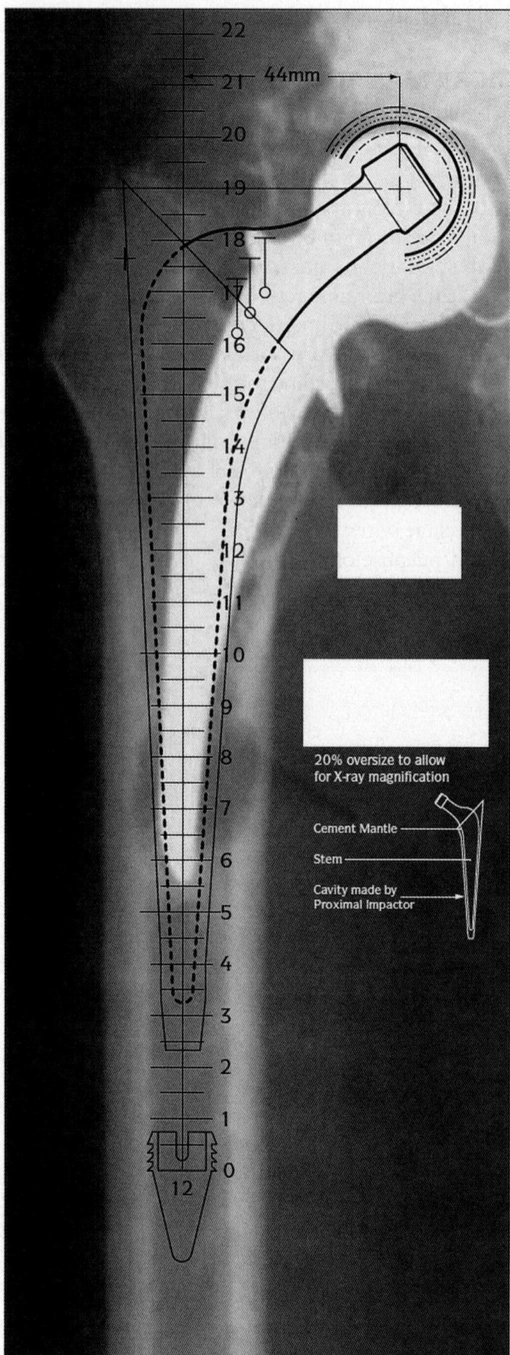

FIG 3 • Templating. (Image reproduced with the kind permission of The Exeter Hip Unit publishers.)

Preoperative Planning

- Elimination of infection is often difficult preoperatively, although every effort should be made to do so.
- Analysis of bone deficiencies—the site(s) of major bone stock loss in the femur should be clarified from x-rays, as far as possible, before surgery starts. This will dictate the exposure that is necessary to address these deficiencies.
- Templating—anteroposterior (AP) and lateral films should include the whole of the femoral component and should extend distally down to the normal diaphysis beyond the femoral component (see **FIG 3**). From these films, the following are determined:
  - The position and size of the distal plug. This should be preferably two cortical diameters beyond the most distal lytic area in the femur.
  - The distance of the plug down the femoral canal against an appropriate anatomic landmark, for example, the tip of the greater trochanter. The distance can be measured using the plug templates and is used with the plug introducer and guidewire to position the plug at the appropriate depth.
  - An estimate of the size of the stem to be used, which can be done by superimposing the stem template on the plug template with the stem at the appropriate position. Final stem sizing is best delayed until the situation is clarified intraoperatively.

Positioning

- The technique of impaction bone grafting is generally more effective if the greater trochanter can be retained. Retention of the trochanter improves proximal stability of the graft and the femoral component.
- Generally, positioning the patient in the lateral decubitus position is appropriate. This will allow exposure of the posterior, lateral, and anterior aspects of the hip by suitable modifications and extensions to the usual posterior or direct lateral approaches.
- A pegboard positioner or a Montreal frame can be used along with an axillary roll to provide protection for the brachial plexus during surgery.

Approach

- The incision should be made through a preexisting scar wherever possible, although it is extremely important not to let the scar dictate the surgical approach.
- A direct lateral approach to the hip can be performed in the supine or lateral position and is extensile in both the proximal and distal directions should additional exposure be required. It involves a split in the anterior half of the gluteus medius and minimus musculature.
- For the posterior approach, a long incision extending up the lateral aspect of the femur and extending posteriorly from the tip of the greater trochanter is favored.
- Fascial incision—initially, this should be made through an area of the fascia lata that has not been involved in previous exposures of the hip. This may be very distal but allows the development of the subfascial plane that is later important in repairing the fascia. The tendinous part of the gluteus maximus at its insertion into the femur might have to be divided.
- The next important step is to identify and protect the sciatic nerve. Identification should start relatively distal, where the

nerve is usually free of scar tissue, and proceed proximally. When distal exposure is not feasible, the sciatic notch may be identified proximally, with the nerve found where it enters the notch, and then traced distally. Several anatomic variations in the pattern of division of the sciatic nerve have been described; the nerve may run a very tortuous course and can be drawn up very close to the trochanteric ridge at times.

- Aspiration of the hip can be repeated at this stage to obtain fluid for microbiology.
- Dissection is then carried out through the gluteus medius and minimus if a direct lateral approach is used or through the short external rotators if a posterior approach is used.
- If the capsule is very thick and scarred, the deeper portions are excised, leaving a thinner flap that is useful for reattachment to the femur during closure. The psoas tendon might have to be released from the lesser trochanter.
- After mobilization of the capsule, the head of the prosthesis is visible. Further superior, inferior, and anterior resection continues with gradual and gentle mobilization of the femur. A large blunt hook or a long gauze swab can be passed around the neck of the prosthesis and dislocation achieved by lifting the head and neck posteriorly using the hook or the swab rather than by rotating the femur through the lower leg. With serious bone stock deficiencies, this phase of the operation carries a risk of fracture of the femur and great care is needed in achieving dislocation with generous soft tissue release as necessary, especially from the anterior aspect of the femoral neck.

TECHNIQUES

Removal of the Femoral Component and Mobilization of the Femur

- Considerable soft tissue release may be necessary to achieve this safely.
- Any cement or bone lying over the shoulder of the femoral component is removed before attempts are made to extract the latter. Vigorous attempts to extract the component in the presence of obstructing proximal cement or bone may lead to a fracture of the proximal femur.
- In some cases, it may be necessary to perform an extended trochanteric osteotomy to allow safe removal of an implant and protect the abductors in a straight lateral approach. If such an osteotomy is performed, the femoral canal integrity should be restored using cerclage wires or cables before commencing impaction grafting to ensure containment of the graft.
- It is always essential to achieve adequate mobilization and delivery of the proximal femur. Superiorly and inferiorly, this is usually straightforward. Often, with gross capsular thickening, much of the capsule requires excision rather than incision. Anteriorly, it might be difficult, especially where scarring has been marked. It is wise to expose the anterior aspect of the femur and excise the anterior capsule under direct vision.
- Anterior femoral deficiencies can be exposed by externally rotating the leg and reflecting the vastus lateralis by taking it off the anterior aspect of the femur below the trochanteric level.
- The proximal part of the greater trochanter must be exposed sufficiently to allow the insertion of the guidewire down the medullary canal, in the midline axis of the canal, and the subsequent insertion of the proximal impactor to prevent a false passage. This means that the neomedullary canal that is formed by the graft is in neutral alignment within the femur and not in varus or valgus. This often requires opening of the trochanteric overhang laterally by around 1 cm to accommodate the introduction of instruments in the correct alignment without risking fracture of the trochanter (**TECH FIG 1**).

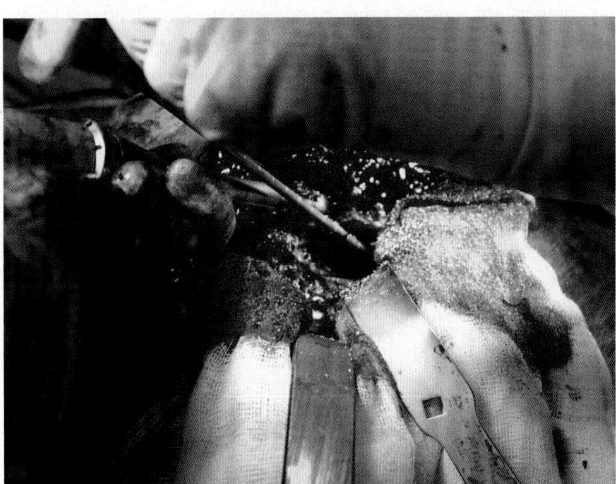

TECH FIG 1 • Burring the overhanging trochanter, allowing the guidewire to lie in neutral alignment. (Image reproduced with the kind permission of The Exeter Hip Unit publishers.)

Preparation of the Graft

- The optimal method of graft preparation is a subject of significant debate.
- Ideally, the preparation should render the tissue safe from disease transmission without compromising its structural integrity. Proponents of fresh frozen graft site improved biologic and biomechanical characteristics relative to irradiated or other secondarily processed bone, whereas fear of bacterial or viral transmission[7,8] warrants some to favor secondarily processed graft.
- Fresh frozen cancellous allograft is recommended. ABO compatibility between graft donor and recipient is not necessary. Rhesus compatibility is important when the patient is a Rhesus-negative woman of child-bearing age. Autogenous cancellous chips may be mixed with the allograft if the surgeon so wishes.
- Allograft chips are prepared by using a bone mill after removal of any soft tissue and sclerotic subchondral bone. The size of the chips should be large enough to give the compressed chips some body (eg, 4 to 6 mm). Bone slurry is not satisfactory because its consistency is too low. Larger chips up to 10 mm in size can be mixed with the smaller chips for packing of the proximal femoral canal around the phantom.
- At least two femoral heads should be available and more if femoral bone stock loss is severe. Strut grafts might be necessary to address significant segmental bone defects.

Preparation of the Femoral Canal

- Cement removal must be complete with one exception: If the existing distal cement plug is greater than two cortical diameters beyond the most distal lytic area in the femur and is solidly fixed, and there is definitely no infection, it can be left in position to act as a distal plug.
- All granulomata and fibrous membranes must be completely and thoroughly removed followed by copious irrigation of the canal. Membrane remnants can be used for frozen section and microbiologic examination.
- As the success of this revision technique depends on adequate physical constraint for the graft, structural defects in the femoral diaphysis must be converted to contained defects before impacting the graft.
- It is essential that the proximal femur is reconstructed up to a level that corresponds to the level of neck section preferred at a primary hip replacement. As a guide, the femoral component should never be positioned so that the lowest of the marks on the anterior and posterior aspects of the base of the neck lie above the level of the graft.
- Prophylactic cerclage wiring of the femur is recommended where the femoral cortex is especially flimsy. Under such circumstances, vigorous packing of the canal can produce a split in the diaphysis. This is more easily managed if cerclage wires have been applied before the split occurs. Overtightening of the wire may crush the femur when its structure is seriously compromised.

Repair of Femoral Cortical Defects

- Diaphyseal defects—if these are small and completely sealed at their margins by soft tissues, they can be ignored and simply packed with chips from within. Larger defects should be exposed surgically, their margins clearly defined, and all associated granulomatous material and fibrous tissue removed. These defects are repaired using a combination of malleable stainless steel mesh (**TECH FIG 2A–C**) and cables or monofilament cerclage wires. Once the defects has been closed in this way, the operation proceeds as though no defect were present. Cortical healing can be anticipated. Large defects, particularly near the tip of the prosthesis, should be bridged either by a long-stem implant, a femoral plate, or strut grafts (**TECH FIG 2D**).
- Metaphyseal defects—these are best repaired following trial reduction and performing the reconstruction with the proximal impactor in position, ensuring an adequate gap between mesh and prosthesis. The defect must be repaired in such a way that the proximal allograft chips can be fully constrained and thus able to take some load and augment rotational stability.

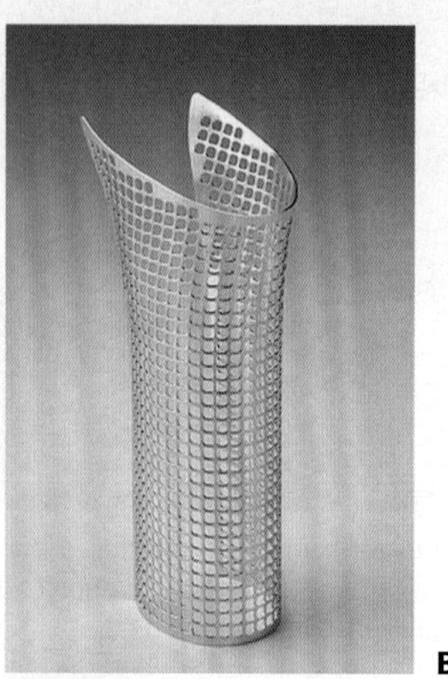
A

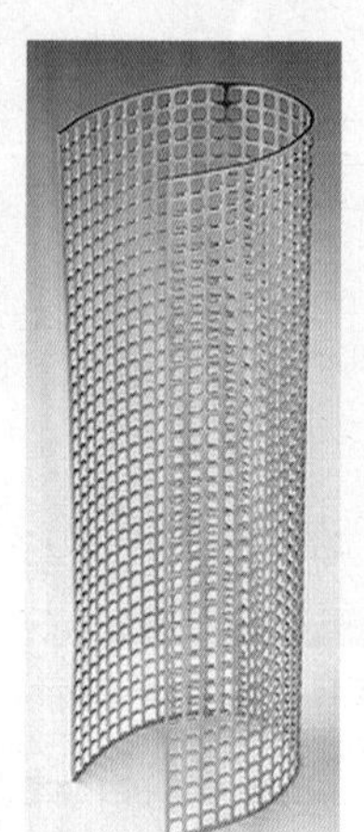
B

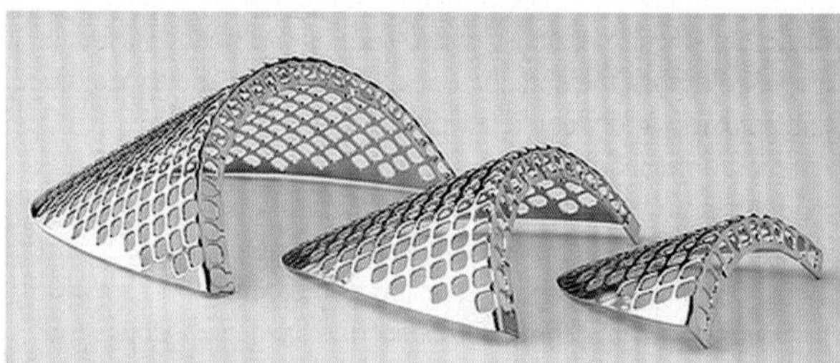
C

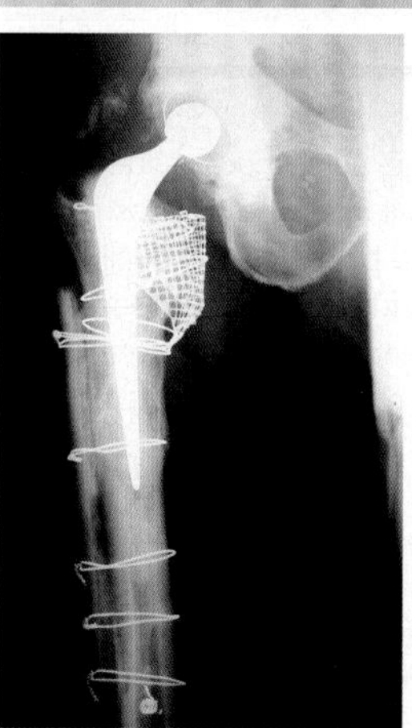
D

TECH FIG 2 • Mesh for large proximal (**A**) and diaphyseal femoral defects (**B**) and rim meshes for lesser proximal defects (**C**). **D.** A strut graft bypassing a cortical defect. (Images reproduced with the kind permission of The Exeter Hip Unit publishers.)

Distal Occlusion of the Femur

- This can be done in a variety of ways.
- Where a new intramedullary (IM) plug is to be used, a threaded plug of the templated size is screwed onto an IM-guide rod and inserted into the medullary canal with a cannulated introducer sleeve, coupled with a slap hammer (**TECH FIG 3A**). The plug is introduced at the templated level, which should be at least two cortical diameters distal to the most distal lytic area, and the introducer removed. The guidewire remains in situ (**TECH FIG 3B**) for cannulated instruments to pass over during impaction grafting (**TECH FIG 3C**).
- Where a new threaded IM plug is required beyond the isthmus, a 2-mm K-wire is drilled through both cortices at the desired level. The pointed end of the plug is cutoff to make a flat end. It is then inserted into the canal and placed on top of the K-wire. If the plug migrates during the impaction process, it can be skewered with a transverse K-wire.
- Where there is a suitable cement plug that is to be left in situ, the largest impactor that will fit is placed down at the level of the plug to act as a drill centralizer. The IM drill is then passed through the impactor and the cement drilled to a depth of 6 mm. The guidewire is passed through the impactor and screwed into the predrilled hole and the impactor is removed.

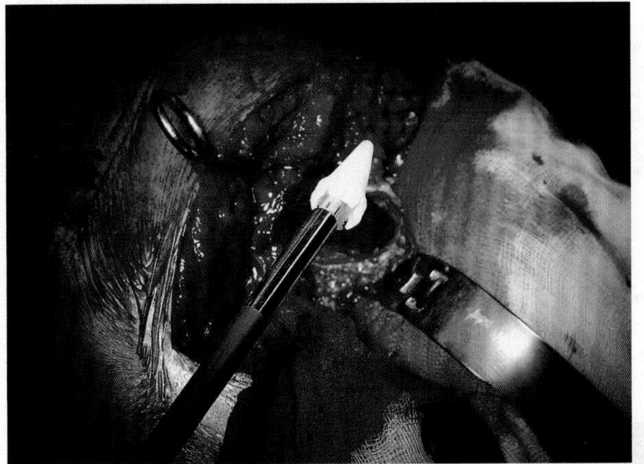

A

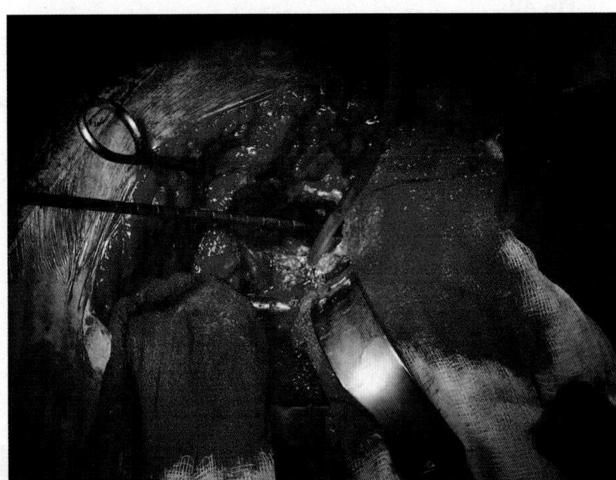

B

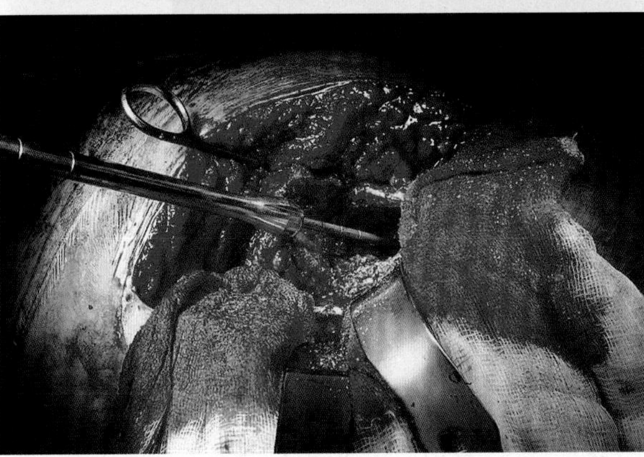

C

TECH FIG 3 • **A.** An IM canal plug. **B.** Guidewire in position. **C.** Cannulated instrument passing over guidewire. (Images reproduced with the kind permission of The Exeter Hip Unit publishers.)

Sizing the Proximal Impactors

- The plug introducer sleeve is removed and the canal sized for proximal impaction.
- Starting with the largest proximal impactor and inserting progressively smaller proximal impactors, the first one that falls easily into the canal is the correct size for use.
- Care should be taken that the guidewire is not driven into varus as the proximal impactor is inserted. If it is, further development of the slot into the trochanter is necessary until neutral alignment of the proximal impactor can be achieved.

Graft Impaction

- Carefully wash and suck out the distal canal to remove any debris.
- Sizing the distal impactors—before using the impactors to impact the bone chips, it is important to establish the distance that each sized impactor can be passed into the femoral canal without jamming against the walls of the canal. Driving the impactors beyond this point runs the risk of splitting the femur. Take each impactor in turn and pass it over the wire, noting the depth of insertion by clipping a marker (**TECH FIG 4A**) onto the groove opposite the tip of the greater trochanter or equivalent mark. Subsequently, when impacting the bone chips, it is important not to drive each impactor beyond its marker clip (**TECH FIG 4B**).
- Introduce allograft chips (**TECH FIG 4C**) proximally around the guidewire. Push as far distally as possible using your fingers and use the large impactors to push the bone chips further down the canal. One centimeter of graft should be packed on top of the plug by using the distal impactors by hand before starting to use the slap hammer. This helps prevent distal migration of the plug. At this stage, the impactor should be carried on the handle assembly, and the slap hammer is used. Continue this process by introducing and impacting more chips using progressively larger impactors in relation to canal diameter (**TECH FIG 4D**). Check the depth of the guidewire after each instrument has been used to make sure the plug is not migrating. Continue this process of packing until the distal impactor cannot be introduced beyond the distal impaction line.
- The distal impaction line is the depth that the tip of the stem will reach on implantation. Its distance from the eventual center of the femoral head will depend on the make and the length of the stem being used. It is important not to continue with distal impaction other than by hand beyond the distal impaction line as this might make it impossible to insert the proximal impactor at the correct depth.
- Once the distal impaction line is reached, the appropriate phantom is mounted on the hand assembly and passed over the guidewire (**TECH FIG 4E**). Load graft into the proximal femur. Using the sliding hammer, drive the phantom distally into the chips to force them up against the walls of the canal. The handle assembly is used to control the rotational position of the phantom and ensure that the neomedullary canal formed is in the correct anteversion. The phantom should be driven vigorously into the bone chips.
- Withdraw the phantom from over the guidewire, insert more chips, and impact them using the distal impactors by hand. Continue to use the distal impactors, alternating them with the proximal impactor, until the graft in the midstem region is adequately packed.
- As the canal is filled from below proximally, continue to insert the phantom over the guidewire, and again drive the phantom into the chips using the slap hammer. The phantom should become progressively tighter. If not, then look for fractures.
- The phantom should be driven into the desired depth as indicated by templating. If the graft is so tight that the proximal impactor cannot be introduced fully, use one size smaller for

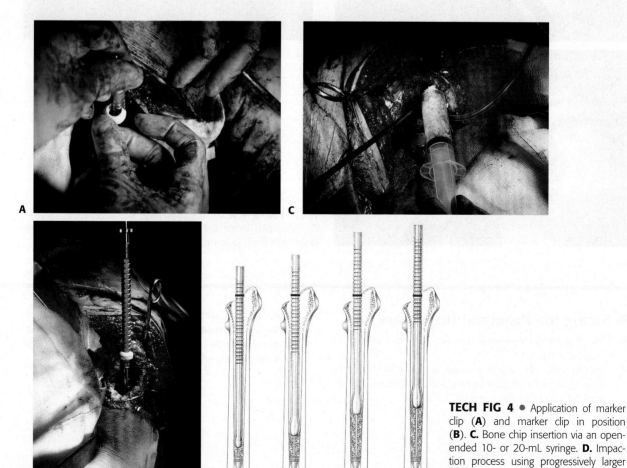

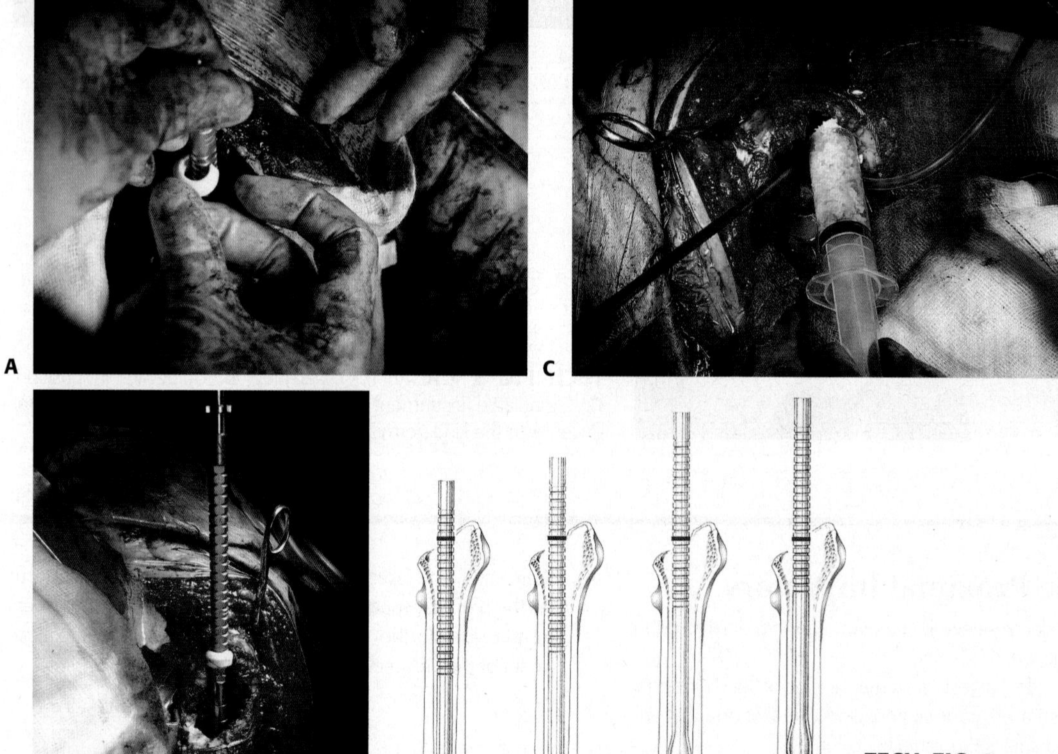

TECH FIG 4 • Application of marker clip (**A**) and marker clip in position (**B**). **C.** Bone chip insertion via an open-ended 10- or 20-mL syringe. **D.** Impaction process using progressively larger impactors. *(continued)*

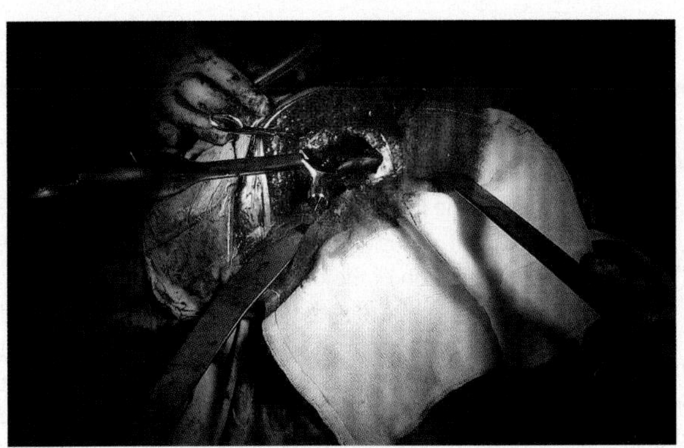
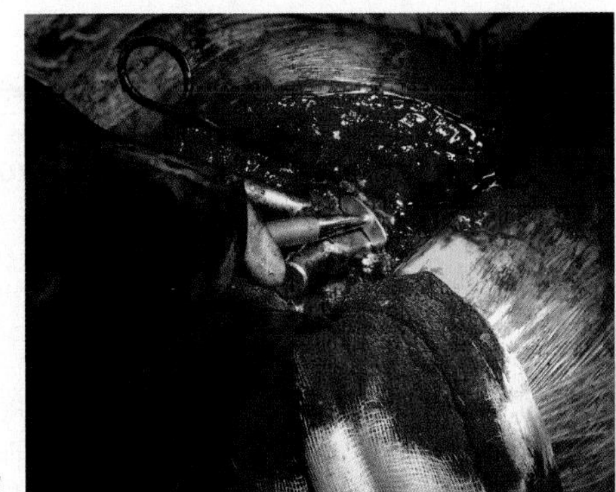

TECH FIG 4 • *(continued)* **E.** Phantom being driven to the marked depth. **F.** Proximal tamping packers. (Images reproduced with the kind permission of The Exeter Hip Unit publishers.)

final impaction. Larger chips should be mixed with the smaller chips for final proximal packing. The proximal tamping packers are used to introduce these chips around the seated phantom, first by hand and then impacted with a mallet (**TECH FIG 4F**). This is continued until no further chips can be introduced. Select the stem size on the basis of the size of the phantom that is used for the final packing.

- The surgeon must ensure absolute axial and rotational stability of the phantom at the conclusion of packing. Several blows with the slap hammer should result in minimal axial advancement of the phantom (<1 mm) and it should be impossible to withdraw the proximal impactor without using the slap hammer.
- It is normally possible to perform a trial reduction with the guidewire in place. If not, the guidewire is unscrewed from the plug and withdrawn from the femur.
- Once the reconstruction is completed, the position of the phantom is marked in relation to the bone or mesh using methylene blue.

Trial Reduction

- Trial reduction allows assessment of stability and leg length and acts as a further guide for the depth of stem insertion.
- The hip is reduced with the appropriate trial head in place.
- Any changes to the depth of insertion of the stem can now be estimated using the relative leg lengths of the patient. If the leg is short, impaction is continued to further build up the femur.
- Carefully redislocate the hip and remove the trial head.
- Once satisfied with the stem position and trial reduction, remove the guidewire and mark the depth and rotation of the trial implant.
- If a calcar or a proximal femoral deficiency is present, these can be reconstructed using the appropriate metal meshes, for example, acetabular rim mesh if reconstruction is required at the level of the lesser trochanter, or an anatomic calcar mesh if the lesser trochanter is involved, keeping the phantom in situ while this is done (**TECH FIG 5A**). The meshes are secured with cerclage wires or cables (**TECH FIG 5B**). Cables may be used distally but are avoided proximally because of the potential risk of intra-articular debris from fretting.
- Carefully remove the stem introducer. Ensure that the connection on the shoulder of the phantom is clear of bone graft debris or soft tissue and replace the impactor connector in preparation for removal of the phantom prior to cement insertion.

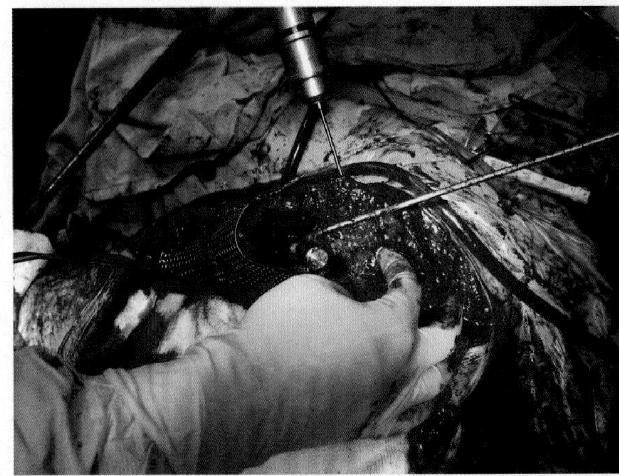
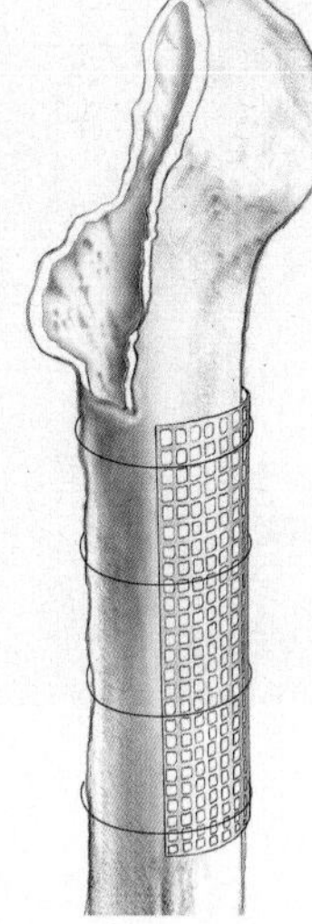

TECH FIG 5 • **A.** Calcar reconstruction. **B.** Mesh secured with cables or monofilament cerclage wires to contain any diaphyseal defects or perforations. (Images reproduced with the kind permission of The Exeter Hip Unit publishers.)

Cement and Stem Insertion

- The phantom must be left in place until just before cement insertion. This keeps the graft compressed and the canal can be sucked dry by a catheter placed down the trial lumen (**TECH FIG 6A**).
- A wingless centralizer is used on the stem tip to minimize graft disruption.
- Low-viscosity cement is inserted in a retrograde fashion using a revision cement gun with a tapered or narrow nozzle to ensure that the graft is not disrupted (**TECH FIG 6B,C**). The timing of insertion will depend on the type of cement being used. Relatively low-viscosity cement is recommended to ensure adequate penetration of the graft. Two 40-g mixes are required to allow adequate cement for continuous pressurization prior to stem insertion.
- Once the canal has been filled retrograde, apply the proximal femoral seal, cut off the nozzle at the level of the seal, and pressurize the cement into the graft (**TECH FIG 6D,E**).
- Maintain pressurization until the viscosity of the cement is appropriate for stem insertion.
- Insert the stem at its predetermined position, paying strict attention to its alignment during insertion and the previously placed methylene blue mark. It is important to obscure the medial aspect of the femoral neck throughout insertion to occlude cement and graft extrusion from the medullary canal, thus maintaining pressurization of the cement throughout insertion.
- As soon as the desired insertion depth is achieved, the stem introducer is removed, and a horse collar seal is applied around the proximal femur in order to maintain pressure on the cement and graft while the cement polymerizes (**TECH FIG 6F,G**). Maintain a constant pressure on the stem to ensure that it does not back out during polymerization.

A
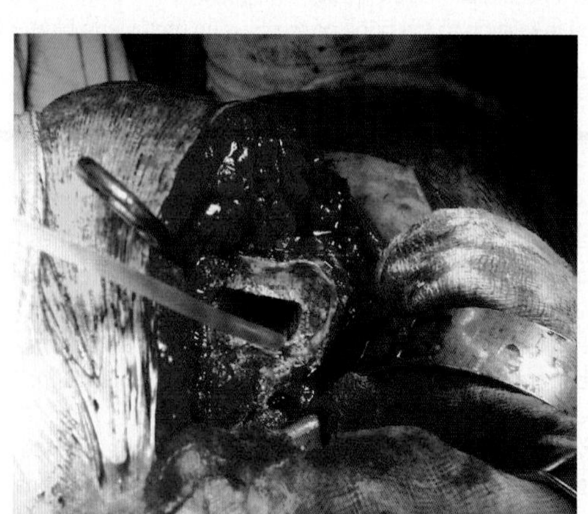
B
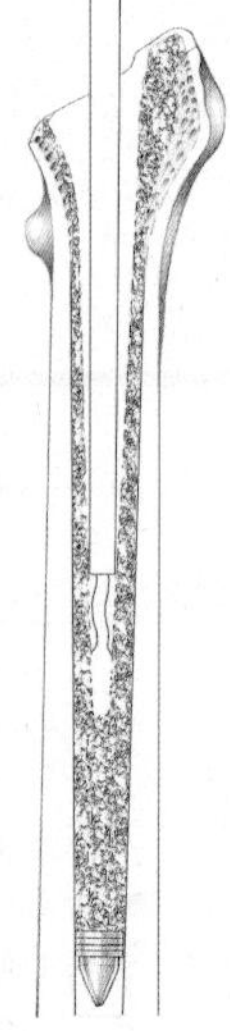
C
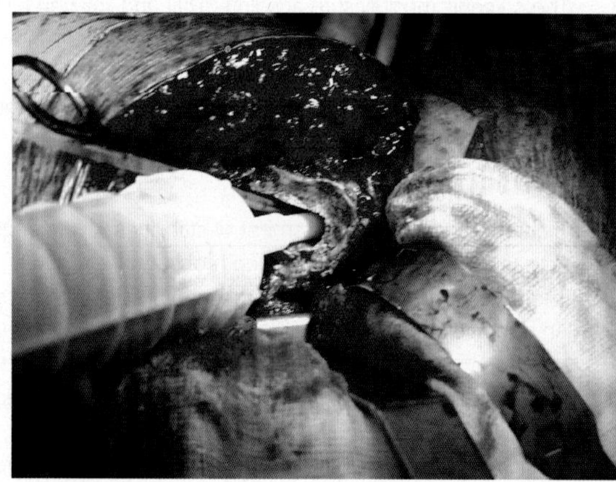
D
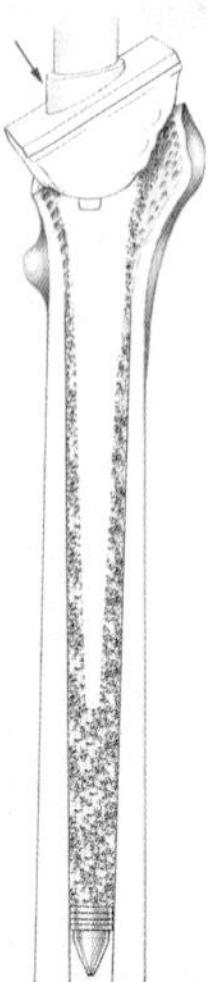
E
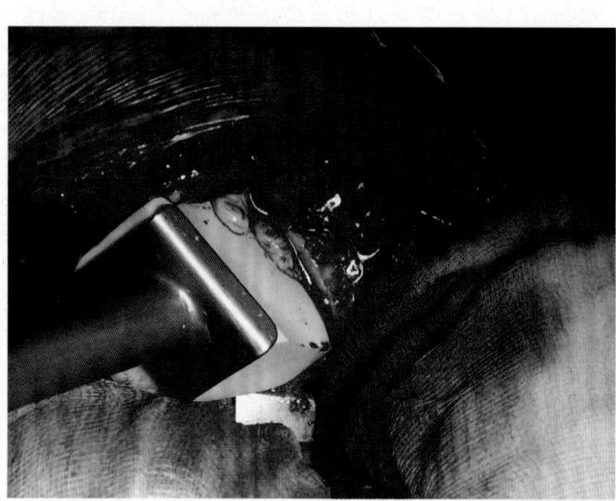

TECH FIG 6 • **A.** Impacted canal with suction catheter. **B.** Impacted canal showing retrograde filling of cement. **C.** Cement insertion using a tapered or narrow nozzle. **D.** Diagram and photo (**E**) of pressurization of cement. *(continued)*

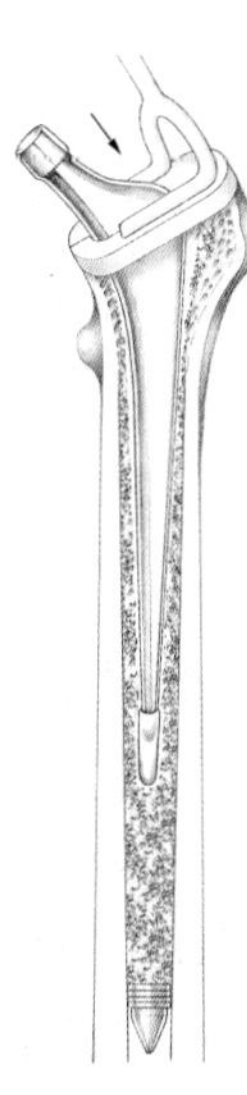

F

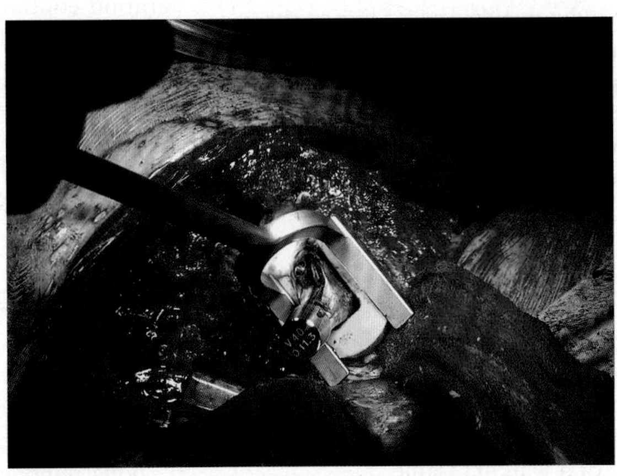

G

TECH FIG 6 • *(continued)* **F.** Diagram and photo (**G**) of pressurization maintained by the horse collar seal. (Images reproduced with the kind permission of The Exeter Hip Unit publishers.)

Reduction and Closure

- These are carried out according to the surgeon's usual practice.
- A layered closure is important along with adequate drainage.

PEARLS AND PITFALLS

Surgical exposure	■ In the presence of severe bone stock deficiencies, dislocation of the hip carries a significant risk of fracture of the femur and great care is needed in achieving dislocation with generous soft tissue release as necessary, especially from the anterior aspect of the femoral neck. ■ If it is necessary to perform an extended trochanteric osteotomy to facilitate safe removal of an implant, the femoral canal should be reconstructed using cerclage wires or cables before commencing impaction grafting.
Femoral canal preparation	■ The success of this revision technique depends on adequate physical constraint for the graft. Structural defects in the femoral diaphysis must therefore be converted to contained defects before impacting the graft. ■ It is vital that the proximal femur is reconstructed at a level that corresponds to the level of neck resection preferred at a primary hip replacement. ■ Prophylactic cerclage wiring of the femur is recommended where the femoral cortex is particularly flimsy.
Repair of femoral cortical defects	■ When segmental defects exist, they must be contained with some type of mesh material or allograft struts and cables to create a continuous femoral tube. ■ Large defects, particularly those near the tip of the prosthesis, should be bridged either by a long-stem implant, a femoral plate, or strut grafts. ■ Cortical lytic areas or femoral defects must be bypassed by at least one, and preferably two, cortical diameters to reduce the risk of postoperative femoral fracture.
Distal occlusion of the femur	■ The IM plug must be a tight fit and should be impacted to a depth of at least two cortical diameters distal to the most distal lytic area. ■ If it is noticed that the plug is migrating during the impaction process, it can be skewered with a percutaneous K-wire.
Graft impaction	■ Before starting the impaction process, it is extremely important to establish the distance that each size of impactor can be passed into the femoral canal without jamming against the walls of the canal, as driving the impactors beyond this point runs the risk of splitting the femur. ■ If at any time during the impaction, driving a phantom to the required level is easier than on the previous occasion, then a femoral burst fracture is present and must be identified and stabilized with cerclage wires. ■ There should be no rotational torque on the femur during impaction.
Prerequisite for success	■ Absolute axial and rotational stability of the phantom must be ensured at the conclusion of packing. ■ It should be impossible to withdraw the phantom without using the slap hammer.

POSTOPERATIVE CARE

- Postoperative care should be individualized according to the differing circumstances of each revision.
- AP pelvis and full-length femoral radiographs are obtained prior to mobilization, which takes place as soon as the patient is comfortable enough to do so.
- Where major reconstruction has been performed, touch or partial weight bearing on crutches is advised for the first 6 weeks.
- If at 6 to 8 weeks there is less than a millimeter of migration of the stem within the cement mantle, the patient is allowed to progress with weight-bearing mobilization, building up to full weight bearing at 12 weeks.
- In the very elderly, where mobility would be compromised by restricted weight bearing, full weight bearing is permitted at an early stage with the use of a walking frame.
- Clinical and radiographic surveillance is carried out at 6 weeks, 6 months, 1 year, 2 years, and then every 2 years indefinitely.

OUTCOMES

- Several factors influence the success of this revision technique, including patient factors (preoperative femoral defects and potency of allograft remodeling), technical factors (degree of bone impaction, allograft bone chip size, and cementing technique), and postoperative rehabilitation factors.
- The short-term clinical results of impaction grafting in 56 hips followed for a period of 1.5 to 4 years reported by Gie et al[2] were encouraging. Radiologic results and histologic data demonstrated bone graft incorporation and partial reconstitution of the bone stock.
- Halliday et al[4] have reported on longer term follow-up from the same center. They reported a stem survivorship of 90.5% at 10 years in 226 hips treated with femoral impaction allografting. Fourteen stems required revision: 2 for infection, 10 for femoral fractures, and 2 for loosening.
- The longest follow-up results have been published by Ornstein et al[10] from the Swedish Arthroplasty Register. They reported their experience with 1188 revisions with a follow-up from 5 to 18 years. The re-revision rate was 5.9%. The survivorship at 15 years was 94.0% for women and 94.7% for men, using any reason for revision as an end point. Survivorship at 15 years was 99.1% for aseptic loosening, 98.6% for infection, 99% for subsidence, and 98.7% for fracture.
- The optimal stem design for use in impaction grafting of the femur is a subject of ongoing debate. The original proponents of the technique advocated the use of a highly polished, collarless, double-tapered cemented stem to allow for controlled subsidence.
- However, Leopold et al[6] demonstrated 92% survivorship at 6 years in 29 hips treated with a precoated, collared, cemented stem, and Fetzer et al[1] found no radiographic loosening in 26 collared stems at an average follow-up of 6 years.
- Several authors have reported on radiostereometric analysis[9] used to study stem migration and the influence of certain factors such as the extent of femoral bone defects and the presence of cement mantle defects on stem migration (micromotion). They concluded that although femoral impaction grafting seems to yield good clinical results, migration continues to a minor degree even 2 years after the revision procedure.
- Cement mantle defects[9] have been shown to be clinically relevant and caused by poor instrumentation. This stresses the importance of good instrumentation, which is absolutely vital to make this technically demanding technique effective in creating a stable stem-allograft construct in the defective femoral canal.

COMPLICATIONS

- Fracture
  - Intraoperative—usually technique-related and avoidable
  - Postoperative—usually related to the poor quality of bone that this procedure attempts to address and perhaps to the bone remodeling process. Two strategies that might help to reduce these are the use of cortical struts and longer stem lengths.
- Migration/subsidence—can be technique- or implant-related, for example, force-closed or taper slip stem designs that rely on a taper to transfer the load to the cement at the stem-cement interface; and stem migration to increase the frictional forces and balance the external forces to maintain mechanical equilibrium at the stem-cement interface. In contrast, shape-closed or composite beam designs transfer a large portion of the axial load directly to the cement, thereby contributing to the mechanical stability of the implant even after debonding of the stem-cement interface.[5] The incidence of massive stem subsidence is low in most large series, suggesting that surgical technique (density of impacted bone, restoration of a cortical tube, and a longer stem) is a key factor in the success of the approach.
- Infection—one of the most serious complications of joint reconstruction with associated bone grafting. However, data to date have not demonstrated a high rate of reinfection when bone grafts are required for a subsequent reconstruction of a previously infected joint.
- Disease transmission—although the risk of disease transmission from the donor and contamination at retrieval or during processing are major concerns, the number of reported incidents of disease transmission after the implantation of allograft bone has been low, given the large number of grafts implanted worldwide.[7,8,13,14]

REFERENCES

1. Fetzer GB, Callaghan JJ, Templeton JE, et al. Impaction allografting with cement for extensive femoral bone loss in revision hip surgery: a 4- to 8-year follow-up study. J Arthroplasty 2001;16(8 suppl 1): 195–202.
2. Gie GA, Linder L, Ling RS, et al. Impacted cancellous allografts and cement for revision total hip arthroplasty. J Bone Joint Surg Br 1993;75:14–21.
3. Gie GA, Ling RS, Timperley AJ. Stryker X-change Revision Surgical Protocol. Montreux, Switzerland: Stryker, 2004.
4. Halliday BR, English HW, Timperley AJ, et al. Femoral impaction grafting with cement in revision total hip replacement. Evolution of the technique and results. J Bone Joint Surg Br 2003;85(6): 809–817.
5. Huiskes R, Verdonschot N, Nivbrant B. Migration, stem shape, and surface finish in cemented total hip arthroplasty. Clin Orthop Relat Res 1998;(355):103–112.
6. Leopold SS, Berger RA, Rosenberg AG, et al. Impaction allografting with cement for revision of the femoral component. A minimum

four-year follow-up study with use of a precoated femoral stem. J Bone Joint Surg Am 1999;81:1080–1092.

7. Lord CF, Gebhardt MC, Tomford WW, et al. Infection in bone allografts. Incidence, nature, and treatment. J Bone Joint Surg Am 1988;70(3):369–376.
8. Mankin HJ, Hornicek FJ, Raskin KA. Infection in massive bone allografts. Clin Orthop Relat Res 2005;(432):210–216.
9. Nelissen RG, Valstar ER, Pöll RG, et al. Factors associated with excessive migration in bone impaction hip revision surgery: a radiostereometric study. J Arthroplasty 2002;17(7):826–833.
10. Ornstein E, Linder L, Ranstam J, et al. Femoral impaction bone grafting with the Exeter stem—the Swedish experience: survivorship analysis of 1305 revisions performed between 1989 and 2002. J Bone Joint Surg Br 2009;91(4):441–446.
11. Sloof TJ, Buma P, Schreurs BW, et al. Acetabular and femoral reconstruction with impacted graft and cement. Clin Orthop Relat Res 1996;324:108–115.
12. Spangehl MJ, Masri BA, O'Connell JX, et al. Prospective analysis of preoperative and intraoperative investigations for the diagnosis of infection at the sites of two hundred and two revision total hip arthroplasties. J Bone Joint Surg Am 1999;81(5):672–683.
13. Sutherland AG, Raafat A, Yates P, et al. Infection associated with the use of allograft bone from the north east Scotland Bone Bank. J Hosp Infect 1997;35:215–222.
14. Tomford WW. Transmission of disease through transplantation of musculoskeletal allografts. J Bone Joint Surg Am 1995;77(11):1742–1754.
15. Ullmark G, Obrant KJ. Histology of impacted bone graft incorporation. J Arthroplasty 2002;17:150–157.

27 CHAPTER

Revision Total Hip Arthroplasty with Femoral Bone Loss: Fluted Stems

Patrick O'Toole and Gregory Deirmengian

DEFINITION

- A fluted femoral stem is designed to provide diaphyseal rotational stability through multiple longitudinally oriented flutes with varying numbers and positions, depending on the manufacturer. These fluted stems may be a useful reconstructive option in one or more of the following situations:
  - Proximal femoral cavitary or segmental defects
  - Abnormal femoral anatomy/femoral deformity
  - Periprosthetic femoral fracture
  - Osteopenic proximal femoral bone secondary to stress shielding
  - Sclerotic bone secondary to prior fracture fixation

ANATOMY

- The proximal femoral anatomy can be quite abnormal in the setting of revision total hip arthroplasty (THA) or complex THA. The proximal femoral bone may be deficient with cavitary or segmental loss and the remaining bone may be osteopenic secondary to stress shielding. The typical bony landmarks used by the orthopaedic surgeon, such as the lesser and greater trochanters, can be abnormal or absent. Higher grades of proximal femoral bone loss can involve the upper femoral diaphysis, which may limit the type of femoral prosthesis that can be used at the time of revision arthroplasty.
  - The proximal aspect of the femur is composed of the head, neck, and greater and lesser trochanters.
  - Important soft tissues include the iliotibial band and muscles that insert into it (tensor fascia lata and gluteus maximus), gluteal muscles (maximus, medius, and minimus), short external rotator muscles (especially when a posterior approach to the revision hip surgery is contemplated), iliopsoas, quadriceps, and hip joint capsule (**FIG 1A**).
  - Vascular and neurologic structures include the femoral artery, vein, and nerve; the sciatic nerve; and the lateral cutaneous nerve of the thigh when a more anterior approach is used.
- The American Academy of Orthopaedic Surgeons' classification of femoral bone loss[6] (Table 1; **FIG 1B**)
- The Paprosky classification of femoral bone loss[19] (Table 2)

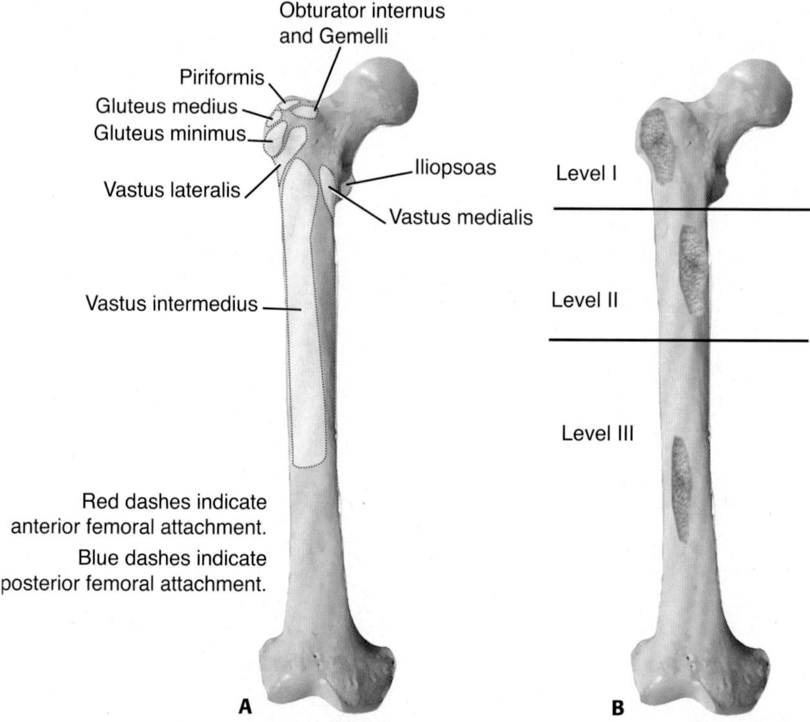

FIG 1 • **A.** Femoral anatomy. **B.** Level of femoral defect.

Table 1 American Academy of Orthopaedic Surgeons' Classification of Femoral Bone Loss

Classification	Description
Type of defect	
Type I	Segmental defects or lesions in the supporting shell, further categorized as proximal, intercalary, or involving the greater trochanter
Type II	Cavitary defects, categorized as cancellous (mild), cortical (moderate), and ectatic (medullary expansion)
Type III	Combined segmental and cavitary defects
Type IV	Malalignment
Type V	Femoral stenosis
Type VI	Femoral discontinuity or fracture
Level of defect	
Level I	Defect proximal to the inferior border of the lesser trochanter
Level II	Defect <10 cm distal to the inferior border of the lesser trochanter
Level III	Defect >10 cm distal to the inferior border of the lesser trochanter
Grade of bone loss	
Grade I	Minimal bone loss with maintenance of bone–implant interface that does not require bone grafting
Grade II	Some loss of bone–implant interface with sustained support of implant
Grade III	Marked loss of bone–implant interface that required structural grafting

PATHOGENESIS

- Osteolysis, from polyethylene wear particles, results in bone loss and ultimate component loosening, leading to premature THA failure. This has led to the consideration of alternative bearing surfaces including metal-on-metal and ceramic-on-ceramic bearings. Highly cross-linked ultra-high-molecular-weight polyethylene has, in recent times, become the polyethylene of choice for use in THA owing to it's enhanced wear resistant properties. Ionizing radiation is used to increase the number of cross-links within the polyethylene, leading to a reduction in the amount of wear debris created during cyclical loading of the prosthetic joint.[13] A reduction in wear rates is as great as 80% when compared to conventional polyethylene for the 28 and 32 mm head sizes.[10]

NATURAL HISTORY

- Uncemented femoral components loosen as a result of progressive osteolysis and bone loss.
- Cemented femoral components fail as a result of osteolysis at the cement–bone interface.
- Micromotion resulting from loose components causes further bone loss.
- Cortical thinning may occur.

Table 2 Paprosky Classification of Femoral Bone Loss

Paprosky Grade	Femoral Bone Loss
Type 1	Minimal loss of metaphyseal cancellous bone with an intact diaphysis, for example, remaining bone after removal of a cementless femoral component that did not osteointegrate
Type 2	Extensive loss of metaphyseal cancellous bone with an intact diaphysis, for example, remaining bone after removal of a cemented femoral component
Type 3A	Nonsupportive and damaged metaphysis with >4 cm of intact diaphyseal bone available for distal fixation, for example, after removal of a grossly loose cemented femoral component
Type 3B	Nonsupportive and damaged metaphysis with <4 cm of intact diaphyseal bone available for distal fixation, for example, with substantial distal osteolysis
Type 4	Extensive metaphyseal and diaphyseal bone loss in conjunction with a widened femoral canal. The isthmus is nonsupportive.

- Varus deformity of the proximal femur may occur.
- Periprosthetic femoral fracture.
- Eventual failure of the prosthesis.

PATIENT HISTORY AND PHYSICAL FINDINGS

- A complete and focused patient history should be obtained. Specific questions in relation to pain include the following:
  - Rest and/or night pain (infection)
  - Pain with weight bearing (infection, aseptic loosening)
  - Start-up pain (aseptic loosening)
  - Severe acute pain (periprosthetic femur fracture, hip dislocation)
- A complete medical and surgical history is necessary to document all information pertaining to the index procedure, including the initial diagnosis, date of surgery, complete operative notes with detailed descriptions of the components used, and the dates of any postoperative complications. All component identifiers (component stickers) should be obtained where possible, as operative reports are sometimes inaccurate.[8]
- Relevant past medical and surgical history should be obtained and appropriate preoperative consultations sought when needed. A decision can also be taken regarding the most suitable form of thromboprophylaxis and whether the patient's current medications are optimized prior to revision surgery.
- The physical examination should include the following:
  - Gait evaluation. A painful THA will result in a shortened stance phase during the gait cycle. A Trendelenburg gait or abductor lurch may raise concern regarding hip abductor function either from injury to the abductor muscle itself or from altered hip joint biomechanics that can limit the success of revision.
  - Trendelenburg test is considered positive when the pelvis on the nonstance side moves into a position of relative adduction (the pelvis on the normal side dips toward the

floor in the patient with unilateral disease). It may indicate abductor weakness, superior gluteal nerve injury, or a loss of effectiveness of the abductor mechanism (eg, greater trochanteric nonunion).[9]
  - Hip abductor strength may indicate abductor weakness, trochanteric bursitis, abductor avulsion, trochanter fracture, or a loose femoral component.
  - Hip joint range of motion should be pain free. Pain suggests a mechanical dysfunction. A palpable or audible click or clunk may indicate femoral head subluxation.
  - Leg lengths should be assessed. Progressive true leg length discrepancy suggests implant subsidence.
  - "Apparent leg length discrepancy may be caused by muscle atrophy, obesity, spinal disease, pelvic obliquity, or asymmetric positioning of the legs, which may be correctable or fixed as in the case of hip adductor contractures.
  - The skin around the hip should be inspected for previous scars, evidence of poor wound healing, and superficial soft tissue infection.
- A complete neurovascular examination of the limb in question should be performed as well as a complete lower limb peripheral neurologic examination to rule out causes of hip pain that are referred from the spine.[21] This examination will also serve as a baseline for comparison with the initial postoperative examination.

Neurovascular Structures

- The sciatic nerve is frequently encased in scar tissue during revision hip surgery. It is located 1 to 2 cm posterior to the posterior rim of the acetabulum and should not be exposed routinely during revision THA if the surgeon is careful with retractor placement and positions the leg appropriately during hip exposure.
- If the surgeon needs to expose the nerve, it is best identified posterior to the gluteal sling and followed proximally toward the hip joint.

Radiographic Examination

- Preoperative radiographic views should include an anteroposterior (AP) pelvis as well as a lateral of the hip in question. The entire implant should be visualized on radiographs. The surgeon should have a low threshold for obtaining full-length femur radiographs. The acetabular and femoral component position and fixation should be assessed and any radiolucent lines about the components or any bony deficits noted. The greater trochanteric anatomy and quality should be reviewed, as this may have a direct effect on the ability to reconstruct the abductor mechanism and limit postoperative instability. Eccentric polyethylene wear and evidence of osteolysis should also be noted. Radiographic evidence of heterotopic ossification should alert the surgeon about the need for a more difficult dissection and approach to the hip joint.
- The amount of competent proximal femoral bone needs to be assessed, as proximal bone deficiencies in this area can be so profound that a fluted stem is not suitable for femoral revision, and a fully porous-coated stem for diaphyseal fixation is preferable.
- Diaphyseal defects in the femur are identified so that during preoperative planning, the proposed femoral component can be templated to bypass the bony defect by at least two cortical diameters.
- A series of older radiographs should be reviewed (if available) so that the progression of radiolucencies and femoral component subsidence can be accurately calculated.

Laboratory Tests

- Erythrocyte sedimentation rate (ESR) and C-reactive protein (CRP) levels should be assessed before any revision procedure to rule out infection. In a series of 202 revision arthroplasties, all patients with deep sepsis had either an ESR above 30 mm or a CRP above 10 mg/L.[18]
- Intra-articular preoperative aspiration should also be performed if either the ESR or CRP is elevated. The white cell count and differential of the aspirate should be measured. A portion of the aspirate should also be sent for culture and sensitivity.
- A technetium 99m bone scan hydroxymethylene diphosphonate (HDP) bone scan may demonstrate increased bony metabolism that can represent loosening, increased stress, or infection. However, a technetium bone scan can produce both false-positive and false-negative results and the surgeon should not base the decision to revise solely on this test. A gallium scan and/or an indium-labeled white cell scan can be performed to detect infection in THA. However, these tests are rarely used.

HIP PAIN POST TOTAL HIP ARTHROPLASTY DIFFERENTIAL DIAGNOSIS

- Infection
- Component loosening (septic or aseptic)
- Periprosthetic fracture
- Component impingement
- Psoas tendon irritation
- Leg length discrepancy
- Trunionosis/corrosion
- Greater trochanteric bursitis
- Lumbosacral pathology

NONOPERATIVE MANAGEMENT

- Nonoperative management is usually not an option and is reserved for patients who are deemed to have too high a risk for anesthesia.
- Nonoperative measures in specific cases include the following:
  - Assistive ambulatory devices
  - Suppressive antibiotics for septic loosening may help control pain or progressive infection in a nonoperative patient.
  - Hip pain due to bursitis may be improved with nonoperative treatments, including physical therapy, nonsteroidal anti-inflammatory drugs, and injections.

SURGICAL MANAGEMENT

- Revision THA can be performed in a single sitting in the absence of periprosthetic joint infection.
- Most fluted femoral stems have a proximal sleeve of varying lengths and configurations that allow for optimal offset and "fit and fill" of the proximal femur. The flutes increase distal fill and resistance to rotational stress.

Preoperative Planning

- Templating should be performed using a current AP radiograph of the pelvis and a lateral of the affected hip. Full-length AP and lateral radiographs of the femur should also be considered (Table 3).
- Additional preoperative planning includes the following:
  - A pathologist must be available to look at intraoperative frozen sections.
  - Previous operative reports
  - Polyethylene liner exchange options
  - Revision acetabular components (even if the socket looks stable)
  - Fully porous-coated femoral component if proximal fixation is insufficient for use of a fluted stem
  - Structural allografts and cables

Positioning

- Following administration of regional anesthesia and insertion of a urinary catheter, the patient should be positioned supine on a gel bump that is centered on the anterior superior iliac spine.
- Supine positioning, the authors' preferred technique, allows the surgeon to accurately assess the patient's leg lengths and to accurately assess the position of the acetabular component.
- The groin and the ipsilateral foot should be isolated with nonsterile drapes, and the entire limb should be prepped. An impervious stockinette can be rolled up to the level of the knee.

Approach

- The approach to the hip in revision surgery should be easily extensile.
- Direct lateral approach
- Posterior approach (patient needs to be in lateral decubitus position)

Soft Tissue

- The hip abductors require careful preoperative evaluation and intraoperative inspection because they are critical to postoperative hip stability and gait. Prior hip surgery may result in a weakened gluteus medius. There can often be a defect in the abductor tendon encountered in the approach for revision surgery in a patient who previously underwent a direct lateral approach.
- The vastus lateralis may be elevated from its posterior border or split in continuity with the distal extend of the gluteus medius tendon split to give the surgeon access to the femoral shaft for correction of bony deformity, fracture repair, and cable placement.
- The posterior hip joint capsule and the short external rotators are often adherent when a previous posterior approach was used. These structures can be tagged and preserved for later repair if a posterior approach to the hip is used for the revision surgery.
- The gluteal sling refers to the insertion of the gluteus maximus on the posterolateral border of the proximal femoral shaft. The 5 cm insertion frequently needs to be partially or completely released to gain exposure of the femur in a posterior approach. This should be repaired to its tendon stump at the end of the case with care taken to avoid suturing the sciatic nerve.

Neurovascular Structures

- The sciatic nerve is frequently found to be encased in scar tissue during revision hip surgery. It is located 1 to 2 cm posterior to the posterior rim of the acetabulum and should not be exposed routinely during revision hip surgery.
- If exposure of the nerve is necessary, it can be identified posterior to the gluteal sling and followed proximally toward the hip joint.

Table 3 Step-by-Step Procedure for Templating Prior to Revision Hip Arthroplasty with a Modular, Fluted Stem[a]

Step	Primary Objective	Instructions
1	Mark and measure leg lengths	Compare location of the lesser trochanter of the operative and nonoperative leg in relation to either the transischial or transobturator lines. Be sure to measure with a magnified ruler.
2	Identify acetabular landmarks	Assess position of the teardrop, superolateral lip, and the medial wall (Kohler line).
3	Template acetabulum	Assess the size and proposed location/orientation of the acetabular component and whether bony defects will require the availability of specialized acetabular components including augments, jumbo cups, cages, or customized implants.
4	Determine center of rotation	Lateralized acetabular implants can be used to compensate for medial bone loss. Mark center of rotation of the proposed hip joint.
5	Assess proximal femoral anatomy	The anatomic axis of the femur should be drawn and any deviations noted, for example, varus remodeling of the proximal femur seen with a loose stem.
6	Select stem diameter	The specific fluted stem system that is being used should be templated allowing for the fact that templating, even in the most experienced hands, can be inaccurate by up to one to two sizes in each direction. Stem diameter selection alerts the surgeon to an extremely narrow or capacious femoral canal.
7	Select stem length	Full-length femur radiographs should be available. Any cortical defect should be bypassed, using the fluted stem by at least two femoral cortical diameters.
8	Position stem and select neck	Modularity on the femoral side allows the surgeon to build up the femoral component so that the normal hip center of rotation and femoral offset is restored.
9	Modular components	Different neck lengths, offsets, and sizes can be templated as well as femoral head sizes.

[a]Prior to templating, the surgeon should be familiar with the templating software and the correct calibration (manual/automatic) should be performed.

Routine Revision without Diaphyseal Defect

- Carefully assess the proximal femur above the lesser trochanter.
- An extended trochanteric osteotomy (ETO) may be used to expose the proximal femur and allows removal of the cement mantle or removal of a fully porous-coated femoral stem.
- Reaming and insertion of the different fluted femoral stem systems vary greatly between manufacturers and the surgeon should be aware of the nuances of each system.
- Perform straight reaming of the proximal diaphysis until cortical chatter is achieved. Reaming should be done to a depth determined by comparing a line on the reamer to the tip of the greater trochanter[1] (**TECH FIG 1A**).
- The diameter of the last reamer will determine the size of the implant and reflects the diameter of the distal end of the implant.
- Prepare the metaphysis with the conical reamers that correspond with the last straight reamer. Cone reaming should stop whenever contact with structurally sound cortical bone is obtained. Care should be taken in osteoporotic bone not to overream the femoral diaphysis. A fresh reamer battery should be used when nearing the end reaming of so that the reamer does not get trapped in the femoral canal.
  - If using the S-ROM system, use the calcar miller to prepare the femur for the triangular modular sleeve (**TECH FIG 1B**).

Implant Placement

- After placing the trial sleeve and femoral stem, perform trial reduction in order to assess version, range of motion, and stability. The modular system allows complete freedom to vary anteversion regardless of proximal femoral geometry (**TECH FIG 2A–D**).
- Insert sleeve and finish by inserting femoral stem (**TECH FIG 2E**).

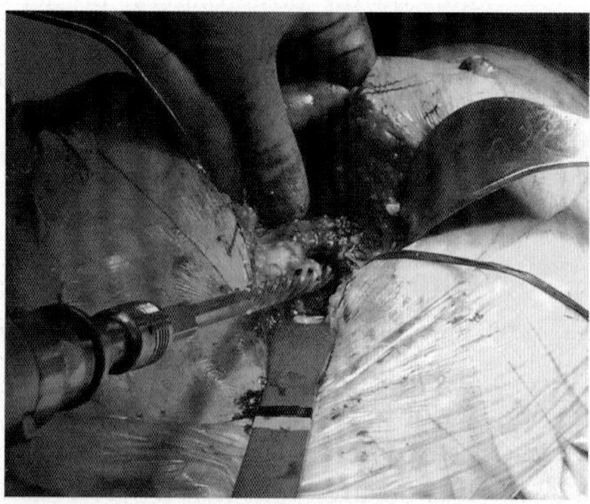
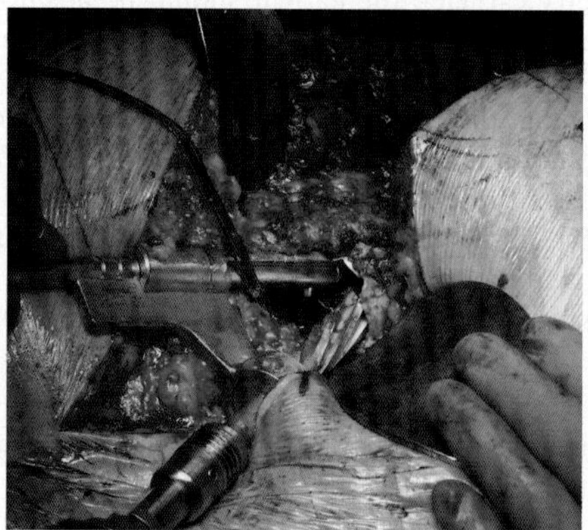

TECH FIG 1 • **A.** Straight reaming of the femur is carried out until contact with diaphysis is obtained. **B.** Calcar miller used for preparation of the proximal femur as part of this prosthesis.

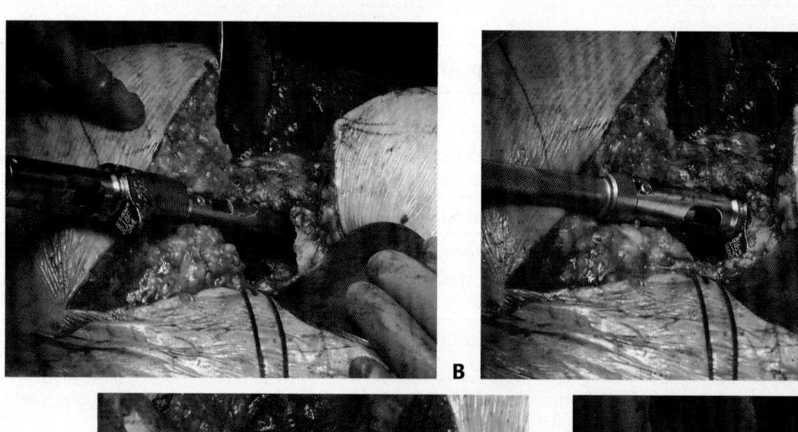
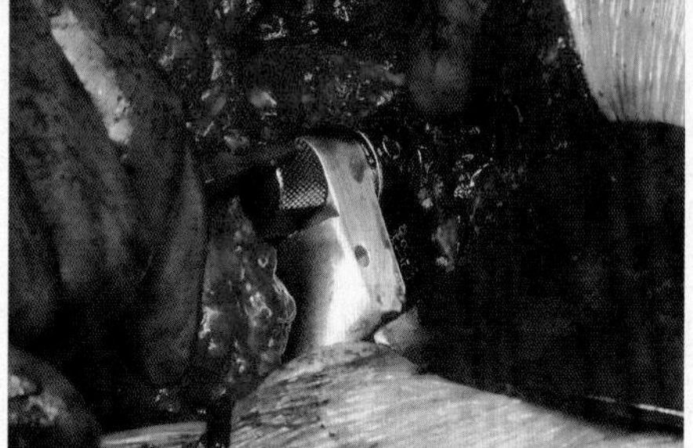
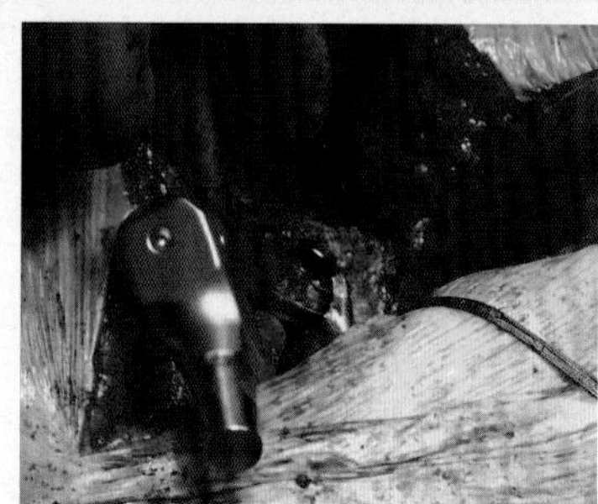
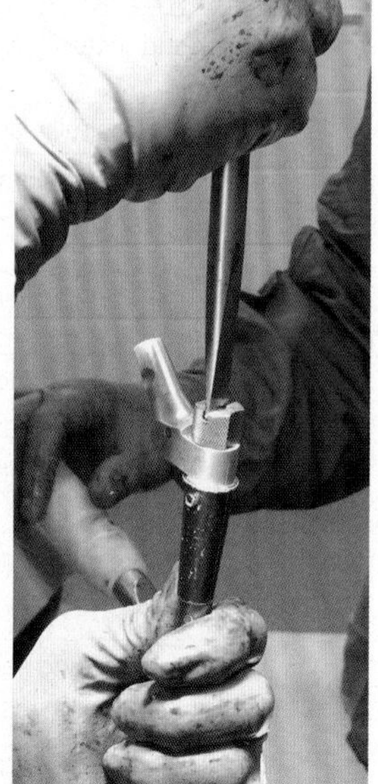

TECH FIG 2 • Placement of trial implants. The sleeve is inserted first (**A**) until it is completely seated (**B**). The trial is assembled on the back table with the appropriate neck anteversion (**C**) and then inserted into the sleeve (**D**). **E.** Insertion of the final component.

Routine Revision with Diaphyseal Defect

- Plan to bypass the diaphyseal defect by two cortical diameters with the fluted femoral stem.
- A long guidewire can be passed into the medullary canal of the femur to ensure that there are no holes in the cortical bone and to guide the flexible reamer down the canal.
- Reamers are used until there is diaphyseal chatter. Reaming is usually 1 to 2 mm greater than the diameter of the final fluted stem, but this varies among different manufacturers.
- Conical and miller reaming is performed in the manner described in the previous section.
- Place trial implants.
- Struts are usually not needed, although they can be used to improve bone stock.

Extended Trochanteric Osteotomy Needed or Diaphyseal Osteotomy or Open Reduction and Internal Fixation of a Periprosthetic Fracture Distal to a Loose Stem

- Remove stem and cement if necessary through the proximal femur or through the fracture site if present.
- Perform exposure posterior to the vastus lateralis (or vastus split) to expose the femoral shaft.
- The diaphysis can be reamed through the fracture site if present. Use bone clamps to gain control of the proximal segment and reduce the fracture or osteotomy and complete the reaming process. Prophylactic protective cerclage cables can be placed prior to reaming to prevent iatrogenic femoral fracture.
- Place the trial implant, crossing the fracture or osteotomy site.
- Reduce the hip and assess leg lengths, offset, stability, and soft tissue tension. Rotational stability will not be obtained at the fracture or osteotomy site at this time, so a true stability examination is not possible.
- Structural allograft maybe required, and if so, it can be secured using cerclage cables.
- Remove trial and place implant. It may be necessary to further ream the distal femur if there is a tight fit to avoid inadvertent fracture (**TECH FIG 3**).

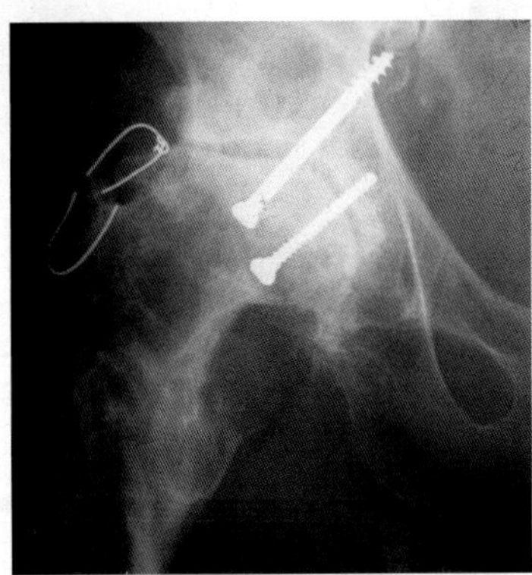
A

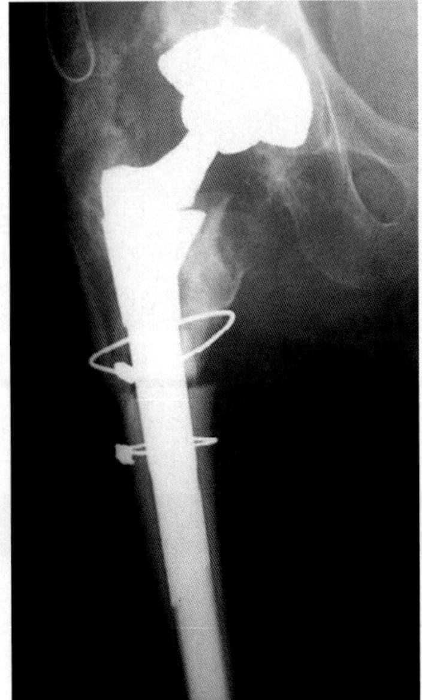
B

TECH FIG 3 • A,B. Preoperative and postoperative AP radiographs of a patient with severe proximal femoral deformity that necessitated a cortical osteotomy for insertion of the prosthesis, allowing femoral realignment.

Use of a Fluted Stem with a Proximal Femoral Allograft

- Choose a large proximal femoral allograft (critical).
- Decide on the level of the graft–host junction and divide the femur at that level. A step cut is not necessary if a bowed and slotted stem is used, as this will give rotational stability.
- Ream the distal diaphysis with a straight or flexible reamer until cortical chatter is achieved in the normal way. The last reamer determines the size of the implant.
- The allograft is prepared with an appropriate neck cut and reamed. Conical reaming and proximal milling then occur on the proximal femoral allograft.
- Make a provisional distal cut of 1 cm on the allograft.
- Make a longitudinal cut on the proximal native femur to open it up so the allograft can be inserted within it. Do not remove any soft tissue attachments from the native proximal femur.
- Perform a trial reduction by placing the trial within the allograft and inserting the distal portion of the stem into the native femoral diaphysis. Attempt to reduce the hip and assess leg lengths, soft

tissue tension, and stability. Remove bone from the distal tip of the allograft to equalize leg lengths. Make sure there is good bony contact at the allograft–host bone junction. The native greater trochanter should be placed in an anatomic position overlying the allograft.

- Pass two cables through the lesser trochanter; these will later be used with a claw to secure the native greater trochanter to the allograft.
- Downsize the sleeve to allow for a cement mantle and assemble the stem and sleeve on the back table.
- Cement the fluted stem and sleeve into the allograft, making sure that all of the cement is wiped off the distal portion of the stem. Keep cement off the distal portion of the allograft to allow complete contact with the host distal femur.
- Insert the allograft–stem composite into the native femur. Rotational stability at the graft–host junction should be complete at this time (**TECH FIG 4A**).
- A claw is used to secure the native greater trochanter to the allograft (**TECH FIG 4B**).

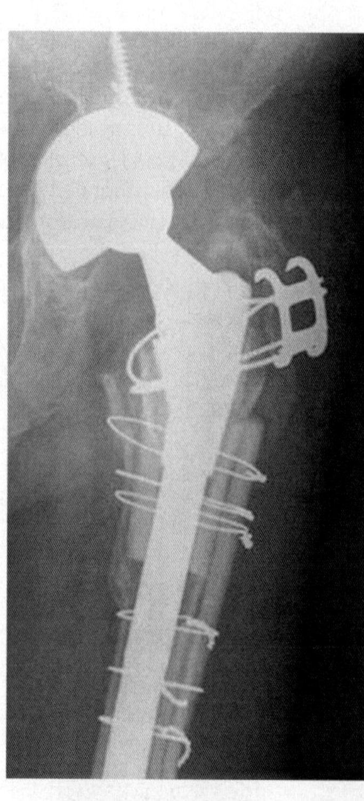

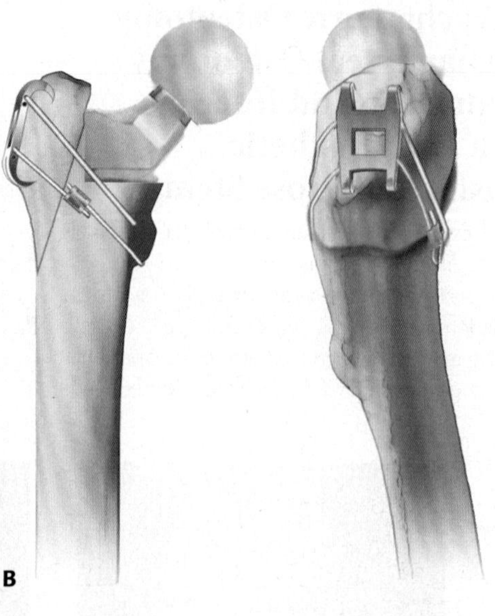

TECH FIG 4 • A. AP radiograph showing use of a fluted stem with proximal femoral allograft. **B.** Claw system technique used to reattach reattach the greater trochanteric fragment.

PEARLS AND PITFALLS

ETO should be used to access the femoral diaphyseal canal for cement removal or for removal of a well-fixed, extensively porous-coated cementless component.	■ ETO should be performed in a controlled fashion using multiple osteotomes to "open the door" in order to avoid fragment fracture.
Complete cement removal is essential.	■ Incomplete cement removal can lead to eccentric femoral canal reaming and cortical perforation or fracture.
An extensile approach should be used so that the femur can be directly inspected if cortical perforation has occurred.	■ Using an intramedullary guidewire can help guide reamers into the distal femur.
Consider an AP and lateral radiograph of the femur at the end of the case to confirm the absence of a fracture distal to the tip of the fluted prosthesis.	■ All cortical perforations and potential stress risers should be bypassed with the new fluted stem by at least two cortical diameters.
Consider the use of larger femoral heads to help prevent instability.	■ Dislocation risk is higher with revision surgery and reconstruction of a normal hip center of rotation and abductor function is essential.

POSTOPERATIVE CARE

- Assisted weight bearing initially with a walking frame, progressing to crutches and eventually a walking stick over the first 6 to 8 weeks for more straightforward revisions.
- Increasing weight bearing may be more gradual with more complex cases.
- Bracing can be used for recurrent instability, but reoperation may be required to increase the level of constraint of the acetabular component.
- Standard postoperative protocols should be adhered to, including thromboprophylaxis, antibiotic treatment, early mobilization, and the use of nonsedating analgesia.
- Any intraoperative tissue and fluid culture results should be obtained.

OUTCOMES

- The majority of studies in the literature on the use of modular femoral stems in revision THA have relatively short follow-up periods.[15]
- The use of modular, tapered, fluted, titanium stems in femoral revision with associated bone loss has been shown to facilitate proximal femoral bone reconstitution with improvement in clinical and quality of life measures and survivorship.[7,11,12,14,16]
- When used for proximal femoral bone loss or other complex revisions, previous authors have reported excellent radiographic and clinical outcomes with the S-ROM system, including no evidence of osteolysis, a mean postoperative Harris hip score of 82, and 84% patient satisfaction.[3,5]
- The S-ROM system has been reported to have a 5-year survival rate of 96%, with a 5% rate of mechanical failure.[17,20]
- Inferior outcomes have been associated with the use of large stem diameters with persistent thigh pain associated with stems[3] greater than 17 mm.
- Stem diameters greater than 16 mm have been correlated with a significantly increased incidence of stress shielding as well as a lack of bony ingrowth.[20]
- Re-revision rates for any reason have been reported from less than 1% to 14%.[2,4]

COMPLICATIONS

- Infection
- Loosening of components
- Dislocation and instability
- Leg length discrepancy
- Periprosthetic fracture
- Osteotomy nonunion
- Greater trochanteric bursitis
- Neurologic deficit

REFERENCES

1. Bolognesi MP, Pietrobon R, Clifford PE, et al. Comparison of a hydroxyapatite-coated sleeve and a porous-coated sleeve with a modular revision hip stem. A prospective, randomized study. J Bone Joint Surg Am 2004;86(12):2720–2725.
2. Bono JV, McCarthy JC, Lee J, et al. Fixation with a modular stem in revision total hip arthroplasty. Instr Course Lect 2000;49:131–139.
3. Chandler HP, Ayres DK, Tan RC, et al. Revision total hip replacement using the S-ROM femoral component. Clin Orthop Relat Res 1995;(319):130–140.
4. Christie MJ, DeBoer DK, Tingstad EM, et al. Clinical experience with a modular noncemented femoral component in revision total hip arthroplasty: 4- to 7-year results. J Arthroplasty 2000;15(7): 840–848.
5. Cossetto DJ, McCarthy JC, Bono JV, et al. Minimum four-year radiographic and clinical evaluation of results following femoral revision surgery with the S-ROM modular hip system. Acta Orthop Belg 1996;62(suppl 1):135–147.
6. D'Antonio JA, Capello WN, Borden LS, et al. Classification and management of acetabular abnormalities in total hip arthroplasty. Clin Orthop Relat Res 1989;(243):126–137.
7. Garbuz DS, Toms A, Masri BA, et al. Improved outcome in femoral revision arthroplasty with tapered fluted modular titanium stems. Clin Orthop Relat Res 2006;453:199–202.
8. Goyal N, Diaz-Ledezma C, Tripathi M, et al. Do previous operative reports provide the critical information necessary for revision total hip arthroplasty? J Arthroplasty. 2012;27(6):1023–1026.
9. Hardcastle P, Nade S. The significance of the Trendelenburg test. J Bone Joint Surg Br 1985;67(5):741–746.
10. Hermida JC, Bergula A, Chen P, et al. Comparison of the wear rates of twenty-eight and thirty-two-millimeter femoral heads on cross-linked polyethylene acetabular cups in a wear simulator. J Bone Joint Surg Am 2003;85(12):2325–2331.
11. Kwong LM, Miller AJ, Lubinus P. A modular distal fixation option for proximal bone loss in revision total hip arthroplasty: a 2- to 6-year follow-up study. J Arthroplasty 2003;18(3 suppl 1):94–97.
12. McInnis DP, Horne G, Devane PA. Femoral revision with a fluted, tapered, modular stem seventy patients followed for a mean of 3.9 years. J Arthroplasty 2006;21(3):372–380.
13. Muratoglu OK, Bragdon CR, O'Connor DO, et al. A novel method of cross-linking ultra-high-molecular-weight polyethylene to improve wear, reduce oxidation, and retain mechanical properties. Recipient of the 1999 HAP Paul Award. J Arthroplasty 2001;16(2): 149–160.
14. Ovesen O, Emmeluth C, Hofbauer C, et al. Revision total hip arthroplasty using a modular tapered stem with distal fixation: good short-term results in 125 revisions. J Arthroplasty 2010;25(3):348–354.
15. Park MS, Lee JH, Park JH, et al. A distal fluted, proximal modular femoral prosthesis in revision hip arthroplasty. J Arthroplasty 2010;25(6): 932–938.
16. Rodriguez JA, Fada R, Murphy SB, et al. Two-year to five-year follow-up of femoral defects in femoral revision treated with the link MP modular stem. J Arthroplasty 2009;24(5):751–758.
17. Smith JA, Dunn HK, Manaster BJ. Cementless femoral revision arthroplasty. 2- to 5-year results with a modular titanium alloy stem. J Arthroplasty 1997;12(2):194–201.
18. Spangehl MJ, Younger AS, Masri BA, et al. Diagnosis of infection following total hip arthroplasty. Instr Course Lect. 1998;47:285–295.
19. Valle CJ, Paprosky WG. Classification and an algorithmic approach to the reconstruction of femoral deficiency in revision total hip arthroplasty. J Bone Joint Surg Am 2003;85(suppl 4):1–6.
20. Walter WL, Walter WK, Zicat B. Clinical and radiographic assessment of a modular cementless ingrowth femoral stem system for revision hip arthroplasty. J Arthroplasty 2006;21(2):172–178.
21. Wilkins RH, Bodyia. Lasègue's sign. Arch Neurol 1969;21(2):219–221.

Revision Total Hip Arthroplasty with Femoral Bone Loss: Proximal Femoral Replacement

Pouya Alijanipour and Javad Parvizi

DEFINITION

- Proximal femur replacement is a salvage limb-sparing surgery for nononcologic and oncologic indications that in the past used to be treated with a major amputation.
- The magnitude of complexity of revision reconstruction of the femur depends mainly on the quantity and quality of femoral bone. During the past decade, remarkable advances in the field of revision hip reconstruction have been made. One such improvement has been the introduction of second-generation modular prosthetic components (**FIG 1**), which provide improved ability to restore limb length and achieve optimal soft tissue tension, both of which may reduce the incidence of instability that often follow insertion of a monolithic megaprosthesis. A new generation of megaprostheses also provides a better environment for soft tissue reattachment and the ability to reapproximate the retained host bone to the prosthesis.

ANATOMY

- Abductors (gluteus medius, gluteus minimus, tensor fascia lata muscles, and iliotibial band) are important stabilizers of the hip and are innervated mainly by the superior gluteal nerve. The nerve exits the pelvis via the suprapiriform portion of the sciatic foramen along with the superior gluteal vessels. Palsy results in abductor lurch, a Trendelenburg gait. The adductors include adductor brevis, adductor longus and gracilis muscles, and the anterior part of the adductor magnus muscle. The external rotators are the piriformis, quadratus femoris, superior gemellus, inferior gemellus, obturator internus, and obturator externus muscles.

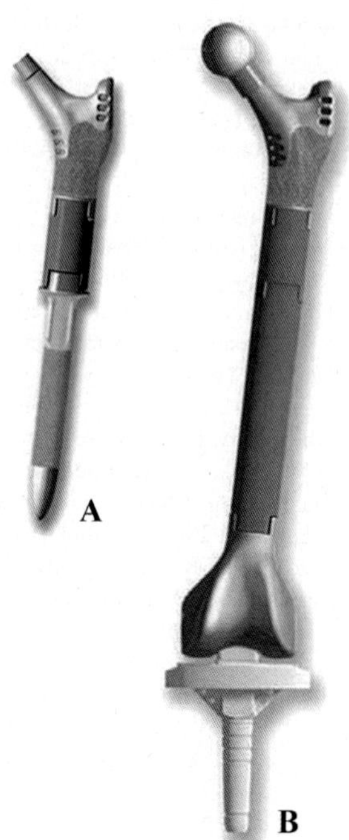

FIG 1 • New generation of modular proximal femoral (**A**) and total femoral replacement prostheses (**B**) Global Modular Replacement System (GMRS; Stryker Orthopaedics, Mahwah, NJ).

PATHOGENESIS

- Femoral bone loss is a constantly rising and predominantly complex and challenging problem in revision arthroplasty. Numerous factors may contribute to the loss of femoral bone stock encountered in revision total hip arthroplasty (THA):
  - Osteolysis secondary to particle debris
  - Stress shielding with adaptive bone remodeling
  - Previous infection
  - The natural processes of aging
  - Periprosthetic fracture
  - Multiple reconstructive procedures with insertion and removal of implants, which adversely affect the integrity and function of the abductor muscles

PATIENT HISTORY AND PHYSICAL FINDINGS

- Assessment of history, physical examination, laboratory tests, and radiographic findings lead to correct diagnosis of hip pathology in most patients.
- History should begin with evaluation of the chief complaint. Identifying the location and nature of pain can be helpful for proper diagnosis. Intra-articular and acetabular pathology usually present as groin pain. Thigh pain (especially start-up pain) is more indicative of a loose femoral stem. Patients may present with referred pain in their knees and should be evaluated for hip pathology.
- Thorough evaluation of past medical history along with a complete review of systems will help identify any potential factors that may lead to perioperative complications. Patients should be optimized for nutritional status and any underlying medical condition prior to surgery. This should include identification and adequate treatment of sources of potential or concurrent infection. Patients with history of chronic venous stasis ulcers, previous vascular bypass surgery, or absent distal pulses should be evaluated by a vascular surgeon.
- The physical examination should begin with analysis of the patient's gait. Antalgic gait can result from pain in any phase of ambulation with weight bearing and is characterized by a shortened stance phase. A Trendelenburg gait or abductor lurch indicates either paralysis or loss of continuity

of the abductor musculature and is identified by shift of the patient's center of gravity over the affected extremity during the stance phase of gait. Use of ambulatory assistive devices and existence of any deformity or limp should be documented. Previous surgical incisions should be routinely inspected. Planning surgical incision is important in determining the appropriate surgical approach for reconstruction. Although skin flap necrosis after hip surgery is rare, the maximum distance and angle is recommended to avoid this complication. Active and passive range of motion of the hip along with strength of the hip girdle musculature should also be recorded. A positive Trendelenburg test indicates abductor muscle weakness with inability of the patient to stabilize the pelvis during ipsilateral single-leg stance. Leg length should be assessed for apparent or functional discrepancy, which may be due to pelvic obliquity, muscular contracture, or scoliosis. Thomas test is performed by maximal flexion of hip and knee toward the chest and serves to evaluate contralateral hip flexion contracture. Provocative tests serve to localize the origin of the pain. Stinchfield test is positive when groin pain is reproduced with resisted ipsilateral hip flexion at 15 to 30 degrees and is highly suggestive for intra-articular hip pathology. If passive straight-leg raise causes radicular pain along the extremity and below the knee, a lower lumbar disc origin of the pain should be suspected. Physical examination should also include evaluation of neurovascular structures, spine, and abdomen to exclude sources of groin pain other than hip such as neuropathies, vascular claudication, spinal stenosis, or intra-abdominal pathologies.

- Erythrocyte sedimentation rate and serum C-reactive protein concentration should be determined. Elevated levels of these markers along with a history of previous infection are indications for joint aspiration and fluid analysis. Negative hip aspiration does not completely rule out infection; if significant risk of infection exists, aspiration should be followed by fresh frozen section evaluation and microbiologic culture of intraoperative tissue samples.

IMAGING AND OTHER DIAGNOSTIC STUDIES

- Proximal and total femur resections are major surgical procedures that necessitate a detailed preoperative evaluation. Patients with femoral bone deficiency due to malignant tumors should undergo adequate staging workup prior to reconstructive surgery. Most complications can be avoided by anticipating them before surgery and modifying the surgical technique accordingly.
- Imaging studies aid in determining the extent of bone loss; dimensions of the required prosthesis; proximity of the scarred-in femoral vessels, femoral nerve, and sciatic nerve to the surgical area; extent of soft tissue resection; and reconstruction possibilities.
- Plain radiographs of the entire femur are used to evaluate the extent and level of bone destruction. However, they may underestimate bone loss. If needed, computed tomography scanning can be added for further delineation of the femur and acetabulum bone structure.
- Magnetic resonance imaging is used to evaluate the medullary canal and soft tissue around the hip joint.
- Three-phase bone scan is essential to determine the presence of metastatic bone disease.
- Angiography of the iliofemoral vessels is essential before proximal femoral replacement if distortion of the anatomy due to previous surgeries is suspected.

DIFFERENTIAL DIAGNOSIS

- Infection including osteomyelitis and periprosthetic joint infection
- Primary bone tumors such as multiple myeloma and chondrosarcoma
- Metastatic lesions
- Periprosthetic fracture
- Osteolysis
- Aseptic loosening
- Paget disease
- Metabolic disease

CLASSIFICATION

- Multiple classification systems have been developed for femoral bone loss in revision arthroplasty. These include those devised by Mallory,[23] the American Academy of Orthopaedic Surgeons,[7] Gross et al,[11] Saleh et al,[39] and Weeden and Paprosky.[45] Of these, Weeden and Paprosky's classification seems to be the most widely used because it is simple and guides the surgeon in how to reconstruct the deficient femur. The basic principle for this classification is that as proximal metaphysis becomes deficient and unsupportive, diaphysis should be considered for reliable fixation of the stem (Table 1).[45]

NONOPERATIVE MANAGEMENT

- In most of the conditions discussed in this chapter, surgical intervention is considered the most reasonable option. However, nonsurgical modalities such as braces may be considered if surgery should not be performed on patients with serious underlying medical problems.

SURGICAL MANAGEMENT

- The objective of revision surgery is to improve function through a biomechanically restored hip by preserving as

Table 1 Paprosky Classification System for Femoral Defects

Type	Description
I	Minimal metaphyseal bone loss
II	Extensive metaphyseal bone loss and an intact diaphysis
IIIA	Extensive metadiaphyseal bone loss with availability of a minimum of 4 cm of intact cortical bone at the isthmus
IIIB	Extensive metadiaphyseal bone loss with availability of less than 4 cm of intact cortical bone at the isthmus
IV	Extensive metadiaphyseal bone loss and a nonsupportive diaphysis

From Blackley HR, Davis AM, Hutchison CR, et al. Proximal femoral allografts for reconstruction of bone stock in revision arthroplasty of the hip. A nine to fifteen-year follow-up. J Bone Joint Surg Am 2001;83-A(3):346–354.

much of bone and soft tissue as possible, augmenting deficient bone, and creating a stable construct.[24]

- The presence of active superficial or deep infection around the hip is an absolute contraindication for any reconstructive procedure. Relative contraindications can be noncooperative patients with increased risk of dislocation, vascular insufficiency that may impose healing problem, and nonoptimized medical comorbidities with unreasonably high risk for anesthesia.
- Options available for dealing with severe femoral bone loss are long cemented or press-fit stems,[6,17,20,30,31,42,44] allograft impaction,[8,13,21,36,37] allograft prosthetic composite (APC),[24,35,47] megaprosthesis,[34] and resection arthroplasty.[40] Age and activity level are important factors in determining the most appropriate reconstructive procedure.
- Allograft impaction is indicated for contained femoral defects in young patients where the diameter of femoral canal is too much expanded and the length of distal intact diaphysis is inadequate to achieve a press-fit for a cementless stem.[24,25,46] This technique is relatively straightforward in concept but time-consuming and technically demanding, with a steep learning curve.[14,27,28] Histologic analysis of biopsies taken from 19 patients 1 to 48 months after revision arthroplasty with this technique confirmed its ability to progressively restore bone stock.[43] However, its technical complexity and its potential complications limit its use.
- An important prerequisite for the use of prosthetic femoral replacement and APC is the availability of sufficient distal femoral length (at least 10 cm) for secure fixation of the cemented or uncemented femoral stem. If distal bone is severely deficient, total femoral replacement should be considered.
- An APC consists of cementing a long-stem prosthesis into a proximal femoral allograft.[24] Distally, the stem can be press-fit or cemented into native bone. However, if it is to be cemented, extreme caution should be taken not to allow the cement interpose into the graft–bone interface. This procedure is best reserved to restore femoral bone mass in younger, active patients.[35] It potentially increases bone stock in the proximal part of the femur and provides sites for soft tissue attachment, including the abductor muscles. However, it is a technically demanding and lengthy procedure that imposes significant physiologic stress on the patient. Moreover, its use is limited due to complications that are not uncommon with this procedure and include infection, junctional nonunion, dislocation, aseptic loosening, graft resorption, and fracture.[14,24]
- Proximal and total femoral replacement with a megaprosthesis (**FIGS 2** to **4**) is probably more available and technically less demanding than an APC for most surgeons. It is a valuable option for extensive circumferential bone loss of femur in elderly patients, particularly if their general medical condition does not allow other lengthier and more complex reconstructive procedures.[24,34] This type of prosthesis has been reported to have an unacceptably high failure rate in young patients and is not recommended for this patient population. However, it is indicated in elderly patients for whom immediate mobilization and weight bearing is of utmost importance in their recovery.[12,33,41] Potential complications include early loosening due to inadequate fixation to distal femur, stress shielding, fatigue fracture, and instability due to poor condition of the surrounding soft tissue.[5,34]

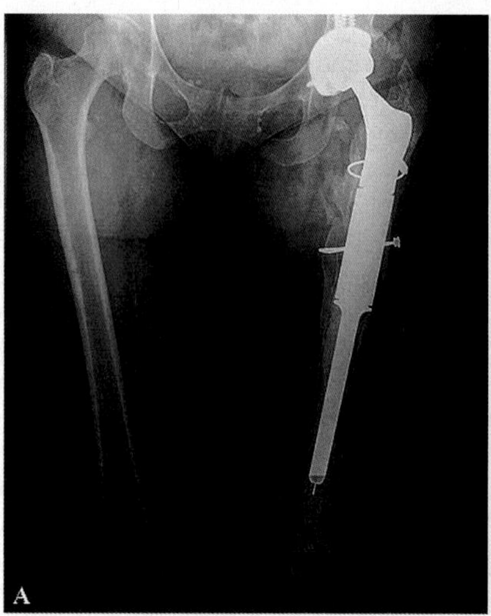

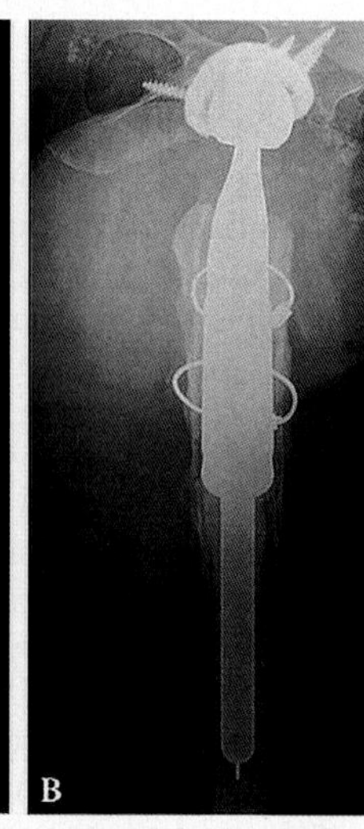

FIG 2 • Anteroposterior (**A**) and lateral (**B**) radiographs of a patient who underwent two-exchange revision arthroplasty at the age of 66 years due to periprosthetic joint infection. The patient had history of revision surgery due to periprosthetic fracture of the femur. Proximal femoral replacement was performed as the second stage of exchange arthroplasty because of massive proximal femoral bone loss.

Preoperative Planning

- The importance of preoperative planning in THA in general, and in proximal femur reconstruction in particular, cannot be overstated. These cases can be technically demanding, requiring meticulous attention to detail to achieve success.

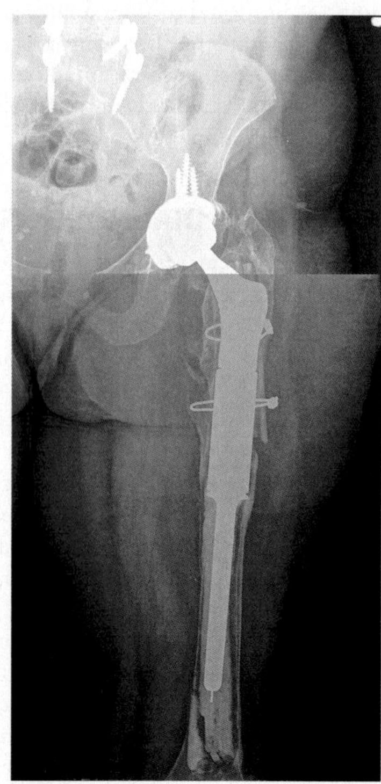

FIG 3 • Same patient as **FIG 2**, 5 years later. The patient presented with progressive thigh pain and loosening of proximal femoral replacement. Perioperative diagnostic workup was negative for periprosthetic joint infection (PJI).

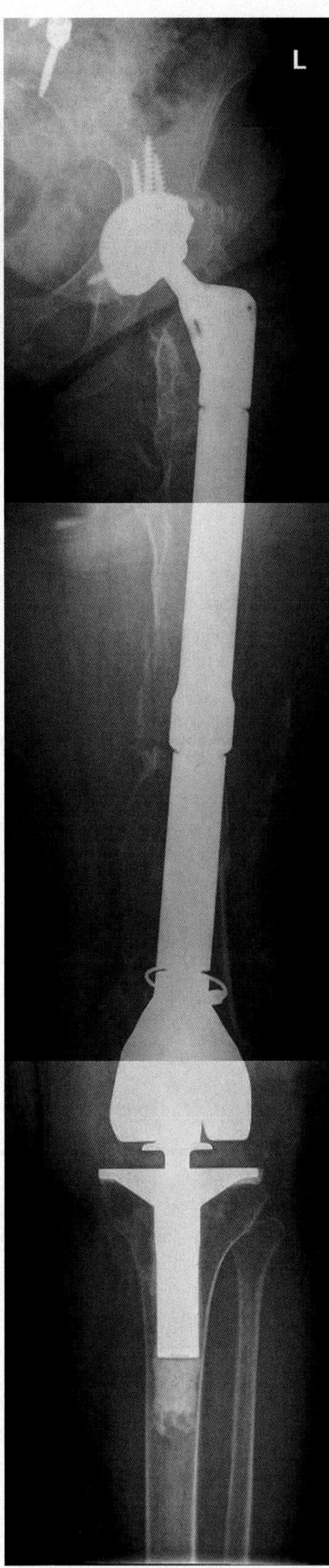

FIG 4 • Same patient as **FIGS 2** and **3**. Reconstruction with total femoral replacement with constrained total knee replacement was carried out to address extensive femoral bone loss. The patient did well after surgery and 1 year later underwent primary THA of the contralateral hip.

- Proximal femur reconstruction is performed for metaphyseal–diaphyseal lesions that extend below the lesser trochanter, cause extensive cortical destruction, and spare at least 10 cm of the distal femoral diaphysis. Total femur resection is performed for diaphyseal lesions that extend proximally to the lesser trochanter and distally to the distal diaphyseal–metaphyseal junction and cause extensive bone destruction.
- Preoperative clinical and radiographic (standing films) assessment of limb length should be carried out. Preoperative templating to select the appropriate stem length and diameter is essential. Even with the most accurate preoperative measurements, a variety of prosthesis sizes should be available in the operating room because intraoperative changes in the anticipated size of the prosthesis are common. A representative of the manufacturing company of the prosthesis to be used should be present in the operating room.
- Intraoperative monitoring of the sciatic and femoral nerves may be required in patients in whom extensive limb lengthening (>4 cm) is anticipated.
- Problems with removal of existing hardware, specific need for acetabular reconstruction, the potential need for insertion of constrained liners, and determining the absence of previous infection should be anticipated and addressed appropriately. Unexpected situations should always be considered. Even with accurate and detailed preoperative planning, the surgeon should allow for flexibility and consider the possibility of intraoperative modifications.
- The surgical team, including anesthesia personnel, should be experienced. Regional anesthesia is preferred over general anesthesia because it is reportedly associated with lower incidence of perioperative complications. These patients are often elderly and frail, and because of the possibility of large-volume blood loss, invasive monitoring methods such as an arterial line or pulmonary artery catheter are often warranted. Therefore, blood conservation strategies such as preoperative blood donation,[32] preoperative administration of erythropoietin,[3] and use of cell saver[9] should be considered in these patients.

Positioning

- Place the patient in the lateral decubitus or supine position.
- Nonpermeable U-drapes are used to isolate the groin.
- The distal third of the extremity is isolated from the field using impermeable drapes. The knee must be included in the operative field, even in patients undergoing proximal femoral replacement.
- Extension of the incision and arthrotomy of the knee to address intraoperative problems such as fractures extending distally is not uncommon.
- The skin is scrubbed with povidone-iodine solution, alcohol, and DuraPrep (3M, St. Paul, MN) before application of Ioban (3M).

Approach

- We use the direct lateral approach (Hardinge approach) or the posterolateral approach with trochanteric slide osteotomy to gain access to the hip and maintain a low threshold to extend the incision as needed.

Exposure

- Meticulous soft tissue handling facilitates tissue healing and minimizes postoperative complications.
- Deep tissue specimens for frozen section and culture are obtained in all cases. Thorough débridement is carried out to remove previous metal debris and hardware around the femur, if present.
- Extensile surgical approaches that allow for wide visualization should be employed. Modified Hardinge or posterolateral Moore approaches are recommended for proximal femoral replacement. Vastus slide osteotomy, as described by Head et al,[15] can be used to mobilize the gluteus minimus and medius, vastus lateralis, and vastus intermedius muscles anteriorly in unison to expose anterior and lateral aspects of the femur (**TECH FIG 1**).
- When the posterolateral approach is used for proximal femur resections, the incision can be extended to the anterolateral aspect of the patellar tendon if a total femur resection is required. After the external rotators and their interval with the abductors are identified, they are transected through their tendinous attachments and retracted posteriorly, exposing the hip joint and acetabulum. The vastus lateralis is reflected distally from its origin and the posterior perforating vessels are ligated. The vastus lateralis must be preserved because of its role in soft tissue coverage of the prosthesis; it is advanced proximally and sutured to the abductors. Care is taken not to ligate its main pedicle, which crosses anteriorly and obliquely along the rectus femoris fascia.

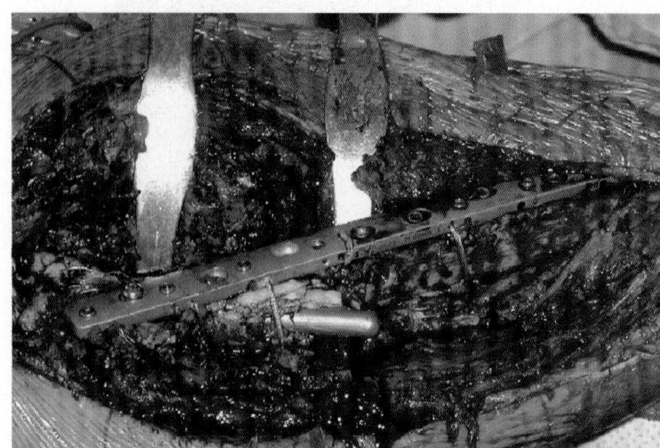

TECH FIG 1 • Exposure of the femur in a patient who sustained a periprosthetic fracture.

Allograft Prosthetic Composite

- If the patient's abductor mechanism remains functional, a sliding trochanteric osteotomy for future incorporation into the allograft is preferred. Distally, a step-cut osteotomy is performed to increase rotational stability of the APC–host bone junction.
- The proximal femoral graft should be smaller in diameter than the host bone and larger than the required length.[19] Irradiated fresh frozen allografts at −70° C that can be thawed in 5% povidone-iodine solution are preferred. However, use of nonirradiated fresh allografts stored above 0° C have also been reported.[37] Osteomy of the neck of allograft is performed 1 cm above the lesser trochanter. Distally, the graft is osteotomized and trimmed to match the receptive surface on the host bone, taking into account that ideally the APC should be telescoped 1 to 2 cm into distal host bone. The graft is reamed and the femoral component is cemented into the graft, ensuring adequate anteversion of the prosthesis. Cerclage cables can be used to secure the composite. Finally, the greater trochanter is attached to the APC through the use of cerclage wires.[19]

Proximal Femoral Replacement

- If the femur is intact, an osteotomy to split the proximal femur may be required to facilitate removal of the previous prosthesis or hardware.
- A transverse osteotomy is first made at the most proximal area of bone with good circumferential quality. Because the outcome of this procedure is influenced directly by the length of the remaining femur, maximum length of the native femur is maintained at all costs.[22,33] We use a longitudinal Wagner type of coronal plane osteotomy to split the proximal femur if the bone quality is poor.
- Soft tissue attachments to the proximal femur—particularly the abductor mechanism, if present—should be retained if at all possible. Once the femur is exposed, the distal portion of the canal is prepared through successive broaching. The cancellous bone, when present, is preserved for better cement interdigitation.
- Both cemented or noncemented stems are viable options, although cemented stems are believed to provide more predictable and secure fixation.[35]
- After completion of femoral preparation and determination of the size of best-fit broach, trial components are inserted, and the stability of the hip is examined.
- A distal cement restrictor is used whenever possible. The restrictor is introduced and advanced distally to allow for at least 2 cm of bone cement at the tip of the stem.
- The cement is pressurized and the final component implanted, with care taken to ensure that the porous-coated portion of the stem is placed directly and firmly against the diaphyseal bone with no interpositioning cement.
- The prosthesis can be assembled and then cemented distally or, alternatively, the stem can be cemented and the body assembled onto it.
- Extreme care must be exercised to prevent rotational malpositioning (**TECH FIG 2**). To mark the rotation, we use a sharp osteotome to scratch the distal femoral cortex once the trial component is appropriately positioned. The rotation of the component cannot be changed once the distal stem is cemented in place.

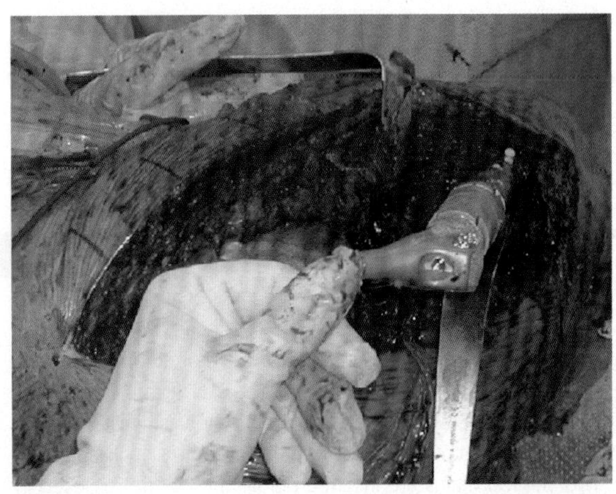

TECH FIG 2 • How the rotational positioning or version of the femoral component is determined. The version of the femoral stem is judged by appropriate positioning of the knee.

Total Femur Replacement

- Indications for total femoral replacement are rare and generally include conditions in which stem fixation is precluded due to inadequate length (<10 cm) or quality of distal femoral bone.
- Once exposure of the femur is completed using a lateral vastus reflecting approach, the entire femur is split longitudinally in the coronal plane. Again, even if bone is of extremely poor quality, as much of it with its soft tissue attachment is retained as possible.
- Total femoral replacement includes an arthrotomy of the knee to allow prosthetic replacement of the knee. The subvastus approach is extended to include a lateral or medial arthrotomy of the knee and eversion of the patella.
- The amount of tibial bone resected is kept to a minimum, but it must be of adequate thickness to allow implantation of the components and insertion of polyethylene without elevating the joint line. The tibia is prepared in the same manner as for total knee arthroplasty. Once appropriate tibial component size is determined, preparation of the tibia followed by insertion of the trial component is carried out.
- A full-length trial femur is assembled, ensuring that appropriate limb length is restored. Unless constrained liners are to be used, we prefer to use a large femoral head size to improve arc of motion and minimize instability.
- The tibial polyethylene is usually between 15 and 20 mm thick, but it may be necessary to adjust the thickness to obtain appropriate length of the extremity and restore the joint line.
- A linked articulated knee design is necessary because of loss of the stabilizing ligamentous structures. Once the prosthesis is assembled, a trial reduction is carried out to test for stability.
- We usually do not resurface the patella unless severe wear of the articular cartilage is noted.

Intraoperative Determination of Length of Femoral Component

- There are two methods for intraoperative determination of the length of the femoral component. In any case, tension of soft tissue is the main determinant of the appropriate length of the femoral prosthesis.[33]
  - The first method is to apply traction to the limb with measurement from the cup to the host bone osteotomy site (for proximal femoral replacement).
  - The second and preferred method is to place a Steinmann pin in the iliac crest to measure a fixed point on the femur before dislocation.
- With the long-stem trial prosthesis in place, proper leg length can be accurately restored. For patients with total femur replacement, radiographs of the opposite, normal femur may be obtained preoperatively and used for accurate templating for length.
- The length of the prosthesis usually equals the length of the resected bone, although in many patients, the integrity of the bone has been breached and the anatomy markedly altered.
- Ultimately, the femoral prosthesis length depends on the soft tissue tension around the hip. Balancing tension, restoring limb length, and avoiding excessive tension on the sciatic nerve are of utmost importance if complications are to be avoided.

Acetabular Reconstruction

- The acetabulum is exposed at the beginning of the operation and examined carefully. If a previous acetabular component is in place, the stability and positioning of the component are scrutinized. If the component is appropriately placed and stable, the liner is exchanged. If a previous acetabular component is not in place, a new component is inserted in a press-fit manner with or without screw fixation.
- The type of acetabular liner is determined after reconstruction of the femur has been completed because it may be necessary to use constrained liners in patients with poor soft tissue tension

and a high probability of instability. The constrained liners can be either snap-fit or cemented into the shell, depending on the type of the acetabular component implanted. In our experience, constrained liners are required in approximately half of patients receiving a megaprosthesis. Absolute indication for the use of a constrained liner is for patients with properly positioned components and equal or near-equal leg length who have intraoperative instability secondary to soft tissue deficiency.

- More complex acetabular reconstruction, such as the use of an antiprotrusio cage, is occasionally needed.

Closure

- The femur, however poor in quality, is maintained and wrapped around the megaprosthesis at the conclusion of implantation.
- The muscle–tendon attachments are preserved whenever possible.
- The soft tissues—especially the abductors, if present—are meticulously secured to the prosthesis (**TECH FIG 3**).
- Multiple loops of nonabsorbable sutures are passed around the trochanter remnant and the attached soft tissue.
- The leg is brought to abduction and the trochanter firmly fixed onto the proximal portion of the prosthesis by passing the sutures through the holes in the prosthesis or around the proximal body and the deep tissues.
- We occasionally suture the abductors to the vastus lateralis, the tensor fascia lata, or the host greater trochanter, if available.
- Two surgical drains are inserted before the wound is closed in layers using interrupted absorbable sutures. Meticulous skin closure, with excision of hypertrophic prior scar if necessary, is carried out to minimize postoperative wound drainage.

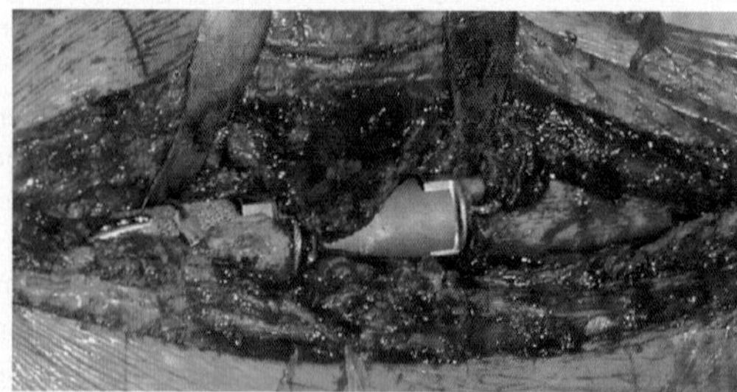

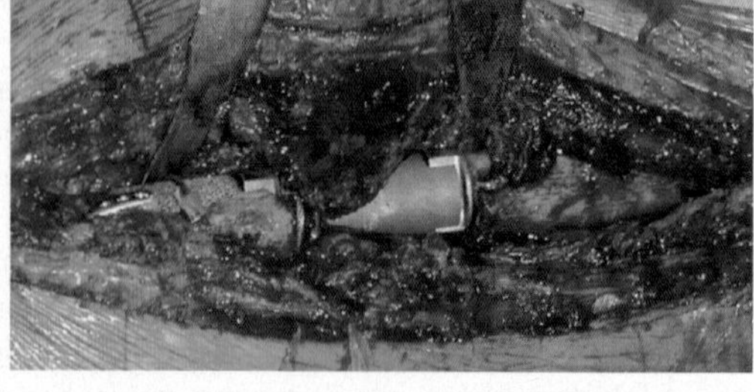

A

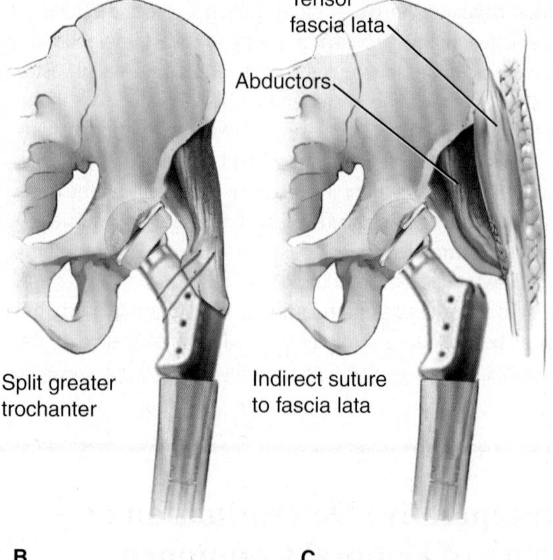

TECH FIG 3 • Soft tissue closure around the femoral stem. **A.** Proximal bone and soft tissue, however poor in quality, must be reapproximated to the stem as meticulously as possible. To achieve this, the greater trochanter with the abductors can be split and attached to the prosthesis (**B**) or the abductors can be indirectly sutured to the fascia lata, among other options (**C**).

PEARLS AND PITFALLS

Preoperative	■ Examine the patient thoroughly. Note previous scars, the status of the abductors, and limb length. ■ Discuss the procedure with the patient and help him or her form realistic expectations. ■ Perform detailed preoperative templating. ■ Have the manufacturer representative available to review your templating and ensure that correct components and neighboring sizes are available on the day of surgery. ■ Ask for an experienced scrub and anesthesia team.
Intraoperative	■ Minimize soft tissue dissection of the native bone and retain as much of the host bone as possible. ■ Restore appropriate leg length and soft tissue tension. ■ Have a low threshold for the use of constrained liners. ■ Ensure good hemostasis and perform a meticulous wound closure.

POSTOPERATIVE CARE

- Intravenous prophylactic antibiotics are given and maintained until final cultures are obtained. Thromboembolic prophylaxis also is administered for 6 weeks.
- Patients are allowed to commence protected weight bearing on postoperative day 1. We recommend use of an abduction orthosis for all patients and protected weight bearing for 12 weeks until adequate soft tissue healing occurs. Patients are usually able to ambulate with the use of a walking aid during this time. In patients who undergo the APC procedure, protected weight bearing for several months should be maintained and serial x-rays should be taken until radiographic evidence of union is observed.
- Daily physical therapy for assistance with ambulation and range-of-motion exercise for the knee are recommended. Patients receiving total femur replacement may require the use of continuous passive motion machines for rehabilitation of the knee replacement.

OUTCOMES

- APC: According to various studies, APC can provide durable long-term results. In a meta-analysis regarding the outcome of APC, 16 studies with a minimum follow-up of 2 years and mean follow-up of 8 years were included. The pooled success rate was reported to be 81%.[37] Two different studies reported a 10-year survival rate of 69%[1] and a 15-year survival rate of 82%.[38] Moreover, based on the analysis by Babis et al,[1] survivorship is significantly affected by baseline bone defects and the number of previous surgeries.
- The first experience with use of a megaprosthesis for reconstruction of the proximal femur in nonneoplastic conditions was reported in 1981.[41] Although all 21 patients in that cohort had significant pain relief, there were two failures. One patient required acetabular component revision and the second needed revision of the femoral component for recurrent instability.
- Two studies have been published regarding proximal femoral replacement in nonneoplastic conditions. Malkani et al[22] reported the outcome of 50 consecutive prosthetic femoral replacements in 49 patients treated for nonneoplastic conditions. All patients had massive proximal bone loss and some had multiple failed attempts with other reconstructive procedures. The mean follow-up was 11 years. The mean preoperative Harris hip score of 43 ± 13 points improved significantly to 80 ± 10 points at 1 year and to 76 ± 16 points at the latest follow-up. Before surgery, 86% of the patients had moderate to severe pain. Pain relief was achieved in 88% of patients at 1 year and 73% of patients at the latest follow-up. However, there was some deterioration in all parameters over time. Detailed radiographic analysis revealed an increase in the incidence of progressive radiolucent lines on the femoral and acetabular sides. Progressive radiolucency was seen in 37% of the acetabular components and 30% of the femoral components. Aseptic loosening was the main reason for revision surgery. Using revision as an end point, overall survivorship in this series was 64% at 12 years. The most common complication was dislocation, with an overall rate of 22%.
- In another study, Parvizi et al[34] reported on 48 patients from two institutions (mean age 73.8 years) who underwent placement of a modular megaprosthesis with or without bone grafting for the following nonneoplastic indications: periprosthetic fracture (20 patients), reimplantation because of a deep infection (13 patients), failed arthroplasty (13 patients), nonunion of an intertrochanteric fracture (1 patient), radiation-induced osteonecrosis with a subtrochanteric fracture (1 patient). Three died before the minimum 2-year follow-up interval had elapsed and 2 additional patients were lost to follow-up. The mean duration of follow-up for the remaining study group of 43 patients was 36.5 months. At the time of follow-up, there was a significant improvement in function as measured with the Harris hip score. The major complications were instability (8 patients), failure of the acetabular component (4 patients), and infection (1 patient). Of the 8 patients with instability, 6 required reoperation because of dislocation and 2 with subluxation required no further intervention. With revision used as the end point, the survivorship of the implant was 87% at 1 year and 72% at 5 years.
- The results of 11 patients undergoing total femur replacement at the Mayo Clinic were recently evaluated. Six of these patients had total femur reconstructions performed for multiple failed ipsilateral total knee arthroplasty and THA. Five patients, 4 of whom had pathologic fractures, underwent total femur replacement as limb salvage for musculoskeletal malignancy. Of the 6 patients who had total femoral replacement for failed arthroplasties, hip instability in 2 necessitated conversion to a constrained acetabular liner. Of 2 patients with previous infections, 1 developed recurrent infection despite staged total femoral reimplantation, and 1 had an elevated sedimentation rate on chronic antibiotic suppression but no evidence of clinical infection. All patients ambulated with either a walker or a cane. Of the 5 patients who had total femoral replacement for treatment of tumor, 1 developed hip and knee pain within 3 years, had wear of the knee hinge bushings, and sought disability. One patient developed wound dehiscence and postoperative sepsis and died. Two patients ambulated with a cane and 3 did not have the routine use of any gait aides.
- Blackley et al[5] reported the outcomes of revision THA with use of a proximal femoral replacement in a cohort of patients who had a Vancouver type B3 periprosthetic fracture. A modular femoral replacement with proximal porous coating was used in all cases. Twenty-one patients (mean age 78.3 years; range 52 to 90 years) were included in the cohort. At follow-up (mean 3.2 years), all but one of the patients were able to walk and had minimal to no pain. Complications included persistent wound drainage that was treated with incision and drainage (two patients), dislocation (two hips), refracture of the femur distal to the stem (one patient), and acetabular cage failure (one hip).
- Zehr et al[47] conducted a comparative study among 33 consecutive patients who required reconstructive surgery following resection of neoplasms of the proximal femur. Functional outcome and survivorship of the allograft prosthesis composite were not found to be significantly different from proximal femoral replacement, and the authors concluded that both procedures do equally well.

COMPLICATIONS

- Instability, infection, aseptic loosening, and fracture (prosthetic component, allograft, or host bone) are major common complications after proximal femoral reconstruction.

- Allograft prosthesis composites are associated with the risk of disease transmission, graft resorption, and nonunion. Graft resorption can occur in various degrees and does not commonly lead to failure of the construct.[38] Symptomatic junctional nonunion may require osteosynthesis and/or bone grafting.
- The major complications encountered following the use of a megaprosthesis are early dislocation and aseptic loosening. The cause of instability in this group of patients is multifactorial. First, these patients often have had multiple previous reconstructive procedures that have led to compromised abductors around the hip. Furthermore, the inability to achieve a secure repair of the residual soft tissues to the prosthesis predisposes these patients to instability.[10] The problem is further exacerbated in patients in whom the proper leg length and appropriate soft tissue tension is not achieved. The rate of dislocation with megaprostheses has been reported to be between 20% and 30% in previous studies.[12,16,22] Bickels et al[4] reported an exceptionally lower rate of dislocation of 1.7% in their series with mean follow-up of 6.5 years and attributed this low rate to acetabular preservation, Dacron-type capsulorrhaphy, and elaborate reconstruction of the iliopsoas, gluteus medius, gluteus maximus, and vastus lateralis tendons. We have implemented changes in our practice to minimize instability. These include the use of constrained cups in selective cases, routine use of a postoperative abduction brace, and augmentation of the proximal bone with the use of strut allograft, which imparts more rigidity for soft tissue attachment. It is conceivable that the problem of soft tissue to metal attachment may be better addressed in the future with the use of trabecular metals such as tantalum, which has excellent potential for soft tissue ongrowth. The use of a modular prosthesis has been a better strategy for dealing with this problem. The proximal femoral bone, however poor in quality, should be retained and reapproximated to the prosthesis to minimize dislocation. In addition, all efforts should be made to achieve equal limb lengths and to obtain acceptable soft tissue tension. Another important factor in the prevention of instability is the use of larger femoral heads in less active, elderly patients if instability is encountered intraoperatively.
- The other common complication of megaprosthesis reconstruction is acetabular and femoral radiolucency, which has a relatively high reported incidence.[12,18,22,47] The reason for this complication lies in the biomechanical aspect of this reconstructive procedure. Diaphyseal cement fixation predisposes the bone-cement-prosthesis unit to high torsional and compressive stresses, leading to early loosening. Cemented long-stem revision implants are known to have limited success and currently are recommended only for elderly and sedentary patients.[26] As expected, the incidence of radiolucency after the use of press-fit or proximally or extensively coated ingrowth stems is markedly lower than that with a megaprosthesis.[2,29] The incidence of radiolucency after megaprosthesis reconstruction at our institution has declined somewhat. This may be the result of improved cementing techniques, namely, the use of pulse lavage and plugging of the canal for better cement interdigitation. However, the more likely explanation for the reduction in the incidence of radiolucency is that we have narrowed the indications for the use of megaprosthesis to elderly and sedentary patients who place lower demands on the prosthesis.

REFERENCES

1. Babis GC, Sakellariou VI, O'Connor MI, et al. Proximal femoral allograft-prosthesis composites in revision hip replacement: a 12-year follow-up study. J Bone Joint Surg Br 2010;92(3):349–355.
2. Berry DJ, Harmsen WS, Ilstrup D, et al. Survivorship of uncemented proximally porous-coated femoral components. Clin Orthop Relat Res 1995;(319):168–177.
3. Bezwada HP, Nazarian DG, Henry DH, et al. Preoperative use of recombinant human erythropoietin before total joint arthroplasty. J Bone Joint Surg Am 2003;85-A(9):1795–1800.
4. Bickels J, Meller I, Henshaw RM, et al. Reconstruction of hip stability after proximal and total femur resections. Clin Orthop Relat Res 2000;(375):218–230.
5. Blackley HR, Davis AM, Hutchison CR, et al. Proximal femoral allografts for reconstruction of bone stock in revision arthroplasty of the hip. A nine to fifteen-year follow-up. J Bone Joint Surg Am 2001; 83-A(3):346–354.
6. Böhm P, Bischel O. The use of tapered stems for femoral revision surgery. Clin Orthop Relat Res 2004;(420):148–159.
7. D'Antonio J, McCarthy JC, Bargar WL, et al. Classification of femoral abnormalities in total hip arthroplasty. Clin Orthop Relat Res 1993;(296):133–139.
8. Duncan CP, Masterson EL, Masri BA. Impaction allografting with cement for the management of femoral bone loss. Orthop Clin North Am 1998;29(2):297–305.
9. Esper SA, Waters JH. Intra-operative cell salvage: a fresh look at the indications and contraindications. Blood Transfus 2011;9(2):139–147.
10. Giurea A, Paternostro T, Heinz-Peer G, et al. Function of reinserted abductor muscles after femoral replacement. J Bone Joint Surg Br 1998;80(2):284–287.
11. Gross AE, Hutchison CR, Alexeeff M, et al. Proximal femoral allografts for reconstruction of bone stock in revision arthroplasty of the hip. Clin Orthop Relat Res 1995;(319):151–158.
12. Haentjens P, De Boeck H, Opdecam P. Proximal femoral replacement prosthesis for salvage of failed hip arthroplasty: complications in a 2-11 year follow-up study in 19 elderly patients. Acta Orthop Scand 1996;67(1):37–42.
13. Halliday BR, English HW, Timperley AJ, et al. Femoral impaction grafting with cement in revision total hip replacement. Evolution of the technique and results. J Bone Joint Surg Br 2003;85(6):809–817.
14. Hartman CW, Garvin KL. Femoral fixation in revision total hip arthroplasty. J Bone Joint Surg Am 2011;93(24):2311–2322.
15. Head WC, Mallory TH, Berklacich FM, et al. Extensile exposure of the hip for revision arthroplasty. J Arthroplasty 1987;2(4):265–273.
16. Ilyas I, Pant R, Kurar A, et al. Modular megaprosthesis for proximal femoral tumors. Int Orthop 2002;26(3):170–173.
17. Isacson J, Stark A, Wallensten R. The Wagner revision prosthesis consistently restores femoral bone structure. Int Orthop 2000;24(3):139–142.
18. Johnsson R, Carlsson A, Kisch K, et al. Function following mega total hip arthroplasty compared with conventional total hip arthroplasty and healthy matched controls. Clin Orthop Relat Res 1985;(192):159–167.
19. Kellett CF, Boscainos PJ, Maury AC, et al. Proximal femoral allograft treatment of Vancouver type-B3 periprosthetic femoral fractures after total hip arthroplasty. Surgical technique. J Bone Joint Surg Am 2007;89(suppl 2, pt 1):68–79.
20. Kwong LM, Miller AJ, Lubinus P. A modular distal fixation option for proximal bone loss in revision total hip arthroplasty: a 2- to 6-year follow-up study. J Arthroplasty 2003;18(3 suppl 1):94–97.
21. Mahoney CR, Fehringer EV, Kopjar B, et al. Femoral revision with impaction grafting and a collarless, polished, tapered stem. Clin Orthop Relat Res 2005;(432):181–187.
22. Malkani AL, Settecerri JJ, Sim FH, et al. Long-term results of proximal femoral replacement for non-neoplastic disorders. J Bone Joint Surg Br 1995;77(3):351–356.
23. Mallory TH. Preparation of the proximal femur in cementless total hip revision. Clin Orthop Relat Res 1988;(235):47–60.
24. Mayle RE Jr, Paprosky WG. Massive bone loss: allograft-prosthetic composites and beyond. J Bone Joint Surg Br 2012;94(11 suppl A):61–64. doi:10.1302/0301-620X.94B11.30791.

25. Meding JB, Ritter MA, Keating EM, et al. Impaction bone-grafting before insertion of a femoral stem with cement in revision total hip arthroplasty. A minimum two-year follow-up study. J Bone Joint Surg Am 1997;79(12):1834–1841.
26. Morris HG, Capanna R, Del Ben M, et al. Prosthetic reconstruction of the proximal femur after resection for bone tumors. J Arthroplasty 1995;10(3):293–299.
27. Oakes DA, Cabanela ME. Impaction bone grafting for revision hip arthroplasty: biology and clinical applications. J Am Acad Orthop Surg 2006;14(11):620–628.
28. Ornstein E, Atroshi I, Franzén H, et al. Early complications after one hundred and forty-four consecutive hip revisions with impacted morselized allograft bone and cement. J Bone Joint Surg Am 2002;84-A(8):1323–1328.
29. Paprosky WG. Distal fixation with fully coated stems in femoral revision: a 16-year follow-up. Orthopedics 1998;21(9):993–995.
30. Paprosky WG, Aribindi R. Hip replacement: treatment of femoral bone loss using distal bypass fixation. Instr Course Lect 2000;49:119–130.
31. Paprosky WG, Greidanus NV, Antoniou J. Minimum 10-year-results of extensively porous-coated stems in revision hip arthroplasty. Clin Orthop Relat Res 1999;(369):230–242.
32. Parvizi J, Chaudhry S, Rasouli MR, et al. Who needs autologous blood donation in joint replacement? J Knee Surg 2011;24(1):25–31.
33. Parvizi J, Sim FH. Proximal femoral replacements with megaprostheses. Clin Orthop Relat Res 2004;(420):169–175.
34. Parvizi J, Tarity TD, Slenker N, et al. Proximal femoral replacement in patients with non-neoplastic conditions. J Bone Joint Surg Am 2007;89(5):1036–1043.
35. Parvizi J, Vegari DN. Periprosthetic proximal femur fractures: current concepts. J Orthop Trauma 2011;25(suppl 2):S77–S81.
36. Pekkarinen J, Alho A, Lepistö J, et al. Impaction bone grafting in revision hip surgery. A high incidence of complications. J Bone Joint Surg Br 2000;82(1):103–107.
37. Rogers BA, Sternheim A, De Iorio M, et al. Proximal femoral allograft in revision hip surgery with severe femoral bone loss: a systematic review and meta-analysis. J Arthroplasty 2012; 27(6):829–836.e1.
38. Safir O, Kellett CF, Flint M, et al. Revision of the deficient proximal femur with a proximal femoral allograft. Clin Orthop Relat Res 2009;467(1):206–212.
39. Saleh KJ, Holtzman J, Gafni A, et al. Reliability and intraoperative validity of preoperative assessment of standardized plain radiographs in predicting bone loss at revision hip surgery. J Bone Joint Surg Am 2001;83-A(7):1040–1046.
40. Sharma H, De Leeuw J, Rowley DI. Girdlestone resection arthroplasty following failed surgical procedures. Int Orthop 2005;29(2):92–95.
41. Sim FH, Chao EY. Hip salvage by proximal femoral replacement. J Bone Joint Surg Am 1981;63(8):1228–1239.
42. Sporer SM, Paprosky WG. Femoral fixation in the face of considerable bone loss: the use of modular stems. Clin Orthop Relat Res 2004;(429):227–231.
43. Ullmark G, Obrant KJ. Histology of impacted bone-graft incorporation. J Arthroplasty 2002;17(2):150–157.
44. Wagner H. Revision prosthesis for the hip joint in severe bone loss [in German]. Orthopade. 1987;16(4):295–300.
45. Weeden SH, Paprosky WG. Minimal 11-year follow-up of extensively porous-coated stems in femoral revision total hip arthroplasty. J Arthroplasty 2002;17(4 suppl 1):134–137.
46. Wraighte PJ, Howard PW. Femoral impaction bone allografting with an Exeter cemented collarless, polished, tapered stem in revision hip replacement: a mean follow-up of 10.5 years. J Bone Joint Surg Br 2008;90(8):1000–1004.
47. Zehr RJ, Enneking WF, Scarborough MT. Allograft-prosthesis composite versus megaprosthesis in proximal femoral reconstruction. Clin Orthop Relat Res 1996;(322):207–223.

29 CHAPTER

Revision Total Hip Arthroplasty with Acetabular Bone Loss: Impaction Allografting

Matthew J. Wilson and A. John Timperley

DEFINITION

- The loss of acetabular bone stock remains a major challenge in revision hip surgery.
- The three main causes of acetabular bone loss encountered in revision hip surgery are aseptic loosening due to osteolysis, bone loss due to infection, and iatrogenic loss encountered during implant removal.
- The use of large amounts of bone cement in isolation for the reconstruction of acetabular defects in revision hip surgery has poor results, with high rates of early loosening.
- Impaction grafting has the ability to restore anatomy and bone stock with histologic incorporation of graft.
- Acetabular impaction grafting (AIG) is defined as vigorous forceful impaction of cancellous bone chips using specially designed instruments to achieve a solid bed of bone into which polymer bone cement can be pressurized prior to insertion of a polyethylene acetabular component.
- True AIG requires the use of a cemented polyethylene acetabular component. Graft used in combination with uncemented shells serves only as a void filler and cannot be loaded in the same physiologic manner.
- Impaction bone grafting is ideal for cavitary defects and can be used in extensive segmental defects, providing that stable containment of the graft can be achieved.
- Stainless steel mesh fixed with small fragment screws can be used to convert segmental defects (medial wall or peripheral) into contained cavitary defects suitable for impaction grafting. Alternatively, porous metal wedges may be used to create a contained defect.[6]
- Adequate pressurization of cement into impacted bone graft creates a composite with immediate mechanical stability, promoting bone remodeling, and restoration of bone stock.
- AIG has shown good long-term results.[5,12–15,18]
- Standard implants and modern cementing techniques are used.

ANATOMY

- The acetabulum is a complex three-dimensional structure with two thick columns of bone, one anteriorly and one posteriorly, and thinner walls superiorly and medially, which contain the socket.
- It is important to identify relevant landmarks intraoperatively, such as the transverse acetabular ligament, the true floor (medial wall), anterior and posterior walls and columns, and superior dome (**FIG 1**).
- AIG combined with a cemented polyethylene cup allows for the restoration of the hip center and normal hip biomechanics.

PATHOGENESIS

- Although autograft is the ideal material for AIG, a limited natural supply necessitates the use of allograft.
- Animal studies show that impacted, morselized fresh frozen allograft bone incorporates into new bone.[11]
- Twenty-four acetabular bone biopsy specimens were obtained from 20 patients who had undergone acetabular reconstruction with impaction bone grafting.[16]
    - Biopsy specimens were obtained at 3 months to 15 years.
    - Histology showed rapid revascularization of the graft followed by osteoclastic resorption and woven bone formation on the graft remnants.
    - A mixture of graft, new bone, and fibrin remodeled completely into a new trabecular structure, with normal lamellar bone and only scarce remnants of graft material.
    - Localized areas of nonincorporated bone graft surrounded by fibrous tissue remained despite the follow-up period.
    - Large nonincorporated fragments of cartilage were also found in cases in which femoral head bone chips were produced by a bone mill.
- Allograft is an osteoconductive material, acting as a scaffold for new bone formation. However, histologic studies have shown that new bone forms within the stromal tissue, indicating that osteoinduction may also play a role, although the exact mechanism by which this occurs is unclear.
- Despite the contact between bone graft and cement, the bone graft retains its biologic and mechanical viability and healing potential.[9]
- Reports on AIG show promising intermediate and long-term results.[5,8,12–15,18]

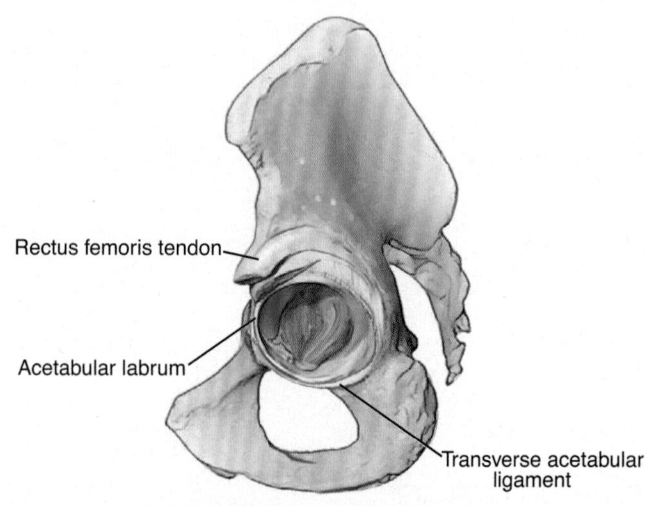

FIG 1 • Anatomy of the acetabulum.

PATIENT HISTORY AND PHYSICAL FINDINGS

- As usual, a thorough history and examination is essential, including a clear understanding of the previous hip surgery and the reasons behind failure.
- Infection is considered a relative contraindication and any suspicion of this should be thoroughly investigated in the usual fashion. Rudelli et al[10] reported their series of the use of impaction bone grafting in one-stage revisions. They reported the following:
  - A 6.2% recurrence of infection at 8.6 years in 32 patients
  - Of these patients, 25 underwent impaction grafting of both the femur and acetabulum, and half required the use of mesh to contain the graft.
  - These results are similar to those reported using a two-stage procedure.
- Physical examination should include examination for previous incisions, sinus tracts, range of motion, contractures, leg length discrepancy, and neurovascular status.
- Records of previous surgeries should be obtained, including details of previous implants.

IMAGING AND OTHER DIAGNOSTIC STUDIES

- The initial diagnostic imaging examination should begin with standard anteroposterior (AP) pelvis and AP and lateral radiographs of the affected hip.
- Oblique Judet views can be extremely useful to assess column and wall defects.
- A computed tomography (CT) scan may be helpful in identifying bone loss and structural defects, although metal artifacts can make interpretation difficult.
- The actual bone defects or bone loss may be more severe than preoperative radiographic studies reveal.[17]
- A preoperative workup for infection should be performed, including aspiration or biopsy as required.

NONOPERATIVE MANAGEMENT

- Nonoperative management is only considered for patients who are not able to tolerate a revision operation or able to comply with the postoperative instructions. In these cases, excision arthroplasty with removal of any loose components may be a reasonable option as a pain-relieving procedure.
- Alternative methods of fixation include cemented acetabular revision, revision with structural allograft, uncemented acetabular components with structural allograft, uncemented components with metal augments, jumbo acetabular components, and trabecular metal acetabular components.
- In cases of pelvic discontinuity or severe anterior or posterior column defects, alternative techniques of reconstruction such as cages, plates and screws, or trabecular metal implants may be necessary.

SURGICAL MANAGEMENT

Preoperative Planning

- One of the benefits of AIG is the ability to recreate anatomy by restoring the center of rotation to the correct level.
- Precise preoperative templating is necessary to plan the requirement for reconstruction of segmental defects and to assess cavitary defects in order to ensure anatomic positioning of the acetabular component.

Positioning

- The patient is positioned according to the surgeon's preference and planned surgical approach. This technique is applicable to most patient positions and surgical techniques.

Approach

- Any surgical approach that allows full acetabular exposure can be used. It is important that the surgeon uses an approach that is both familiar and extensile.
- Extensile approaches that allow good visualization of the posterior column are favored, as this facilitates the reconstruction of segmental defects.

TECHNIQUES

Acetabular Exposure

- Circumferential exposure of the acetabulum for the assessment of bony deficiencies is essential.
- Releases that may facilitate acetabular exposure include release of gluteus maximus tendon from the femur, release of the iliofemoral ligament and reflected head of rectus from the superoanterior acetabulum, and release of iliopsoas tendon.
- Removal of the femoral stem can also facilitate exposure. Cemented taper slip femoral stem can be tapped out of the intact mantle and replaced following reconstruction using a cement-in-cement technique.[3]
- The previous acetabular components are removed using traditional implant removal techniques. Particular attention must be taken to avoid additional bone loss.
- All residual cement and fibrous tissue must be removed using small burrs and curettes, taking care to preserve the thin acetabular walls (**TECH FIG 1**).
- In the cases of medial defects, the membrane here can be left intact as removal may risk damaging intrapelvic structures.

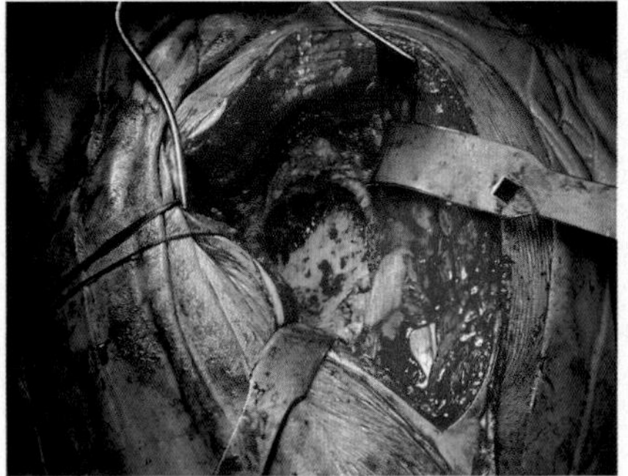

TECH FIG 1 • The acetabulum cleared of soft tissue prior to assessment.

- Identification of the transverse acetabular ligament, if present, can be a useful landmark for positioning of the revised component.
- Following exposure, the bony anatomy is assessed and acetabular defects are identified.
- As soon as the defect has been assessed and its suitability for AIG is confirmed, it is advisable to remove the autograft femoral heads from the freezer and allow these to defrost in warm saline.

Acetabular Preparation

- The use of acetabular reamers should be kept to a minimum to avoid removing host bone and damaging thin acetabular walls. Areas of sclerotic bone that are not bleeding can be burred gently or drilled with a 2-mm drill bit to encourage bleeding, which may improve graft incorporation.
- In order to assess acetabular defects and to determine whether containment is required, it is useful to hold a trial component in the intended inclination and anteversion at the level of the transverse acetabular ligament (**TECH FIG 2A**).
- For purely cavitary defects, no further reconstruction with mesh is required and impaction can begin.
- Peripheral segmental defects require containment using stainless steel rim meshes (X-change Revision Instrument System, Stryker Orthopaedics, Mahwah, NJ) that can be cut to size, ensuring sharp edges are not placed posteriorly where they might risk injury to the sciatic nerve, and secured to the acetabular rim using multiple small fragment screws placed at 1-cm intervals along the acetabular wall. It is useful to secure the mesh at the apex initially and, after rotating the mesh to the correct anteversion, screws can be placed at the anterior and posterior corners and then in the intervals (**TECH FIG 2B**).
- Porous metal wedges may be used in peripheral defects to create a contained defect for impaction grafting.
- When securing peripheral meshes, it is useful to place an appropriately sized impactor in the acetabulum to ensure the mesh or wedge is appropriately oriented and the defect is adequately contained.
- Medial segmental defects are common and require reinforcement prior to impaction. Specific medial meshes can be cut to size and gently impacted medially. The placement of a thin wafer of femoral head or cancellous bone chips can be placed medially to stabilize the mesh. If required, additional stability can be achieved using two or three small fragment screws.

A

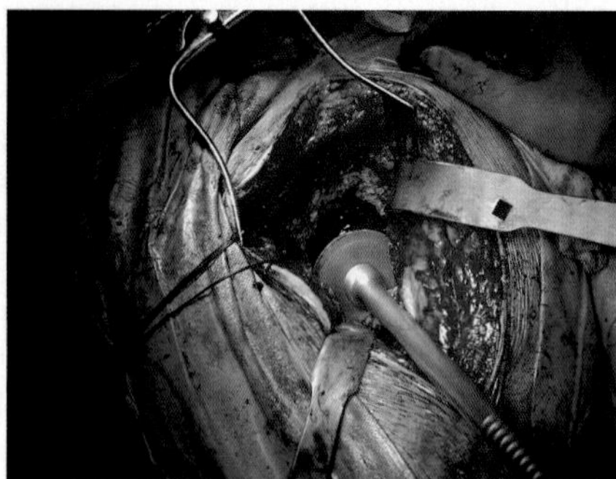

B

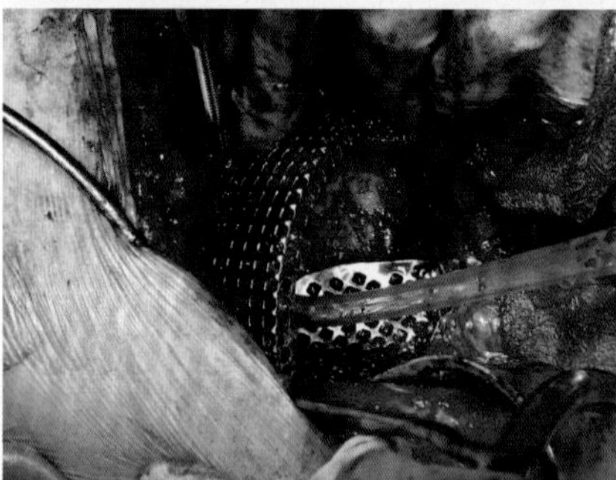

TECH FIG 2 • **A.** Acetabular impactor in position within the socket to help define the defect. **B.** Large superior mesh being secured. An anterior mesh has previously been placed.

- Anterior wall defects can also be contained with a small mesh, although in these circumstances, the mesh is secured to the inner surface of the acetabulum.
- Large defects that require use of the large rim mesh should be carefully assessed, as results have shown higher failure rates with larger rim meshes, probably due to the difficulty in achieving stable containment.[5,18] Alternative methods of reconstruction may be required in these cases.

Preparation of Bone Graft

- In revision cases, sufficient autograft is rarely available. In these cases, fresh frozen femoral heads are the preferred choice.
- The graft can be prepared either by hand, using large rongeurs, or using a commercially available bone mill as long as appropriate size chips can be produced.
- Better stability has been shown with larger bone chips and a 7- to 10-mm bone chip is recommended,[1] in contrast to the smaller bone graft size used with femoral impaction grafting.
- Most commercially available bone mills are not capable of producing bone chips of this larger size; therefore, we recommend handmade bone chips.
- In addition to larger chip size, pulsatile lavage can be used to clean the graft after morselization and this has also been shown to improve stability of the impacted graft.[1,4]

Acetabular Bone Reconstruction

- Bone chips are introduced into the acetabulum and impacted in layers.
- It is important to fill superior defects first (**TECH FIG 3A**) using small impactors to fill small cavitary defects and work around any screws that may be passing across the defect.
- It is a technical mistake to place too much graft medially, resulting in lateralization of the final acetabular component.
- Reverse reaming with an acetabular reamer should not be used. This technique has demonstrated inferior results with less graft stability.[2]
- Impaction using hemispherical acetabular impactors needs to be vigorous—forceful enough to ensure a stable bed of graft but not so forceful as to fracture the acetabulum.

- Once the main defect has been filled, more chips should be placed at the periphery and impacted. Impaction in the periphery should continue until it is no longer possible to insert more bone chips (**TECH FIG 3B**). In order to facilitate this, the final impactor can be backed off by 1 or 2 mm. Once peripheral impaction is complete, hammer the impactor back into place.
- The final impactor should be 4 to 6 mm larger than the outer diameter of the planned acetabular component to allow for an adequate cement mantle.
- Following final impaction, the bone bed should have the consistency of cortical bone (**TECH FIG 3C**).
- Pulse lavage can be used to clean the graft bed, but the graft should be protected using a mesh or slotted spoon.

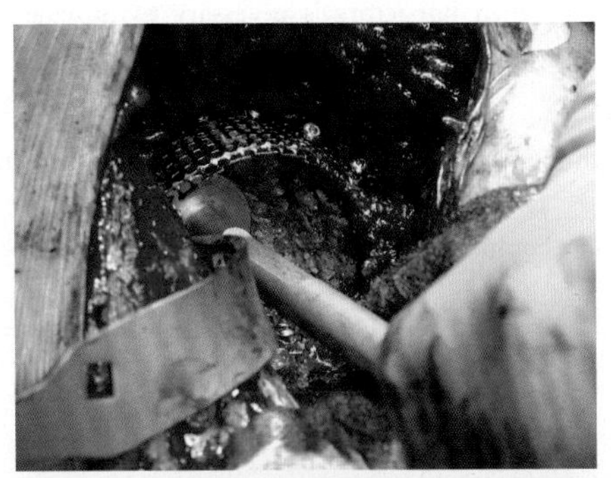
A

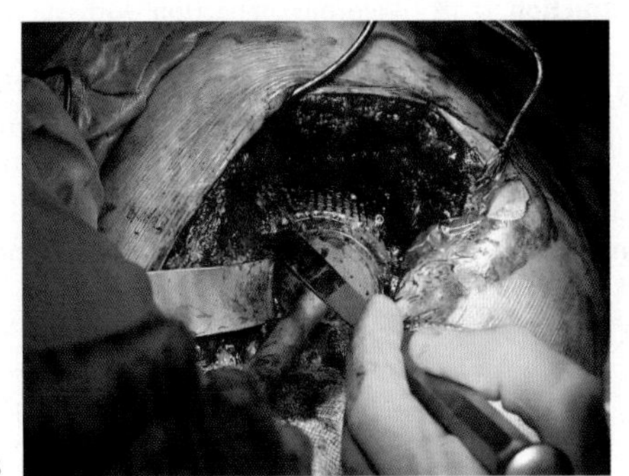
B

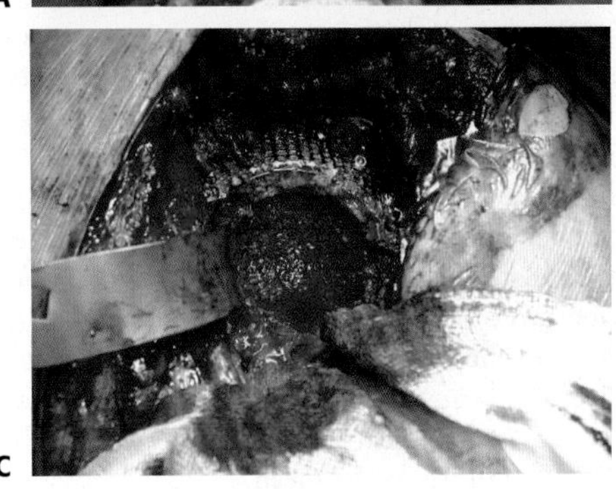
C

TECH FIG 3 • **A.** Graft being placed superiorly under the mesh. **B.** Peripheral impaction underway with impactor held in socket. **C.** Completed impaction prior to washing and cementation.

Cemented Cup Insertion

- Hydrogen peroxide–soaked gauzes can be placed in the acetabulum to clean the graft surface while the polymethylmethacrylate (PMMA) bone cement is mixed.
- The PMMA cement is inserted into the acetabulum once it has reached the correct consistency and is pressurized for a minute prior to cup insertion.
- The authors prefer a flanged all-polyethylene acetabular component.
- Following insertion, pressure is maintained on the acetabular component until the PMMA cement has polymerized (**TECH FIG 4**).

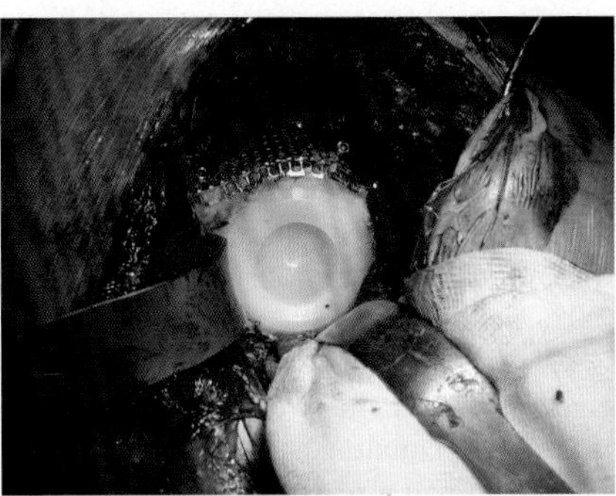

TECH FIG 4 • Completed reconstruction following socket insertion.

PEARLS AND PITFALLS

Acetabular exposure	▪ Good exposure of the entire bony acetabular rim is essential to ascertain the extent of the defect.
Acetabular preparation	▪ Defects requiring the use of a large rim mesh may be better managed with alternative techniques. ▪ Stability of the mesh and therefore the graft is the key to success. ▪ Impacted bone should have the consistency of cortical bone.
Bone graft preparation	▪ Fresh frozen femoral head is considered the gold standard. ▪ Remove all soft tissue and cartilage. ▪ Bone graft chips should be 7–10 mm.[4] ▪ Commercial bone mills often produce smaller graft sizes.
Acetabular bone reconstruction	▪ Vigorous impaction with specially designed impactors is necessary to provide initial mechanical stability of the graft. ▪ Overimpaction may cause fractures. ▪ Reverse reaming with acetabular reamers should not be used with this technique. ▪ Extrusion of PMMA cement through the superolateral graft and mesh construct suggests inadequate packing.
Cemented cup insertion	▪ Late insertion of a flanged acetabular component into well-pressurized PMMA bone cement is the gold standard.

POSTOPERATIVE CARE

- Postoperative protocols are according to the surgeon's preference. Perioperative antibiotics are recommended.
- Prophylaxis for heterotopic ossification should be considered.
- Patients are toe-touch weight bearing for 6 weeks, followed by partial weight bearing with crutches or a walker for another 6 weeks.
- Interval-appropriate radiographs are recommended.

OUTCOMES

- Schreurs et al[12] reported on 62 consecutive acetabular revisions in 58 patients with acetabular impaction bone grafting and a cemented cup at an average follow-up of 16.5 years and found an overall survival rate of 79% and an 84% survival rate when aseptic loosening was used as an end point.
- Schreurs et al[13] reported a 20-year survival rate of 91% with aseptic loosening as an end point in patients younger than 50 years of age. The overall survival in this patient population was 80% when acetabular revision for any reason was evaluated.
- Schreurs et al,[15] using a similar technique in 35 hips in patients with rheumatoid arthritis, demonstrated a prosthetic survival rate of 90% at 8 years, with aseptic loosening as the end point.
- Pitto et al[8] reported on 81 patients treated with impaction bone grafting and reinforcement rings. At an average of 6.5 years, only one patient had a revision because of dislocation. All grafts demonstrated graft incorporation at 3 months.
- Gilbody et al[5] reported on a minimum 10-year follow-up of 304 hips revised using AIG. The mean follow-up was 12.4 years and the survival rate with revision for aseptic loosening as the end point was 85.9%.

COMPLICATIONS

- Complications generally related to revision hip arthroplasty, such as infection, instability, hematoma, and neurovascular injury are risks of surgery.
- Wide acetabular exposure puts neurovascular structures such as the superior gluteal nerve and vessels at risk.
- Intraoperative fractures may occur with vigorous packing of the bone graft. If this occurs, the fracture should be stabilized prior to completion of the impaction procedure.
- Socket migration can occur, but radiostereometric analysis (RSA) studies have shown that this reduces in the first postoperative year.[7] The mechanism of failure in large defects is usually shear within the graft substrate; shear is less likely to occur if large bone chips are used. Significant migration in defects reconstructed using large rim meshes may result in fatigue failure of the mesh.

ACKNOWLEDGMENT

All images reproduced with the kind permission of The Exeter Hip Unit publishers.

REFERENCES

1. Arts JJ, Verdonschot N, Buma P, et al. Larger bone graft size and washing of bone grafts prior to impaction enhances the initial stability of cemented cups: experiments using a synthetic acetabular model. Acta Orthop 2006;77:227–233.
2. Bolder SB, Schreurs BW, Verdonschot N, et al. Particle size of bone graft and method of impaction affect initial stability of cemented cups: human cadaveric and synthetic pelvic specimen studies. Acta Orthop Scand 2003;74:652–657.
3. Duncan WW, Hubble MJ, Howell JR, et al. Revision of the cemented femoral stem using a cement-in-cement technique. J Bone Joint Surg Br 2009;91(5):577–582.
4. Dunlop DG, Brewster NT, Madabhushi SP, et al. Techniques to improve the shear strength of impacted bone graft: the effect of particle size and washing of the graft. J Bone Joint Surg Am 2003;85A:639–646.
5. Gilbody J, Taylor C, Bartlett GE, et al. Clinical and radiographic outcomes of acetabular impaction grafting without cage reinforcement for revision hip arthroplasty: a minimum 10 year follow-up study. Bone Joint J 2014;96-B(2):188–194.
6. Gill K, Wilson MJ, Whitehouse SL, et al. Results using Trabecular Metal™ augments in combination with acetabular impaction bone grafting in deficient acetabular. Hip Int 2013;23(6):522–528.

7. Ornstein E, Franzen H, Johnsson R, et al. Five-year follow-up of socket movements and loosening after revision with impacted morselized allograft bone and cement: a radiostereometric and radiographic analysis. J Arthroplasty 2006;21(7):975–984.
8. Pitto RP, Di Muria GV, Hohmann D. Impaction grafting and acetabular reinforcement in revision hip replacement. Int Orthop 1998; 22:161–164.
9. Roffman M, Silbermann M, Mendes DG. Viability and osteogenicity of bone graft coated with methylmethacrylate cement. Acta Orthop Scand 1982;53:513–519.
10. Rudelli S, Uip D, Honda E, et al. One-stage revision of infected total hip arthroplasty with bone graft. J Arthroplasty 2008;23(8): 1165–1177.
11. Schimmel JW, Buma P, Versleyen D, et al. Acetabular reconstruction with impacted morselized cancellous allografts in cemented hip arthroplasty: a histological and biomechanical study on the goat. J Arthroplasty 1998;13:438–448.
12. Schreurs BW, Bolder SB, Gardeniers JW, et al. Acetabular revision with impacted morsellised cancellous bone grafting and a cemented cup: a 15- to 20-year follow-up. J Bone Joint Surg Br 2004;86B:492–497.
13. Schreurs BW, Busch VJ, Welten ML, et al. Acetabular reconstruction with impaction bone-grafting and a cemented cup in patients younger than fifty years old. J Bone Joint Surg Am 2004;86A:2385–2392.
14. Schreurs BW, Slooff TJ, Buma P, et al. Acetabular reconstruction with impacted morsellised cancellous bone graft and cement: a 10- to 15-year follow-up of 60 revision arthroplasties. J Bone Joint Surg Br 1998;80B:391–395.
15. Schreurs BW, Thien TM, de Waal Malefijt MC, et al. Acetabular revision with impacted morselized cancellous bone graft and a cemented cup in patients with rheumatoid arthritis: three to fourteen-year follow-up. J Bone Joint Surg Am 2003;85A:647–652.
16. van der Donk S, Buma P, Slooff TJ, et al. Incorporation of morselized bone grafts: a study of 24 acetabular biopsy specimens. Clin Orthop Rel Res 2002:131–141.
17. Walde TA, Weiland DE, Leung SB, et al. Comparison of CT, MRI, and radiographs in assessing pelvic osteolysis: a cadaveric study. Clin Orthop Relat Res 2005;(437):138–144.
18. Wilson MJ, Whitehouse SL, Howell JR, et al. The results of acetabular impaction grafting in 129 cemented total hip replacements. J Arthroplasty 2013;28(8):1394–1400.

Revision Total Hip Arthroplasty with Acetabular Bone Loss: Antiprotrusio Cage

Patrick Kane, Matthew S. Austin, James J. Purtill, and Brian A. Klatt

DEFINITION

- Acetabular bone deficiency may occur primarily (eg, dysplasia, inflammatory arthritis, or seronegative arthropathy) or secondarily (eg, aseptic or septic loosening of acetabular components, osteolysis, trauma, or iatrogenic loss during removal of well-fixed components).
- The use of antiprotrusio cages is indicated in situations where an uncemented porous-coated acetabular component will not gain reliable initial stability.

ANATOMY

- The confluence of the ilium, the ischium, and the pubis forms the hemispherically shaped acetabulum, each contributing to the anterior and posterior walls and columns.
- Surgical landmarks include the anterior and posterior walls, dome, and medial wall "teardrop."
- The acetabulum is normally oriented with 45 degrees of inclination and 15 degrees of anteversion relative to the pelvic plane.

PATHOGENESIS

- Acetabular bone deficiency may occur primarily due to dysplasia. This type of deficiency usually does not require the use of an antiprotrusio cage.
- Certain conditions (eg, rheumatoid arthritis, juvenile rheumatoid arthritis, ankylosing spondylitis, or Paget disease) may predispose patients to acetabular protrusio but usually do not require the use of an antiprotrusio cage.
- The antiprotrusio cage is used most often in cases of secondary bone stock deficiency so massive that the use of a cementless press-fit acetabular component is precluded.

NATURAL HISTORY

- The natural history of massive acetabular bone defects that would require an antiprotrusio cage is not known. Patients usually require revision surgery to return to functional activities.

PATIENT HISTORY AND PHYSICAL FINDINGS

- The history should be conducted to determine whether the source of pain is extrinsic or intrinsic.
- The patient's pain may be extrinsic (eg, lumbar radiculopathy or intrapelvic pathology), in which case revision surgery may fail to relieve pain completely.
  - Pain usually, but not always, is located in the groin.
- Infection must always be assessed with careful questioning about previous infections, fevers, chills, wound drainage, and pain at rest.
- Start-up pain is an indication of loosening.
- Medical comorbidities must be assessed to determine the presence of any that may compromise the outcome of the surgery or place the patient at increased risk of complications.
- The skin should be inspected visually for placement of prior incisions and signs of infection.
  - The appropriate incision for the surgical approach must be used with an adequate (6 cm) skin bridge.

IMAGING AND OTHER DIAGNOSTIC STUDIES

- Plain radiographs, including anteroposterior (AP) of the pelvis and AP and true lateral of the hip, should be obtained to classify bone loss and to adequately plan preoperatively (**FIG 1**).
- Computed tomography (CT) scans may be used to assess the remaining bone stock.
  - This is especially important in cases of superior or posterior bone loss that may require allograft reconstruction.
  - The CT scan can help determine the need to have allograft bone available to reconstruct the defect and may help dictate the approach if a posterior column reconstruction or plating is necessary.
- CT scans with intravascular contrast are useful in situations in which a prior implant is medial to Kohler line and proximity of the implant to the vessels and intra-abdominal contents is unknown.
- Erythrocyte sedimentation rate (ESR) and C-reactive protein (CRP) are useful screening tools to detect infection.
- Aspiration of the hip to assess for infection is valuable if the ESR, CRP, or clinical suspicion is elevated.

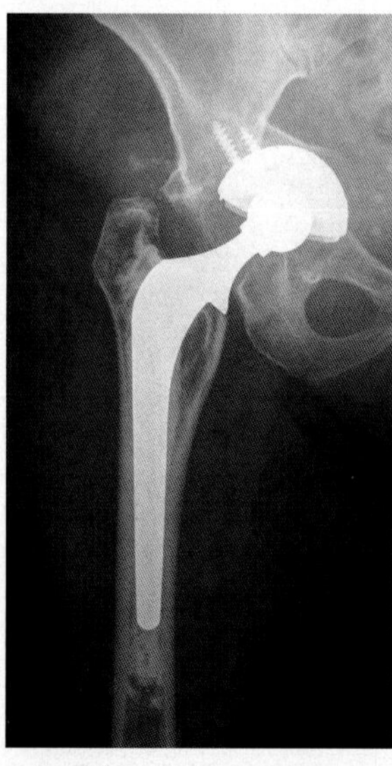

FIG 1 • AP radiograph of the hip demonstrates medial migration of the acetabular cup with significant loss of acetabular bone stock.

- Nuclear medicine studies such as technetium 99 methylene diphosphonate in combination with gallium citrate, indium 111–labeled leukocyte scans, positron emission tomographic scans with ^{18F}fluorodeoxyglucose, and sulfur colloid scans may help differentiate aseptic from septic loosening.

DIFFERENTIAL DIAGNOSIS

- The following conditions may contribute to pain and may be the cause of continued pain after the surgery:
  - Lumbar radiculopathy
  - Spinal stenosis
  - Sacroiliac degenerative joint disease
  - Intra-abdominal pathology
  - Intrapelvic pathology
  - Neuropathy
  - Meralgia paresthetica
  - Complex regional pain syndrome
  - Vascular claudication
  - Primary bone tumors
  - Metastasis

NONOPERATIVE MANAGEMENT

- Nonoperative management of severe acetabular bone loss is reserved for those patients in whom surgical management is contraindicated. This includes patients with substantial medical comorbidities and those with active infection.

SURGICAL MANAGEMENT

- Surgical management begins with preoperative planning.
- The radiographs are assessed and it is determined whether the defect can be reconstructed with a cementless acetabular component or will require an antiprotrusio cage.
- The surgical approach is planned.
  - If posterior column plating is anticipated, a posterior approach is indicated.
  - If this is not required, a direct lateral or posterior approach may be used, according to the surgeon's preference.
- The acetabulum is exposed, bone loss is assessed, and determination about the appropriate reconstructive choice is made.

Preoperative Planning

- Planning for the antiprotrusio cage begins with appropriate radiographs.
  - The radiographs allow for classification of the defect and aid in planning for the reconstruction.
- We have found the Paprosky classification to be helpful in defining bone deficiency and predicting the method of reconstruction[3] (**FIG 2**).
  - Paprosky type 1 acetabular defects have minimal bone loss and can usually be reconstructed using only a cementless component.
  - Type 2A defects have an intact superior rim and the acetabulum is oval in shape. The anterior and posterior columns are intact. The implant has migrated less than 2 cm. These defects may be reconstructed with so-called jumbo cups or cementless reconstruction with additional bone grafting or trabecular metal augments. The socket may also be placed in a more superior position to attain greater contact with host bone.
  - Type 2B defects are similar to type 2A defects, with the exception of loss of the superior rim. The implant has migrated less than 2 cm. The superior rim can be reconstructed with an uncemented socket in association with bone grafting or trabecular metal augments.
  - Type 2C defects involve medial bone loss with intact anterior and posterior columns. Medial bone loss may be reconstructed with bone graft or trabecular metal augments.
  - Type 3A defects generally migrate more than 2 cm superolaterally. The medial wall and ischium usually are still present but damaged. These defects can be reconstructed with bone grafting or trabecular metal augments and an uncemented socket.
  - Type 3B defects generally migrate more than 2 cm superomedially. There is loss of the teardrop and severe damage to the ischium. Pelvic discontinuity should be suspected. These defects can be reconstructed with bulk allograft, trabecular metal, an antiprotrusio cage, or a combination. Posterior column plating may be needed in cases of acute discontinuity. If this is a possibility, then a posterior approach should be selected.

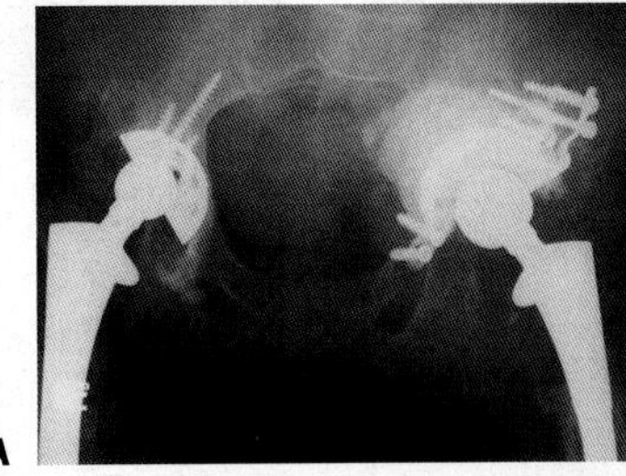
A

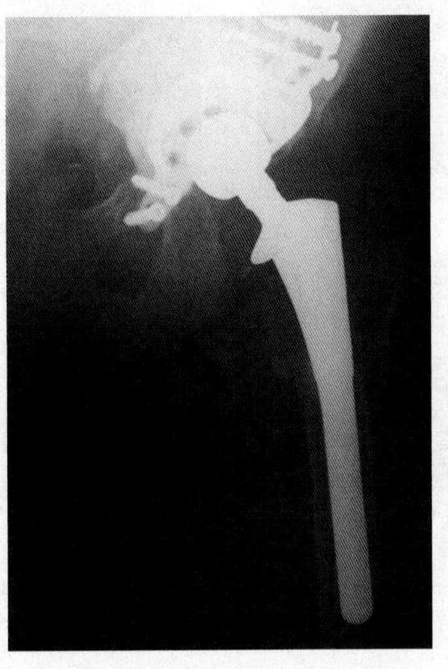
B

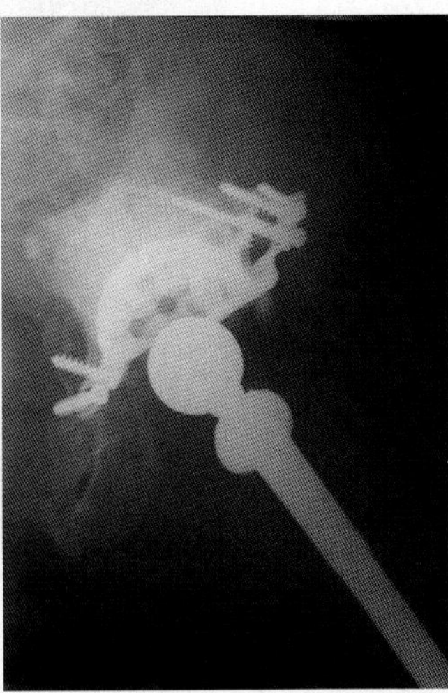
C

FIG 2 • Preoperative radiographs of a patient with severe acetabular bone loss due to superior and medial migration of construct as well as pelvic discontinuity (Paprosky type 3B defect). An AP radiograph of the pelvis (**A**), an AP view of the hip (**B**), and a frog-leg lateral view of the hip (**C**) are obtained. Occasionally, more specialized views of the pelvis, such as the Judet view, may be necessary to assess integrity of the acetabular columns.

- Pelvic discontinuity should be suspected if a fracture is noted that involves both the anterior and posterior columns, the inferior hemipelvis has migrated medial to the superior hemipelvis, or the inferior hemipelvis is rotated in relation to the superior hemipelvis.
- Large posterior column defects may predispose to cage failure and reconstruction of the defect should be included in preoperative planning.
- An appropriate device should be selected.
  - The flanges should be malleable to allow the cage to be shaped to the bone.
  - The implant must have sufficient strength.
  - We believe that an inferior flange that gains fixation in or on the ischium is superior to a hook that gains fixation on the teardrop.

Positioning

- The patient is positioned according to surgeon preference and as dictated by the surgical approach. The hip should be draped to allow wide surgical exposure.

Approach

- The surgeon should select a posterior approach if he or she anticipates the need for posterior column plating or reconstruction. Otherwise, the surgeon should select the approach that is most familiar and comfortable.
- A trochanteric osteotomy, either conventional or extended, may improve exposure of the acetabulum and pelvis.
- Exposure of the sciatic nerve (posterior approach) is left to the judgment of the surgeon.

TECHNIQUES

Acetabular Exposure

- The acetabulum is exposed and the failed construct and any soft tissue that interferes with visualization should be retracted or removed (**TECH FIG 1A–E**).
- The anterior and posterior walls/columns, superior dome/rim, medial wall, teardrop, and ischium are identified and bone loss is noted (**TECH FIG 1F–H**).

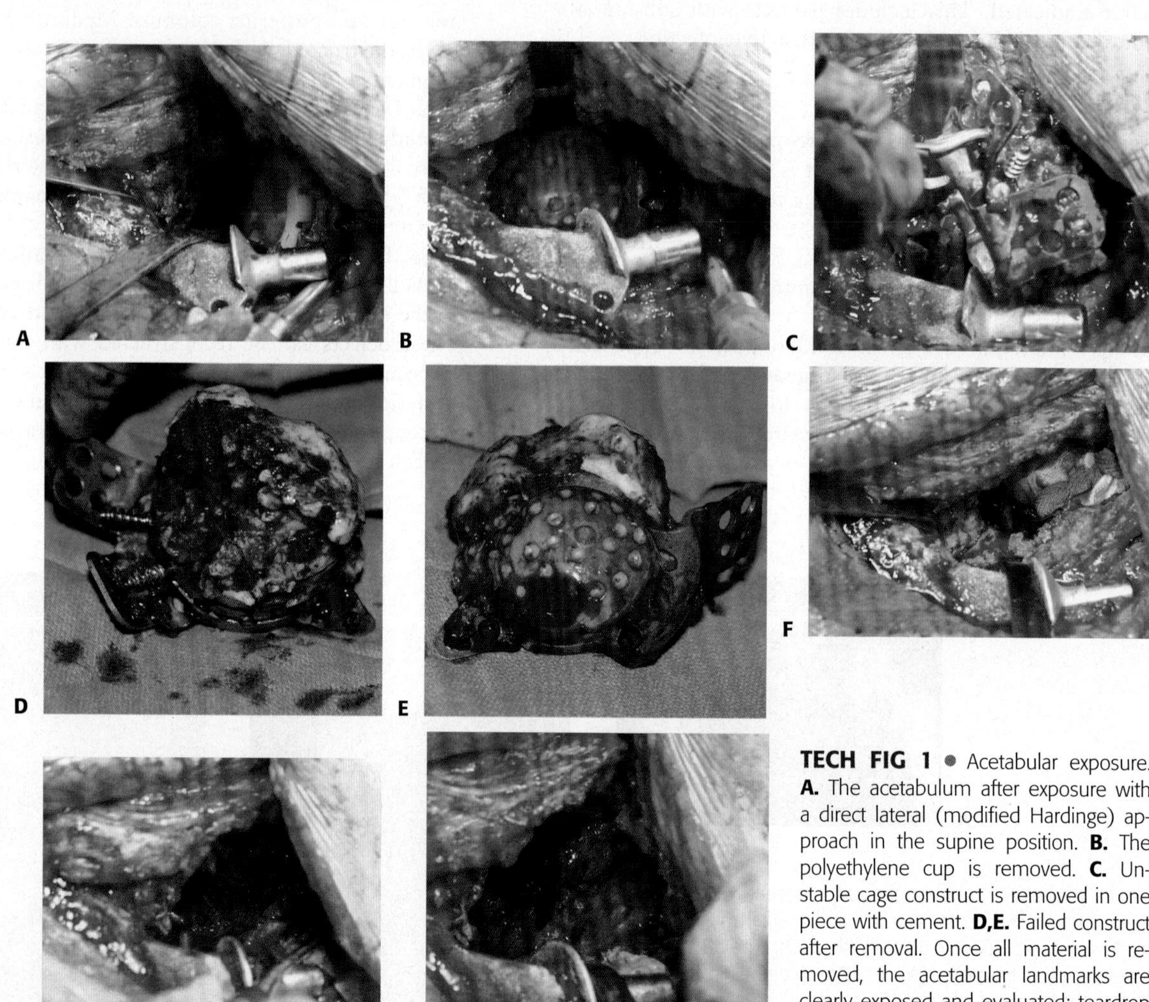

TECH FIG 1 • Acetabular exposure. **A.** The acetabulum after exposure with a direct lateral (modified Hardinge) approach in the supine position. **B.** The polyethylene cup is removed. **C.** Unstable cage construct is removed in one piece with cement. **D,E.** Failed construct after removal. Once all material is removed, the acetabular landmarks are clearly exposed and evaluated: teardrop (**F**), posterior column (**G**), and superior dome/rim (**H**).

Intraoperative Determination of Reconstructive Technique

- The remaining bone stock is assessed and corroborated with the preoperative assessment of bone loss.
  - Paprosky types 1, 2A, 2B, 2C, and 3A defects can usually be reconstructed with an uncemented acetabular component with or without bone grafting or trabecular metal augments.
  - All acetabuli, especially Paprosky type 3B defects, should be tested for pelvic discontinuity.
- If pelvic discontinuity exists (**TECH FIG 2**), the surgeon may elect to use an antiprotrusio cage with or without posterior column plating or additional bone grafting.
  - Alternatively, the surgeon may elect to distract the discontinuity with an uncemented socket and bridge the defect in this manner.
- The acetabulum should be assessed for the remaining bone's ability to support an uncemented component. To support an uncemented cup, the remaining bone stock should allow for at least partial inherent stability of the reamer or trial.
  - Reamers or trials that are inherently unstable may not be appropriate for cementless reconstruction.
- The reamers are not used initially to shape the acetabulum but are used to assess the ability of the remaining bone to support a socket.
- If it is determined that the remaining bone stock cannot support a socket, then an antiprotrusio cage should be used.

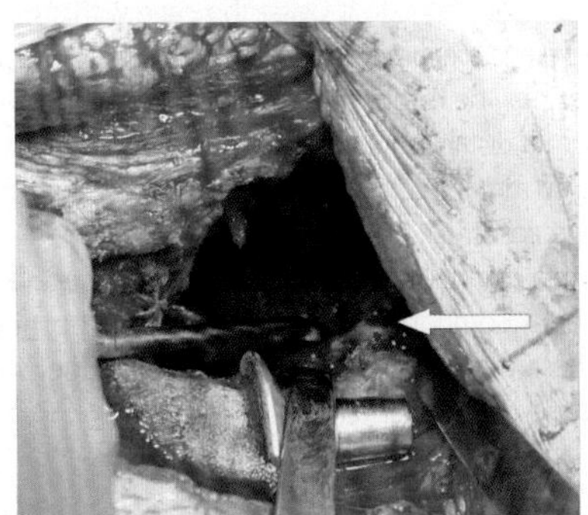

TECH FIG 2 • Intraoperative determination of reconstructive technique. A large central defect is visible where the cage was removed. Pelvic discontinuity is demonstrated (*arrow*) with a fracture of the posterior column.

Bone Preparation

- The ilium must be exposed with care to avoid the superior gluteal neurovascular bundle (**TECH FIG 3A**).
- The size of the defect can be assessed with a standard acetabular reamer. The reamer can then be used to remove small amounts of bone that may prevent complete seating of the cage (**TECH FIG 3B**).
  - It should not be necessary to remove significant bone because the indication for use of this device is severe bone loss.
- The outer diameter of the reamer that best fits the acetabulum determines the outer diameter of the cage.
  - The trial cage or the actual implant can be used to determine the removal of small amounts of bone that interfere with complete seating of the cage (**TECH FIG 3C**).

A
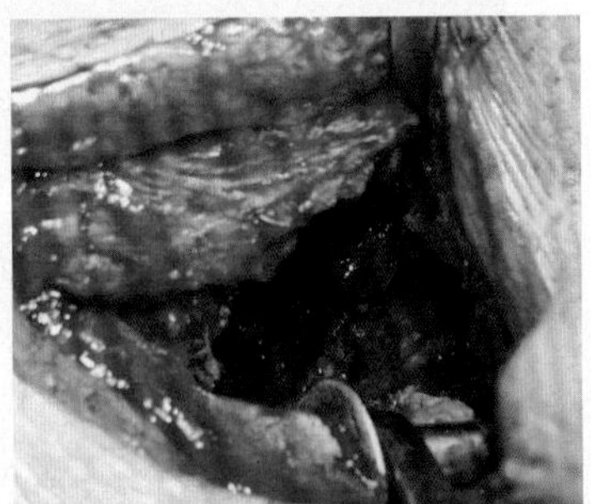
B
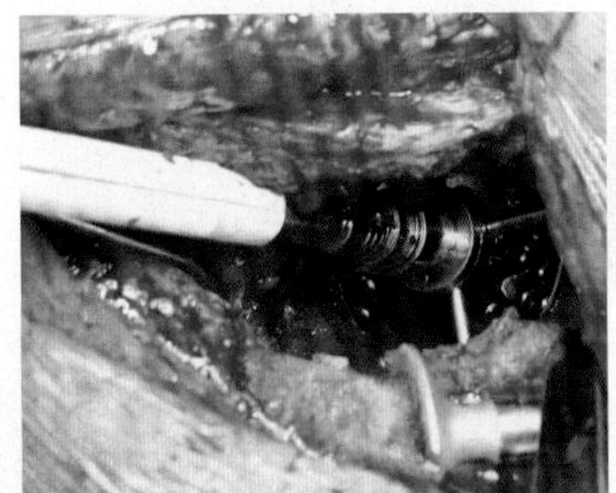
C
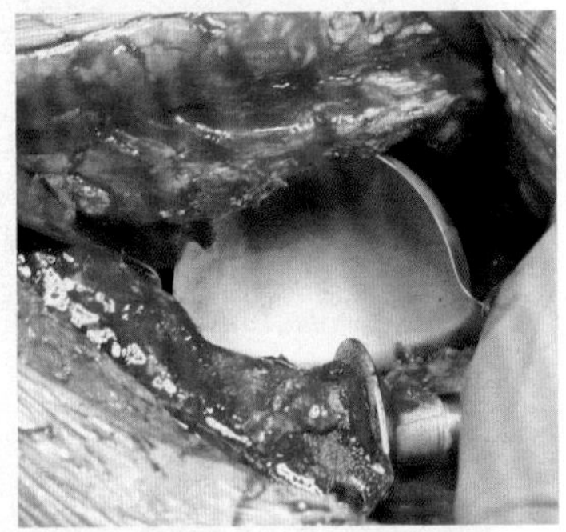

TECH FIG 3 • Bone preparation. **A.** The ilium is exposed. **B.** Minimal reaming is performed to allow the cage to seat. **C.** A trial cage is seated to determine whether the actual cage will seat. Small amounts of bone that interfere are removed.

Bone Graft and Trabecular Metal Augmentation

- The cage may not be stable in situations with severe superior dome or posterior bone loss.
  - It may be necessary to augment the acetabulum with either structural or particulate bone graft (**TECH FIG 4**) or trabecular metal to provide the cage with support.
  - Severe superior dome or posterior wall or column bone loss may be reconstructed with structural allograft fashioned from a distal femur, proximal tibia, or acetabular allograft.
- Trabecular metal acetabular components can be used in the cup–cage construct.
  - It may be necessary to support the trabecular metal acetabular component with a cage if native host bone contact is less than 50%. However, this technique is beyond the scope of this chapter.

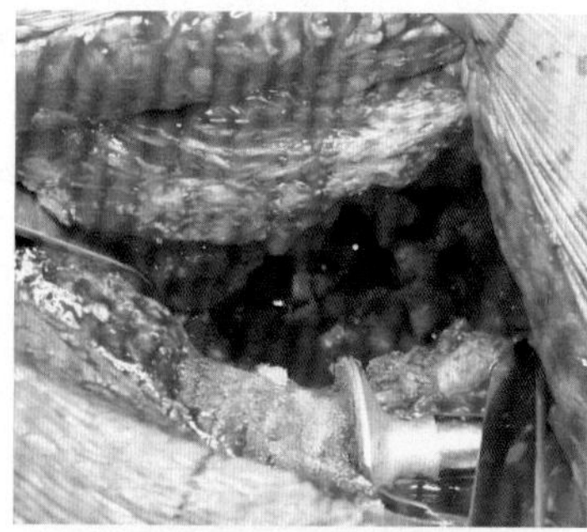

A

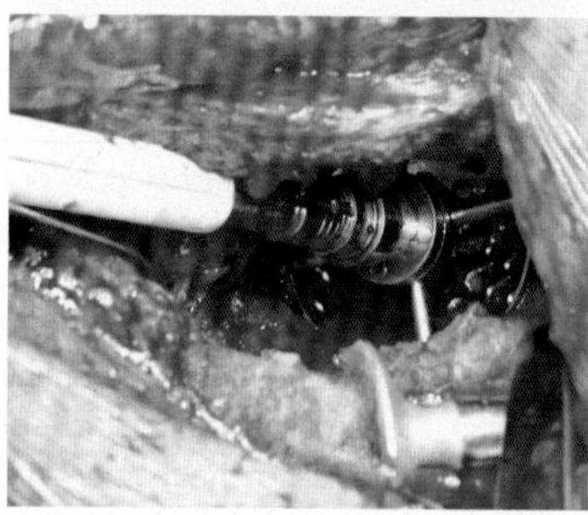

B

TECH FIG 4 • Bone graft and trabecular metal augmentation. **A.** Allograft cancellous bone is placed into the prepared acetabulum. **B.** Large reamer is used in reverse to crush and distribute the graft.

Cage Implantation

- The ischial flange can be placed on or in the ischium (**TECH FIG 5A,B**).
  - The advantage of placing the flange on the ischium is that screws can be used to fix the cage to the ischium (**TECH FIG 5C,D**).
  - The advantage of blade-plating the flange in the ischium is avoidance of the sciatic nerve (**TECH FIG 5E**).
  - Both methods allow for stable fixation.
- The cage is shaped to the contour of the ilium and ischium while allowing for seating of the socket portion of the cage into the remaining acetabulum. Usually, the ischial flange must be bent laterally to follow the contour of the ischium.

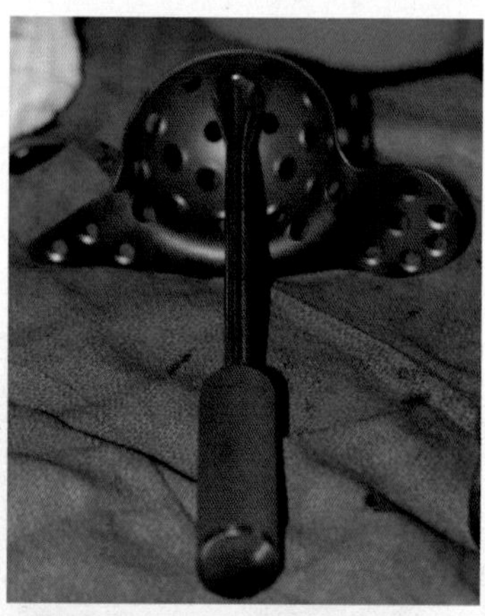

A

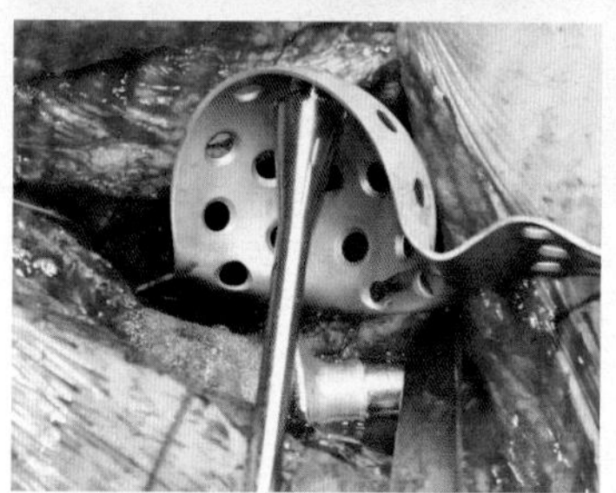

B

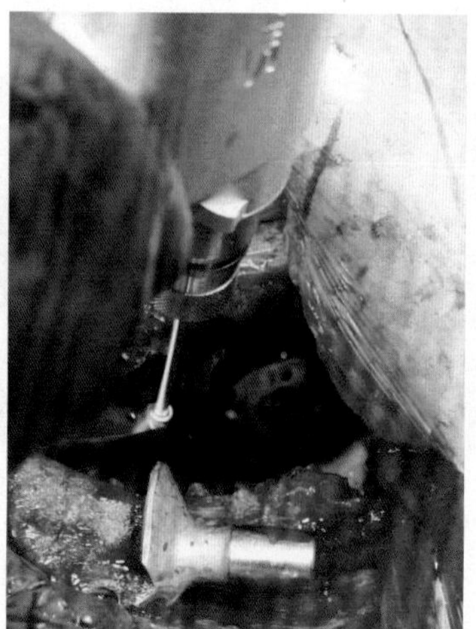

C

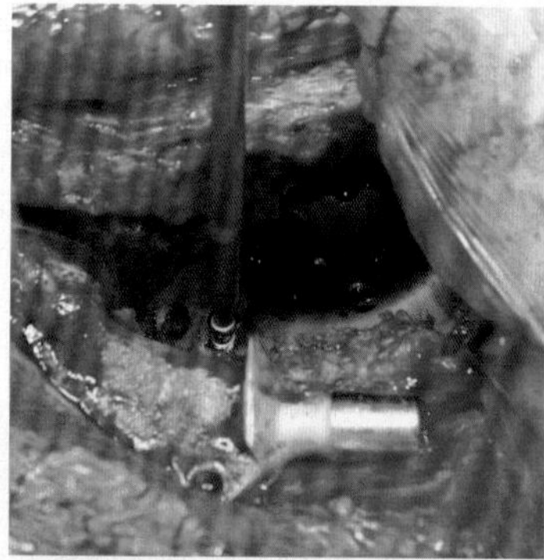

D

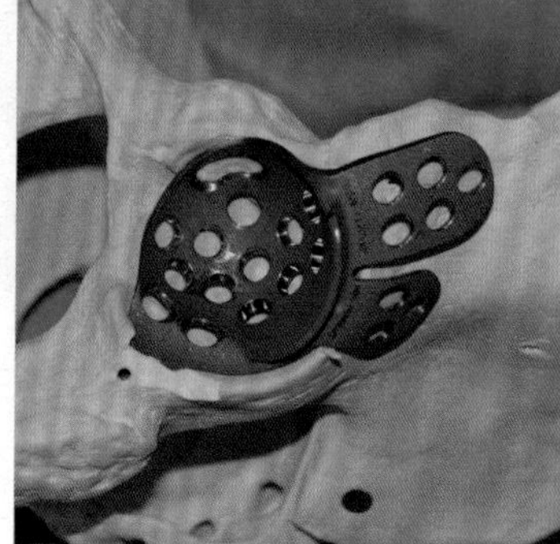

E

TECH FIG 5 • Cage implantation. **A.** The cage is shown in the orientation in which it will be inserted. **B.** Cage being inserted. **C,D.** Screw fixation to ischium. **E.** Blade plate fixation of the ischium flange. *(continued)*

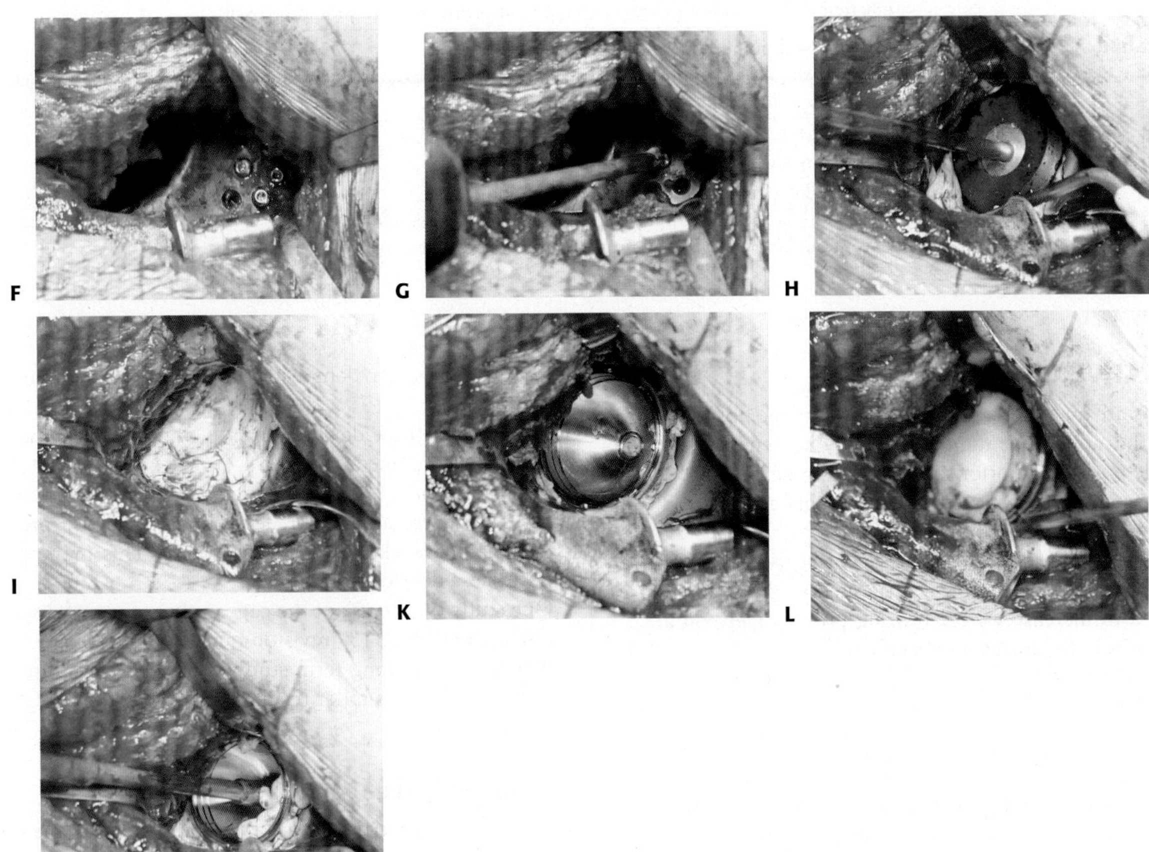

TECH FIG 5 • *(continued)* **F,G.** Screw fixation to the ilium. **H.** Cement pressurization. **I.** Cement after pressurization. **J,K.** Cup cemented in place. **L.** Polyethylene liner placed into cup.

- The ischial flange is fixed to or in the ischium using the surgeon's preferred method.
- The socket portion of the cage must be fully seated within the acetabulum to maximize the stability of the construct.
- The flange must be contoured to the ilium to minimize cage motion. Usually, this requires the flange to be bent medially with some rotation.
- Once the cage is appropriately contoured to the ischium, ilium, and acetabulum and fixed to the ischium, it is fixed with screws through the dome of the cage.
  - Fixation usually can be obtained in the posterior and anterior columns, with care to stay within the recognized safe zones.
- Additional screws should then be passed through the superior flange into the ilium (**TECH FIG 5F,G**). The number of screws is limited by the amount of bone that can safely provide fixation.
- A polyethylene liner is then cemented into the cage construct.
- The cement is placed in the socket and pressurized (**TECH FIG 5H–K**).
- A liner designed for cementation or a liner appropriately modified for cementation is then cemented into place in the appropriate position (**TECH FIG 5L**).
- A 2-mm cement mantle is desirable.
- Care must be taken not to leave large areas of the liner uncovered.

PEARLS AND PITFALLS

Preoperative planning	■ Thorough preoperative planning enables the surgeon to have the appropriate instrumentation, implants, bone graft, staff, and assistants available. ■ A complete plan includes contingency plans in case the primary plan is inadequate or the bone loss is worse than anticipated.
Preoperative workup	■ Infection must be excluded. ■ The patient's medical status must be optimized. ■ The patient must be compliant.

Intraoperative bone assessment	■ The remaining acetabulum must be assessed for ability to support an uncemented socket. If partial inherent stability is not possible, then an antiprotrusio cage should be used.
Bone preparation	■ Minimal additional bone should be removed. ■ The cage should be supported by adequate superior and posterior bone, which may require augmentation to be achieved.
Cage fixation	■ The ischial flange may be fixed on or in the ischium. ■ The socket portion of the cage must be fully seated. ■ The ilial flange must be contoured to the ilium. ■ Screws should be passed through the dome and ilial flange. ■ Care should be taken to remain within the "safe zones."

POSTOPERATIVE CARE

- Radiographs are taken to confirm appropriate cage positioning (**FIG 3**). Intraoperative radiographs may be beneficial to confirm cage positioning prior to final fixation of the device.
- The patient is allowed protected weight bearing as tolerated if bone augmentation was not necessary.
- The patient is restricted to toe-touch weight bearing for 6 to 12 weeks if bone augmentation was necessary. He or she is then allowed to increase weight bearing progressively on a schedule that is individualized to each patient.

OUTCOMES

- The survivorship of antiprotrusio cages has been acceptable in short- to midterm follow-up.
  - Several series have shown 100% survivorship at both 5 and 7.3 years[1,7] and 93.4% survivorship at 10.9 years.[3]
  - However, because most of these devices cannot achieve biologic fixation, it is assumed that they will loosen over time. Long-term results have been mixed, with one series reporting 92% survivorship at 21 years,[6] whereas another more recent study demonstrating a 61.75% survivorship at 14 years.[5]
- The success of these devices depends on the environment in which they are placed.
  - Most surgeons in North America use these devices only in cases of severe acetabular deficiency in which a press-fit uncemented socket is not appropriate. This may predispose these devices to failure.
  - One study on the use of the cage in the setting of discontinuity revealed a 31% revision rate at 46 months.[2]
  - A more recent, long-term study in patients with discontinuity has shown similar results with a 72.2% survival rate at 16.6 years.[4]

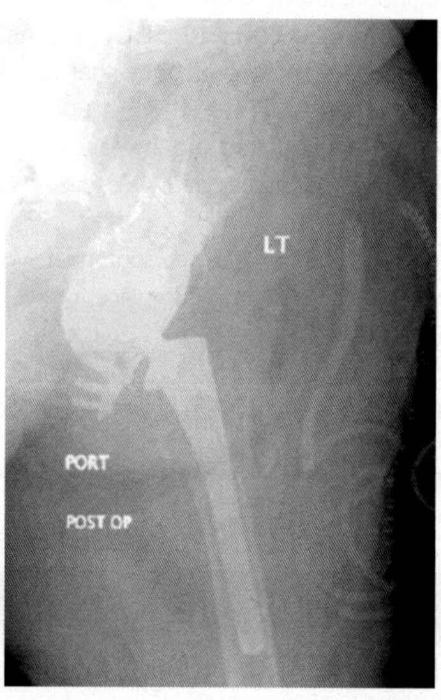

FIG 3 • Postoperative radiographs are taken to verify the position of the cage.

COMPLICATIONS

- The use of antiprotrusio cages is accompanied by the complications inherent to significant revision surgery:
  - Blood loss
  - Infection
  - Neurovascular injury
  - Construct failure
  - Anesthetic and medical complications

REFERENCES

1. Lamo-Espinosa J, Duart Clemente J, Diaz-Rada P, et al. The Burch-Schneider antiprotrusio cage: medium follow-up results. Musculoskelet Surg 2013;97:31–37.
2. Paprosky WG, Sporer S, O'Rourke MR. The treatment of pelvic discontinuity with acetabular cages. Clin Orthop Relat Res 2006;453: 183–187.
3. Pieringer H, Auersperg V, Bohler N. Reconstruction of severe acetabular bone-deficiency: the Burch-Schneider antiprotrusio cage in primary and revision total hip arthroplasty. J Arthroplasty 2006;21:489–496.
4. Regis D, Sandri A, Bonetti I, et al. A Minimum of 10-year follow-up of the Burch-Schneider cage and bulk allografts for the revision of pelvic discontinuity. J Arthroplasty 2012;27(6):1057–1063.
5. Symeonides PP, Petsatodes GE, Pournaras JD, et al. The effectiveness of the Burch-Schneider antiprotrusio cage for acetabular bony deficiency. J Arthroplasty 2009;24(2):168–174.
6. Wachtl SW, Jung M, Jakob RP, et al. The Burch-Schneider antiprotrusio cage in acetabular revision surgery: a mean follow-up of 12 years. J Arthroplasty 2000;15(8):959–963.
7. Winter E, Piert M, Volkmann R, et al. Allogeneic cancellous bone graft and a Burch-Schneider ring for acetabular reconstruction in revision hip arthroplasty. J Bone Joint Surg Am 2001;83A:862–867.

Revision Total Hip Arthroplasty: Pelvic Discontinuity

Paul B. McKenna and Matthew S. Austin

DEFINITION

- Pelvic discontinuity occurs when there is loss of continuity between the superior and inferior aspects of the pelvis as a result of disruption of both the anterior and posterior columns.

ANATOMY

- See **FIG 1**.

PATHOGENESIS

- Present in 0.9% of revision total hip arthroplasty procedures[1]
- Bone loss leading to a pelvic discontinuity can be the result of osteolysis secondary to polyethylene wear particles in combination with migration of the acetabular component.
- Other causes include trauma, stress fractures, infection, iatrogenic fractures, and aggressive reaming in either primary or revision surgery.
- Risk factors include female sex, rheumatoid arthritis, previous radiation exposure, and massive pelvic bone loss.

NATURAL HISTORY

- A pelvic discontinuity leads to motion between the superior and inferior hemipelvis. Pelvic discontinuities rarely heal without surgical intervention.[1,12]

PATIENT HISTORY AND PHYSICAL FINDINGS

- History should include all prior hip operations performed; reason for revision; and details of the surgery, outcomes, and complications.

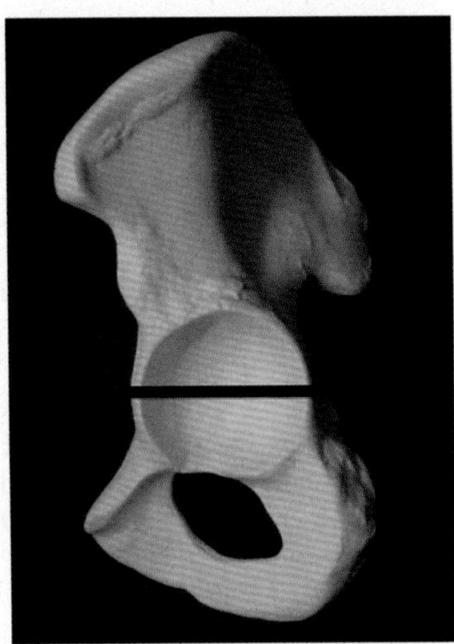

FIG 1 • A pelvic discontinuity is defined as a loss of continuity between the superior and inferior hemipelvis.

- It is particularly important to obtain information about prior surgeries, with particular attention paid to risk factors for infection such as prolonged wound drainage.
- The patient should be queried regarding a history of trauma.
- Obtaining prior operative reports is paramount; information including the approach used, surgical findings, and details of the prosthesis in situ should be sought.
- Pain can often be quite significant, especially in acute discontinuities, and usually is located in the groin but may also present in the buttock or thigh.
- A history of unexplained fevers and rest pain should alert the physician to the possibility of infection.
- The neurovascular status of the extremity should be assessed and documented. Patients with vascular compromise should be referred to vascular specialists for evaluation.
- Abductor function should be assessed. Nonfunction of the abductors may occur from disruption of the abductors; a shortened lever arm secondary to superior migration; and/or medialization of the acetabular component, superior gluteal nerve injury, or pain inhibition.
- Leg lengths should be measured and recorded. The patient should be counseled regarding postoperative leg length inequality and reasonable expectations.

IMAGING AND OTHER DIAGNOSTIC STUDIES

- Pelvic discontinuity can be identified on plain radiographs; however, it can be unrecognized preoperatively and one must maintain an index of suspicion with certain bone loss patterns. Paprosky et al[13] noted, in a series of 147 patients with discontinuity, that 11% were diagnosed at operation and not detected by radiographs.
- Anteroposterior (AP) pelvis (**FIG 2**) radiographic findings suggestive of pelvic discontinuity include the following:
  - A visible fracture line or bone defect that includes both columns of the acetabulum
  - A medial shift or rotation of the inferior hemipelvis in relation to the superior hemipelvis
  - Asymmetry of the obturator foramen in a well-centered radiograph
- Iliac oblique (**FIG 3**) and false-profile views of Lequesne should also be obtained to increase sensitivity for the detection of discontinuity as opposed to a single AP view of the pelvis.[24]
- Computed tomography (CT) studies with a metal artifact suppression technique can be useful in confirming the presence of a discontinuity, further defining the extent of bone loss, aiding in preoperative planning, and for the design of custom implants, if needed (**FIG 4**).
- For components that have migrated medial to Kohler line, contrast CT can define the proximity of the intrapelvic contents to the implant.

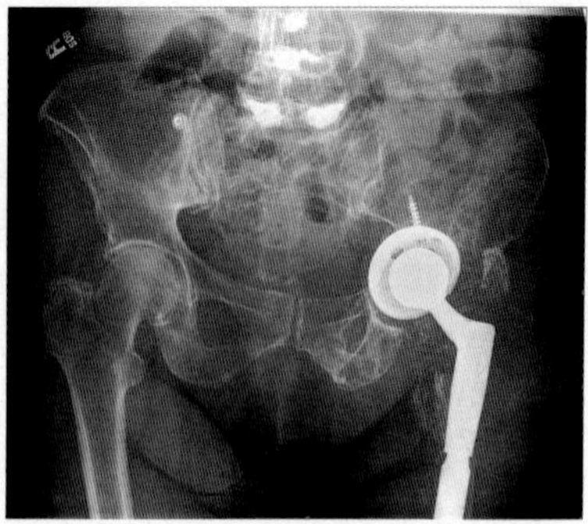

FIG 2 • AP pelvis of pelvic discontinuity. Note the superomedial migration of the acetabular component, obliteration of Kohler line, ischial osteolysis, and the asymmetry of the obturator foramen. These x-ray findings should alert the surgeon to the possible presence of a discontinuity.

- Patients should be screened for infection with serology (erythrocyte sedimentation rate [ESR] and C-reactive protein [CRP]). If either ESR or CRP is significantly elevated, image-guided aspiration should be performed to obtain synovial white blood cell count, differential, and culture.

DIFFERENTIAL DIAGNOSIS

- Pelvic discontinuity can occur from aseptic loosening, osteolysis as a result of particulate wear, iatrogenic damage, trauma, infection, or tumor.

NONOPERATIVE MANAGEMENT

- Can be used in cases of massive bone loss, resulting in a defect that cannot be reconstructed
- Also useful in cases where there is an unacceptable surgical risk
- Conservative management includes walking aids and/or wheelchairs for mobility, shoe modifications for leg length discrepancy, and analgesia medications.

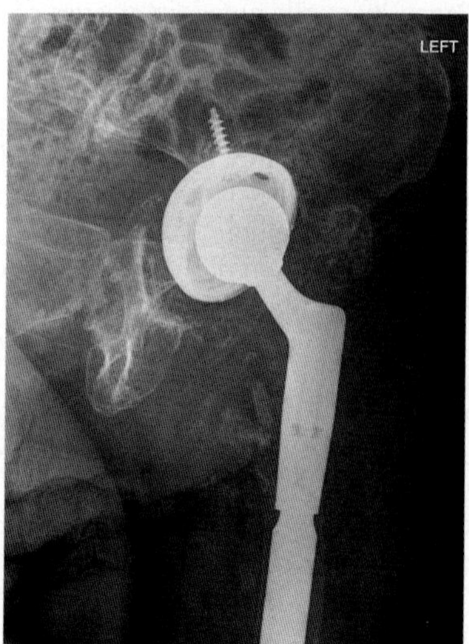

FIG 3 • Iliac oblique view of discontinuity further demonstrates migration of the acetabular component. There is a massive amount of bone loss at the medial wall of the acetabulum and no evidence of bony contact between the inferior and superior hemipelvis.

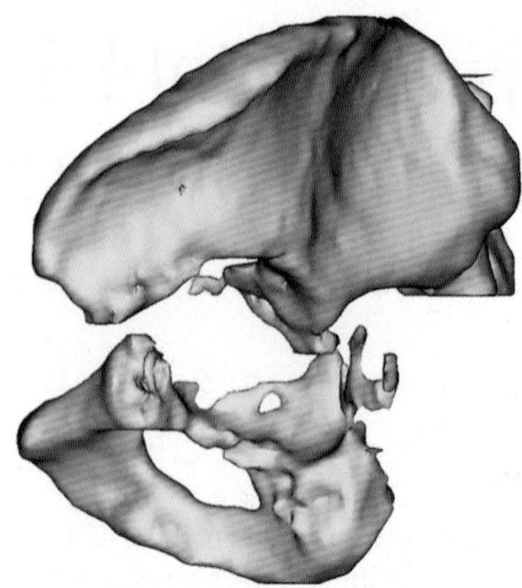

FIG 4 • Metal subtraction CT scan demonstrating massive bone loss and pelvic discontinuity.

SURGICAL MANAGEMENT

- The goals of surgical management of a pelvic discontinuity are as follows:
  - Stabilization of the hemipelvis
  - Achievement of stable acetabular component fixation
  - Restoration of hip biomechanics
  - Appropriate soft tissue balancing
  - Leg length optimization

Preoperative Planning

- Treatment and prognosis differs depending on the type and degree of bone loss and the length of time the discontinuity has been present.
  - Acute (healing potential)
  - Chronic (reduced healing potential)
- An AP of the pelvis can be used to define the extent of the majority of the bony defects. There are four factors that help classify acetabular bone loss:
  - Presence and degree of superior migration of the hip center
  - Presence and degree of ischial osteolysis
  - Presence of "teardrop" osteolysis
  - Position of the acetabular component in relation to Kohler line
- These factors allow the surgeon to anticipate the degree and location of bone loss as well as plan the reconstruction.
- The Paprosky classification is one of the more commonly used classification systems and is useful to define bone loss and guide subsequent reconstruction.[13]
- The Paprosky classification does not have a specific pelvic discontinuity subclassification; however, the majority of pelvic discontinuities are Paprosky type IIIB, in which radiographs demonstrate extensive ischial osteolysis and obliteration of the teardrop, more than 3 cm of superomedial migration of the acetabular component, and a break in Kohler line. There is typically less than 50% of host bone available for osseointegration.
- Several surgical techniques for dealing with pelvic discontinuity have been reported. The technique of choice is based on the degree of bone loss, the chronicity of the discontinuity, and cost.

- Intrapelvic hardware may require a retroperitoneal approach to extract the hardware and avoid iatrogenic damage to vital structures.
- Surgical techniques include the following:
  - Posterior column plating and a cementless acetabular component with or without porous metal augments/structural bone graft
  - Acetabular distraction
  - The use of an off-the-shelf reconstruction cage with or without porous metal augments/structural bone allograft with or without posterior column plating
  - The use of a triflange prosthesis (custom)
  - The use of cup–cage constructs

Positioning

- The patient should be positioned according to surgeon preference and in accordance with standard surgical principles.
- Draping should allow for extensile exposure, allowing for the possible need for a retroperitoneal approach in case of a vascular complication.

Approach

- The approach is chosen based on the surgeon's preference but may also be dictated by the pattern of the bone loss and reconstructive plan.
- The acetabulum, including the ilium, ischium, and pubis, can be adequately exposed through the following approaches:
  - Posterior
  - Direct lateral (Hardinge)
  - Transtrochanteric
- A posterior approach may facilitate exposure of the posterior column for plating.
- A trochanteric slide or extended trochanteric osteotomy may be helpful to maneuver the femur out of the way.

TECHNIQUES

Posterior Column Plating and a Cementless Acetabular Component with or without Porous Metal Augments and/or Structural Allograft

- Plating may be more useful in acute as opposed to chronic discontinuity.
- Plating relies on the ability of the bone to heal, but in the case of a chronic discontinuity with a large amount of bone loss and an unfavorable biologic environment, nonunion is a common outcome.[1]
- Open reduction and internal fixation of the posterior column is performed primarily.
- Acetabular reamers are placed in position to restore the hip center. The reamer/trial should achieve two points of fixation (anterior to posterior, anteroinferior to posterosuperior, or anterosuperior to posteroinferior).
- Porous metal augments or structural allograft may be used to restore a rim to enhance press-fit fixation. The location and orientation of the augments depends on the pattern of the bone loss. The available size and shape of porous metal augments allows for significant flexibility. The augments may be applied either before or after the acetabular component is implanted. To reduce fretting between the augments and the acetabular component, it is recommended that the interface between the two be fixed with bone cement.
- Particulate bone graft may then be placed in any remaining crevices or defects.
- Screws are recommended to supplement acetabular component fixation.

Acetabular Distraction

- Acetabular distraction is an option in the presence of chronic pelvic discontinuity. In chronic discontinuity, there is often both poor bone stock and an inadequate biologic environment for bone healing, leading to high failure rates of internal fixation and cage techniques.[7,14,16]
- The principle of acetabular distraction depends on the elastic nature of the pelvis. The discontinuity is distracted and the elasticity of the pelvis provides some intrinsic stability of the component that is wedged between the superior and inferior hemipelvis. Osseointegration then provides long-term fixation of the component.[16]
- All fibrous tissue is removed from the acetabulum to reveal bleeding, viable bone.
- Hemispherical reamers are placed in the acetabulum in a position to restore the native hip center. The reamers are sequentially increased in size until contact is made between the superior and inferior hemipelvis. It is important to avoid aggressive reaming as the goal is not to remove bone but achieve two-point fixation. This provides for initial stability of the component and stabilization of the discontinuity.
- Porous metal augments or structural allograft may be helpful to fill any large cavitary defects or augment initial stability of the acetabular component.
- Particulate bone graft may be used to fill cavitary defects as well.
- It is recommended to use bone cement to fix the interface of the porous metal augment and the acetabular component to avoid fretting.
- A porous metal acetabular component 6 to 8 mm larger than the last reamer is chosen and impacted into place by positioning the inferior aspect of the component against the ischium. The implant is then rotated into proper position while keeping the inferior aspect of the component secured against the ischium. The oversized implant generates a distracting force against the elasticity of the pelvis and creates initial stability (**TECH FIG 1**).
- Supplemental fixation with multiple screws is recommended.
- A polyethylene component can be cemented into the shell. Cementation allows the screws to function as a fixed-angle device, aiding the stability of the construct.

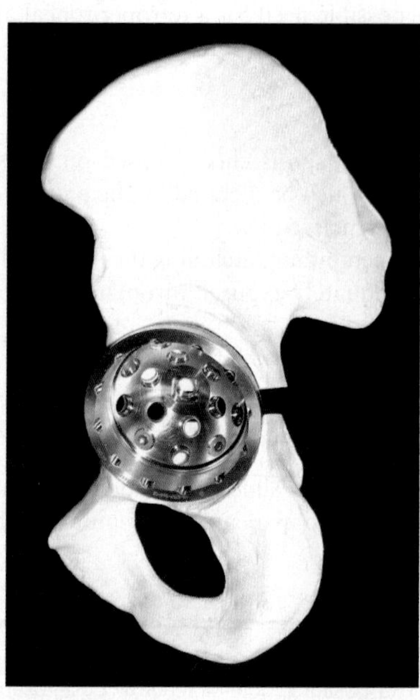

TECH FIG 1 • The acetabular distraction method relies on the elastic nature of the superior and inferior hemipelvis. A cup 6 to 8 mm larger than the last reamer is inserted, distracting the acetabulum. Multiple screws supplement fixation.

Off-the-Shelf Reconstruction Cages with or without Porous Metal Augments/Structural Bone Allograft with or without Posterior Column Plating

- Cages are relatively affordable and easily available.
- These are large metallic cups that have malleable flanges with screw holes for fixation in the ilium and ischium (**TECH FIG 2A**).
- Cages are often used in conjunction with bone allograft or posterior plating and serve to mechanically protect the construct while incorporation of the allograft and/or healing of the discontinuity occurs.
- The cages can also serve as internal fixation devices, especially in acute discontinuity.
- Potential disadvantages include the following:
  - Limited or no osseointegration potential
  - Malleable flanges predispose the construct to fatigue failure.
  - Predetermined shapes and sizes do not readily conform to the host bone, creating increased areas of strain and additional intraoperative work.

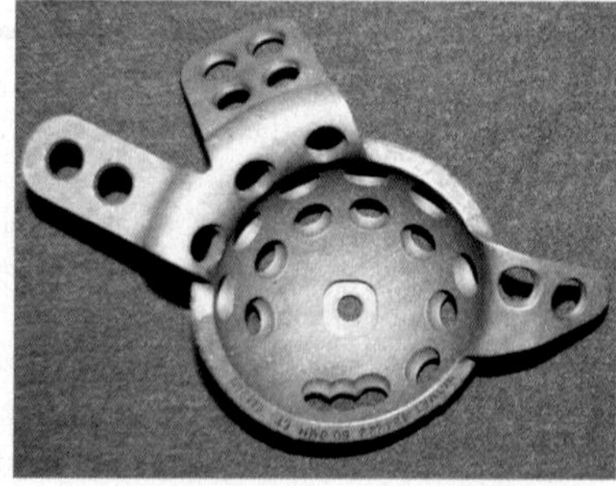

A

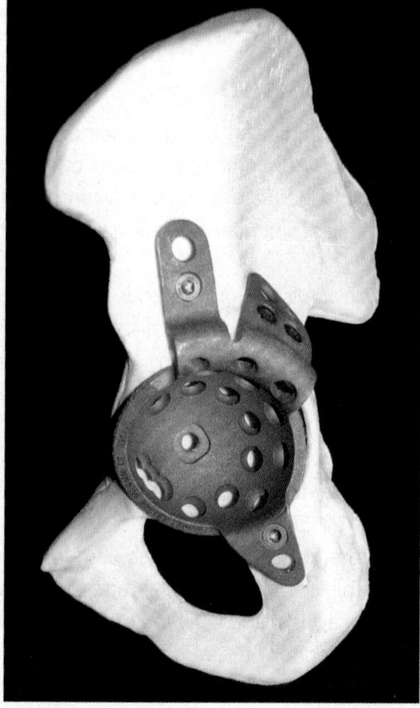

B

TECH FIG 2 • **A.** Acetabular cage. This off-the-shelf cage has multiple screw holes for fixation, along with malleable flanges (Max-*Ti* protrusion cage; Biomet, Warsaw, IN). **B.** Acetabular cage fixation. The ischial flange can either be fixated with screws (as shown) or through a slot in the ischial bone. Care must be taken in the insertion of any screws into the ischium as sciatic nerve palsy is a risk.

- The acetabulum must be exposed to allow visualization of the ilium, ischium, inferior cotyloid fossa, and remainder of the columns.
- Care must be taken when exposing the ilium so as not to endanger the superior gluteal nerve and artery. The deep branch of the superior gluteal artery and superior gluteal nerve traverse deep to the gluteus medius, roughly 4 to 6 cm superior to the acetabular rim.
- All fibrous tissue should be removed from the acetabulum.
- If structural allograft is required, it should be prepared at this time.
  - The remaining ilium, which provides support to the allograft, is identified.
  - Acetabular reamers are used to size the extent of the cavity and help identify the amount and position of potentially supportive bone.
  - The structural allograft is prepared to provide support for the superior aspect of the cage.
  - The allograft is secured to the ilium using multiple large fragment screws with washers.
  - A porous metal augment can be used in the same fashion as allograft.
  - An appropriately sized cage is chosen to fit the reconstructed acetabulum and bridge the ilium and ischium, thereby protecting the allograft/augment.
- The flanges can be bent so as to ensure maximum bone contact. Care should be taken to minimize the number of times that the flange is bent as excessive bending results in metal fatigue and leads to early failure.
- The ischial flange can be fixated either by the use of a slot in the ischium or with a screw. Slotted fixation is safer as there is an increased rate of screw fracture associated with migration of the cage and sciatic nerve palsy.[2,7]
- To create the slot for the ischial flange, the ischium needs to be exposed. Care must be taken to protect the sciatic nerve during this maneuver due to its close proximity.
- A drill is used to place a hole posteroinferiorly in the optimum direction for the flange. This hole is widened with a small osteotome to allow the inferior flange to slot into the bone.
- Ischial fixation is paramount to avoid cage failure.
- The ilial flange is secured with multiple bicortical screws. Care must be taken to avoid intrapelvic penetration of drills or screws. Dome screws in the acetabular portion of the cage are recommended. There may be limited bone available for screw fixation (**TECH FIG 2B**).
- A polyethylene liner can then be cemented into the cage. Care must be taken to achieve correct inclination and version.

Custom Triflange Component

- The custom triflange component is most often used in type IIIB defects with an associated pelvic discontinuity.
- The advantages of the custom triflange over the noncustom cage are as follows:
  - Potential improved conformity with host bone
  - Greater construct rigidity and less chance of fatigue failure
  - Porous ongrowth surface to allow for osseointegration (some noncustom cages have limited coating as well)
- The disadvantages of the triflange include the following:
  - Limited availability; requirement for advanced imaging, manufacture time, and expense
  - Inability to modify the cage intraoperatively
- The goal of acetabular reconstruction with the triflange cage is to achieve initial stable fixation through intimate contact between structural host bone and the ilial, ischial, and pubic flanges augmented with multiple screws.
- The design of the triflange component is a customized process based on a metal subtraction, implant-specific CT scan sequence (**TECH FIG 3A**).

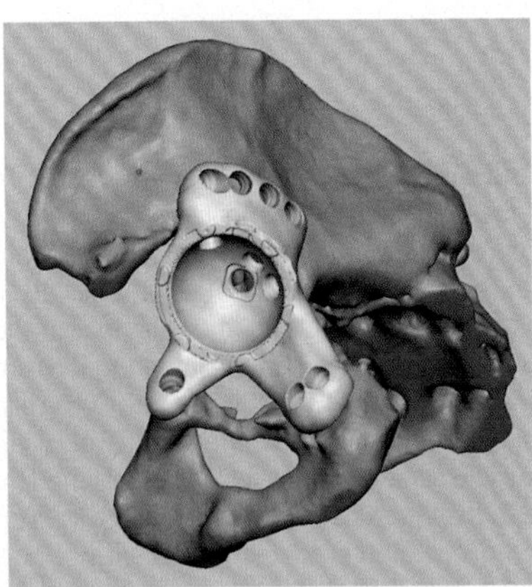
A

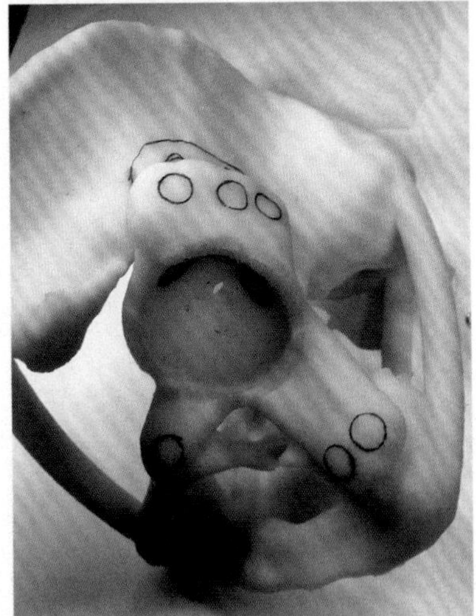
B

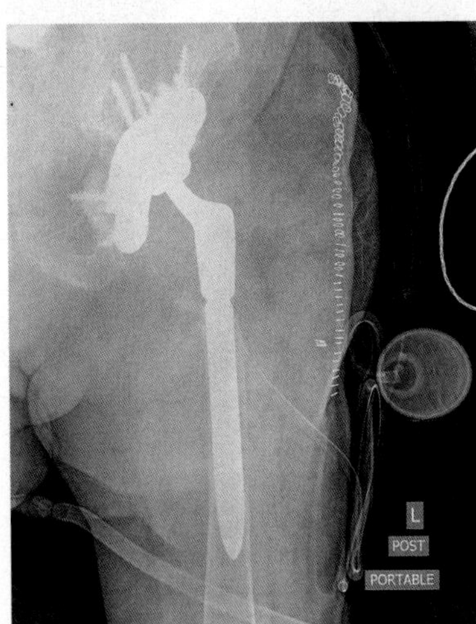

C

TECH FIG 3 • **A.** A three-dimensional metal subtraction CT scan is used to design a custom triflange implant. The size and position of the implant takes into account the remaining bone stock and orientation of the pelvis. **B.** A physical model of the proposed construct is created. Screw hole position and direction can be determined to maximize host bone contact. Both the manufacturer and surgeon have input into the production of the true component. **C.** Radiograph of custom triflange. Note the multiple screw fixation, maximizing the limited remaining host bone.

- A three-dimensional computer generated one-to-one physical model of the patient's hemipelvis is created (**TECH FIG 3B**).
- From the remaining landmarks (ilium, obturator foramen, and pubic ramus), the patient's hip center, cup orientation, and flange geometry are determined. A minor amount of host bone may need to be removed to allow the implant to seat appropriately. This is detailed on the model.
- Screw hole positioning in the cup and flanges is determined and is available in either standard or locking configurations.
- The exposure of the acetabulum is similar to that previously mentioned. All fibrous tissue in the remaining acetabular bone is removed. The iliac wing and ischium need to be adequately visualized to ensure the flanges are seated. As mentioned, a small amount of host bone may need to be removed to allow the implant to seat appropriately.
- Bone allograft can be placed at this point.
- The ischial flange is placed on the surface of the ischium and secured with screws. Care must be taken to avoid iatrogenic damage to the sciatic nerve.
- It is recommended that the first ilial screw be nonlocking, pulling the flange into intimate contact with the host bone, helping reduce the discontinuity, and rotating the inferior half of the hemipelvis into the correct orientation. Pubic screws are then placed (**TECH FIG 3C**).

Cup–Cage Construct

- The rationale for the cup–cage construct is to use the ilioischial cage to provide initial stability to a pelvic discontinuity and to protect a porous metal acetabular component from mechanical forces, allowing for biologic stabilization from both the superior and inferior aspects of the hemipelvis into the porous metal component. This biologic fixation gives the construct its long-term stability.
- Exposure and confirmation of the discontinuity are the same as for the previous techniques.
- Exposure of the ilium should be performed with care to avoid damage to the superior gluteal nerve and artery.
- The acetabulum is reamed sequentially until two-point contact is made and bleeding bone is seen (usually anterosuperior and posteroinferior). This is similar to the technique described in the posterior column plating and cementless acetabular component section earlier. However, this technique is only used in cases with more extensive bone loss.
- Particulate bone graft is packed into the defects and reverse reamed. Care should be taken to ensure that the pelvis is not breached.
- The acetabulum is sized for the appropriate porous metal acetabular component. It is preferred to use a nonmodular porous metal component to allow for the cup portion of the off-the-shelf cage to fit inside the porous metal acetabular component. The cage then spans the defect from ilium to ischium.
- The porous metal component is impacted and supplemental fixation is achieved with screws. If necessary, new drill holes can be made in the porous metal cup adjacent to bone (**TECH FIG 4A**).
- If press-fit cannot be achieved due to the severity of the bone loss, or if a large portion of the superior cup is uncovered, a porous metal augment may be placed to supplement fixation and act as a buttress.
- The cage is then placed in position, ensuring bony contact with both the ilial and ischial flanges using the techniques described earlier. Additionally, screws are used to transfix the cage through the porous metal cup (**TECH FIG 4B**).
- The polyethylene component is cemented into the cage. The cement needs to be pressurized so that any gaps between the cage and the trabecular metal acetabular component are eliminated. This reduces micromotion between the hemispherical parts of the cage and the acetabular component.

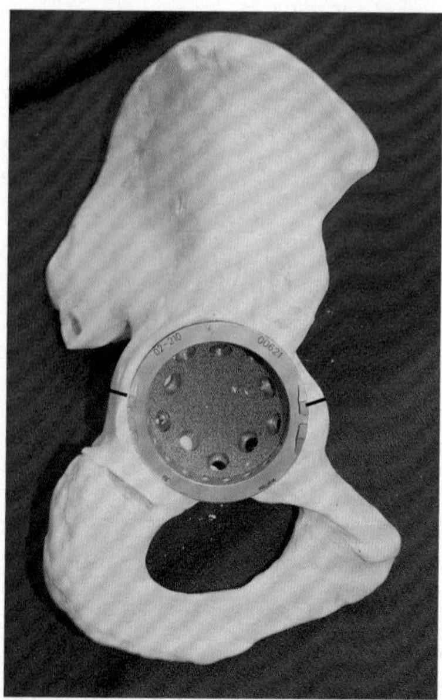
A

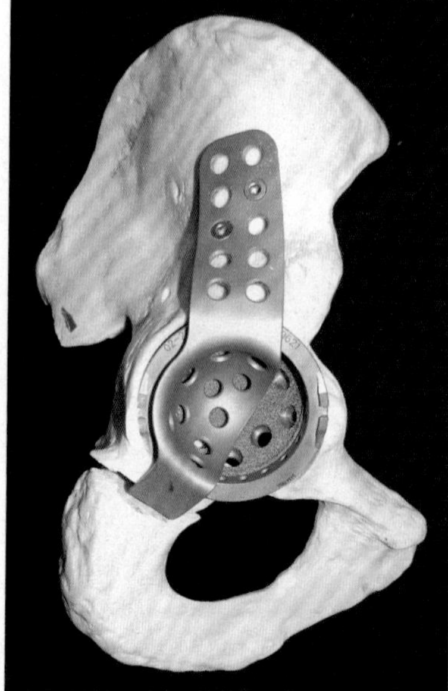
B

TECH FIG 4 • A. Cup–cage construct. A porous metal cup is impacted into the defect, ensuring that two points of contact are achieved. Eventual bony ingrowth will occur in both hemispheres of the cup to achieve eventual stability. Note the slot in the ischium for fixation of the ischial flange. **B.** Cup–cage construct. A cage is inserted and fixed with multiple screws. A polyethylene cup is then inserted with the correct inclination and version and fixed with cement. The cement not only fixates the polyethylene cup but also eliminates any micromotion between the cage and the porous metal cup, along with the screws.

PEARLS AND PITFALLS

Preoperative planning is invaluable.	■ Classifying bony defects and anticipating equipment needs are essential in efficiently and effectively dealing with pelvic discontinuity. Develop a sequential, stepwise plan for the reconstruction.
Adequate exposure is paramount.	■ Failure to expose the ilium, ischium, and pubis increases the difficulty of the case and may lead to component malpositioning.
The fibrous interface must be removed from the acetabulum.	■ Failure to remove the fibrous interface may lead to lack of appreciation of the bony defects and failure of osseointegration.
It is critical to obtain rigid fixation.	■ Failure to obtain rigid fixation may lead to early failure of the construct.
Spatial awareness is essential.	■ Routine landmarks may be obscured or missing. This may lead to iatrogenic damage to bone or soft tissue structures.
Plan for the worst.	■ It may be necessary to have a general or vascular surgeon available if components are intrapelvic.

POSTOPERATIVE CARE

- Depending on the construct, weight bearing may be restricted for 6 to 12 weeks. Gradual increase in weight bearing is then permitted. The degree and duration of weight bearing is individual according to bone defect, bone quality, and surgeon preference.
- We recommend hip precautions during the acute postoperative period secondary to the large surgical dissection usually required. Hip precautions are specific to approach.
- Patients are followed at routine intervals after surgery. The authors prefer follow-up at 6 weeks, 3 months, 6 months, and annually.

OUTCOMES

- There is no perfect solution for to the difficult problem of a pelvic discontinuity, especially in the situation where there is a large bone stock deficiency. Each discontinuity has its own "personality," and no one solution can be used for all types. The outcomes of surgical treatment of pelvic discontinuity include the following:
  - A high rate of complications
  - Early and late implant failure
  - Failure to consistently restore bone stock
- Compression plating of the posterior column with 3.5-mm reconstruction plates, supplemented by porous metal shell in the acute fracture setting, has seen relatively positive results, with survivorship at 18 to 36 months of up to 100%.[15,18,20] This suggests that, in acute discontinuity, the bone does indeed possess fracture healing potential.
- Chronic pelvic discontinuities have traditionally had high failure rates (14% to 50%), particularly in the presence of Paprosky type IIIB bone loss.[1,5,7,9,14] This failure is largely believed to occur due to nonunion.
- Noncustom off-the-shelf acetabular cages are designed to bridge the defect. They are often used in conjunction with large structural allografts to help restore bone stock. Osseointegration potential is often limited to none, and failure due to micromotion and fatigue occur. Failure rates of 50% to 60% have been reported due to mechanical loosening or fatigue failure of the flange.[7,16,25] This usually occurs in the first 18 months after implantation and is evident on radiographs. Typically, the failure pattern is loosening of the ischial screws and disengagement of the ischial flange. The addition of posterior column plates or structural allograft does not seem to improve the results. In a series by Goodman et al[7] of 10 pelvic discontinuities fixed with bulk allograft and a support cage, 5 were unsuccessful. Three of these became loose, two continued to have a pelvic dissociation, two flanges fractured, and three patients experienced hip instability.
- The relatively poor results of using noncustom cages and the lack of biologic ingrowth into the supporting structures led to the use of custom triflange components. Their increased mechanical stability and porous ongrowth surface make them an attractive option. There are reports of success with this technique.[3,4,22] Taunton et al[22] described a large series of 57 patients treated with a custom triflange. At a minimum follow-up of 2 years, only 1 of the 57 (1.7%) had signs of loosening and 81% had radiographic evidence of stable components with a healed pelvic discontinuity. At an average of 10 years follow-up, DeBoer et al[4] demonstrated healing of the discontinuity in 18 of 20 hips. These results are encouraging. However, expense and the time to create the models for implants are drawbacks to routine use of these constructs.
- Failure of allograft and autograft bone grafting techniques have driven surgeons to find other materials, such as porous metal, that can span the discontinuity and provide internal fixation to the superior and inferior hemipelvic fragments. Surgeons have used porous metal to span the superior and inferior aspects of the pelvis (cup–cage construct or distraction) with some success.[4,10,15,17,19,22]
- The cup–cage technique, which was first described by Hanssen and Lewallen,[8] does not try to restore bone stock with bone but porous metal. The cage is seen as a temporary fixation measure, whereas the trabecular metal cup achieves union with both the superior and inferior aspects of the pelvis, giving it long-term stability. Midterm results have been generally positive. Kosashvili et al[10] reported no component migration in 88.5% of their 26 cases at a mean follow-up of 44 months. Rogers et al[15] reported an 86.3% survivorship rate at 8 years in nine patients.

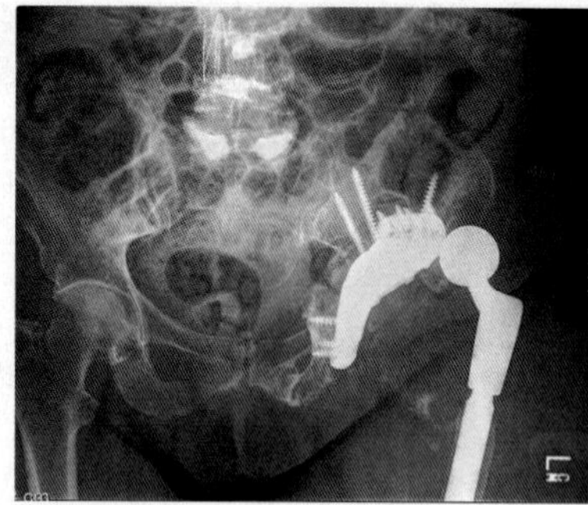

FIG 5 • Dislocation can occur in as high as 30% of cases. Some authors have recommended the liberal use of constrained liners for certain cases.

- In the presence of a pelvic discontinuity, achieving initial stability of a trabecular metal cup can be difficult because of the relative motion between the two segments of the acetabulum and the degree of bone loss. An alternative technique, which has gained recent favor, is acetabular distraction, first described by Sporer et al[17] In their original series, 19 of 20 patients were radiologically stable at an average of 4 years follow-up and 17 of these were reported to be pain free. Four of the original 20 did have some early component migration that later became stable and asymptomatic. The majority in this series (13) were hips with a Paprosky type IIIB bone defect.

COMPLICATIONS

- High complication rates have been reported for reconstruction for pelvic discontinuity, ranging from 25% to 80%.[3,5,7] The most frequent complications are dislocation, infection, nerve injury, and loss of fixation or implant failure.
- Dislocation may occur in up to 15% to 30% of cases (**FIG 5**).[3,4,6,22,23] Secondary to these high rates, some authors have reported the use of constrained liners in all revisions with an associated pelvic discontinuity.[6] The potential drawback of constrained liners in this setting is increased strain on the construct and perhaps an increased chance of nonunion and failure.
- Others have proposed a more selective use of constrained liners, such as in cases with severe abductor insufficiency or extensive soft tissue scarring and damage, a deficient proximal femur, nonunion of the greater trochanter, or history of recurrent dislocation.[3,23]
- Neurologic injury is a concern, with injury to either the superior gluteal nerve or the sciatic nerve.
- Superior gluteal nerve injury can be the result of surgical dissection or by placement of the component. This may be an etiology of postoperative Trendelenburg gait, poor abductor function, and instability of the hip.
- Sciatic nerve injury most commonly occurs during exposure of the ischium for fixation of the inferior flange of a cage.
- Reported rates of infection associated with pelvic discontinuity reconstruction range from 6% to 10%.[1,7,11,14,19,21]

REFERENCES

1. Berry DJ, Lewallan DG, Hanssen AD, et al. Pelvic discontinuity in revision total hip arthroplasty. J Bone Joint Surg Am 1999;81:1692–1702.
2. Chahal J, McCarthy T, Safir O, et al. Late presentation of sciatic neuropathy after failure of acetabular reconstruction rings in revision hip arthroplasty: a report of two cases. Curr Orthop Pract 2008;19:688–690.
3. Christie MJ, Barrington SA, Brinson MF. Bridging massive acetabular defects with the triflanged cup: 2 to 9 years result. Clin Orthop Relat Res 2001;393:216–227.
4. DeBoer DK, Christie MJ, Brinson MF, et al. Revision total hip arthroplasty for pelvic discontinuity. J Bone Joint Surg Am 2007;89:835–840.
5. Eggli S, Muller C, Ganz R. Revision surgery in pelvic discontinuity. Clin Orthop Relat Res 2002;398:136–145.
6. Garbuz D, Morsi E, Mohamed N, et al. Classification and reconstruction in revision acetabular arthroplasty with bone stock deficiency. Clin Orthop Relat Res 1996;(324):98–107.
7. Goodman S, Sastamoinen H, Shasha N. Complications of ilio-ischial reconstruction rings in revision total hip arthroplasty. J Arthroplasty 2004;19:436–446.
8. Hanssen AD, Lewallen DG. Modular acetabular augments: composite void fillers. Orthopedics 2005;28:971–971.
9. Holt GE, Dennis DA. Use of custom triflanged acetabular components in revision total hip arthroplasty. Clin Orthop Relat Res 2004;429:209–214.
10. Kosashvili Y, Backstein D, Safie O, et al. Acetabular revision using an anti-protrusion (ilio-ischial) cage and trabecular metal acetabular component for severe acetabular bone loss associated with pelvis discontinuity. J Bone Joint Surg Br 2009;91:870–876.
11. Lietman SA, Bhawnani K. The partial pelvic replacement cup in severe acetabular defects. Orthopedics 2001;24(12):1131–1135.
12. Moed BR, McMichael JC. Outcomes of posterior wall fractures of the acetabulum. J Bone Joint Surg Am 2007;89:1170–1176.
13. Paprosky WG, Perona PG, Lawrence JM. Acetabular defect classification and surgical reconstruction in revision arthroplasty. A 6-year follow-up evaluation. J Arthroplasty 1994;9:33–44.
14. Paprosky WG, Sporer S, O'Rourke MR. The treatment of pelvic discontinuity with acetabular cages. Clin Orthop Relat Res 2006;453:183–187.
15. Rogers BA, Whittingham-Jones PM, Mitchell PA, et al. The reconstruction of periprosthetic pelvic discontinuity. J Arthroplasty 2012;27:1499–1506.
16. Sembrano JN, Cheng EY. Acetabular cage survival and analysis of factors related to failure. Clin Orthop Relat Res 2008;466:1657–1665.
17. Sporer SM, Bottros JJ, Hulst JB, et al. Acetabular distraction. Clin Orthop Relat Res 2012;470:3156–3163.
18. Sporer SM, O'Rourke M, Paprosky WG. The treatment of pelvic discontinuity during acetabular revision. J Arthroplasty 2005;20(4)(suppl 2):79–84.
19. Sporer SM, Paprosky WG. Acetabular revision using a trabecular metal acetabular component for severe acetabular bone loss associated with a pelvic discontinuity. J Arthroplasty 2006;21:87–90.
20. Springer BD, Berry DJ, Cabanela ME, et al. Early postoperative transverse pelvic fracture: a new complication related to revision arthroplasty with an uncemented cup. J Bone Joint Surg Am 2005;87(12):2626–2631.
21. Stiehl JB, Saluja R, Diener T. Reconstruction of major column defects and pelvic discontinuity in revision total hip arthroplasty. J Arthroplasty 2000;15:849–857.
22. Taunton MJ, Fehring TK, Edward P, et al. Pelvic discontinuity treated with custom triflange component: a reliable option. Clin Orthop Relat Res 2012;470:428–434.
23. Udomkiat P, Dorr LD, Won YY. Technical factors for success with metal ring acetabular reconstruction. J Arthroplasty 2001;16:961–969.
24. Wendt MC, Adler MA, Trousdale RT, et al. Effectiveness of false profile radiographs in detection of pelvic discontinuity. J Arthroplasty 2012;27:1408–1412.
25. Winter E, Piert M, Volkmann R, et al. Allogeneic cancellous bone graft and a Burch-Schneider ring for acetabular reconstruction in revision hip arthroplasty. J Bone Joint Surg Am 2001;83:862–867.

32

CHAPTER

Hemiarthroplasty of the Hip

Hari P. Bezwada

DEFINITION

- Femoral neck fractures are classified according to the Garden classification (Table 1).[9]
  - This classification divides these fractures into displaced or nondisplaced fractures. Guidelines for treatment of nondisplaced femoral neck fractures are beyond the scope of this chapter.
- The indications for a hemiarthroplasty of the hip include displaced femoral neck fractures and salvage for massive acetabular osteolytic defects in revision total hip arthroplasty (THA). Ideally, hemiarthroplasty should be reserved for elderly patients with low functional demands with displaced femoral neck fractures. Younger, more active patients may have improved outcomes with THA.[16]
- Published reports suggest that bipolar hemiarthroplasty has poor outcomes when used as a primary prosthesis for failures with degenerative joint disease, and this technique currently is not recommended. Similarly, poor results have been noted in osteonecrosis of the femoral head.[11]
- The two types of hemiarthroplasty implants are the unipolar type (eg, Austin Moore; **FIG 1A**) and the bipolar type (**FIG 1B**).
  - The bipolar prosthesis has been favored because of its theoretical reduction of wear on the acetabular side. Motion between the inner and outer heads of the prosthesis leads to less motion at the acetabulum–implant interface.[13]

ANATOMY

- The neck–shaft angle is about 130 ± 7 degrees in adults and does not vary significantly between genders.
- The femoral neck is anteverted 10.4 ± 6.7 degrees with respect to the femoral shaft in Caucasians.
  - Some ethnic groups (eg, Asians) have a propensity for higher degrees of anteversion, up to 30%.
- Femoral head diameters range from 40 to 60 mm.
- Femoral neck length and shape vary considerably.
  - In cross-section, the femoral neck is cam-shaped, with a shorter anteroposterior (AP) than mediolateral diameter.

Table 1 Garden's Classification of Femoral Neck Fractures

Grade	Description
I	Incomplete fracture with varus malalignment
II	Nondisplaced fracture through femoral neck
III	Incompletely displaced fracture through femoral neck
IV	Completely displaced fracture with no engagement of fragments

- The calcar femorale is a condensed, vertically oriented area of bone that originates superiorly toward the greater trochanter and fuses with the cortex at the posterior aspect of the femoral neck.
- The major vascular supply of the femoral head comes from the lateral epiphyseal branch of the medial femoral circumflex artery.
  - Other contributing vessels include the inferior metaphyseal artery, arising from the lateral femoral circumflex artery, and the medial epiphyseal artery through the ligamentum teres, arising from the obturator artery.

PATHOGENESIS

- In elderly persons, a femoral neck fracture is usually the result of a fall.
- Several mechanisms have been proposed:
  - A direct blow to the lateral aspect of the greater trochanter from a fall
  - A sudden increase in load with the head fixed in the acetabulum along with a lateral, rotatory force. This causes impaction of the posterior neck on the acetabulum.
  - A fatigue fracture that precedes and causes a fall
  - The incidence of femoral neck fractures increases as bone density falls to osteoporotic levels.
- Femoral neck fractures in young patients typically are the result of high-energy mechanisms.
  - The mechanical explanation is axial loading of the distal femur or the foot if the knee is extended.
  - The amount of bony displacement and associated soft tissue injury can be much higher.

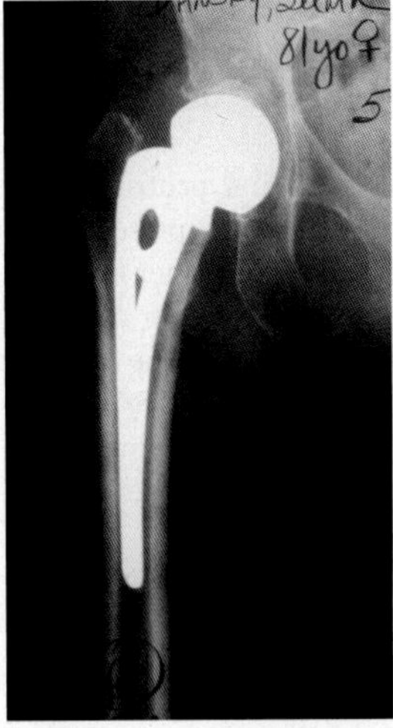

A

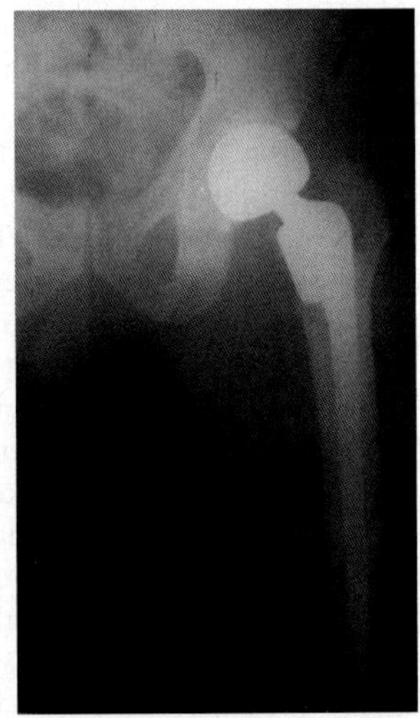
B

FIG 1 • **A.** Austin Moore prosthesis. **B.** Cemented bipolar prosthesis.

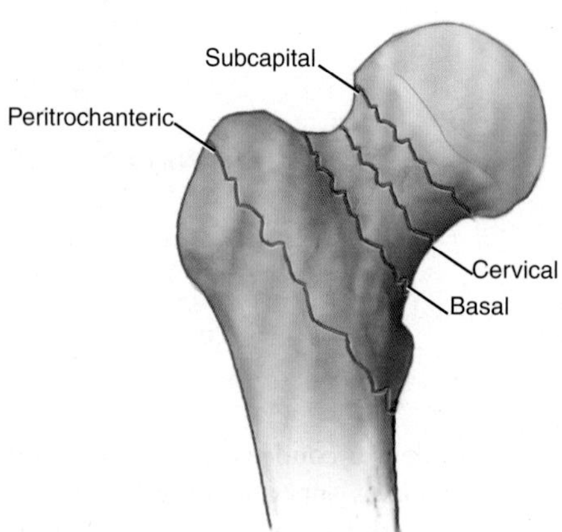

FIG 2 • Geography of proximal femoral fractures.

- Displacement of a femoral neck fracture can lead to disruption of the vascular supply of the femoral neck.
  - This vascular compromise may contribute to the high incidence of avascular necrosis (AVN) with this injury.
- If femoral neck fracture occurs, the intraosseous cervical vessels are disrupted.
  - The risk of AVN generally corresponds to the degree of displacement of the fracture of the femoral neck on initial radiographs.
  - In displaced fractures, most of the retinacular vessels are disrupted. Femoral head blood supply is then dependent on remaining retinacular vessels and those functioning vessels in the ligamentum teres.
  - The role of early fixation and joint capsulotomy in prevention of AVN remains controversial.
- The incidence of nonunion following a displaced fracture is as high as 60% with nonoperative treatment in some reports.
- Femoral neck fractures can be divided into subcapital, transcervical, and basicervical types, based on the location of the injury.
  - Basicervical fractures can often be treated in a manner similar to intertrochanteric fractures with regard to fracture fixation (**FIG 2**).

NATURAL HISTORY

- Femoral neck fractures are most commonly seen in patients older than age of 50 years.[14]
- Patients with a single femoral neck fracture have an increased risk of sustaining a second hip fracture.
- Bateman[2] and Gilberty[10] reported the use of a bipolar prosthesis.
  - The rationale was that less erosion and protrusion of the acetabulum would occur because motion is present between the metal head and polyethylene socket's inner bearing.
  - Acetabular wear is diminished by reduction of the total amount of motion that occurs between the acetabular cartilage and metallic outer shell with interposition of the second low-friction inner bearing within the implant.
  - Overall hip motion also may be greater because of the compound bearing surface.
- Barnes et al[1] showed that mortality in the first month postoperatively was substantial: as high as 13.3% in men and 7.4% in women.
  - More importantly, delaying surgery beyond 72 hours led to a substantial increase in the mortality rate.
- Factors influencing mortality in cemented bipolar hemiarthroplasty include cardiac history, residence in a nursing home, chronic pulmonary disease, elevated serum creatinine, pneumonia, history of myocardial infarction, duration of surgery, and gender.[8]
- Associated injuries may include subdural or epidural hematoma and ipsilateral upper extremity injury for low-energy fractures.
  - High-energy fracture patterns have a higher incidence of associated injury, including closed head injury, pneumo- or hemothorax, spinal fracture, visceral injury, and ipsilateral lower extremity bony injury.[5]

PATIENT HISTORY AND PHYSICAL FINDINGS

- A complaint of groin, proximal thigh, or, rarely, lateral hip pain following a fall in an elderly patient should raise suspicion for a low-energy femoral neck fracture.
- If a patient has fallen on the floor and is unable to ambulate, that should also raise suspicion for a femoral neck fracture.
- The patient's preinjury ambulatory status must be ascertained when the history is taken. His or her preoperative activity level can help determine the most appropriate type of surgical management.
- Care must be taken to evaluate other possible sources of injury about the hip as well as associated ipsilateral injury.
  - Pelvic fracture: Associated injury to the pelvic rami is common. Radiographs are useful in diagnosing these associated injuries.
  - Acetabular fracture: In a low-energy injury, acetabular fracture is an uncommon association with a femoral neck fracture. However, this is not the case in high-energy injury patterns. Thin-slice computed tomography (CT) may be useful for diagnosing this injury.
  - Inter- and subtrochanteric fracture: Injury to the intertrochanteric area is commonly seen about the hip in elderly patients. Subtrochanteric fractures are less common. Usually, the limb is held in extension, not in a flexed, externally rotated position. Radiographs again are useful for establishing the diagnosis.
- A thorough physical examination should include the following:
  - Observation of the lower extremity. If it is shortened, externally rotated, and painful to move, a joint effusion secondary to fracture hematoma is most likely responsible, which increases the available space in the joint capsule.
  - Logroll maneuver, which is the most sensitive physical finding. A positive result elicits pain at the groin due to the side-to-side movement of the lower extremity, which creates shear forces across a femoral neck fracture, leading to exquisite pain.
  - Axial load test, which is positive if the maneuver elicits pain at the groin. This test is less specific than the logroll test.
  - Range-of-motion tests. Pain at the end points of the range of motion may be the only clue to detect a nondisplaced occult fracture.

IMAGING AND OTHER DIAGNOSTIC STUDIES

- Plain radiographs of the AP pelvis and injured hip should be obtained.
  - If possible, the legs should be immobilized in internal rotation for the film.

- A shoot-through lateral radiograph is useful for determining the degree of displacement of the fracture fragment, especially for fractures that appear minimally displaced on an AP view.
- A radiograph taken while applying axial traction is helpful to determine location of the fracture along the femoral neck if displacement of the fracture fragments obscures a view of the fracture pattern.
- CT scanning is useful for identifying nondisplaced fractures when clinically suspected as well as associated injuries. However, it usually is not employed for an isolated, low-energy femoral neck fracture.
- Radionucleotide uptake bone scans are helpful in identifying occult femoral neck fractures but may take up to 72 hours to be apparent on film.
- Magnetic resonance imaging is more sensitive to identifying occult femoral neck fractures than CT scan or bone scan within the first 72 hours.
  - It also is highly sensitive to identifying occult fractures at the ipsilateral intertrochanteric area.

DIFFERENTIAL DIAGNOSIS

- Intertrochanteric fracture
- Subtrochanteric fracture
- Pelvic fracture
- Acetabular fracture
- Hip contusion or traumatic trochanteric bursitis

NONOPERATIVE MANAGEMENT

- Femoral neck fractures are rarely managed nonoperatively. Both nondisplaced and displaced fracture patterns have better functional and overall outcomes when treated surgically.
  - Nonoperative management may be relatively indicated in the patient with severe medical comorbidities who is unable to tolerate anesthesia for surgical intervention.
  - Because nondisplaced fractures can be internally fixed with percutaneous techniques under local anesthetic and monitored sedation, nonoperative treatment is usually not indicated for this fracture type.
- In most cases, nonoperative treatment should be limited to initial management of the injury before surgical stabilization.
  - A soft pillow should be placed under the patient's knee and leg to keep them in a comfortable position.
- All patients with femoral neck fractures should be placed on strict bed rest with a Foley catheter and intravenous fluids on admission.
- Axial traction of the injured lower extremity is contraindicated for femoral neck fractures because it can increase displacement of the fracture fragments.

SURGICAL MANAGEMENT

- The best method of surgical fixation of femoral neck fractures is controversial. The debate between internal fixation versus hemiarthroplasty versus THA continues and is beyond the scope of this chapter.
- General indications for surgical management using hemiarthroplasty include the elderly patient with low functional demands or poor bone quality not amenable to internal fixation.
- Hemiarthroplasty is indicated for patients with displaced femoral neck fractures who meet the following criteria:
  - Reasonable general health
  - Pathologic hip fractures
  - Neurologic diseases including Parkinson disease, previous stroke, or hemiplegia
  - Physiologic age older than 75 to 80 years
  - Severe osteoporosis with loss of primary trabeculae in the femoral head
  - Inadequate closed reduction
  - Displaced fracture
  - Preexisting hip disease on the femoral side, namely osteonecrosis, without any acetabular disease
- Contraindications include the following:
  - Preexisting sepsis
  - Young age
  - Failure of internal fixation devices, mainly because of acetabular damage that often occurs in that situation
  - Preexisting acetabular disease. Even patients with normal preoperative cartilaginous space may become symptomatic after about 5 years due to degradation caused by friction between the metal and the acetabular cartilage.
- Indications for cementing a femoral stem vary from surgeon to surgeon and institution to institution.
  - Primary candidates for this approach are patients with poor bone quality, such as those with a stovepipe femur or Dorr type C femur.[6] These patients can be difficult to manage with uncemented implants because they require either massive, canal-filling, uncemented implants that often produce significant stress shielding of the femur or have proximally filled implants that can make accurate adjustment of limb lengths very difficult.
  - Antibiotic-impregnated cement may be advisable for certain high-risk groups of patients. Some patients, such as those on dialysis, may be more prone to sepsis, and use of antibiotic-impregnated cement may be considered appropriate.
    - Appropriate antibiotics include tobramycin, vancomycin, cefazolin, and erythromycin.
  - Cemented stems also should be considered for patients with pathologic fractures. For these patients, the use of cement with a bone-replacing prosthesis may be the preferred treatment, regardless of age or bone quality.
  - The first-generation cementing technique involved finger-packing without the use of pressurization and a reduction of porosity. Modern cementing techniques use a medullary brush, cement restrictor, medullary pulsatile lavage, the insertion of epinephrine-soaked sponges, reduction of cement porosity (ie, vacuum mixing), cement centralizers, and a cement gun for retrograde cement insertion, after which pressurization can be performed with a surgeon's gloved finger or, alternatively, with a wedge-shaped pressurization device.
  - Because of the embolic load secondary to pressurization, many surgeons avoid cemented components in patients with a history of cardiopulmonary disease.

Preoperative Planning

- It is important that the preoperative x-rays are reviewed and templated for appropriate size and for fixation.
- Appropriate implant selection should be undertaken, whether to proceed with a tapered stem, a fully coated medullary-locking stem, or a cemented stem.

- The patient should undergo an appropriate preoperative workup including medical, cardiac, and anesthesia evaluations.
  - Banked blood should also be available.
  - Important preoperative laboratory studies include complete blood counts, electrolytes, and coagulation studies.
  - Additional blood tests could include total protein, albumin, and appropriate liver studies to evaluate the patient's overall nutritional status.
- Electrocardiogram, chest radiograph, and possibly, further cardiac studies, including echocardiogram, may be appropriate preoperatively.
- The femoral head size must be evaluated to establish the correct component size.
  - If the component is too large, equatorial contact occurs, which can result in a tight joint with decreased motion and pain.
  - If the component is too small, polar contact occurs, leading to increased contact stresses, and, therefore, to greater erosion and possible superomedial migration.
- It is also important to template neck length and offset.
  - If the neck length is too long, reduction can be difficult, and the increased soft tissue tension could lead to increased pressure on the acetabular cartilage.
  - The offset should be reproduced postoperatively. It can be created by evaluating the distance between the center of the femoral head and the greater trochanter, thereby restoring the length of the abductor mechanism and decreasing postoperative limp.
- These procedures can be performed under spinal or combined spinal and epidural anesthesia because hypotensive anesthesia can have the benefit of reducing blood loss.
- Prophylactic antibiotics are administered before the surgery.
- The procedure must be performed in a clean operating room with laminar flow. Vertical laminar airflow in conjunction with operating suite and body exhaust systems is helpful.
- Associated injuries should be addressed concurrently if possible.

Positioning

- Patient positioning is important and should be done very carefully.
- General positioning principles include padding all bony prominences, positioning the patient in a stable position for implant placement, and creating a range-of-motion arc so that implant position and stability can be tested intraoperatively.

Supine Position for Direct Approach (Smith-Petersen) Approach

- Once the patient is adequately anesthetized, he or she is placed in a supine position, which allows for direct measurement of leg length.
- The operating table is placed in a flat position.
- The patient is brought down the table so the leg break is at the level of the midthigh. In order to facilitate this positioning, the headpiece is often placed at the foot of the bed.
- A bump is placed beneath the sacrum. This sacral pad is constructed of folded sheets or a gel bump approximately 1.5 to 2 inches in height and rectangular with an approximate dimension of 12 × 10 inches (**FIG 3**).
  - The modest elevation of the sacrum allows the femur to drop posteriorly when sizing and inspecting the acetabulum.
  - It also allows hip stability to be evaluated in extension.

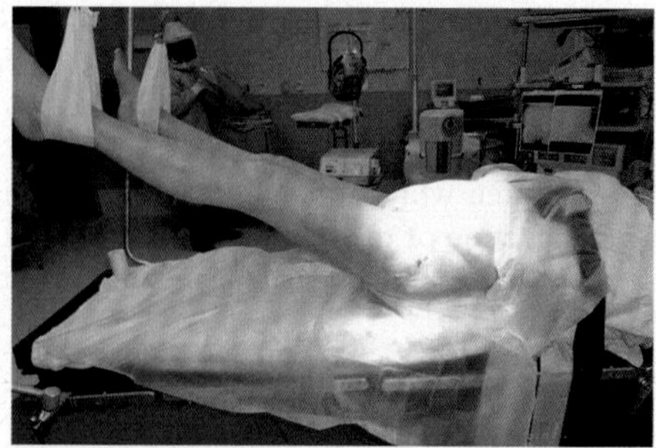

FIG 3 • Positioning with sacral bump.

- Both arms are placed on arm boards secured at 90 degrees of abduction.

Supine Position for Direct Lateral (Modified Hardinge) Approach

- Once the patient is adequately anesthetized, he or she is placed in a supine position, which allows for direct measurement of leg length.
- The operating table is placed in a flat position.
- The patient is brought to the edge of the table so that the operative hip slightly overhangs the edge of the table.
- A bump is placed beneath the sacrum. This sacral pad is constructed of folded sheets or a gel bump approximately 1.5 to 2 inches in height and rectangular with an approximate dimension of 12 × 10 inches.
- The modest elevation of the sacrum allows the fat and soft tissues from above the trochanter to fall posteriorly away from the incision, thereby minimizing the amount of tissue that must be dissected in a lateral approach.
  - It also allows hip stability to be evaluated in extension.
- A footrest is fixed to the operating table, so that the surgical hip is flexed 40 degrees.
- Both arms are placed on arm boards secured at 90 degrees of abduction.
- The operating room table is inclined 5 degrees away from the operating surgeon to improve visualization of the acetabulum.

Lateral Position

- The lateral position is used for a posterolateral approach to the hip and can also be used for an anterolateral approach.
- Once the patient is adequately anesthetized and a Foley catheter is inserted, they are placed in the desired position in a gentle, organized fashion.
  - The anesthesiologist controls the patient's head and neck, holding the endotracheal tube securely.
  - One surgical team member controls the patient's hands and shoulders, and another controls the patient's hips.
- The ipsilateral arm is positioned in no more than 90 degrees of forward flexion and slight adduction.
- An axillary pad is placed by lifting the patient's chest and positioning the pad distal to the contralateral axilla.
- The contralateral arm must be kept in no greater than 90 degrees of forward flexion.
- Extremities are padded over all bony protuberances.
- The operating room table must be kept in an absolute horizontal position, parallel to the floor.

- A number of holders can be used to hold the patient in a lateral decubitus position.
  - A beanbag can be used, although it is not as rigid as a variety of other types of holders. The pubis and sacrum must be secured in the holder.
  - Placement of the pubic clamp must be done cautiously, with the pad directly against the pubic symphysis.
    - Placement of the pad more inferiorly causes occlusion or compromise of the femoral vessels in the opposite limb, which may go unrecognized.
    - Placement of the pad superiorly may compromise ipsilateral femoral vessels and may prevent adequate flexion and adduction of the operated hip.
- A sacral pad is placed over the midsacrum. It should be at least 3 to 5 inches away from the most posterior end of the skin incision (**FIG 4A**).
- When the patient is securely positioned in lateral decubitus, the position of the pelvis is checked to make sure that it is not tilted in the AP direction (**FIG 4B**).
- A chest positioner and pillows between the arms are helpful in preventing anterior displacement of the torso.
- The perineum is isolated using an adhesive U-shaped plastic drape.

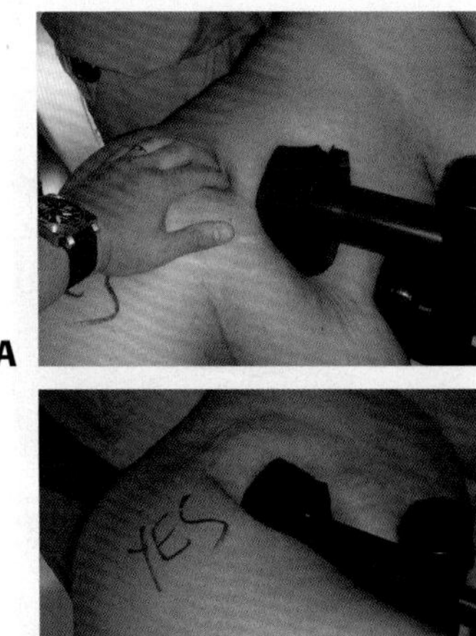

FIG 4 • **A.** Palpation of ASIS for lateral position. **B.** Adequate range of motion must be ensured after positioning.

Approach

- Hemiarthroplasty can be performed through a number of different approaches.
- There are four commonly employed approaches to the hip joint:
  - Anterior (Smith-Petersen)
    - This approach uses the interval between the sartorius and the tensor fascia superficially and between the rectus femoris and tensor fascia deeply.
    - Risks include injury to the lateral femoral cutaneous nerve.
    - Allows the surgeon direct access to the anterior hip capsule
    - Femoral preparation may be more challenging and require traction, hip extension, and the use of a hook to deliver the femur anteriorly for preparation.
  - Anterolateral (Watson-Jones)
  - Lateral (modified Hardinge)
  - Posterior (Southern)
- Choice of approach is highly dependent on surgeon preference.
  - I use a modification of the direct anterior as described by Smith-Petersen, Heuter, and Judet. Previously, I preferred a lateral muscle-splitting approach to the hip, as originally described by Hardinge, and the use of a cementless tapered stem.[3]
- A cemented stem can be implanted through a number of surgical exposures.

Anterior Approach (Modified Smith-Petersen)

Preparation of the Surgical Site

- Both lower extremities are prepped into the surgical field. Plastic adhesive drapes are used to isolate the operative field from the perineum and adjacent skin.
  - A large U-drape is placed, isolating the perineum and abdomen from the hip and repeated for the opposite side.
  - A second drape is placed transversely above the level of the iliac crest, completing the isolation of the wound area from the abdomen and thorax. This is also done for the nonoperative side but to a lesser degree.
  - The excess drapes are debulked down the center (perineum) with silk tape.
- Both lower extremities are scrubbed with a chlorhexidine brush, followed by a preparation with chlorhexidine and alcohol (**TECH FIG 1A**).
- The incision area is dried to allow better adherence of Ioban drapes (3M, St. Paul, MN).
- A down sheet is placed and a surgical towel is placed over the crotch and perineum. Both limbs are removed from the leg holders and the surgeon grasps the foot with a double-thickness stockinette.
  - Impermeable drape is placed across of the bottom of the operating table up to the level of the patient's buttock. This U-drape is placed bilaterally. A second U-drape is placed only on the operative side. A bar drape seals the upper portion of the surgical site (**TECH FIG 1B**).
  - The stockinette is unrolled to the level of the upper thigh and higher on the nonoperative side. A bilateral extremity drape is placed over both legs, not to exceed the stockinettes. The stockinettes are secured with a Coban dressing (3M) (**TECH FIG 1C**).
- A rectangular window is cut off the drape over the surgical site and the sides are secured with staples. The surgical site is additionally prepped with a chlorhexidine and alcohol or Betadine and alcohol solution (**TECH FIG 1D**).

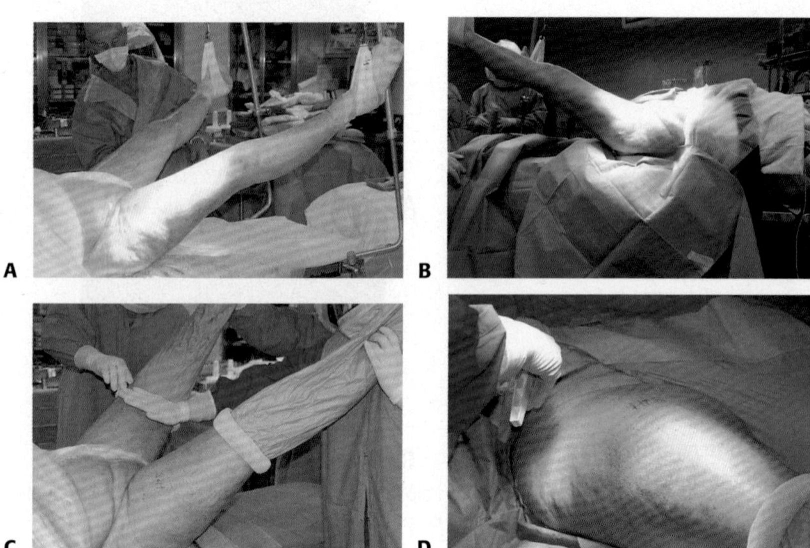

TECH FIG 1 • **A.** Both legs prepped. **B.** First sterile U-drape. **C.** Bilateral stockinettes. **D.** Operative side isolated.

Skin Incision

- The anterior superior iliac spine (ASIS) and greater trochanter are marked and an oblique skin incision approximately 3 to 4 inches in length and starting a finger's breadth distal and lateral to the ASIS is outlined. This window is then sealed with Ioban drapes (**TECH FIG 2A**).
- The skin incision is taken down through subcutaneous tissue to the tensor fascia. The fascia over the muscle is identified. The fascial incision is directly over the tensor muscle not directly in the interval. Too medial is over the interval and too lateral is over the fascia lata (**TECH FIG 2B**).
- The fascia is incised and elevated bluntly medially with a pickup and finger dissection. The finger must wrap around the tensor medially, dropping into the interval between the tensor and rectus. This should be done bluntly (**TECH FIG 2C**).
- A blunt Hohmann retractor is placed around the lateral side of the femoral head and a second double-angled Hohmann retractor is placed around the lateral femur (greater trochanter). Hibbs retractors are placed medially retracting the rectus. Ascending branches of the lateral femoral circumflex vessels are identified and coagulated or tied (**TECH FIG 2D**).
- The distal fascia between the rectus and tensor is released, allowing the rectus to slide medially and allowing a second blunt

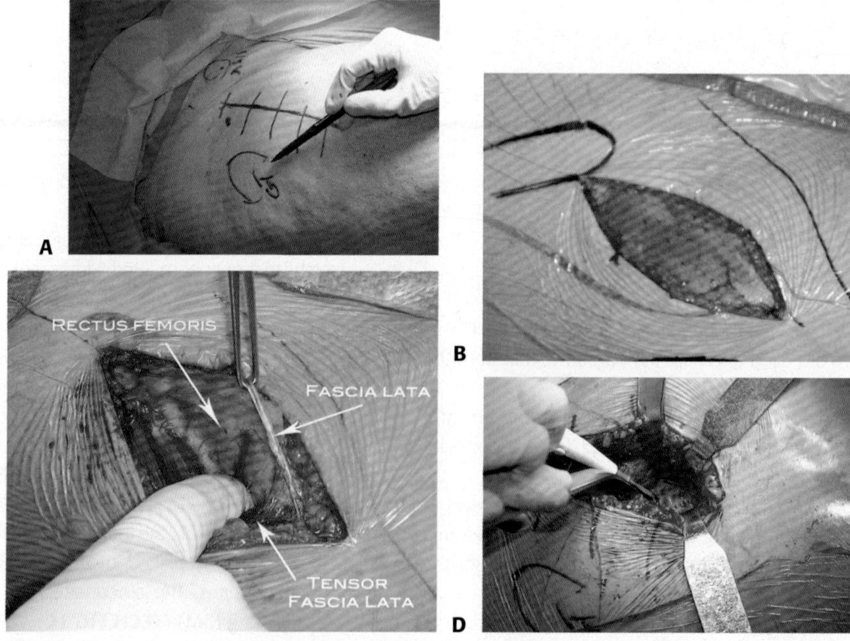

TECH FIG 2 • **A.** Skin markings of ASIS, greater trochanter, and skin incision. **B.** Fascia overlying tensor muscle belly. **C.** Elevating fascia off the tensor and blunt finger dissection into the Smith-Petersen interval between tensor and rectus. **D.** Identifying the ascending branches of the lateral femoral circumflex vessels. (**B,D:** Courtesy of Jonathan Yerasamides, MD.)

Hohmann retractor to be placed around the medial side of the femoral neck. The rectus is then dissected from the anterior hip capsule with a Cobb elevator and a final blunt cobra retractor is placed on the anterior column.

Acetabular Preparation

- The anterior hip capsule is fully exposed. Perforating vessels are coagulated. The capsule is opened in an H fashion and excised. Both blunt Hohmann retractors are placed intracapsularly. The femoral neck fracture is identified. A femoral neck osteotomy is performed distal to the fracture, using the saddle as reference at a 45-degree angle. Typically, a blunt osteotome can be used at both the osteotomy and fracture site to remove the fractured neck segment. A more proximal osteotomy may be performed as well in the subcapital area, if necessary, to remove that segment. The femoral head is removed with a power corkscrew.
- The leg is then placed in a figure-4 position with a pointed Hohmann retractor below the lesser trochanter in order to assess the osteotomy level and perform medial capsular release (capsule above the lesser trochanter is released from the calcar). Once the level is determined to be satisfactory, the leg is placed back in a neutral position. Additional neck resection is performed if necessary.
- Three retractors are placed around the acetabulum. A blunt cobra retractor is placed on the anterior column above the labrum and beneath the capsule and rectus. A double-angled Hohmann retractor is placed at the level of the transverse acetabular ligament. A pointed Aufranc retractor is placed along the posterior acetabulum (**TECH FIG 3**).
- The acetabulum should be inspected to remove any bony fragments and debris and then should be sized. The acetabulum should be sized with a trial bipolar or unipolar component to ensure that there will be good fit without overfilling the acetabulum.

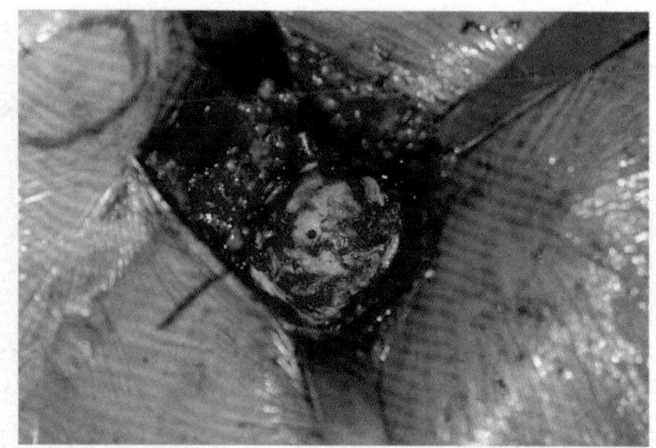

TECH FIG 3 • Acetabular exposure with three retractors.

- This can be achieved with a good suction-tight feel with placement of the trial component.

Femoral Preparation

- Attention is then placed to the femur.
  - The leg of the table is then extended 30 degrees. The nonoperative leg is placed on a padded Mayo stand. The operative leg is placed in a figure-4 position under the nonoperative leg (**TECH FIG 4A**).
  - The second assistant places a hand on the knee, pushing down and adducting the leg, thereby creating external rotation, extension, and adduction of the operative femur. A double-footed retractor is placed along the posterior femoral neck and a double-angled retractor is placed along the anterior femoral neck (**TECH FIG 4B**).
- The next step is to perform the femoral releases in order to prepare the femur. The releases include the superior or lateral capsule, which is draped in front of the inside of the greater trochanter when the leg is in externally rotated position. The medial

A

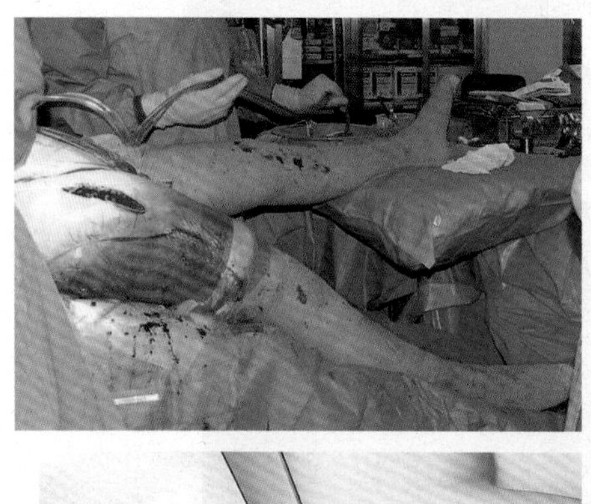

B

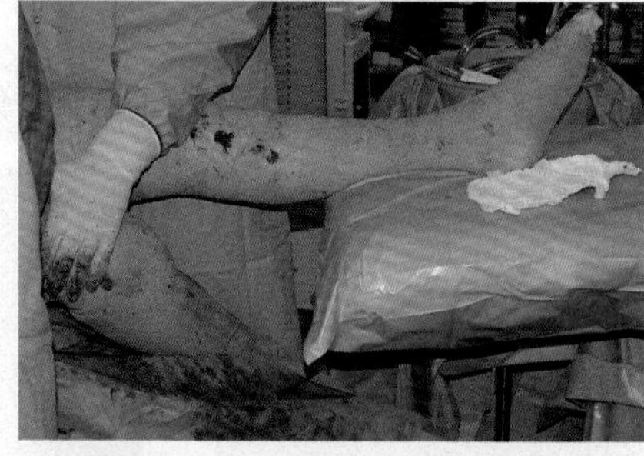

C

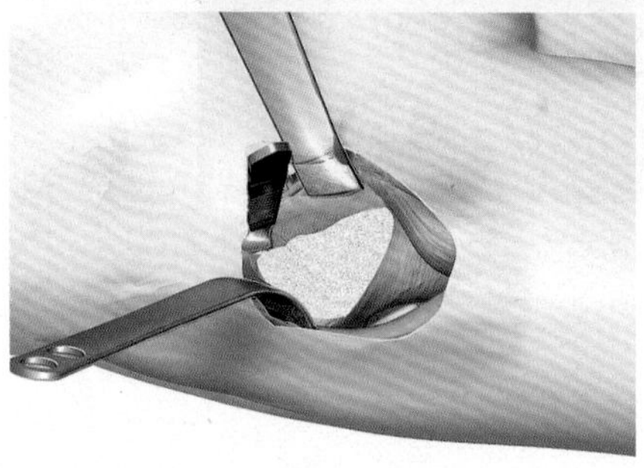

D

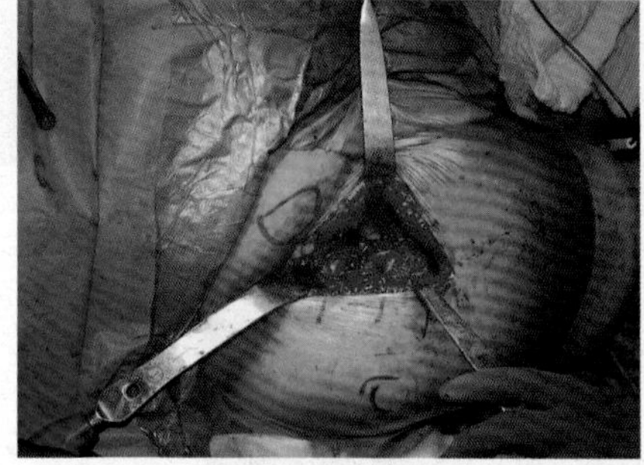

TECH FIG 4 • **A.** Table position for femoral preparation. **B.** Position of nonoperative leg and second assistant maneuvering operative leg. **C.** Diagram representing superior capsular release for a right hip. **D.** Exposure of proximal femur after releases. *(continued)*

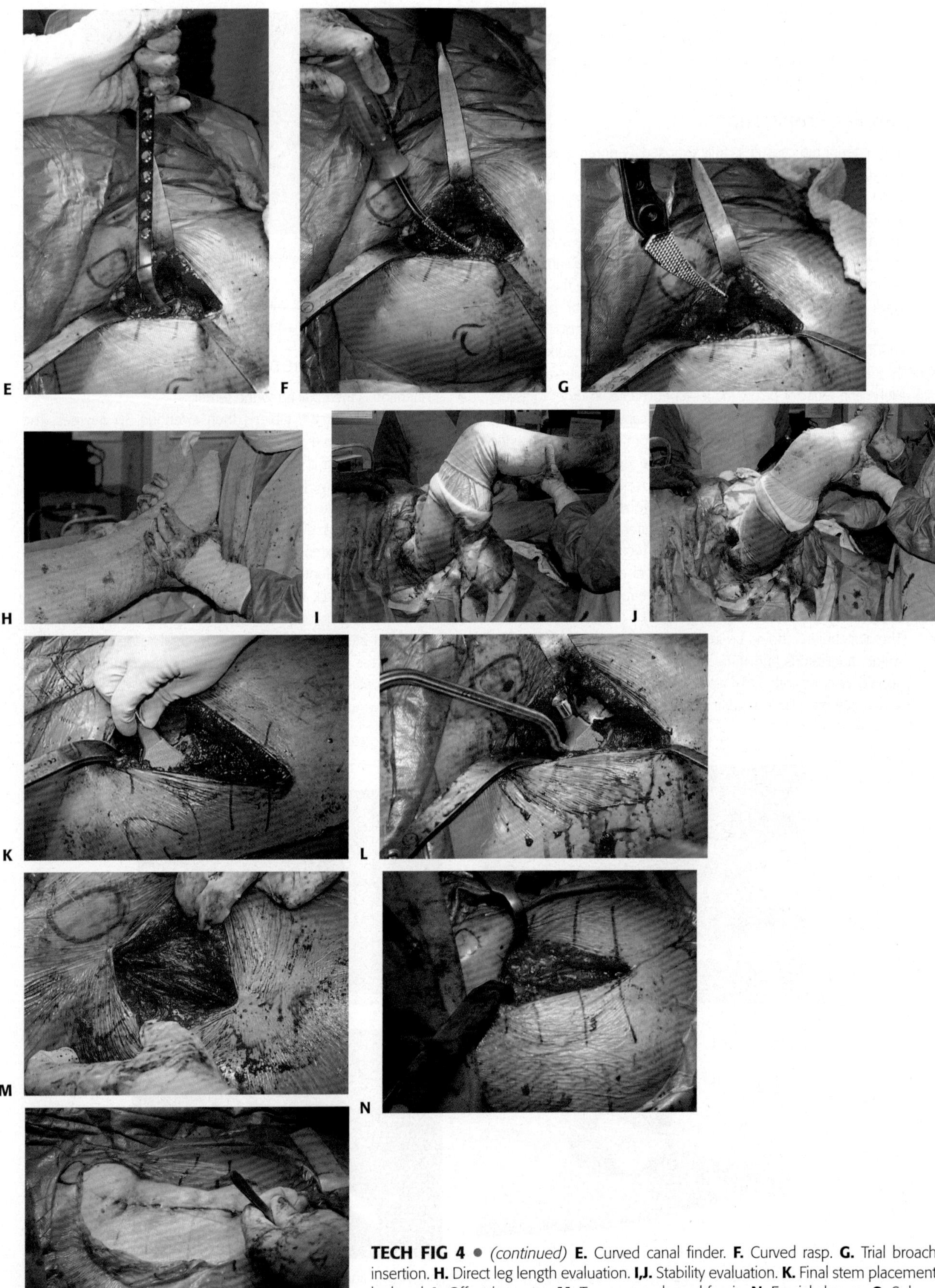

TECH FIG 4 • *(continued)* **E.** Curved canal finder. **F.** Curved rasp. **G.** Trial broach insertion. **H.** Direct leg length evaluation. **I,J.** Stability evaluation. **K.** Final stem placement by hand. **L.** Offset impactor. **M.** Tensor muscle and fascia. **N.** Fascial closure. **O.** Subcutaneous closure.

aspect of the greater trochanter should be exposed. Additionally, the conjoint tendon, which consists of the inferior gemellus, obturator internus, and superior gemellus, may need to be released. Occasionally, the piriformis tendon may need to be released in a contracted hip (**TECH FIG 4C**).
  - Once the proximal femur is adequately exposed, the proximal femur is sometimes opened with an offset box osteotome. More commonly, it is opened with a curved canal finder, a curved rasp, and a rongeur to further open the canal. A curette can be used to clear the medial side of the trochanter and the rongeur again in this area. The curved rasp should be used to open the canal as well as feel the cortices and appreciate the orientation of the femur (**TECH FIG 4D–F**).
  - The canal is sequentially broached until there is a tight feel. The broach should be stable to rotation.
    - The femoral broach is introduced in a neutral position and neutral version of the rotation is judged in relation to the position of the knee and the calcar as well as the posterior femoral neck (**TECH FIG 4G**).
- Broaching is begun with the smallest broach and then increased until appropriate fit and fill is achieved. This can be gauged by preoperative templating and tactile feedback.
- The broach is introduced each time to its full depth.
  - If significant resistance is met, broaching should continue with a series of small inward and then outward taps.
  - Broaching is continued until full cortical seating has been accomplished. This is indicated by an upward change in pitch as the broach is being seated.
- Final seating and sizing is determined by pitch, tactile feedback, and lack of progression.
- Trial reduction is performed with a minus neck trial and a standard neck offset to start. The head should be carefully reduced. This will require flexion, traction, and internal rotation. The surgeon must carefully turn the bipolar head so that it may be reduced under the rectus and anterior soft tissue sleeve. If it is a difficult reduction, then the trial construct is typically too long and a smaller broach needs to be countersunk and the femoral neck recut. If it reduces too easily, then the trial construct may be too short or have inadequate offset.
- Once a reasonable trial construct has been established, leg lengths are measured directly near the medial malleoli and heels. Anterior stability is checked with external rotation and extension in a neutral and adducted position. Posterior stability is checked with flexion and internal rotation. Once satisfactory stability is achieved, the final components are placed (**TECH FIG 4H–J**).
  - The final stem is placed by hand and impacted until final seating. The final bipolar hemiarthroplasty is assembled on the back table and impacted onto a clean trunnion (**TECH FIG 4K,L**).
  - The final prosthesis is reduced with flexion, traction, and internal rotation. The table is placed in a level position with a new downsheet. The wound is thoroughly irrigated and a medium Hemovac drain placed with a distal exit site.
- Wound closure begins with interrupted absorbable sutures in the tensor fascia. Interrupted absorbable sutures are used for the subcutaneous tissues. Skin staples are applied to the skin, sealed with Dermabond and a final sealed hydrofiber dressing (**TECH FIG 4M–O**).

Lateral Approach (Modified Hardinge)

Preparation of the Surgical Site

- Plastic adhesive drapes are used to isolate the operative field from the perineum and adjacent skin.
  - A large U-drape is placed, isolating the perineum and abdomen from the hip.
  - A second drape is placed transversely above the level of the iliac crest, completing the isolation of the wound area from the abdomen and thorax.
  - The foot also is sealed with a plastic 10 × 10 drape, isolating the foot above the level of the ankle.
- The operative field is scrubbed with a chlorhexidine brush, followed by a preparation with chlorhexidine and alcohol (**TECH FIG 5A**).
  - The incision area is dried to allow better adherence of Ioban drapes.
- The limb is removed from the leg holder and the surgeon grasps the foot with a double-thickness stockinette.
  - An impermeable drape is placed across of the bottom of the operating table up to the level of the patient's buttock.
  - The stockinette is unrolled to the level of the midthigh and secured with a Coban dressing.
- The limb is draped sterilely using two full-sized sheets brought beneath the leg and buttock and held above the level of the iliac crest.
  - A double sheet is placed transversely across the abdomen above the level of the iliac crest.

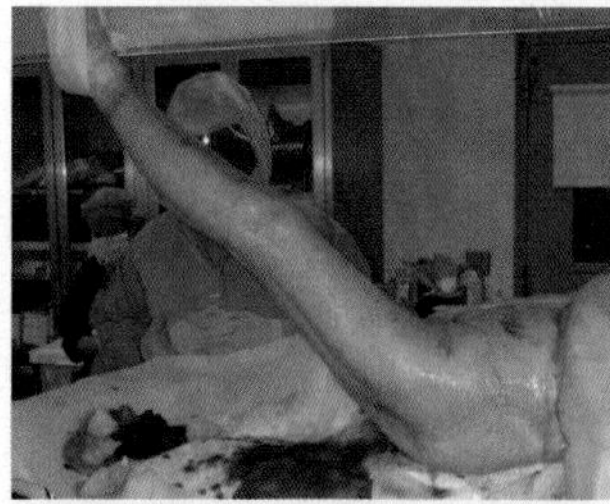
A

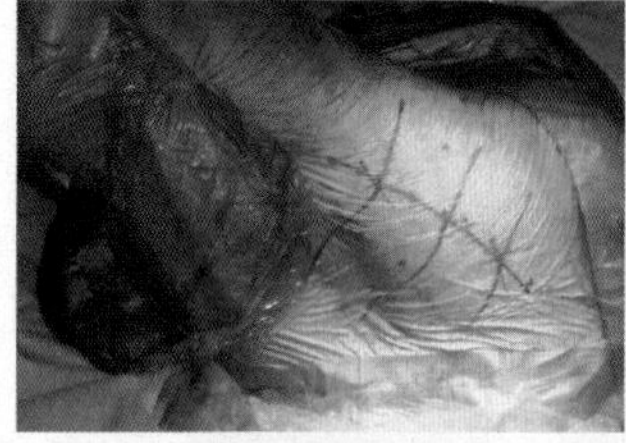
B

TECH FIG 5 • **A.** Skin preparation for lateral (Hardinge) approach to the hip. **B.** Lateral skin incision.

- A clean air room is sealed at the head of the operating table with sterile adhesive drape.
- The hip area is marked using a sterile pen.
  - The greater trochanter is outlined.
  - The iliac crest and femoral shaft are palpated, and the skin incision, centered over the trochanter and slightly anterior, is drawn with large cross-hatchings (**TECH FIG 5B**).
- The hip is flexed to 40 degrees and slightly adducted. The foot is placed on the footrest.

Incision

- The skin incision is approximately 5 inches in length.
  - It is slightly anterior to the apex of the vastus ridge.
  - The length of the incision also depends on the patient's degree of obesity.
- The skin incision is taken sharply through subcutaneous tissues down to the tensor fascia lata (TFL) (**TECH FIG 6A**).
- The fascia is exposed to a small degree to allow the incision and subsequent closure.
  - Hemostasis is achieved in the subcutaneous tissue with electrocautery and bayonet forceps.
- The incision through the fascia lata is in line with the skin incision.
  - A scalpel is used to penetrate the fascia lata and allow a safe entrance to the compartments.
  - The incision is continued with the use of heavy Mayo-Noble scissors. It is not undermined beyond the skin incision or distal or proximal to the skin incision (**TECH FIG 6B**).

Proximal Dissection

- More proximally, the fibers of the gluteus maximus muscle are split using firm thumb dissection.
  - A Hibbs retractor is used to retract the anterior flap of the fascia lata.
  - Once that is done, the gluteus medius, greater trochanter, and vastus lateralis are clearly visualized.

A
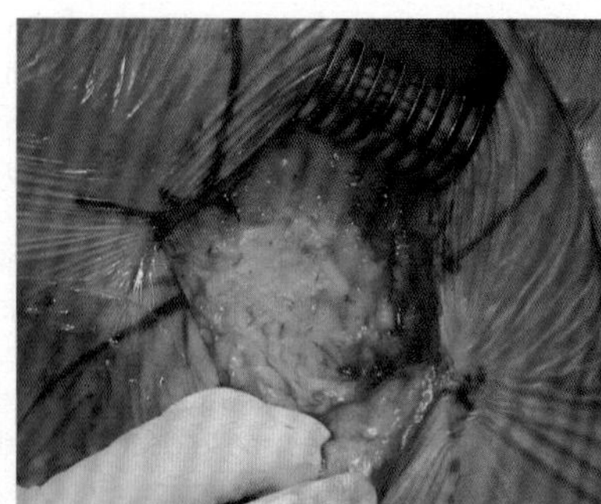

B
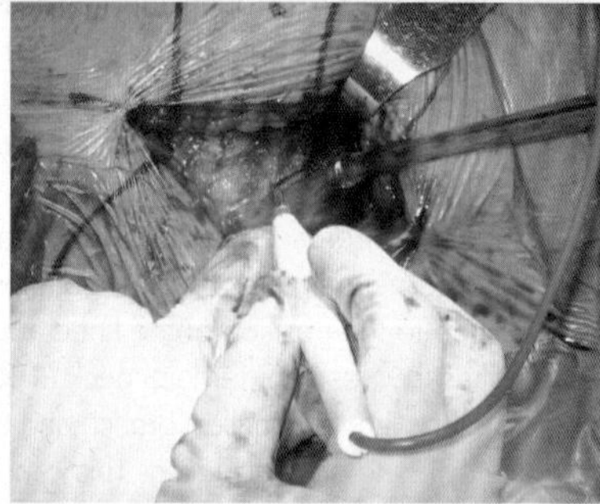

TECH FIG 6 • **A.** The TFL exposed. **B.** An incision is made into the tensor fascia.

- The abductor mass is split.
  - The basic premise of the modified Hardinge approach is to develop an anterior flap, composed of the anterior portion of the vastus lateralis, anterior capsule, anterior third of the gluteus medius muscle, and most of the gluteus minimus muscle to allow exposure of the hip joint.
  - The muscle split is usually located in the anterior third of the gluteus medius.
  - The muscle split is made using electrocautery through the gluteus medius (**TECH FIG 7A,B**).

A
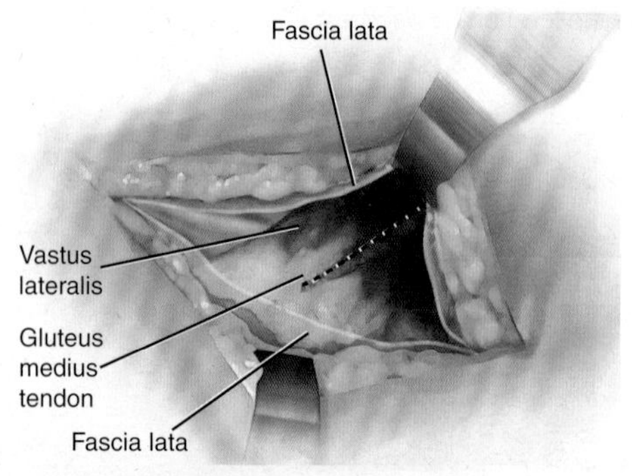

B
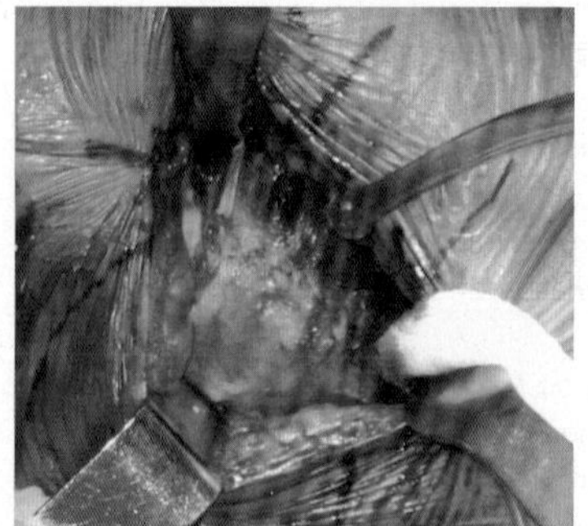

C
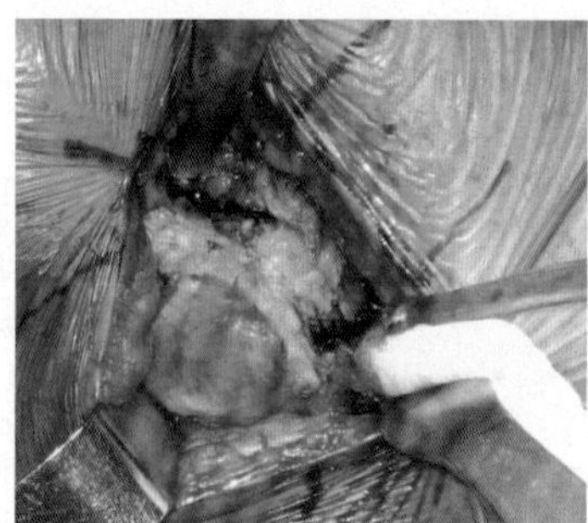

D
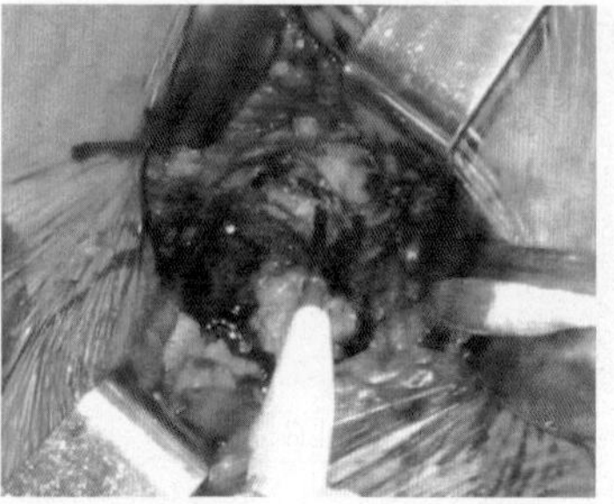

TECH FIG 7 • **A.** Diagram of the splitting of the abductor mass. **B.** The abductor mass exposed. **C.** Detachment of the abductor mass. **D.** Exposure of the femoral neck.

- Once the gluteus medius is penetrated, the surgeon encounters a fatty layer, beneath which is found the gluteus minimus.
  - The gluteus minimus is isolated and a more posterior incision is made with the electrocautery through the gluteus minimus and the capsule onto the acetabulum (**TECH FIG 7C**).
- A blunt Hohmann retractor is placed posteriorly to expose the gluteus minimus and capsule. The blunt end of the Hibbs retractor is used to retract the anterior aspect of the gluteus medius.
- The capsule then is visualized in the depths of the wound.
  - The capsule is incised parallel to the superior aspect of the femoral neck and the incision is extended to the bony rim of the acetabulum with care not to damage the labrum.
  - This area is then packed with an E-tape sponge (**TECH FIG 7D**).

Distal Dissection

- Attention is turned to the more distal aspect of the wound and the vastus lateralis.
- The anterior third of the vastus lateralis is incised longitudinally using electrocautery, beginning at the trochanteric ridge and extending 2 to 3 cm beyond.
- Once this is dissected subperiosteally in the anterior direction, a blunt Hohmann retractor is placed around the femur medially to reflect the vastus lateralis anteriorly.
- An anterior bridge of soft tissue remains along the greater trochanter between the incision in the vastus lateralis and the incision in the gluteus medius and superior capsule. This bridge consists of the anterior fibers of the gluteus medius, minimus, and capsule.
  - This bridge is incised through the tendon in a gentle arc along the anterior aspect of the greater trochanter, connecting the incisions.
  - Healthy soft tissue must be present on both sides of this arc to allow effective repair during closure.
- The bridge is dissected using electrocautery in the anterior aspect of the greater trochanter to develop a flap in continuity consisting of the anterior portion of the gluteus minimus and going around the gluteus medius, anterior hip capsule, and gluteus minimus. This exposes the femoral neck and head.
  - The dissection is carried medially until the medial aspect of the neck is exposed (**TECH FIG 8**).

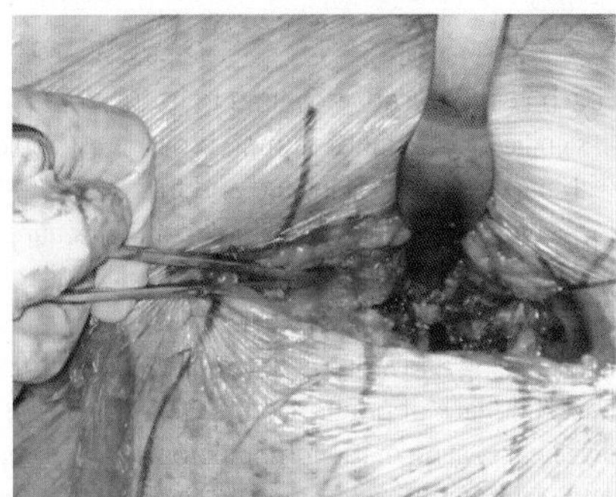

TECH FIG 8 • More proximal femoral exposure.

- Exposure is usually adequate to allow for dislocation of the hip, femoral neck, or proximal femur.
  - A bone hook is placed around the neck of the femur anteriorly and the leg is externally rotated to allow for dislocation of the hip (ie, the hip is placed in the figure-4 position).
- At this point, with a femoral neck fracture, the proximal femur will often dissociate from the femoral neck.
- An initial rough cut of the femoral neck can be performed in line with appropriate preoperative templating.
  - Two blunt-tip retractors are placed around the femoral neck to protect the soft tissues.
  - Electrocautery is used to mark the femoral neck and an initial cut of the femoral neck is made with an oscillating saw.

Placement of Acetabular Retractors

- Attention is turned to the acetabulum.
  - The first retractor is placed in the anterior acetabulum.
  - A small plane is created between the anterior wall of the acetabulum and the anterior capsule using a Cobb elevator.
- A blunt-tip Hohmann retractor is placed in the 12 o'clock position anterior to the acetabulum beneath the capsule.
  - An assistant can then easily retract the anterior soft tissues.
- The second spiked Mueller acetabular retractor is placed in the superior aspect of the acetabulum, retracting the superior capsule in the cranial direction.
  - The retractor is placed at 10 o'clock position for the right hip and 2 o'clock position for the left hip.
  - The exact placement of the retractor is outside the labrum and inside the capsule.
- Using the impactor mallet, the surgeon drives this retractor into the ilium in a slightly cranial direction.
  - The tip is not driven perpendicular to the axis of the body because it may perforate the dome of the acetabulum.
- To facilitate appropriate exposure prior to placement of the third retractor and to allow posterior mobilization of the proximal femur, a medial capsular release must be performed.
  - A curved hemostat is placed between the iliopsoas and capsule, anterior and in line with the pubofemoral ligament.
  - The capsule is incised medial to lateral, thereby increasing the mobilization of the femur in a posterior direction.
- A third, double-angled acetabular retractor is placed inferiorly in the ischium.
  - It is placed with the blade of the retractor resting on the neck of the femur rather than on the cut surface.

Femoral Head Removal and Implant Sizing

- At this point, the femoral head and neck are clearly visualized in the acetabulum.
- The femoral head and neck fracture can be removed using a corkscrew in combination with a Cobb elevator or a tenaculum.
  - This should be done carefully so as not to damage the acetabular cartilage or the labrum (**TECH FIG 9A,B**).
- Once the femoral head is removed, it should be measured to enable the surgeon to estimate the size of the acetabulum.

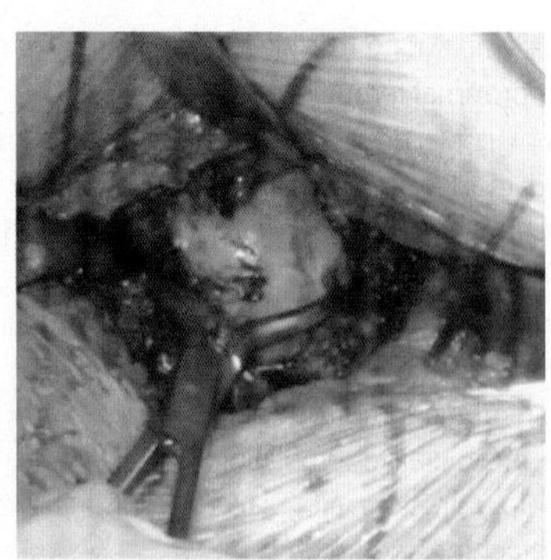

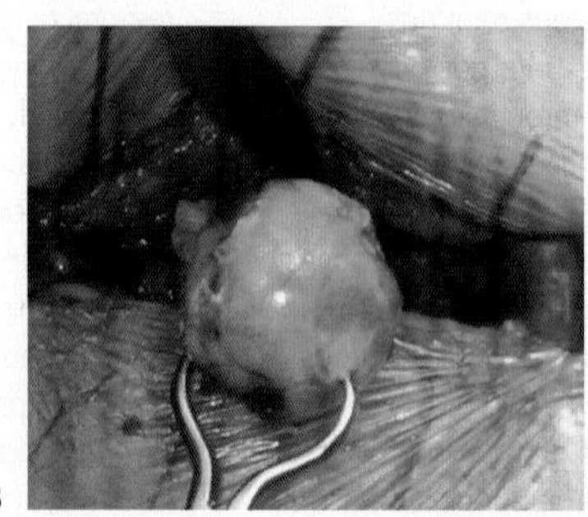

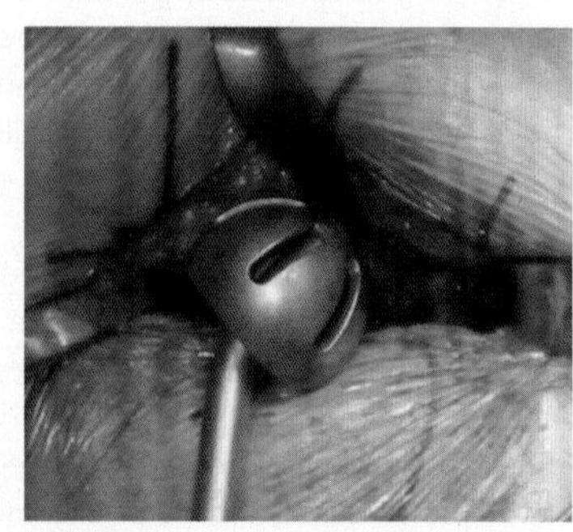

TECH FIG 9 • A. Placement of point-to-point clamp around the femoral head. **B.** Removal of femoral head from acetabulum. **C.** Insertion of prosthesis head sizer.

- The acetabulum should be sized with a trial bipolar or unipolar component to ensure that there will be good fit without overfilling the acetabulum.
  - This can be achieved with a good suction-tight feel with placement of the trial component.
  - It should move freely without resistance.
  - If it floats freely in the acetabulum, the trial component is undersized (**TECH FIG 9C**).

Femoral Reaming

- The femur is exposed with the use of two double-footed retractors, one beneath the greater trochanter and a second retractor medially in the area of the calcar.
- The leg is placed in a figure-4 position, crossed over the opposite thigh.
  - The femur should be easily exposed.
  - If there is difficulty in this exposure, the leg should be placed in a greater degree of figure 4 and rotation.
- Excess soft tissue is removed from the tip of the greater trochanter to allow for reaming and broaching. This will prevent varus positioning of the component.
- A large rongeur is used to open the femoral canal slightly.
- A small, straight curette is introduced into the femoral canal in neutral orientation.
  - The second assistant should use his or her hand to create a target at the distal femur in line with the femur.
  - As the surgeon places the small curette, he or she can place his or her opposite hand on the patient's knee to help direct the small metal curette in the appropriate orientation (**TECH FIG 10A**).
- An entry reamer is then introduced into the femoral canal, pushed into valgus, and worked into the trochanter to ensure appropriate component positioning (**TECH FIG 10B**).
- The bone within the area of the greater trochanter in the lateral aspect of the femoral canal is removed using a lateral rasp or a curette (**TECH FIG 10C**).

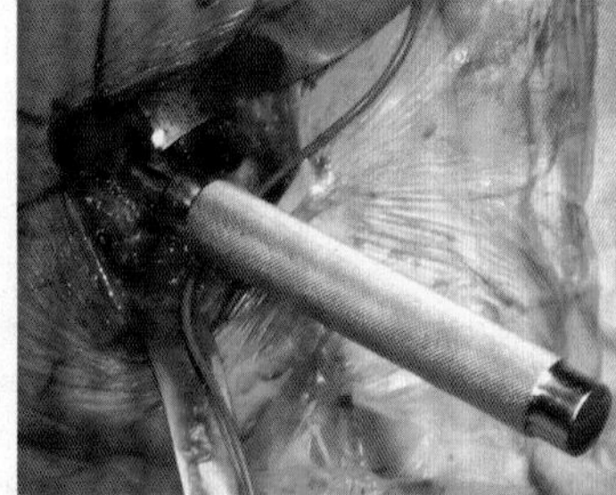

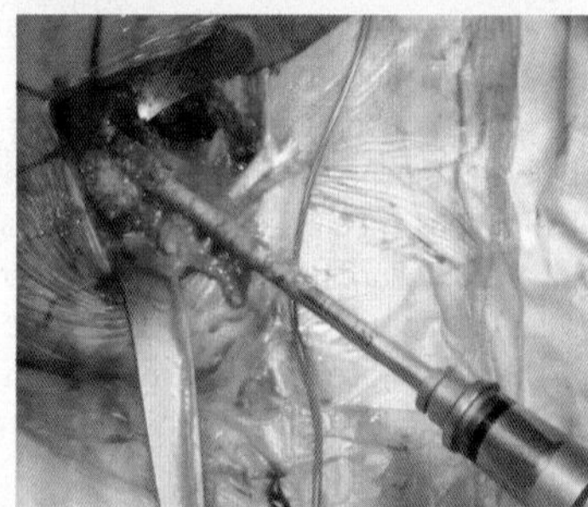

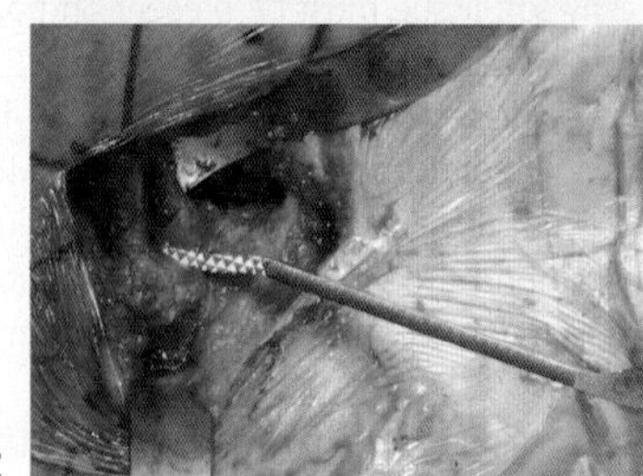

TECH FIG 10 • A. Use of a curette for femoral orientation. **B.** Reaming of the femoral canal. **C.** Lateralization of the femoral canal with a lateral rasp.

Femoral Broaching

- The femoral broach is introduced in neutral position and neutral version of the rotation is judged in relation to the position of the knee.
- Broaching is begun with the smallest broach and then increased until appropriate fit and fill is achieved. This can be gauged by preoperative templating and tactile feedback.
- The broach is introduced each time to its full depth.
  - If significant resistance is met, broaching should continue with a series of small inward and then outward taps.
  - Broaching is continued until full cortical seating has been accomplished. This is indicated by an upward change in pitch as the broach is seated.
  - Final seating and sizing is determined by pitch, tactile feedback, and lack of progression (**TECH FIG 11A**).
- Once the final seating of the femoral broach is accomplished, an initial reduction with the appropriate-sized hemiarthroplasty bipolar or unipolar trial component is performed (**TECH FIG 11B**).

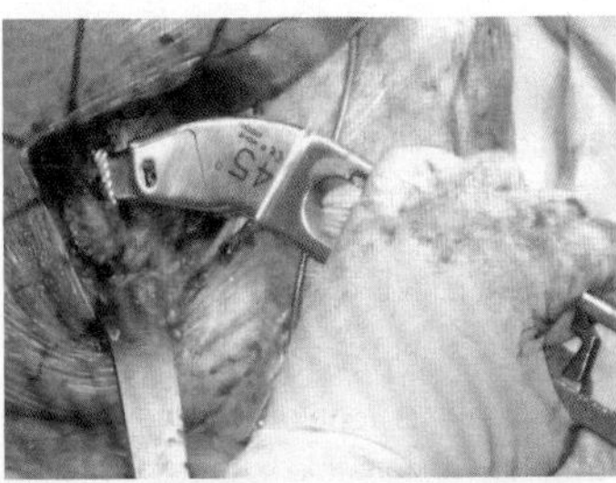

A

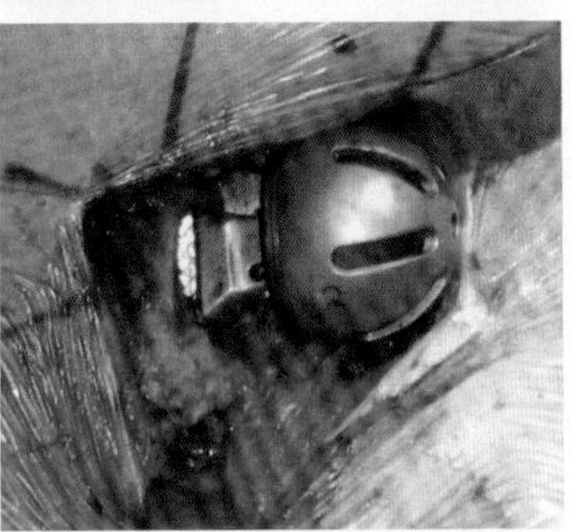

B

TECH FIG 11 • **A.** Broaching of the femoral canal. **B.** Placement of trial head onto trial femoral prosthesis.

Evaluation of Trial Prosthesis

- The hip is reduced for evaluation.
  - Hip stability is evaluated in full flexion and in internal and external rotation.
  - One finger is kept in the joint to evaluate for anterior impingement.
  - Anterior stability is evaluated with external rotation, adduction, and extension.
  - Leg lengths are measured directly.
  - The position of the pelvis, shoulders, and knees must be evaluated as the assistants help with orientation (**TECH FIG 12**).
- Stability also is evaluated with a longitudinal shuck test, with a goal of 1 or 2 mm of shuck.
  - Excessively tight soft tissues about the hip cause difficult or incomplete extension of the hip; excessive laxity leads to increased shuck.
  - For inadequate soft tissue tension and appropriate leg length restoration, a lateral offset can also be used.

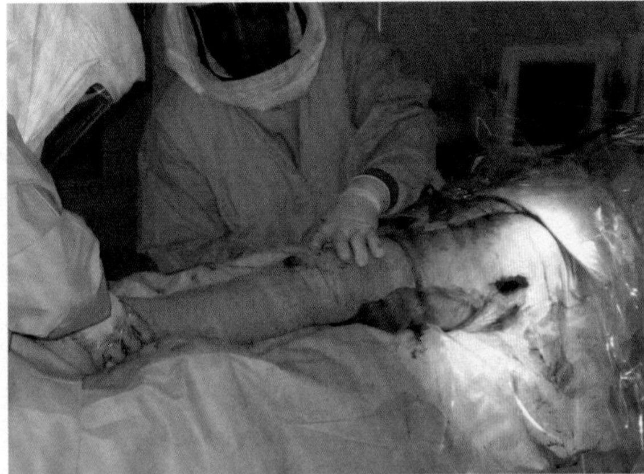

TECH FIG 12 • Intraoperative evaluation of trial prosthesis leg length.

  - It is important to achieve stability, which takes precedence over leg length.

Placement of the Femoral Stem

- Once stability is satisfactory, the trial components are removed.
- The wound and the femur are irrigated with pulsatile lavage.
  - Excessive debris is removed.
  - The femur is prepared again with the curette only, to clear any soft tissue debris from the lateral aspect of the femur.
  - The femoral canal must be copiously irrigated.
  - The surgeon and assistant change outer gloves.
- The appropriately sized femoral component is placed in the femoral canal with the use of an impactor.
  - Varus positioning must be avoided. It can be prevented with appropriate valgus positioning of the stem on insertion, with attention paid to maintaining the appropriate version.
  - The femoral component is seated into position using firm taps with a mallet.
  - A pause between taps may allow some plastic deformation of the femur.
  - Final seating is determined in relation to the last broach, tactile feedback, pitch change, and lack of progression (**TECH FIG 13**).

Completion of Implant Placement

- Once the stem is placed, a second trial reduction can be performed with the trial next segment and trial bipolar shell, or a

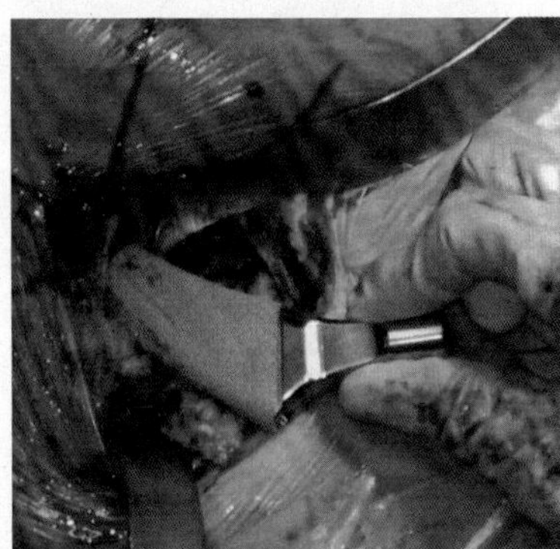

A

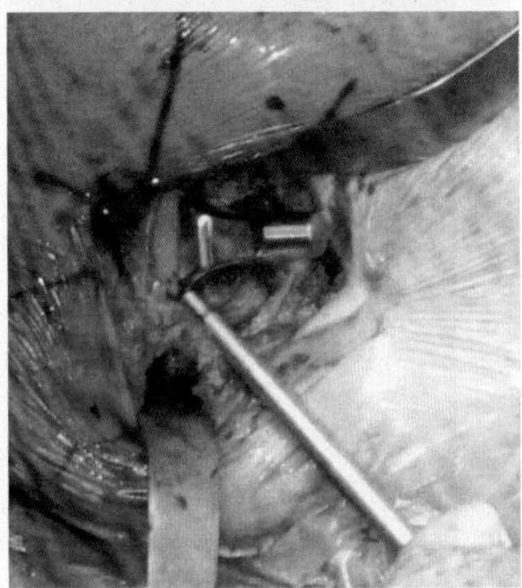

B

TECH FIG 13 • **A.** Placement of final femoral stem. **B.** Impaction of femoral stem.

final component can be placed if the broach and stem achieve the same position.

- If the trial bipolar shell is desired, trial reduction is performed again.
- The reduction is performed with the patient held in position by the second assistant and the first assistant.
- The surgeon reduces the hip with distraction, internal rotation, and adduction.
- The surgical technician can assist the reduction with longitudinal traction.

- The bipolar is assembled on the back table with the outer acetabular bipolar shell impacted on the appropriately sized head.
  - This can be a 22-, 28-, or 32-mm head, depending on the implant system, with a polyethylene insert and bipolar shell that sits over it (**TECH FIG 14A**).
- Once that is assembled on the back table, the trunnion is cleaned and dried and the bipolar shell is impacted on to the trunnion of the neck of femoral prosthesis.
- The acetabulum is checked one last time before final reduction for any debris or any soft tissue (**TECH FIG 14B**).
- Once it is checked and cleared, the hip is reduced, and the bipolar shell is reduced and checked for appropriate position, after which the wound is thoroughly irrigated and copiously irrigated with pulsatile lavage (**TECH FIG 14C**).
- At this point, drains can be used according to the preference of the surgeon. I prefer not to use drains.

Wound Repair and Closure

- The abductor mass is repaired.
- The vastus lateralis is repaired to the remaining tissue sleeve with interrupted absorbable sutures in figure-8 fashion with no. 1 Vicryl.
- The gluteus medius tendon and capsule are repaired to the tissue sleeve on the bridge of the trochanter.
  - This is done with heavy absorbable sutures in figure-8 fashion.
  - The repair is done at the corner of the gluteus medius tendon and then extended into the proximal split with simple sutures (**TECH FIG 15A**).

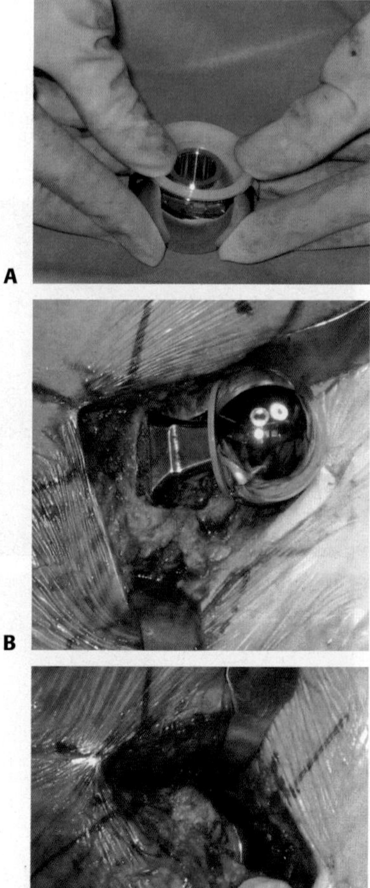

TECH FIG 14 • A. Assembly of bipolar head. **B.** Placement of bipolar head onto femoral stem. **C.** Relocation of the prosthetic hip into the native acetabulum.

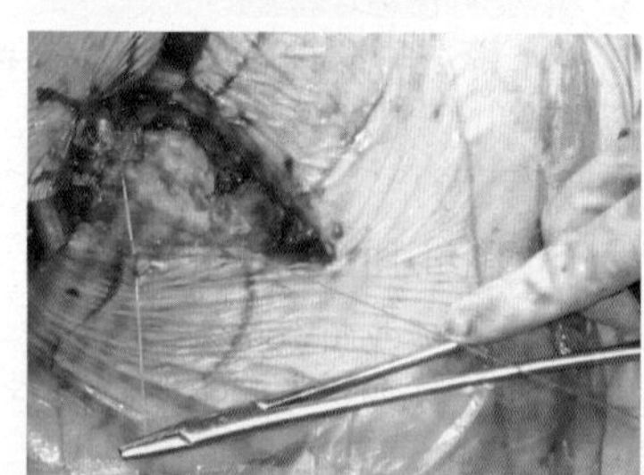

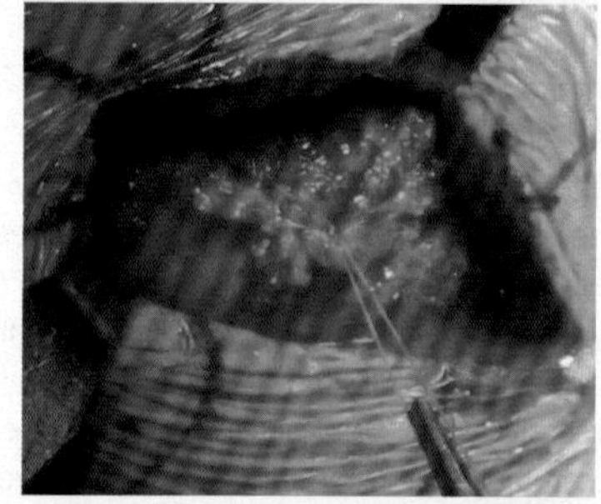

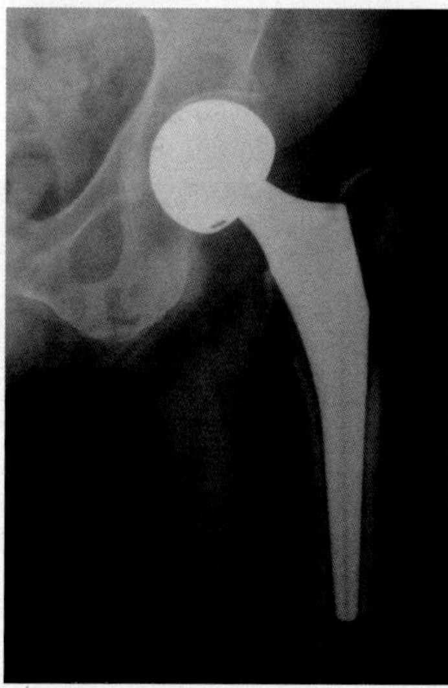

TECH FIG 15 • A. Repair of the abductor mass. **B.** Repair of the TFL. **C.** AP radiograph of an implanted bipolar prosthesis.

- Once the hip abductor is adequately repaired, the TFL is approximated with absorbable sutures in figure-8 fashion.
  - This must be done to both the proximal and distal extents of the fascia lata.
- The potential dead space is obliterated with heavy absorbable sutures, and smaller absorbable 2-0 sutures are placed in subcutaneous tissue (**TECH FIG 15B**).
- Skin staples are applied.
- Sterile dressing is applied with Microfoam surgical tape (3M).
- An abduction pillow is placed between the legs and loosely secured.
- The patient is awakened from anesthesia and brought to the recovery room if, or as soon as, his or her condition is stable.
- Postoperative radiographs are taken in the recovery room (**TECH FIG 15C**).

Posterior Approach (Southern)

Incision and Dissection

- Exposure of the hip begins with appropriate identification of the bony landmarks.
  - The posterolateral corner of the greater trochanter and the anterior and posterior borders of the proximal femoral shaft are marked 10 cm below the greater trochanter (**TECH FIG 16A,B**).
- The incision begins at this point and extends obliquely over the posterolateral corner of the greater trochanter, continuing proximally, so that the acetabulum is centered in the incision.
  - The incision usually is 15 to 20 cm, although this will vary depending on the patient's body habitus (**TECH FIG 16C**).
- Once the subcutaneous tissue is divided, the fascia lata is identified and incised in line with the incision.
  - The fibers of the gluteus maximus belly are bluntly separated with firm finger pressure (**TECH FIG 16D,E**).

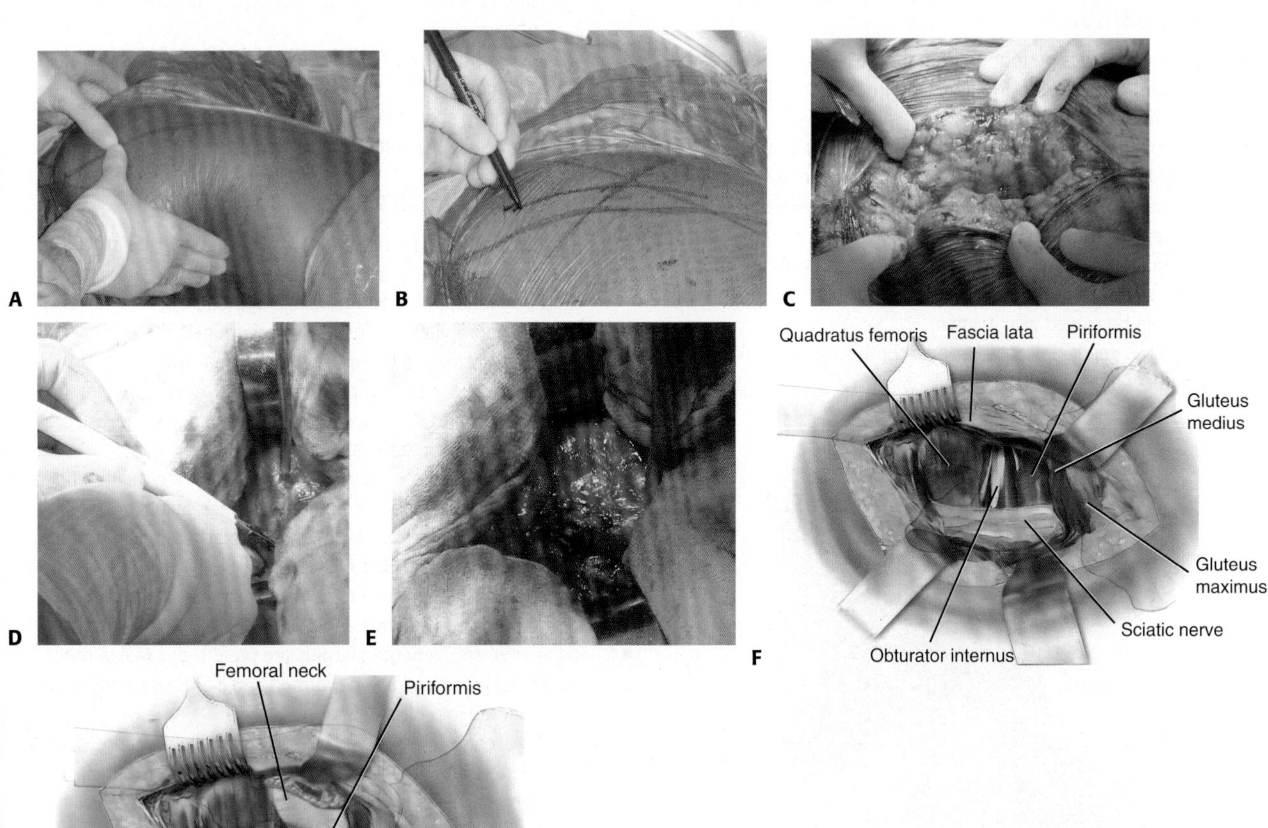

TECH FIG 16 • **A.** Palpation of bony landmarks for posterior approach. This is created by the midpoint of the ASIS and the ischial tuberosity. **B.** Incisional line. Note its placement with respect to the axis of the femur, the proximal extent of the greater trochanter, and the previous line created by bony palpation. **C.** Skin incision. **D.** Identification and incision of the TFL. **E.** Exposure of the deep posterior structures of the hip after blunt separation of the gluteus maximus. **F.** Deep posterior structures of the hip. **G.** Reflection of the short external rotators. (**A–E:** Courtesy of Norman A. Johanson, MD.)

- A Charnley self-retaining retractor is placed to retract the gluteus maximus and tensor fascia. The gluteus maximus tendon may be released from the femur.
- The hip is internally rotated to offer exposure to the posterior structures.
- The piriformis tendon is identified by palpation and a curved retractor is placed deep into the abductors just superior to the piriformis (**TECH FIG 16F**).
  - A cobra retractor is placed inferior to the femoral neck.
- The short external rotators and piriformis may be released separately from the capsule and tagged.
  - The piriformis and conjoint tendons should be divided as close to their insertions as possible.
  - Alternatively, the external rotators and capsule can be taken down as one continuous sleeve off the trochanter and femoral neck (**TECH FIG 16G**).
- Following the reflection of the short external rotators, the capsule is isolated by repositioning the superior and inferior retractors.
  - The curved superior retractor is placed deep to the gluteus minimus just over the superior femoral neck and capsule.

Site Preparation

- A capsulotomy is performed from this posterosuperior acetabulum and continued to the tip of the trochanter in line with the posterior border of the abductors.
- It is continued inferiorly along the femoral neck instead of making oblique posterior limit of the capsulotomy in favor of reflecting this capsule as continuous sleeve to the level of the lesser trochanter (**TECH FIG 17**).
- The quadratus femoris can be released along with the capsule, leaving a small muscular cuff with later reattachment. The capsule can be tagged with a suture.
- The hip is gently dislocated using a combination of flexion, internal rotation, and adduction.

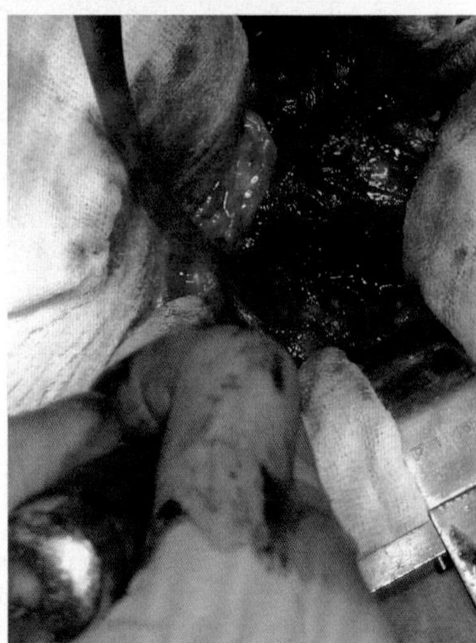

TECH FIG 17 • Exposure of the hip capsule. (Courtesy of Norman A. Johanson, MD.)

- The leg is held at 90 degrees of internal rotation so that the femoral neck is parallel to the ground.
- At this point, the proximal femur usually dissociates from the femoral neck and head, which often remain in the acetabulum.
  - Two retractors can be placed around the proximal femur and a fresh cut of the femoral neck can be performed with an oscillating saw.
  - Alternatively, if this is a low femoral neck fracture, this area can be smoothed with a rongeur and attention turned to the acetabulum.
- At this point, the retractors are placed around the acetabulum. Initially, a curved retractor is placed anteriorly, retracting the proximal femur out of the view of the acetabulum.
  - The operated extremity is placed in slight flexion, which aids in exposure.
  - Occasionally, the reflected head of the rectus femoris must be released.
- A Steinmann pin can be placed in the ilium to reflect the abductors and a small capsulotomy can be made inferiorly to allow for placement of a cobra retractor deep to the transverse acetabular ligament.
  - A bent Hohmann retractor can be placed posteriorly, taking care to first palpate the sciatic nerve to ensure that it is out of harm's way.
- At this point, the acetabulum is exposed and the femoral head can be removed again with a corkscrew and a Cobb elevator.
  - This step should be done very carefully to avoid damaging the acetabular cartilage.

Component Placement

- The femoral head is measured. A trial shell can be placed in the acetabulum for appropriate sizing, which is performed as described for the modified Hardinge approach.
- Once an appropriate size has been determined, the leg is flexed and internally rotated to expose the proximal femur.
  - The leg is held at approximately 90 degrees of internal rotation and 70 degrees of flexion, bringing the osteotomized neck into the surgeon's view.
  - A trochanteric elevator is placed with the teeth under the anterior aspect of the femoral neck, lifting it out of the wound. This allows for unencumbered preparation of the femoral neck (**TECH FIG 18A**).
- The femur is then prepared in a fashion similar to that described for the modified Hardinge approach (**TECH FIG 18B–F**).
- In cases where cemented femurs are preferred, a trial of reduction for leg lengths can be performed and a final component can be cemented into place.
  - The component must be cemented in the appropriate version and the neck of the prosthesis must sit on the femoral neck, which can be additionally prepared with a calcar planer.

Completion of the Procedure

- Once the final components are placed and the hip is reduced, two drill holes can be made in the posterior aspect of the greater trochanter for repair of the capsular and short external rotators.

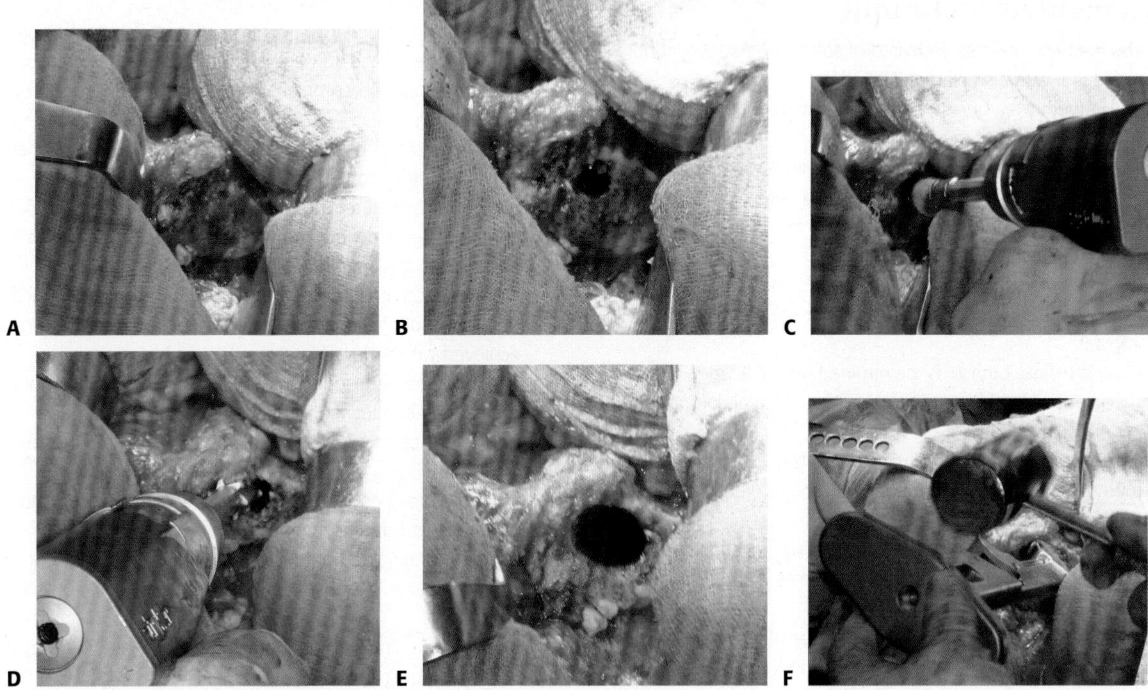

TECH FIG 18 • **A.** Presentation of the proximal femur. **B.** Pilot hole for femoral preparation. **C.** Reaming of the femoral shaft. **D.** Lateralization of the femoral shaft using a reamer. **E.** Reamed femoral shaft. Note the lateralization of the canal. **F.** Broaching of the femoral shaft. (Courtesy of Norman A. Johanson, MD.)

- Two nonabsorbable sutures are placed in the capsular flap.
  - The capsular and external rotator tagging sutures are brought through the drill holes and the greater trochanter tied in layers.
  - The quadratus femoris and gluteus maximus tendon also can be repaired if that is the surgeon's preference (**TECH FIG 19**).
- Subsequently, the Charnley retractor is removed and the TFL and gluteus maximus fascia are reapproximated.
- Dead space is closed with absorbable sutures in the subcutaneous fat and absorbable sutures are placed in the subcutaneous tissue.
- Skin staples and a sterile compressive dressing are applied at the skin level.
- The hip must be held in an abducted position. An abduction pillow is placed and the patient is moved from the lateral position to the supine position at the end of the operation.

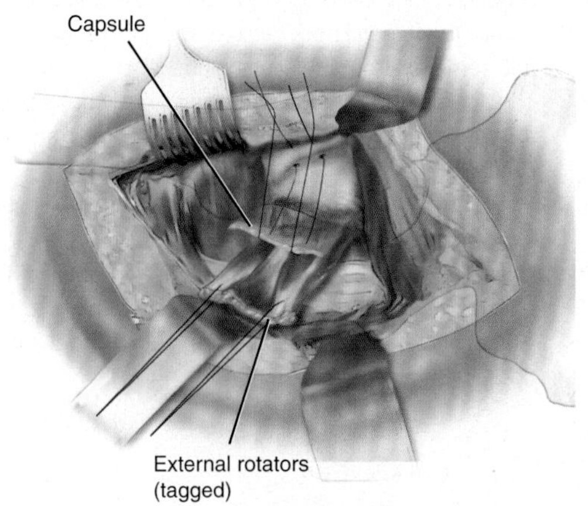

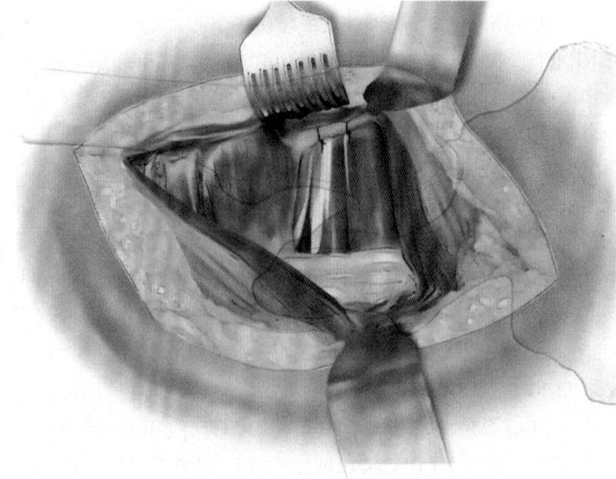

TECH FIG 19 • Approximation and repair of the short external rotators.

Cemented Technique

- The trochanteric fossa is cleared of soft tissue and a pilot hole is made in it with a small metal curette.
  - An entry reamer is inserted along this pilot hole to seek the long access of the femoral canal.
- The residual femoral neck is cleared with a rongeur or box osteotome. Sometimes, a lateralizing reamer is used to ensure direct access to the femoral canal and minimize the possibility of varus implantation.
- Broaches often are oversized relative to the final implant size, thereby ensuring a minimum cement mantle all around the implant.
  - The final broach is determined when it adequately fills the proximal femur; it also serves as a trial component for reduction.
- Once the stability, limb length, and offset are satisfactory, cementation can be performed. The canal is gently curetted to remove any loose cancellous bone.
- The canal is irrigated with a long, pulsating, irrigating tip.
  - High-quality cancellous bone remains in the femoral canal following this preparation.
  - It is important to centralize the prosthesis to ensure an uninterrupted cement mantle around the implant.
- A plug is placed after the canal is irrigated.
  - I prefer to allow 1 to 2 cm of cement below the tip of the implant so that the plug may be placed at that level.
  - It must be secure enough to withstand pressurization.
  - Three 40-g packs of cement are typically mixed with a vacuum system.
- The canal is packed with sponges to keep it dry during the cementation. Alternatively, continuous suction may be used.
- The viscosity of the cement is an important consideration. The cement should be somewhat doughy and delivered through a cement gun.
  - Appropriate cement viscosity has been reached when the cement no longer sticks to the surgical gloves.
- Once the cement reaches the appropriate viscosity, the packing sponges are removed and the canal is suctioned. Cement is delivered in a retrograde fashion into the canal.
- Once the canal is filled with cement, a pressurizing unit can be placed over the proximal femur, or pressurization can be achieved with a gloved finger.
- The prosthesis is inserted into the doughy mass of cement with the centralizer attached to the tip.
- The leg is placed in a secure position and the prosthesis is inserted.
  - The prosthesis must be inserted with the appropriate anteversion from insertion all the way down.
  - It is preferable not to rotate the femoral component within the canal because this will create undesirable cement voids.
  - The prosthesis must be inserted with great care to avoid varus malpositioning.
- All the excess cement is removed and the stem is held in place until the cement has fully hardened. The femoral trunnion should be cleaned at this point and the hemiarthroplasty component should be inserted onto the stem.
- The hip is then reduced and the appropriate closure is performed.

Anterolateral (Watson-Jones) Technique

- One major difficulty with the Watson-Jones technique is dealing with the gluteus medius and minimus.
  - The hip abductors lie over anterior hip capsule and could be damaged in an effort to obtain adequate exposure.
  - The original approach used by Charnley placed the patient in a supine position and required a trochanteric osteotomy. This approach is used less commonly now because of problems associated with trochanteric reattachment.
- The skin incision is made 2.5 cm behind the ASIS to the tip of the greater trochanter and extended vertically along the anterior margin of the trochanter.
- The intraneural interval is between the TFL and gluteus medius. An incision is made in the underlying iliotibial band, after which the TFL is retracted medially and the gluteus medius is retracted laterally.
- Deep dissection may require release of the anterior parts of the gluteus medius and minimus, which are raised from the femur and retracted posteriorly.
  - The upper part of the capsule at the hip joint is seen with a reflected head of the rectus femoris attached to the upper part of the acetabular rim.
  - It can then be detached with greater exposure of the capsule, which may be incised.
- The ascending branch of the lateral femoral circumflex artery and the accompanying veins run deep to the muscles and must be ligated.
- A longitudinal incision is made in the joint capsule along the femoral neck and transversely from the proximal femur.
- A bone hook can be used to apply a direct lateral force to disimpact the femoral neck fracture. The femoral head can be carefully removed from the acetabulum.
- The acetabulum is then sized as previously described.
- After the femur is externally rotated, adducted, and extended, it can be prepared.
  - Femoral preparation in this approach may require specialized instruments.
- Consider detaching or splitting along the anterior third of the gluteus medius to eliminate the risk of damage to the superior gluteal nerve, which passes 4.5 cm above and 2 cm behind the tip of the greater trochanter.

PEARLS AND PITFALLS

Acetabular reaming	▪ Not recommended for hemiarthroplasty because it leads to poor results. Appropriate femoral head size should be chosen intraoperatively to avoid reaming.
Varus malalignment	▪ Care should be taken to broach the lateral cortex of the proximal femur adequately to prevent varus malalignment of the implant.
Implant orientation (anteversion)	▪ Ideally, the patient's hip should be reoriented to its native position. Ideal anteversion of the hip in adults is 10–30 degrees, depending on multiple patient-specific factors. If the patient has pathology that affects hip orientation (eg, developmental displacement of the hip), a modular THA implant could be considered.
Cement technique	▪ I recommend the use of uncemented, proximal-fit, porous-coated implants in most patients, if possible. The presence of poor bone quality, stovepipe proximal femoral metaphysis and shaft, and angular/rotational deformities of the proximal femur argue for use of a cemented implant. Proper cement technique includes vacuum mixing of cement, pressurized cement delivery, proper canal preparation, placement of a cement restrictor plug, finger pressurization of cement, and stable implant pressurization of the cement. An ideal cement mantle is 2 mm circumferentially around the implant.
Posterior approach	▪ Careful retractor placement is essential to avoid errant sciatic or femoral nerve injury. Enhanced posterior capsular repair is important to reduce the risk of dislocation.

POSTOPERATIVE CARE

- All patients are placed into a soft hip abduction pillow, and bilateral thromboembolic stockings are put on with sequential venous compression devices.
- Antiembolic prophylaxis is started according to the surgeon's preference.
  - Extended prophylaxis may be considered for these patients.

OUTCOMES

- Bipolar hemiarthroplasty was introduced in the 1970s in an effort to prevent or retard acetabular wear.
  - These femoral prostheses have a 22- to 32-mm head that articulates with a polyethylene liner.
  - The liner is covered with a polished metal outer shell that articulates with the acetabular cartilage.
  - Depending on implant design, about 45 degrees of angular motion is achieved before the prosthetic neck impinges on the liner and axial rotation is restricted.
- Theoretically, hip motion occurs primarily at the prosthetic joint and only secondarily at the metal-cartilage interface.
  - The polyethylene liner may help to protect the native acetabular cartilage by cushioning the high-contact pressures that occur across the bearing.
- LaBelle et al[13] reported no acetabular protrusio or articular cartilage wear greater than 2 mm in 49 femoral neck fractures treated with cemented bipolar hemiarthroplasties at 5- to 10-year follow-up.
- Wetherell and Hinves[15] reported a 50% reduction in acetabular erosion for patients treated with a cemented bipolar prosthesis when compared to those treated with a unipolar prosthesis.
- Research attempting to demonstrate that motion occurs within a bipolar prosthesis has yielded conflicting results.
  - Drinker and Murray[7] fluoroscopically evaluated 13 hips in 10 young patients following bipolar reconstruction for AVN and noted that only a minor amount of motion occurred at the inner bearing and that motion tended to decrease over time.
  - They further demonstrated that in this group most implants functioned as a unipolar prosthesis and concluded that motion will occur at the interface where there is the least frictional resistance. They found that this location is not the same in arthritic hips as in fractured hips.
  - In patients with acute hip fractures with normal articular cartilage, primary intraoperative or intraprosthetic motion occurred in only 25% and most implants functioned as unipolar.
- Brueton et al[4] whose radiographic analysis of 75 bipolar prostheses compared 32-mm and 22-mm heads, showed that the smaller head was associated with more motion.

COMPLICATIONS

- Thromboembolism (eg, deep vein thrombosis or pulmonary embolism)
- Kenzora et al[12] reported a mortality rate of 14% during the first year following hip fracture.
  - When compared to 9% mortality in a population of similar age, the mortality after hemiarthroplasty is 10% to 40%.
- The incidence of intraoperative femur fracture is 4.5%. Most are nondisplaced and involve either the trochanter or calcar.
  - When an intraoperative femur fracture occurs, treatment options include methylmethacrylate combined with long-stem prosthesis or, alternatively, a fully coated cementless stem and cables.
- The rate of dislocation is less than 10%. Dislocation is more common with incorrect version, posterior capsulectomy, and excessive postoperative flexion or rotation with the hip adducted.
- Postoperative sepsis has been reported to range from 2% to 20% and may be more common with the posterior surgical approach. Infections may be superficial or deep.
- Loosening or migration may be suspected with the presence of a radiolucent line around the prosthesis.
  - If clinical signs and symptoms are present, or loosening or migration is present, a revision arthroplasty may be considered.

- Cementation presents some hazards, and, in some cases, the application of pressurized cement is associated with an embolization phenomenon with cement elements (ie, monomer, polymethylmethacrylate elements, or fat). Embolization of these materials may result in hypoxia, cardiac arrest, or death.
  - The risk factors include older age or patent foramen ovale.
  - The use of pulsatile lavage can reduce that risk by removing fat and marrow from the femoral canal.
  - In older patients with substantial medical comorbidities, it may be wise to avoid pressurization of the cement within the canal because the risk of acute embolization may be high.

REFERENCES

1. Barnes JT, Brown JT, Garden RS, et al. Subcapital fractures of the femur: a prospective review. J Bone Joint Surg Br 1976;58:2–24.
2. Bateman JE. Single assembly total hip prosthesis preliminary report. Orthop Dig 1974;2:15.
3. Bezwada HP, Shah AR, Harding SH, et al. Cementless bipolar hemiarthroplasty for displaced femoral neck fractures in the elderly. J Arthroplasty 2004;19(7 Suppl 2):73–77.
4. Brueton RN. Effect of femoral component head size on movement of the two-component hemi-arthroplasty. Injury 1993;24:231–235.
5. Dedrick DK, Mackenzie JR, Burney RE. Complications of femoral neck fractures in young adults. J Trauma 1986;26:932–937.
6. Dorr LD, Faugere MC, Mackel AM, et al. Structural and cellular assessment of bone quality of proximal femur. Bone 1993;3:231–242.
7. Drinker H, Murray WR. The universal proximal femoral endoprosthesis: a short-term comparison with conventional hemiarthroplasty. J Bone Joint Surg Am 1979;61:1167–1174.
8. Eiskjaer S, Ostgard SE. Risk factors influencing mortality after bipolar hemiarthroplasty in the treatment of fracture of the femoral neck. Clin Orthop Relat Res 1991;270:295–300.
9. Garden RS. Stability and union in subcapital fractures of the femur. J Bone Joint Surg Br 1964;46:630–647.
10. Gilberty RP. Bipolar endoprosthesis minimizes protrusio acetabuli, loose stems. Orthop Rev 1985;14:27.
11. Ito H, Matsuno T, Kaneda K. Bipolar hemiarthroplasty for osteonecrosis of the femoral head. A 7-18 year followup. Clin Orthop Relat Res 2000;(374):201–211.
12. Kenzora JE, McCarthy RE, Lowell JD, et al. Hip fracture mortality. Relation to age, treatment, preoperative illness, time of surgery, and complications. Clin Orthop Relat Res 1984;186:45–56.
13. LaBelle LW, Colwill JC, Swanson AB. Bateman bipolar arthroplasty for femoral neck fractures. A five- to ten-year follow-up study. Clin Orthop Relat Res 1990;251:20–25.
14. Robinson CM, Court-Brown CM, McQueen MM, et al. Hip fracture in adults younger than 50 years of age—epidemiology and results. Clin Orthop Relat Res 1995;312:238–246.
15. Wetherell RG, Hinves BL. The Hastings bipolar hemiarthroplasty for subcapital fractures of the femoral neck. J Bone Joint Surg Br 1990;72:788–793.
16. Yu L, Wang Y, Chen J. Total hip arthroplasty versus hemiarthroplasty for displaced femoral neck fractures: meta-analysis of randomized trials. Clin Orthop Relat Res 2012;470:2235–2243.

Resection Arthroplasty and Spacer Insertion

33

CHAPTER

Mark J. Spangehl and Christopher P. Beauchamp

DEFINITION

- Resection arthroplasty and insertion of a spacer is used for the management of chronic deep periprosthetic infection of the hip.
- This chapter discusses the diagnosis and management of late chronic infections. Acute infections, described in the following text, have a different presentation, methods of diagnosis, and management algorithm.
- Antibiotic-loaded spacers are an adjuvant treatment for the management of deep infection by providing elusion of antibiotics into the local tissues.[6]
  - Historically, deep periprosthetic infection was treated by resection arthroplasty alone.
  - However, depending on the type used, spacers allow for improved function between resection and reimplantation when compared with resection arthroplasty alone by providing soft tissue tension and an articulating surface and, in most cases, allow weight bearing through the lower extremity.
- Spacers can be grouped into articulating spacers or nonarticulating (static) spacers.
  - Articulating spacers can resemble either a total hip replacement, with antibiotic-loaded implants inserted on the acetabular and femoral sides, or a hemiarticulating spacer, with an antibiotic-loaded implant inserted only on the femoral side.
  - Static spacers are blocks and dowels of antibiotic-loaded cement placed into the acetabulum and femoral canal after removal of the implants.

ANATOMY

- The pertinent anatomy of the hip is shown in **FIG 1**.
- The fasciae lata cover the musculature of the hip.
  - Distally, the fibers condense and form the iliotibial band, which inserts onto the lateral aspect of the proximal tibia (Gerdy tubercle).
  - Proximally, the fascia splits and envelops the gluteus maximus (inferior gluteal nerve) and the tensor fascia lata (superior gluteal nerve).
- Deep to the fascia lata, over the lateral aspect of the hip, are the major abductors: the gluteus medius and minimus (superior gluteal nerve).
- More posteriorly, deep to the gluteus maximus, are the short external rotators.
  - From proximal to distal: piriformis (branches from S1 and S2), superior gemellus (nerve to obturator internus), obturator internus (nerve to obturator internus), inferior gemellus (nerve to quadratus femoris); slightly deeper is the obturator externus (posterior branch obturator nerve); distally is the quadratus femoris (nerve to quadratus femoris).
- The sciatic nerve usually emerges from the lower border of the piriformis and is posterior to the short external rotators.
  - When approaching the hip posteriorly, retracting the short rotators posteriorly will provide some protection to the sciatic nerve.

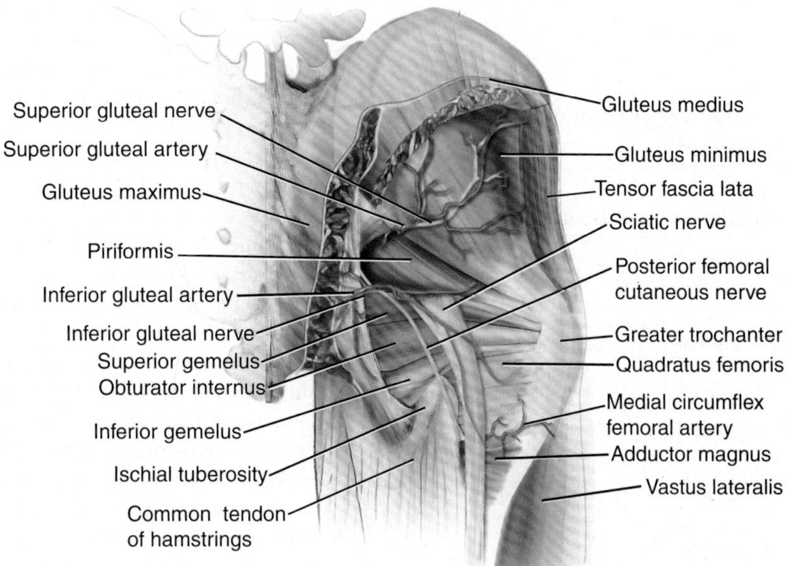

FIG 1 • Anatomy of the posterolateral aspect of the hip joint.

- An ascending branch from the medial femoral circumflex courses over the posterior aspect of the quadratus femoris; this may produce bleeding during dissection.
- Anterior to the hip capsule is the iliopsoas tendon on which the femoral nerve lies as it crosses under the ilioinguinal ligament and enters the thigh.
  - Retractors placed over the anterior wall need to be placed directly on bone to avoid injury to the nerve.

PATHOGENESIS

- Periprosthetic infections are classified as acute or chronic infections (Table 1).[9,30]
- Acute infections are either acute postoperative infections or acute hematogenous (late) infections.
  - If diagnosed early, acute infections can be managed with débridement and irrigation with component retention.
- Chronic infections generally present in a delayed manner, usually months or occasionally years after the index procedure. The infection has likely been present since the original procedure, but because of the low virulence of the infecting organism, classic signs of infection are lacking, and hip pain may be the only presenting symptoms.
- Chronic infections also include a missed or delayed diagnosis of an acute infection. A missed or delayed diagnosis of an acute infection must now be treated as a chronic infection.

NATURAL HISTORY

- Chronic periprosthetic infection will continue to cause pain and disability.
- The severity of symptoms depends on the virulence of the organism, the overall health or comorbidities of the patient, and fixation of the implants and status of the surrounding soft tissues.
- Low-virulence organisms (eg, coagulase-negative *Staphylococcus*) may present with chronic pain, whereas more virulent organisms (eg, *Staphylococcus aureus*) or hosts that are immunocompromised may present with more obvious signs of infection.
- Untreated patients are at risk for seeding other joint replacements. The incidence is unknown and likely depends on the virulence of the organism and the host's medical comorbidities.

Table 1 Classification of Deep Periprosthetic Infection (Based on Timing of Presentation)

Type of Infection	Timing of Presentation	Treatment
Acute postoperative infection	Up to 4 wk after index operation	Débridement and component retention
Acute hematogenous /late infection	Sudden onset of pain in well-functioning joint	Débridement and component retention
Late chronic infection	Infection presenting >1 mo after index operation (includes missed or delayed diagnosis of acute infection)	Removal and reimplantation

- Patients who have multiple medical comorbidities or are infected with more virulent organisms may be at greater risk for signs or symptoms of systemic infection and, subsequently, seeding of other joints by hematogenous spread.
- With time, chronic infection can cause bone loss and loosening of implants.
  - In addition to increased pain from implant loosening, the osteolysis, which may be secondary to both infection and loose implants, can result in an increased risk of periprosthetic fracture.

PATIENT HISTORY AND PHYSICAL FINDINGS

- In most cases, a careful history will lead to suspicion of a diagnosis of chronic infection.
- Often, patients give a history of poor wound healing, with prolonged drainage, prolonged antibiotic use, or surgical débridement.
  - These cases represent missed or failed treatment for acute postoperative infections. Missed acute hematogenous (late) infections, which are now chronic, present with a history of sudden deterioration in hip function, without other obvious mechanical causes of failure.
- Another subset of patients with chronic infection present only with pain. Often, it has been present since the time of the initial index procedure.
  - There may also be a history of poor wound healing or prolonged drainage.
  - The pain is usually different in character than preoperative activity-related arthritic pain. It may be more constant, present at rest, and consist of a dull ache. The pain may worsen with activity but tends to be more constant than pure mechanically related pain from a loose implant.
- The physical examination is often nonspecific in the setting of chronic infection.
  - The examination findings range from nearly normal, with only mild pain with range of motion, to more obvious signs of infection, such as a chronically draining sinus.
- Examinations to perform include the following:
  - Observe gait pattern. Pain or muscle weakness may cause limp. Trunk may shift over affected hip.
  - Trendelenburg sign. A positive result may indicate abductor dysfunction, pain, or a neurologic problem (superior gluteal nerve or L5 nerve root).
  - Inspect any old incision sites and surrounding skin. Plan to incorporate all or as much of the old incisions as possible. A draining sinus indicates a deep infection.
  - Examine the soft tissue for thickness and compliance. Poor tissue compliance may compromise closure and wound healing. Poor tissue integrity may require rotation flap for closure.
  - Passive range of motion. Significant stiffness may make surgical exposure more difficult. Excessive motion may increase the risk of instability.
  - Straight-leg raising may be limited by pain from infection, loose implants, or hip flexor tendonitis.
  - Assess true and apparent leg lengths.
  - Perform a neurovascular examination. Check and document the status of motor group function, sensation, and pulses preoperatively in case of any change following surgery.

IMAGING AND OTHER DIAGNOSTIC STUDIES

- Radiographs
  - In most cases, radiographs do not show signs of chronic infection. Radiographs are necessary to exclude other causes of aseptic failure and for surgical planning.
  - Radiographs from patients with long-standing chronic infection will show signs of deep infection. A periosteal reaction is considered pathognomonic for deep infection. Sinus tracks, extending through bone, may rarely be seen (**FIG 2**).
- Laboratory investigations
  - The most useful laboratory tests, both to confirm and to exclude a suspected diagnosis of deep infection, are the erythrocyte sedimentation rate (ESR) and C-reactive protein (CRP).
    - Various values have been considered positive (indicative of infection). It is generally accepted that an ESR above 30 mm per hour and a CRP above 10 mg/L are indicators of potential infection, provided the patient does not have other diagnoses that lead to elevated inflammatory markers.[27]
    - The sensitivity of the ESR or CRP, used individually, is diminished in the setting of nonvirulent chronic indolent infections.[22] However, when used in combination, if both values are strongly negative (low normal), it is unlikely that the patient is infected, and other diagnoses should be considered.
  - White blood cell count is rarely abnormal in chronic infection and is not helpful for diagnosing deep infection.
  - Hip aspiration for culture and synovial white blood cell count is indicated if there is any clinical suspicion of infection or if there is elevation of either the ESR or CRP. Any antibiotics that the patient may be receiving should be discontinued at least 2 to 3 weeks before aspiration to reduce the risk of false-negative cultures.[2]
    - The specimen should be separated into two, or preferably three, specimens for culture. If all cultures are positive for the same organism and the results correlate with the clinical presentation and elevation of inflammatory markers, then the diagnosis is confirmed.
    - The aspiration is routinely sent for aerobic and anaerobic cultures. In patients who have been previously investigated or managed for presumed infection with negative cultures or in patients who are immunosuppressed (eg, transplant patients, HIV-positive patients, or cancer patients undergoing chemotherapy), the specimen is also sent for fungal and mycobacterial cultures.
  - Synovial white blood cell count has become a useful method to help diagnose deep infection. Synovial cell count values diagnosing infection are mostly based on knee aspiration results, with only one study reporting data from hip aspirations. Although results vary, generally, a synovial white blood cell count of greater than 3000 cells/μL or over 70% polymorphonuclear leukocytes is suggestive of infection.[15,23,29]
- Frozen section is a helpful intraoperative test, but as with other investigations, it must be interpreted within the context of the clinical presentation and the results of other investigations; no single test is 100% reliable. The sensitivity and specificity of frozen section are approximately 0.80 and 0.90, respectively.[25]
  - Tissue for frozen section should be obtained from the areas that look most inflamed. A positive result, indicative of infection, is considered when there are more than five polymorphonuclear leukocytes per high-power field.[18]
- Intraoperative Gram stain should not be used to determine the presence or absence of infection. In late chronic infection, it has an extremely poor sensitivity.[26]
- In 2010, the American Academy of Orthopaedic Surgeons[1] (AAOS) published the first set of Clinical Practice Guidelines on the Diagnosis of Periprosthetic Joint Infections of the Hip and Knee. The diagnostic workup algorithms are based on the pretest probability of infection. The pretest probability of infection (either high or low) is based on the clinical presentation of the patient. The guideline recommendations and investigation algorithms are available on the AAOS website.[1]
- The diagnosis of chronic periprosthetic infection is made by the interpretation of clinical findings and the investigations mentioned earlier. The Musculoskeletal Infection Society established criteria for the diagnosis of periprosthetic joint infection.[20] Recently, these criteria were updated at the International Consensus Meeting on Periprosthetic Joint Infection.[33] The updated definition of periprosthetic joint infection is outlined in Table 2.

A
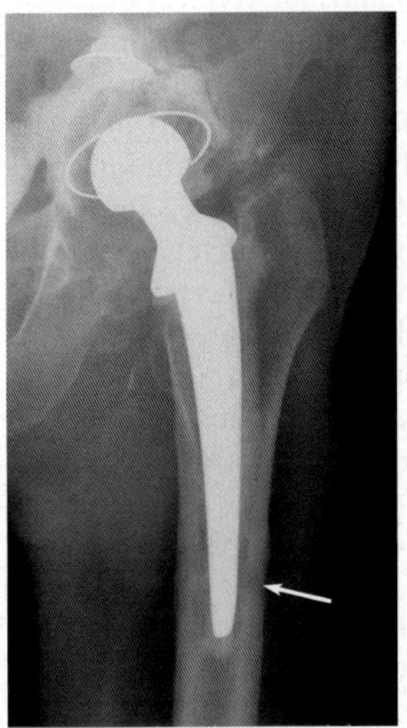
B
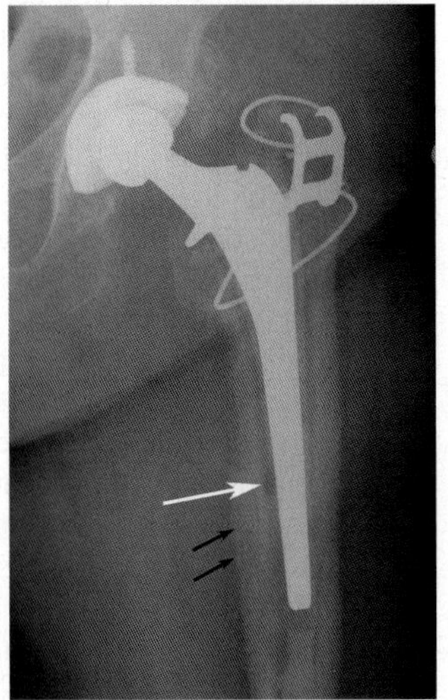

FIG 2 • **A.** Anteroposterior (AP) radiograph of infected total hip replacement showing a sinus tract through the lateral cortex (*arrow*). **B.** AP radiograph of infected total hip replacement showing periosteal reaction (*black arrows*) and sinus tract (*white arrow*) through posteromedial cortex.

Table 2 International Consensus Meeting on Periprosthetic Joint Infection Definition of Periprosthetic Joint Infection

Two positive periprosthetic cultures with phenotypically identical organisms
A sinus track communication with the joint
Three of the following minor criteria:
- Elevated serum ESR (>30 mm/hr) or CRP (>10 mg/L)
- Elevated synovial fluid WBC (>1100 cells/μL knees; >3000 cells/μL hips)
- Elevated synovial neutrophil percentage (>64% knees; >80% hips)
- Positive histologic analysis of periprosthetic tissue
- A single positive culture

ESR, erythrocyte sedimentation rate; CRP, C-reactive protein; WBC, white blood cell.
From Zmistowski B, Della Valle C, Bauer TW, et al. Workgroup 7: diagnosis of periprosthetic joint infection. In: Parvizi J, Gehrke T, eds. *Proceedings of the International Consensus Meeting on Periprosthetic Joint Infection*. Brooklandville, MD: Data Trace Publishing, 2013:158.

DIFFERENTIAL DIAGNOSIS

- Intrinsic
  - Aseptic loosening
  - Fibrous ingrowth (uncemented implants)
  - Polyethylene wear with synovitis
  - Modulus mismatch
  - Tendinitis (eg, psoas tendon impingement)
  - Bursitis or degenerative abductor avulsion
  - Heterotopic ossification
  - Stress fracture
- Extrinsic
  - Spinal pathology (eg, L2 nerve root impingement)
  - Vascular claudication
  - Hernia
  - Lateral femoral cutaneous nerve impingement

NONOPERATIVE MANAGEMENT

- In established cases of chronic infection, nonoperative management is rarely indicated for definitive treatment.
- Once the organism has been identified, antibiotic suppressive therapy may be used as a temporizing measure.
  - Antibiotic treatment may be able to suppress the infection and will likely prevent bacteremia if surgical treatment has to be delayed.
  - Antibiotic suppression may be considered in patients with very limited life expectancy who have a reasonably well-functioning joint, provided that the infecting organism has been identified and the infection can be suppressed with a well-tolerated oral antibiotic.
  - The use of antibiotics alone will not eradicate an established chronic infection, and antibiotic therapy alone should not be used if curing the infection is the goal.

SURGICAL MANAGEMENT

- The favored method of management of chronic periprosthetic hip infection is a two-stage exchange: removal of all implants and foreign material, followed by delayed reimplantation.
  - The time between stages allows the surgeon to observe the patient's response to therapy, thereby allowing him or her to assess for the possibility of recurrence of infection after the antibiotics have been stopped and before reimplantation.
- The principles of surgical management during the first stage are removal of the implants and all foreign material, thorough débridement of the joint, and insertion of a high-dose antibiotic cement spacer (either articulating or static).
- The patient is then treated with the appropriate antibiotic therapy, in addition to medical and nutritional management. This is ideally followed by a period of time off all antibiotics to ensure clinical resolution of infection, after which the second-stage reimplantation is performed.
- The principles of reconstruction during the second stage are as for aseptic revisions and are independent of the infection.
  - If infection is suspected at the time of reimplantation, definitive reconstruction should not be performed and the patient should instead be treated with repeat débridement and insertion of a spacer.
  - Otherwise, if the pre-reimplantation workup is negative and if there is no suspicion of infection at the time of reimplantation, it is assumed that the patient is free of infection, and reconstruction should be performed in a manner that is likely to give stable fixation of the implants and the best chance for good long-term functional outcome.
- In most cases, an uncemented reconstruction is favored.[7,8,17,19,28] The use of cement is not specifically indicated for the second stage of reconstruction when a two-stage approach is used.
- A variety of techniques have been described to create spacers after removal of the implants.[3,7,8,11,16,24] The common practice involves using high-dose antibiotics in the bone cement to obtain high local antibiotic concentrations.
  - Prefabricated commercially available spacers currently contain only low doses (generally considered prophylactic levels) of antibiotics. When used, these spacers are often inserted with the addition of high-dose antibiotic-loaded cement. Currently, we recommend against the use of these spacers and favor making spacers intraoperatively with high-dose antibiotics tailored to the organism.
  - We use the prosthesis with antibiotic-loaded acrylic cement (Prostalac [Depuy Synthes, Warsaw, Indiana]) molds,[5] which are described later. The technique can be adapted to other mold systems, however.

Preoperative Planning

- Preoperative planning is similar to any revision hip replacement procedure. Planning the steps used for managing the infection and inserting an antibiotic spacer is also required.
  - These steps include ensuring that the patient is medically stable to undergo the procedure, having the appropriate equipment available to remove the implants (eg, high-speed burrs, thin blade saws, ultrasonic cement removal equipment, trephines, or acetabular removal systems), and having equipment on hand for making the antibiotic-loaded spacer intraoperatively.
- Management of a chronically infected total hip replacement requires that every reasonable attempt be made to identify the organism preoperatively.
  - In most cases, the antibiotics used in the bone cement will be the same, although occasionally, an atypical organism will be identified preoperatively, requiring alteration in the content of antibiotics mixed into the bone cement.
- It is unlikely that nonimmunosuppressed patients with chronic infections will become bacteremic if antibiotics are stopped for a short period of time. Therefore, antibiotics that the patient may be receiving preoperatively should be discontinued about 2 to 4 weeks before surgery to improve the yield of positive cultures at the time of surgery.
  - Occasionally, a second organism or an organism with a different antibiotic sensitivity profile than that obtained preoperatively will be identified from intraoperative cultures.
- The appropriate molds and antibiotics to be mixed into the cement need to be available to make the spacer intraoperatively.
  - The most commonly used antibiotics are vancomycin and gentamicin or tobramycin. Other antibiotics can be used as well (Tables 3 and 4).
- Intrapelvic cement, if present, needs to be identified preoperatively.
  - Small amounts can be removed from the defect within the floor of the acetabulum.

Table 3 Antibiotics Used in Antibiotic-Impregnated Cement

Can Be Mixed with Cement	
Amikacin	Erythromycin
Amoxicillin	Gentamicin (powder)
Ampicillin	Lincomycin
Bacitracin	Methicillin
Cefamandole	Novobiocin
Cefazolin	Oxacillin
Cefuroxime	Penicillin
Cefuzonam	Polymyxin B
Cephalothin	Streptomycin
Ciprofloxacin	Ticarcillin
Clindamycin (powder)	Tobramycin
Colistin	Vancomycin
Daptomycin	
Decreased Activity Because of Heat from Cement	
Chloramphenicol	
Colistimethate	
Tetracycline	
Adversely Affect Curing of Cement	
Rifampin	
Liquid antibiotics (gentamicin, clindamycin) because of aqueous content	

Adapted from Joseph TN, Chen AL, Di Cesare PE. Use of antibiotic-impregnated cement in total joint arthroplasty. J Am Acad Orthop Surg 2003;11:38–47.

- Large amounts of cement require a preoperative contrast computed tomography (CT) scan to assess the location of cement relative to intrapelvic structures. A separate retroperitoneal approach may be required and should be planned.
- Radiolucent bone cement also requires CT evaluation preoperatively to determine its distal extent within the femoral canal or within the pelvis.

Table 4 Doses of Antibiotics Used in Antibiotic-Impregnated Cement (per 40 g of cement)

Antibiotic	Dose for Spacer	Dose for Prosthetic Fixation
Amikacin	2 g	1 g
Cefazolin	4–8 g	Not reported
Cefotaxime	Not reported	3 g
Cefuroxime	Not reported	1.5–3 g
Clindamycin	4–8 g	Not reported
Erythromycin	Not reported	0.5–1 g
Gentamicin	2–5 g	1 g
Ticarcillin	5–13 g	Not appropriate
Tobramycin	2.4–9.6 g	1.2 g
Vancomycin	3–9 g	1 g

Adapted from Joseph TN, Chen AL, Di Cesare PE. Use of antibiotic-impregnated cement in total joint arthroplasty. J Am Acad Orthop Surg 2003;11:38–47.

Positioning

- Patients are positioned as for other revision hip procedures.
- The lateral decubitus position, with the affected hip upward, is favored. The extremity is freedraped with sufficient exposure of skin to allow for extension of the incision as required.
- If a retroperitoneal approach is required for removal of medial cement, the patient is positioned supine for this portion of the procedure.

Approach

- The approach depends on the fixation status of the implants, length of the cement column if present, quality of bone, and stiffness of the hip joint.
- The primary goals of the exposure are to allow for safe, efficient, and thorough removal of the implants and cement or other foreign material and to allow for thorough débridement of the joint.
- An extended trochanteric osteotomy is usually used. This provides for excellent exposure of the acetabulum and allows for safe removal of the femoral component.
- If the femoral component is loose or has minimal proximal fixation, a standard approach can be used. Radiographs must be carefully inspected to ensure that removal of the femoral component can be accomplished from above.
- Varus remodeling of the proximal femur, or cement that is wider distally than proximally and still well fixed to the implant within the canal, impedes removal of the femoral component and increases the risk of fracture (**FIG 3**).
  - A posterior approach is favored as it is more extensile and allows for an osteotomy if removal of implants becomes more difficult than expected.
- The skin incision should be made through the previous incision, unless the old incision significantly compromises the exposure of deep structures. A portion of the old incision can usually

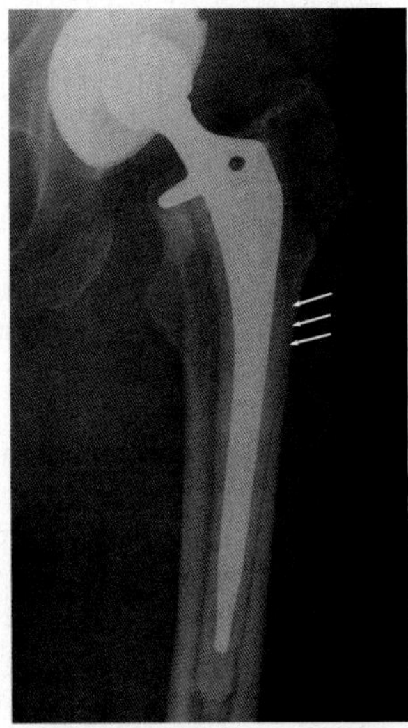

FIG 3 • AP radiograph of loose femoral component. The stem has failed at the bone–cement interface and the cement is still well fixed to the implant. Removal from above would be difficult as the cement becomes wider in the metaphyseal region (*white arrows*). An extended trochanteric osteotomy is required to remove the stem safely.

be incorporated; however, when joining the old incision, avoid acute angles to reduce the risk of wound edge necrosis.
  - The old incision can be excised to give fresh, nonscarred skin edges that may improve wound healing.
- Sinus tracts should be excised elliptically.
- Once the joint has been exposed, at least three samples are obtained for culture.
- Removal of the implants is then carried out as per the techniques of nonseptic revision cases and will not be detailed here (please see corresponding chapters).
  - Removal of implants and débridement is more thorough than in aseptic revisions and every attempt should be made to remove all foreign and potentially infected material.

Articulating Antibiotic Spacer

- After exposure and removal of the implants, the joint is thoroughly débrided. It is important to remove all foreign material, which is potentially infected.
  - Retention of cement or other foreign material is associated with an increased failure rate for curing the infection.
- Intraoperative radiographs can be used to look for retained cement. An arthroscope passed down the femoral canal can also be used to inspect the canal for remaining cement.
- The steps to using a system of molds to make an articulating spacer and to maximize efficiency are as follows:
  - Remove infected femoral component (and cement if applicable).
  - Size and make the antibiotic-loaded femoral implant in the appropriate mold.
  - While the cement for the femoral component is hardening in the mold, remove and débride the acetabulum.
  - Cement the acetabular component into the acetabulum with antibiotic-loaded cement.
  - Remove the femoral component from the mold and insert into the femoral canal.
  - Perform trial reduction.
  - If the femoral component is not stable within the femoral canal and if there is obvious rotation or risk of significant subsidence, a third batch of antibiotic-loaded cement is mixed. When doughy, the cement is placed around the proximal portion of the femoral spacer as it is reinserted into the femoral canal to the desired level to provide rotational and axial stability to the implant. Ensure that not too much cement stays laterally, which may impede closure of the osteotomy if used.
  - Reduce the hip and close.

Spacer Creation

- For most infections, including methicillin-resistant organisms, the antibiotic mixture used in the cement is 3.6 g of gentamicin or tobramycin, 3 g of vancomycin, and 2 g of cefazolin per pack (40 g) of cement. Palacos is favored, as most studies have indicated superior elution compared with other cements.[21] The use of Cefazolin is optional. It is added as a porogen to increase elusion of other antibiotics. It may also provide additional efficacy for methicillin-sensitive organisms.
- Most cases require a total of two mixes of cement (one for the acetabulum and one for the femoral mold). If more than two batches are required and the patient is renally impaired (serum creatinine above 1.5 mg/dL), the dose is decreased to 2.4 g of gentamicin (or tobramycin), 2 g of vancomycin, and 2 g of cefazolin per batch of cement.
- The Prostalac molds are available in variety of sizes and lengths (120, 150, 200, and 240 mm). The length of implant used depends on the length of the extended trochanteric osteotomy (if used), the amount of bone loss, and the size of the canal.
  - In most cases, a middle (200 mm) or long (240 mm) stem is chosen as a longer length also helps achieve better rotational and axial stability within the canal.
- Antibiotics are mixed with one batch of cement in a mixing bowl and then placed into the mold.
- The mold is closed but not fully tightened (to allow for cement to extrude) and the stem is inserted. The mold is then fully tightened and extruded cement is removed from its outer aspect (**TECH FIG 1**).
- Alternatively, after filling the open mold with cement, the implant is laid into the mold, which is closed over the implant.

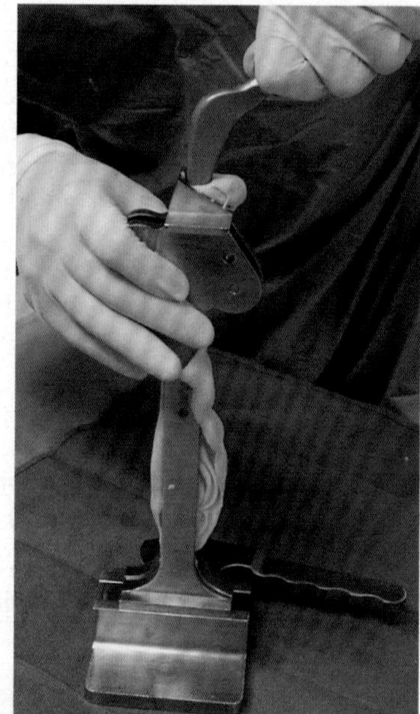

A

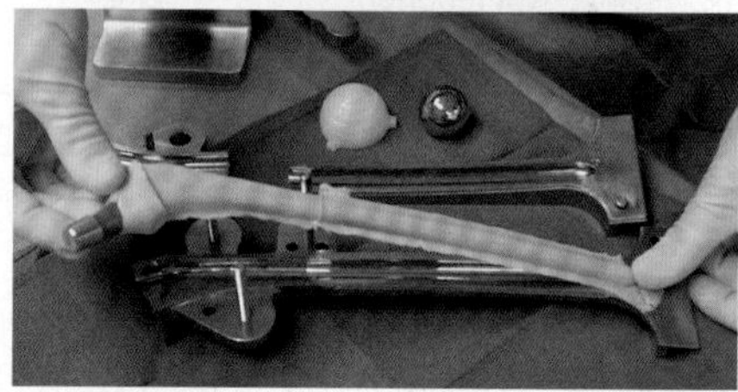

B

TECH FIG 1 • **A.** The femoral component is inserted into the mold, which has been filled before closing with antibiotic-loaded cement. **B.** The femoral component is removed from the mold. The extruded cement seen on the implant medially and laterally can be removed with a rongeur.

Implant Placement

- While the cement is hardening in the femoral mold, the infected acetabular component is removed and the socket débrided. Acetabular reamers can be used to help with débridement, but excessive bone loss from reaming should be avoided.
- A second mix of antibiotic-loaded cement is prepared, and when in a doughy phase, the polyethylene acetabular implant is cemented into the socket.
  - A "perfect cement technique" should be avoided because this can make removal at the time of reimplantation more difficult.
  - Waiting until the cement is doughy and applying some but not excessive force when cementing in the liner will provide a stable cup that can be readily removed.
- If there are large acetabular defects, leftover cement from the femoral mold can be shaped over a reamer of approximate size to make an "antiprotrusio-like" cup that can be placed into the floor of the acetabulum before cementing in the polyethylene cup (**TECH FIG 2A**).
  - Warm saline can be poured into the acetabulum to decrease the setting time.
- Once the acetabular cement has hardened, the femoral component is removed from the mold (see **TECH FIG 1B**) and inserted into the femoral canal.
- In many cases, the stem is press-fitted into the canal, good rotational and axial stability is obtained, and no further adjustment is required.
- In some cases, the fit may be too tight and the antibiotic-loaded implant will not fully seat to the desired level.
  - A high-speed burr is used to remove high points or areas of impingement to allow the stem to seat at the desired level. Alternatively, flexible reamers can be used to increase the opening of the femoral canal, provided there is ample bone stock.
- In other cases, especially with significant bone loss or very large canals, the femoral component is loose within the femoral canal.
  - A trial reduction is performed to estimate leg lengths, and the desired position of the stem within the femoral canal is noted.
  - An additional batch of antibiotic-loaded cement is mixed, and when of a doughy consistency, cement is packed around the proximal portion of the femoral spacer and the implant is reinserted to the desired level. The additional cement provides rotational and axial stability (**TECH FIG 2B–D**).
- Once the stem is stable within the femoral canal, a trial reduction can be performed to assess leg lengths and stability.
- The appropriate femoral head is then placed onto the stem and the hip is reduced and closed.
- The Prostalac articulating antibiotic spacer uses a snap-fit all-polyethylene acetabular implant into which the femoral head is snap-fitted into the cup when reduced, enhancing hip stability (**TECH FIG 2E**).
  - The snap-fit poly liner may reduce the risk of dislocation, particularly in situations of proximal femoral bony or soft tissue deficiency.

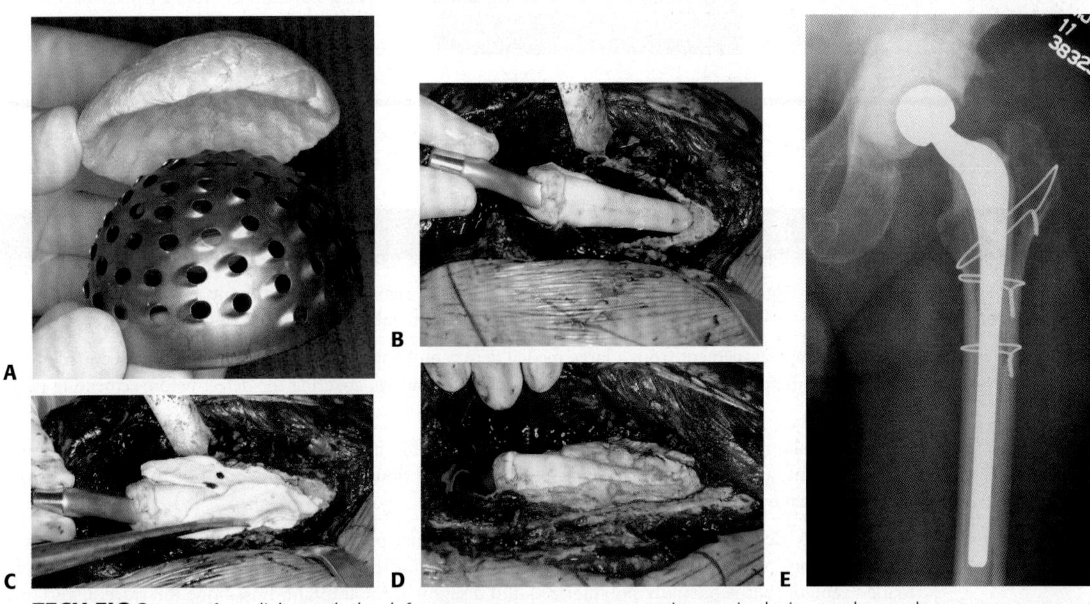

TECH FIG 2 • **A.** If medial acetabular defects are present, a cement antiprotrusio device can be made to prevent cement from escaping into the pelvis at the time the acetabular implant is inserted. This device can be made by using leftover cement from the femoral component and shaping it over an appropriate-sized acetabular reamer. **B.** The femoral component within the femoral canal. In this case, a large femoral canal resulted in the component's being axially and rotationally unstable. **C.** Antibiotic-loaded cement is packed around the proximal portion of the implant to provide axial and rotational stability. **D.** Once the cement has hardened and the stem is stable, a final trial reduction is performed. The stem is axially and rotationally stable within the femoral canal. **E.** Postoperative AP radiograph of a Prostalac articulating spacer.

Nonarticulating Antibiotic Spacer Block

- The initial steps for using a nonarticulating spacer are as for the articulating spacer.
  - This involves ensuring that all the foreign material is removed and the hip is thoroughly débrided.
- The same antibiotic concentrations are used in the bone cement.
  - For an unusual organism, the antibiotics can be adjusted to be organism-specific, but for most infections, the mixture is outlined earlier.
- Two mixes of antibiotic-containing bone cement are required: one for the acetabulum and one for the femur.
- Once the hip is débrided, one mix of antibiotic-loaded cement of a partially polymerized doughy consistency is placed into the socket. It is molded into the acetabulum, matching the bony contour to give some stability to the cement block to prevent it from migrating or dislodging spontaneously.
- The second mix is made into a tapered dowel. Once hardened, the dowel is placed down the femoral canal.
- It is important to make a taper so that the dowel can be easily extracted at the time of reimplantation.
  - The nozzle from a cement gun can be used to make a long tapered dowel (**TECH FIG 3**).
  - An alternative method is to wrap cement around a threaded pin, again making sure that a taper is created with cement larger proximally to keep the dowel from migrating down the canal.
- Once the spacers are inserted, the hip is closed.

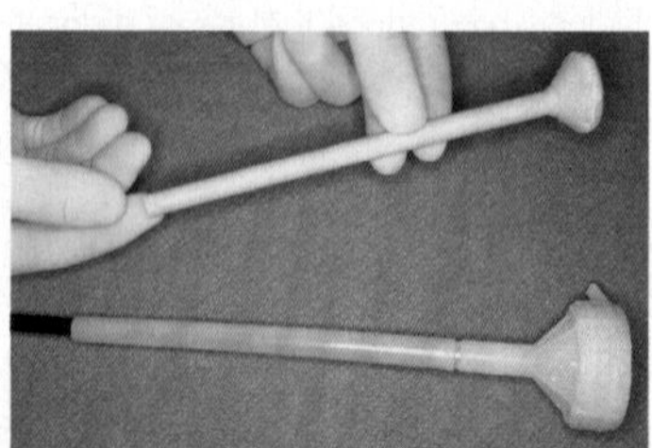

A

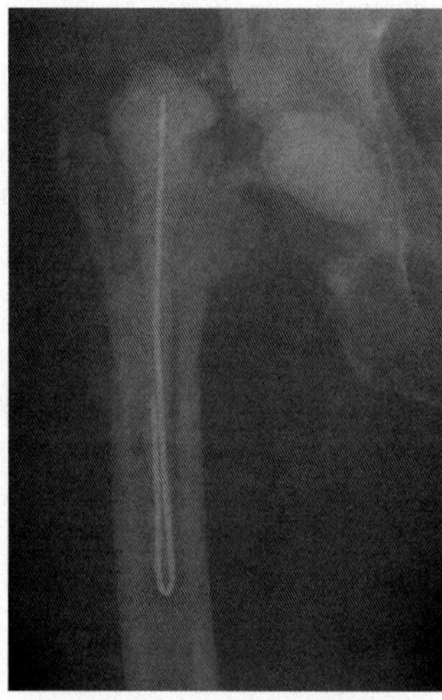

B

TECH FIG 3 • **A.** A nonarticulating static spacer can be made from the nozzle of a cement gun. The nozzle provides a gentle taper and a larger area of cement proximally to prevent the cement dowel from migrating down the femoral canal. **B.** AP radiograph of a nonarticulating static spacer. Note the antibiotic-loaded cement block within the acetabulum and the cement around the Steinmann pin within the femoral canal.

PEARLS AND PITFALLS

Cementing polyethylene liner for articulating spacer	▪ Avoid overly aggressive pressurization, which can make removal more difficult. ▪ Apply modest insertion pressure to the poly cup with partially polymerized doughy cement.
Large medial acetabular defect	▪ To avoid intrapelvic cement from a large medial defect, an "antiprotrusio" cement block can be made by shaping cement over an appropriate-sized reamer. Place into acetabulum, covering the defect before cementing poly cup in place.
Femoral stem that is rotationally unstable	▪ Femoral implant may be rotationally or axially unstable in very large canals. Mix additional antibiotic-loaded cement, and when it is partially polymerized and doughy, pack it around the proximal portion of the implant to make it rotationally and axially stable.
Severe proximal femoral bone loss	▪ With severely deficient or absent proximal femoral bone, place the implant at the desired position during trial reduction. After redislocation, position the implant at the noted position, and place a mix of antibiotic-loaded cement that is partially polymerized and doughy at the implant–host bone interface. Overlap cement onto host bone to make the implant rotationally and axially stable (**FIG 4**).
Femoral dowel for nonarticulating spacer	▪ The nozzle of a cement gun has a slight taper that allows it to be used as a mold for a femoral dowel.

Mixing antibiotics into cement	■ When mixing high-volume antibiotics into cement, depending on which antibiotics are used (eg, tobramycin [Nebcin], which is a very high-volume powder), the handling properties can become difficult because of poor viscosity. The cement has a very dry, powdery feel, making it difficult to handle. ■ To improve the handling properties, three techniques are helpful: ■ Add a few extra milliliters of monomer liquid from an extra package of cement. ■ Use slightly less than a full batch of polymer powder (approximately 7/8 of a package) to increase the fluid-to-powder ratio. ■ Mix slightly cooled monomer and polymer together. When well mixed but still in a very liquid phase, add the antibiotic powder to the mixed cement.

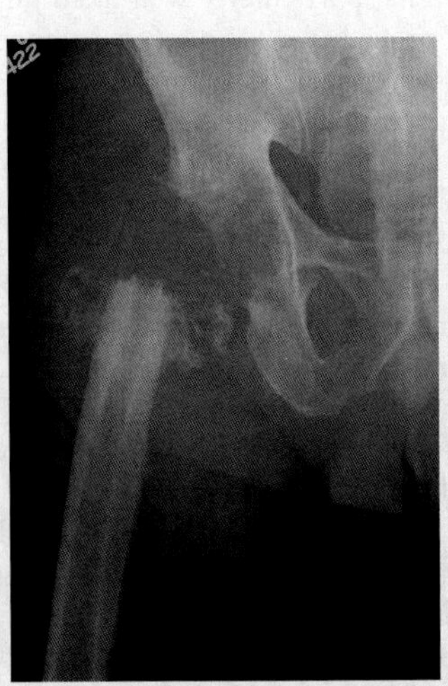

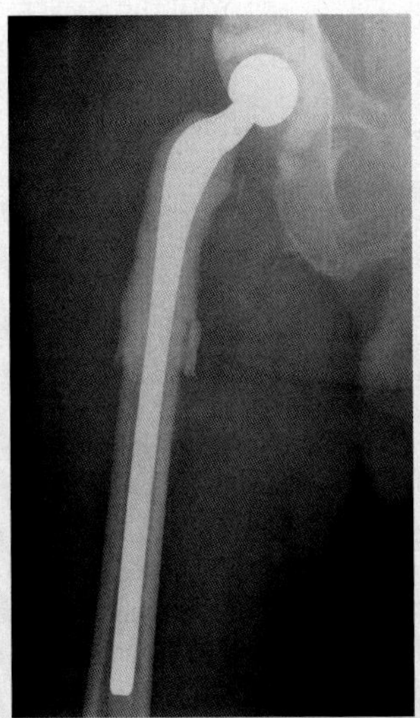

FIG 4 ● An example of severe proximal femoral bone loss with deep infection. **A.** Preoperative radiograph showing severe proximal bone loss with infected bone. **B.** Postoperative articulating spacer radiograph. The femoral component is placed at the desired level and an extra mix of antibiotic-loaded cement is placed at the bone–implant junction to provide rotational and axial stability.

POSTOPERATIVE CARE

Management of the Infection

- Infection management consists of medical and nutritional support and appropriate antibiotics to treat the infecting organism(s).
- The optimal duration and regimen of antibiotics remain controversial.
  - Most authors recommend 6 weeks of intravenous antibiotic therapy, although there is considerable variability in published reports, ranging from 0 to 9 weeks of intravenous antibiotics and none to more than 2 years of oral antibiotics.[14]
  - The choice of antibiotics depends on the organism, but there is a tendency (such as with methicillin-resistant staphylococcal infections) to use multiple antibiotics for synergistic effect (eg, vancomycin and rifampin).[12]
- We favor 6 weeks of antibiotics, at which time the antibiotics are discontinued. Inflammatory markers (ESR and CRP) are repeated at 6 weeks (at the time the antibiotics are stopped). The inflammatory markers often return to normal or trend markedly downward, and reimplantation is planned for around 3 months from insertion of the spacer.
- If the ESR and CRP remain elevated at 6 weeks, we favor stopping the antibiotics and following the patient's course clinically.
  - The ESR and CRP are repeated at 4-week intervals. If they return to normal or have markedly decreased from very high levels preoperatively to near normal, and there are no clinical signs of ongoing infection, then reimplantation can be planned for 3 to 4 months after insertion of the spacer.
- If the inflammatory markers remain elevated at 3 months, the options are as follows:
  - Continue to follow the patient clinically, particularly if he or she is functioning well with an articulating spacer, and reinvestigate prior to the planned reimplantation with repeat ESR and CRP as well as a hip aspiration for cell count.
  - Repeat the débridement and insertion of a new antibiotic spacer.
- Multiple débridements at short intervals, based solely on elevated inflammatory markers, should be avoided.
- Routine reaspiration for culture is of limited value as periprosthetic antibiotic levels are often still above minimum inhibitory concentrations at 3 months. Synovial white blood cell count differential may be of greater value to determine the presence or absence of infection prior to reimplantation, although data supporting routine use of this are limited.[24]

Management of the Hip (Spacer)

- Postoperative weight bearing and mobility depend on the type of spacer used.
- Most patients with an articulating spacer are very functional between stages, often having minimal pain and ultimately ambulating near full weight bearing with a cane or walker prior to reimplantation.
- Patients with articulating antibiotic spacers that have a stable press-fit with good rotational stability are allowed to

mobilize with partial weight bearing (50%) for 6 weeks, followed by weight bearing as tolerated, particularly if follow-up radiographs at 6 weeks show no significant change in implant position.

- If there is concern about the stability of the femoral component within the femoral canal (eg, large canal with difficulties getting good rotational or axial stability of the implant in the canal), then the patient is maintained at 50% weight bearing until the time of reimplantation.
- If a nonarticulating spacer is used, then patients generally cannot bear weight through the lower extremity and are kept touch weight bearing until reimplantation.

OUTCOMES

- The overall success for curing periprosthetic hip infection using a two-stage exchange technique is approximately 89% to 93%.[3,4,7,8,10,14,17,31,32]
- Numerous variables influence the success of treatment:
  - Depth of infection
  - Time from index operation
  - Prosthetic status (fixation and position)
  - Soft tissue status
  - Host status (medical comorbidities)
  - Pathogen (virulence)
  - Surgeon capabilities
  - Patient expectations
- Without the use of antibiotic-loaded cement spacers and without antibiotic-loaded cement at the time of reimplantation, the cure rate for infection using two-stage (delayed) reconstruction is approximately 82%.[10]
  - This cure rate is also similar to a one-stage (direct) exchange in which antibiotic-loaded cement is used at the time of the direct exchange. This implies that delayed reconstruction and the use of antibiotic-loaded spacers are in part responsible for the improved success rate when treating infected total hip replacements.
- Combining a series of patients treated with a two-stage (delayed) reconstruction without antibiotic spacers but with antibiotic-loaded cement at the time of reimplantation reveals a success rate of approximately 90%.[10]
  - Patients treated with a two-stage (delayed) reconstruction using antibiotic-loaded spacers and uncemented reconstruction show a similar success rate to those treated with spacers and antibiotic-loaded cement at the time of reconstruction. This success rate is approximately 89% to 93%.[3,4,10,31,32]
  - Uncemented reconstruction at the time of reimplantation, when used with antibiotic-loaded spacers, has not resulted in a lower infection cure rate.[7,8,17] Also, uncemented reconstruction will likely result in a better long-term mechanical survival.
- Using the articulating Prostalac antibiotic-loaded spacer has an infection cure rate of 93% (45/48 patients).[32] In this series of patients, three became reinfected—two with new organisms and one with the same organism.
- The use of the articulating spacer allows patients to be more functional and thereby reduces the urgency to proceed with reimplantation. This delay between resection and reimplantation allows the surgeon to monitor the patient and assess for possible recurrence after the antibiotics have been stopped.
- The optimal time from resection to reimplantation remains controversial; however, the longer the patient remains clinically free of infection between insertion of the spacer and reimplantation, the more likely that the infection has been cured.

COMPLICATIONS

- General medical complications are similar to those of other revision procedures (eg, thromboembolic disease, postoperative ileus, or cardiac ischemia) and will not be further detailed.
- Local complications can occur with removal of the implants or with the spacer.
  - Removal of the implants, particularly well-fixed implants (as in other revision procedures), can result in bone loss, fracture, or canal perforation. These complications are not reported to be any greater in septic versus aseptic revisions.
- Complications related to the spacer depend on the type of spacer used.
  - Static spacers, in addition to functional problems experienced by the patient, can result in difficulties at the time of reimplantation because of contractures or excessive shortening. Excessive shortening may make reestablishment of leg lengths more difficult.
  - Articulating spacers may cause polishing or sclerosis of the endosteum, resulting in bone that is less suitable for cementing should a cemented reconstruction be chosen at the time of reimplantation. However, cementless reconstruction is widely used and is not associated with an increased risk of infection. We rarely use cemented femoral reconstruction at the time of reimplantation and reserve its use for very low-demand patients with limited life expectancy.
  - Articulating spacers, as with conventional hip replacements, can lead to hip instability. This may be more common if there is bony or soft tissue deficiency. A snap-fit polyethylene liner used in the Prostalac system can markedly reduce this problem.
- Complications of the infection are failure to cure the infection and side effects or toxicity related to antibiotic use. Although there is some variation in the literature, it can be concluded that the rates for curing the infection are about 89% to 93%.[4,7,8,17,31,32]
  - The ability to cure the infection relates to a number of factors: the status of the local soft tissues, systemic comorbidities, the virulence of the organism, and surgical technique.
- The surgeon can improve outcomes by identifying the organism, performing a thorough débridement, and using appropriate high-dose antibiotics in the spacer. As noted earlier, the dose of antibiotics in cement may require adjustment in patients with renal insufficiency. Proper medical and nutritional support may also improve the outcome. Depending on which systemic antibiotics are used, monitoring serum levels is required to avoid toxicity.

REFERENCES

1. American Academy of Orthopaedic Surgeons. Clinical practice guidelines on the diagnosis of periprosthetic joint infections of the hip and knee. http://www.aaos.org/research/guidelines/PJIguideline.asp. Published June 18, 2010. Accessed February 11, 2014.
2. Barrack RL, Jennings RW, Wolfe MW, et al. The value of preoperative aspiration before total knee revision. Clin Orthop Relat Res 1997;345:8–16.

3. Ben-Lulu O, Farno A, Gross AE, et al. A modified cement spacer technique for infected total hip arthroplasties with significant bone loss. J Arthroplasty 2012;27(4):613–619.
4. Biring GS, Kostamo T, Garbuz DS, et al. Two-stage revision arthroplasty of the hip for infection using an interim articulated Prostalac hip spacer: a 10 to 15 year follow-up study. J Bone Joint Surg Br 2009;91:1431–1437.
5. Duncan CP, Beauchamp C. A temporary antibiotic-loaded joint replacement system for management of complex infections involving the hip. Orthop Clin North Am 1993;24:751–759.
6. Duncan CP, Masri BA. The role of antibiotic-loaded cement in the treatment of an infection after a hip replacement. J Bone Joint Surg Am 1994;76A:1742–1751.
7. Fehring TK, Calton TF, Griffin WL. Cementless fixation in 2-stage reimplantation for periprosthetic sepsis. J Arthroplasty 1999;14: 175–181.
8. Haddad FS, Muirhead-Allwood SK, Manktelow AR, et al. Two-stage uncemented revision hip arthroplasty for infection. J Bone Joint Surg Br 2000;82B:689–694.
9. Hanssen AD, Osmon DR. Evaluation of a staging system for infected hip arthroplasty. Clin Orthop Relat Res 2002;403:16–22.
10. Hanssen AD, Spangehl MJ. Treatment of the infected hip replacement. Clin Orthop Relat Res 2004;420:63–71.
11. Hsieh PH, Shih CH, Chang YH, et al. Two-stage revision hip arthroplasty for infection: comparison between the interim use of antibiotic-loaded cement beads and a spacer prosthesis. J Bone Joint Surg Am 2004;86A:1989–1997.
12. Isiklar ZU, Demirors H, Akpinar S, et al. Two-stage treatment of chronic staphylococcal orthopaedic implant-related infections using vancomycin-impregnated PMMA spacer and rifampin-containing antibiotic protocol. Bull Hosp Jt Dis 1999;58:79–85.
13. Joseph TN, Chen AL, Di Cesare PE. Use of antibiotic-impregnated cement in total joint arthroplasty. J Am Acad Orthop Surg 2003;11: 38–47.
14. Kuzyk PR, Dhotar HS, Sternheim A, et al. Two-stage revision arthroplasty for management of chronic periprosthetic hip and knee infection: technique, controversies and outcomes. J Am Acad Orthop Surg 2014;22:153–164.
15. Mason JB, Fehring TK, Odum SM, et al. The value of white blood cell counts before revision total knee arthroplasty. J Arthroplasty 2003;18:1038–1043.
16. Masri BA, Duncan CP, Beauchamp CP. Long-term elution of antibiotics from bone-cement: an in vivo study using the prosthesis of antibiotic-loaded acrylic cement (PROSTALAC) system. J Arthroplasty 1998;13:331–338.
17. Masri BA, Panagiotopoulos KP, Greidanus NV, et al. Cementless two-stage exchange arthroplasty for infection after total hip arthroplasty. J Arthroplasty 2007;22:72–78.
18. Mirra JM, Amstutz HC, Matos M, et al. The pathology of joint tissues and its clinical relevance in prosthesis failure. Clin Orthop Relat Res 1976;117:221–240.
19. Mitchell PA, Masri BA, Garbuz DS, et al. Cementless revision for infection following total hip arthroplasty. Instr Course Lect 2003;52:323–330.
20. Parvizi J, Zmistowski B, Berbari EF, et al. New definition for periprosthetic infection. From the Workgroup of the Musculoskeletal Infection Society. Clin Orthop Relat Res 2011;469:2992–2994.
21. Penner MJ, Duncan CP, Masri BA. The in vitro elution characteristics of antibiotic loaded CMW and Palacos-R bone cements. J Arthroplasty 1999;14:1141–1145.
22. Sanzen L, Sundberg M. Periprosthetic low-grade infection hip infections: erythrocyte sedimentation rate and C-reactive protein in 23 cases. Acta Orthop Scand 1997;68:461–465.
23. Schinsky MF, Della Valle CJ, Sporer SM, et al. Perioperative testing for joint infection in patients undergoing revision total hip arthroplasty. J Bone Joint Surg Am 2008;90(9):1869–1875.
24. Shukla SK, Ward JP, Jacofsky MC, et al. Perioperative testing for persistent sepsis following resection arthroplasty of the hip for periprosthetic infection. J Arthroplasty 2010;25(6)(suppl 1):87–91.
25. Spangehl MJ, Masri BA, O'Connell JX, et al. Prospective analysis of preoperative and intraoperative investigations for the diagnosis of infection at the sites of two hundred and two revision total hip arthroplasties. J Bone Joint Surg Am 1999;81A:672–683.
26. Spangehl MJ, Masterson E, Masri BA, et al. The role of intraoperative Gram stain in the diagnosis of infection during revision total hip arthroplasty. J Arthroplasty 1999;14:952–956.
27. Spangehl MJ, Younger AS, Masri BA, et al. Diagnosis of infection following total hip arthroplasty. Instr Course Lect 1998;47:285–295.
28. Toms AD, Davidson D, Masri BA, et al. The management of periprosthetic infection in total joint arthroplasty. J Bone Joint Surg Br 2006;88B:149–155.
29. Trampuz A, Hanssen AD, Osman DR, et al. Synovial fluid leukocyte count and differential for the diagnosis of prosthetic knee infection. Am J Med 2004;117:556–562.
30. Tsukayama DT, Estrada R, Gustilo RB. Infection after total hip arthroplasty. A study of the treatment of one hundred and six infections. J Bone Joint Surg Am 1996;78A:512–523.
31. Wentworth SJ, Masri BA, Duncan CP, et al. Hip prosthesis of antibiotic-loaded acrylic cement for the treatment of infections following total hip arthroplasty. J Bone Joint Surg Am 2002;84A(suppl 2):123–128.
32. Younger AS, Duncan CP, Masri B, et al. The outcome of two-stage arthroplasty using a custom-made interval spacer to treat the infected hip. J Arthroplasty 1997;12:615–623.
33. Zmistowski B, Della Valle C, Bauer TW, et al. Workgroup 7: diagnosis of periprosthetic joint infection. In: Parvizi J, Gehrke T, eds. *Proceedings of the International Consensus Meeting on Periprosthetic Joint Infection*. Brooklandville, MD: Data Trace Publishing, 2013:158.

34

CHAPTER

Hip Reimplantation Surgery

Peter N. Misur, Winston Y. Kim, and Bassam A. Masri

DEFINITION

- *Hip reimplantation* refers to the insertion of another prosthesis after removal of the original, infected prosthesis. This may be performed as a single- or two-staged procedure, using either cemented or uncemented components.

ANATOMY

- Hip reimplantation surgery is most commonly performed via the posterolateral or direct lateral (transgluteal) approaches. Either approach may be combined with a trochanteric osteotomy to provide further exposure.
- The sciatic nerve is at risk during the posterolateral approach to the hip. In patients with severe scarring, it may be necessary to formally expose the nerve before proceeding with the implantation itself. The sciatic nerve typically emerges deep and inferior to the piriformis muscle and then passes superficial to the obturator internus muscle. However, the sciatic nerve is prone to significant variation in its course and, in some patients, may emerge proximal to, or even emerging through, the piriformis muscle belly.
- In a direct lateral approach, the function of the abductors may be compromised if sufficient care is not taken to avoid injury to the superior gluteal nerve, located on average 5 cm proximal to the greater trochanter.
- For acetabular reconstruction, screw fixation is often necessary. The safest zone for the insertion of acetabular screws, so as to avoid neurovascular structures, is the posterior superior quadrant.[18]

PATHOGENESIS

- The prevalence of infection is 0.7% to 2% following primary hip arthroplasty and 3% to 4% for revisions.[1,10]
- The organisms most commonly isolated in infected total hip replacements are *Staphylococcus aureus*, *S. epidermidis*, and gram-negative bacteria, with an increasing prevalence of antibiotic-resistant bacteria.[2,19]
- Infected prostheses may be classified as one of the following subtypes:[17]
  - Type I—positive intraoperative cultures in an otherwise grossly normal joint
  - Type II—early postoperative infection (occurring within 4 weeks of the primary surgery)
  - Type III—acute hematogenous (occurring in a patient with otherwise well-functioning joint with <4 weeks of symptoms)
  - Type IV—late chronic infections (>4 weeks of symptoms)
- Patients with unexpected positive intraoperative cultures may initially be treated with antibiotics alone. Types II and III infections can frequently be successfully treated with débridement of the joint, liner exchange, and retention of the implant. Type IV (ie, chronic) infections generally indicate removal of all implants and complete revision.
- This difference in management, based on the chronicity of the infection, is due to the predictable establishment of a bacterial biofilm on the implants, which may prohibit effective clearance of the infection without prosthesis removal. The development of biofilms occurs to a degree that varies depending on the particular bacterial species involved. The surgical management described in the following text is concerned with cases in which prosthesis revision is required.

PATIENT HISTORY AND PHYSICAL FINDINGS

- The main presenting symptom of patients with a periprosthetic infection is pain, which is often present at rest.
- Delayed wound healing, persistent wound drainage, and a history of superficial wound infection after the primary procedure are highly suggestive of infection.
- Risk factors for infection include a history of diabetes mellitus, chronic skin lesions, the use of corticosteroids, any type of immunocompromisation, and the duration of the primary surgery.[1]
- Initial assessment should begin with a general hip examination.
- The hip wound is examined for warmth, erythema, fluctuance, discharging sinuses, and the presence of any hematoma.
- The abductors are palpated and their function assessed.
- Pulses are palpated and a full neurologic examination is performed with particular attention to the function of the sciatic nerve.

IMAGING AND OTHER DIAGNOSTIC STUDIES

- Infection is monitored by serial assessment of the erythrocyte sedimentation rate (ESR) (normal <30 mm per hour) and C-reactive protein (CRP) (normal <10 mg/L). A normal CRP has a negative predictive value for infection of over 95%.[16]
- ESR and CRP may be elevated if the patient has other inflammatory systemic diseases (eg, rheumatic disease) and these tests therefore may not be completely reliable in such cases.
- A hip aspiration with a white cell count of greater than 3000 cells/μL and more than 80% neutrophils is highly predictive for infection. Gram stain has a very low sensitivity for infection.[5]
- Three samples are obtained at the time of hip aspiration. A positive culture result is considered to be one in which growth is obtained in two separate specimens.
- Radiographs are obtained, including an anteroposterior (AP) view of the pelvis, lateral view of the hip, and Judet views, if necessary, to assess the integrity of the acetabular columns (**FIG 1**). In some cases, AP and lateral views of the full length of the femur may be necessary. Bone defects

FIG 1 • Preoperative radiographs. **A.** Pelvis. **B.** AP view of the femur. **C.** Obturator oblique view. **D.** Iliac oblique view.

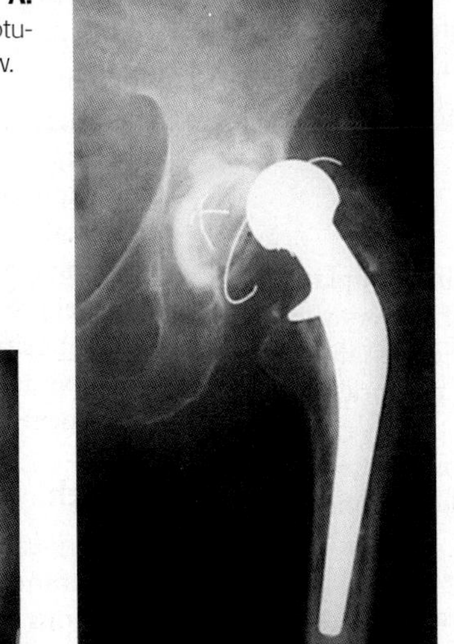

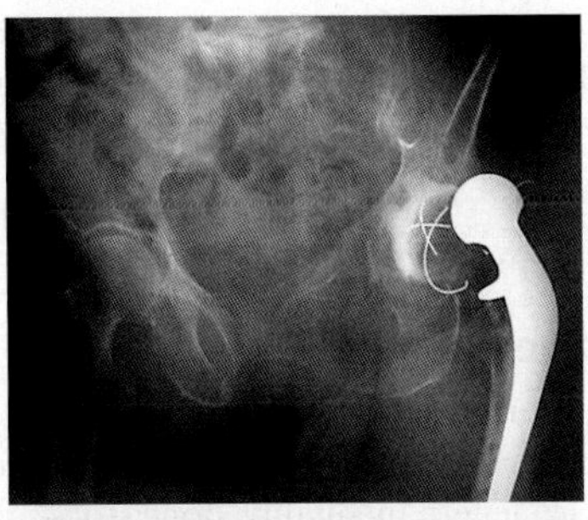

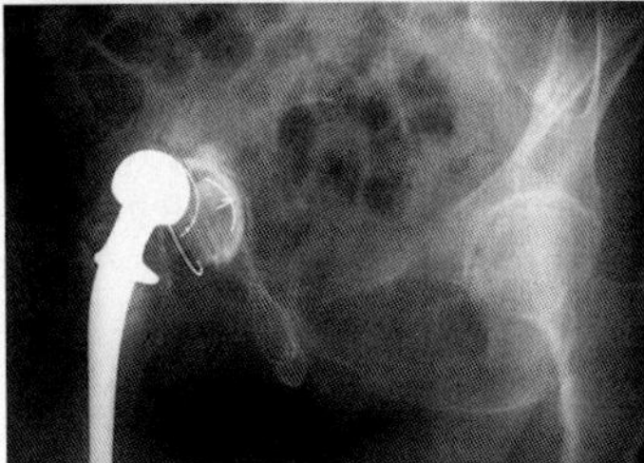

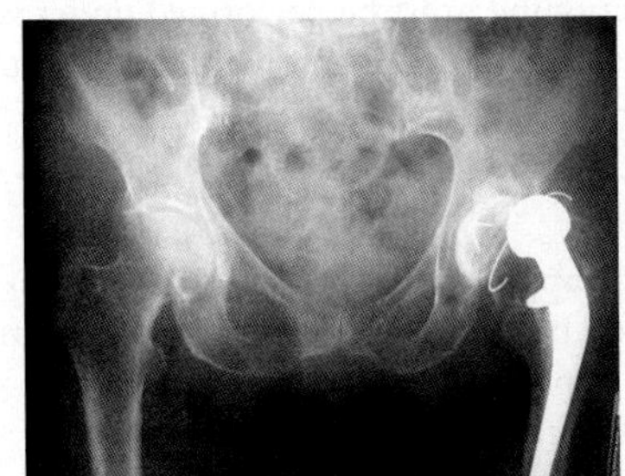

should be estimated on plain radiographs and appropriate reconstructive prostheses made available.

- Computed tomography scans are helpful to ascertain the magnitude of acetabular bone defects.

DIFFERENTIAL DIAGNOSIS

- Adverse reactions to metal ions can manifest with symptoms and signs similar to those of an infected prosthesis, although these cases can typically be differentiated on the basis of serologic testing, imaging studies, and joint aspiration.

NONOPERATIVE MANAGEMENT

- For some patients with significant comorbidities or previous multiple failed reimplantations, further surgery may not be a viable option. In such cases, the decision may be made to leave the infected prosthesis in situ and to use long-term suppressive antibiotic therapy.

SURGICAL MANAGEMENT

- The aims of surgical treatment are to eradicate infection, minimize morbidity, and restore function.
- Prosthetic reimplantation may be performed as a single operation, immediately following the removal of an infected implant, or as a two-stage procedure, weeks or months after removal of the initial infected components. In either case, it is essential to ensure a sterile surgical field prior to hip reimplantation.
- In a one-stage procedure, at least one of the implants, typically the femoral component, needs to be inserted with antibiotic-loaded bone cement.
- Many surgeons favor a two-stage approach to hip reimplantation surgery, typically with an antibiotic-loaded spacer in situ, between the two procedures. An articulating spacer can be used both as a vehicle to deliver high-dose local antibiotics and as a means of preserving the articular space while preserving overall limb function ahead of the definitive reimplantation (**FIG 2**).
- In two-stage procedures, the definitive hip reimplantation surgery can be scheduled once the patient has completed their antibiotic course and demonstrated a trend toward normalization of their inflammatory markers. A routine preoperative hip aspiration is not required in most cases.
- The selection of prostheses for both femoral and acetabular reconstruction is determined by a number of factors, including the quality and quantity of remaining host bone

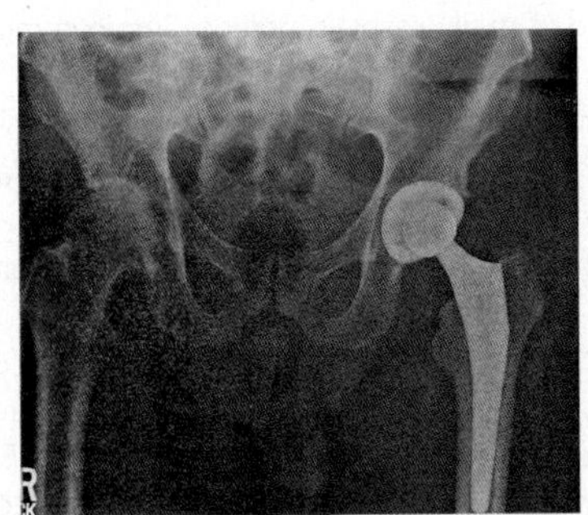

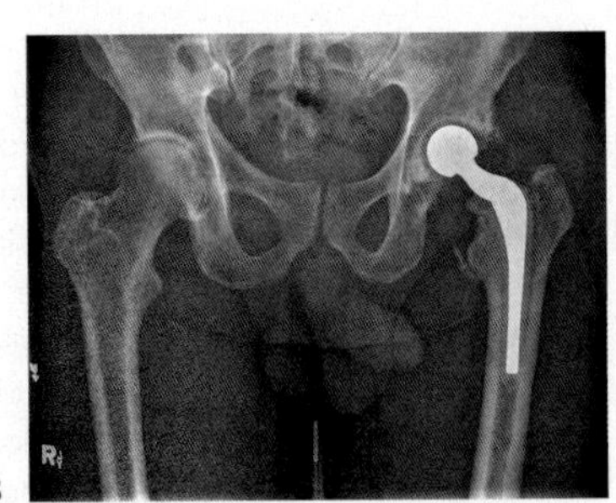

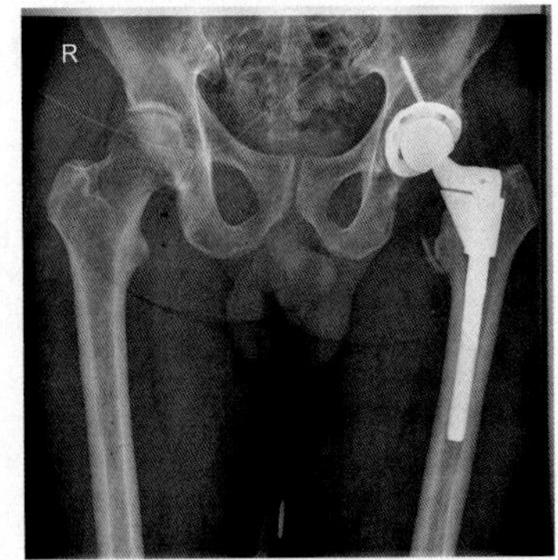

FIG 2 • **A.** AP pelvis radiograph demonstrating infected primary prosthesis. **B.** The temporary articulating spacer with antibiotic-impregnated cement. **C.** Second-stage revision in the same patient, using a modular prosthesis. Note that minimal additional bone loss has occurred between the primary surgery and the final revision procedure.

for osseointegration or cementation, the status of the surrounding soft tissues, and the surgeon's preference.
- In some low-demand patients and those with a history of previous failed reimplantation surgery, a resection arthroplasty may be considered.

Preoperative Planning

- It is important to anticipate the need for specialized implants and instruments before surgery, taking note of factors such as offset, leg length inequality, bone stock, and joint stability.
- Careful preoperative templating is essential to anticipate implant size, length, and offset (**FIG 3**).
- Insufficiency of hip abductors may require a constrained acetabular implant, larger diameter femoral head components, or a dual mobility cup.
- The pathology laboratory should be informed of the possibility that intraoperative frozen section analysis may be required in equivocal cases of persistent infection. These tissue samples are taken at the soft tissue interface adjacent to the removed spacer implant. In addition, if intraoperative cultures are obtained, the microbiology laboratory should be alerted for the need for a prolonged incubation of 14 days.
- Alternative surgical plans are useful to have at hand in case of unexpected intraoperative findings or complications, which may include the need to reinsert an antibiotic spacer prosthesis if there is evidence of ongoing infection.

Positioning

- The patient is positioned in the lateral decubitus position with anterior and posterior supports (**FIG 4**).
- The pelvis must be vertical, and it must be confirmed that the supports are stable. The patient's back is kept straight with their shoulders vertical.
- A clinical note is made of any leg length discrepancy prior to prepping the limb. This allows for intraoperative monitoring of leg length adjustments.
- Patient positioning must be performed under surgeon supervision because errors in positioning may result in acetabular component malalignment.

Approach

- The surgical approach is chosen after careful preoperative consideration of important factors, including the following:
  - Previous approach
  - Anatomic location and extent of bone loss
  - Anticipated instability
  - Function of the abductors
  - Surgeon preference and training
- The main options are as follows:
  - Posterolateral approach
  - Direct lateral (transgluteal) approach
  - Trochanteric osteotomy
  - Trochanteric slide osteotomy
  - Extended trochanteric osteotomy (ETO)

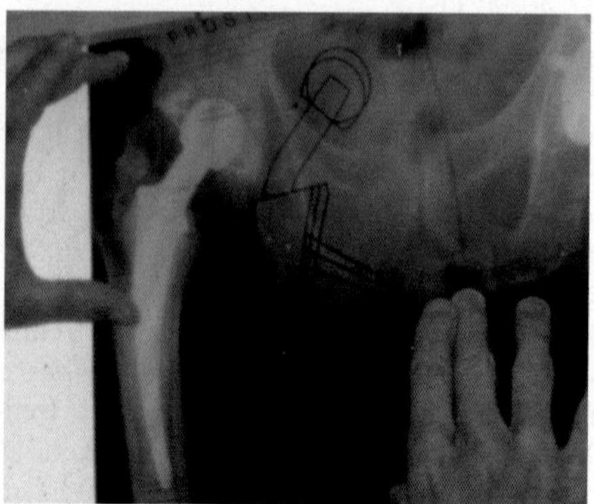

FIG 3 • Preoperative templating is essential to determine the diameter and length of the implant that may be needed.

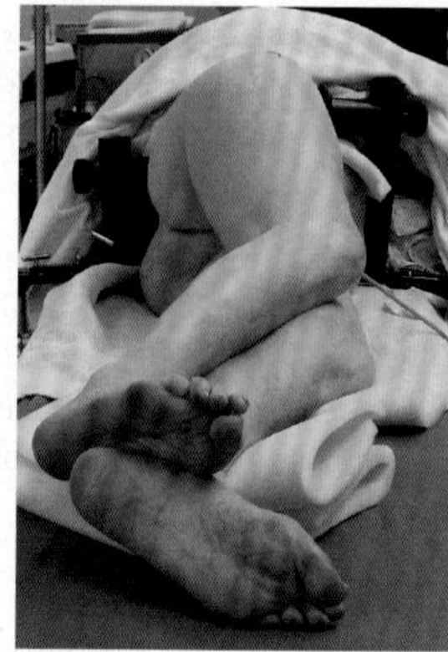

FIG 4 • Patient positioned in the lateral decubitus position.

TECHNIQUES

Hip Exposure and Removal of Antibiotic Spacers

- The posterior approach is often used for surgical exposure.
- The sciatic nerve is identified and protected throughout the procedure. This is facilitated by placement of the foot on a padded stand with the knee in flexion and the hip in slight abduction during the exposure.
- Initial visualization of the nerve is often obscured by scar tissue from previous operations and care should be taken to verify the nerve's precise location.
- The short external rotators and posterior capsule are identified and incised as a composite flap. These are tagged with sutures for later repair. The gluteus maximus tendon insertion is released in many cases in order to improve mobilization of the femur.
- Tissue samples are obtained from within the hip joint and sent for microbiology. We do not recommend obtaining frozen sections routinely.
- The hip is dislocated, with flexion and internal rotation of the femur.
- Anterior capsular scar tissue may need to be debulked to improve exposure. Exposure is further aided by releasing the anterior femoral capsule, with a femoral retractor placed to displace the femur anteriorly within the wound (**TECH FIG 1A**).

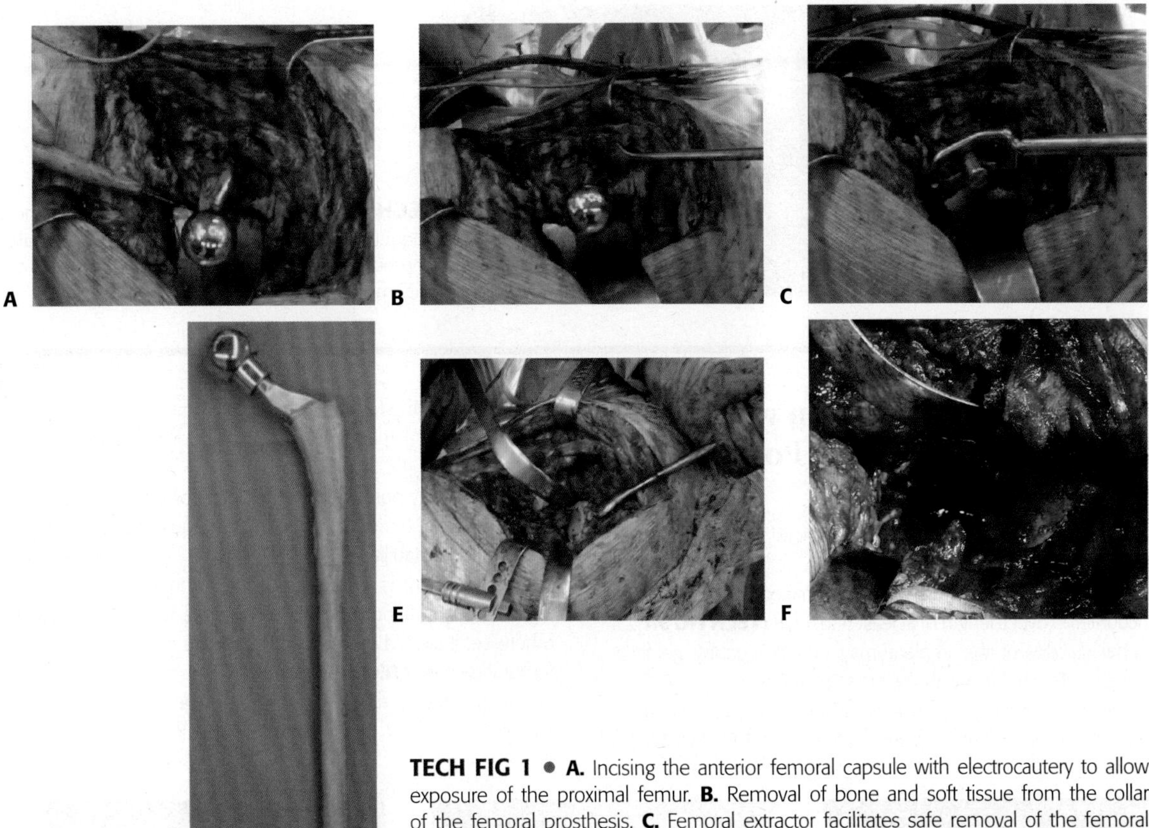

TECH FIG 1 • A. Incising the anterior femoral capsule with electrocautery to allow exposure of the proximal femur. **B.** Removal of bone and soft tissue from the collar of the femoral prosthesis. **C.** Femoral extractor facilitates safe removal of the femoral component. **D.** Complete removal of the antibiotic cement-coated femoral prosthesis is confirmed. **E.** Safe removal of the acetabular antibiotic spacer with a Cobb elevator. **F.** The acetabulum is fully exposed after complete débridement.

- Removal of cement, soft tissue, and bone from the shoulder of the prosthesis and greater trochanter facilitates removal of the preexisting antibiotic implant spacer and reduces the risk of greater trochanter fracture (**TECH FIG 1B**).
- A femoral extractor should be used to remove the femoral antibiotic spacer (**TECH FIG 1C**), ensuring complete removal of all cement (**TECH FIG 1D**).
- The acetabular antibiotic spacer is carefully removed, with an osteotome to break the cement and a gouge to remove the liner if present. Care is taken to ensure no further bone loss (**TECH FIG 1E**).
- Femoral débridement is performed with reverse hooks, curettes and brushes, and pulsed lavage.
- Acetabular débridement is performed using a combination of curettes, rongeurs, and Cobb elevators to remove any residual soft tissue, ensuring complete exposure of the acetabulum (**TECH FIG 1F**).
- The bone stock of the posterior acetabular walls is verified by palpation.

Acetabular Reimplantation

- The acetabulum is reamed incrementally to obtain a concentric, hemispheric surface, taking care to preserve the rim of the acetabulum (**TECH FIG 2A**).
- An implant 1 to 2 mm larger than the diameter of the last reamer is used in order to obtain a press-fit.
- The implant is inserted in 40 degrees of lateral inclination and 15 to 20 degrees of anteversion (**TECH FIG 2B**).
- Ascertain that the component is uniformly in contact with the underlying host bone.
- Supplementary screw fixation is required in most cases, with placement in the posterior superior quadrant of the cup.
- The appropriate trial liner is placed into the acetabulum for later trial reduction after femoral canal preparation.

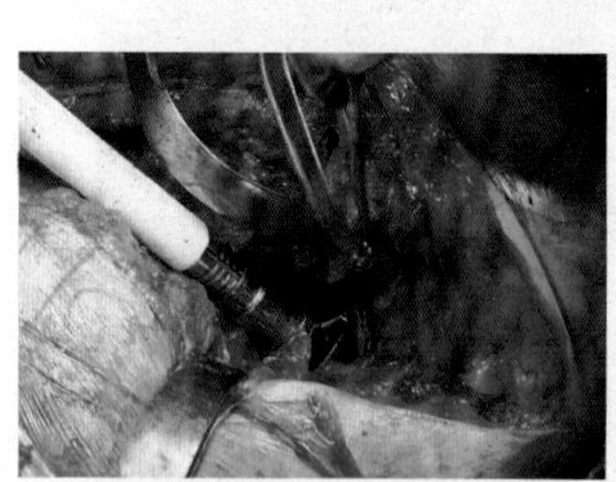

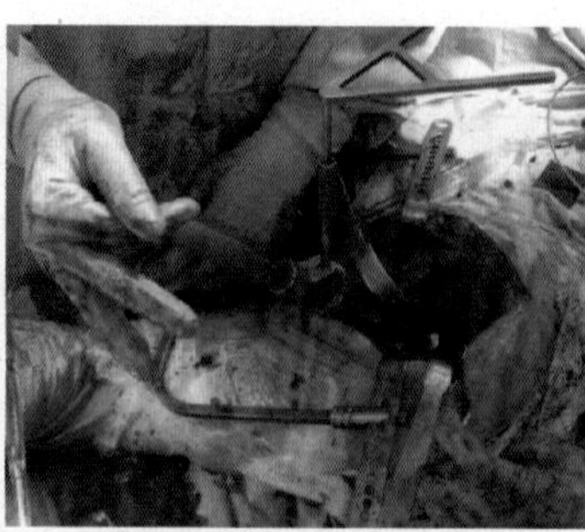

TECH FIG 2 • A. The acetabulum is reamed sequentially. **B.** Alignment of the acetabular component is confirmed with use of an external alignment jig.

Two-Stage Reimplantation with an Uncemented, Extensively Porous-Coated Femoral Stem

- The diameter, offset, and length of the femoral implant are anticipated by careful preoperative templating.
- The femoral canal is sequentially reamed until cortical resistance is encountered over a length of at least 5 to 6 cm (**TECH FIG 3A**).
- Torsional stability of the implant may be ensured by gently torquing the femoral trial with the broach handle.
- Trial reduction is performed, ensuring satisfactory leg lengths, soft tissue tension, range of motion, and a stable hip (**TECH FIG 3B**).
- Under-reaming the femoral canal by 0.5 mm compared with the diameter of the actual femoral implant is confirmed by checking with a "hole gauge."
- In an extensively porous-coated femoral component, 5 to 6 cm of diaphyseal fit (so-called scratch fit) is required to provide axial and rotational stability.
- The final implant is inserted into the femoral canal. It should be inserted by hand as close as possible to its final position; otherwise, it should be reamed line to line to avoid inadvertent femoral fracture (**TECH FIG 3C**).
- The final implant seating is achieved by gentle impaction with a mallet.

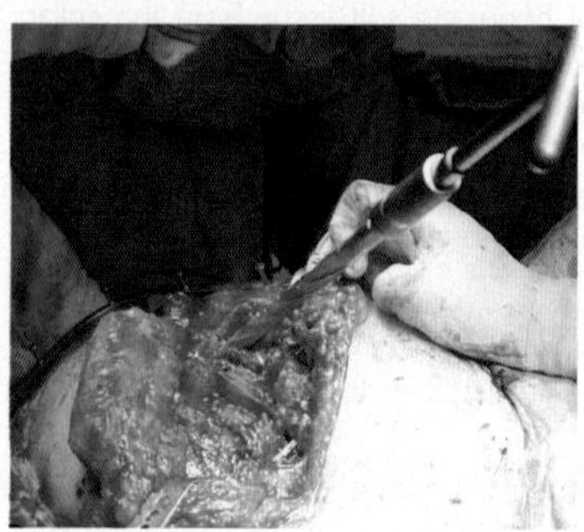

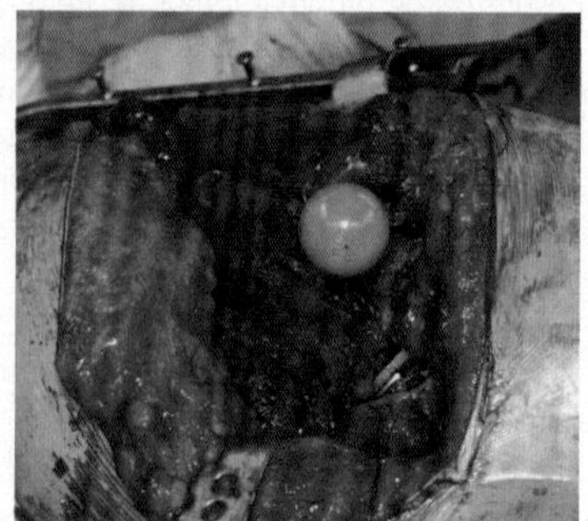

TECH FIG 3 • A. Femoral canal preparation with reamers. **B.** Trial components inserted. **C.** Insertion of the definitive, extensively coated femoral implant.

Two-Stage Reimplantation with Uncemented, Tapered, Fluted Femoral Stem

- Curettes and reverse hooks are used to débride fibrous tissue from the femoral canal (**TECH FIG 4A**).
- Femoral canal reaming is performed with tapered reamers, with the depth and diameter guided by preoperative templating, until endosteal contact is made (**TECH FIG 4B**).
- The aim of diaphyseal reaming is to ensure implant stability, which will resist stem subsidence.
- The length of the stem, as determined by preoperative templating, should be at least two cortical diameters distal to any potential stress risers, for example, the tip of an ETO.
- Unlike fully porous-coated cylindrical stems, under-reaming the femoral canal by 0.5 mm compared with the diameter of the actual femoral implant is not recommended. Line-to-line reaming is preferred.
- Proximal femoral preparation is then performed using conical reamers.
- Torsional stability of the implant may be ensured by gently torquing the femoral trial with the broach handle.
- Trial reduction is performed for assessment of correct femoral stem anteversion, limb length, soft tissue tension, range of motion, and hip stability (**TECH FIG 4C**).
- The modularity of the uncemented tapered fluted femoral stem allows independent adjustment of femoral anteversion (**TECH FIG 4D**).

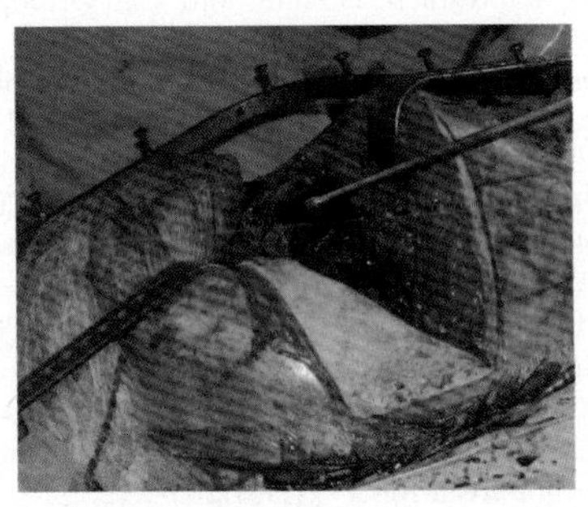

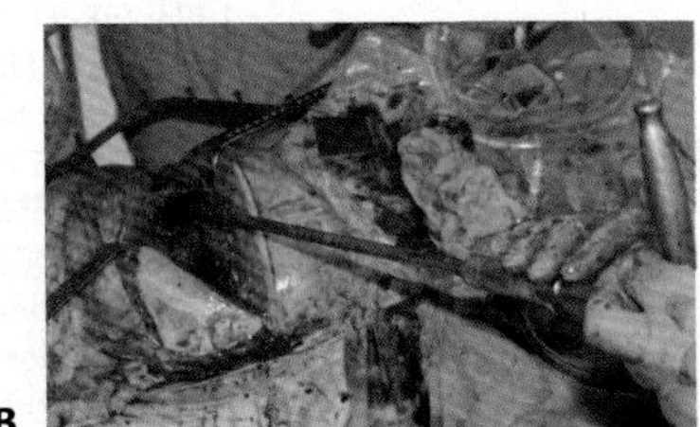

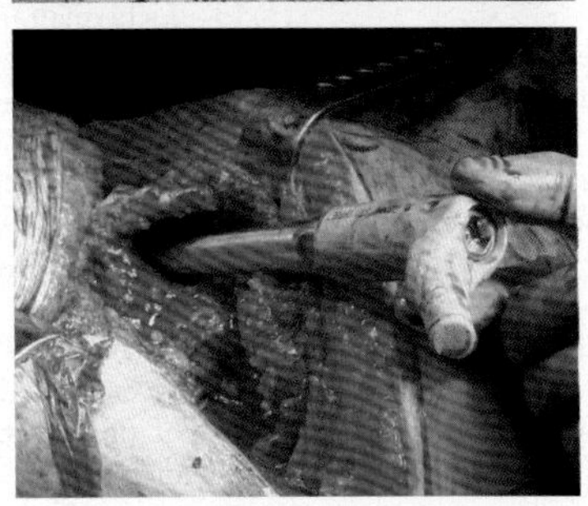

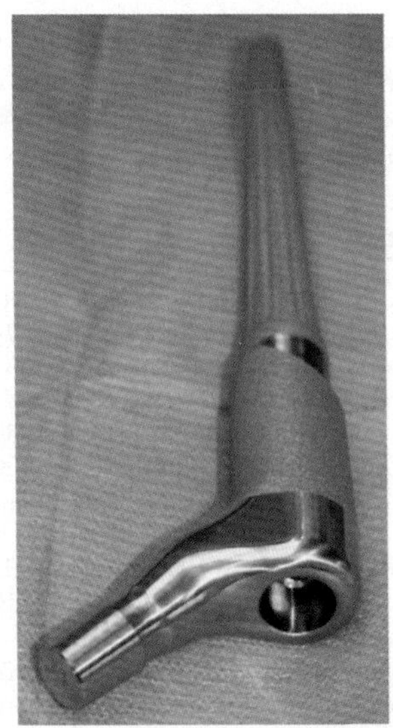

TECH FIG 4 • A. Femoral canal débridement. **B.** Femoral canal preparation with reamers. **C.** Trial components inserted. **D.** The modular uncemented, tapered, fluted stem.

PEARLS AND PITFALLS

Implant removal and acetabular reconstruction	■ Removal of acetabular cement may require sequential pie-crusting of cement beginning at the cement–bone interface. ■ Gentle acetabular reaming can be used as a means of mechanical débridement.
Femoral reimplantation with extensively porous-coated femoral stem	■ Concentric and central reaming of the femoral canal is crucial during femoral preparation. ■ A minimum of 5–6 cm of "scratch fit" is required to provide immediate initial component stability. ■ The use of a hole gauge to confirm any differences between the femoral implant and final reamer diameters can reduce the rate of intraoperative femoral fractures.
Femoral reimplantation with uncemented, tapered, fluted stem	■ Sufficient bone stock in the diaphyseal region is a prerequisite for an uncemented fluted stem. ■ Fixation of two cortical diameters distal to any potential stress risers is crucial to ensure implant fixation. ■ Uncemented stems require rigid torsional stability, which can be confirmed by torquing the femoral trail while an assistant holds the leg still.
Cemented reimplantation surgery	■ Performed as a single- or two-staged procedure (see Outcomes) ■ The preferred method of hip reimplantation in some units in Europe but rarely performed in North America

POSTOPERATIVE CARE

- Postoperative care is individualized, depending on the precise nature of the reimplantation procedure.
- The quality of implant fixation, severity of preoperative bone loss, intraoperative stability, and patient compliance influence the amount of weight bearing permitted and the specific restrictions on hip range of movement.
- If a transgluteal (direct lateral) approach was used, restriction of active abduction may be necessary.
- Clear postoperative instructions and frequent communication with the multidisciplinary team are essential. Instructions include postoperative blood work, deep venous thrombosis prophylaxis, and perioperative antibiotic requirements.
- All intraoperative specimens sent for microbiology at the time of reimplantation must be carefully monitored for any positive culture growths.

OUTCOMES

- An uncemented two-stage procedure may successfully eradicate infection in 89% to 93% of cases.[2,7,8,11]
- Single-stage reimplantation with the use of antibiotic-loaded cement has a success rate of 77% to 91%.[3,4,6,15]
- A two-stage procedure with the use of antibiotic-containing bone cement in the reimplantation procedure attains a success rate of 90% to 95%.[9,13]

COMPLICATIONS

- Recurrent infection after reimplantation is a devastating complication and is associated with a poor outcome.[14]
- Infection with a methicillin-resistant organism is associated with a higher rate of treatment failure.[12]
- Recurrent infection may be either recurrence of the initial infection or a new infection by a different organism, which

is often due to multiple patient risk factors and indicates host failure.[11]

- Hip dislocation, leg length discrepancy, venous thromboembolism, nerve and vessel injury, fracture, and a small mortality risk are potential complications, as they are for any revision arthroplasty.

REFERENCES

1. Aggarwal VK, Tischler EH, Lautenbach C, et al. Mitigation and education. J Arthroplasty 2014;29(2 suppl):19–25.
2. Biring GS, Kostamo T, Garbusz DS, et al. Two-stage revision arthroplasty of the hip for infection using an interim articulated Prostalac hip spacer. J Bone Joint Surg Br 2009;91B:1431–1437.
3. Buchholz HW, Elson RA, Engelbrecht E, et al. Management of deep infection of total hip replacement. J Bone Joint Surg Br 1981;63B: 342–353.
4. Callaghan JJ, Katz PR, Johnston RC. One-stage revision surgery of the infected hip: a minimum 10-year follow-up study. Clin Orthop Relat Res 1999;369:139–143.
5. Dinnenn A, Guyot A, Clements J, et al. Synovial fluid white cell and differential count in the diagnosis or exclusion of prosthetic joint infection. Bone Joint J 2013;95-B:554–557.
6. Elson RA. One-stage exchange in the treatment of the infected total hip arthroplasty. Semin Arthroplasty 1994;5:137–141.
7. Faddad FS, Muirhead-Allwood SK, Manktelow AR, et al. Two-stage uncemented revision hip arthroplasty for infection. J Bone Joint Surg Br 2000;82B:689–694.
8. Fehring TK, Calton TF, Griffin WL. Cementless fixation in 2-stage reimplantation for periprosthetic sepsis. J Arthroplasty 1999;14: 175–181.
9. Garvin KL, Evans BG, Salvati EA, et al. Palacos gentamicin for the treatment of deep periprosthetic hip infections. Clin Orthop Relat Res 1994;298:97–105.
10. Garvin KL, Hanssen AD. Infection after total hip arthroplasty: past, present, and future. J Bone Joint Surg Am 1995;77:1576–1588.
11. Kraay MJ, Goldberg V, Fitzgerald SJ, et al. Cementless two-staged total hip replacement for deep periprosthetic infection. Clin Orthop Relat Res 2005;441;243–249.
12. Leung F, Richards CJ, Garbuz DS, et al. Two-stage total hip arthroplasty: how often does it control methicillin-resistant infection? Clin Orthop Relat Res 2011;469:1009–1015.
13. Lieberman JR, Callaway GH, Salvati EA, et al. Treatment of the infected total hip arthroplasty with a two-stage reimplantation protocol. Clin Orthop Relat Res 1994;301:205–212.
14. Pagnano MW, Trousdale RT, Hanssen AD. Outcome after reinfection following reimplantation hip arthroplasty. Clin Orthop Relat Res 1997;338:192–204.
15. Raut VV, Siney PD, Wroblewski BM. One-stage revision of total hip arthroplasty for deep infection: long-term follow-up. Clin Orthop Relat Res 1995;321:202–207.
16. Spangehl MJ, Masri BA, O'Connell JX, et al. Prospective analysis of preoperative and intraoperative investigations for the diagnosis of infection at the sites of two hundred and two revision total hip arthroplasties. J Bone Joint Surg Am 1999;81-A:672–683.
17. Tsukayama DT, Estrada R, Gustilo RB. Infection after total hip arthroplasty. A study of the treatment of one hundred and six infections. J Bone Joint Surg Am 1996;78(4):512–523.
18. Wasielewski RC, Cooperstien LA, Kruger MP, et al. Acetabular anatomy and the transacetabular fixation of screws in total hip arthroplasty. J Bone Joint Surg Am 1990;72A:501–508.
19. Zimmerli W, Moser C. Pathogenesis and treatment concepts of orthopaedic biofilm infections. FEMS Immunol Med Microbiol 2012;65:158–168.

Upper Tibial Osteotomy (High Tibial Osteotomy)

35 CHAPTER

Tomoyuki Saito, Yasushi Akamatsu, and Ken Kumagai

DEFINITION

- High tibial osteotomy (HTO) is realignment surgery, which has developed for treating medial compartment osteoarthritis (OA) of the knee.[7]
- One of the main etiologic factors of knee OA is excessive biomechanical stress loaded on a focal area due to varus deformity of the lower limb alignment.
- Excessive biomechanical stress is loaded onto either compartment of the knee joint; consequently, such overload is more likely to give rise to degeneration of articular cartilage with aging.
- The aim of HTO is to correct malalignment of the limb, resulting in a transfer of weight bearing from the degenerated medial compartment to the relatively healthy lateral compartment.
- Correction to appropriate knee alignment provides stability of the affected knee, subsidence of synovitis, and cease of cartilage degeneration.
- The indications for HTO include medial compartmental knee OA with or without instability and osteonecrosis of the knee.

ANATOMY

- The proximal tibial portion for osteotomy has several important anatomic landmarks to obtain successful results and avoid complications.
- On the anterior aspect of the proximal tibia, the tibial tuberosity is the most prominent feature. The osteotomy should be carried out at the proximal level of the tuberosity.
- Gerdy tubercle is located at 2 to 3 cm lateral to the tibial tubercle, which is the insertion of the iliotibial tract. Gerdy tubercle is the most suitable place to place fixative devices because of the thick cortical bone.
- On the medial aspect of the proximal tibia, there are insertions of the pes anserinus, the gracilis, and semitendinosus covered with the fascia, and on the posteromedial portion, the superficial layer of the medial collateral ligament is attached. In cases of medial soft tissue tightness, these sometimes need to be elevated subperiosteally.
- The anterior aspect of the proximal tibia and the fibula is the origin of the tibialis anterior, extensor digitorum longus, and peroneus longus muscles.
- On the lateral side, the common peroneal nerve runs on the lateral side of the neck of the fibula. On excision of the fibular head or division of the proximal tibiofibular ligament in closing wedge osteotomies, much attention should be paid to avoid nerve injury.
- The posterior neurovascular structure, including the popliteal artery and vein and tibial nerve, should be protected while the posterior portion of the tibia is osteotomized.
- The cross-section of the proximal tibia has a triangular shape. In opening wedge high tibial osteotomies (OW-HTO), the posterior portion of the osteotomized site should be opened more than the anterior portion to avoid an expected increase of the tibial slope.
- When performing fibular osteotomy in closing wedge high tibial osteotomies (CW-HTO), the fibular shaft can be resected safely at the level of about 16 cm distal to the fibular head.

PATHOGENESIS

- Knee OA is a common joint disorder in elderly people that leads to progressive dysfunction of a knee joint.
- Knee OA develops and progresses due to risk factors including heredity, weight, age, gender, repetitive stress injury, and high-impact sports.
- Although the etiology of knee OA is multifactorial, medial compartmental knee OA reveals varus deformity, the mechanical axis passes through far medial side from a knee joint, and excessive mechanical stress loaded on the medial cartilage are considered to be main causative factors.
- Excessive overload is more likely to give rise to degeneration of articular cartilage, and cartilage fragments entrapped by synovium induce synovial inflammation, resulting in further degeneration of articular cartilage.
- Synovial inflammation is marked around the degenerated articular cartilage and related to joint swelling and provocation of pain.

NATURAL HISTORY

- Once a knee joint is affected by OA, the disease advances with time, and osteoblastic changes, including subchondral bone sclerosis and osteophyte formation, are clearly visible. Further cartilage degeneration occurs, resulting in joint space narrowing or obliteration.
- Range of motion (ROM) is gradually limited. Flexion contracture or restriction of the knee appears.
- However, quadriceps strengthening exercise or reducing body weight can modify the clinical course of the disease. These measures may stabilize a knee joint and reduce overload applied on the cartilage-degenerative portion, providing good relief of pain.
- As the disease progresses, loss of articular cartilage brings about varus–valgus instability, so-called "lateral thrust." This instability promotes further cartilage degeneration, producing bony wear at the medial femorotibial articulation, and varus deformity increases.
- Osteophytes formed around intercondylar notch and may cause anterior cruciate ligament (ACL) deficiency, and the disease expands to the lateral and the patellofemoral compartment.
- A knee joint is destructed and knee function is markedly disabled due to severe pain and limited ROM.

HISTORY AND PHYSICAL FINDINGS

- Diagnosis of knee OA can be made based on patient-reported symptoms and physical and radiologic examination.
- Clinical examination of the knee should start with complete history of the symptoms; past history, including previous trauma such as fracture or meniscus tear; medical diseases, including diabetes mellitus or hypertension; and occupational history.
- Knee pain is a crucial clinical sign of knee OA. Patients experience pain around a knee joint when standing up from a chair and starting to walk. This pain modality, called *starting pain*, is very specific for knee OA. Pain is also aggravated by physical activities such as descending or ascending stairs.
- Some patients complain of pain at night and morning stiffness.
- Asking patients about the onset of pain, the duration and frequency, and physical activities that aggravate pain is essential to help make differential diagnosis.
- The physical examination should cover posture, gait pattern, the involved limb, the joints on either side of the knee, the spine, and, particularly, the hip joint, which can also cause knee pain.
- Observation shows that a significant varus deformity at the knee, antalgic gait, and lateral thrust in early stance phase of gait visualized joint effusion and quadriceps muscle atrophy.
- Palpitation indicates the exact location of pain around the tibiofemoral and patellofemoral joints. Tender zones are easily determined by asking patients to point to painful sites with one finger. When joint effusion exists, a ballotable patella is noticed. Crepitation, defined as a cracking or grinding sound, is identified when the patient with knee OA experiences a sensation in the joint during physical examination.
- Pain is often provoked at the medial joint space by valgus-stressed maneuvers because more marked synovitis and osteophyte formation are present in medial compartmental knee OA.

IMAGING AND OTHER DIAGNOSTIC STUDIES

- Routine radiographic examination of knee OA consists of standing (weight bearing) anteroposterior (AP) and lateral views and tangential axial views. Other views include the tunnel view, 45-degree flexed weight-bearing posteroanterior (PA) view, varus or valgus stress views, and a full-length standing radiograph (a mechanical axis view).
  - A standing AP view provides more accurate assessment of knee alignment and joint space width than one taken in the supine position (**FIG 1A**).
  - A lateral view depicts the status of the extensor mechanism, including the patella height (patella alta or baja), the quadriceps and patellar tendon, the tibial posterior slope, the distal end of the femur, and the proximal end of the tibia.
  - Morphologic changes of the patellofemoral joint can be assessed using a tangential axial view (the Merchant view).
  - The tunnel view demonstrates osteophytes formed on the posterior aspect of the intercondylar notch.
  - The flexed, weight-bearing PA view of the knee reveals the joint space width of the more posterior aspect of the femorotibial joint. Early degenerative changes of the articular cartilage can be detected with this view.
  - A mechanical axis view provides exact alignment of the whole lower extremity. This view is commonly used in preoperative planning of HTO (**FIG 1B**).
  - The varus and valgus stress views are helpful to visualize the stability of medial and lateral laxity in medial knee OA and to confirm that the lateral compartment is almost intact (**FIG 1C**).
- Magnetic resonance imaging (MRI) provides multiplanar assessment of the pathology of the whole structure of a knee joint, including cartilage, synovium, ligaments, menisci, and bone marrow.

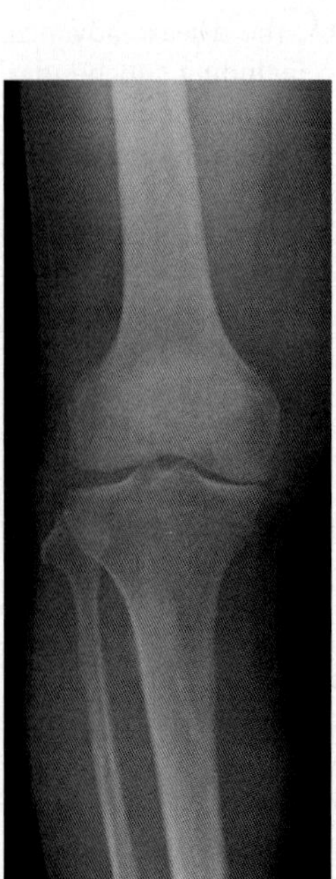

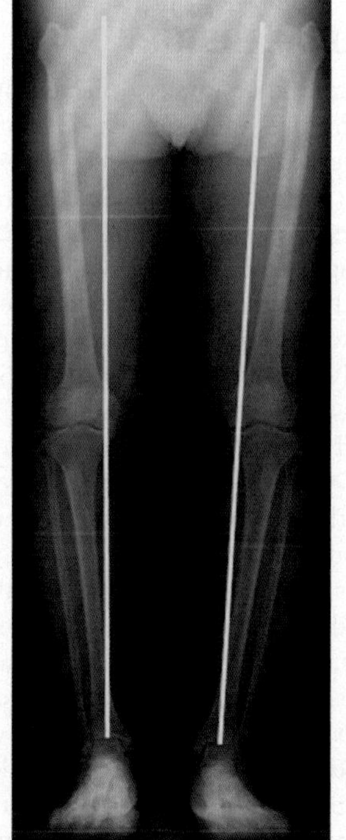

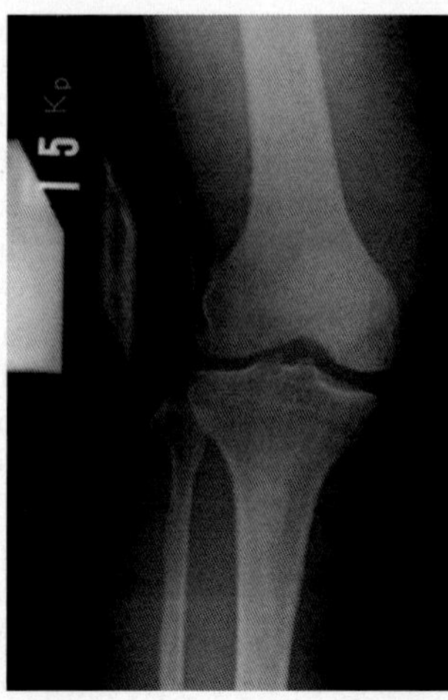

FIG 1 • Preoperative radiographs. **A.** AP radiograph of the right knee showing significant narrowing of the medial joint space with osteophyte formation. **B.** Mechanical axis view of the bilateral lower extremities showing bilateral varus deformities of the lower extremity. Note that mechanical axis is obtained as follows: (1) Mark the center of the femoral head. (2) Mark the center of the ankle. (3) Draw a straight line between them (ie, the most medial line on the illustration). **C.** Valgus-stressed AP radiograph showing presence of full-thickness articular cartilage with intact lateral joint space.

- In medial compartmental knee OA, MRIs can satisfactorily depict the morphologic changes of articular cartilage from an irregular surface as the disease progresses, synovial hyperplasia, thick subchondral bone, the degenerative process of the medial meniscus, the condition of the ACL and medial collateral ligament, and bone marrow edema indicating overload applied to the articular surface.
- Other diagnostic imaging tools include bone scintigraphy and positron emission tomography scan using fluorodeoxyglucose or 18F-sodium fluoride (18F-NaF).

DIFFERENTIAL DIAGNOSIS

- Osteonecrosis of the femoral condyle
- Osteonecrosis of the tibial plateau
- Charcot joint
- Idiopathic joint apoplexy
- Elderly onset rheumatoid arthritis
- Crystal-induced arthritis
- Pyogenic arthritis

NONOPERATIVE MANAGEMENT

- Employment of a combination of pharmacologic and nonpharmacologic treatment is recommended for clinical practice (Osteoarthritis Research Society International recommendations for the management of hip and knee OA).[25]
- Patients should be instructed about the purpose of treatment and the importance of changes in lifestyle, pacing of activities, weight reduction, and the need for walking aids to reduce overload to the joint.
- A knee brace can reduce pain in knee OA with mild or moderate instability. Lateral-wedged insoles provide symptomatic relief for some patients with medial compartmental knee OA.
- As pharmacologic treatments, acetaminophen is commonly used as an analgesic. Nonsteroidal anti-inflammatory drugs (NSAIDs) are recommended to be used at the lowest effective dose to prevent the increase of gastrointestinal risks. COX-2 selective agents should be used with caution in patients with cardiovascular risk factors. Glucosamine or chondroitin and weak opioids and narcotic analgesics may provide symptomatic benefits for patients with knee OA.
- Intra-articular injections with corticosteroids or hyaluronate can be used in the treatment of knee OA.

SURGICAL MANAGEMENT

Indications

- The main indication for HTO is medial compartment knee OA, which does not provide adequate pain relief and functional improvement from a combination of nonpharmacologic and pharmacologic treatment.[17,18]
- Patients with knee OA with lateral thrust are likely candidates for HTO.
- Patients with osteonecrosis of the knee are also good candidates for HTO.
- The ideal patients are physiologically young (younger than 55 years). However, a higher failure rate in obese or elderly patients of older than 65 years is not always identified. Old age and overweight patients are not contraindications for HTO.
- Medial compartmental knee OA with less than 15 degrees of anatomic varus angulation and fixed flexion deformity of less than 15 degrees is indicated for OW-HTO. For other cases, CW-HTO should be considered as a surgical option.
- To perform HTO, the ACL must be functionally intact rather than insufficient. CW-HTO can decrease the tibial posterior slope and should be selected for ACL-deficient knee OA.
- Inflammatory knee arthritis or knee OA with involvement of both the medial and lateral compartment is not indicated for HTO.

Preoperative Planning

- At the beginning of preoperative planning, it is extremely important to check that the lateral joint space width is maintained in valgus-stressed AP knee radiographs because the postoperative main weight-bearing portion becomes the lateral compartment.
- In planning for osteotomy, it is a basic principle to determine the location and direction of the osteotomy line and the desired angle of correction.
- Using a standing AP knee radiograph, a single osteotomy line is drawn from 35 mm of the point of the medial tibial cortex distal to the medial joint line to the proximal tibiofibular joint.
- The desired postoperative knee alignment is 170 degrees of standing femorotibial angle (SFTA), which was proposed by Bauer and associates[4] (10 degrees of anatomic valgus angulation). The desired angle of correction ($\theta°$) is the angle calculated by subtraction of 170 degrees from the SFTA of the affected knee.
- From a point of intersection of the osteotomy line to the lateral tibial cortex, the base of a triangle (θ) is drawn, and the distance from the initial point of the osteotomy line to the point of intersection to the medial cortex is measured, which indicates the tibial width for opening the gap during operation.

Positioning

- The patient is positioned supine on the operating table with a sandbag inserted into the ipsilateral buttock region to place the lower extremity in neutral position (**FIG 2**).

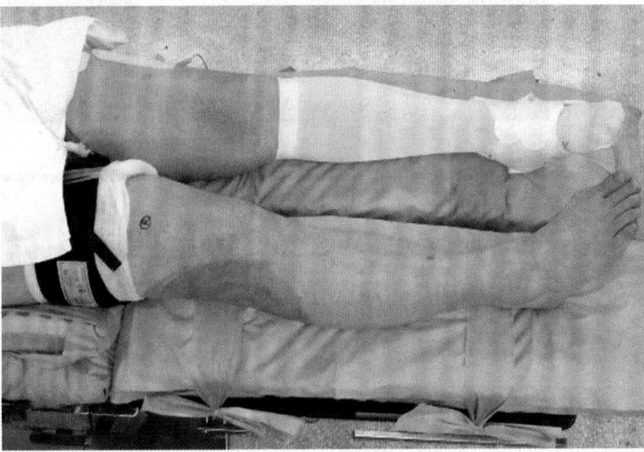

FIG 2 • Positioning. Patient is in the supine position. A tourniquet is placed at the upper thigh area.

- A pneumo-tourniquet is applied to the upper thigh area.
- Under preoperative fluoroscopy, it is necessary to check that the center of the femoral head, the ankle, and the position of the knee joint can be visualized.

Approach

- The approach for OW-HTO is a medial parapatellar incision from the lower part of the patella to 3 cm distal to the tibial tuberosity (**FIG 3**).
- When arthrotomy is needed for intra-articular procedures, including resection of osteophytes and resourcing articular cartilage, a longer skin incision is made from the upper part of the patella to distal to the tibial tuberosity, and the subvastus approach is commonly used.

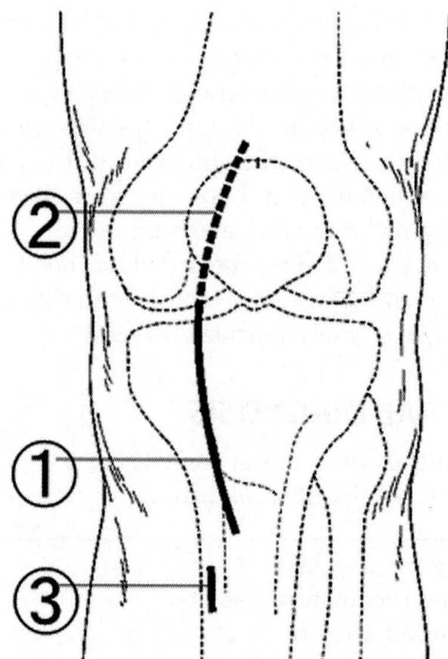

FIG 3 • Approach for opening wedge HTO. (*1*) Slightly oblique skin incision parallel to the medial border of the patellar ligament beginning at the level of the inferior pole of the patella and extending distally to the level of the tibial tuberosity. (*2*) Proximally extended skin incision for intra-articular procedures. (*3*) Separate incision for distal screws with the minimally invasive plate osteosynthesis (MIPO) technique.

Arthroscopy

- A routine arthroscopic examination is performed through the anteromedial or anterolateral portal to determine the intra-articular pathology.
- It is important to check the status of the articular surface of the lateral compartment because derangement of the articular cartilage influences the long-term clinical outcomes of HTO (**TECH FIG 1A,B**).
- The condition of the ACL and the patellofemoral compartment are also investigated because OW-HTO is feasible to exacerbate the patellofemoral arthritis.
- During arthroscopy, free body can be removed and meniscus tears are débrided if necessary. Bone marrow stimulation can be performed using a Kirschner wire or an ice pick.

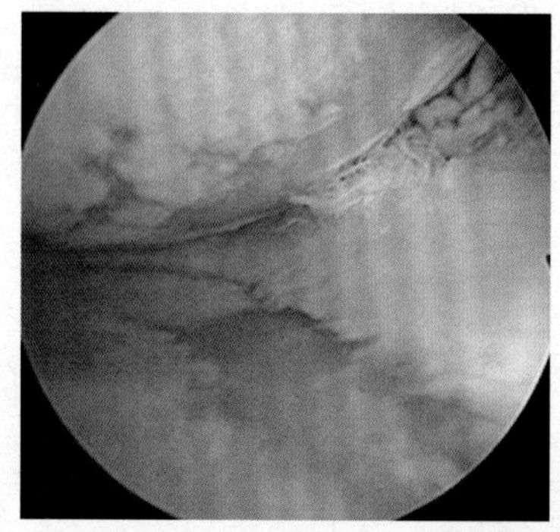

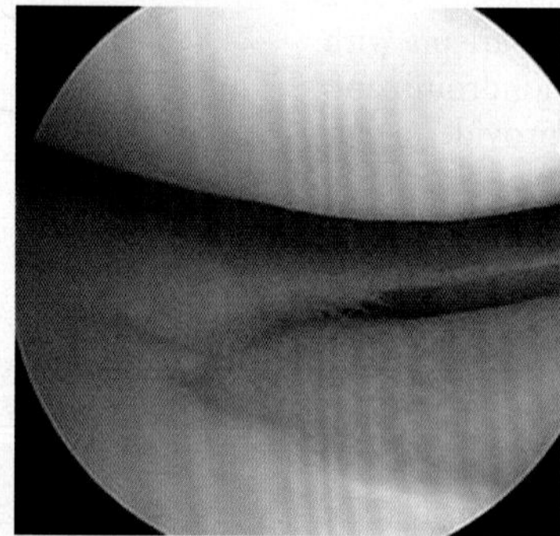

TECH FIG 1 • Arthroscopy. **A.** Arthroscopic image of the medial compartment with exposure of subchondral bone on the medial femoral condyle and tibia. **B.** Arthroscopic image of the lateral compartment with intact articular surface.

Opening Wedge High Tibial Osteotomy

Initial Dissection

- Bony anatomic landmarks, including relief of the patella tendon, the tibial tuberosity, a joint line, and Gerdy tubercle, are marked with a skin marker.
- The medial parapatellar oblique skin incision is made from the lower part of the patella to 3 cm distal to the tibial tuberosity.
- The incision is made through the skin and subcutaneous dissection is carried out until the anterior aspect of the proximal tibia covered by the sartorius fascia is exposed.
- The fascia is longitudinally incised along both the medial and lateral margin of the patella tendon and the posterior insertion of the tendon is cleared for making a flange at the tibial tuberosity.

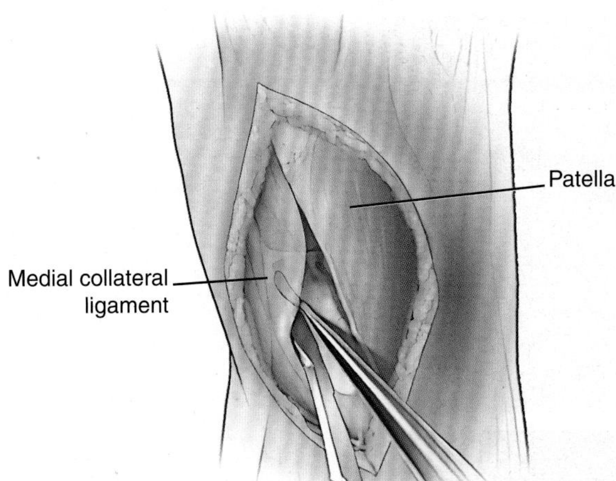

TECH FIG 2 • Subperiosteal elevation. Subperiosteal elevation of the superficial layer of the medial collateral ligament from the medial to the posterior portion.

The anterior aspect of the lateral side of the proximal tibia is also subperiosteally released for osteotomy (**TECH FIG 2**).

- Insertion of hamstrings and superficial medial collateral ligament are released subperiosteally and the periosteum at the proximal tibia is elevated using a Cobb elevator from the medial to the posterior portion until the knee becomes slightly genu recurvatum.
- The periosteum of the posterior portion of the tibia is thick and firm. The periosteum, associated with the muscle and soft tissue, is satisfactorily elevated to avoid unexpected neurovascular injury.

Placing Guide Pins

- Under fluoroscopic image control, two Kirschner wires (2 mm in diameter) are inserted at the medial cortex, which is 3.5 cm below the medial joint surface (**TECH FIG 3A**) and directed in almost parallel line to the proximal tibiofibular joint, making an osteotomy plane (**TECH FIG 3B**).

Osteotomy

- When performing osteotomy, the medial and anterior cortical cut is made along the two Kirschner wires using a small oscillating bone saw (**TECH FIG 4A**), and the posterior, posterolateral and anterolateral cortical cut is made with thin osteotomes (**TECH FIG 4B**). The osteotomy is deepened. At this time, the lateral tibial cortex should remain intact.
- At the tibial tuberosity, an L-shaped osteotomy is performed to make a flange of about 2 cm in height. The height is determined based on the opening. Then incomplete osteotomy is achieved.
- An opener is inserted from the osteotomized site (**TECH FIG 4C**) and to less than 10 mm of the lateral cortex (**TECH FIG 4D**). The separation of the proximal and the distal bone fragment is gradually accomplished with the use of an opener until the width of the gap is same as the distance measured in the preoperative radiograph (**TECH FIG 4E**). The limb alignment is supposed to be corrected to 170 degrees of SFTA (10 degrees of anatomic valgus angulation). The corrected alignment can also be used to check that the mechanical axis passes through the 62% coordinate along the tibial plateau using electrocautery.

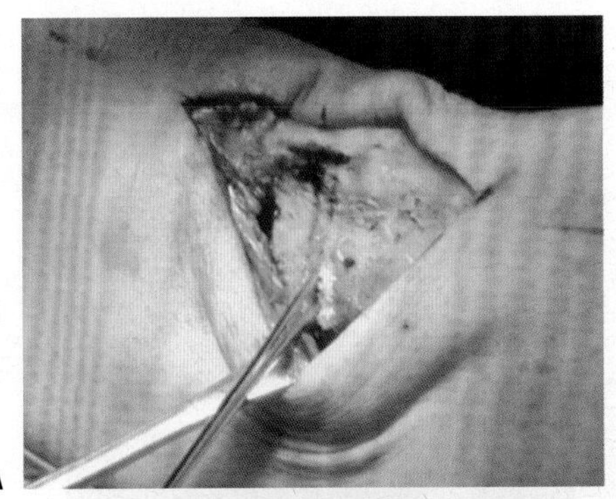

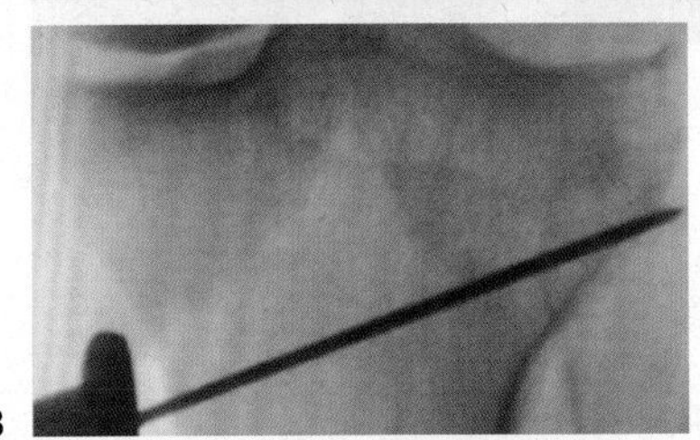

TECH FIG 3 • Placing guide pins. **A.** Two Kirschner wires placed in parallel from the medial side at 35 mm distal from the articular level of the femorotibial joint to the upper third of the proximal tibiofibular joint. **B.** Confirmation of parallel insertion of two wires under fluoroscopic image control.

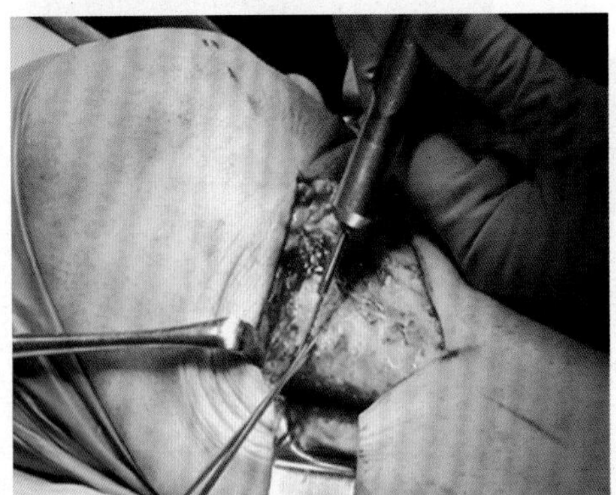

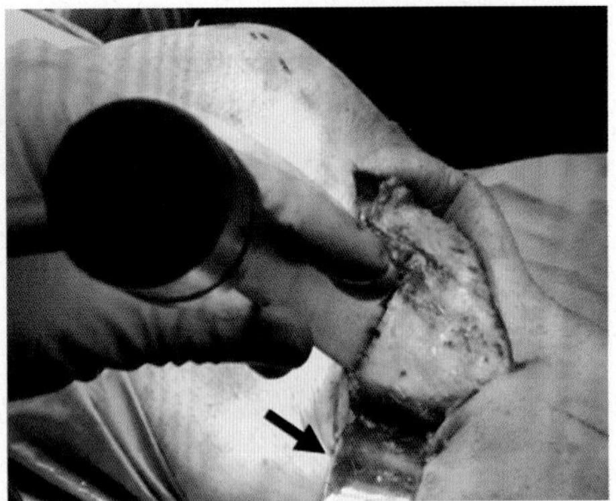

TECH FIG 4 • Osteotomy and opening of osteotomy gap. **A.** An oblique osteotomy using an oscillating bone saw along the Kirschner wire guide. **B.** Note that posterior portion should be protected by retractor (*arrow*). *(continued)*

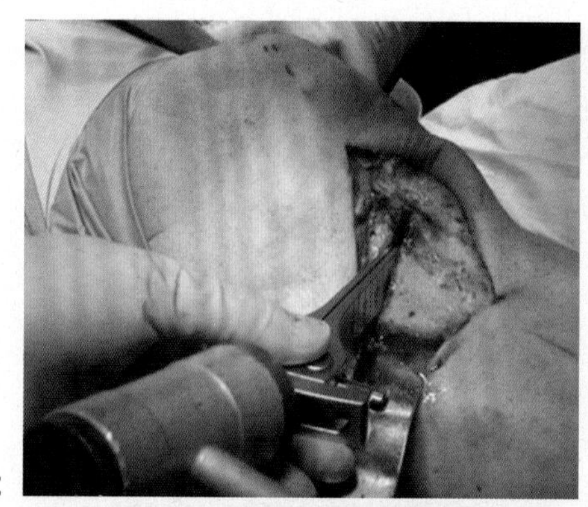

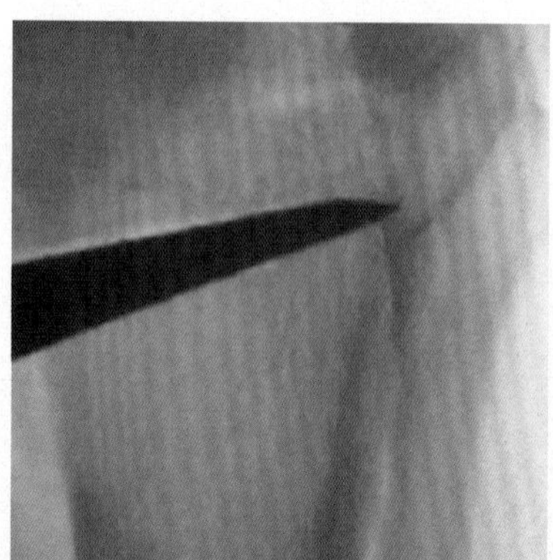

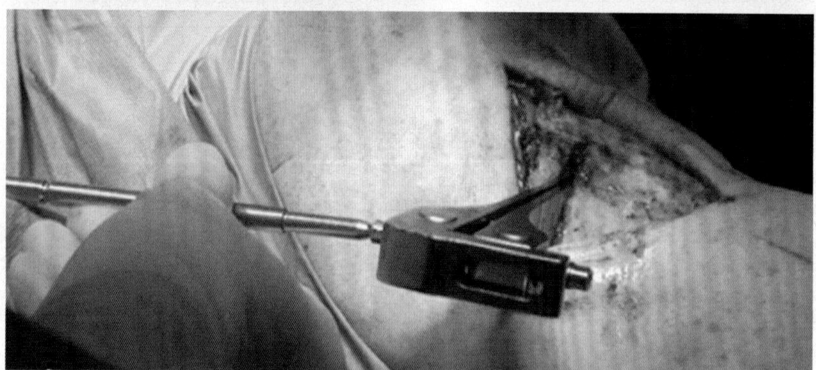

TECH FIG 4 • *(continued)* **C.** Insertion of opener. **D.** Note that insertion of opener should be ended 5 mm from the lateral cortical margin, leaving lateral cortex intact. **E.** Gradual opening of the osteotomized gap using an opener until the preoperatively planned opening distance is obtained.

Bone Grafting

- The space is maintained with two spreaders inserted in the anterior and posterior side (**TECH FIG 5A,B**). Two wedge-shaped bone substitutes made of β-TCP (tricalcium phosphate) with 60% of porosity or bone grafts taken from the iliac crest are inserted into the opening space in order to reinforce mechanical strength against weight bearing and keep the corrected alignment (**TECH FIG 5C,D**).
- To maintain the natural tibial posterior slope, the first wedge-shaped bone substitute or allograft should be placed at the most posterior corner, and with knee extension, the base of wedge should be higher posteriorly than anteriorly (**TECH FIG 5E**). The size-adjusted second bone substitute or bone graft is inserted.

Plate Fixation and Closure

- The periosteum is sutured as it was before separation and TomoFix plate (Synthes, Paoli, PA) with a locking mechanism is placed over the periosteum. Both the distal and the proximal fragment are fixed with screws (**TECH FIG 6A,B**). About 2 cm of additional incision above the distal end of the plate is often necessary for the distal screw fixation.
- A medium Hemovac drain is placed in the osteotomized site and the subcutaneous tissue and the operative wound are closed in the standard fashion. A sterile dressing is applied. Knee immobilizers are not necessary.

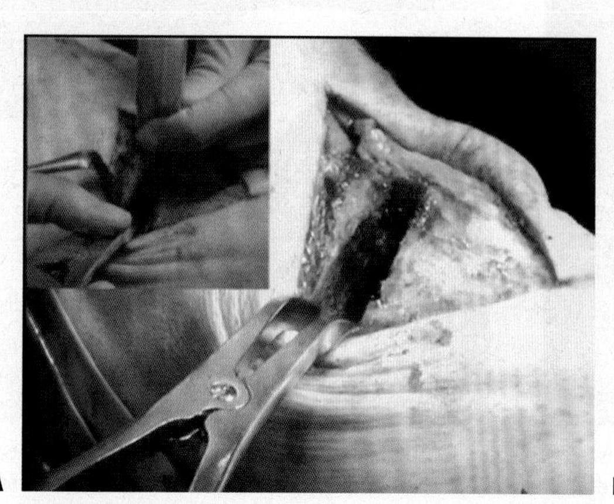

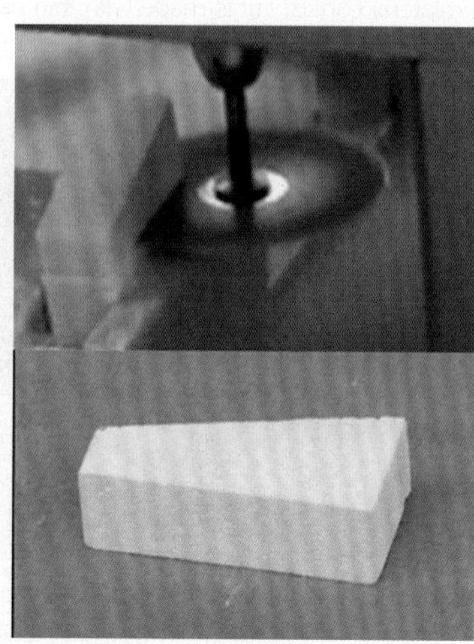

TECH FIG 5 • Osteotomy gap maintained with spreader. **A.** Maintenance of osteotomy gap after opening. **B.** Wedge-shaped bone substitutes are made from a rectangular one. *(continued)*

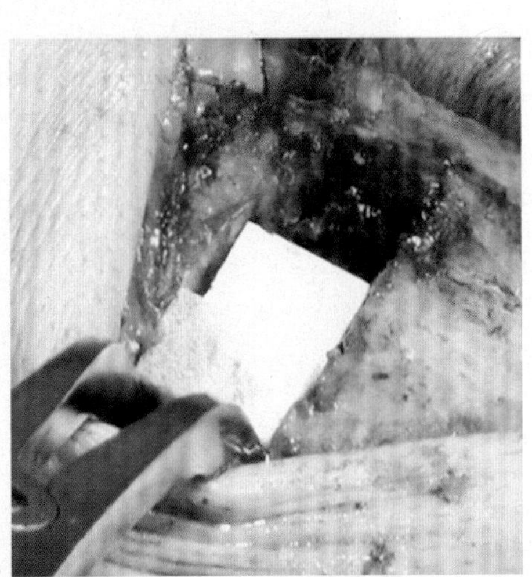

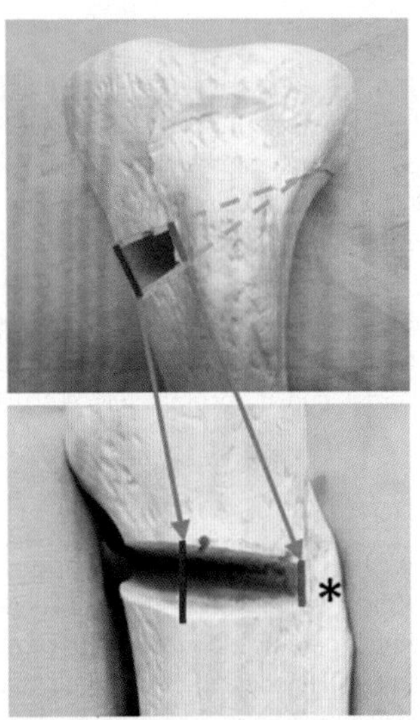

C D

TECH FIG 5 • *(continued)* **C.** Two wedge-shaped bone substitutes are inserted into the opening gap. **D.** Note that care was taken to keep the anterior opening gap approximately two-thirds of the posterior opening gap to avoid unintended increase of posterior slope in sagittal plane (*asterisk*).

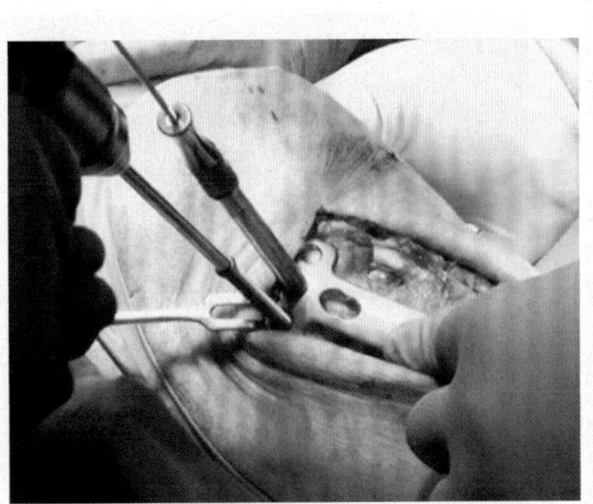

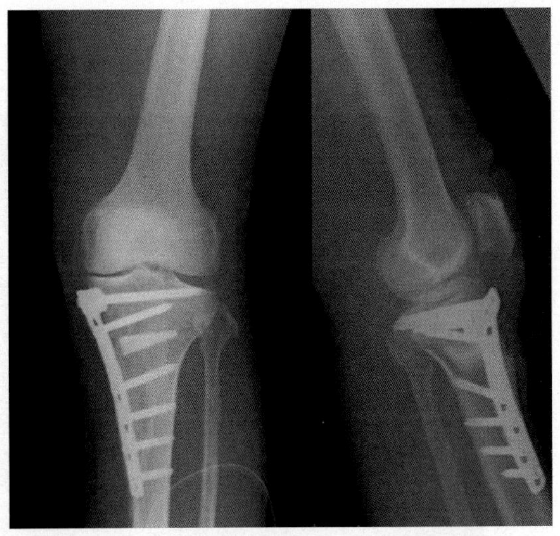

A B

TECH FIG 6 • Fixation of bone fragments. **A.** Subcutaneous fixation of osteotomy site with TomoFix plate and locking screws. **B.** Postoperative AP and lateral radiographs.

Application of Opening Wedge High Tibial Osteotomy to Another Pathologic Conditions of the Knee

Dual Osteotomy for the Medial Compartmental Knee Osteoarthritis Associated with Patellofemoral Osteoarthritis

- Combined medial OW-HTO and tibial tuberosity anteromedialization osteotomies

Approach

- A midline longitudinal skin incision is made starting at the superior pole of the patella and ending nearly 5 cm distal to the tibial tuberosity.
- Subcutaneous tissue is retracted medially and the medial retinaculum is released at the medial border of the patellar ligament. Distally, the incision is extended along with medial border of the tibial tuberosity and the medial collateral ligament and pes anserinus are subcutaneously elevated.
- The lateral retinaculum is sharply dissected to release completely from the patella to the level of the vastus lateralis.

Osteotomy

- The first osteotomy is a medial opening wedge oblique osteotomy, leaving the tibial tuberosity intact. Starting posterior to the patellar tendon insertion, an osteotomy of the proximal tuberosity is performed parallel to the anterior tibial cortex.
- The second osteotomy is made as a tibial tuberosity anteromedialization after completing the opening wedge technique. An osteotomy is performed extending to 4 to 5 cm distal from the patellar ligament insertion with 8- to 10-mm thickness at proximal site. The distal end is incompletely cut with intact periosteum.

Bone Grafting and Osteosynthesis

- The proximal part of the tibial tuberosity is transferred medially on its periosteal distal hinge. The distance of medialization depends on the extent of patellar subluxation. The proximal part is then elevated 10 mm anteriorly and the wedged-shaped artificial bone substitute with two holes for screws is placed under the partly detached bony fragment of the tibial tuberosity. Finally, the bony fragment is fixed with two 4.5-mm cannulated cortical screws (**TECH FIG 7**).

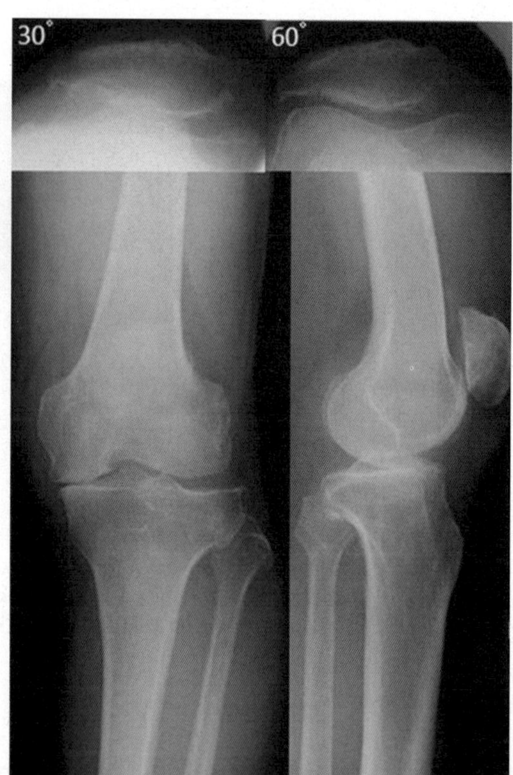

A

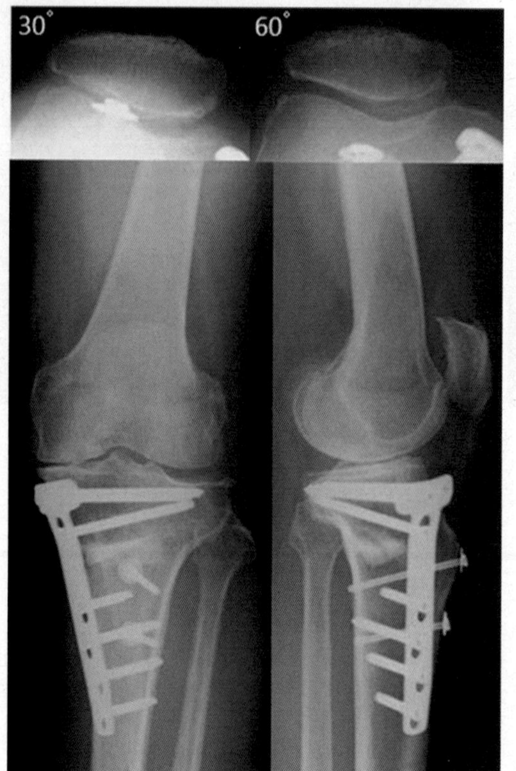

B

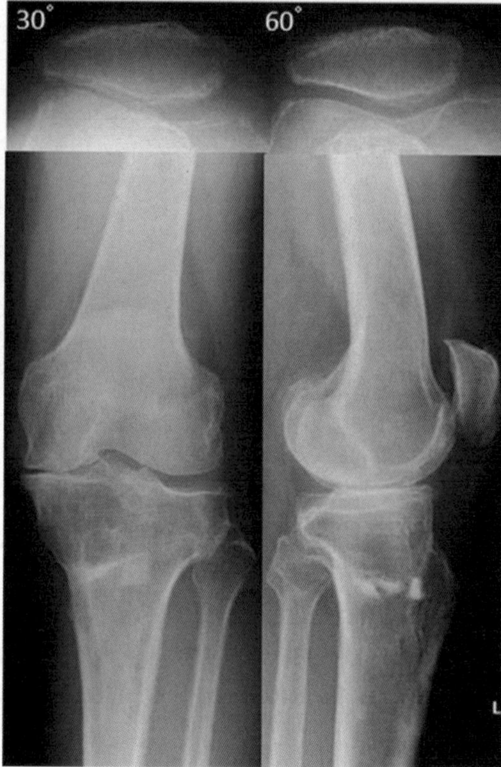

C

TECH FIG 7 • OW-HTO associated with advancement of the tibial tuberosity. **A.** Preoperative radiographs showing medial compartment OA and patellofemoral OA with patellar subluxation. **B.** Radiographs of postoperative 1 year showing valgus corrected knee with anteromedialized patella. **C.** Radiographs of postoperative 3 year showing maintained patellofemoral congruence.

Opening Wedge High Tibial Osteotomy Associated with Mosaicplasty for Osteonecrosis of the Knee with a Large Cartilage Defect

Approach

- In addition to skin incision for simple OW-HTO, a medial parapatellar skin incision is extended to the proximal pole of the patella.
- Articular surface is exposed through subvastus arthrotomy.

Donor Harvest

- The commonly used donor sites are the areas with less weight bearing, including the medial and lateral margins of the femoral trochlea.
- Several small cylindrical osteochondral plugs of 20 mm depth are manually harvested using tubular chisels.

Graft Insertion

- Remnants of residual cartilage and subchondral lesion are removed from the defect.
- With the knee flexed, the recipient holes perpendicular to the articular surface are created using a drill.
- A press-fit transplantation of the donor osteochondral plugs is performed. All plugs should be placed at the same level of the healthy cartilage (**TECH FIG 8**).

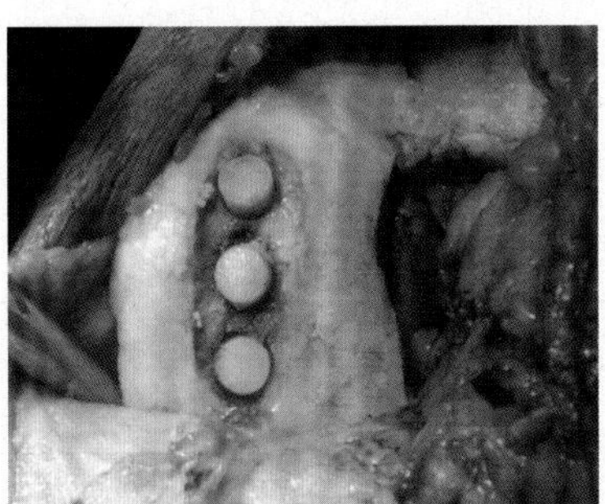

TECH FIG 8 • Cartilage restoration procedure. Photograph showing the medial femoral condyle treated with autologous osteochondral mosaicplasty.

PEARLS AND PITFALLS

Exposure and dissection	■ Be sure to expose the entire anterior surface of the proximal tibia. ■ Release the thick periosteum of the posterior portion of the tibia in line with the planned osteotomy line. ■ Insert a retractor in the posterior side to protect the neurovascular structures.
Osteotomy	■ Insert two Kirschner wires on the extended knee and check that they are parallel using an image intensifier. ■ Make a flange with enough length to bridge the gap between the proximal and distal fragment. ■ Be sure that osteotomy site can open with a slight valgus stress when incomplete osteotomy is accomplished.
Opening gap	■ Insert an opener as close to the lateral cortex as possible to prevent breach of the lateral side of the tibial plateau. ■ With the medial soft tissue still tight to hamper opening, add multiple small incisions with a scalpel to release this tightness. ■ Place the first wedge of artificial substitute in the most posterior corner of the base of the gap. ■ Make the length of the anterior gap two-thirds of that of the posterior gap to keep the natural tibial posterior slope with gentle knee extension.
Plate fixation	■ Place a TomoFix plate over the periosteum. ■ Do not protrude the tip of screws into the joint space or the posterior cortex. ■ Selection of the proper length of screws is essential. ■ Extend a knee joint on screwing the distal fragment to achieve full knee extension.

POSTOPERATIVE CARE

- In immediate postoperative care, patients receive a femoral nerve block set at anesthesia with a patient-controlled ropivacaine injection for the first night.
- After removal of the catheter, NSAIDs are used for pain control.
- Sequential compression devices including foot pump (A-V Impulse System, Covidien, Mansfield, MA) are used during hospitalization to reduce the risk of deep venous thrombosis.
- The drain is removed within 48 hours postoperatively and active ROM exercise is started the day after the operation.
- Straight-leg raising and setting exercises are allowed, and full knee extension is observed.
- Patients can walk non–weight bearing using crutches and partial weight bearing is allowed 1 week after the operation.
- Walking exercise with full weight bearing using a T-cane starts 1 week after surgery.
- Patients are allowed to be discharged from the hospital when they achieve the rehabilitation level of walking up and down stairs.

OUTCOMES

- Many studies reported that HTO provided a good functional outcome for knee OA and postoperative clinical results were satisfactorily maintained for a long-term follow-up period, especially in cases with adequate postoperative limb alignment.[20]

Table 1 Clinical Outcomes with Opening Wedge High Tibial Osteotomy

Study	Cases	Follow-up (y)	Results
Asik et al, 2006	65	1.5–5 (mean 2.8)	Mean Knee Society knee score of 85.6
Benzakour et al, 2010	118	5–27 (mean 15)	Mean Knee Society scoring (knee score and function score) of 101/200 at 15 y
Brosset et al, 2011	51	1.8–2.1 (mean 2)	Mean IKS knee score of 90
DeMeo et al, 2010	20	8.3, mean	70% survivorship with 42% of patients rating their knees as good or excellent at 8 y
El-Azab et al, 2011	50	2.5–3.8 (mean 3)	Mean Lysholm score of 85
Floerkemeier et al, 2013	533	2.4–4.7 (mean 3.6)	Mean Oxford Knee Score of 43 (0: worst, 48: best)
Haviv et al, 2012	22	6.3, mean	Mean Oxford Knee Score of 37
Hernigou et al, 1987	93	10–13 (mean 11.5)	90% good to excellent at 5 y, 45% good to excellent at 10 y
Kolb et al, 2009	51	2.8–5.5 (mean 4.3)	82% good to excellent results at final follow-up
Niemeyer et al, 2010	69	3-y minimum	Mean International Knee Documentation Committee score of 72.7
Saito et al, 2014	78	5–10 (mean 6.5)	Mean Knee Society knee score of 88.1

IKS, International Knee Society.

- Correction of the varus deformity reduces synovial inflammation and induces regeneration in the involved articular cartilage following HTO.
- However, HTO has several potential disadvantages, such as limited patient selection, technical difficulty, short longevity (5 to 7 years),[1,24] and possibility of neurovascular injury.
- Recently, OW-HTO has become more popular because of its surgical simplicity, intraoperative fine-tuning of correction, quick and safe exposure of the bone without any muscle attachment, and no risk for peroneal nerve palsy.
- Previous studies on OW-HTO have demonstrated promising clinical and functional short-term and midterm results (Table 1).[3–6,8,9,11,13–15,19,21]

COMPLICATIONS

- HTO is considered to be a technically demanding surgery; its complication rates are relatively high and vary depending on the experience of the surgeon, surgical procedures, and postoperative management.

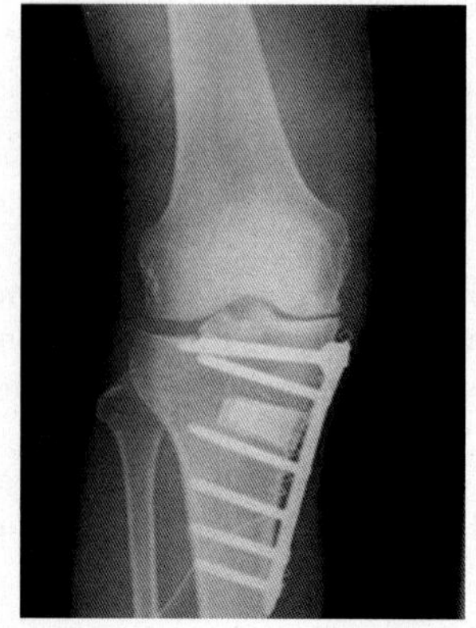

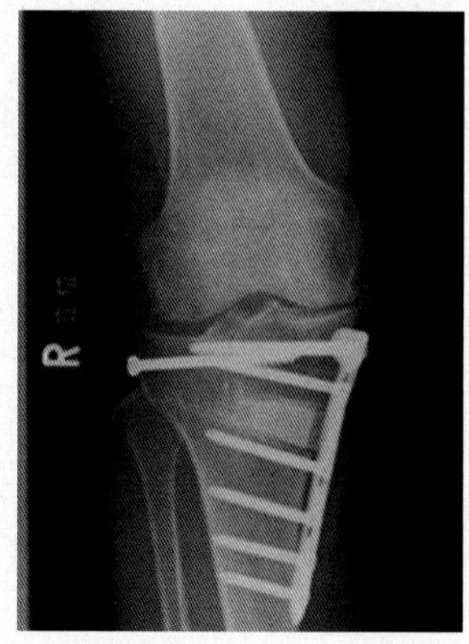

FIG 4 • Case with the lateral plateau fracture during surgery. **A.** 69-year-old man. The lateral plateau fracture is observed on the anteroposterior radiograph taken just after OW-HTO. **B.** Cancellous screw is inserted from the lateral side of tibia. Callus formation and osseous consolidation in the osteotomy site is observed in the radiograph taken at 6 months after surgery without loss of correction angle.

Intraoperative Complications

- Malalignment
  - Undercorrection or overcorrection causes unsatisfactory postoperative clinical and functional outcomes.
- Fracture of the medial or lateral cortex
  - A high incidence of lateral hinge fracture was reported in OW-HTO (**FIG 4**).[23]
- Unexpected increase of the tibial posterior slope in OW-HTO
- Unexpected intra-articular protrusion of the screw
- Peroneal nerve palsy or blood vessel injury in CW-HTO
  - Rates were reported to be between 2% and 16% for paresis of the peroneal nerve and 0.4% in vessel injury.[10,12]

Immediate Postoperative Complications

- Hematoma
- Early infection
  - In a systematic literature review, superficial infections occurred in 1% to 9% and deep infections in 0.5% to 4.7%.[2,16]
- Compartment syndrome
- Venous thromboembolism
  - Reports of venous thromboembolism after HTO are quite limited. The rate of deep vein thrombosis was 12.5% and that of asymptomatic pulmonary embolism was 9.4% with the use of a tourniquet in our recent study.

Late Postoperative Complications

- Patella baja
- Pseudarthrosis
  - The rate of pseudarthrosis is reported to be between 0.7% and 4.4%.[22]
- Implant failure
- Correction loss and recurrence of varus deformity

REFERENCES

1. Aglietti P, Buzzi R, Vena LM, et al. High tibial valgus osteotomy for medial gonarthrosis: a 10- to 21-year study. J Knee Surg 2003;16:21–26.
2. Anagnostakos K, Mosser P, Kohn D. Infections after high tibial osteotomy. Knee Surg Sports Traumatol Arthrosc 2013;21:161–169.
3. Asik M, Sen C, Kilic B, et al. High tibial osteotomy with Puddu plate for the treatment of varus gonarthrosis. Knee Surg Sports Traumatol Arthrosc 2006;14:948–954.
4. Bauer GC, Insall J, and Koshino T. Tibial osteotomy in gonarthrosis (osteo-arthritis of the knee). J Bone Joint Surg Am 1969;51:1545–1563.
5. Benzakour T, Hefti A, Lemseffer M, et al. High tibial osteotomy for medial osteoarthritis of the knee: 15 years follow-up. Int Orthop 2010;34:209–215.
6. Brosset T, Pasquier G, Migaud H, et al. Opening wedge high tibial osteotomy performed without filling the defect but with locking plate fixation (TomoFix) and early weight-bearing: prospective evaluation of bone union, precision and maintenance of correction in 51 cases. Orthop Traumatol Surg Res 2011;97:705–711.
7. Cass JR, Bryan RS. High tibial osteotomy. Clin Orthop Relat Res 1988;230:196–199.
8. DeMeo PJ, Johnson EM, Chiang PP, et al. Midterm follow-up of opening-wedge high tibial osteotomy. Am J Sports Med 2010;38: 2077–2084.
9. El-Azab HM, Morgenstern M, Ahrens P, et al. Limb alignment after open-wedge high tibial osteotomy and its effect on the clinical outcome. Orthopedics 2011;34:e622–e628.
10. Flierl S, Sabo D, Hornig K, et al. Open wedge high tibial osteotomy using fractioned drill osteotomy: a surgical modification that lowers the complication rate. Knee Surg Sports Traumatol Arthrosc 1996;4:149–153.
11. Floerkemeier S, Staubli AE, Schroeter S, et al. Outcome after high tibial open-wedge osteotomy: a retrospective evaluation of 533 patients. Knee Surg Sports Traumatol Arthrosc 2013;21:170–180.
12. Georgoulis AD, Makris CA, Papgeorgiou CD, et al. Nerve and vessel injuries during high tibial osteotomy combined with distal fibular osteotomy: a clinically relevant anatomic study. Knee Surg Sports Traumatol Arthrosc 1999;7:15–19.
13. Haviv B, Bronak S, Thein R, et al. Mid-term outcome of opening-wedge high tibial osteotomy for varus arthritic knees. Orthopedics 2012;35:e192–e196.
14. Hernigou P, Medevielle D, Debeyre J, et al. Proximal tibial osteotomy for osteoarthritis with varus deformity. A ten to thirteen-year follow-up study. J Bone Joint Surg Am 1987;69:332–354.
15. Kolb W, Guhlmann H, Windish C, et al. Opening-wedge high tibial osteotomy with a locked low-profile plate. J Bone Joint Surg Am 2009;91:2581–2588.
16. Koshino T. The treatment of spontaneous osteonecrosis of the knee by high tibial osteotomy with and without bone grafting or drilling of the lesion. J Bone Joint Surg Am 1982;64(1):47–58.
17. Marti RK, Verhagen RA, Kerkhoffs GM, et al. Proximal tibial varus osteotomy. Indications, technique, and five to twenty-one-year results. J Bone Joint Surg Am 2001;83-A:164–170.
18. Matthews LS, Goldstein SA, Malvitz TA, et al. Proximal tibial osteotomy. Factors that influence the duration of satisfactory function. Clin Orthop Relat Res 1988;229:193–200.
19. Niemeyer P, Schmal H, Hauschild O, et al. Open-wedge osteotomy using an internal plate fixator in patients with medial-compartment gonarthritis and varus malalignment: 3-year results with regard to preoperative arthroscopic and radiographic findings. Arthroscopy 2010;26:1607–1616.
20. Odenbring S, Egund N, Hagstedt B, et al. Ten-year results of tibial osteotomy for medial gonoarthrosis: the influence of overcorrection. Arch Orthop Trauma Surg 1991;110:103–108.
21. Saito T, Kumagai K, Akamatsu Y, et al. Five- to ten-year outcome following medial opening-wedge high tibial osteotomy with rigid plate fixation in combination with an artificial bone substitute. Bone Joint J 2014;96-B:339–344.
22. Spahn G. Complications in high tibial (medial opening wedge) osteotomy. Arch Orthop Trauma Surg 2003;124:649–653.
23. Takeuchi R, Ishikawa H, Kumagai K, et al. Fractures around the lateral cortical hinge after a medial opening-wedge high tibial osteotomy: a new classification of lateral hinge fracture. Arthroscopy 2012;28: 85–94.
24. Yasuda K, Majima T, Tsuchida T, et al. A ten- to 15-year follow-up observation of high tibial osteotomy in medial compartment osteoarthritis. Clin Orthop Relat Res 1992;282:186–195.
25. Zhang W, Moskowitz RW, Nuki G, et al. OARSI recommendations for the management of hip and knee osteoarthritis, Part II:OARSI evidence-based, expert consensus guidelines. Osteoarthritis Cartilage 2008;16:137–162.

36 CHAPTER

Unicondylar Knee Arthroplasty

Danielle Y. Ponzio, Eric A. Levicoff, Robert J. Ponzio, and Jess H. Lonner

DEFINITION

- Unicondylar knee arthroplasty (UKA) is a surgical treatment alternative to total knee arthroplasty (TKA) for replacement of either the medial or lateral tibiofemoral compartment of the knee in selected patients with painful focal arthritis or osteonecrosis.[4]
- The primary objectives of UKA are pain relief and improvement in lower extremity alignment and function.
- UKA implant designs, polyethylene quality, and implant alignment and fixation methods continue to evolve. Adherence to strict surgical indications and appropriate patient selection, combined with meticulous surgical execution, optimizes the functional outcomes and survival rates of UKA.[10]
- Although UKA has numerous potential clinical advantages, the technical challenges in achieving consistent, accurate component alignment and soft tissue balance have prompted advances in the development and use of computer and robotic technologies.[13,15,16,25]

ANATOMY

- The knee has three compartments: the medial and lateral tibiofemoral compartments and the patellofemoral compartment.
- The alignment of the knee joint is described relative to the mechanical axis of the lower extremity, which is a straight line from the center of the femoral head to the center of the ankle joint.
  - When the center of the knee lies on the mechanical axis, the knee is in neutral alignment, which allows for appropriate load distribution between the medial and lateral compartments of the knee.
  - If the mechanical axis passes medial to the knee center, a varus deformity is present; if the axis passes lateral to the knee center, a valgus deformity is present.
- Normal knee joint alignment is defined by asymmetric bony anatomy, which creates a tibiofemoral angle of approximately 5 to 7 degrees valgus, ligamentous tension, and a uniform joint space throughout the medial and lateral compartments through the full range of motion of the knee.[19,38]
  - The proximal articular surface of the tibia is oriented approximately 3 degrees varus to the mechanical axis of the tibia.
  - In the sagittal plane, the tibia is sloped posteriorly approximately 5 to 7 degrees to accommodate femoral rollback during knee flexion.
  - The distal femoral condyles are oriented approximately 3 degrees valgus to the mechanical axis of the femur and 9 degrees valgus to the anatomic axis of the femur.
  - In flexion, the medial femoral condyle extends more posteriorly than the lateral femoral condyle.[34]
- The goal of UKA is to restore the affected tibiofemoral joint line by implanting a prosthesis that matches the thickness of the bone and cartilage lost or resected, thereby correcting or partially correcting the deformity with balanced soft tissues so that there is 1 to 2 mm of laxity through the full range of motion of the knee.

PATHOGENESIS

- The etiologies of articular cartilage degeneration include primary osteoarthritis (OA), osteonecrosis, and arthritis secondary to trauma, infection, or an inflammatory process.
- The degenerative process causes deterioration and loss of the bearing surface of the knee joint, characterized by cartilage and osteochondral junction breakdown, subchondral microfractures and cyst formation, and increased osseous stresses leading to the development of osteophytes.[1]
- When isolated to the medial or lateral tibiofemoral compartment, articular degeneration reduces the joint space in the affected compartment, causing overall malalignment of the knee joint.
- In medial compartment OA with an intact anterior cruciate ligament (ACL), the cartilage loss is typically anteromedial, whereas the posterior tibial and femoral cartilage are preserved.[17,39]
  - Posteromedial tibial wear suggests ACL insufficiency and may be a contraindication for UKA.
- In lateral compartment OA, the wear is typically on the posterior (flexion) surface of the lateral femoral condyle, with preservation of the distal femoral cartilage.
- Unicompartmental arthritis most commonly involves the medial compartment, causing a varus deformity.

NATURAL HISTORY

- Cartilaginous degeneration of the knee joint is progressive as described by the Outerbridge grading system.
  - Grade I: soft superficial discoloration
  - Grade II: fragmentation less than 1.3 cm^2
  - Grade III: fragmentation greater than 1.3 cm^2
  - Grade IV: erosion to subchondral bone (eburnation)
- Angular malalignment of the lower extremity accentuates stress on the damaged articular cartilage, causing pain, progression of unicompartmental arthritis, and increased angular deformity of the knee.[20]
  - For a single-leg stance with a neutral mechanical axis, the load across the medial compartment is approximately 60%. The load increases progressively up to 90% in the presence of a varus deformity of 4 to 6 degrees.[19]
- In the most advanced stages, the degenerative process leads to ligamentous instability with failure of the ACL perpetuating

joint incongruity and the progression of arthritis to the posterior aspect of the tibiofemoral articulation and, at the end-stage of the disease, to the adjacent compartments of the knee.[17]

- However, many cases (approximately 15% to 35%) will never progress beyond one compartment.[5]

PATIENT HISTORY AND PHYSICAL FINDINGS

- The most common presenting symptom of unicompartmental knee arthritis is activity-related pain confined to the affected compartment and relieved by rest.[20]
  - Associated symptoms include swelling, instability, stiffness, and restriction of activity.
  - Diffuse knee pain and rest pain suggest multiple compartment involvement and more advanced arthritis.
  - Anterolateral pain with stair climbing, prolonged sitting, or squatting suggests patellofemoral involvement.
  - Mechanical symptoms such as locking or catching may be related to articular surface irregularity, loose bodies, or meniscal pathology, which are commonly seen in conjunction with arthritis.
  - Knowledge of response to previous treatments such as nonsteroidal anti-inflammatory drugs (NSAIDs), injections, or bracing is helpful to direct further management.
- Physical examination findings consistent with unicompartmental knee arthritis may include joint line tenderness, joint effusion, crepitus, malalignment, and pseudolaxity.
  - Unicompartmental medial or lateral degeneration may cause varus or valgus deformity about the knee, respectively.
    - Medial compartment arthritis amenable to UKA presents with a varus deformity of up to 10 degrees, which is passively correctable toward neutral alignment in zero degrees of knee flexion.
    - Lateral compartment arthritis conducive to UKA presents with a valgus deformity of up to 15 degrees, which is passively correctable toward neutral alignment and does not increase in magnitude with further valgus stressing (indicative of incompetence of the medial collateral ligament).
  - Range of motion and the presence and degree of flexion contracture are assessed.
    - UKA requires a minimum of 90 degrees of flexion and no more than a 5- to 10-degree flexion contracture.[23]
  - Ligamentous stability must be present for consideration of UKA.
    - ACL deficiency without functional instability is not a contraindication for UKA. However, functional ACL instability during activities and posterior tibial wear due to anterior tibial subluxation is a contraindication for UKA.[17]
  - Other physical examination considerations include the following:
    - Previous incisions
    - Patellofemoral or adjacent tibiofemoral tenderness or crepitus
    - Body habitus
    - Indications of spine or ipsilateral hip pathology
    - Neurovascular status

IMAGING AND OTHER DIAGNOSTIC STUDIES

- Preoperative radiographs include weight-bearing anteroposterior (AP), midflexion posteroanterior (PA), lateral, and skyline patellar views to assess tibiofemoral alignment and the condition of the remaining compartments of the knee (**FIG 1A–D**).
  - Radiographic findings of unicompartmental knee arthritis may include joint space narrowing, subchondral sclerosis and cystic change, osteophytes, and malalignment of the affected lower extremity.
  - Small patellar osteophytes or peripheral osteophytes of the other tibiofemoral compartment may be seen in the absence of cartilage wear in those compartments and are not contraindications to UKA.

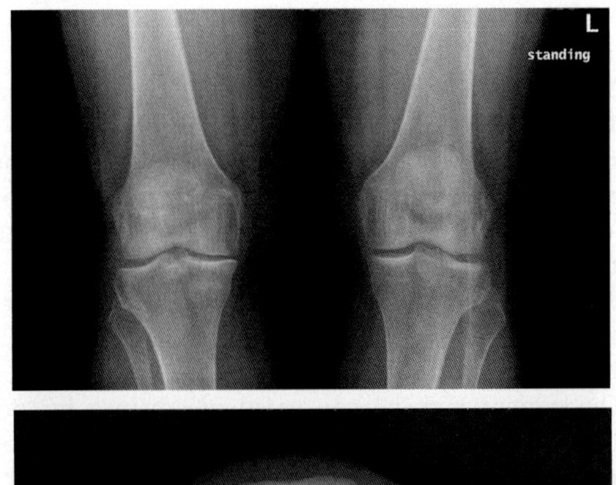

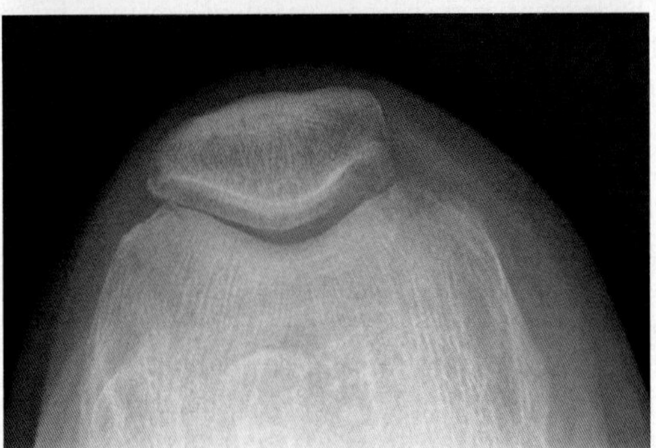

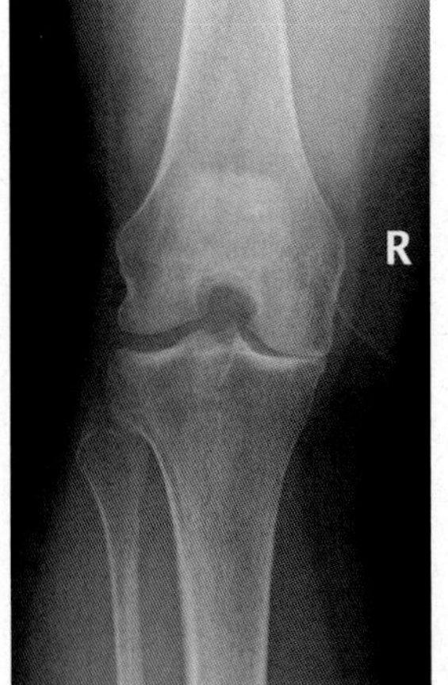

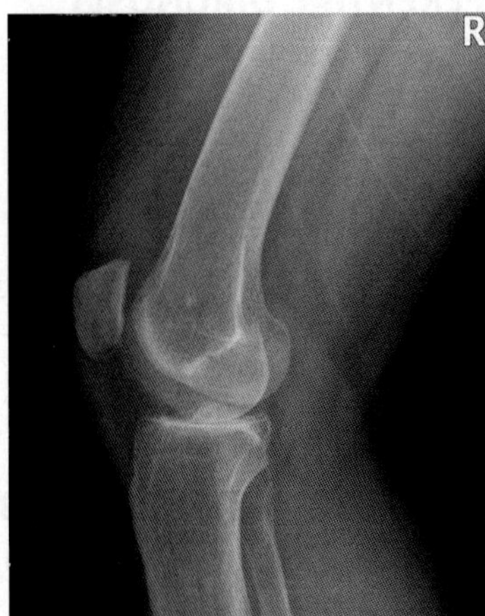

FIG 1 • Preoperative radiographs. **A.** AP view demonstrates right knee medial joint space narrowing and varus deformity. **B.** PA view. **C.** Lateral view demonstrates preservation of the posterior tibiofemoral joint space. **D.** Skyline patellar view.

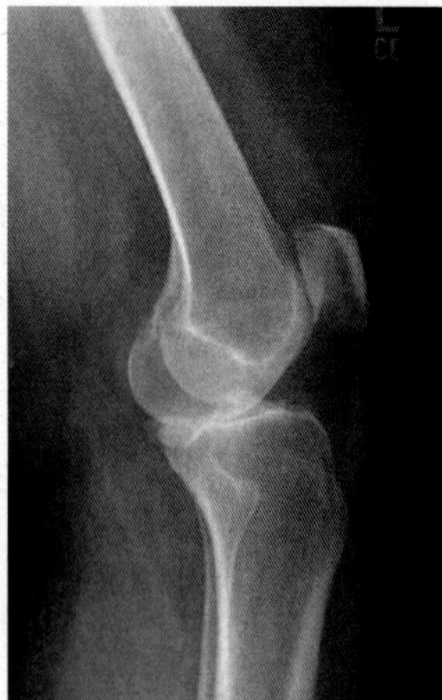

FIG 2 • Posteromedial tibial wear shown on a lateral radiograph of the knee suggests ACL insufficiency, which may be a contraindication for UKA.

- Large subchondral cysts would exclude UKA due to potentially compromised osseous support.
- Tibiofemoral contact is assessed on the lateral radiograph and is an indirect indicator of the functional integrity of the ACL. Concave erosion on the anterior two-thirds of the tibial plateau is indicative of an intact ACL (95% probability). Posterior contact and wear are characteristic of chronic ACL laxity (**FIG 2**).[17]
- Some surgeons perform stress view radiographs to identify whether there is occult full-thickness cartilage loss in the unaffected tibiofemoral compartment as well as to determine how correctible the deformity is.
- Magnetic resonance imaging (MRI) and computed tomography (CT) are infrequently used in the standard workup of patients suspected of having unicompartmental arthritis, unless there is a significant discrepancy between history and physical examination findings and the findings on plain radiographs.

DIFFERENTIAL DIAGNOSIS

- Unicompartmental OA
- Bi- or tricompartmental OA
- Osteonecrosis
- Meniscal tear
- Osteochondral injury
- Pes anserine bursitis
- Iliotibial band syndrome
- Saphenous neuritis
- Septic arthritis
- Hip or spine pathology

NONOPERATIVE MANAGEMENT

- Multiple nonoperative management options are available for treatment of unicompartmental knee OA, each with varying degrees of success.[4] These include the following:
  - Lifestyle modifications including weight loss and low-impact exercise
  - NSAIDs
  - Analgesic medications
  - Physical therapy
  - Ambulatory assistive devices
  - Unloader braces
  - Viscosupplementation injections
  - Intra-articular corticosteroid injections
  - Glucosamine and chondroitin sulfate supplements

SURGICAL MANAGEMENT

- UKA is a surgical treatment alternative to TKA or periarticular osteotomy in selected patients with painful unicompartmental knee degeneration.
- Adherence to sound indications and patient selection criteria is a key determinant of successful outcome following UKA.
  - Conservative data suggest that 6% to 15% of arthroplasty patients are candidates for UKA, although these numbers may be as high as 30% or more.[5,32,37]
- Classic indications and prerequisites for UKA include the following:[9,10,23,27,35]
  - Diagnosis of noninflammatory unicompartmental OA or spontaneous osteonecrosis with symptoms resistant to nonoperative management
  - Radiographic evidence of preservation of alternate compartments of the knee
  - No pain and no exposed bone in alternate compartments of the knee
  - Low-demand patients
  - Age older than 60 years
  - Weight less than 82 kg (181 pounds)
  - A minimum range of motion of 90 degrees
  - Flexion contracture of less than 5 degrees
  - Intact ACL
  - Angular deformity of the knee of a maximum of 10 degrees varus or 15 degrees valgus and partially passively correctable
- Expanded indications for UKA include the following[6,30]:
  - Younger, more active patients as a bridge procedure
  - Moderate obesity (body mass index 35 to 40 or less)
    - UKA is used cautiously in the morbidly obese due to more diffuse disease and a potentially increased risk of aseptic loosening and wear (debated in the literature).[6,7,11]
    - Recent studies have not supported a correlation between weight and poor outcome following UKA.[11]
  - ACL deficiency, if there is no functional instability and the tibiofemoral contact is anterior[17]
  - Asymptomatic grade IV patellofemoral chondromalacia, if the lateral facet and lateral trochlea are spared
- Additional considerations include age and occupational or recreational demands. The decision to proceed with UKA requires a prudent risk–benefit analysis based on multiple factors.[24]
- Although the decision to proceed with UKA is most often made prior to surgery, the patient's suitability for UKA is ultimately confirmed after arthrotomy.
  - The patient may be consented in advance for possible TKA or combined UKA and patellofemoral arthroplasty in cases where it is not completely clear in advance that UKA is appropriate.

Preoperative Planning

- High-quality radiographs allow for proper preoperative evaluation, including standing AP, midflexion PA, lateral, sunrise, and stress views (at the surgeon's discretion).
- A full-length, weight-bearing AP radiograph from the hip to the ankle is helpful in determining the mechanical and anatomic axes of the lower extremity and assessing unusual

bowing or deformity, as well as occult pathology of the hip or ankle, although this radiograph is not used routinely.
- Template overlay can be used to estimate component size and bone defects.

Positioning

- The patient is positioned supine on the operating table with a bump, roller, or dynamic leg positioner secured to the table to support the patient's heel when the knee is flexed.
- A thigh tourniquet is applied as proximally as possible on the operative lower extremity.
- Surgical drapes are applied to isolate the sterile surgical field.
- If a tourniquet is used, the lower extremity is exsanguinated by application of an elastic compressive wrap and inflation of the tourniquet.

Approach

- Note: For purposes of this chapter, the primary emphasis of surgical details will focus on the more common medial UKA.
- With the knee in moderate flexion, a skin incision is made from just proximal to the medial margin of the proximal pole of the patella to the medial aspect of the tibial tubercle (**FIG 3**). The underlying extensor mechanism and joint capsule are exposed.
- The knee joint is accessed via a medial parapatellar arthrotomy from the proximal patella to just medial to the tibial tubercle. Great care is taken along the superior portion of the arthrotomy to avoid damage to the intact cartilage of the trochlea. A cuff of capsular tissue is left intact along the medial border of the patella for later wound closure.
  - Alternatively, and less commonly, a lateral incision and lateral parapatellar capsulotomy can be used for UKA of the lateral compartment. The lateral arthrotomy must extend more proximally to allow medial subluxation of the patella.[31]
  - In a very tight or muscular knee, extending the incision more proximally, incising the medial capsule transversely for 1 cm just below the vastus medialis muscle, or formalizing a midvastus or subvastus approach may help facilitate surgical exposure.

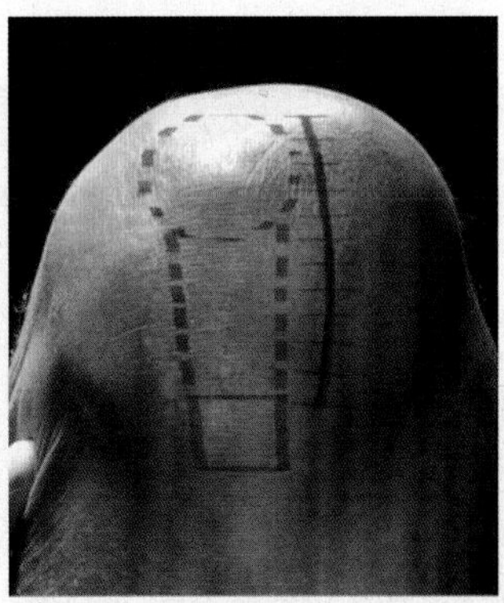

FIG 3 • The surgical approach to UKA is through a longitudinal, straight skin incision from the medial margin of the proximal pole of the patella to adjacent to the medial aspect of the tibial tubercle.

Exposure

- After the arthrotomy, all three compartments of the knee are inspected to confirm the decision to proceed with UKA.
- The patella is subluxated laterally as the knee is brought into flexion to achieve exposure of the medial joint.
- A portion of the retropatellar fat pad is excised to facilitate visualization.
- The coronary ligament is incised at the anterior horn of the medial meniscus and a sharply dissected subperiosteal sleeve of soft tissue that includes the deep medial collateral ligament is elevated from the anteromedial aspect of the tibia along the joint line.
  - For replacement of the lateral compartment, the coronary ligament is incised lateral to the midline and a periosteal sleeve is elevated from the anterolateral aspect of the tibia, as far as Gerdy's tubercle.
- An osteotome or rongeur is used to remove notch and marginal osteophytes that may cause impingement or interfere with proper collateral ligament balancing.

Distal Femoral Condyle Resection

- With the knee flexed to 90 degrees, an entry hole is drilled in the distal femur 1 cm anterior to the origin of the posterior cruciate ligament (PCL) and just anterior to the intercondylar notch to accommodate an intramedullary femoral alignment and resection guide (**TECH FIG 1A**).
- The intramedullary guide is inserted into the femoral medullary canal, in line with the anatomic axis of the femur. The resection guide is flush with the distal femoral condyle, rotationally parallel to the resected tibial surface, and perpendicular to the tibial shaft (**TECH FIG 1B**).
- A distal femoral cutting block is attached to the intramedullary guide and allows for adjustment of the cut angle relative to the anatomic axis of the femur (**TECH FIG 1C**).
  - The anatomic angle of the distal femoral cut is typically 4 to 7 degrees valgus.
  - An alternative method of distal femoral resection is to use a spacer block technique, which ensures parallelism to the tibial cut.
- With retractors positioned to protect the collateral ligament and soft tissues, a narrow, oscillating or reciprocating saw blade is used to cut the distal femoral condyle through the appropriate slot of the cutting block (**TECH FIG 1D**).
- An 8-mm spacer block is inserted into the extension space to ensure adequate spacing without overstuffing or overcorrection.

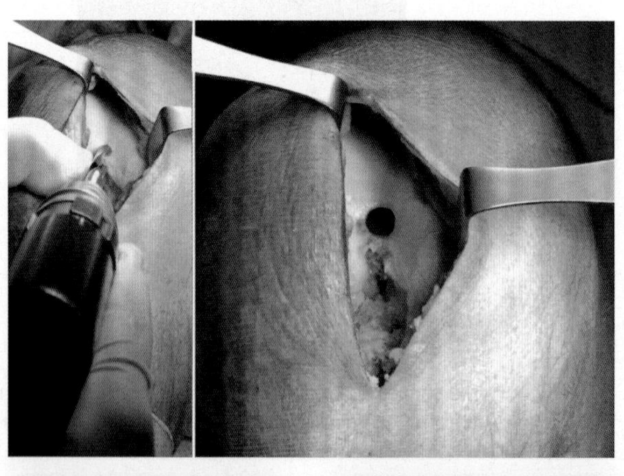

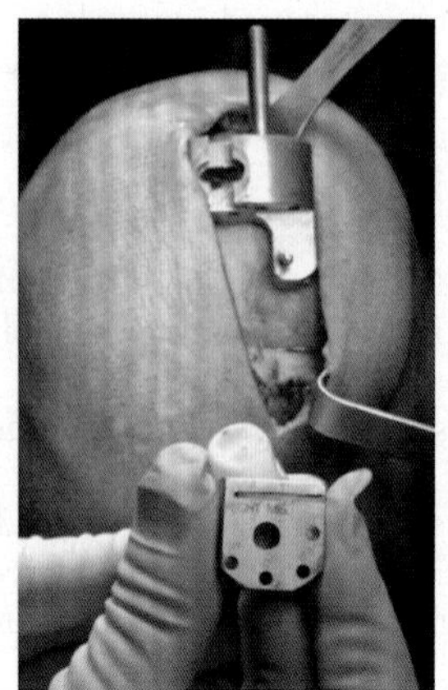

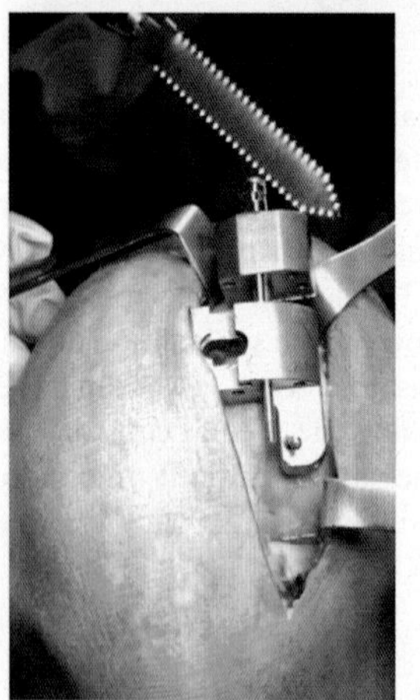

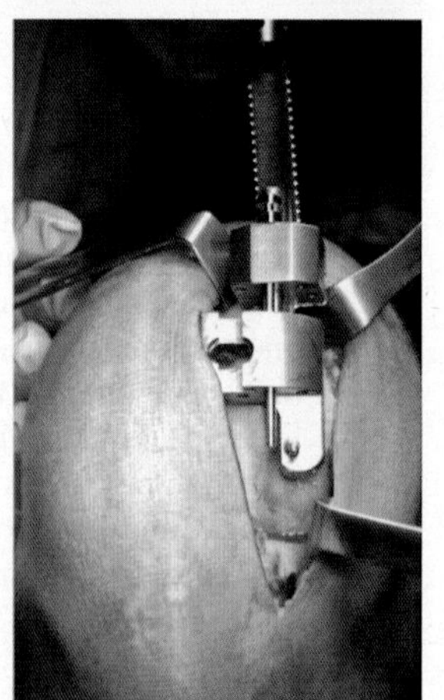

TECH FIG 1 • **A.** An entry hole is drilled in the distal femur 1 cm anterior to the origin of the PCL and just anterior to the intercondylar notch. **B.** The intramedullary femoral alignment and resection guide is inserted into the medullary canal, thus aligned with the anatomic axis of the femur. The distal femoral resection guide is flush with the distal femoral condyle, parallel to the tibial articular surface and perpendicular to the tibial shaft in preparation for attachment of the distal femoral cutting block. **C.** The distal femoral cutting block is attached to the intramedullary guide and allows for adjustment of the cut angle relative to the anatomic axis of the femur. **D.** The distal femoral condyle cut is made through the appropriate slot of the cutting block.

Posterior Femoral Condyle Resection

- An insertion handle is attached to a femoral sizing and posterior resection guide to position its flat surface on that of the cut distal femoral condyle (**TECH FIG 2A**).
- Various guides are trialed to select the proper size, so that when the guide is positioned on the posterior femoral condyle, 2 mm of bone is exposed between the anterior edge of the guide and the cartilage tidemark (**TECH FIG 2B**). This minimizes the risk of patellar impingement on the femoral component as the knee flexes.
- The posterior/chamfer resection guide is secured in position with the posterior surface of the guide parallel to the intended proximal tibial cut. It is lateralized toward the intercondylar notch to centralize the femoral component on the tibia.
- The anterior and posterior lug holes are drilled.
- The posterior femoral condyle and chamfer cuts are made through the cutting slots in the guide, with a retractor in place to protect the collateral ligament (**TECH FIG 2C**).

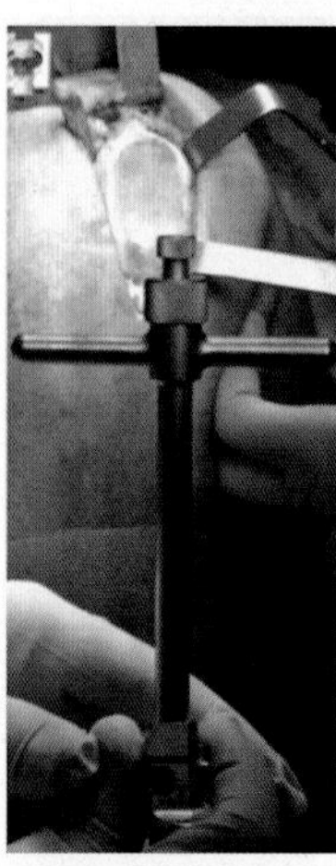

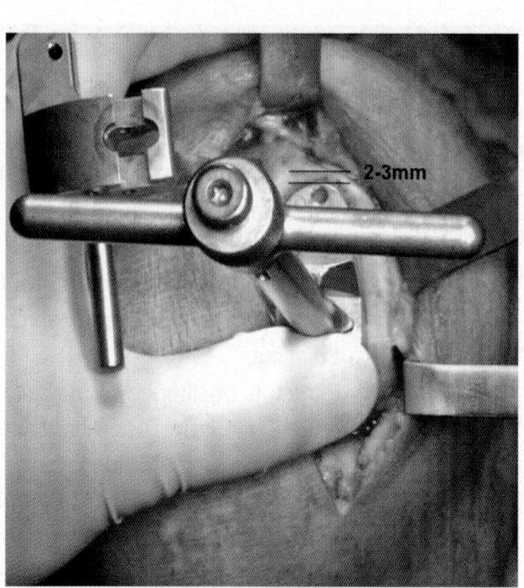

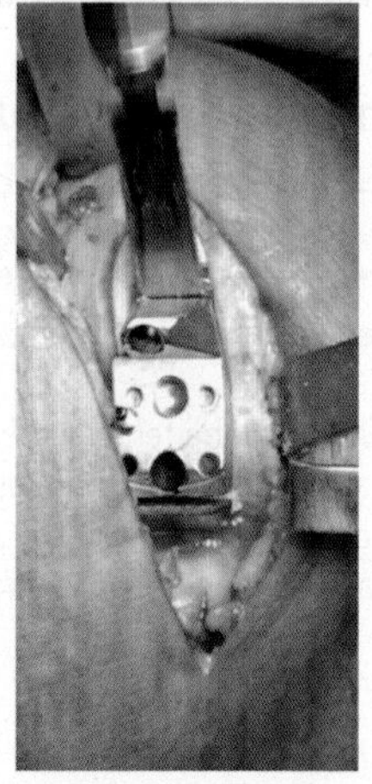

TECH FIG 2 • **A.** An insertion handle is attached to a femoral sizing and posterior resection guide to position its flat surface on that of the cut distal femoral condyle. **B.** The guide is shifted anteriorly until it contacts the posterior condyle with 2 mm of bone exposed at the anterior edge of the guide. **C.** The posterior chamfer and posterior femoral condyle cuts are made through the cutting slots of the guide, and lug holes are drilled.

Proximal Tibial Resection

- The anterior aspect of the tibia is exposed in the distal part of the wound from the margin of the tibial plateau to the tibial tubercle.
- An extramedullary tibial alignment and resection guide is positioned with its resector stem parallel to the mechanical axis of the tibia in the coronal plane, so that the stem is directly over the medial third of the tibial tubercle proximally and the tibial crest distally.
  - Although ideally the guide is parallel to the entire tibial crest, this is not possible in the setting of tibial bowing.
  - With the ankle clamp secured distally, the guide often points to the second metatarsal of the neutrally positioned foot.
- The posterior slope of the resection guide is set to mimic the native slope of the tibial plateau.
  - The sagittal slope should be measured on preoperative radiographs, and if the slope is greater than 7 degrees, the posterior slope should be limited to no more than 7 degrees (**TECH FIG 3A**).[18]
- With the knee flexed 90 to 100 degrees, a narrow, reciprocating saw blade is used to make a vertical tibial cut in the sagittal plane parallel to and just off the peak of the tibial eminence (**TECH FIG 3B**).
  - The cut should not extend deep to the intended level of the horizontal cut as this could cause tibial plateau fracture.
  - Care is taken to avoid disrupting the ACL or PCL attachment.
- With a retractor positioned to protect the collateral ligament and soft tissues, a conservative horizontal cut is made with an oscillating saw blade perpendicular to the mechanical axis of the tibia in the coronal plane and with a slight posterior slope as described (**TECH FIG 3C**).
  - The level of proximal tibial resection is guided by the depth of tibial erosion so that the cut removes the sclerotic surface and extends approximately 2 to 4 mm below the deepest part of erosion.
  - In the presence of large osteophytes and more extreme but partially correctable deformity, less of the tibia (2 mm) is typically resected. When there are minimal osteophytes, slightly more tibial resection (4 mm) may be necessary.
  - In lateral UKA, tibial resection should be highly conservative.
- A tibial alignment rod dropped from the cut tibial plateau surface in alignment with the mechanical axis of the tibia confirms proper orientation of the tibial cut (**TECH FIG 3D**).
  - The goal is to produce a parallel relationship between the distal femoral condyle cut and the proximal tibial cut in full extension and flexion.
- The meniscus and any remaining osteophytes are removed.

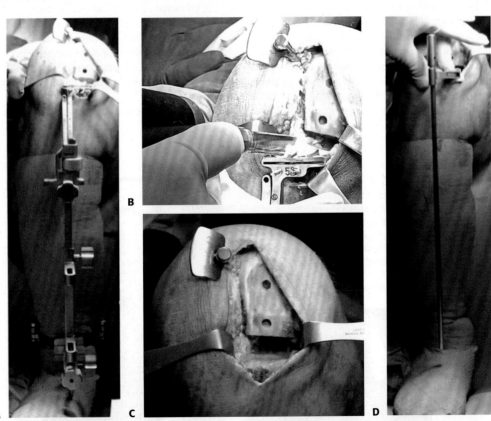

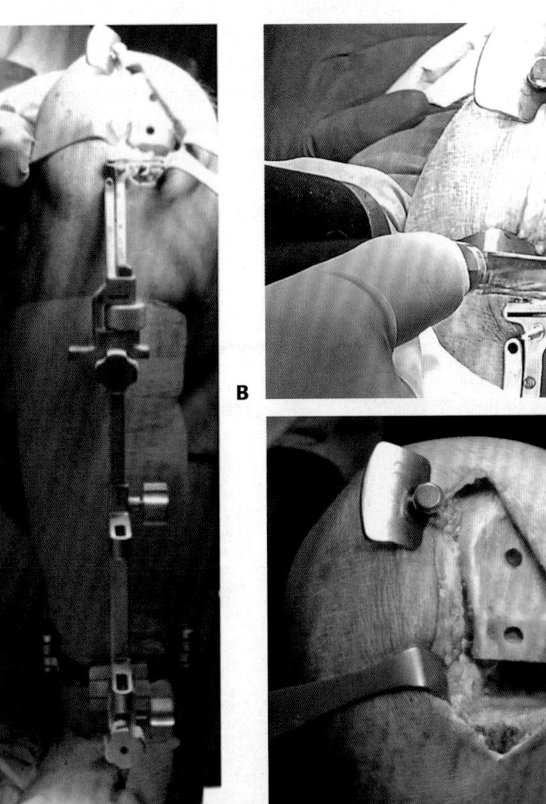

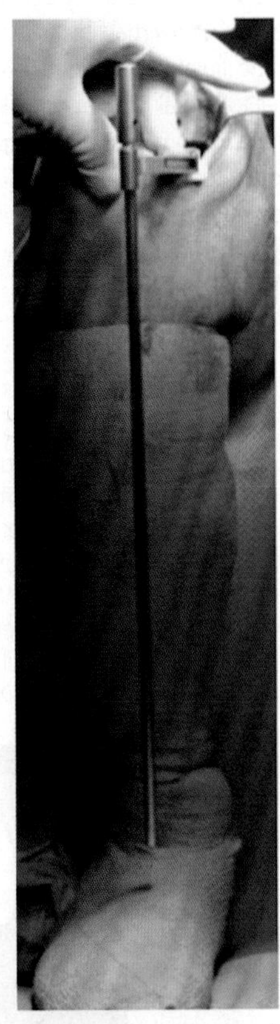

TECH FIG 3 • **A.** An extramedullary tibial alignment and resection guide is positioned with its resector stem parallel to the mechanical axis of the tibia in the coronal and sagittal planes. The ankle clamp at the distal end of the guide is centered over the distal tibia at approximately 40% of the intermalleolar distance from the medial malleolus. **B.** With the knee flexed, a vertical tibial cut is made in the sagittal plane at the base of the tibial eminence and parallel to the eminence in the AP plane. **C.** After a horizontal cut is made perpendicular to the mechanical axis of the tibia in the coronal plane and in slight posterior tilt in the sagittal plane, there is a parallel relationship between the distal femoral condyle cut and the proximal tibial cut in the coronal plane. **D.** A tibial alignment rod dropped from the cut tibial plateau surface confirms alignment with the mechanical axis of the tibia and thus proper orientation of the tibial cut.

Balancing the Flexion and Extension Gaps

- All retractors and implants are removed.
- Gap spacers corresponding to the various tibial articular surface thicknesses are used to assess the flexion and extension gaps.
- If the joint space is symmetrically tight in flexion and extension, additional tibial bone is resected or the polyethylene insert is downsized.
- If the joint space is symmetrically loose in flexion and extension, the thickness of the polyethylene insert is progressively increased.
- If the joint space is asymmetrically tight in extension and acceptable in flexion, additional distal femur is resected or the posterior tibial slope is reduced by removing some anterior tibial bone.
- If the joint is asymmetrically tight in flexion and acceptable in extension, the posterior slope of the tibial resection is increased or the femoral component is downsized with resection of additional posterior femoral condyle.
- After any adjustment or additional resection, the flexion and extension gaps are rechecked.
- Care is taken to not overstuff the operative compartment. One to 2 mm of laxity is appropriate following proper balancing of the flexion and extension gaps. Overstuffing may limit motion and/or overcorrect the alignment and cause overloading of the opposite tibiofemoral compartment.

Trial Component Insertion and Reduction

- To determine proper tibial component size, a tibial sizing tray is positioned on the cut surface of the proximal tibia with the straight edge against the flat sagittal surface along the tibial spine.
  - The tray size should be selected to maximize coverage of the resected proximal tibial surface while minimizing overhang.
  - If the tibial component covers the tibial surface from medial to lateral but not completely from anterior to posterior, the component should be positioned on the anterior tibial cortex to try to reduce the risk of anterior tibial subsidence.
- The properly sized trial tibial baseplate is positioned onto the cut surface of the tibia, and the impactor engages the central fin into the bone so that the baseplate sits flush on the tibial surface, along the sagittal cut of the tibial eminence, and positioned translationally from anterior to posterior so the anterior surface is aligned with the anterior cortex (**TECH FIG 4A**).
- The trial femoral component is impacted in place (**TECH FIG 4B**).
- A trial tibial articular insert is snapped into the tibial baseplate.
- With the trial bearing in place, the knee is manipulated through a full range of motion to demonstrate stability of the joint, balanced flexion and extension gaps, 1 to 2 mm of laxity, restoration of alignment (without overcorrection), security of the bearing (in the case of mobile bearings), acceptable contact of the femoral component on the tibial component, and absence of patellar impingement on the leading edge of the prosthesis.
- Once trial reduction is complete, all trial components are extracted.

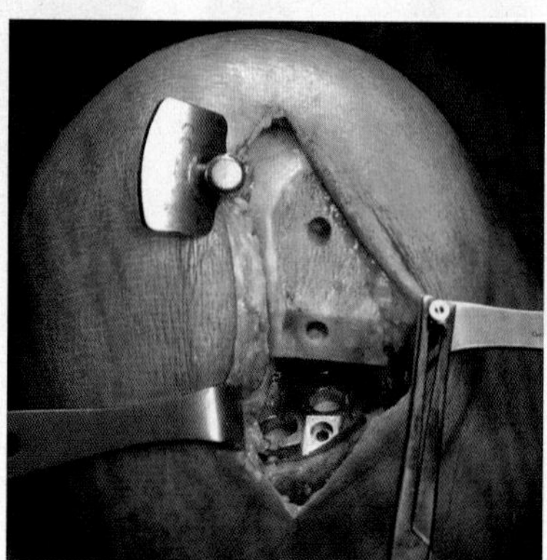

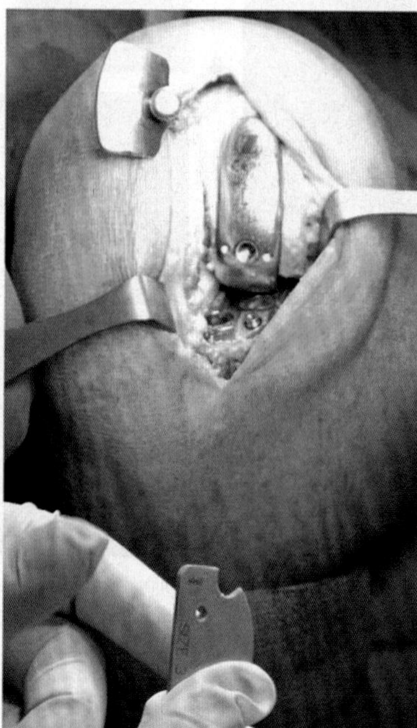

TECH FIG 4 • **A.** The properly sized trial tibial baseplate is positioned onto the cut surface of the tibia and impacted to sit flush on the tibial surface and perpendicular to the long axis of the tibia in the coronal plane. **B.** The trial femoral component is positioned in the center of the femoral condyle. The trial tibial articular component can be inserted into the tibial baseplate.

Implanting the Final Components

- The femoral and tibial bone surfaces are irrigated using pulsatile lavage and then dried.
- Polymethylmethacrylate is used for fixation of the final components.
- The knee is flexed and the tibia externally rotated to optimize exposure of the proximal tibia for cementing.
- A very thin layer of cement is pressurized into the tibia and a small amount is applied to the undersurface of the tibial component. The tibial component is pressed down and impacted into place, first posteriorly and then anteriorly, so that excess cement is preferentially extruded anteriorly. Excess extruded cement is cleared from the margin of the metal tibial tray (**TECH FIG 5A**).
- The dried femoral surface is covered with cement, and a small amount is applied to the undersurface of the femoral component. It is impacted into place (**TECH FIG 5B**), and excess extruded cement is removed from the margin of the femoral component.
- The joint space is irrigated and the tibial tray dried before snapping the polyethylene tibial articular component into the tibial baseplate (**TECH FIG 5C,D**).
- The knee is maintained in approximately 30 degrees of flexion to concentrically load the components while the cement hardens. A 1- to 2-mm spacer can help pressurize the components while the cement cures.
  - Keeping the knee fully extended during cement curing may cause the components to lift up slightly posteriorly and should be avoided.
- After the cement has cured, the joint is reassessed to ensure that no visible cement is present beyond the margins of the implants. The knee is irrigated to ensure that no bone or cement particles remain.
- The knee is again evaluated through a full range of motion to demonstrate stability of the joint, security of the bearing (if a mobile bearing is used), and absence of impingement.
- Routine closure of the wound follows.

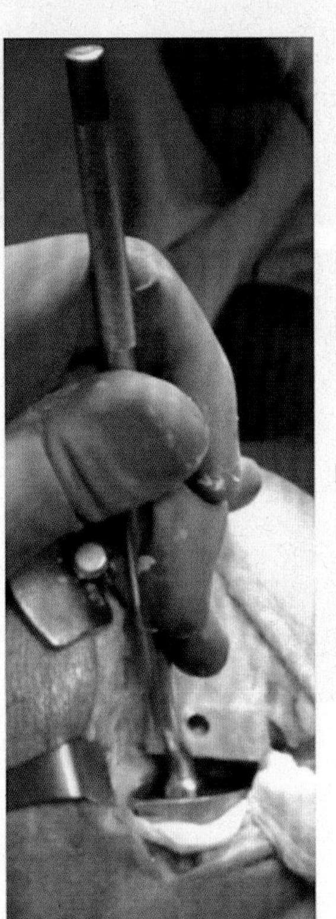

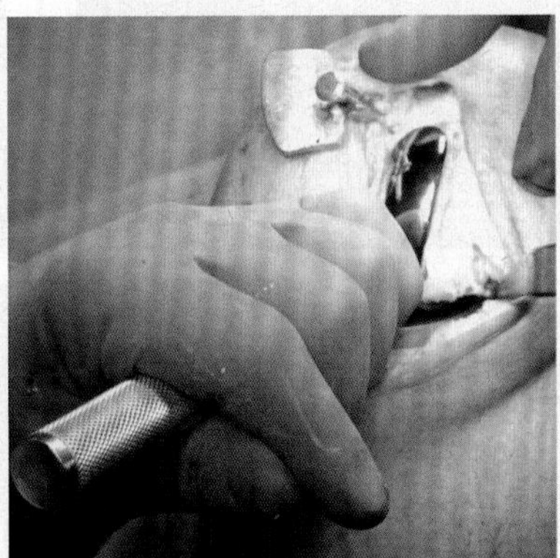

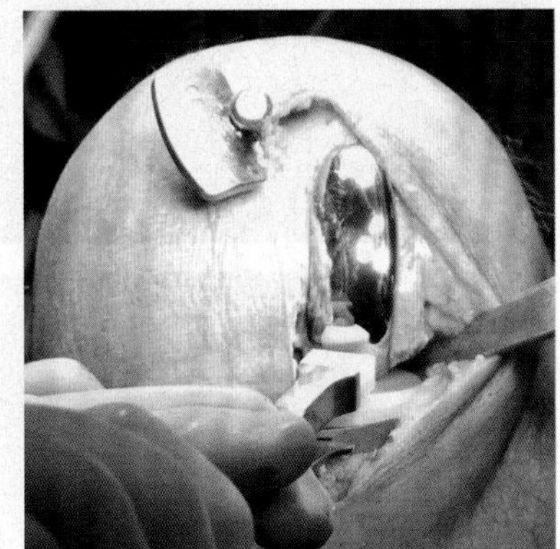

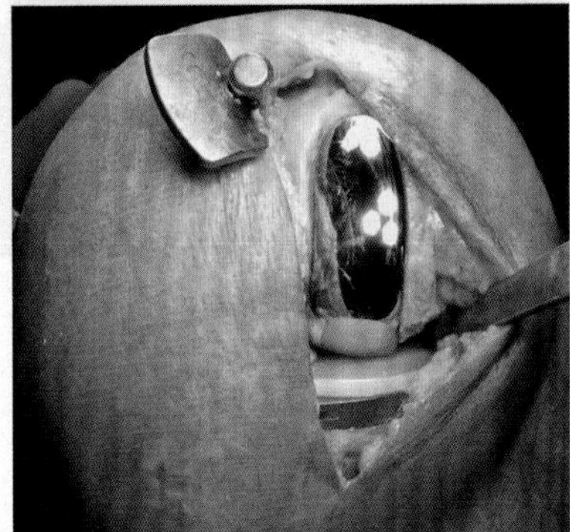

A B C D

TECH FIG 5 • **A.** Cement is applied to the tibial component, which is pressed down, first posteriorly and then anteriorly, so that excess cement is extruded anteriorly. **B.** The femoral component is cemented, positioned on the femoral condyle, and impacted. **C.** After the cement has cured, the polyethylene tibial articular component is snapped onto the tibial baseplate. **D.** Final components are shown.

Robotic-Assisted Unicondylar Knee Arthroplasty

- Robotic assistance has been shown to enhance the accuracy of bone preparation, implant component alignment, and soft tissue balance in UKA.[13,15,21,25,36,37,26]
  - It has yet to be determined whether this improved accuracy translates to improved clinical performance or longevity of the UKA implant; however, midterm data have shown a revision rate at a minimum of 2-year follow-up of less than 1%.[25]
- Depending on the system used, a preoperative CT scan may be needed for preoperative mapping.
- Newer generation, image-free robotic technology, Navio Precision Freehand Sculpting system (NavioPFS, Blue Belt Technologies, Inc., Plymouth, MN), allows accurate bone preparation and soft tissue balancing without the need for a preoperative CT scan (**TECH FIG 6A,B**).
- Implant planning, development of the cutting zone, and gap balancing takes place entirely intraoperatively through accurate registration and mapping of anatomic landmarks and determination of knee kinematics.

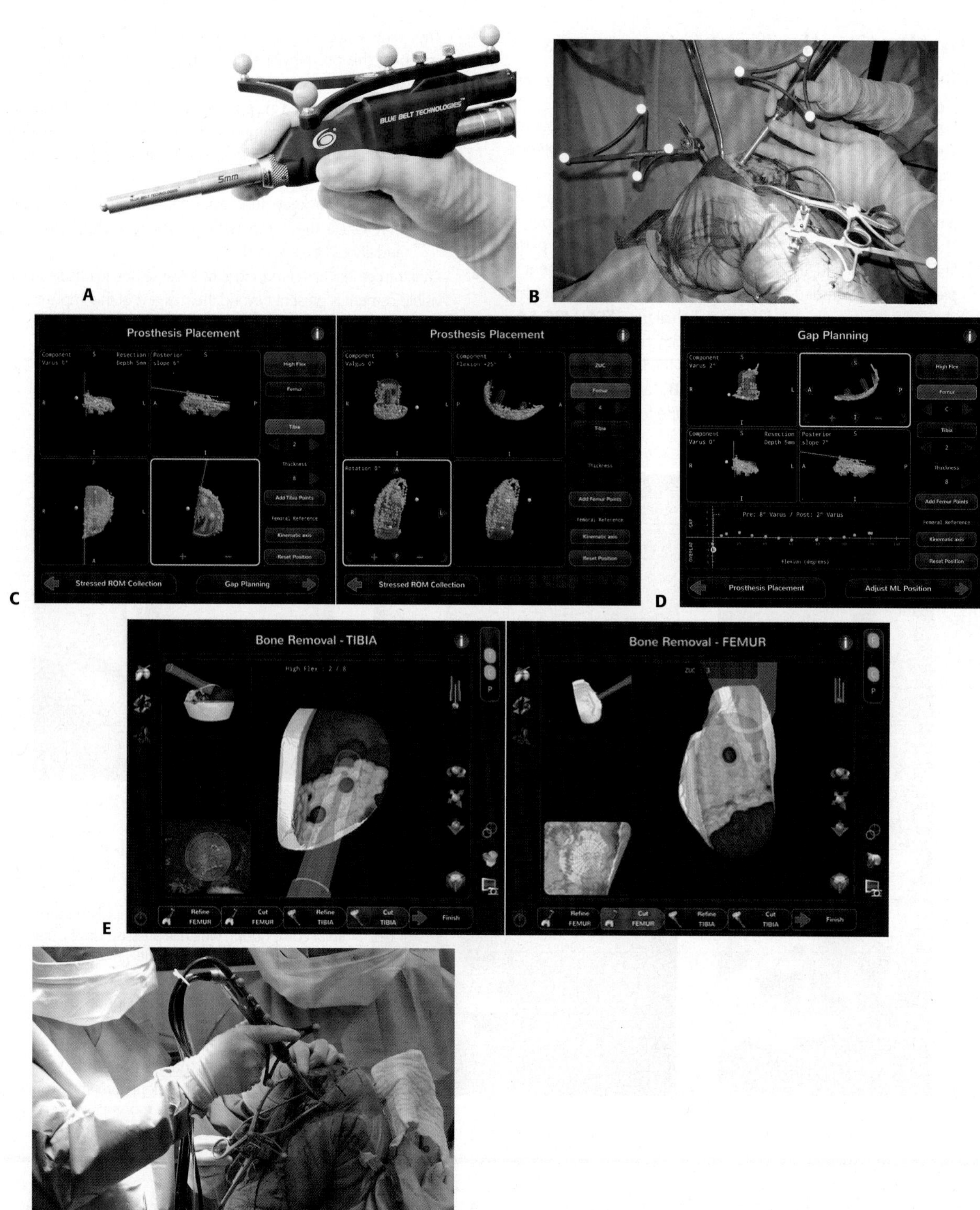

TECH FIG 6 • A. The NavioPFS handheld sculpting instrument. **B.** Intraoperative setup and use of handheld sculpting instrument. **C.** The surgeon selects the implant size which best fits the patient's anatomy and closely matches the size of the condyle to be replaced as well as its position in the coronal, sagittal, and rotational planes. **D.** The surgeon determines parameters for gap and ligament balancing. **E.** Tibial and femoral resection are displayed virtually. **F.** The arthritic cartilage and bone are methodically removed using the NavioPFS handheld sculptor.

- Intraoperative data are used by the system's software algorithms to determine the coronal, sagittal, and axial bone axes and morphology.
- The surgeon selects the implant size that best fits the patient's anatomy and closely matches the size of the condyle to be replaced as well as its position in the coronal, sagittal, and rotational planes (**TECH FIG 6C**).
- Subsequent steps are directed at determining gap and ligament balance after virtual implant positioning, removal of osteophytes, and stressing of the ligaments and soft tissues (**TECH FIG 6D**). Adjustments in implant position and size can be made to optimize soft tissue balance, component tracking, and position before beginning bone preparation.
- After planning for size, position, alignment, bone volume, and gap balancing, the arthritic cartilage and bone are methodically removed using the NavioPFS handheld sculptor (**TECH FIG 6E,F**).
  - Unlike first-generation technologies that provided haptic constraint via a robotic arm, this newer system works with a combination of speed and exposure control safeguards applied through a lightweight, handheld, surgeon-driven, semiautonomous robotic sculpting tool.
- Once the desired bone has been resected, the robotic burr either retracts into the guard when on exposure mode or stops spinning if in speed mode.
- Despite relying entirely on intraoperative surface registration and mapping, the NavioPFS provides accuracy equivalent to earlier robotic devices (Table 1).[26]

Table 1 Root Mean Square Errors of Robotic and Conventional Techniques in Unicondylar Knee Arthroplasty

	NavioPFS (Lonner et al[26])	MAKO Rio (Dunbar et al[15])	Acrobot (Karia et al[21])	Conventional (Dunbar et al[15])
Flexion/extension (deg)	1.7	2.1	1.7	6.0
Varus/valgus (deg)	2.4	2.1	2.1	4.1
Internal/external rotation (deg)	1.7	3.0	3.4	6.3
Medial/lateral (mm)	1.3	1.2	1.0	2.6
Anterior/posterior (mm)	1.3	1.6	1.8	2.4
Proximal/distal (mm)	1.0	1.0	0.6	1.6

PEARLS AND PITFALLS

Lengthen the incision as necessary.	■ Use of a minimally invasive approach with conventional UKA instrumentation may cause difficulty in accurate positioning and alignment of the components. ■ Malalignment may cause aseptic loosening of the implant.
Avoid overcorrection of the lower extremity alignment.	■ Overcorrection results in excess load transfer to the adjacent tibiofemoral compartment with potential for accelerated cartilaginous degeneration.
Avoid "overstuffing" the joint space.	■ Adjusting component thickness to allow for 1 to 2 mm of joint laxity on varus or valgus stress is ideal for protecting the adjacent compartment and the polyethylene from increased stresses.
Avoid anterior placement of the femoral component.	■ An oversized femoral component increases the risk that the anterior edge of the component may extend past the tidemark with the potential for patellar impingement and progressive patellofemoral pain and deterioration.
Preserve bone stock.	■ Excessive bone resection can result in insufficient prosthetic replacement. It is also important to preserve bone stock so that possible future revision TKA does not excessively lower the joint line.

POSTOPERATIVE CARE

- For most patients, surgery is performed on an outpatient basis.
- Prophylactic intravenous antibiotics are administered.
- Standard venous thromboembolism prophylaxis is implemented.
- Pain management is optimized to facilitate active and accelerated rehabilitation.
- Immediately following surgery, patients may weight bear as tolerated and initiate physical therapy with a focus on active-assisted muscle strengthening and range-of-motion exercises.
- Routine follow-up in the office is arranged for initial postoperative care and radiographic assessment of component and limb alignment (**FIG 4A–C**).

OUTCOMES

- UKA is a predictable surgical option, and its potential advantages over TKA in properly selected patients include the following[33]:
  - More conservative surgical procedure
    - Less extensive surgical approach and dissection
    - Preservation of native anatomy and bone stock
    - Decreased blood loss
    - Fewer complications
  - Improved rehabilitation
    - Increased postoperative range of motion (**FIG 5**)
    - Decreased rate of manipulation under anesthesia
    - Preserved kinematics and proprioception
    - Improved gait

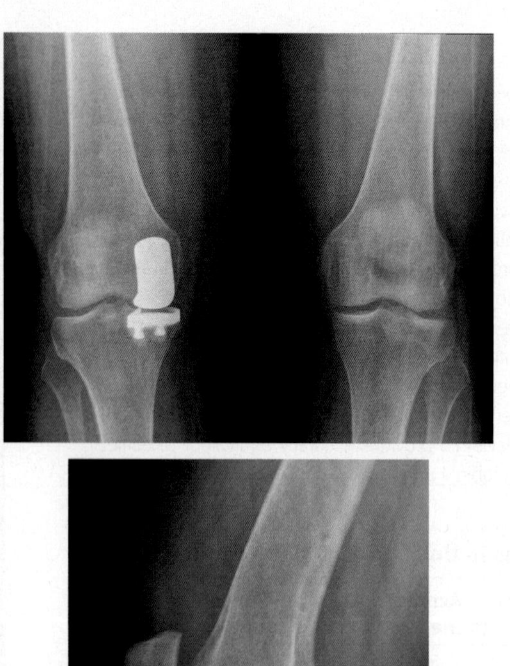

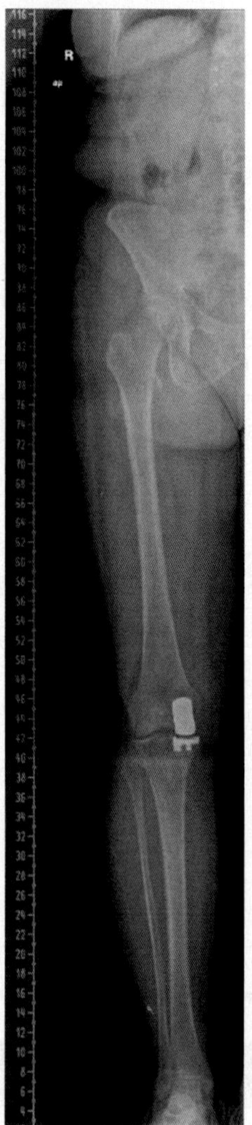

FIG 4 • Postoperative radiographs. **A.** AP view. **B.** Lateral view. **C.** Full-length, weight-bearing AP radiograph.

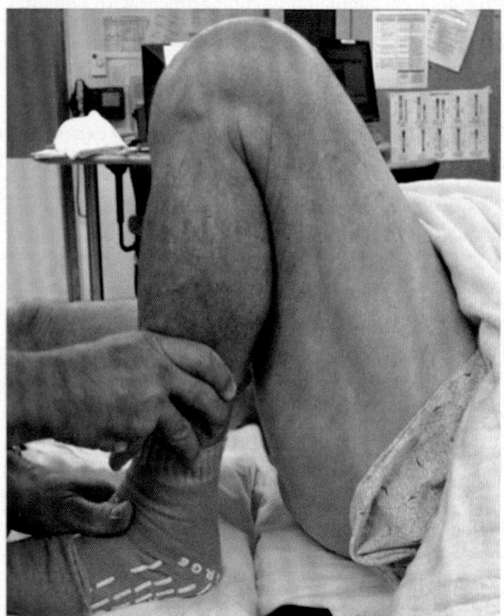

FIG 5 • Patients typically enjoy rapid recovery following UKA, achieving high flexion with normal knee kinematics.

- Improved logistics
  - Shorter hospital stays and often performed in the outpatient setting
  - More commonly discharged to home
  - Decreased readmission rate
  - Decreased cost
- Patients report better satisfaction and fewer residual symptoms with UKA versus TKA in comparison studies.[14]
- The 10-year survival rate of UKA is greater than 90% (Table 2).

COMPLICATIONS

- Tibial and femoral component and/or limb malalignment is poorly tolerated in UKA and can jeopardize long-term survival of the implant due to increased polyethylene wear, disease progression to the adjacent compartments, and component loosening.[12]
  - Polyethylene wear is the major cause of osteolysis and is minimized by the following[2,3]:
    - Use of a polyethylene thickness greater than 6 mm
    - Use of highly cross-linked, oxidatively stable polyethylene
    - Appropriate component position

Table 2 Unicondylar Knee Arthroplasty Survival Rates

Year	Authors	Prosthesis	N	Survival Rate
2005	Berger et al[8]	Miller-Galante (Zimmer, Warsaw, IN)	62	98% at 10 y 95.7% at 13 y
2004	Keblish and Briard[22]	Low Contact Stress (LCS) (Johnson & Johnson/DePuy, Warsaw, IN)	177	82% at 11 y
2004	Naudie et al[28]	Miller-Galante (Zimmer, Warsaw, IN)	113	94% at 5 y 90% at 10 y
2005	O'Rourke et al[29]	Marmor (Richards, Memphis, TN)	136	84% at 20 y 72% at 25 y
2004	Rajasekhar et al[32]	Oxford (Biomet, Warsaw, IN)	135	96.73% at 5 y 94.04% at 10 y

- Adjacent compartment degeneration is caused by the following[33]:
  - Progression of disease
  - Component impingement (patellofemoral)
  - Overcorrection of the mechanical axis of the lower extremity
- Aseptic loosening is related to the following[12]:
  - Poor cement technique
  - Component malalignment
  - Excessive tibial slope
- Other potential complications include the following:
  - Infection
  - Fracture
  - Polyethylene dislocation (mobile-bearing UKA)
  - Venous thromboembolism

REFERENCES

1. Adouni M, Shirazi-Adl A. Evaluation of knee joint muscle forces and tissue stresses-strains during gait in severe OA versus normal subjects. J Orthop Res 2014;32(1):69–78.
2. Argenson JA, O'Connor JJ. Polyethylene wear and meniscal knee replacement. J Bone Joint Surg Br 1992;74:228–232.
3. Argenson JA, Parratte S. The unicompartmental knee: design and technique considerations in minimizing wear. Clin Orthop Rel Res 2006;452:137–142.
4. Argenson JA, Parratte S, Bertani A, et al. The new arthritic patient and arthroplasty treatment options. J Bone Joint Surg Am 2009;91(suppl 5): 43–48.
5. Arno S, Maffei D, Walker PS, et al. Retrospective analysis of total knee arthroplasty cases for visual, histological, and clinical eligibility of unicompartmental knee arthroplasties. J Arthroplasty 2011;26(8):1396–1403.
6. Berend KR, Lombardi AV Jr, Adams JB. Obesity, young age, patellofemoral disease, and anterior knee pain: identifying the unicondylar arthroplasty patient in the United States. Orthopaedics 2007; 30(5 suppl):19–23.
7. Berend KR, Lombardi AV Jr, Mallory TH, et al. Early failure of minimally invasive unicompartmental knee arthroplasty is associated with obesity. Clin Orthop Relat Res 2005;440:60–66.
8. Berger RA, Menegini RM, Jacobs JJ, et al. Results of unicompartmental knee arthroplasty at a minimum of ten years of follow-up. J Bone Joint Surg Am 2005;87:999–1006.
9. Billante MJ, Diduch DR. Knee replacement in aging athletes. In: DeLee JC, Drez D, Miller MD, eds. DeLee and Drez's Orthopaedic Sports Medicine, ed 3. Philadelphia: W.B. Saunders, 2009: chap 23.
10. Borus T, Thornhill T. Unicompartmental knee arthroplasty. J Am Acad Orthop Surg 2008;16:9–18.
11. Cavaignac E, Lafontan V, Reina N, et al. Obesity has no adverse effect on the outcome of unicompartmental knee replacement at a minimum follow-up of seven years. Bone Joint J 2013:95-B(8):1064–1068.
12. Collier MB, Eickmann TH, Sukezaki F, et al. Patient, implant, and alignment factors associated with revision of medial compartment unicondylar arthroplasty. J Arthroplasty 2006;21(6 suppl 2): 108–115.
13. Conditt MA, Roche MW. Minimally invasive robotic-arm-guided unicompartmental knee arthroplasty. J Bone Joint Surg Am 2009;9(1 suppl 1):63–68.
14. Dalury DF, Fisher DA, Adams MJ, et al. Unicompartmental knee arthroplasty compares favorably to total knee arthroplasty in the same patient. Orthopaedics 2009;32(4).
15. Dunbar NJ, Roche MW, Park BH, et al. Accuracy of dynamic tactile-guided unicompartmental knee arthroplasty. J Arthroplasty 2012; 27(5):803–808.
16. Fitz W. Unicompartmental knee arthroplasty with use of novel patient-specific resurfacing implants and personalized jigs. J Bone Joint Surg Am 2009;9(1 suppl 1):69–76.
17. Goodfellow JW, O'Connor JJ. The anterior cruciate ligament in knee arthroplasty. Clin Orthop Relat Res 1992;276:245–252.
18. Hernigou P, Deschamps G. Posterior slope of the tibial implant and the outcome of unicompartmental knee arthroplasty. J Bone Joint Surg Am 2004;86:506–511.
19. Hsu RW, Himeno S, Coventry MB, et al. Normal axial alignment of the lower extremity and load-bearing distribution at the knee. Clin Orthop Relat Res 1990;255:215–227.
20. Iorio R, Healy WL. Unicompartmental arthritis of the knee. J Bone Joint Surg Am 2003;85:1351–1364.
21. Karia M, Masjedi M, Andrews B, et al. Robotic assistance enables inexperienced surgeons to perform unicompartmental knee arthroplasties on dry bone models with accuracy superior to conventional methods. Adv Orthop 2013;2013:481039.
22. Keblish PA, Briard JL. Mobile-bearing unicompartmental knee arthroplasty: a 2-center study with an 11-year (mean) follow-up. J Arthroplasty 2004;19(7 suppl 2):87–94.
23. Kozinn SC, Scott R. Unicondylar knee arthroplasty. J Bone Joint Surg Am 1989;71:145–150.
24. Laskin RS. Unicompartmental knee replacement: some unanswered questions. Clin Orthop Relat Res 2001;392:267–271.
25. Lonner JH, John TK, Conditt MA. Robotic arm-assisted UKA improves tibial component alignment: a pilot study. Clin Orthop Relat Res 2010;468:141–146.
26. Lonner JH, Smith JR, Picard F, et al. High degree of accuracy of a novel image-free handheld robot for unicondylar knee arthroplasty in a cadaveric study. Clin Orthop Relat Res 2015;473(1):206–212.
27. Mihalko WM. Arthroplasty of the knee. In: Canale ST, Beaty JH, eds. Campbell's Operative Orthopaedics, Vol 1, ed 12. Philadelphia: Mosby, 2012:chap 7.
28. Naudie D, Guerin J, Parker DA, et al. Medial unicompartmental knee arthroplasty with the Miller-Galante prosthesis. J Bone Joint Surg Am 2004;86:1931–1935.
29. O'Rourke MR, Gardner JJ, Callaghan JJ, et al. Unicompartmental knee replacement: a minimum twenty-one-year followup, end-result study. Clin Orthop Relat Res 2005;440:27–37.

30. Pandit H, Jenkins C, Gill HS, et al. Unnecessary contraindications for mobile-bearing unicompartmental knee replacement. J Bone Joint Surg Br 2011;93(5):622–628.
31. Pennington DW, Swienckowski JJ, Lutes WB, et al. Lateral unicompartmental knee arthroplasty: survivorship and technical considerations at an average follow-up of 12.4 years. J Arthroplasty 2006;21:13–17.
32. Rajasekhar C, Das S, Smith A. Unicompartmental knee arthroplasty 2- to 12-year results in a community hospital. J Bone Joint Surg Br 2004;86:983–985.
33. Ritter MA, Faris PM, Thong AE, et al. Intra-operative findings in varus osteoarthritis of the knee: an analysis of pre-operative alignment in potential candidates for unicompartmental arthroplasty. J Bone Joint Surg Br 2004;86(1):43–47.
34. Scott RD, Santore RF. Unicondylar unicompartmental replacement for osteoarthritis of the knee. J Bone Joint Surg Am 1981;63(4):536–544.
35. Servien E, Merini A, Lustig S, et al. Lateral unicompartmental knee replacement: current concepts and future directions. Knee Surg Sports Traumatol Arthrosc 2013;21:2501–2508.
36. Sisto DJ, Blazina ME, Heskiaoff D, et al. Unicompartment arthroplasty for osteoarthritis of the knee. Clin Orthop Relat Res 1993;286:149–153.
37. Smith JR, Picard F, Rowe PJ, et al. The accuracy of a robotically-controlled freehand sculpting tool for unicondylar knee arthroplasty. J Bone Joint Surg Br 2013;95B(suppl):68.
38. Stern SH, Becker MW, Insall JN. Unicondylar knee arthroplasty: an evaluation of selection criteria. Clin Orthop Relat Res 1993;286:143–148.
39. White SH, Ludkowski PF, Goodfellow JW. Anteromedial osteoarthritis of the knee. J Bone Joint Surg Br 1991;73:582–586.

Cemented Total Knee Arthroplasty

Eric A. Levicoff and Robert P. Good

37
CHAPTER

DEFINITION

- Total knee arthroplasty (TKA) is a successful surgical procedure that provides excellent and durable relief of pain and improvement in functional status for patients with degenerative joint disease (DJD) of the knee.
- Cement fixation is currently the most popular method of fixation for TKA.

ANATOMY

- The knee is a synovial hinge joint with little rotational motion.
- The stability of the joint is provided by both bony and soft tissue constraints, particularly the collateral and cruciate ligaments.
- The mechanical axis of the lower extremity is a straight line drawn from the center of the femoral head to the center of the tibiotalar joint, and constitutes the weight-bearing axis for the lower extremity.
- In the tibia, the mechanical and anatomic axes are the same, whereas in the femur, the two are different by approximately 6 degrees (**FIG 1A**).
  - The exact difference between the mechanical and anatomic axes of the femur differs slightly based on femoral neck offset and femoral length (ie, shorter femurs with higher offset will result in a greater difference).
  - This creates a femorotibial valgus angle with respect to the intramedullary (IM) canals of the femur and the tibia of approximately 6 degrees.
  - The epicondylar axis of the femur is perpendicular to the mechanical axis.
  - At the condylar level, there is an additional 3 degrees of tibia vara and compensatory femoral valga, resulting in a total of 9 degrees of valgus between the condylar joint line and the femoral shaft.
- The varus orientation of the joint line, combined with the offset of the hip center of rotation, results in the weight-bearing surface of the tibia being parallel to the ground during a single-leg stance.
- The asymmetry of the distal femoral condyles is also carried over to their posterior surfaces. When the normal knee is flexed, the joint remains parallel to the floor. For this relationship to be maintained on the varus tibial surface, there must be an asymmetry of the posterior dimensions of the femoral condyles. When observed in flexion, the medial femoral condyle extends more posterior than the lateral femoral condyle by approximately 3 degrees.
- The sagittal alignment of the tibial articular surface is also important. In the sagittal plane, the tibia is sloped posteriorly about 5 to 7 degrees (**FIG 1B**). In the normal knee, the asymmetry of the bony anatomy maintains the alignment of the joint and ligamentous tension.[2]

PATHOGENESIS

- Arthritis of the knee can be generally divided in osteoarthritis (OA) and inflammatory arthritis (RA):
  - OA, the most common type of DJD, can be subdivided into two major categories:
    - Primary OA: articular degeneration without any apparent underlying reason
    - Secondary OA: articular degeneration resulting from another primary etiology (eg, posttraumatic arthritis) (**FIG 2**)
    - In primary OA, the medial compartment is most often affected, whereas lateral compartment disease is thought to arise from trauma or aberrant anatomy, frequently hypoplasia of the lateral femoral condyle.
  - RA is a systemic inflammatory condition that commonly affects multiple joints earlier on in life.

NATURAL HISTORY

- The natural history of DJD is typically a progression of disease leading to increasing pain and disability. Although the intensity of clinical symptoms may vary, they usually become more severe, frequent, and debilitating over time. The rate of progression varies from patient to patient.
- Whereas medications can help control the progression of RA and other inflammatory conditions, no proven disease-modifying agents for the treatment of knee OA currently exist.

PATIENT HISTORY AND PHYSICAL FINDINGS

- Historical findings of DJD typically include the following:
  - Pain that is typically better with rest and worse with increased activities
  - Stiffness
  - Swelling
  - Subjective instability or giving way of the knee
  - Night pain and rest pain can be indicative of more severe disease
  - History of prior knee injury or surgery
  - Progressive bowing of the knees or "knock knees"
- Physical examination findings typically include the following:
  - Varus or valgus knee deformities, particularly with weight bearing
  - Limp
  - Muscle atrophy
  - Effusion
  - Joint line or patellofemoral tenderness to palpation
  - Painful, limited range of motion (ROM)
  - Crepitus

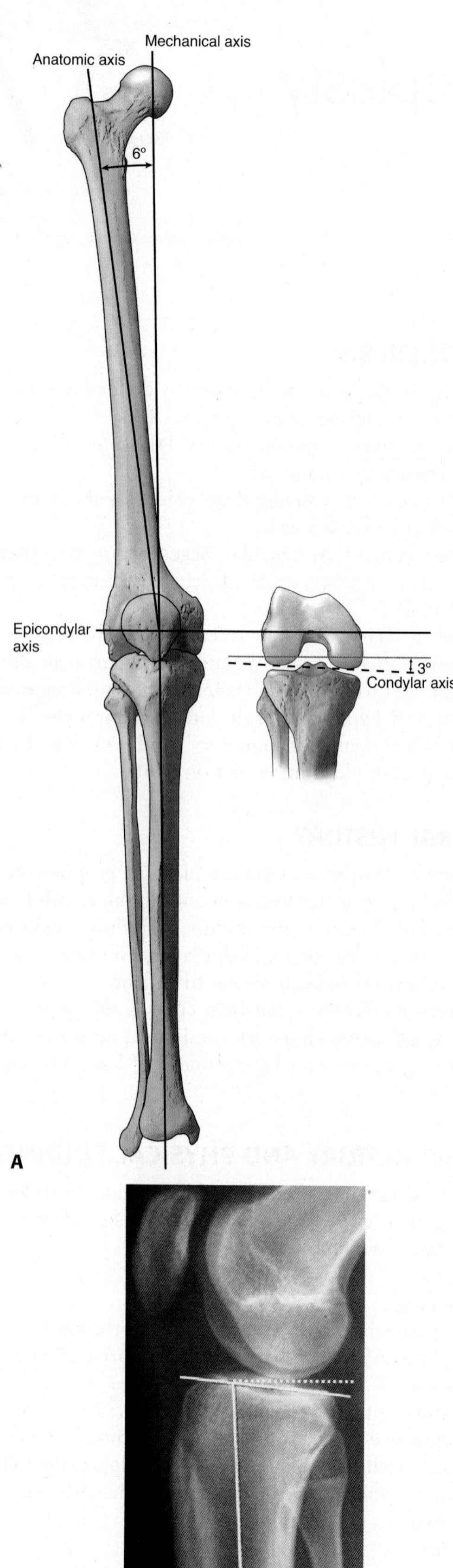

FIG 1 • A. Mechanical and anatomic axes of the lower extremity. **B.** The posterior slope of the tibial plateau in the sagittal plane is approximately 5 to 7 degrees.

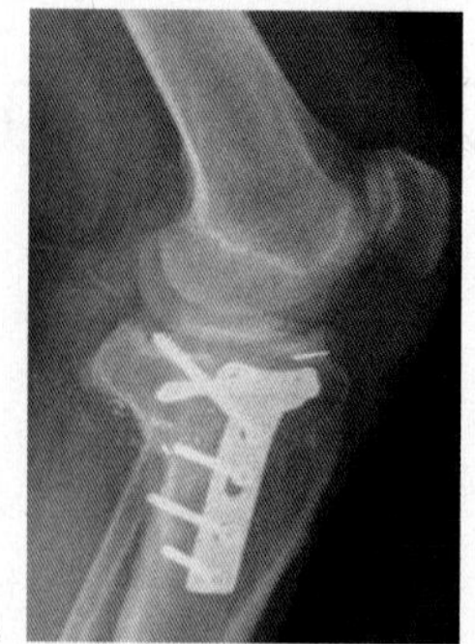

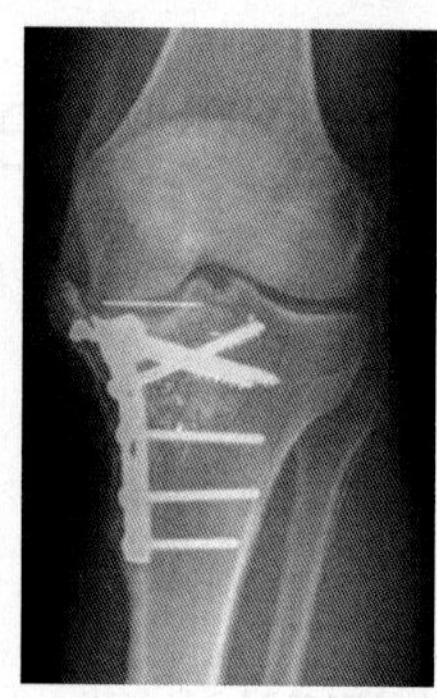

FIG 2 • A,B. AP and lateral radiographs showing posttraumatic arthritis following medial tibial plateau injury.

- When considering knee replacement surgery, it is also important to observe for the following:
  - Skin condition, including old scars or psoriatic lesions
  - Ligamentous stability
  - Active and passive ROM
  - Varus or valgus deformities
  - Muscle strength
  - Neurovascular status
- Specific tests for examining the osteoarthritic knee before arthroplasty include the following:
  - A Q-angle of more than 15 degrees is often the cause of patellar subluxation/dislocation or patellofemoral pain and arthritis.
  - Anterior drawer test: Increased anterior translation of the tibia compared to the other side plus an indefinite end point indicates anterior cruciate ligament (ACL) deficiency.
  - Posterior drawer test: Translation of the tibia more than 10 mm posterior to the femoral condyle is highly suggestive of multiligamentous knee injury and deficiency of the posterior cruciate ligament (PCL).
  - Varus and valgus stress test: Instability at 30 degrees of flexion suggests isolated collateral ligament injury. Instability at both 0 and 30 degrees is suggestive of a multiligamentous injury.
  - Patellar apprehension test: A patient with a history of patellar instability may report a sensation that his or her patella feels as if it is about to dislocate.
  - Patellar tilt test: More than 15 degrees of lateral tilt is suggestive of laxity. Lack of patellar tilt is suggestive of a tight lateral constraint.
  - The patellar grind test reveals pain or crepitus.
  - Quadriceps active test: Forward translation of the tibia after attempted knee extension is positive for PCL insufficiency (reduction of posterior tibial sag).
- It is critical to evaluate both the ipsilateral hip and lumbar spine to rule out hip or spine pathology as a major contributor to knee pain. Evidence of possible hip or spine pathology includes the following:
  - Poorly localized knee pain or thigh pain
  - Radiation of symptoms into the leg or foot
  - Worsening pain with prolonged sitting or lying down
  - Concomitant numbness or tingling
  - Trendelenburg gait pattern (ie, leaning over the affected extremity during the stance phase)
  - Reproduction of knee pain with hip ROM or passive straight-leg raise testing

- Lack of knee swelling or tenderness to palpation on examination
- Absent or diminished reflexes
- Pain out of proportion to radiographic examination findings

IMAGING AND OTHER DIAGNOSTIC STUDIES

- Standard radiographs include the following:
  - Standing anteroposterior (AP), which reveals joint space narrowing and dynamic instability, presence or absence of marginal osteophytes, subchondral sclerosis, and angular deformities
  - Standing posteroanterior (PA), typically taken in 30 to 45 degrees of flexion, which reveals chondral wear in the functional zones of the femoral condyles as well as occult deformity not seen on the AP view
  - Standing lateral in extension to reveal patella, posterior tibial and posterior femoral condyle osteophytes, native tibial slope, and patellar height
  - Merchant view, which demonstrates patellar position, patellofemoral joint space and osteophytes, and evidence of trochlear hypoplasia
- Additional radiographs that may be necessary include the following:
  - Full-length standing films, particularly in cases of prior long bone injury or deformity
  - Hip and spine films if suspicion exists for referred pain
- Advanced imaging studies such as computed tomography, magnetic resonance imaging, and bone scan are typically not necessary, unless history and physical examination findings are strongly suggestive of pathology with negative plain films.

DIFFERENTIAL DIAGNOSIS

- Any potential cause of local or diffuse knee pain should be considered in the differential diagnosis of knee OA, including the following:
  - Hip arthritis
  - Low back pain/spinal stenosis
  - Patellofemoral syndrome
  - Meniscal tear
  - Bursitis
  - Infectious arthritis
  - Gout or pseudogout
  - Iliotibial band syndrome
  - Collateral or cruciate ligament injury

NONOPERATIVE MANAGEMENT

- A wide range of nonoperative modalities are available for treatment of knee OA. These interventions do not alter the underlying disease process but may substantially diminish pain and disability.
  - Health and behavior modifications, including patient education, physical therapy, weight loss, and knee braces
  - Pharmacotherapy includes acetaminophen, nonsteroidal anti-inflammatory drugs, and glucosamine and/or chondroitin sulfate.
- Intra-articular injections
  - Corticosteroid injections in knees with considerable inflammation (eg, swelling) are useful.
  - Hyaluronic acid (viscosupplementation)

SURGICAL MANAGEMENT

- Osteotomy may be indicated for unicompartmental knee OA associated with malalignment or for correction of symptomatic posttraumatic malunions about the knee.
- Arthroscopic débridement and lavage has a minimal role in the treatment of knee OA, except in cases where mechanical symptoms (eg, locking and catching) constitute the vast majority of symptoms.
- Arthroplasty: partial or total knee arthroplasty

Indications

- TKA is a valuable intervention for patients who have severe daily pain along with radiographic evidence of arthritis.
- TKA is typically reserved for those patients who have failed several methods of nonsurgical treatment.

Contraindications

- Absolute
  - Active or latent (<1 year) knee sepsis
  - Presence of active infection elsewhere in the body
  - Incompetent quadriceps muscle or extensor mechanism
- Relative
  - Neuropathic arthropathy (eg, Charcot arthropathy)
  - Poor soft tissue coverage or skin conditions such as uncontrolled psoriatic lesions in the vicinity of the incision
  - Well-functioning and painless knee ankylosed in a good position
  - Morbid obesity (body mass index >40 kg/m^2)
  - Noncompliance due to major psychiatric disorders, including dementia, hostile personality, or alcohol or drug abuse
  - Insufficient bone stock for reconstruction
  - Poor health or presence of comorbidities that make the patient an unsuitable candidate for major surgery and anesthesia
  - The patient has poor motivation or unrealistic expectations.
  - Severe peripheral vascular disease

Preoperative Planning

- A comprehensive medical and drug history is mandatory to confirm that the patient is an appropriate candidate for major surgery and anesthesia.
- Good-quality radiographs must be obtained, as described earlier.
- Template overlay is used to estimate component size and bone defects as well as the potential need for augmentation.

Positioning

- The skin around the knee is shaved using clippers shortly before the procedure in a holding area outside the room where the procedure will be performed. Shaving should be performed in such a manner that skin integrity is preserved.
- The patient is positioned supine on the operating table. The upper torso is secured with a protective belt to allow tilting of the table as needed. A roller or a bump is securely taped to the table so that it supports the heel when the patient's knee is flexed and frees the assistant's hands (**FIG 3A**).

- A lateral post and/or a sacral bump may be used to prevent intraoperative hip abduction or external rotation.
- A tourniquet is applied snugly and as far proximally as feasible to the upper thigh. In obese or short-limbed patients, it may be necessary to use a sterile tourniquet to ensure adequate access to the surgical field.
- The heel is suspended in a leg holder (**FIG 3B**).
- An adhesive drape is put in place distal to the tourniquet to prevent antimicrobial solutions from dripping under the tourniquet.
- Preoperative antibiotics are administered 30 to 60 minutes before the skin incision is made and 5 to 10 minutes before the tourniquet is inflated. Typically, these include first-generation cephalosporins. Alternatives such as vancomycin or clindamycin are sometimes used, particularly in patients with beta-lactam allergies.
- Surgical skin preparation is begun using a broad-spectrum germicidal agent.
- A meticulous and secure draping technique is important to reduce the risk of infection. Bulky drapes obscure the palpable bony landmarks, such as malleoli or metatarsal bones, which are routinely used for accurate bone cuts, rotation, and alignment in knee arthroplasty.
- The incision is marked on the front of the knee along with several horizontal lines that will be used to align the skin properly during closure (**FIG 3C**).
  - Classically, an anterior longitudinal midline incision is used for TKA. This incision may sacrifice the infrapatellar branch of the saphenous nerve, causing an area of lateral numbness; the patient should be warned about this possibility before the surgery.
  - Principles of incisions for TKA include the following:
    - Blood is primarily supplied to the skin of the anterior aspect of the knee from the medial side.
    - Prior scars should be taken into consideration to preserve skin vascularity.
    - Preexisting anterior longitudinal scars should be incorporated when possible.
    - When parallel anterior longitudinal scars are present, the most lateral one should be used if possible.
    - If it is not possible to use a prior incision, a wide bridge of intact skin at least 8 cm should be allowed between the new incision and the previous scar.
    - Horizontal scars can be crossed at right angles, and short oblique scars may be ignored.
    - Avoid acute angles of intersection.

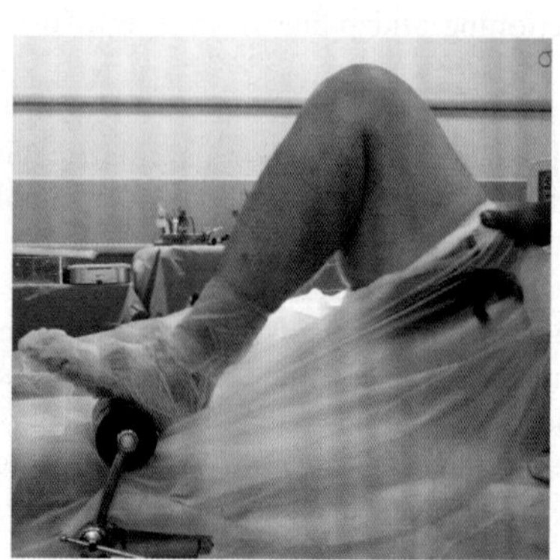
A

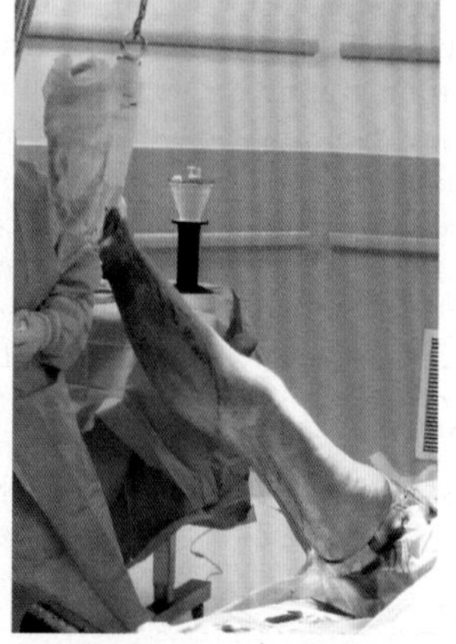
B

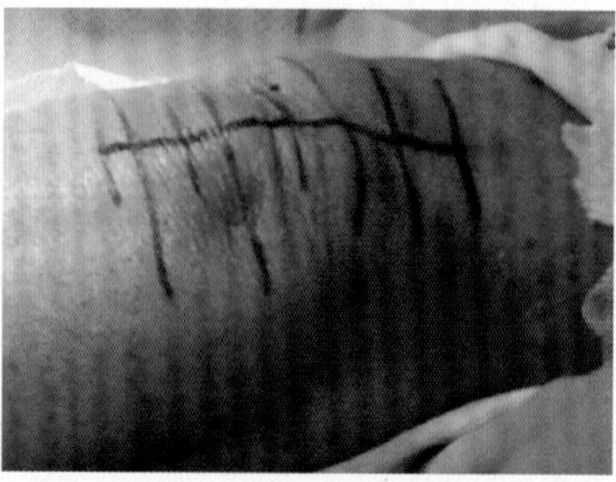
C

FIG 3 • **A.** A bump is taped to the table so that it supports the heel when the knee is flexed. **B.** The heel is suspended in a leg holder for surgical skin preparation. **C.** The incision is marked on the front of the knee along with several horizontal lines.

TECHNIQUES

Initial Exposure

- If using a tourniquet, the lower extremity is exsanguinated and the tourniquet inflated.
- The incision is classically made from the superior edge of the quadriceps tendon proximally (one handbreadth above the superior pole of the patella) to the inferomedial aspect of the tibial tuberosity (**TECH FIG 1**).
- The skin, fat, and fascia are incised directly down to the extensor mechanism, and the medial and lateral flaps are reflected only as far as necessary to have adequate exposure while preserving their blood supply.
  - Full-thickness skin flaps are created to minimize risks of skin necrosis.
- Once the deep fascia is opened, the prepatellar bursa is incised and retracted medially and laterally. The paratenon of the patellar tendon should be exposed and protected.

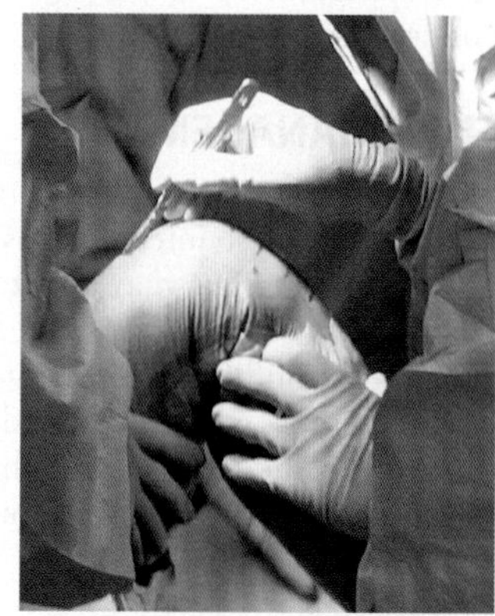

TECH FIG 1 • The incision is made with the knee either straight or in flexion.

Arthrotomy

- The arthrotomy can be performed using the medial parapatellar, subvastus (Southern), or midvastus approaches (**TECH FIG 2**).
- The most current data indicates that the results following TKA using any of these three approaches are similar.[3,16]

Medial Parapatellar Approach

- The quadriceps tendon is cut longitudinally from proximal to distal along its medial border, leaving a cuff of tendon approximately 5 to 10 mm wide. Then the incision is carried further, skirting along the medial border of the patella and patellar tendon.
- The arthrotomy incision is made through the medial retinaculum, capsule, and synovium, leaving a 5-mm cuff of retinaculum attached to the patella to facilitate repair at the end of the procedure. Distally, the incision should stop at the inferior aspect of the patellar tendon insertion, proximal to the insertion of the pes anserine tendons on the superomedial tibia.

Subvastus (Southern) Approach

- Blunt dissection is carried from the medial intermuscular septum. Care should be taken to avoid damaging the intermuscular septal branch or the articular branch of the descending genicular artery. This can be accomplished by limiting proximal dissection to 10 cm or less.
- A transverse incision is made at the midpatella through the medial retinaculum and inferior to the vastus medialis.
- This incision is stopped once the patellar tendon is reached, and a second incision is made along the medial border of the patellar tendon approximately 1 cm along the medial border to the tibial tubercle.

Midvastus Approach

- Blunt finger dissection is begun at the superomedial pole of the patella in the midsubstance and through the full thickness of the vastus medialis muscle, and is extended parallel to its fiber, to a maximum of 4 cm proximal medial to this starting point. By doing this, the incision does not extend far enough medially to violate the saphenous nerve to the vastus medialis obliquus. The medial superior genicular artery and the muscular branches of the descending genicular artery are similarly preserved.

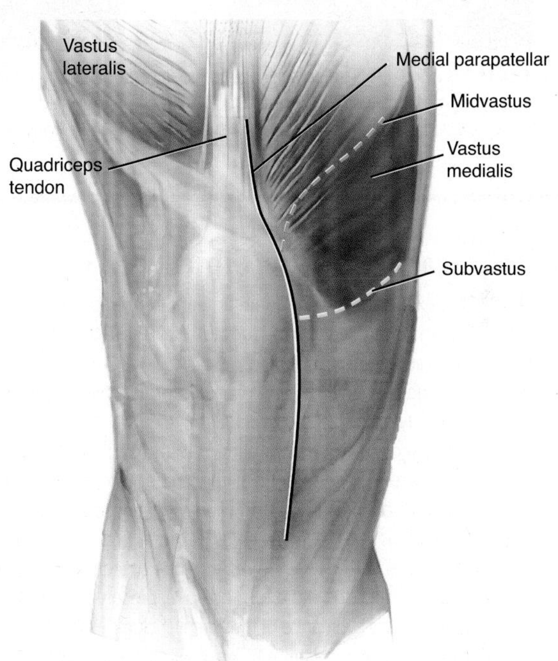

TECH FIG 2 • Planes of dissection for the medial parapatellar midvastus and subvastus approaches.

Knee Joint Exposure

- The soft tissue sleeve is dissected from the proximal medial tibial metaphysis (**TECH FIG 3A**) by taking the amount of varus or valgus deformity into account.
  - More extensive dissection is performed for knees with varus deformity and limited or no dissection for knees with valgus deformity.
- With sharp dissection or cautery, a subperiosteal layer that includes the deep medial collateral ligament (MCL) is raised carefully from the medial tibial flare to the sagittal midline of the tibia. The dissection must not be extended more than 2 to 3 cm distal to the medial joint line.
- A portion of the anterior synovium over the supracondylar area is excised to facilitate visualization of the anterior femoral cortex and permit appropriate sizing on the femoral component.
- A portion of the retropatellar fat pad is excised to permit full exposure of the lateral tibial plateau.
- The patella is either everted or subluxated laterally into the lateral gutter (**TECH FIG 3B,C**), and the knee is flexed.
  - Current data do not support any difference in outcomes with respect to patellar eversion during TKA.[13,23]
- The medial flap of the quadriceps must be reflected medially off the face of the femur. There should be no undue tension at the patellar tendon insertion. Placing one smooth pin in the tibial tuberosity may provide some protection against tendon avulsion in very tight knees but is typically not necessary in primary TKA.
  - Release of a portion of the medial portion of the patellar tendon and elevation of a small cuff of periosteum immediately adjacent to the patellar tendon insertion can be helpful.
- A retractor is inserted lateral to the lateral meniscus.
- A second retractor is placed along the medial joint line for medial exposure.

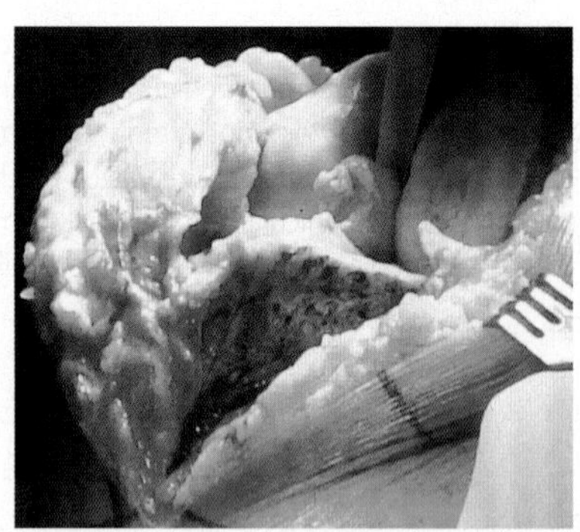
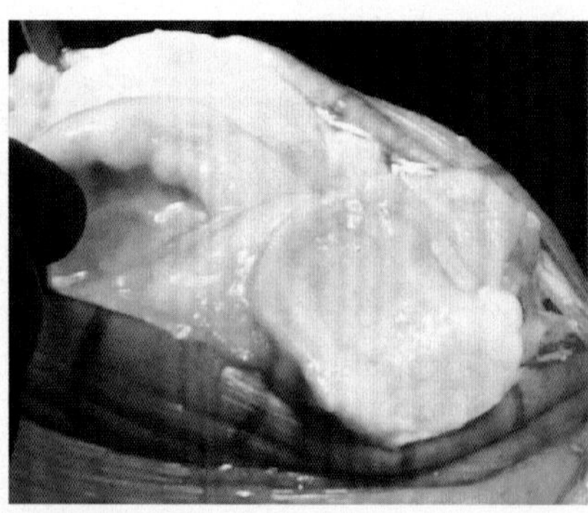
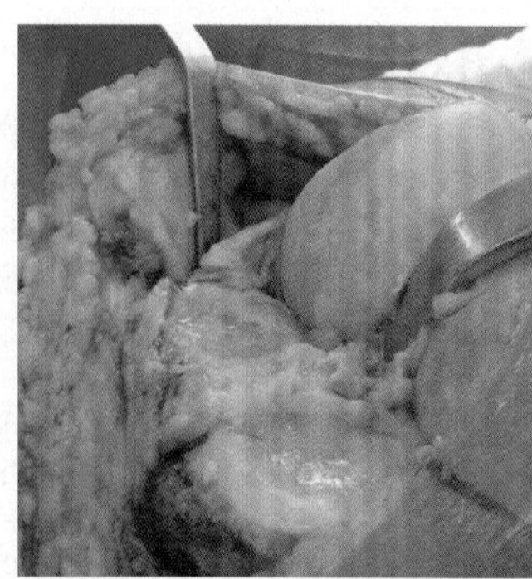

TECH FIG 3 • **A.** The soft tissue sleeve is dissected from the proximal medial tibial metaphysis as much as necessary for the correction of a varus deformity of the knee. **B.** The patella is everted, and the knee is flexed. **C.** The patella is subluxated, and Hohmann retractors are inserted laterally for soft tissue retraction and posteriorly to deliver the tibia anteriorly.

Preparation of the Tibia

- The ACL is excised, allowing further anterior translation of the tibia.
- The PCL can be preserved (in cruciate-retaining TKA) or excised (in cruciate-substituting TKA).
  - This choice depends on surgeon's preference, degree of deformity, and status of the PCL.
  - Advantages to PCL-substituting TKA include ease of exposure (increased anterior tibial translation), more predictable "rollback" of the femur, and fewer ligamentous structures involved in TKA balancing.
  - Advantages to PCL-retaining TKA include preservation of femoral bone stock (no need for a box cut), preservation of native anatomy, and avoidance of the "patellar clunk" phenomenon.
  - However, data comparing PCL-substituting and PCL-retaining knee do not indicate the superiority of one versus the other.[9,24]
- Complete anterior subluxation of the tibia from beneath the femur is accomplished with hyperflexion and external rotation of the tibia, providing complete exposure of the tibial plateau and posterior horn attachments of the menisci.
  - This maneuver may be blocked by osteophytes or incomplete release of medial capsular structures.
- A retractor is placed posteriorly to aid in anterior dislocation of the tibial plateau and to protect the popliteal fossa during the proximal tibial osteotomy.
- With the tibia completely subluxated anteriorly, the medial and lateral menisci are excised and the PCL exposed, released, or excised, as the surgeon prefers. The popliteus tendon is protected during all soft tissue and bone resection.
- If adequate exposure of the tibia cannot be obtained, the femoral cuts can be made first, allowing easier access to the back of the joint.

Bone Cuts

- The five standard bone cuts for any TKA are as follows:
  - Transverse proximal tibial resection
  - Distal femoral condylar resection
  - Anterior and posterior condylar resections
  - Anterior and posterior chamfer resections from the distal femur
  - Retropatellar cut (in patellar resurfacing)
- The sixth step of the intercondylar box or box cut is performed only for posterior stabilized designs.
- Either the femoral or the tibial cut is performed first, depending on surgeon preference and technique.
- Bone cuts can be made using open or slotted cutting guides (**TECH FIG 4**).
- Classically, bone cuts are made to align the implanted knee joint perpendicular to the mechanical axis of the lower extremity,

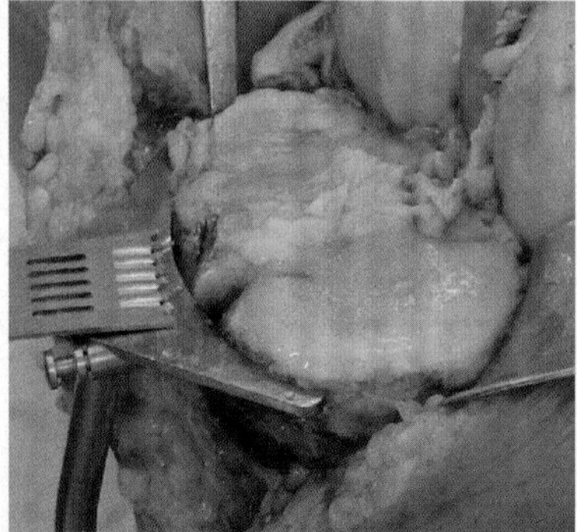
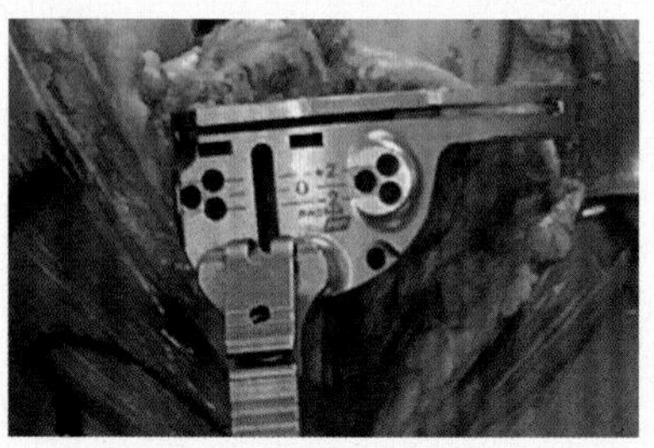

TECH FIG 4 • **A.** Open and (**B**) slotted cutting guides.

thereby distributing weight-bearing forces evenly between the medial and lateral compartments.
  - This technique uses both native bony anatomy or computer assistance and cutting guides to properly align the knee.
  - The clinical success and survivorship of TKA using this technique has been linked to correct orientation of the components with respect to the mechanical axis.
  - Greater than 3 degrees of malalignment in the coronal plane has been associated with an increased failure rate.
- More recently, some surgeons have advocated bone cuts made relative to a three-dimensional kinematic axis of the knee.
  - This technique seeks to restore the native tibia vara and femoral valga as opposed to referencing the mechanical axis of the lower extremity.
  - Bony preparation in these cases often uses preoperative advanced imaging and creation of patient-specific cutting guides.
  - Although the short-term results of TKA using this technology demonstrate feasibility, long-term data regarding survivorship are currently lacking.[8]
- The following paragraphs describe bone cuts made using the classic mechanical alignment technique, which is the authors' current preferred method.

Proximal Tibial Cut

- The goal of the proximal tibial resection is to create a flat surface perpendicular to the mechanical axis of the tibia.
- Because the mechanical axis typically parallels the anatomic axis of the tibia, either an IM or extramedullary (EM) alignment rod can be used to help align this resection, provided that there is no deformity, bowing, offset to the tibial shaft, or blockage in the medullary canal.
  - EM rods are advantageous because they limit fat emboli and can be used even in the presence of significant tibial bowing or obstruction.
  - IM rods can be particularly useful when external bony landmarks are difficult to palpate such as in obese patients.
- When using an EM guide
  - Attach the strap of the distal end of the alignment guide above the ankle and pin the proximal end to the upper tibial metaphysis. Adjust the alignment guide to sit on the medial third of the tibial tubercle proximally and parallel the tibial crest, which serves as a landmark for the mechanical axis of the tibia (**TECH FIG 5A**).
  - Set the proximal part to obtain 3 to 5 degrees of posterior slope in the sagittal plane (**TECH FIG 5B**).
  - When sufficient anatomic landmarks exist, an "angel wing" placed along the proximal medial tibial plateau can be used to set the slope to match the patients native slope.
    - Particularly with PCL-substituting TKA, it is important to avoid excessive tibial slope, as too much slope can cause flexion instability and impingement of the femoral box on the post in extension.
- Fit the proximal cutting block snugly up against the tibial cortex to improve the accuracy of the resection.
- Remove an appropriate amount of cartilage and bone from the tibial plateau.
  - The bone resected should have approximately the same thickness as the final tibial component, including the metal base plate and polyethylene liner.
  - When judging depth of the resection, it is often useful to reference the least involved portion of the tibial plateau, as this provides a more constant reference point.
- When using an IM guide
  - Accurately choose the pilot hole that is at the junction of the tibial insertion of the ACL and the anterior horn of the lateral meniscus (**TECH FIG 5C**).
    - Irrigation and aspiration of the canal; insertion of a fluted, hollow rod; and drilling a hole slightly larger than the size of the IM rod to allow egress of material can reduce the risk of fat embolization.
  - Insert the IM rod and fix the cutting block in the desired position, then remove the rod together with its outrigger.
- Carefully protect the MCL and lateral collateral ligament (LCL) through proper insertion of retractors.
- Use an oscillating saw to cut the bone. To protect the posterior neurovascular bundle, stop cutting the last few millimeters of bone by saw and crack the rest afterward by levering or using an osteotome.

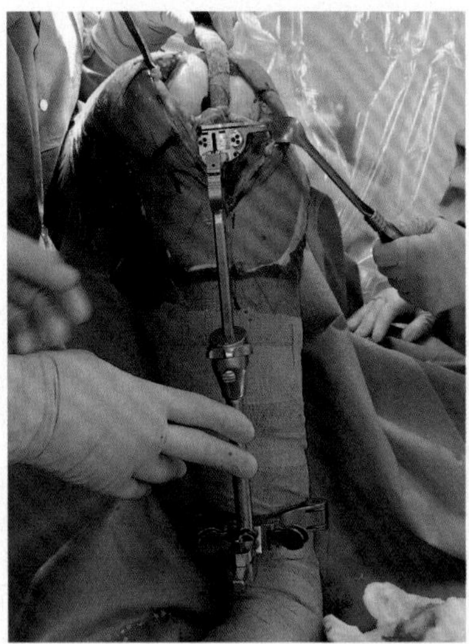
A

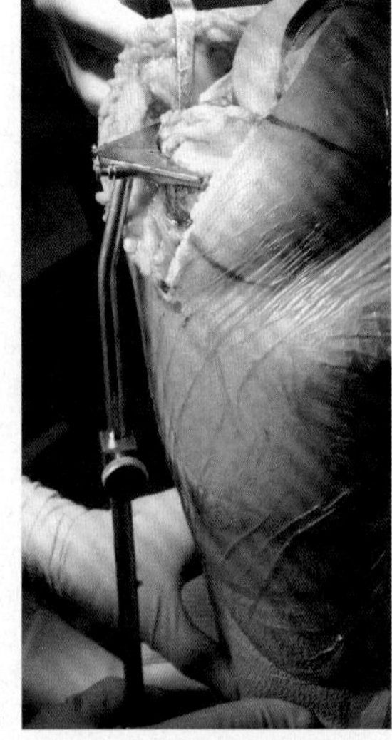
B

TECH FIG 5 • **A,B.** The strap of the distal end of the EM alignment guide is attached above the ankle, tunings are done, and the proximal end is pinned to the upper tibial metaphysis. *(continued)*

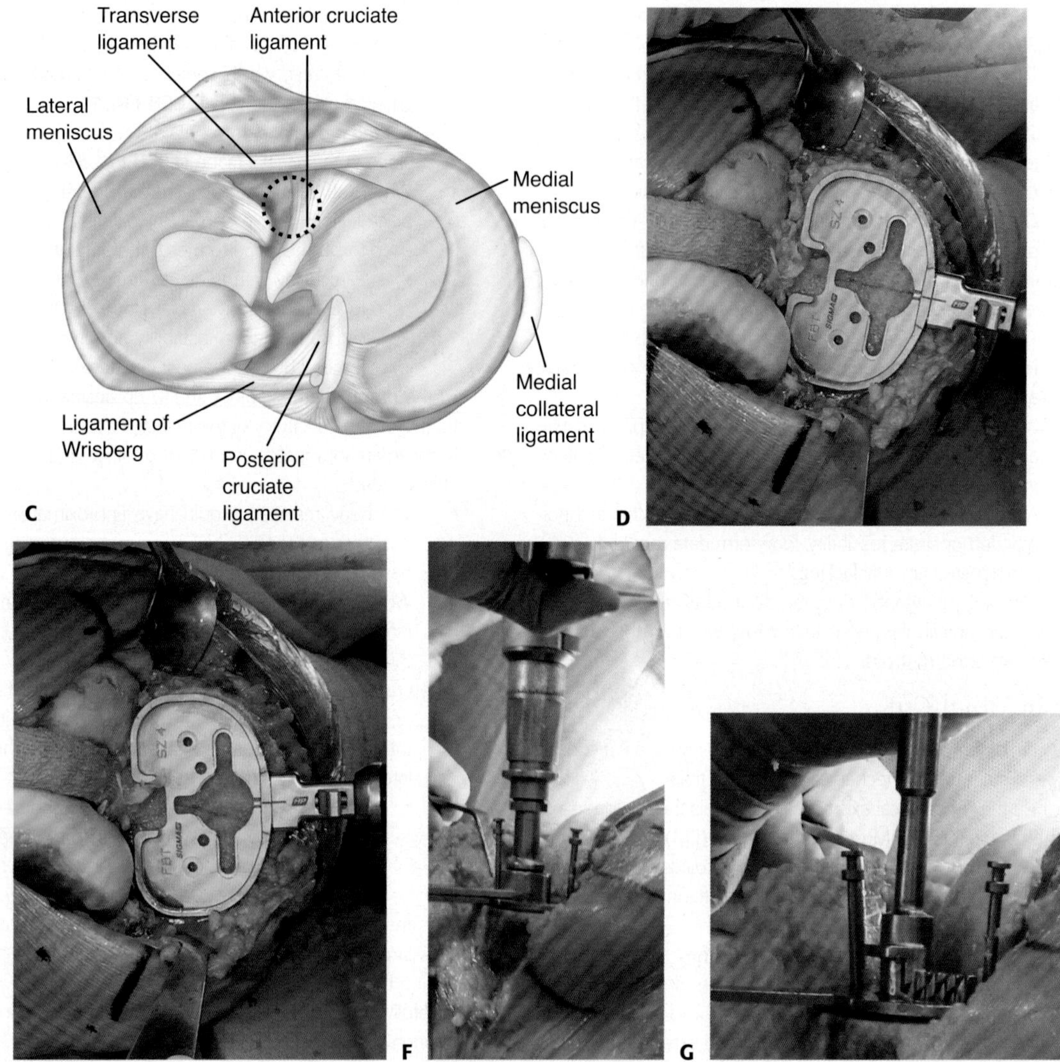

TECH FIG 5 • *(continued)* **C.** Entry hole for the IM guide at the junction of the tibial insertion of the ACL and the anterior horn of the lateral meniscus. **D.** Proper alignment of the tibial rotational guide, with the apex of rotation pointing to the medial one-third of the tibial tubercle. **E.** A malaligned proximal tibial rotational guide, pointing well medial to the tibial tubercle. **F.** Drilling for the stem. **G.** Impacting the broach to the proper depth.

- Remove the osteotomized bone along with the remnants of menisci. Establish the anatomic boundary of the tibial metaphysis by removing the osteophytes.
  - Proximal tibial osteophytes can often resemble true articular surfaces, but all osteophytes must be removed to facilitate proper balancing of the knee.
- The proximal tibia is then sized appropriately, and the rotation is set by aligning the tibial axis with the junction of the medial and middle third of the tibial tubercle (**TECH FIG 5D**).
- Alternatively, tibial rotation may be achieved by "floating" the tibial component during the trial phase and allowing the fixed femoral component articulation to set the rotation of the tibial component.
  - No matter how rotation is set, it is important to avoid internal rotation of the tibial component, as this can result in significant patellar tracking problems (**TECH FIG 5E**).
- If necessary, place the appropriately sized stem drill guide on the sizing tray and drill for the stem (**TECH FIG 5F**).
- Assemble the proper size of tibial broach on the broach impactor. Seat the impactor on the tray and impact the broach to the proper depth (**TECH FIG 5G**). Impact the stemmed tibial trial to ensure proper fit before implanting the final prosthesis.

Distal Femur Cuts

- Because of a lack of reliable palpable external landmarks, the IM alignment guide is superior to the EM guide for preparation of the femur, except in cases of excessive femoral bowing, previous fracture, Paget disease, or an ipsilateral long-stemmed total hip replacement.
- Drill an entry hole 1 cm anterior to the origin of the PCL, slightly medial to the midportion of the intercondylar notch (**TECH FIG 6A**). Touching the anterior surface of the femoral shaft with the other hand can be a good guide to the direction of drilling.

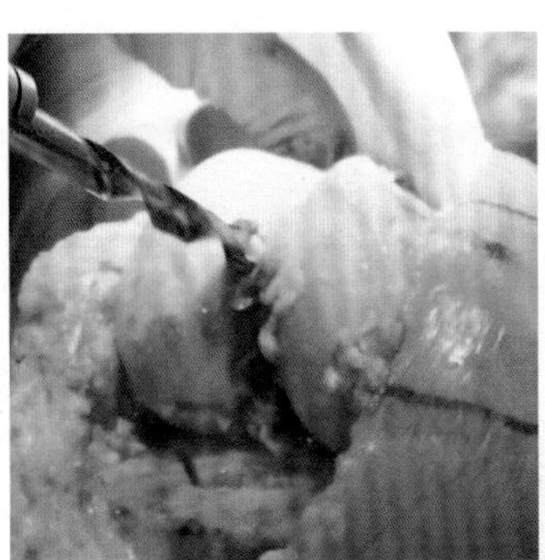
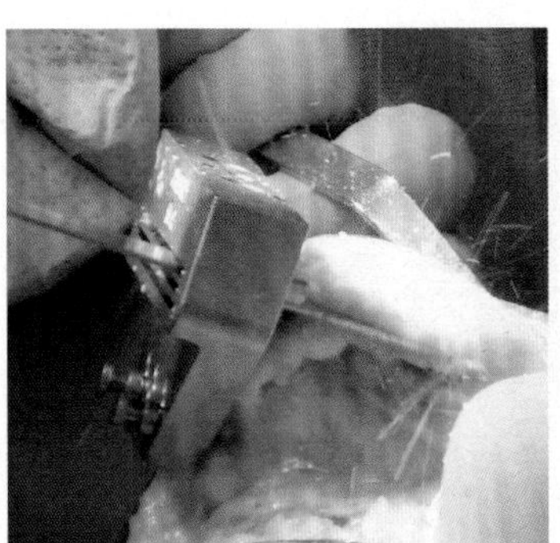
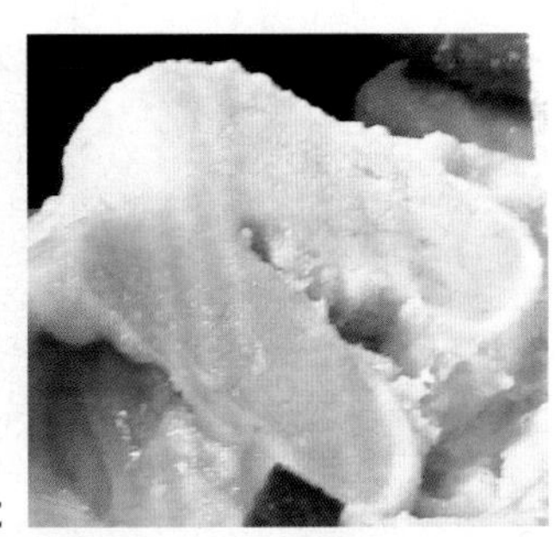

TECH FIG 6 • A. Entry hole of the femoral IM guide 1 cm anterior to the origin of the PCL, slightly medial to the midportion of the intercondylar notch. **B,C.** Osteotomy of the distal femur.

- As with IM tibial rods insertion, slight overdrilling using a fluted IM guide and aspiration of the marrow contents before insertion of the guide are recommended to decompress the femoral canal and to subsequently reduce the risk of fat emboli.
- Insert the IM guide and pass it directly into the center of the canal without making any contact with the femoral cortices; otherwise, the angle of resection will be changed. Attach the cutting block to the IM rod, adjust it to the desired amount of valgus (typically 5 to 6 degrees), and then fix it in place.
  - The amount of valgus imparted to the distal femoral cut is based on the difference between the mechanical and anatomic axes of the femur.
- Remove the IM rod and cut the bone. It is crucial to prevent the saw blade from bending or going forward in an undesired direction while proceeding through the osteotomy line, particularly during resection of hard and sclerotic bone.
- The amount of bone to be resected should be precisely equivalent to the thickness of the final femoral component. In the sagittal plane, the distal femur should be cut at 90 degrees to the femoral mechanical axis and, after soft tissue balancing, should be parallel to the resected surface of the proximal tibia with the knee in extension (**TECH FIG 6B,C**).

Anterior and Posterior Femoral Condylar Cuts

- Making accurate cuts is essential to obtain proper size and rotation of the final femoral component.
  - This step is critical with respect to balancing the flexion gap and achieving appropriate patellar tracking.
- There are four basic techniques to setting femoral rotation, three of which use femoral anatomic landmarks:
  - Using the posterior condyles as a reference, align the AP cutting block in 3 degrees of external rotation relative to the posterior condylar axis.
    - This accounts for the asymmetry of the native posterior condyles.
    - Increased external rotation may be necessary, particularly in valgus knees with hypoplasia of the lateral femoral condyle.
  - Align the AP cutting block parallel to the epicondylar axis of the femur.
  - Align the cutting block perpendicular to Whiteside line, which is a line drawn from the top of the intercondylar notch to the deepest part of the femoral trochlea.
- These are known as *measured resection techniques* for achieving appropriate femoral rotation.
  - The advantages of these procedures include technical ease and the ability to use either a tibia first or a femur first work flow.
  - Their disadvantages include inconsistency of anatomic landmarks.
- The fourth technique is known as a *gap balancing technique*, is independent of femoral anatomic landmarks, and uses the flat proximal tibial resection and ligament balance to set femoral rotation.
  - Once the proximal tibia and distal femoral cuts are made, the knee is balanced in extension by performing appropriate resection of osteophytes and any necessary ligament releases.
  - The knee is flexed, the collateral ligaments are tensioned using a spacer block, and the femur is allowed to freely rotate.
  - The femoral AP cutting block is then situated parallel with the flat tibial surface.
  - The advantages of this technique include no reliance on possibly inconsistent femoral anatomy and insurance of a congruent flexion gap.
  - The disadvantages of this technique include technical difficulty in achieving both a balanced extension *and* flexion gap prior to making posterior femoral cuts and dependence on a perfectly flat proximal tibial resection.
- Using a combination of all four techniques and multiple reference points (ie, appreciating that the posterior cut should be parallel to the transepicondylar line, perpendicular to the Whiteside line, and parallel to the upper tibial cut) can help the surgeon reduce any error in the rotation of the femoral component (**TECH FIG 7A–C**).
- Adjust the stylus that indicates where the anterior cut exits the femur to size the knee.
- Sizing of the femoral component can be done in one of two ways:
  - In an anterior referencing technique (top down), the anterior position of the femoral component is set to be flush with the anterior femoral cortex and held constant, and upsizing or downsizing of the component changes the flexion gap.
    - The main advantage of this technique is avoidance of femoral notching.
    - The main disadvantage of this technique is the potential to create an asymmetric flexion gap.

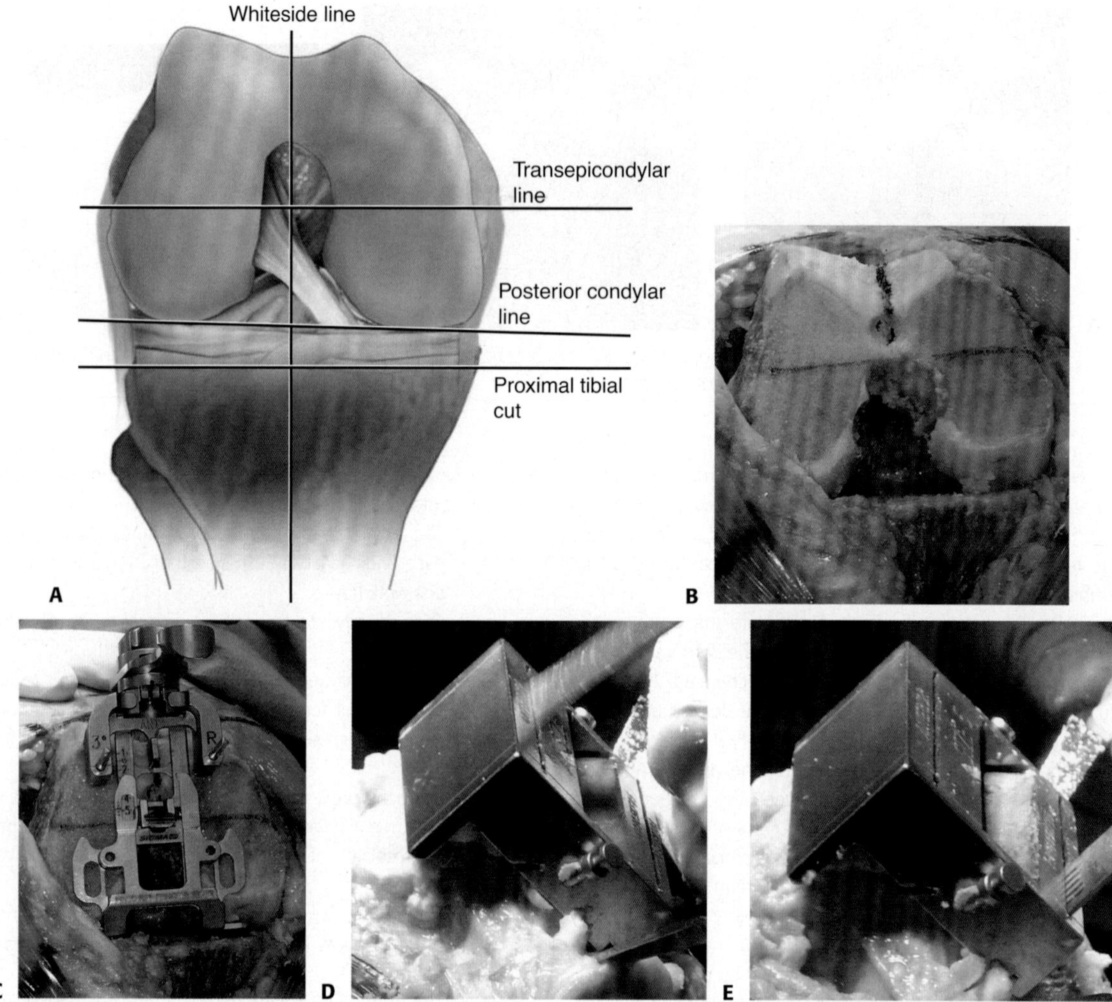

TECH FIG 7 • A. Femoral component rotation is determined by reference lines used for performing the distal femoral cut. **B.** An intraoperative view of the reference lines. **C.** The alignment guide is placed so that rotational holes are drilled parallel to the epicondylar axis, perpendicular to Whiteside line, and 3 degrees externally rotated to the posterior condyles. **D,E.** Anterior and posterior femoral condylar osteotomies.

- In a posterior referencing technique (bottom up), the posterior position of the femoral component is set and held constant, and upsizing or downsizing the component changes the position of the component relative to the anterior cortex of the femur.
  - The main advantage of this technique is the ability to set and hold constant a predetermined flexion gap.
  - The main disadvantage to this technique is the potential for anterior femoral notching or overstuffing the patellofemoral joint if the component is not sized appropriately.
- Maximally flex the knee to reduce the chance of injury to the posterior neurovascular bundle during posterior sawing and use a saw to make the guided cuts (**TECH FIG 7D,E**).

Anterior and Posterior Chamfer Cuts

- Anterior and posterior chamfer cuts are essential for the prosthesis to fit over the distal femur.
- A chamfer guide is placed on the distal femur. In some systems, this step is integrated into the same block as that used for the anterior and posterior femoral cuts (**TECH FIG 8A,B**).
- When the sawing is complete, use an osteotome to free small remnant portions of uncut bone (**TECH FIG 8C**).
- Once the bony cuts are made, it is important to open up the flexion gap with lamina spreaders and remove any remaining osteophytes, loose bodies, or unresected meniscus and bone from the back of the knee.
  - In a properly balanced knee, the tension on the lamina spreaders will be equal medially and laterally and the flexion gap will be rectangular (**TECH FIG 8D**).
- If necessary, a release of the posterior capsule may be done at this time, taking great care to avoid injury to the popliteal neurovascular structures.
- To accommodate the post–cam mechanism in a posterior stabilized prosthesis, place the finishing guide onto the distal femur to make the intercondylar box cut. Center the guide mediolaterally and secure it firmly by pin or screw.
  - Use a reciprocating saw to resect the bone from the notch. Complete the resection with a chisel or osteotome.
  - Lateralization of the femoral component can help to optimize patellar tracking.

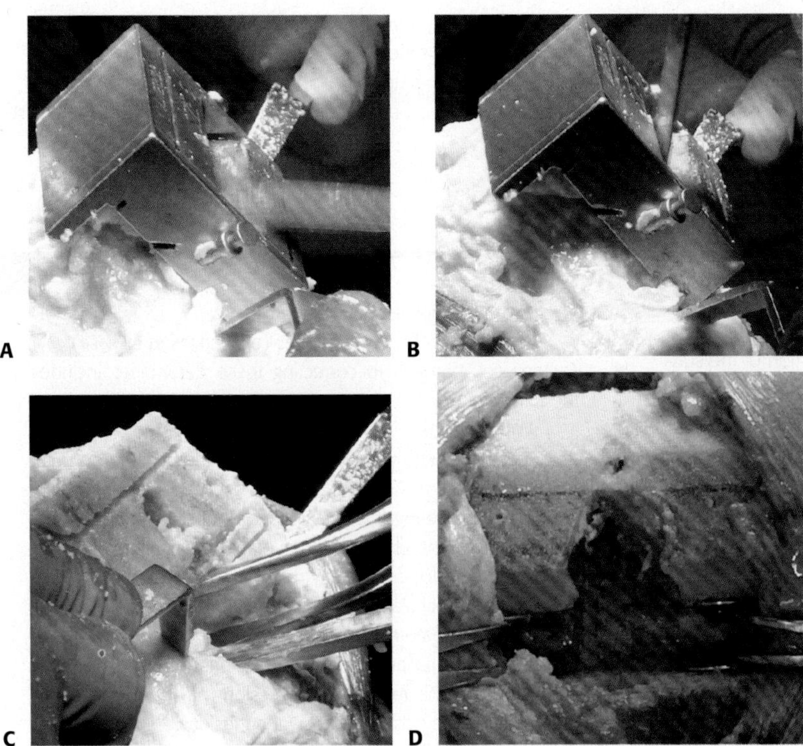

TECH FIG 8 • A,B. Anterior and posterior chamfer cuts. **C.** An osteotome is used to free small remnant portions of uncut bone and removing posterior osteophytes. **D.** Following bony resection, lamina spreaders demonstrate a balanced, rectangular flexion gap.

Patellar Preparation

- Patellar resurfacing is often, but not always, performed during TKA.
- Patellar preparation can be done at any point in the procedure, but is typically done either following both tibial and femoral preparation, or immediately following the initial approach in an effort to facilitate exposure.
- Remove the osteophytes, synovial insertions, and fat to demarcate the anatomic margins of the patella.
- Use a caliper (**TECH FIG 9A**) to assess the patellar thickness before the cut and after the patella is resurfaced to ensure that the patellar thickness is equal to the original thickness and that at least 12 mm of bone stock remains.[20]
  - To obtain an exact measurement of the patellar thickness, the prepatellar bursa should be dissected to completely expose the anterior surface of the patella.
- Use a patellar cutting jig, mill, or freehand technique. Pass the patellar cut parallel to the anterior surface of the patella through

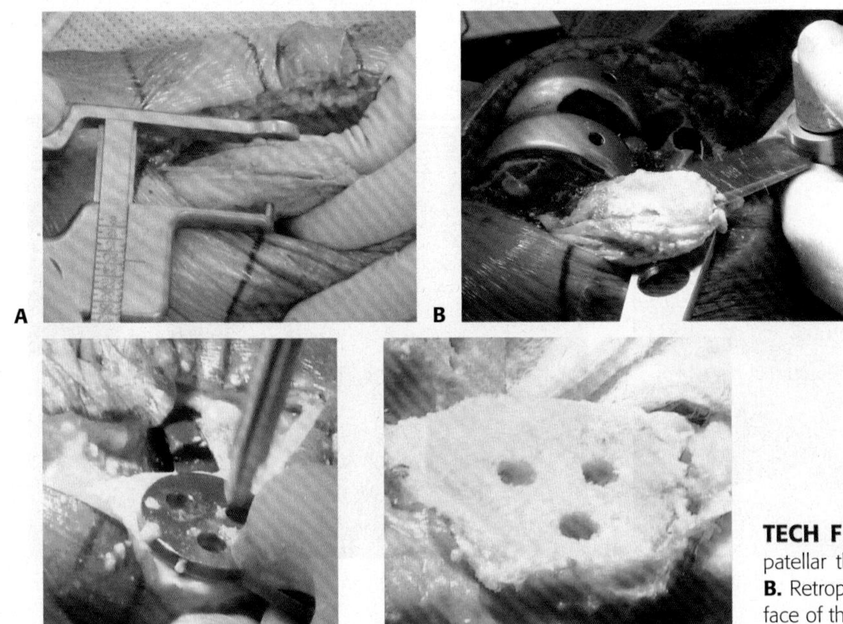

TECH FIG 9 • A. Calipers are used to assess the patellar thickness before the retropatellar osteotomy. **B.** Retropatellar osteotomy parallel to the anterior surface of the patella. **C,D.** Three lug holes are drilled in a triangular pattern.

the chondro-osseous junction, completely resecting both facets (**TECH FIG 9B**). Proximally, the cut passes just superficial to the quadriceps insertion; distally, it passes through the nose of the patella, superficial to the patellar tendon.
  - Make a flat cut, removing any remnants of cartilage.
- Center and firmly hold the appropriate drill guide and drill lug holes to facilitate patellar fixation (**TECH FIG 9C,D**).
  - Placing the patellar button superiorly and medially can help achieve optimal patellar tracking within the femoral trochlea.

Soft Tissue and Ligament Balancing

- Soft tissue and ligament balancing is a vital portion of the surgical procedure.[11,21]
- To achieve proper ligament balance, it is critical to first remove all marginal osteophytes from both the tibial and femoral margins.
- In knees with minimal deformity, balance can often be achieved by performing a minimal soft tissue release, making the bone cuts, and checking the knee through insertion of trial components.
- However, in knees with complex or severe deformity, cautious stepwise release is necessary.
  - Spacer blocks can be used after creation of each gap to check balance in both flexion and extension (**TECH FIG 10A,B**).
  - If no release is necessary, proceed to the next step.
  - Once both the flexion and extension gaps are created and balanced, make sure the gaps are equal in size.
  - If the gaps are asymmetric, augmentation may be necessary (see in the following text).
  - When the deformity is severe and leads to loss of the integrity of the collateral ligaments, a constrained prosthesis may be necessary.

Correction of Preoperative Flexion Contracture

- Preoperative flexion contractures can result from various different sources, often in combination.
  - Posterior femoral or tibial osteophytes
  - Soft tissue contraction
  - Posterior capsular scarring
  - Neuromuscular comorbidities (eg, Parkinson disease)
- A stepwise approach to correcting these deformities includes the following:
  - With the knee in flexion, use a curved osteotome to release and remove osteophytes from the posterior femoral condyles.
  - Upon delivering the tibia anteriorly, observe the posterior margin of the tibia and remove any osteophytes.
  - Make sure to remove any notch osteophytes and all loose bodies, particularly those that become lodged behind the PCL in cruciate-retaining knees.
  - Carefully strip any capsular adhesions from the posterior aspect of the femur. PCL recession may be necessary to fully release posterior capsular adhesions.
  - If there is still a persistent flexion contracture at this point, additional distal femur can be resected.
    - This step should be done only if the preceding steps do not resolve the contracture, as resecting more distal femur can potentially raise the joint line and cause varying degrees of patella baja, impingement, and midflexion instability.
    - Spacer blocks can also be inserted following these maneuvers to ensure no flexion contracture remains prior to insertion of trial and definitive components.
- In knees with severe preoperative flexion contractures, it may be necessary to cut the posterior capsule transversely and release the tendinous origins of the gastrocnemius.

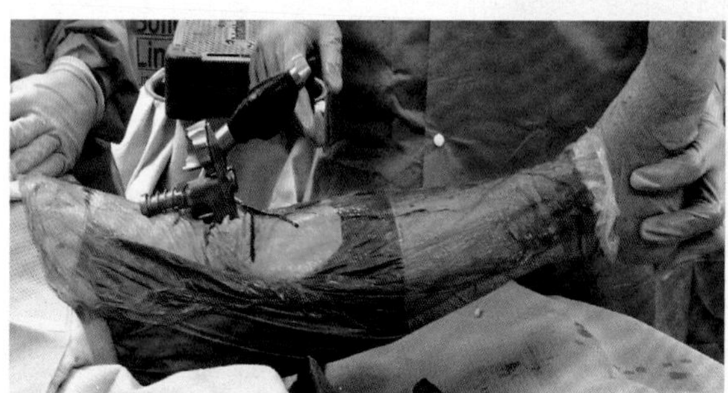
A

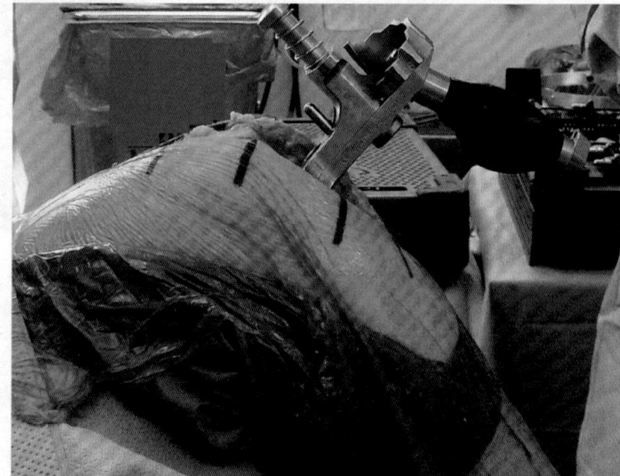
B

TECH FIG 10 • **A,B.** Spacer blocks inserted with the knee in extension (**A**) and flexion (**B**) can help balance gaps prior to insertion of trial components.

Correction of Varus Deformity

- The medial capsulotomy, along with the subperiosteal medial release included in the initial approach and exposure, can correct minimal varus deformities.
- If the knee remains tight medially, balancing it involves the following steps:
  - Make certain that all osteophytes have been removed.
    - Marginal femoral osteophytes can become trapped under the MCL.
    - Marginal tibial osteophytes can resemble articular surface.
  - Extend the medial subperiosteal release for an additional 2 to 3 cm.
  - If the medial knee is tight in flexion only, release the anterior portion of the superficial MCL.
  - If the medial knee is tight in extension only
    - Make sure that the hamstrings have been adequately released from the posterior margin of the tibia.
    - Release the posterior oblique fibers of the superficial MCL.
- It may be necessary to check the proximal tibial cut to make sure the cut is not in valgus.
- If the knee is still tight medially, the MCL can be "pie crusted" or released entirely.
  - If this step is performed, it is often necessary to use a constrained component.

Correction of Valgus Deformity

- It is unusual for the lateral side of the knee to be tight with valgus arthritis.
  - If this situation occurs, the tibial cut should first be checked to make sure the proximal tibia is not in varus.
- When addressing valgus knees that are tight laterally, balancing involves the following:
  - Sequential release of the iliotibial band, popliteal tendon, LCL, and finally the posterior capsule
  - If the lateral knee is tight in extension, release the iliotibial band and then the popliteus.
  - If the lateral knee is tight in flexion, release first the popliteus and then the LCL subperiosteally from the femoral condyle.
- If the knee remains significantly tight laterally, the biceps femoris tendon may be released if necessary.

Correction of Valgus Knee with Incompetent Medial Collateral Ligament

- A valgus knee with an incompetent MCL occurs in knees with severe, long-standing valgus deformity.
- This situation should be identified preoperatively with an appropriate physical examination.
- Treatment strategies include the following:
  - Use of a constrained articulation
  - MCL advancement
  - MCL reconstruction

Component Insertion and Trial Reduction

- Insert provisional tibial, femoral, and patellar components of the correct size (see **TECH FIG 9A**).
  - Avoid overhang of the components.
  - If this is not possible, allow overhang to occur laterally, as medial overhang often results in soft tissue impingement and postoperative pain.
- Insert a spacer of the proper height and reduce the joint. Check the ROM and ligament stability. Apply varus and valgus stresses in flexion, midflexion (approximately 40 degrees), and extension to determine the stability of the knee and the appropriate thickness of the tibial insert.
- It is essential at this point, if not done with spacer blocks earlier in the procedure, to ensure gap symmetry (**TECH FIG 11**).
  - If both gaps are equal, no further adjustments need to be made.
  - If both gaps are loose, a thicker polyethylene insert is necessary.
  - If both gaps are tight, a thinner tibial insert should be used, or more tibial bone should be resected.
  - If the extension gap is tight and the flexion gap is appropriate, correct the flexion contracture with the steps listed earlier.
  - If the extension gap is appropriate, but the flexion gap is tight (often indicated by lifting of the tibial insert in flexion), it may be necessary to either augment the distal femur and use a thinner polyethylene component or anteriorize or downsize the femoral component to achieve gap symmetry.

		Extension gap: Tight	Extension gap: Loose
Flexion gap	Tight	• Use thinner tibial insert • Resect additional tibia	• Augment distal femur • Anteriorize femoral component • Downsize femoral component (anterior referencing system only)
	Loose	• Release posterior soft tissues • Resect additional distal femur • Augment posteriorly	• Use thicker tibial insert

TECH FIG 11 • A chart depicting corrective measures to undertake if the flexion and extension gaps are not symmetric.

Patellar Tracking

- The patella should track centrally in the trochlear groove without lateral subluxation or lateral tilt in full flexion (**TECH FIG 12**).
- Perform the no-thumbs test by reducing the patella and taking the knee through the full flexion arc without closing the medial arthrotomy and without applying any medially directed force with the thumb to keep the patella in position.
- If there is patellar tilting or slight subluxation with the no-thumbs test, reapproximate the medial retinaculum at the superior pole of the patella with a single suture. If the suture does not break through full flexion of the knee, a lateral release is likely not necessary and should not be performed at this point in the procedure.
- The accuracy of evaluations of extensor mechanism balance can be improved by deflating the tourniquet, which can bind the extensor mechanism and result in perceived patellofemoral maltracking.[5]
- Tracking may be improved by the following:
  - Appropriate femoral and tibial rotation
  - Lateralization of the femoral component
  - Medialization and superiorization of the patellar component
- Persistent lift-off or subluxation after tourniquet deflation may require a lateral release.

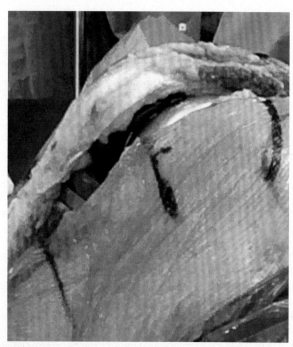

TECH FIG 12 • An intraoperative photograph demonstrating appropriate patellar tracking, with no patellar tilt in full flexion.

Component Fixation

- The setup of all components and basic instruments for component insertion should be done before the cement is prepared (**TECH FIG 13A,B**).
- With a small (1/8 inch) drill bit, drill the sclerotic areas of the tibial plateau (1 to 2 mm deep) to achieve adequate anchorage of the tibial component.
- Plug the IM hole of the distal femur with small pieces of cancellous bone (**TECH FIG 13C**).
- Use pulsatile lavage to thoroughly irrigate the cut surfaces with normal saline in order to remove all debris and increase the depth of cement penetration into the trabecular bone. Dry the bone completely with suction and dry gauze.
- Polymethylmethacrylate is used for fixation of the components in a cemented knee arthroplasty.
  - Vacuum mixing systems are typically used to remove any air bubbles that can impede biomechanical strength of the cement and ensure thorough mixing of cement powder and monomer.
- When the cement is in a doughy state, apply it to the tibial plateau (**TECH FIG 13D**). At this point, finger packing may improve the cement mantle. Add a thin layer of cement and impact the tibial component and polyethylene liner into place (**TECH FIG 13E**).
  - Trim and remove the excess cement as it extrudes from under the plateau.

A 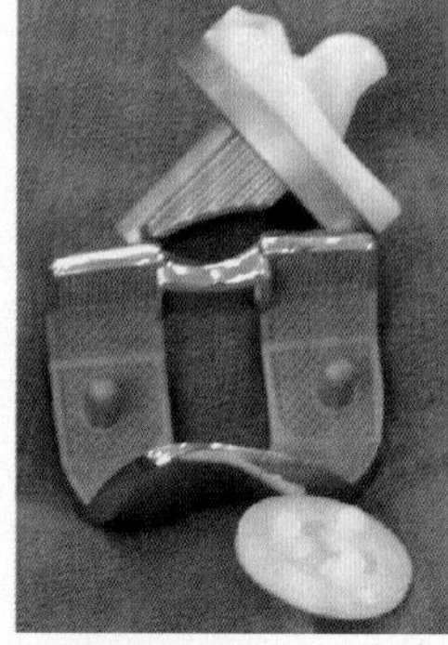

B 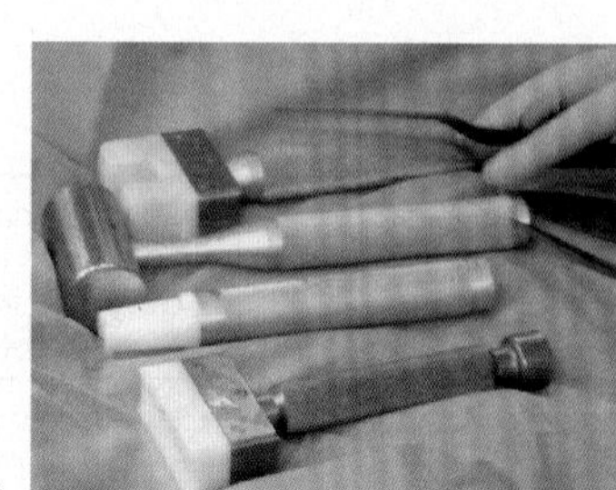

C 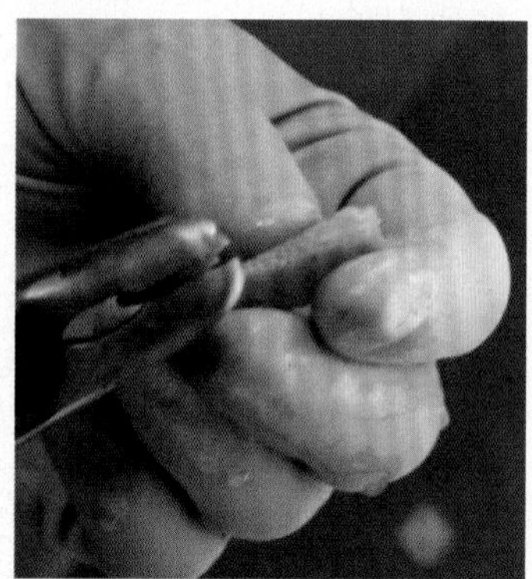

TECH FIG 13 • **A.** All components and (**B**) basic instruments for component insertion are set up in advance of cement preparation. **C.** The IM hole of the distal femur is plugged with small fragments of cancellous bone. *(continued)*

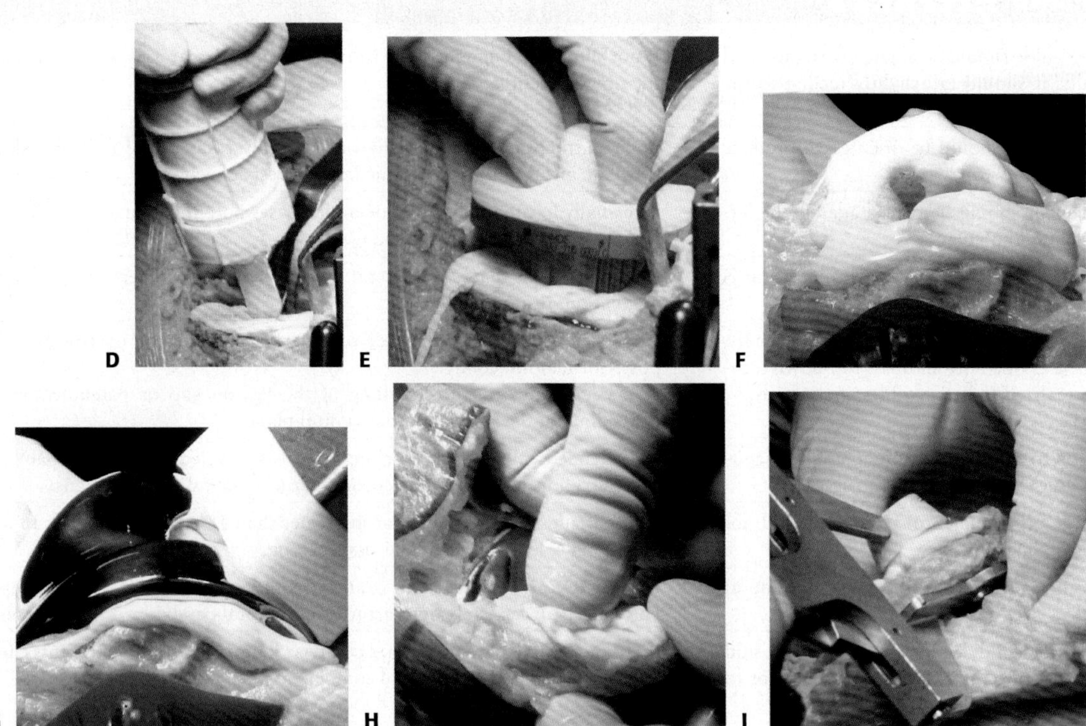

TECH FIG 13 • *(continued)* **D.** Cement is applied to the tibial plateau. **E.** A thin layer of cement is added to the tibial tray, and the tibial component and polyethylene liner are impacted into place. **F.** Cement is applied to the femoral cut surfaces and the femoral component. **G.** The femoral component is impacted into position. **H.** Cement is applied to the patella. **I.** The patellar component is inserted and clamped firmly.

- Apply cement to the femoral cut surfaces (**TECH FIG 13F**).
  - It can be difficult to place cement on the posterior femoral condyles, so cement is often applied directly to the component prior to impaction.
- Impact the femoral component into position and remove the excess cement from around the prosthesis (**TECH FIG 13G**).
- Reduce the knee and bring it to full extension. It may be useful to place a small bump under the ankle to ensure full extension of the knee at this stage.
- With the knee extended, apply cement to the patella (**TECH FIG 13H**). Insert the patellar component and clamp it firmly in place (**TECH FIG 13I**). Trim and remove the excess cement.
- Keep the knee in full extension until the cement is fully cured. Inspect all the corners of the joint, especially the posterior parts, to make certain that no extra cement or loose pieces of bone or cement remain.
- Irrigate the knee thoroughly. For the last time before closing the joint, check the ROM, knee stability, and patellar tracking.

Closure

- Copiously irrigate the knee to ensure that no bone or cement particles remain.
- Identify the formerly placed markings. Close the arthrotomy to produce a watertight seal.
- Place the knee through a full ROM to make sure that the closure is strong enough not to rupture during physical therapy and confirm that the patella is tracking normally.
- Close subcutaneous tissue and superficial fascia with interrupted no. 2 Vicryl stitches or its equivalent in a single layer. (Use a double layer if the patient is obese.)
- Close the skin with a quickly absorbing suture or skin clips.

PEARLS AND PITFALLS

The tibial cutting guide should be aligned with the tibial crest, and distally, it should fall slightly medial to the midpoint of the malleoli.	▪ If not shifted 3–5 mm medially from the intermalleolar axis, varus orientation of the tibial resection will result.
The tibial cutting guide should be oriented to produce 3–7 degrees of posterior slope.	▪ If the cutting guide is internally or externally rotated, the posterior slope will translate into valgus or varus inclination, respectively.
The tibial component should be placed against the lateral margin of the tibial plateau.	▪ A medially located tibial component increases both the Q-angle (causing patellar maltracking) and medial overhang.
The starting point for the femoral IM rod insertion is approximately 1 cm anterior to the PCL insertion.	▪ A starting point that is too lateral or too medial will increase valgus and varus angulation, respectively.
The femoral component should be sized appropriately, and the consequences of a bottom-up or top-down technique should be realized to help avoid complications.	▪ Undersizing introduces the risk of anterior notching or overresection of the posterior femoral condyles. ▪ Oversizing can cause overstuffing of the flexion gap or patellofemoral joint, depending on the position in the sagittal plane.
Pay close attention to the distal femoral cut in the sagittal plane to avoid flexion or extension.	▪ An extended cut will risk notching, whereas a flexed cut can risk patellar maltracking and cam/post impingement in cruciate-substituting designs.
The distal femoral cut in the coronal plane should not exceed 7 degrees of valgus.	▪ Coronal alignment of the femur in greater than 7 degrees of valgus can increase the Q-angle, leading to patellar maltracking.
Use a combination of references for assessing femoral rotation.	▪ Using only one reference can result in malrotation of the femoral component, particularly in cases of valgus arthritis or femoral condyle erosion or hypoplasia.
If using the posterior condylar line as a reference, add an extra degree or two to the external rotation prior to making cuts in valgus knees.	▪ If not recognized, lateral femoral condylar hypoplasia in these patients can cause internal rotation of the femoral component.
Lateralization of the femoral component can help patellar tracking.	▪ Medial overhang of the femoral component can cause significant tissue irritation and patellar maltracking by increasing the Q-angle.
The goal of patellar resection is to remove the same thickness that will be replaced by the component.	▪ Overresection may result in patellar fracture or osteonecrosis. Decreasing the overall thickness of the patella can result in extensor mechanism weakness.
At least 12–14 mm of bone should be left in all cases.	▪ Underresection can result in overstuffing of the patellofemoral joint, leading to excessive lateral soft tissue tension, patellar maltracking, anterior knee pain, and limited flexion.
Medialization and superior positioning of the patellar component can help tracking.	▪ Lateral positioning increases the Q-angle and causes patellar maltracking.

POSTOPERATIVE CARE

- At the conclusion of the operation, a gently compressive bandage may be applied.
- Current analgesic strategies employ a multimodal approach to pain management:
  - Pre- and perioperative use of anti-inflammatories and nerve modulator therapy
  - Intraoperative local analgesic injections or placement of intra-articular pain pumps
  - Postoperative use of intravenous cyclooxygenase (COX) inhibitors and acetaminophen
  - Narcotic and nonnarcotic oral pain medications
- Antibiotics are typically administered for one to two doses postoperatively.
- Initiate appropriate thromboprophylaxis.
- Postoperative rehabilitation protocols vary but typically include the following:
  - Early mobilization and initiation of weight-bearing activities
  - Early ROM
  - Appropriate pain management
  - Allowing sufficient periods of rest to help limit excessive swelling and inflammation.
  - Weaning off assistive devices as tolerated.
- Common therapeutic exercises include the following:
  - Active, active-assisted, and passive ROM exercises
  - Quadriceps sets
  - Straight-leg raises
  - Occupational therapy (eg, transfer training, stair climbing)
- Patients typically are discharged 1 to 3 days after surgery, either to home or to an inpatient rehabilitation facility.
- Early office follow-up concentrates on wound healing and progression of strength and ROM.
  - Early wound complication needs to be followed closely.
  - Early stiffness must be monitored, with manipulation under anesthesia considered at 6 to 8 weeks following surgery if stiffness persists.
- Once strength, mobility, and balance are regained, patients can resume low-impact sport activities (eg, cycling, swimming, gentle aerobic-style exercises, walking, hiking, golf, or bowling).
- Higher impact activities such as basketball, soccer, and football are generally discouraged, but current data do not suggest an absolute contraindication.

OUTCOMES

- TKA is a reliable and predictable surgery, with recently reported survival rates above 95% at 10 years and above 85%

up to 23 years of follow-up. Favorable gains for pain and functionality following TKA are well reported and recognized.[10,14]

- For the vast majority of patients, overall satisfaction with the outcome of the surgery is good to excellent.
- Patients who tend to have lower satisfaction rates and therefore deserve special consideration and counseling prior to surgery include the following[12,19]:
  - Younger patients (age younger than 50 years) with knee arthritis
  - Morbidly obese patients (body mass index >40 kg/m^2)
  - Patients with prior reconstructive knee surgery (eg, osteotomy, patellar realignment)
  - Patients receiving worker's compensation

COMPLICATIONS

- The overall mortality rate following TKA is very low, and this procedure does not considerably reduce the life expectancy in patients with OA.

Infection

- Infection should be considered in any persistently painful TKA or with the acute onset of pain in a previously well-functioning TKA.
- Workup for infection should include at the very least[15]
  - Appropriate history and physical examination
  - Radiographs
  - Lab work, including erythrocyte sedimentation rate (ESR) and C-reactive protein (CRP)
  - Aspirate sent for cell count, gram stain, and culture
- Physical examination findings consistent with infection include the following:
  - Progressive or persistent erythema
  - Persistent drainage, particularly beyond 7 days postoperatively
  - Purulent drainage from the incision
- Radiographic evidence of infection includes the following:
  - Progressive radiolucent lines or periprosthetic lysis
  - Progressive loosening or subsidence
- Lab work studies can be variable but typically demonstrate the following:
  - Elevated CRP and ESR
  - Normal to elevated serum white blood cell count
  - Gram stain and culture can be helpful but have a high false-negative rate.[26]
  - Elevated synovial cell white blood cell count and neutrophil percentage[1,6]
    - In the acute setting (up to 6 weeks postoperatively), a synovial fluid white blood cell count of greater than 20,000 and a neutrophil percentage greater than 89% is highly suspicious for infection.
    - In the chronic setting, a synovial fluid white blood cell count of greater than 1500 and a neutrophil percentage greater than 65% is highly suspicious for infection.
  - Presence of leukocyte esterase in the synovial fluid[18]
- Superficial incisional infection, characterized by erythema, dry wound, nonpurulence, and neither loculation nor induration, may be treated with systemic antibiotics with the understanding that once antibiotic therapy is initiated, the opportunity to accurately diagnose a deep infection may be lost.
  - Drainage for up to 1 week may be observed with local wound care and immobilization, but drainage beyond a week warrants open débridement.
- In contrast, a wound with either drainage or skin necrosis usually benefits from prompt surgical débridement, at which time, reliable culture material may be obtained if antibiotic therapy has not been initiated.[25]

Instability

- Instability after TKA is the cause of failure in 10% to 20% of all failures. Successful outcomes are obtained in many of these cases, but without identifying the cause of instability, the surgeon risks repeating the mistakes that led to the instability after the initial TKA.[17]
- Three types of instability may occur after a TKA:
  - Extension instability
  - Flexion instability
  - Genu recurvatum
- Surgical treatment is generally indicated and is largely aimed at restoring balanced flexion and extension gaps at the time of revision TKA. Selective use of constrained and rotating hinge TKA designs is appropriate for subgroups of patients with instability.[17]

Osteolysis

- The most significant cause for late revision TKA is osteolysis, which occurs as the result of a foreign body response to particulate wear debris from the prosthetic joint, ultimately resulting in loosening of the components.
- Osteolysis is often asymptomatic.
- Symptomatic osteolysis typically indicates a fairly progressed process and presents with the following[7]:
  - Pain, which is often worse at the initiation of gait (start-up pain)
  - Swelling
  - Instability
  - Crepitus
- Depending on the clinical situation, asymptomatic osteolysis can be followed with serial radiographs, whereas symptomatic osteolysis usually necessitates revision surgery.

Vascular Injury

- Popliteal artery injury during TKA is rare but potentially catastrophic.
- The injury may have acute or delayed presentation.
- Causes include the following:
  - Arterial thrombosis due to tourniquet application
  - Arterial kinking during knee manipulation
  - Direct injury to the artery
- Direct, sharp arterial injury is believed to have a better prognosis than arterial thrombosis.
- Prompt recognition of injury by the orthopaedic surgeon and treatment by an experienced vascular surgeon are necessary to achieve a good outcome.[4]

Nerve Injury

- Both the tibial and peroneal nerves may be injured during TKA.
- Preoperative flexion contracture, particularly in the setting of a concomitant valgus deformity, is a risk factor for postoperative nerve palsy.
- Postoperative hematoma also increases the risk of peroneal nerve injury.

- Initial therapy once nerve palsy is recognized includes the following:
  - Knee and hip flexion to 20 to 45 degrees and immediate release of constrictive dressings.
- Surgical exploration of the non-neurolytic nerve can be employed if no functional recovery is noted after 3 months from the onset of the injury.[22]

REFERENCES

1. Bedair H, Ting N, Jacovides C, et al. The Mark Coventry Award: diagnosis of early postoperative TKA infection using synovial fluid analysis. Clin Orthop Relat Res 2011;469(1):34–40.
2. Benjamin J. Component alignment in total knee arthroplasty. Instr Course Lect 2006;55:405–412.
3. Bonutti PM, Zywiel MG, Ulrich SD, et al. A comparison of subvastus and midvastus approaches in minimally invasive total knee arthroplasty. J Bone Joint Surg Am 2010;92(3):575–582.
4. Da Silva MS, Sobel M. Popliteal vascular injury during total knee arthroplasty. J Surg Res 2003;109:170–174.
5. Eisenhuth SA, Saleh KJ, Cui Q, et al. Patellofemoral instability after total knee arthroplasty. Clin Orthop Relat Res 2006;446:149–160.
6. Ghanem E, Parvizi J, Burnett RS, et al. Cell count and differential of aspirated fluid in diagnosis of infection at the site of total knee arthroplasty. J Bone Joint Surg Am 2008;90(8):1637–1643.
7. Gupta SK, Chu A, Ranawat AS, et al. Osteolysis after total knee arthroplasty. J Arthroplasty 2007;22:787–799.
8. Howell SM, Howell SJ, Kuznik KT, et al. Does a kinematically aligned total knee arthroplasty restore function without failure regardless of alignment category? Clin Orthop Relat Res 2013;471(3):1000–1007.
9. Kim YH, Choi Y, Kwon OR, et al. Functional outcome and range of motion of high-flexion posterior cruciate-retaining and high-flexion posterior cruciate-substituting total knee prostheses. A prospective, randomized study. J Bone Joint Surg Am 2009;91(4):753–760.
10. Kim YH, Kim JS, Choe JW, et al. Long-term comparison of fixed-bearing and mobile-bearing total knee replacements in patients younger than fifty-one years of age with osteoarthritis. J Bone Joint Surg Am 2012;94(10):866–873.
11. Lombardi AV Jr, Berend KR. Posterior cruciate ligament-retaining, posterior stabilized, and varus/valgus posterior stabilized constrained articulations in total knee arthroplasty. Instr Course Lect 2006; 55:419–427.
12. McElroy MJ, Pivec R, Issa K, et al. The effects of obesity and morbid obesity on outcomes in TKA. J Knee Surg 2013;26(2):83–88.
13. McPherson EJ. Patellar tracking in primary total knee arthroplasty. Instr Course Lect 2006;55:439–448.
14. Meftah M, Ranawat AS, Ranawat CS. Ten-year follow-up of a rotating-platform, posterior-stabilized total knee arthroplasty. J Bone Joint Surg Am 2012;94(5):426–432.
15. Mihalko WM, Manaswi A, Cui Q, et al. Diagnosis and treatment of the infected primary total knee arthroplasty. Instr Course Lect 2008;57:327–339.
16. Nestor BJ, Toulson CE, Backus SI, et al. Mini-midvastus vs standard medial parapatellar approach: a prospective, randomized, double-blinded study in patients undergoing bilateral total knee arthroplasty. J Arthroplasty 2010;25(6 suppl):5–11.
17. Parratte S, Pagnano MW. Instability after total knee arthroplasty. J Bone Joint Surg Am 2008;90:184–194.
18. Parvizi J, Jacovides C, Antoci V, et al. Diagnosis of periprosthetic joint infection: the utility of a simple yet unappreciated enzyme. J Bone Joint Surg Am 2011;93(24):2242–2248.
19. Parvizi J, Nunley RM, Berend KR, et al. High level of residual symptoms in young after total knee arthroplasty. Clin Orthop Relat Res 2014;472(1):133–137.
20. Patel J, Ries MD, Bozic KJ. Extensor mechanism complications after total knee arthroplasty. Instr Course Lect 2008;57:283–294.
21. Peters CL. Soft-tissue balancing in primary total knee arthroplasty. Instr Course Lect 2006;55:413–417.
22. Schinsky MF, Macaulay W, Parks ML, et al. Nerve injury after primary total knee arthroplasty. J Arthroplasty 2001;16:1048–1054.
23. Umrani SP, Cho KY, Kim KI. Patellar eversion does not adversely affect quadriceps recovery following total knee arthroplasty. J Arthroplasty 2013;28(4):591–594.
24. Verra WC, van den Boom LG, Jacobs W, et al. Retention versus sacrifice of the posterior cruciate ligament in total knee arthroplasty for treating osteoarthritis. Cochrane Database Syst Rev 2013;10:CD004803.
25. Vince K, Chivas D, Droll KP. Wound complications after total knee arthroplasty. J Arthroplasty 2007;22(4 suppl 1):39–44.
26. Zywiel MG, Stroh DA, Johnson AJ, et al. Gram stains have limited application in the diagnosis of infected total knee arthroplasty. Int J Infect Dis 2011;15(10):e702–705.

Fixation of Periprosthetic Fractures Above Total Knee Arthroplasty

38
CHAPTER

Frank A. Liporace and Derek J. Donegan

DEFINITION

- Fractures that occur above or around the femoral component of a total knee arthroplasty (TKA).
- The rates of periprosthetic fractures for TKA vary.
- The incidence is reported to be 0.3% to 5.5% after primary TKA and up to 30% after revision TKA.[3,5,6,13]
- Supracondylar femur fractures are the most common type and the most widely reported with an incidence of 0.3% to 2.5% for primary TKA and 1.6% to 38% for revision TKA.[5,6,8,13]
- Can occur in the setting of a stable prosthesis or an unstable prosthesis
- Periprosthetic fractures can create substantial difficulty with regard to management and outcome.
- Reduction and fixation of these fractures is a complex undertaking, primarily as a result of the preexisting implants that can obstruct reduction and placement of fixation devices.[2]

ANATOMY

- The distal femur is a trapezoidal shape.
- The lateral distal femur is larger in the anteroposterior (AP) diameter than the medial distal femur.
- The lateral femoral condyle has a 10-degree slope.
- The medial femoral condyle has a 25-degree slope (**FIG 1**).
- The origin of the gastrocnemius on the distal femur acts as a deforming force leading to a recurvatum deformity.
- The insertion of the adductors on the distal femur acts as a deforming force leading to a varus deformity (**FIG 2**).

PATHOGENESIS

- Most periprosthetic femur fractures typically result from a low-energy fall in the elderly or a high-energy trauma in a young person.[1]
- Multiple risk factors have been identified.
- Metabolic issues such as osteoporosis are known risk factors for the development of periprosthetic fractures about a TKA.
- Many studies have demonstrated a decrease bone mineral density after TKA.[11]
- Surgical technique has also been implicated, specifically notching of the distal femur.
- Violation of the anterior cortex of the distal femur has been thought to be an important risk factor for periprosthetic distal femur fracture after TKA.
- There is a theoretical increased risk due to the change of the geometry of the femur and the decrease radius of curvature leading to higher stresses on the distal femur.

NATURAL HISTORY

- The goals of treatment, whether surgical or nonsurgical, are fracture healing, restoration and maintenance of knee range of motion, and pain-free function.

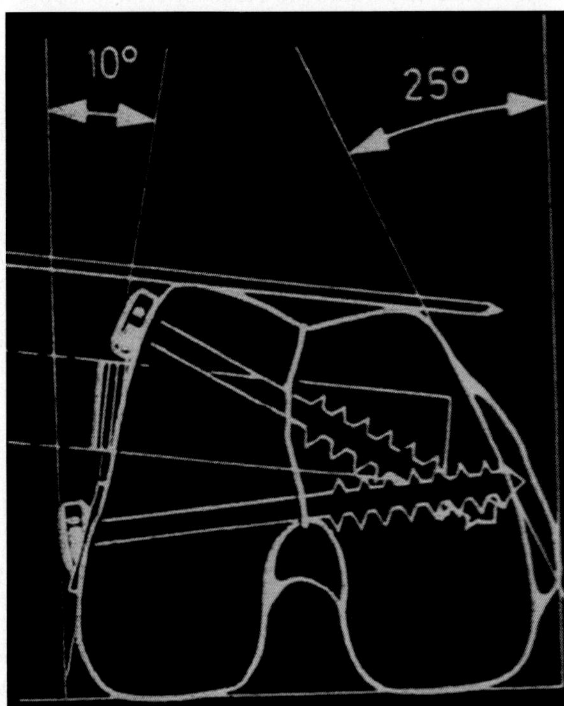

FIG 1 • Schematic representation of axial of distal femoral anatomy. Note the trapezoidal shape and angular differential on lateral versus medial side.

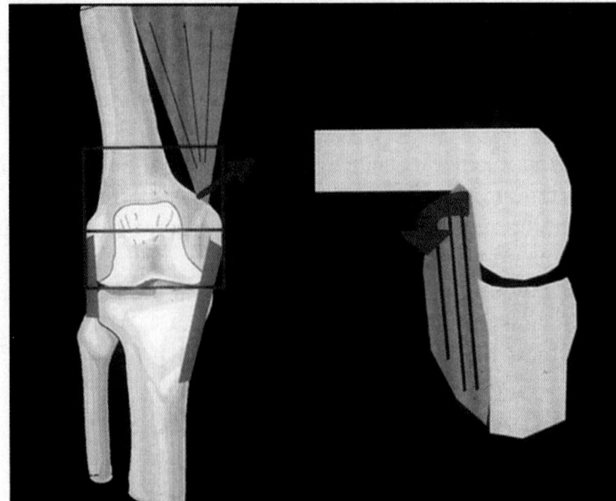

FIG 2 • Schematic representation of main muscular deforming forces to distal femoral fractures (adductors and gastrocnemius, respectively).

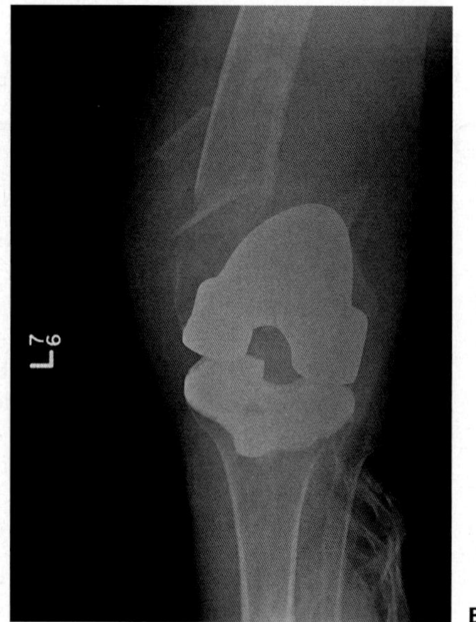

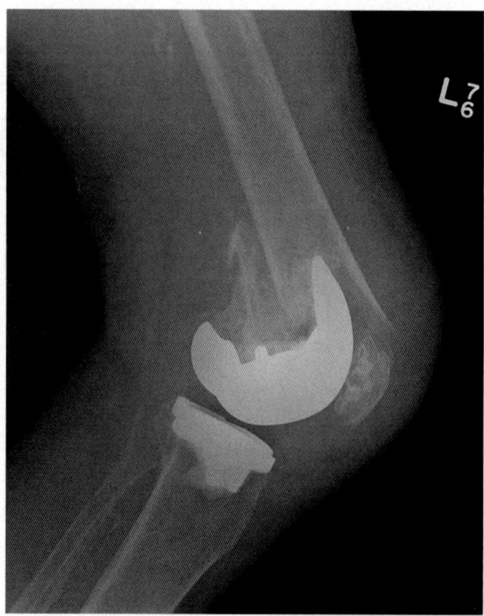

FIG 3 • AP (**A**) and lateral (**B**) radiographs of typical periprosthetic distal femur fracture. Note the fracture occurs at the level of the anterior flange of the total knee replacement and progress posteriorly with variable comminution.

- A good result is a minimum of 90 degrees of knee motion, fracture shortening less than or equal to 2 cm, varus/valgus malalignment less than or equal to 5 degrees, and flexion/extension malalignment less than or equal to 10 degrees.[14]
- Nonsurgical management using skeletal traction, casting, or cast bracing has been used in primary fractures; however, due to the prolonged immobility and risks associated, surgical intervention is preferred unless the patient is too sick to undergo the procedure.

PATIENT HISTORY AND PHYSICAL FINDINGS

- It is important to get a history and try to elicit any preexisting symptoms that may indicate whether or not an implant is loose, such as pain or instability.
- Medical records are helpful to identify surgical approach as well as type of implants.
- If there is suspicion for infection based on preexisting symptoms or preinjury films demonstrating loosening, further investigation should take place to include complete blood count (CBC), erythrocyte sedimentation rate (ESR), and noncardiac C-reactive protein (CRP).
- If the infection workup is suspicious, then intraoperative biopsy or staged procedures should be planned.
- Following a general medical examination, a comprehensive examination of the affected limb should be performed.
- The condition of the skin and neurovascular status should be documented.
- Specifically, ankle–brachial index (ABI) should be performed and documented.
- An ABI less than 0.90 warrants further investigation.[9]

IMAGING AND OTHER DIAGNOSTIC STUDIES

- Standard AP and lateral of the affected extremity should be obtained (**FIG 3**).
- It is also routine practice to get images of the joint above and below the injury.
- Mechanical axis series can also be beneficial in certain instances.
- Advance imaging can be helpful to determine bone stock but are not routinely required (**FIG 4**).

DIFFERENTIAL DIAGNOSIS

- Loose TKA
- Infected TKA
- Periprosthetic tibial fracture
- Periprosthetic patellar fracture
- Periprosthetic fracture around a total hip arthroplasty (THA)

NONOPERATIVE MANAGEMENT

- Indication for nonoperative management include truly nondisplaced fractures with a stable prosthesis or a patient that is too medically unstable for surgery.
- Nonsurgical management includes skeletal traction, casting, or cast bracing.
- Nonsurgical management does eliminate the surgical risks such as bleeding, infection, loss of fixation, and anesthetic complications.
- With nonsurgical management, the extremity should be kept immobilized in extension for 4 to 6 weeks and the patient kept non–weight bearing.

SURGICAL MANAGEMENT

- Once surgical management has been decided, it is crucial to determine if the implant is stable or not.
- Fractures about a stable femoral component are typically treated with intramedullary nailing (IMN) or laterally based locked plating.
- Retrograde IMN represents a good option when there is adequate bone stock and an "open box" TKA femoral component.
- Locked plates represent a significant advance in the treatment of periprosthetic fractures of the distal femur.

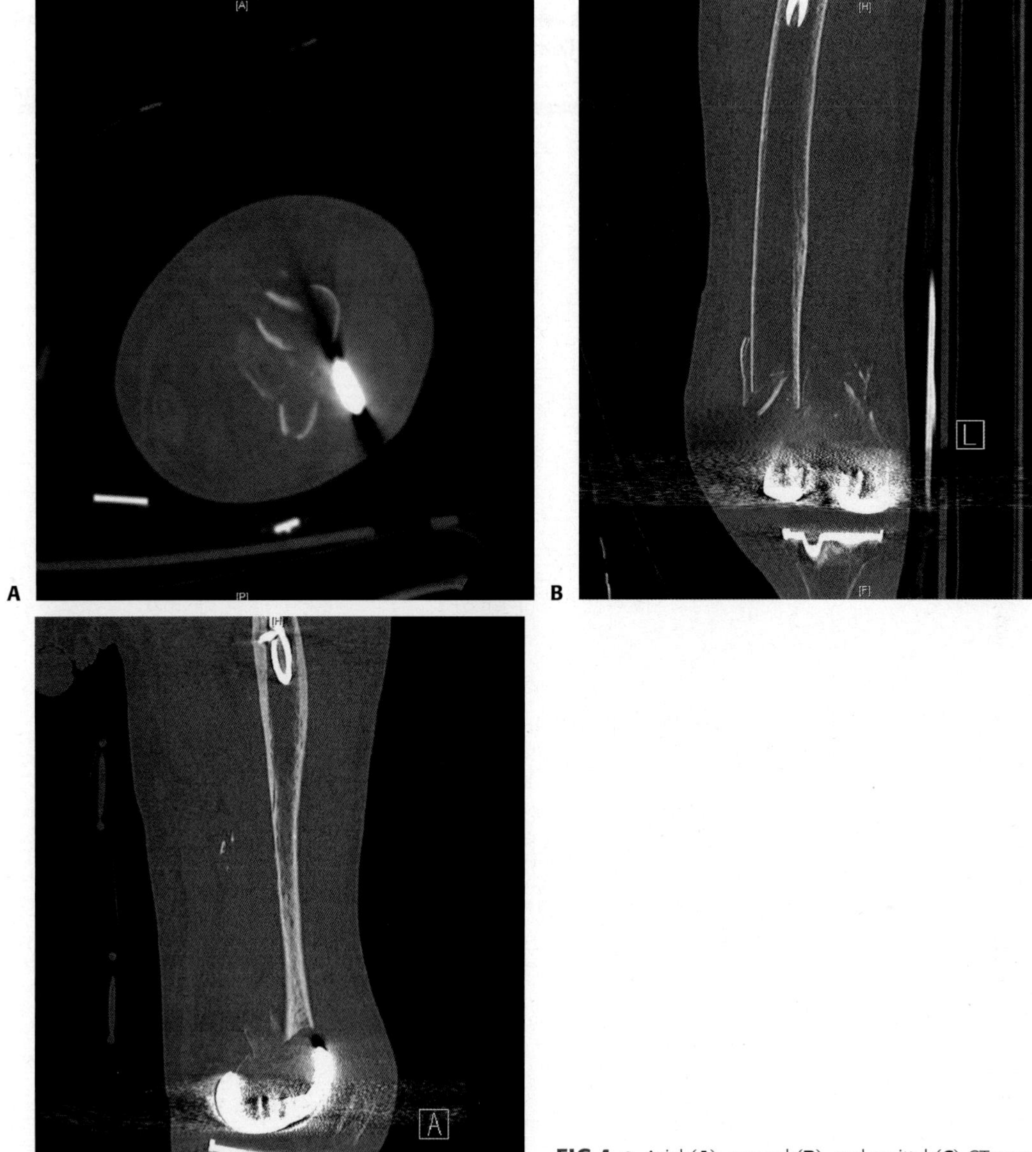

FIG 4 ● Axial (**A**), coronal (**B**), and sagittal (**C**) CT scan of distal femoral periprosthetic fracture that shows location and comminution.

- Advantages of locked plating include the ability for multiple fixed-angle points of fixation in osteoporotic bone, increased biomechanical strength over conventional plates, and the ability for insertion in minimally invasive techniques.[10]
- When minimally invasive techniques are used, it is crucial to avoid the typical malalignment of valgus and hyperextension of the distal fragment.[4]
- When periprosthetic fractures above a TKA are associated with a loose component, revision arthroplasty is the treatment of choice.

Preoperative Planning

- The history and physical is reviewed.
- Preinjury radiographs are reviewed if available to determine if there was any evidence of loosening or infection.
- Evidence of infection requires further workup as mentioned earlier.
- Prior operative reports are obtained and reviewed specifically looking for type of implant to determine if the femoral component is an open box or not (Table 1).
- Injury films are reviewed and classified (Table 2).
- Key factors in decision-making process for operative treatment:
  - Is the bone stock adequate?
  - Does the implant have an open or closed box?
  - Is the implant loose or stable?
- If the implant is stable and there is adequate bone stock, then open reduction and internal fixation (ORIF) is treatment of choice:
  - If implant has open box, then IMN versus laterally based locked plate
  - If implant has closed box, then laterally based locked plate
- If the implant is loose, then revision arthroplasty

Table 1 Chart of Common Manufacturers and Implants with Representative Intercondylar Width That Limits Nail Size Usage for Retrograde Intramedullary Nailing of Distal Femoral Periprosthetic Fracture

Component	Model	Size	Intercondylar Width (mm)
Biomet			
	Maxim Primary		13.3
		PS Open Box	15.2
		PS Closed Box	Closed
	AGC 3000		18.0
		PS	18.0
		HPS	15.4
	Ascent Primary		18.4
		PS Open box	20.3
		PS Closed box	Closed
	Vanguard		
		PS	16.2
		CR	13.3
Smith & Nephew			
	Genesis I		
		CR	20.1
		PS	17.9
	Genesis II		
		CR 1–2	16.0
		CR 3–9	18.5
		PS	16.3
	Profix		
		CR	19.8
		PS	14.6
	Tricon M and C		17.0
Stryker Howmedica			
	Duracon		18.5
	Stabilizer		Stemmed
	Kinemax		
		XS	17.0
		S	18.5
		M	19.5
		L	21.0
		XL	22.5
		XXL	22.5
		Modular Condylar and Plus	Stemmed
		Modular Stabilizer and Plus	Closed
	Kinematic II		21.0
		Condylar	Stemmed
		Stabilizer	Closed
	PCA		
		S	16, 18
		M	15, 18
		M/L	15, 16
		L	13, 15
		XL	12, 15
	Scorpio		
		CR/PS 3	16.5
		CR/PS 5	16.5
		CR/PS 7	18.5
		CR/PS 9	18.5
		CR/PS 11	20.5
		CR/PS 13	20.5
		TS	Stemmed
	Series 7000 PS		20.5
		Modular	Stemmed
		Omnifit	20.5
		PS	Closed
	Triathlon CR/PS		16.0

(continued)

Table 1 *(continued)*

Component			Intercondylar Width (mm)
Zimmer, Centerpulse, Sulzermedica			
	Nexgen CR		
		A	11.9
		B	12.1
		C	12.2
		D	12.5
		E	12.8
		F	12.9
		G	13.3
		H	13.4
	Nexgen PS/LPS		
		A	13.7
		B	13.7
		C	16.6
		D	16.6
		E	17.8
		F	17.8
		G	21.2
		H	21.2
	1/8 I PSCK		
		55	15.7
		58	15.5
		65	17.0
		66	17.1
		70	18.8
	1/8 II PSCK		
		54	15.3
		59	16.7
		64	18.2
		69	19.6
		74	21.0
	M/G 1		
		S	10.6
		S+	10.6
		Reg	12.1
		Reg+	12.3
		L	14.4
		L+	14.3
		L++	17.4
	M/G II		11.9
	Natural Knee I		
		0–1	12
		2	16
		3	19
		4	20
		5	22
	Natural Knee II		17
	Apollo		17
Dow Corning & Wright Medical			
	Axiom Primary		
		55	14
		60	15
		65	17
		70	18
		75	19
		80	20
		85	22
		PS 55	16
		PS 60	18
		PS 65	18
		PS 70	20
		PS 75	21
		PS 80	23
		PS 85	24
		Modular	Closed

(continued)

Table 1 *(continued)*

Component			**Intercondylar Width (mm)**
	Advance Primary		
		PS 1	15
		PS 2	17
		PS 3	18
		PS 4	19
		PS 5	21
		PS 6	22
	Advantium		
		TC	19
		Open house	16
		PS	Closed
	Ortholoc		
		Standard	21
		Large	25
		Ex Large	25
	Ortholoc II		24
Depuy and J&J			
	PFC		
		CR	20
		CS 1	14.3
		CS 2	15.1
		CS 3	17.0
		CS 4-6	20.0
	PFC Sigma		
		CR	12.7, 17.8
		CS	17.8
	AMK		
		CR 1	14.2
		CR 2	16.4
		CR 2+	16.5
		CR 3	18.5
		CR 3+	17.9
		CR 4	17.6
		CR 5	20.6
	CS Congruency		
		1	18.7
		2	19.7
		3	21.9
		4	22
		5	24.8
	LCS Complete CR		
		Sm	14.4
		Sm+	15.7
		Med	16.6
		Std	17.5
		Std+	18.8
		Lrg	20.3
		Lrg+	21.9

Modified from Heckler MW, Tennant GS, Williams DP, et al. Retrograde nailing of supracondylar periprosthetic femur fractures: a surgeon's guide to femoral component sizing. Orthopedics 2007;30(5):345–348.

Positioning

- When performing operative fixation of a periprosthetic femur fracture above a TKA (plate or IMN), the patient is usually positioned supine on a radiolucent flat-top Jackson table (**FIG 5**).
- Position the patient to the ipsilateral side of the table.
- One rolled blanket bump is placed under the ipsilateral hip.
- Tape the ipsilateral arm over the chest.
- Sequential compression devices (SCDs) on contralateral extremity
- Secure the patient with safety belt at abdomen level and 2-inch silk tape over blue towel on contralateral leg.
- Make sure all bony prominences are padded.
- C-arm will enter from contralateral side, perpendicular to the operating room (OR) table.

Table 2 Chart of Classifications Commonly Used for Distal Femoral Periprosthetic Fractures

Supracondylar Periprosthetic Fractures: Classification Systems

Study	Type/Group	Description
Neer et al	Type I	Undisplaced (<5 mm displacement and/or <5 degrees angulation)
	Type II	Displaced >1 cm
	Type IIa	With lateral femoral shaft displacement
	Type IIb	With medial femoral shaft displacement
	Type III	Displaced and comminuted
DiGioia and Rubash	Group I	Extra-articular, undisplaced (<5 mm displacement and <5 degrees angulation)
	Group II	Extra-articular, displaced (>5 mm displacement or >5 degrees angulation)
	Group III	Severely displaced (loss of cortical contact) or angulated (>10 degrees); may have intercondylar or T-shaped component
Chen et al	Type I	Nondisplaced (Neer type I)
	Type II	Displaced and/or comminuted (Neer types II and III)
Lewis and Rorabeck	Type I	Undisplaced fracture; prosthesis intact
	Type II	Displaced fracture; prosthesis intact
	Type III	Displaced or undisplaced fracture; prosthesis loose or failing

Modified from Su ET, DeWal H, Di Cesare PE. Periprosthetic femoral fractures above total knee replacements. J Am Acad Orthop Surg 2004;12(1):12–20.

- When plating, a black ramp can be placed under the ipsilateral leg.
- When nailing, a radiolucent triangle is used to support the femur.
- For difficult fractures to reduce, sterile skeletal traction can be placed and weight hung off the end of the bed over a pipe bender.

Approach

- For lateral locked plating, a standard lateral approach to the femur can be used. This can be extended into a subvastus approach if extension proximally is desired.
- For retrograde IMN, a standard midline incision can be used with a medial parapatellar arthrotomy.

A

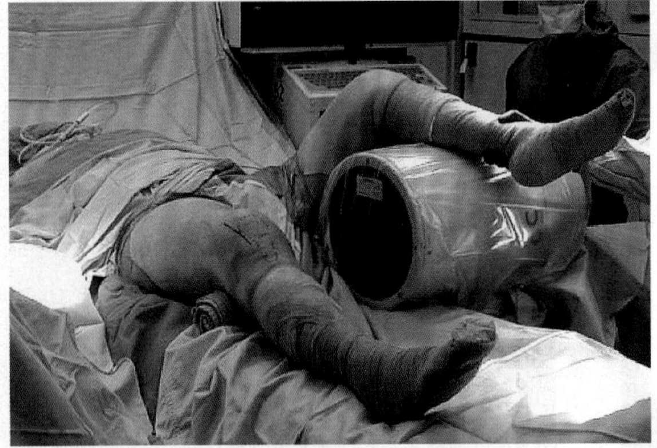

B

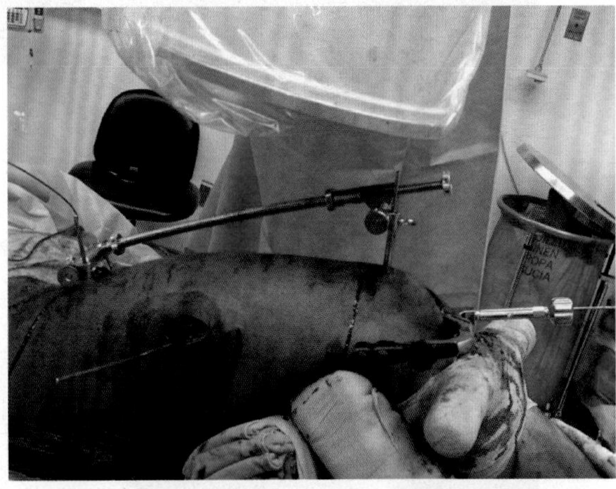

FIG 5 • A. Patient positioning supine for distal femoral plate fixation. Both legs sterile prepped to allow for elevation of nonaffected extremity and prevent movement of operative extremity to allow for accurate lateral fluoroscopy without potential displacement of reduction. Note laterally drawn incision. Note sterile bump under area of fracture site to aid with sagittal reduction. **B.** Positioning for retrograde nail. Note percutaneous reduction incision laterally, femoral distractor for length, proximal tibia pin for manual traction, and bump positioning for sagittal alignment. Femoral distractor placed anteriorly and medially to proposed track of ultimate IMN.

Laterally Locked Plating

Exposure—Lateral Approach to Femur

- Mark out landmarks of joint line and femoral shaft/condyle (**TECH FIG 1A**).
- Mark lateral incision in line with the femoral shaft starting at Gerdy tubercle and extending proximally to include fracture site (**TECH FIG 1A**).
- Incise skin along marked incision down to level of iliotibial (IT) band fascia.
- Incise fascia in line with the skin.
- Expose vermillion border and/or border of femoral component.
- Be mindful to remain extra-articular and avoid violation of the joint capsule.
- If plan to bridge fracture, do not expose fracture site.
- If plan for direct anatomic reduction, extend proximally to subvastus to directly visualize the fracture.

Reduction/Fixation

- Length, alignment, and rotation are assessed using fluoroscopy.
- A bump is used to control the sagittal balance. This should be placed strategically to counteract the forces of the gastrocnemius and the recurvatum deformity (**TECH FIG 1B,C**).
- Length is achieved and maintained by longitudinal traction either manually or with the use of skeletal traction.

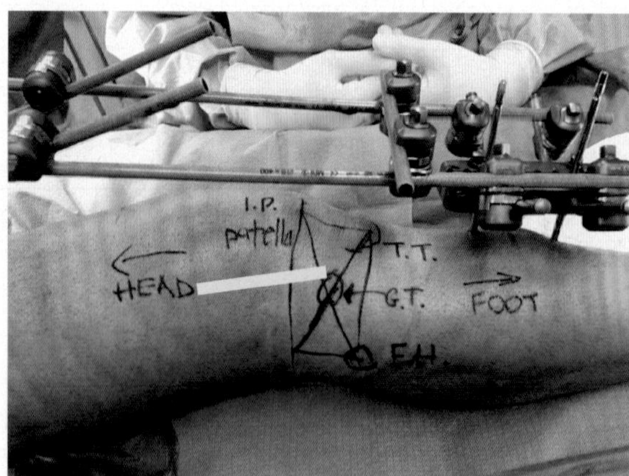

A

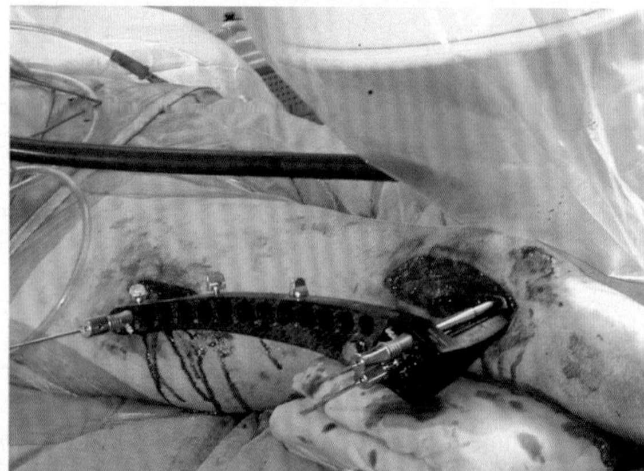

B

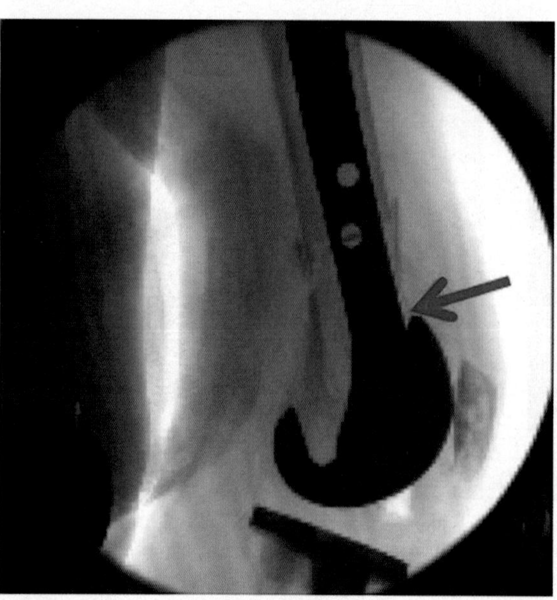

C

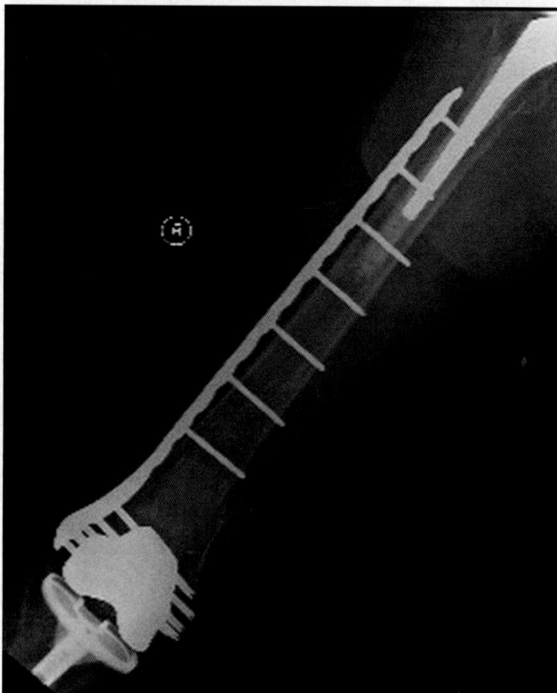

D

TECH FIG 1 • **A.** Gerdy tubercle identification. Central point of "box" of distal pole of patella, fibula head, tibia tubercle, and point in line with perpendicular cross-section of first two landmarks. The yellow line indicates a utilitarian skin incision for plating distal femur fractures, beginning at Gerdy tubercle and extending proximally (about 7 cm). **B.** Laterally based incision distally to allow for passage of plate and proximal provisional fixation through jig to allow for box to be created. **C.** Lateral intraoperative positioning of plate for distal femoral plating. Note plate is sitting as anteriorly as possible to match posterior aspect of anterior flange of implant. This is indicated with the red arrow. **D.** Final AP radiograph of same patient in **C**. Note distal screws in plate parallel to distal femoral condyles to allow for appropriate alignment.

- Once the length, alignment, and rotation are adequate, the appropriate length plate is determined. The goal is to have at least six holes of the plate proximal to the fracture site (**TECH FIG 1D**).
- The plate is then slid submuscularly below the vastus lateralis along the lateral border of the femur. It is important to feel the plate contact the femur throughout the entire course.
- Using AP fluoroscopy, the appropriate plate height is determined.
- The plate is then pinned to the distal segment using a K-wire through the center hole of the plate. Ultimately, this will be replaced with a screw that will be parallel to the distal femoral condyles, aiding in achieving appropriate coronal alignment (**TECH FIG 1D**).
- Using fluoroscopy to get a good lateral, the sagittal plate balance is evaluated and adjusted.
- The plate is then pinned to the proximal femur in the second to last screw hole of the plate using a K-wire through perfect circle technique or an external jig and a stab incision.
- The plate height and balance is then confirmed using AP and lateral fluoroscopy.
- The plate is then secured to bone with a nonlocking screw distally to bring the plate to bone.
- A nonlocking screw is then placed immediately proximal to the fracture site through the plate to bring the plate to bone and make fine adjustments to the coronal balance.
- The overall length, alignment, and rotation, as well as the plate balance, are confirmed.
- The plate is then secured distally using locking screws. It is important to remember the trapezoidal shape of the distal femur as to not place screws that are too long.
- The plate is then secured proximally with hybrid fixation of nonlocked and locked screws spread evenly throughout the shaft of the plate. The most proximal point of fixation is either a unicortical locked screw or a bicortical non-locked screw to ease the transition of stiffness from the plated bone to the remaining host bone. If there is a concomitant hip arthroplasty, then the plate and fixation should overlap by at least 2 femoral cortical diameters (**TECH FIG 1D**).
- Final fluoroscopic evaluation is performed.

Closure

- Place a Hemovac drain if necessary.
- Irrigate wounds.
- No. 1 Vicryl for the fascial layer
- A 2-0 Vicryl for superficial and subcutaneous layers
- A 3-0 nylon mattress for skin
- Sterile dressing and Ace wrap from toes to thigh

Retrograde Intramedullary Nailing

Exposure

- Place a sterile radiolucent triangle under the ipsilateral leg so that the knee is roughly 30 to 40 degrees of flexion.
- Mark out landmarks: inferior pole patella, tibial tubercle, medial and lateral margins of the patellar tendon, previous TKA incision
- Mark out new surgical incision through previous TKA incision roughly 3 cm in length (two fingerbreadths below inferior pole of patella to one fingerbreadth above the inferior pole of the patella).
- Incise skin down to paratenon of patellar tendon.
- Raise small medial and lateral flaps to identify the medial and lateral border of the patellar tendon.
- Make a medial parapatellar arthrotomy to expose the intercondylar notch.
- Débride any scar tissue to clearly visualize the box of the femoral component of the TKA.

Reduction/Fixation

- Length, alignment, and rotation are assessed using fluoroscopy.
- A bump is used to control the sagittal balance. This should be placed strategically to counteract the forces of the gastrocnemius and the recurvatum deformity (see **FIG 5B**).
- Length is achieved and maintained by longitudinal traction either manually or with the use of skeletal traction.
- Insert the guidewire through the incision to the appropriate starting point and confirm fluoroscopically (**TECH FIG 2A,B**).
  - AP view: slightly lateral to midline aiming straight up the intramedullary canal
  - Lateral view: slightly anterior aiming straight up the intramedullary canal
- Insert the guidewire until the pin is past the fracture site and into the metaphyseal region of the femur.
- Confirm location of guidewire and reduction on fluoroscopy.
- Open the distal femur with the appropriate opening reamer. Due to implant designs, it is sometimes necessary to enlarge the box with a metal-cutting burr in order to fit the appropriate size reamers and nail through the box.
- Remove the opening reamer and guidewire.
- Place the ball-tipped guidewire through the entry site and up the entire length of the femur.
- Use the depth gauge and determine the length of the nail.
- Begin reaming with the end-cutting reamer and increase by 0.5 mm until 1 mm over the diameter nail being inserted.
- Assemble the nail and targeting jig on the back table.
- Insert nail over the ball-tipped guidewire as far as possible by hand then advance until fully seated with mallet assistance.
- Be sure nail is buried deep to femoral component.

Locking the Nail

- Insert the trocar assembly through the targeting jig and make small stab incision at the site of screw insertion.
- Drill both cortices with the pilot drill and measure the screw length using the calibrations on the drill it and confirm with a depth gauge. Again, be aware of the trapezoidal shape of the distal femur to avoid long screws.
- Insert the appropriate length screw.
- Repeat this step for two to three interlocking screws depending on the location of the fracture.
- Confirm the length, alignment, and rotation prior to continuing with the proximal interlocking screws.
- Bring the C-arm proximally and obtain perfect circles of the proximal AP interlocking holes.

TECHNIQUES

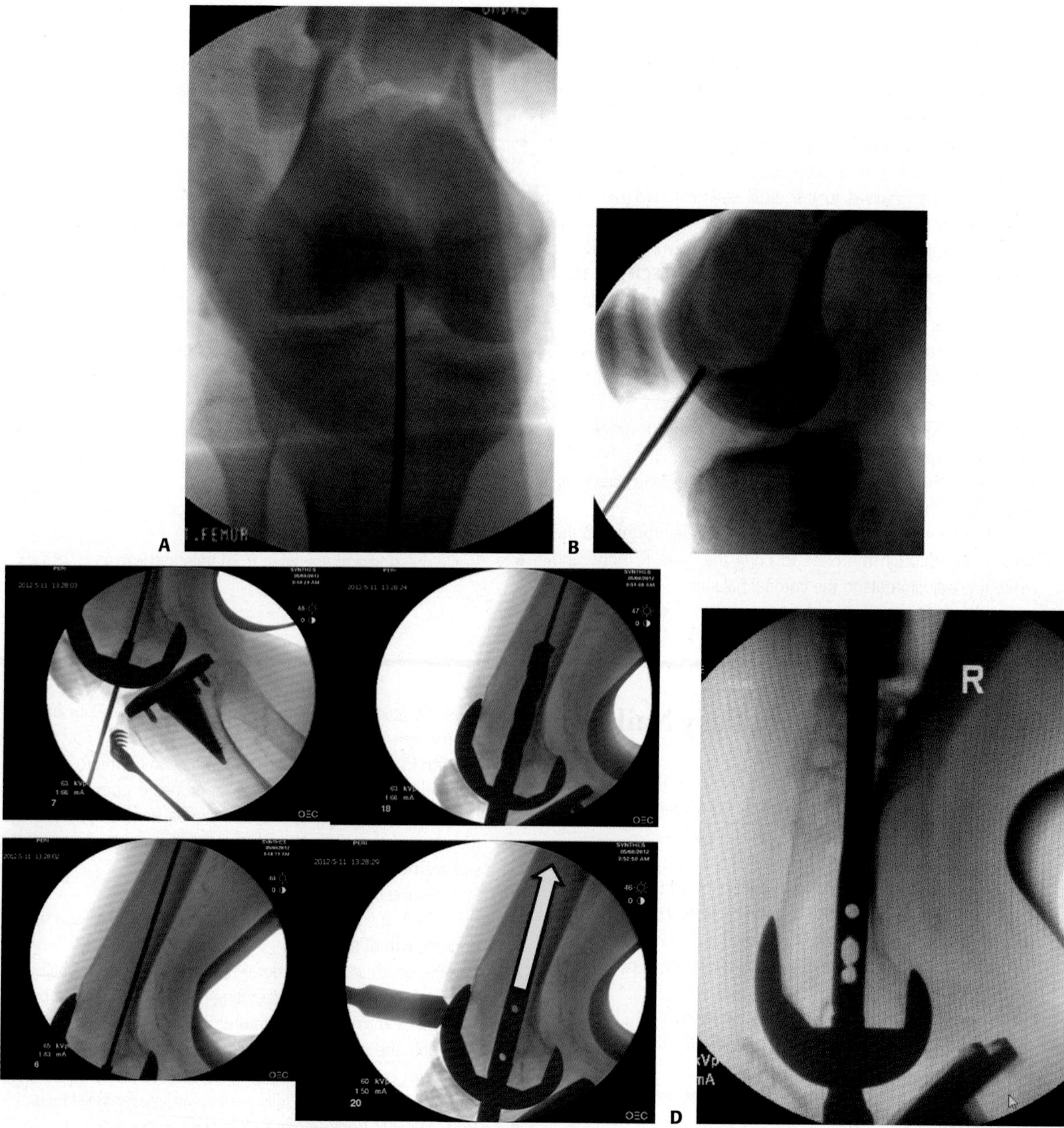

TECH FIG 2 • Typical AP (**A**) and lateral (**B**) starting point for retrograde IMN without total knee replacement. No change in AP positioning if total knee replacement preexist. **C.** Preexisting total knee replacement places the starting point more posterior in the lateral. Even with a cruciate retaining implant, the trochlea part of the component dictates the starting point more posteriorly. **D.** Resultant apex posterior (extension) deformity that is promoted by this posteriorly based starting point with current implants.

- Make small incision at the site of screw insertion. Place drill and confirm with fluoroscopy in two planes the trajectory prior to drilling.
- Drill bicortical hole.
- Use depth gauge and measure screw length and confirm on fluoroscopy.
- Insert appropriate length screws.
- Repeat steps for second interlocking screw.

Closure

- Irrigate wound and be sure to get any debris out of the knee joint to prevent third body wear.
- No. 1 Vicryl to close arthrotomy
- A 2-0 Vicryl for superficial and subcutaneous layer
- A 3-0 nylon for skin
- Sterile dressing and Ace wrap from toes to proximal thigh

PEARLS AND PITFALLS

Obtain complete radiographs including mechanical axis when appropriate.	■ Orthogonal films of femur, knee, and tibia. Consider computed tomography (CT) scan for preoperative planning.
If implants are stable, consider indirect reduction techniques.	■ Obtain history of any pain or difficulties with the TKA prior to injury.
For retrograde IMN, be sure to check box status of implant.	■ Obtain operative reports to identify implant manufacturer.
Use polyaxial locking plates.	■ Allows for multiple points of fixation around the prothesis
Do not accept axis deviation.	■ Evaluate mechanical axis intraoperatively using fluoroscopy versus plain films.
Do not leave loose implants.	■ If implants are loose, revise the TKA in addition to treating the fracture.
Do not use incompetent fixation.	■ Assure adequate fixation and stability. Use locking constructs as determined by bone quality and fracture pattern.
Do not delay postoperative range of motion.	■ Start range of motion immediately postoperatively. Assure appropriate physical therapy orders and consider use of continuous passive motion (CPM).
Do not delay surgery in the elderly.	■ Medically optimize patients to allow surgery as expeditiously as possible. Communicate with medical colleagues regarding urgency of surgical intervention.

POSTOPERATIVE CARE

- Obtain postoperative radiographs in the OR prior to waking the patient up.
- For laterally locked plating, toe-touch weight bearing for 6 weeks
- For retrograde IMN, weight bearing as tolerated
- Knee range of motion as tolerated
- Hinged knee brace for varus/valgus support
- Deep vein thrombosis (DVT) prophylaxis per surgeon preference
- Twenty-four hours of IV antibiotics
- Pain control
- Physical therapy (PT)/occupational therapy (OT)
- Postoperative follow-up
  - Two weeks for wound check
  - Six weeks for x-rays
  - Three months for x-rays
  - Six months for x-rays
  - One year for x-rays

OUTCOMES

- A 16.4% malunion rate with retrograde intramedullary nails[12] (see **TECH FIG 2C,D**)
- A 7.6% malunion rate with locked plating[12]
- A 3.6% nonunion rate with retrograde intramedullary nails[12]
- An 8.8% nonunion rate with locked plating[12]
- A 9.1% secondary surgical procedure rate with retrograde intramedullary nails[12]
- A 13.3% secondary surgical procedure rate with locked plating[12]
- Comparable long-term complication and survival rates compared to primary TKA[7]
- Worse midterm functional outcomes compared to primary TKA[7]

COMPLICATIONS

- Infection
- Malunion
- Nonunion
- Decrease functional outcomes
- TKA failure

REFERENCES

1. Berry DJ. Epidemiology: hip and knee. Orthop Clin North Am 1999;30:183–190.
2. Della Rocca GJ, Leung KS, Pape HC. Periprosthetic fractures: epidemiology and future projections. J Orthop Trauma 2011;25 (suppl 1):S66–S70.
3. Figgie MP, Goldberg VM, Figgie HE III, et al. The results of treatment of supracondylar fracture above total knee arthroplasty. J Arthroplasty 1990;5:267–276.
4. Haidukewych GJ. Innovations in locked plate technology. J Am Acad Orthop Surg 2004;12:205–212.
5. Healy WL, Siliski JM, Incavo SJ. Operative treatment of distal femoral fractures proximal to total knee replacements. J Bone Joint Surg Am 1993;75:27–34.
6. Inglis AE, Walker PS. Revision of failed knee replacements using fixed-axis hinges. J Bone Joint Surg Br 1991;73:757–761.
7. Lizaur-Utrilla A, Miralles-Muñoz FA, Sanz-Reig J. Functional outcome of total knee arthroplasty after periprosthetic distal femoral fracture. J Arthroplasty 2013;28(9):1585–1588.
8. Merkel KD, Johnson EW Jr. Supracondylar fracture of the femur after total knee arthroplasty. J Bone Joint Surg Am 1986;68:29–43.
9. Mills WJ, Barei DP, McNair P. The value of the ankle-brachial index for diagnosing arterial injury after knee dislocation: a prospective study. J Trauma 2004;56(6):1261–1265.
10. Nauth A, Ristevski B, Bégué T, et al. Periprosthetic distal femur fractures: current concepts. J Orthop Trauma 2011;25(suppl 2):S82–S85.
11. Plazter P, Schuster R, Aldrian S, et al. Management and outcome of periprosthetic fracture after total knee arthroplasty. J Trauma 2010;68:1464–1470.
12. Ristevski B, Nauth A, Williams DS, et al. Systematic review of the treatment of periprosthetic distal femur fractures. J Orthop Trauma 2014;28(5):307–312.
13. Ritter MA, Faris PM, Keating EM. Anterior femoral notching and ipsilateral supracondylar femur fractures in total knee arthroplasty. J Arthroplasty 1988;3:185–187.
14. Rorabeck CH, Taylor JW. Periprosthetic fractures of the femur complicating total knee arthroplasty. Orthop Clin North Am 1999;30: 265–277.

Revision Total Knee Arthroplasty with Femoral Bone Loss: Metal Augments

Gwo-Chin Lee

DEFINITION

- The number of revision total knee arthroplasty (TKA) procedures performed is projected to increase at an annual rate of 19.3%.[13]
- Femoral bone defects are uncommon in primary TKA but are very common in revision knee surgery.
- Modular femoral augments are useful for moderate-sized bony defects, allowing the surgeon to maximize bone–prosthesis contact while restoring the joint line and/or posterior condylar offset.
- Improvements in design and biomaterials have increased the usefulness and versatility of metal augments in addressing larger bone defects, particularly those that are uncontained.
- A systematic approach to preoperative planning, intraoperative evaluation, and reconstruction is essential in addressing femoral defects using augments.

ANATOMY

- The most common form of bone defect encountered at the time of revision surgery is bone loss from the distal and posterior femur (Table 1).
- Aside from filling the defect, it is important to restore the femorotibial joint line and posterior condylar offset. Significant alterations in either or both will be detrimental to the function of the prosthesis.

Table 1 Anderson Orthopaedic Research Institute Classification for Femoral Bone Defects

Type	Description	Illustration	Reconstruction
I	Intact metaphyseal bone Minor bone defect not compromising component stability		Cement or morselized bone graft
II	Damaged metaphyseal bone Cancellous bone loss necessitating cement fill, augments, or bone graft to restore reasonable joint line level Defects can involve one condyle (IIA) or both condyles (IIB).		Defects <5 mm: cement or bone graft Defects >5 mm but <10 mm: metallic augments (distal or posterior) with or without bone grafting
III	Deficient metaphyseal bone that compromises a major portion of either condyle, requiring a structural bone graft, hinged implant, or custom component		Unicondylar: metal augments or femoral head allograft Bicondylar: metal augments with or without distal femoral allograft for bicondylar bone loss

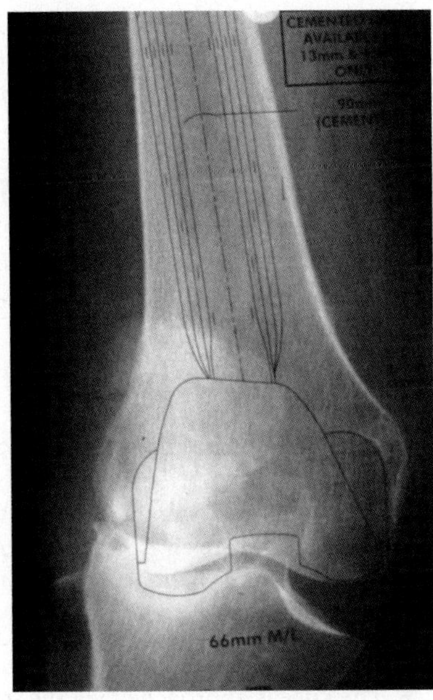

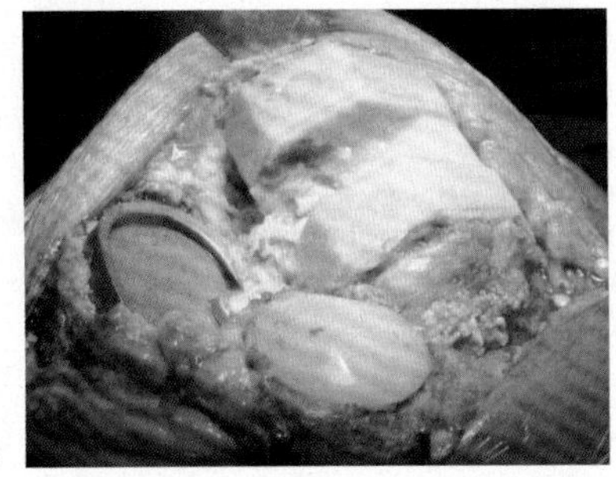

FIG 1 ● **A.** AP radiograph of a knee with severe deformity that has resulted in severe bone loss. **B.** Massive bone loss was encountered during revision surgery with severe osteolysis.

- The joint line typically lies 25 mm distal to the femoral epicondyles and the posterior femoral condyles are offset an average of 25.8 mm from the posterior cortex of the femur.[1,2]

PATHOGENESIS

- In unoperated knees, bone loss on the femoral side can be caused by previous osteochondral defects, avascular necrosis, severe valgus or varus deformity, posttraumatic arthritis, or Charcot arthropathy (**FIG 1A**).
- During revision surgery, osteolysis secondary to wear debris and bone loss secondary to removal of well-fixed components or a cement mantle are the most common causes of femoral bone defects (**FIG 1B**).
- Prior trauma resulting in severe angular deformity may rarely require the use of augments for joint reconstruction and restoration of limb alignment.

NATURAL HISTORY

- Untreated bone defects in the native knee can lead to progressive joint collapse, ligamentous laxity, or progressive bone loss.
- Osteolytic lesions caused by wear debris can progress and lead to loss of implant support and eventual component loosening.
- Intraoperative mismanagement of defects can lead to suboptimal fixation, significant alterations in knee kinematics, instability, or early implant failure.

PATIENT HISTORY AND PHYSICAL FINDINGS

- A complete history and physical examination must be performed before any revision knee surgery is undertaken. The details of the index arthroplasty with regard to pain relief and the interval to failure should be recorded. In addition, problems during the postoperative period such as falls or operative wound complications should be anticipated.
- Patients with loose femoral components often present with painful TKAs. Pain often occurs at start-up, arising from the seated position, and with stair climbing. These patients often may complain of swelling and effusions within the knees.
- An anteroposterior (AP) radiograph of the pelvis and a careful back and hip examination should be performed to rule out coexistent spinal or hip disorder as the cause of the patient's knee pain.

IMAGING AND OTHER DIAGNOSTIC STUDIES

- Plain radiographs of the knee, including standing AP, lateral, and Merchant views of the affected knee, should be reviewed. For patients with deformity, the entire length of the affected bone should be visualized.
- In revision cases, serial radiographs may help assess the progression of osteolysis, radiolucent lines, and implant migration. A knee component is definitely loose when there has been evidence of change of implant position, migration, or subsidence on serial radiographs. An implant is likely loose if there is evidence of progressive radiolucent lines on serial radiographs.
- Computed tomography (CT) scans of the knee permit assessment of component rotation and can help assess the size and location of osteolysis more accurately.[7] Recently, magnetic resonance imaging has been shown to be effective in quantifying osteolytic defects.[14]
- Blood studies, including a complete blood count with differential, erythrocyte sedimentation rate (ESR), and C-reactive protein (CRP), should be obtained to rule out infection.
- Nuclear medicine studies including bone scan (to detect a loose prosthesis) and indium and sulfur colloid scans (to detect the presence of infection) can also sometimes be helpful in the preoperative workup when obvious signs of failure are absent. It is important to remember that these modalities are technique-dependent and a bone scan can continue to show increased activity up to 18 months following index arthroplasty.[10]
- Aspiration should be done when there is any suspicion of infection or elevations in serum inflammatory markers (eg, ESR or CRP). The synovial fluid should be examined for the number and differential of white blood cells and cultured for the presence of microorganisms.[5]

DIFFERENTIAL DIAGNOSIS

- Infection
- Arthritis of the hip and spine
- Flexion instability
- Patellar maltracking and extensor mechanism dysfunction
- Tibial component loosening
- Periprosthetic fractures

NONOPERATIVE MANAGEMENT

- Unless the patient has obvious signs of component malpositioning, loosening, fracture, or infection, a trial of conservative treatment aimed at strengthening the quadriceps musculature with emphasis on the vastus medialis oblique muscle should be the cornerstone of nonoperative treatment.
- Patients who have evidence of late osteolysis and polyethylene wear on plain radiographs but no clinical symptoms or pain should be encouraged to obtain serial radiographs annually to check for progression of the lesion(s).
- No consensus has been reached regarding when it is appropriate to revise or perform bone grafting in an asymptomatic knee with radiographic evidence of osteolysis. However, revision should occur as soon as symptoms present in order to avoid progression and worsening of bone loss.

SURGICAL MANAGEMENT

- A systematic approach is required to reconstruct bone defects successfully during revision surgery.

Preoperative Planning

- Thorough preoperative planning is the key to a successful reconstruction.
- Review of radiographs and CT scans and careful templating allow anticipation of problems that could be encountered during surgery (**FIG 2A,B**).
- Most bone loss can be addressed by the use of metal augments and a stemmed prosthesis (**FIG 2C**). There have been no differences in the clinical outcomes of revisions performed using cemented stemmed components compared to uncemented press-fit implants. Diaphyseal engagement of a press-fit stem is required to minimize the risk of component loosening.[6]
- For larger, uncontained bone lesions, special augments (eg, cones or sleeves), femoral heads, and allografts must be ordered in advance so they are available during reconstruction (see **TECH FIG 4B** and Video 1).
- In all cases of revision, stemmed and constrained implants (or sometimes a hinged prosthesis) must be considered and made available.

Positioning

- The standard position for patients undergoing revision TKA is supine.
- Care is taken to drape a wide surgical field in case a more extensile approach is necessary. A sterile tourniquet applied on the surgical field may be helpful.

Approach

- The knee is approached via the standard medial parapatellar approach.
- Protection of the patellar tendon during this phase of the operation is crucial.
- An extensive synovectomy and débridement of the medial and lateral gutters are critical for decompression of the joint.
- The patella is usually not everted during revision TKA.
- In knees with severe ankylosis, techniques such as the quadriceps snip, lateral release, and tibial tubercle osteotomy are helpful for exposure. The surgeon must know the implications of each of these releases and repair or reconstruct them properly at the end of the procedure.
- The bone defect is addressed by the use of cement (smaller lesions), metal augments, or structural grafts or metaphyseal augments (cones or sleeves) for large uncontained defects. The critical issues are to restore joint line, achieve appropriate alignment, and attain ligamentous balancing. Reconstruction also aims at restoring a stable platform for positioning and fixation of the components.

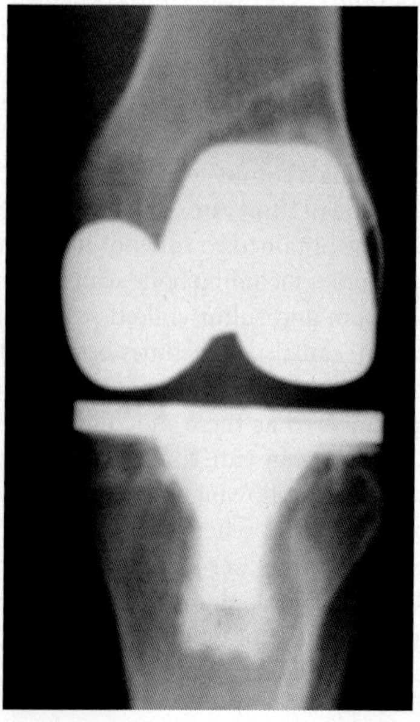

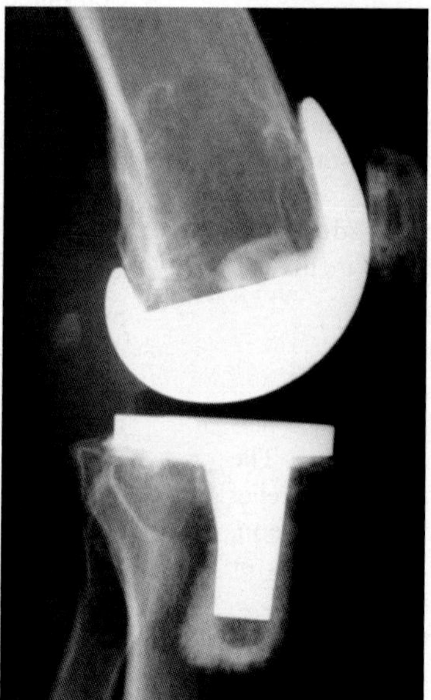

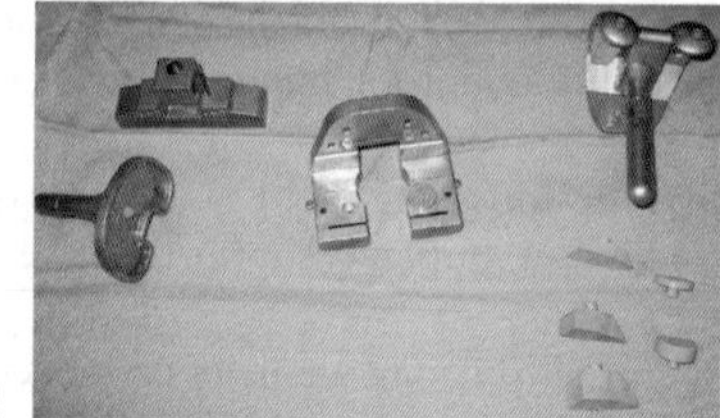

FIG 2 • A,B. AP and lateral radiographs of the knee before revision surgery. Large osteolytic defects involving both the femur and the tibia are visible. Careful preoperative planning is required to address bone loss encountered at the time of arthroplasty. **C.** Most cases of knee revision with bone loss can be addressed with the use of a long-stem prosthesis and metal augments.

Metal Augments

- Modular metal augments allow for restoration of distal, posterior, and even metaphyseal femoral defects.
- For most systems, the largest femoral augments allow for restoration of 8 to 10 mm of bone defect. The use of cemented stacked augments for filling defects up to 30 mm has been reported.[8]
- Most revision systems have intramedullary systems that allow bone cuts to be made relative to a press-fit intramedullary rod.
- The distal femoral cut is freshened to provide a stable platform for the new prosthesis.
- Next, the size of the femoral component is selected. Preoperative templating can give clues to the proper component size. Traditionally, the femoral component is upsized to better fill the flexion gap (**TECH FIG 1A**).
- Determining proper femoral component rotation is critical to a successful reconstruction. The femoral component should be set parallel to the transepicondylar axis of the femur (**TECH FIG 1B**). Other secondary guides include the proximal tibia (parallel) and the femoral intercondylar line (perpendicular).
- Malrotation of the femoral component can also exaggerate the severity of bone loss. Typically, a posterolateral augment and distal femoral augments are required to ensure proper restoration of rotation and joint line.
- The rest of the reconstruction varies according to the revision knee system being used but should follow a systematic approach. In some systems, the trial components have slots that allow bone cuts to be made for more precise fitting of the modular augment (**TECH FIG 1C**).
- A stemmed trial femoral component with the necessary augments is assembled and inserted. Trialing should focus on the overall stability of the knee in extension and flexion as well as patellofemoral tracking (**TECH FIG 1D**).
- The definitive prosthesis is assembled and cemented into place in the standard fashion.

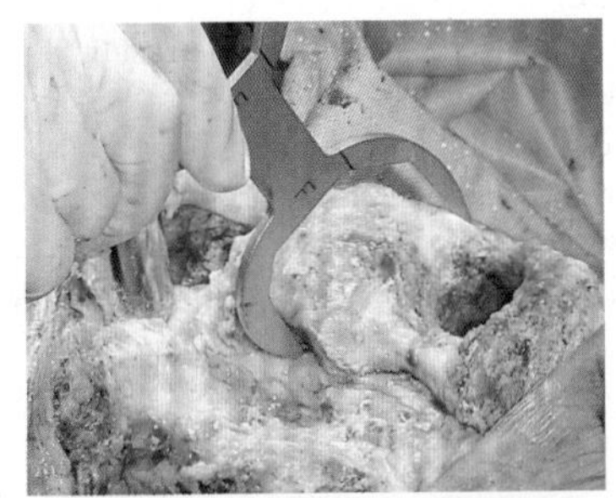
A

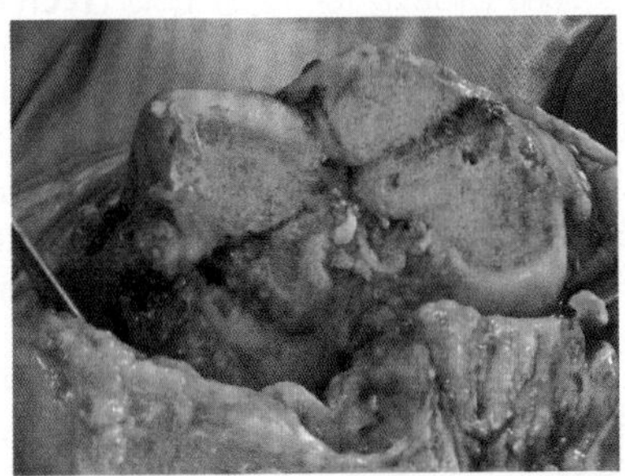
B

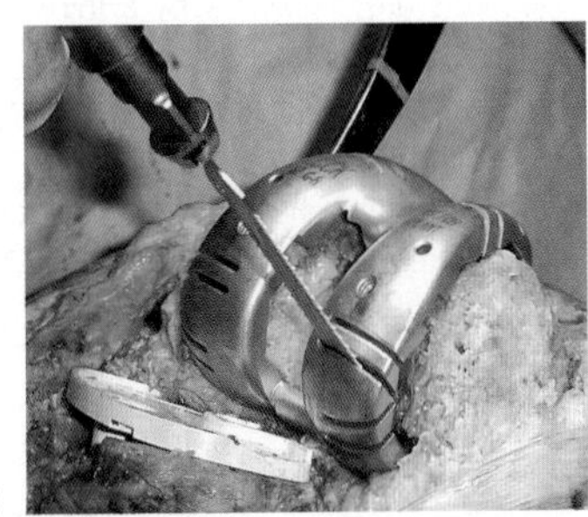
C

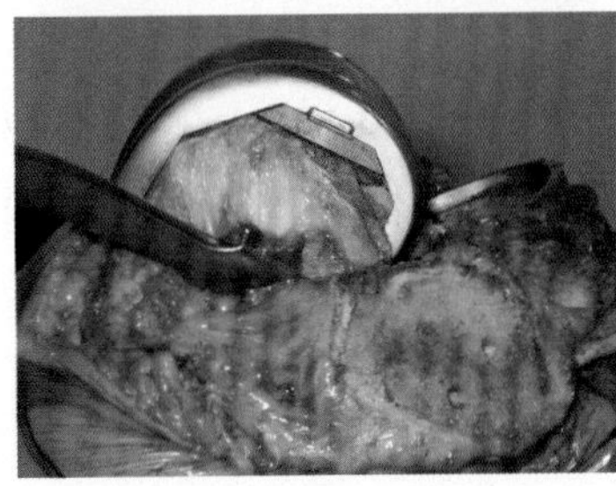
D

TECH FIG 1 • **A.** Sizing the femoral component is an important part of the revision process. **B.** Assessing the appropriate rotation using transepicondylar axis and Whiteside's line. Note the distortion of the posterior condylar line as a result of bone loss. **C.** Some implants have trials with slots, which allow for more precise sizing and preparation for modular augments. **D.** Femoral trial with augments and stem in place.

Bone Cement

- Bone cement is indicated for use in small, preferably contained, bony defects up to 5 mm in depth.
- Its limitations include low modulus of elasticity and that it does not restore bone stock.
- Following removal of the existing prosthesis, all surfaces are thoroughly débrided. There is a membrane that often forms between the old bone–cement interface. Areas of bony sclerosis should be débrided with the aid of a high-speed burr to punctate bleeding.
- The femur is prepared with the revision instrumentation specific to the implant system, paying attention to joint line restoration, rotation, and restoration of the posterior condylar offset. The use of stemmed implants allows for distribution of joint stresses and is almost always required in cases of revision surgery with bone loss.
- The new femoral component is cemented into place separately, and the cement is allowed to harden under direct vision.

Morselized Autograft or Allograft

- Indicated for use in larger contained defects, especially in younger patients. The main advantage of this technique is that it allows for restoration of bone stock.
- Its limitations are that it cannot be used for uncontained defects and does not restore a stable platform capable of supporting the prosthesis.
- Using a curette or a high-speed burr, the host bone is débrided to create a favorable environment for graft incorporation.
  - Visible defects are packed with morselized autograft or allograft.
  - A bone tamp may be used to pack the bone chips tightly.
- Prepare the femur using the revision instrumentation particular to the system being used.
- Once the femur is prepared, insert a stemmed trial femoral component, with or without wedges, onto the femur.
- Before final impaction of the trial component, tightly pack the bone chips around the stems and the posterior condyles. Impacting the trial prosthesis into place will effectively shape the new distal femur.
- The new stemmed femoral component is cemented separately to minimize the chance of component malposition.

Structural Allografts (Femoral Hemicondyle)

- Structural allografts are indicated for large, uncontained defects involving one femoral condyle. The attachments of the collateral ligaments are preserved by a thin shell of bone following removal of the femoral implant.
- The host bone–allograft interface is prepared as previously described.
- Gently, using a hemispherical acetabular reamer, the bony defect is reamed to accept a femoral head (**TECH FIG 2A**).
- Using the corresponding female resurfacing reamer, a femoral head allograft is reamed to remove all cartilaginous debris (**TECH FIG 2B**).
- The femoral head is coupled to the bony defect and secured using two threaded Steinmann pins inserted from proximal to distal (**TECH FIG 2C**).
- The distal femur is then prepared using the instrumentation particular to the system being used.
- The femoral head allograft is fixed to the host bone using 4.5-mm short-thread cancellous screws inserted from proximal to distal (**TECH FIG 2D**).
- Finally, a stemmed femoral component is cemented into place.

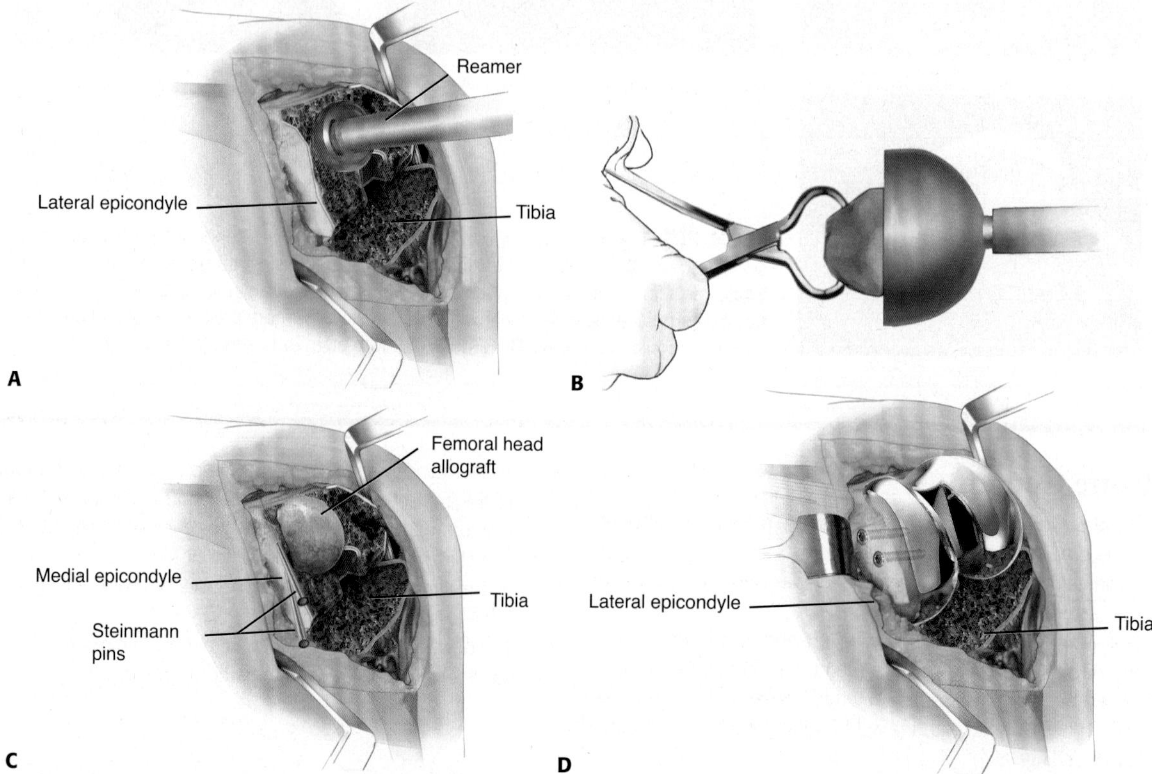

TECH FIG 2 • **A.** A hemispherical reamer is used to prepare the host surface. **B.** Using the matching female reamer, the cartilage of the femoral head allograft is denuded to cancellous bone. **C.** The graft is provisionally fixed using two threaded Steinmann pins. **D.** The allograft is fixed definitively using two short-thread, 4.5-mm cancellous screws from proximal to distal before implantation of the prosthesis.

Distal Femoral Allograft

- Indicated for massive osteolytic defects involving both distal condyles and distal femoral metaphysis. It allows for restoration of bone stock while preserving the collateral ligament insertions.
- In cases in which a distal femoral allograft may be required, preoperative sizing of the host femur and the allograft is crucial.
  - Comparing radiographs of the allograft to the host femur (may size against an unoperated side if available) improves fit and decreases the chances of mismatch.
- The native femur is prepared to accept the allograft by carefully preserving the collateral ligament attachments (**TECH FIG 3A**).
- The allograft is then shaped to allow for intussusception (bone within bone) into the native femur. It is important to obtain a secure fit of the allograft during this step (**TECH FIG 3B**).
- Using traditional distal femoral cutting guides, the femur is prepared to accept a stemmed prosthesis (**TECH FIG 3C–E**).
- Demineralized bone matrix is used to line the host–allograft interface. This allows the filling of gaps and also provides a barrier against cement intrusion (**TECH FIG 3F**).
- A stemmed femoral implant is cemented into place (**TECH FIG 3G,H**).

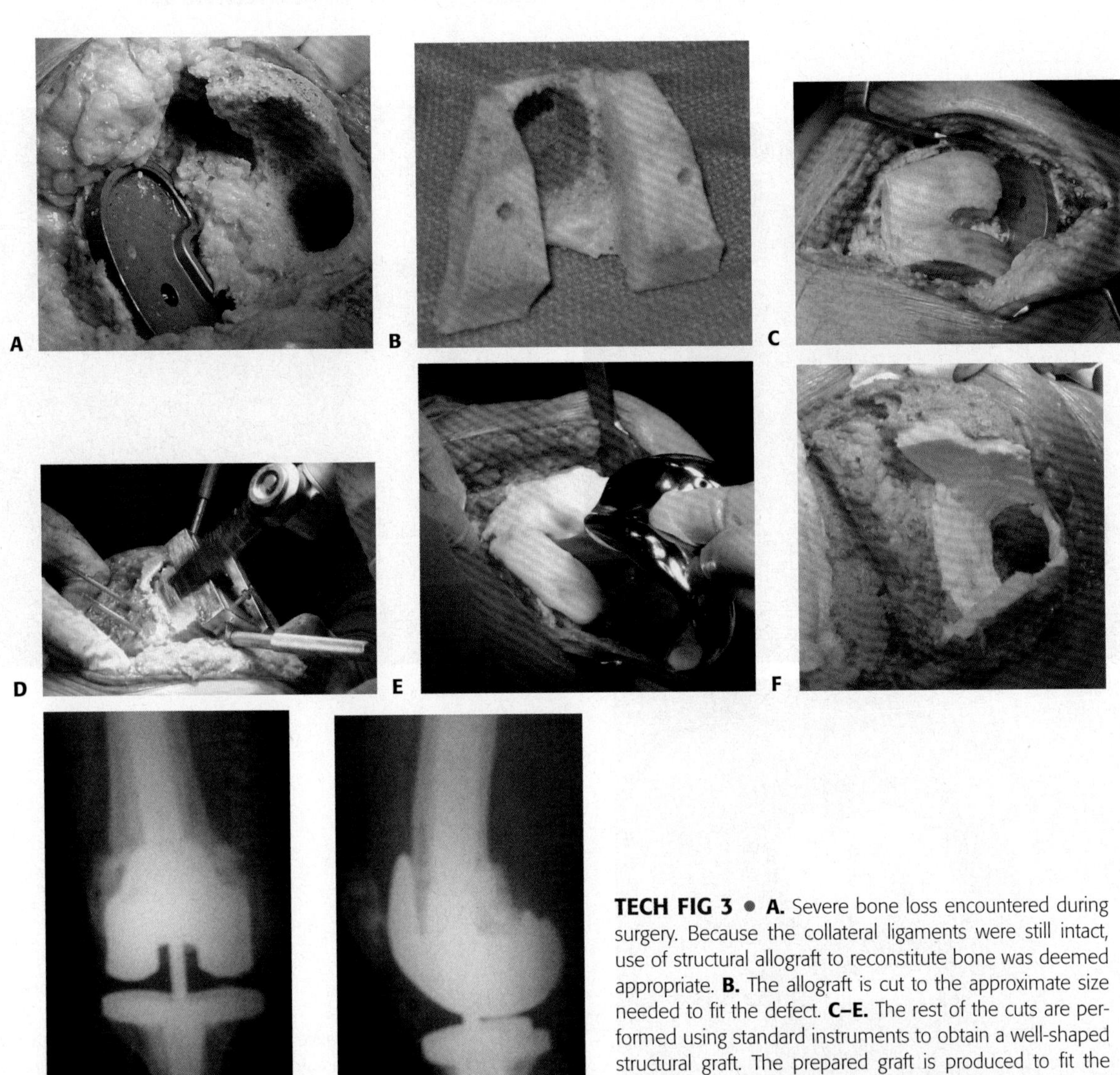

TECH FIG 3 • **A.** Severe bone loss encountered during surgery. Because the collateral ligaments were still intact, use of structural allograft to reconstitute bone was deemed appropriate. **B.** The allograft is cut to the approximate size needed to fit the defect. **C–E.** The rest of the cuts are performed using standard instruments to obtain a well-shaped structural graft. The prepared graft is produced to fit the defect exactly. **F.** Demineralized bone matrix can be used in the interface between allograft and host. **G,H.** The long-stem implant is then cemented over the allograft.

Metaphyseal Augments (Cones and Sleeves)

- Indicated for large, uncontained metaphyseal defects when rotation of the femoral component cannot be achieved using cement, morselized grafts, or other structural grafts.
- Its advantages over structural allografts include instrumentation, no risk for disease transmission, and osteointegration with no risk for graft resorption.
- Following removal of the old femoral component, the host bone is débrided, and the nature, size, and shape of the defect is identified.
- Using a high-speed burr (cones) or broaches (sleeves), the femoral defect is prepared to accept the metaphyseal augment. The augment should fit securely into the host bone to maximize the chance for bone ingrowth (**TECH FIG 4A,B**).
  - Particular attention should be given to the depth of seating of the augment in relation to the joint line and to the rotation of these augments. If the augment is countersunk, it will not allow for support at the proper level in order for proper joint line restoration. Similarly, if the augment or the sleeve is severely malrotated, it will not allow the revised femoral component to properly restore rotation.
- The cone augment is inserted independently prior to femoral component implantation. When a femoral sleeve is used, the augment is united with the femoral component and inserted as part of the final implantation (**TECH FIG 4C**).

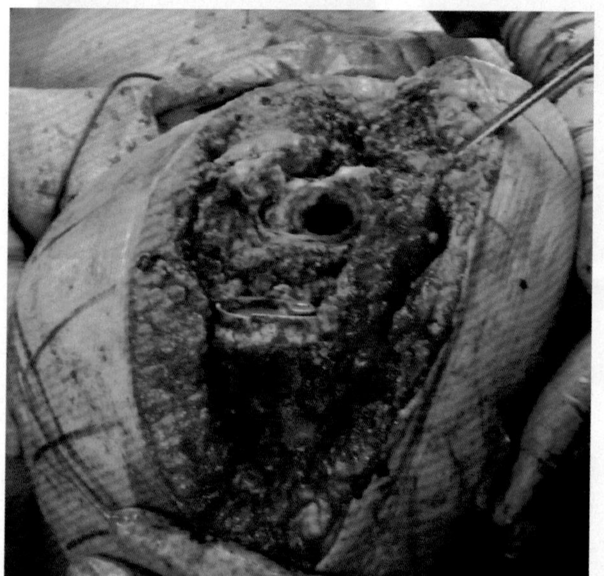

A

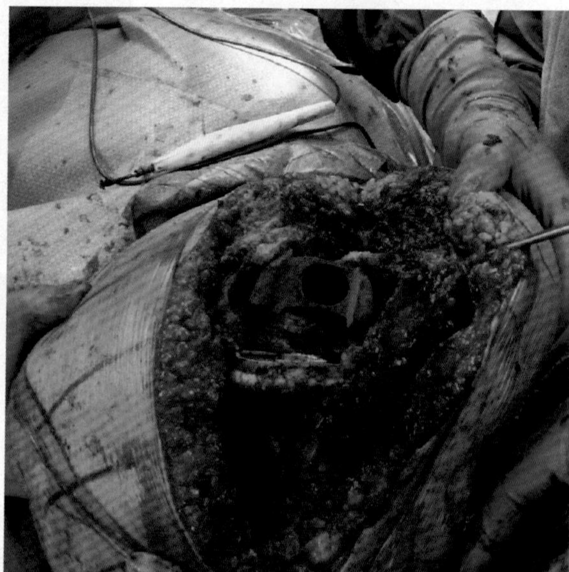

B

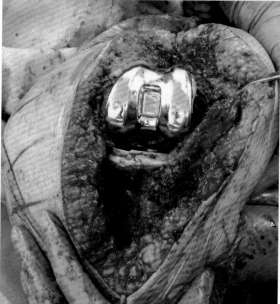

C

TECH FIG 4 • **A.** Intraoperative photograph of a large, uncontained femoral defect. Under these circumstances, restoring structural support for the eventual femoral component is critical for success. **B.** Intraoperative photograph of a porous metal structural augment in a large uncontained, metaphyseal femoral defect. The augment provides the stable foundation for the eventual femoral prosthesis. The position and rotation of the augment are critical as the augment dictates the final position of the femoral component. **C.** Once the augment is in place, the femoral component is cemented into the augment, thus uniting these structures into one.

PEARLS AND PITFALLS

Preoperative planning	■ Comprehensive preoperative evaluation including workup for infection and other causes of knee pain (hip and spine) should be performed in all patients undergoing revision TKA. ■ CT scans of the knee are helpful in assessing component rotation and quantifying the degree of bone loss. ■ Preoperative templating is critical for successful reconstruction.
Exposure	■ Removal of preexisting components is a common cause of bone loss during revision TKA. ■ Careful exposure of the implants with attention to the interface between the posterior phalanges of the prosthesis and the host bone will prevent unnecessary bone loss.
Bone loss	■ Small contained bony defects can be addressed with either cement or morselized bone graft. ■ Metal augments are useful for augmenting distal and posterior femoral defects measuring less than 1 cm and with good structural support. ■ Proper sizing of the femoral component, the use of offset stems, and correct component rotation can minimize smaller defects. ■ Large structural and uncontained femoral defects involving one or both femoral condyles require augmentation with either the metaphyseal cone of sleeve augments or structural allografts.
Reconstruction	■ The host bone should be thoroughly débrided to optimize the interface between the native bone and the allograft bone or cement. ■ Restoration of the joint line and the posterior condylar offset is crucial to the overall success of the revision process. Failure to restore posterior offset can lead to motion loss.[11] ■ When using metallic augments, the decision to use distal femoral augments is made early in the procedure. Revision instrumentation will key off these augments for subsequent bone cuts. ■ When using distal femoral allografts, prepare the allograft by first removing the epicondyles and making a provisional cut on the anterior cortex of the allograft. This will allow the allograft to be impacted into the host bone.
Trial components	■ Whether cementing or press-fitting the stem, the trial femoral component should be assembled using a stem, which confers axial and rotational stability to the femoral trial. ■ Using a marking pen, trace out the anterior phalange of the revision femoral component once a satisfactory trial has been achieved. This will provide a guide to fixation of the definitive prosthesis (**FIG 3**). ■ An intraoperative radiograph can help assess the overall alignment of the implants and their position in relation to the tibiofemoral joint.
Fixation	■ Each component should be cemented separately to prevent inadvertent changes in component position. ■ During final impaction of the definitive prosthesis, pay attention to its position in relation to that of the trial components. Overimpaction of the implants may lead to fracture, loss of fixation of structural bone grafts, and alterations in the flexion and extension gaps.

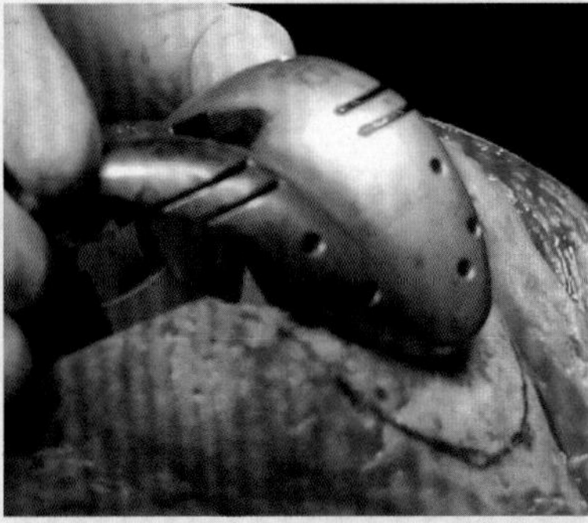

FIG 3 ● Using a marking pen, the trial prosthesis is traced following a satisfactory trial of all the components. This tracing will provide a guide to the depth of seating for the definitive prosthesis.

POSTOPERATIVE CARE

- Early motion is instituted for most patients using a continuous passive motion machine set from 0 to 60 degrees immediately following surgery.
- For patients who have had extensive procedures, a well-padded Robert Jones dressing is applied following the operation. Immobilization is maintained for 24 to 48 hours.
- Following revision TKA, patients are usually allowed to bear weight as tolerated on the prosthesis.
- Alterations of weight-bearing status and limitations on knee flexion are similar to that of other procedures performed at the time of arthroplasty such as tibial tubercle osteotomy, quadriceps snip, or V-Y turndown.

OUTCOMES

- Overall, the survivorship of revision femoral components using metal wedges with or without structural augments is 79.4% at 8 years.[8]
- For knees with small, contained cavitary defects requiring only cement or morselized graft, the 10-year survivorship approaches that of primary TKA.[11]

- Modular femoral augments used for reconstruction of type II defects have an 11-year survival rate of 92%. It is not uncommon to see nonprogressive radiolucent lines surrounding metallic augments.[12]
- Early results of tantalum femoral cones and porous metal sleeves have shown these devices to achieve reliable fixation and osteointegration in complex revision TKAs.[4,9,15]
- Femoral revisions augmented with structural allografts have a 10-year survival rate of 75%.[3]

COMPLICATIONS

- Traditional complications following revision TKA include infection, wound complications, and loosening.
- Patellar maltracking and extensor mechanism dysfunction can also occur, especially if there is component malrotation.
- Knee instability can result from an imbalance in the flexion and extension gaps.
- Resorption of large structural allografts leading to subsequent implant loosening has been described.

REFERENCES

1. Banks SA, Harman MK, Bellemans J, et al. Making sense of knee arthroplasty kinematics: news you can use. J Bone Joint Surg Am 2003;85(suppl 4):64–72.
2. Bellemans J, Banks S, Victor J, et al. Fluoroscopic analysis of the kinematics of deep flexion in total knee arthroplasty. Influence of posterior condylar offset. J Bone Joint Surg Br 2002;84:50–53.
3. Clatworthy MG, Ballance J, Brick GW, et al. The use of structural allograft for unconstrained defects in revision total knee replacement. A minimum five-year review. J Bone Joint Surg Am 2001;83:404–411.
4. Daines BK, Dennis DA. Management of bone defects in revision total knee arthroplasty. Instr Course Lect 2013;62:341–348.
5. Della Valle C, Parvizi J, Bauer TW, et al. American Academy of Orthopaedic Surgeons clinical practice guideline on: the diagnosis of periprosthetic joint infections of the hip and knee. J Bone Joint Surg Am 2011;93(14):1355–1357.
6. Fehring TK, Odum S, Olekson C, et al. Stem fixation in revision total knee arthroplasty: a comparative analysis. Clin Orthop Relat Res 2003;(416):217–224.
7. Gonzalez MH, Mekhail AO. The failed total knee arthroplasty: evaluation and etiology. J Am Acad Orthop Surg 2004;12:436–446.
8. Hockman DE, Ammeen D, Engh GA. Augments and allografts in revision total knee arthroplasty: usage and outcome using one modular revision prosthesis. J Arthroplasty 2005;20:35–41.
9. Howard JL, Kudera J, Lewallen DG, et al. Early results of the use of tantalum femoral cones for revision total knee arthroplasty. J Bone Joint Surg Am 2011;93(5):478–484.
10. Kitchener MI, Coats E, Keene G, et al. Assessment of radionuclide arthrography in evaluation of loosening of knee prostheses. Knee 2006;13(3):220–225.
11. McAuley JP, Engh GA, Ammeen DJ. Revision of failed unicompartmental knee arthroplasty. Clin Orthop Relat Res 2001;(392): 279–282.
12. Patel JV, Masonis JL, Guerin J, et al. The fate of augments to treat type-2 bone defects in revision knee arthroplasty. J Bone Joint Surg Br 2004;86:195–199.
13. Saleh KJ, Rand JA, McQueen DA. Current status of revision total knee replacements: how do we assess results. J Bone Joint Surg Am 2003;85(suppl 1):S18–S20.
14. Vessely MB, Frick MA, Oakes D, et al. Magnetic resonance imaging with metal suppression for evaluation of periprosthetic osteolysis after total knee arthroplasty. J Arthroplasty 2006;21:826–831.
15. Werle JR, Goodman SB, Imrie SN. Revision total knee arthroplasty using large distal femoral augments for severe metaphyseal bone deficiency: a preliminary study. Orthopedics 2002;25:325–327.

Revision Total Knee Arthroplasty with Tibial Bone Loss: Metal Augments

40

CHAPTER

R. Michael Meneghini

DEFINITION

- Bone loss and indications for the use of metallic augments in revision total knee arthroplasty (TKA) usually are guided by classification of the bony defect and the intraoperative findings.
- Probably the most widely used, the Anderson Orthopaedic Research Institute (AORI) bone defect classification system divides bone loss of the distal femur or the proximal tibia into three types, based on the radiographic status of the metaphyseal bone.[5,6]
  - Proximal tibial metaphyseal defects are graded as type I (TI), type II (TII), or type III (TIII).
  - TI defects of the proximal tibia have intact metaphyseal bone with no component subsidence or loss of the primarily reconstructed joint line.
    - Minor defects may be present that will not compromise the stability of the tibial component; primary type reconstruction components may typically be used without augments.
  - TII defects of the proximal tibia have damaged metaphyseal bone with component subsidence or joint line alteration due to loss of metaphyseal bone.
    - Bone loss in TII defects can involve either the lateral or, more commonly, the medial tibial plateau as well as the entire proximal tibia.
    - Defect reconstruction with cement, metal augments, or bone grafting is required and revision stemmed components usually are required.
    - Collateral ligament origins and insertions are preserved in TII-type defects.
  - TIII defects of the proximal tibia have deficiency of the proximal metaphyseal bone that involves a major segment of the proximal tibia.
    - This type of defect may involve the tibial tubercle, with resulting patellar tendon detachment and loss of extensor mechanism function.
    - The medial collateral ligament also may be detached or functionally incompetent as a result of bony deficiency.
    - The broad insertion of the medial collateral ligament on the proximal medial metaphysis of the tibia renders incompetence or frank loss of attachment due to tibial bone loss less likely as compared to femoral condylar bone loss where the origin of the medial collateral has a much smaller area of attachment to the medial epicondyle.
- In summary, proximal tibial bone defects are classified as intact (TI), damaged (TII), and deficient (TIII).
  - By definition, the use of metallic augments is restricted to TII or TIII defects. TIII defects with larger bone voids typically require reconstruction with bulk allograft or the newer highly porous metal metaphyseal augments.

ANATOMY

- Although native knee anatomy is relevant in primary TKA, this chapter will focus on the pertinent anatomy that is relevant in the more complex revision TKA requiring augments.
- The tip of the fibular head is approximately 1 cm below the surface of the lateral tibial plateau[2] and is the most commonly used bony reference for joint line restoration in the revision TKA setting.
  - Improved outcomes are noted if the joint line is elevated less than 8 to 10 mm.[9,12]
- The tibial tubercle is 25 to 40 mm below the joint surface, and the average insertion point of the patellar tendon is 29 mm distal to the tibial plateau.
  - The distal pole of the patella averages 15 mm (range, 12 to 16 mm) above the joint surface.
- Neurovascular injury during primary and revision TKA is rare.
  - The popliteal neurovascular bundle is 3 to 12 mm posterior to the tibia articular surface when the leg is extended and 6 to 15 mm posteriorly when the knee is flexed to 90 degrees.[18]
  - At the level of the tibial resection, the distance is approximately 2 cm posterior to the cut surface and the popliteal artery and vein are anterior to the tibial nerve at this level.[14]
  - Most revisions do not put the tibial artery trifurcation at risk unless more than 30 mm of proximal tibia is resected.
  - Most neurovascular injuries during primary and revision TKA result from tourniquet use in the patient with peripheral vascular disease.
- The proximal tibial anatomy of the TKA requiring revision TKA is highly variable due to the various mechanisms of TKA failure and their effect on the native bone stock through overt loss or remodeling.[17]

PATHOGENESIS

- Proximal tibial bone loss in primary TKA failure can be attributed to the following factors: implant malalignment primarily or due to bony collapse, aseptic loosening with implant migration, osteolysis due to particulate wear debris, bone loss from excessive motion of cement spacers used for staged treatment of chronic infection, or intraoperative bone loss during implant removal.[8]
- If osteolysis is present, its severity is affected by implant design and the quality of polyethylene as well as host response to particulate debris and the quality of the host bone.
- Osteolysis of the proximal tibial bone is a result of the histiocytic and macrophage response to polyethylene particulate debris from wear at the bearing interface as well as "backside" wear.[4]
  - Osteolytic lesions are either focal or expansile, depending on the submicron particle burden as well as the host

Medial or Lateral Block or Step Augment

- Intramedullary reaming is followed by placement of an intramedullary alignment cutting guide, and a minimal transverse proximal tibial "skim" resection is taken after the cutting guide is pinned in place.
- A block augment cutting guide can either be attached separately or will be incorporated into the intramedullary alignment cutting guide that exists in most revision knee systems. Particular attention must be paid to tibial component rotation so that the sagittal block cut will align with the final implant in the correct rotation (**TECH FIG 1A,B**).
- Most surgeons will avoid wedge or sloped augments; it has been shown that block augments are superior to wedges biomechanically in creating an overall more stable and rigid tibial construct.[3]
- Once the proximal tibial surface is adequately prepared, a trial stemmed component that reflects the intramedullary stem to be used with attached augments is trialed.
- When adequate bony support is achieved, the joint surface is restored and flexion and extension gaps are balanced. The component to be implanted then is constructed to match the trial and appropriately cemented into place (**TECH FIG 1C**).

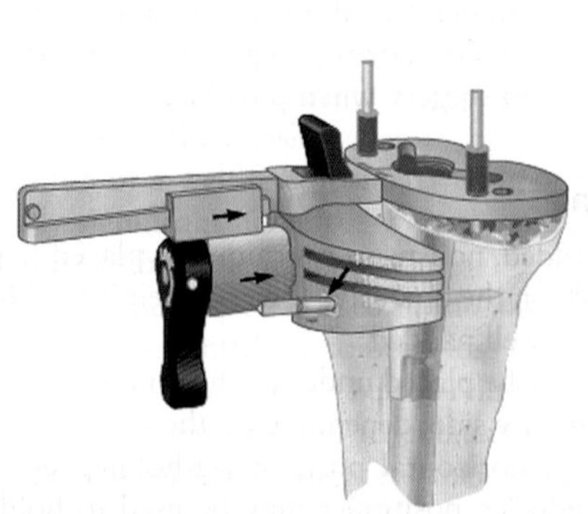
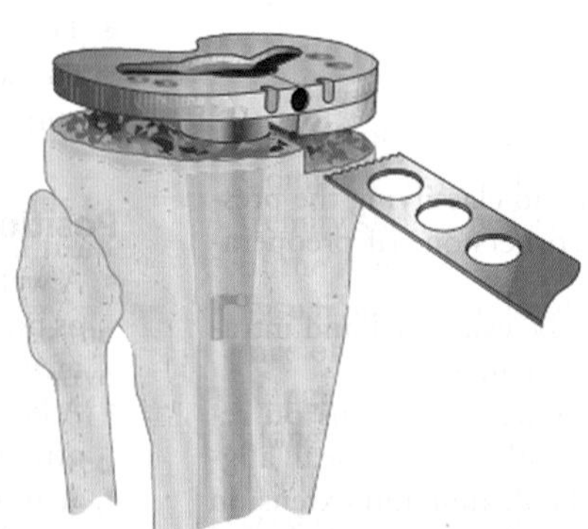
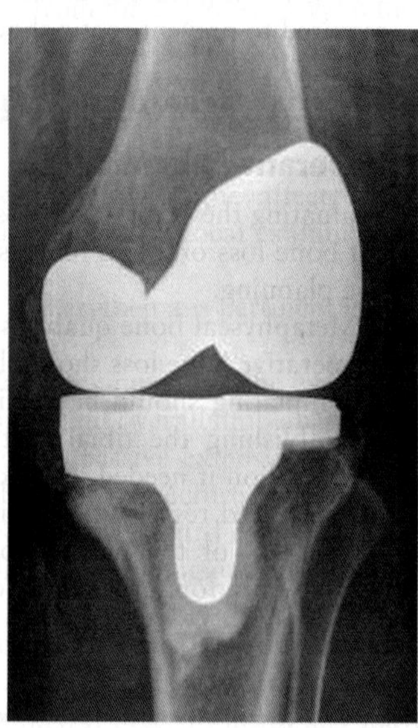
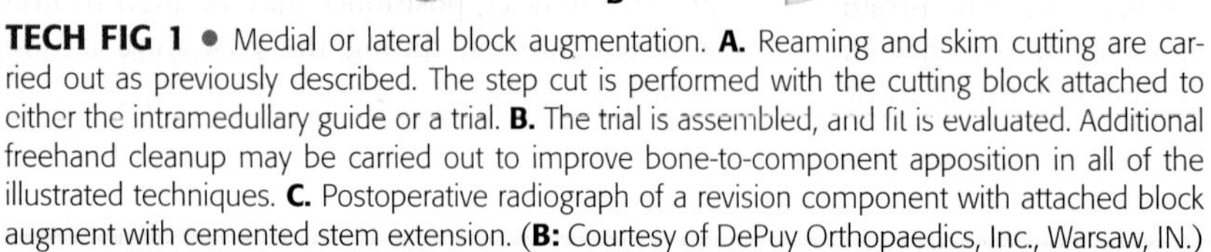

TECH FIG 1 • Medial or lateral block augmentation. **A.** Reaming and skim cutting are carried out as previously described. The step cut is performed with the cutting block attached to either the intramedullary guide or a trial. **B.** The trial is assembled, and fit is evaluated. Additional freehand cleanup may be carried out to improve bone-to-component apposition in all of the illustrated techniques. **C.** Postoperative radiograph of a revision component with attached block augment with cemented stem extension. (**B:** Courtesy of DePuy Orthopaedics, Inc., Warsaw, IN.)

Metaphyseal Cone (Sleeve) Augmentation

- Intramedullary reaming should be carried out to the depth of the stem available in the revision system in use to place the tibial tray at the appropriate level. Most metaphyseal sleeves are used with cementless stem extensions and therefore an intimate fit of the reamer and subsequent stem into the diaphysis is desired.
- Once the appropriate-sized diaphyseal engaging stem is selected, the proximal tibia is sequentially broached with the appropriate-sized trial stem attached to the broach to provide proper alignment (**TECH FIG 2A**).
  - There is some rotational freedom between the metaphyseal sleeve and the tibial tray, so that the surgeon can focus on optimizing metaphyseal fixation. However, the surgeon should be familiar with the degree of rotational freedom within the system to ensure optimal tibial rotation.
  - Broaching is carried out until rotational and axial stability is obtained, which usually occurs when the majority of the metaphyseal defect is filled with the sleeve augment.
- Some systems then use the proximal surface of the broach as the cutting guide. This necessitates placing the broach at the level determined by preoperative planning and intraoperative assessment. Ideally, this position resects 2 mm or less of the proximal tibial metaphysis (**TECH FIG 2B**).
- Once the proximal tibia is resected and broached, a trial metaphyseal sleeve is placed and rotation is marked on the anterior tibia, a properly sized trial tibial tray and stem are assembled and placed through the cone, lack of excessive rotational disparity between the two is verified, and tibial tray rotation is marked.
- Final assembly of the tibial components is done to match the trial, and the tibial cone is impacted onto the Morse taper of the revision tibial baseplate, with care taken to match the trial model cone rotation on the trial stem (**TECH FIG 2C**).
- Cement is applied to the assembled component selectively at the tibial baseplate undersurface only as most cones allow for bony ingrowth with a porous surface coating, and the diaphyseal stem is press-fit and baseplate-cemented to the proximal tibia. The metaphyseal sleeve is allowed to contact the bone to facilitate osseointegration of the porous coating (**TECH FIG 2D,E**).

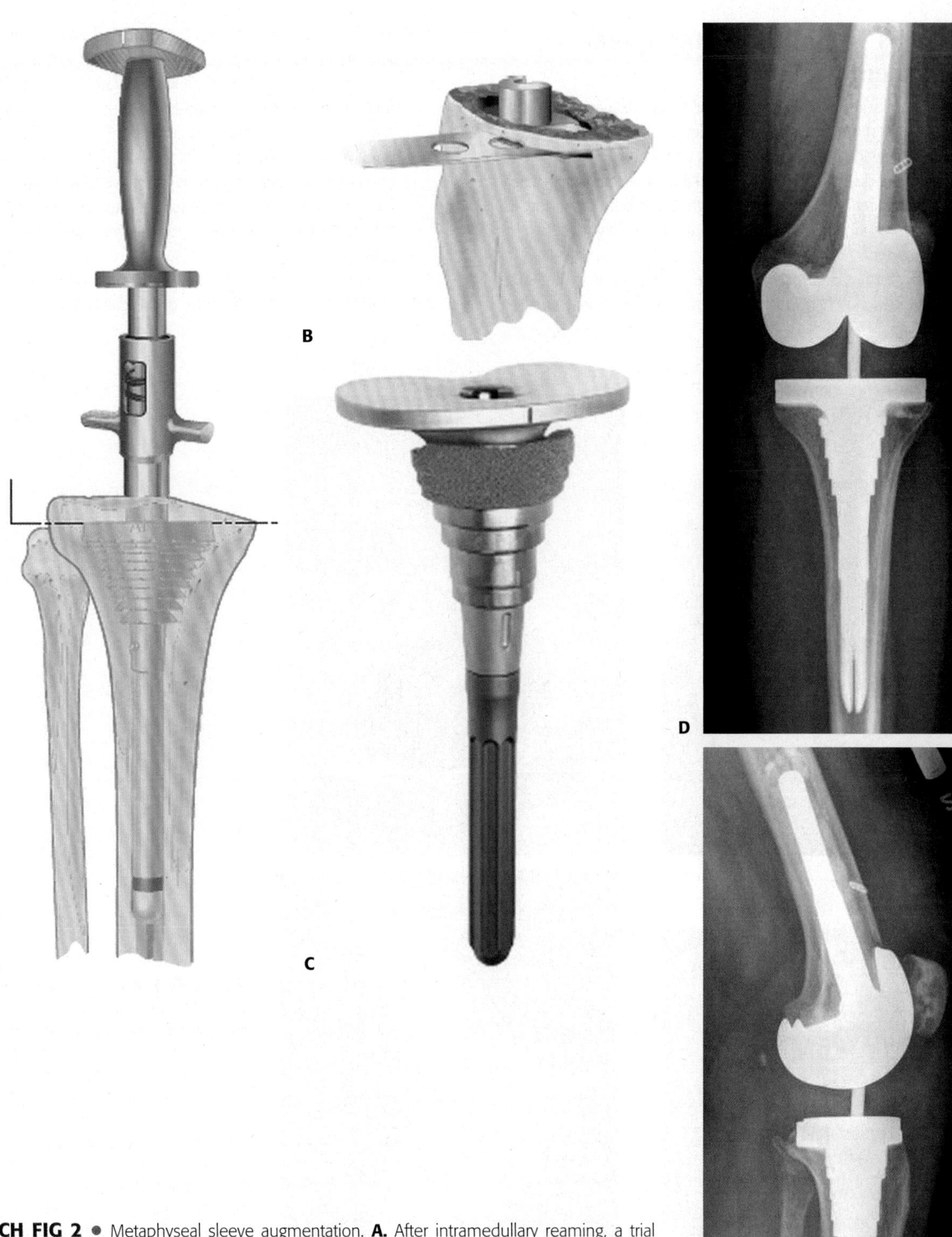

TECH FIG 2 • Metaphyseal sleeve augmentation. **A.** After intramedullary reaming, a trial stem of the appropriate length is attached to the metaphyseal broach. Sequential broaching is carried out until good metaphyseal fill is obtained and the top of the broach is at the level of the planned skim cut. The handle is removed, and the broach is left in place. **B.** A skim cut is taken off the top of the broach. Careful attention should have been taken during broaching to ensure that the proximal surface of the broach rests at the planned level of the "cleanup" cut. **C.** The final component is assembled and shown in this image. Note the porous proximal sleeve that is positioned for bone ongrowth. Care should be taken to keep the metaphyseal cone bone ingrowth surfaces free of cement during component insertion and impaction. **D.** Postoperative AP and lateral (**E**) radiographs demonstrating a well-fixed TKA with metaphyseal sleeve augments required due to the moderate central and contained defects. Note the proximal metaphyseal sleeve is uncemented with isolated tibial baseplate cementation.

Porous Tantalum Metaphyseal Augments

- After a very minimal freshening cut perpendicular to the anatomic axis of the tibia, the cavitary defect of the proximal tibia is curetted clean, and all membrane is removed.
- The size and shape trabecular metal augment that most closely fits the defect is selected, and a high-speed burr is used to remove minimal amounts of bone to allow for a tight press-fit of the augment.
- The augment is impacted into place. In cases in which the augment does not fully contact the surrounding bone, crushed cancellous allograft croutons can be combined with demineralized bone matrix to fill the peripheral void (**TECH FIG 3A**).
  - To minimize the chance of intraoperative periprosthetic fracture, the surgeon should be careful of overly aggressive impaction of the final implant. Tibial metaphyseal bone in the revision setting is typically sclerotic, damaged, mechanically weak, and prone to inadvertent fracture. The frictional coefficient of the actual porous tantalum implant will create greater resistance to insertion and subsequent stability.
- If an offset stem is selected to allow for good tibial coverage, or if the augment is placed off-center of the diaphysis to allow for

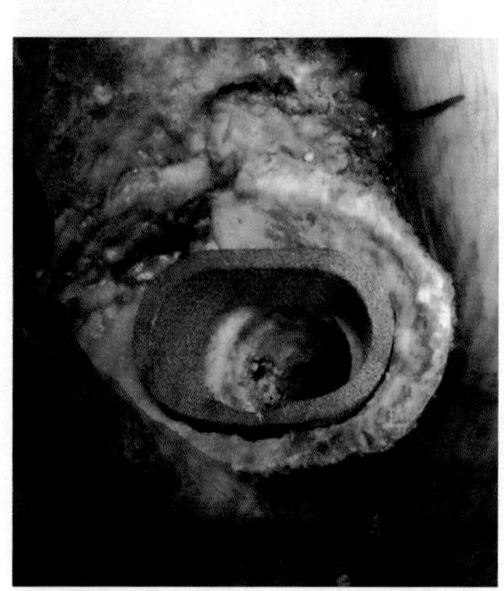

A

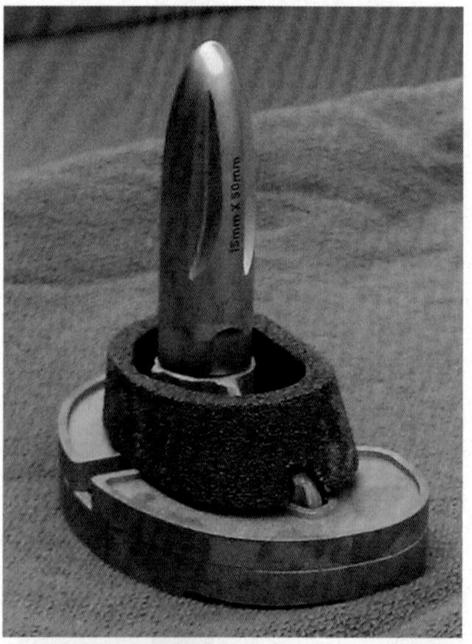

B

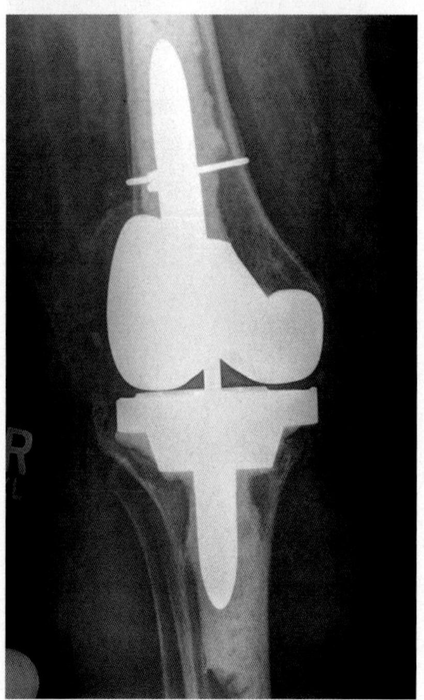

C

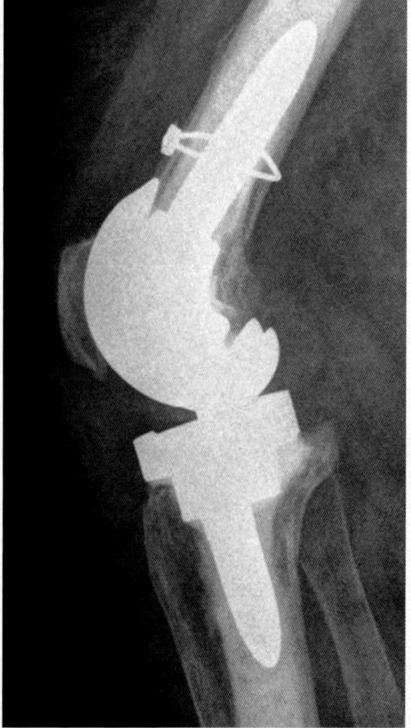

D

TECH FIG 3 • Metaphyseal porous tantalum cone augment. **A.** Once the trials have been inserted and appropriate fit has been achieved, the final augment is gently impacted into place. Excessive force may fracture the proximal tibia. Any defect that remains between the metaphyseal bone and the augment may be grafted to fill the void. Impaction grafting techniques may be used. This intraoperative picture demonstrates stable seating and positioning of the porous tantalum cone. **B.** Porous tantalum metaphyseal cone is shown with medial and lateral slots created with a high-speed, metal-cutting burr. These slots can be created to accommodate a keel to optimize tibial component rotation. **C.** AP and lateral (**D**) radiograph of a well-fixed and osseointegrated porous tantalum metaphyseal cone is used to perform the revision TKA.

best void fill, then a high-speed metal-cutting burr can be used to trim the augment centrally. The metal-cutting burr can also be used to cut slots for the tibial tray and optimized rotation.

- Once clearance is obtained for the augment, the trial tibial stem with baseplate is inserted into the tibial diaphysis through the trabecular metal augment to verify fit (**TECH FIG 3B**).
- When adequate bony support is achieved, the joint surface is restored, and flexion and extension gaps are balanced, the component to be implanted is constructed to match the trial and appropriately cemented into place (**TECH FIG 3C,D**).
- The proximal portion of the tibial stem is cemented to the trabecular metal augment, and the stem is either press-fit in the tibial diaphysis or cemented per the preoperative.
- Newer porous tantalum cones were developed that are smaller in size and can be implanted in the diaphysis or metaphysis. If proximal tibial defects are moderate and contained with an intact peripheral rim and supporting cortical bone but insufficient central metaphysis for rotational control of the tibial implant, the diaphyseal cone can be implanted into the metaphysis for rotational stability.

PEARLS AND PITFALLS

Block augment overhang	■ An augment that overhangs the underlying tibial metaphyseal bone may irritate the medial collateral ligament or soft tissue envelope, particularly about the anterior and medial aspects of the knee. Downsizing of the tibial component or an offset stem may be required.
Joint line elevation	■ Use of medial and lateral augments simultaneously should be an indication to carefully evaluate possible elevation of the joint line. If the joint line is restored, it may be preferable to use medial and lateral augments with a shorter insert to decrease the varus/valgus moment arm on the polyethylene.
Tibial stem to tibial tray mismatch	■ The tibial tray that provides appropriate coverage of the proximal tibial with augmentation may not be centered over the tibial diaphysis. In this case, a central stem will move the tibial tray into an overhanging position or require downsizing that does not allow for adequate coverage of the proximal tibial. Offset uncemented stems or shorter cemented stems are typically required to reconcile this mismatch.
Internal rotation of the tibial component	■ Careful attention must be given to the rotational position of the block augment cutting guide as it is pinned to the tibia. Unlike some primary total knee techniques, rotation cannot be adjusted after the bone cut for the augment is made. All efforts should be made to verify appropriate rotation by anatomic landmarks, including the tibial tubercle, anterior tibial crest, and second metatarsal.
Extensor mechanism/tibial tubercle	■ In the face of significant bone loss in the proximal tibia, the extensor mechanism and its bony attachment should be handled with great care. Exposure of the knee should be accomplished without placing excessive tension on the patellar tendon. When step cuts are made to accommodate block augments, careful attention should be paid to ensure preservation of bone about the tibial tubercle. Prevention of extensor mechanism disruption is of paramount importance.

POSTOPERATIVE CARE

- Postoperative care is directed by the intraoperative findings and the stability of the newly implanted component.
- If a proximally cemented stemmed component is seated on cortical bone with all defects contained after use of an augment, then immediate full weight bearing may be allowed.
- Range-of-motion exercises also may begin immediately if the skin over the anterior knee is in good condition postoperatively and the incision has been closed without tension.
- When the tibial component is not fully supported directly by native metaphyseal bone, then toe-touch weight bearing should be initiated until incorporation of any allograft that was used in conjunction with augmentation.
- When ongrowth cones or porous tantalum metal augmentation is used with less than full bone support, consideration should be given to delaying full weight bearing until ingrowth occurs.
- In cases in which partial weight bearing is initiated postoperatively, progression to full weight bearing can take place at 6 weeks postoperatively.

OUTCOMES

- Several studies have reported successful midterm results with modular metal augments in revision knee arthroplasty.[10,15,16] Patel et al[15] reported the 5- to 10-year results of 102 revision knee arthroplasties in patients with TII defects treated with augments and stems which were studied prospectively.

Average follow-up was 7 years, and nonprogressive radiolucent lines were observed around the augment in 14% of knees but were not associated with decreased survivorship or increased failure of the implants. The overall survivorship of the components was 92% at 11 years.[15]

- Rand[16] prospectively studied 41 consecutive revision TKAs with modular augmentation. Modular augments were used for the distal femur alone in 2 knees, posterior condyles of the femur alone in 16, and both distally and posteriorly in 12 knees. Tibial augmentation was used in 13 knees. At a mean of 3 years follow-up, 96% of the knees demonstrated good to excellent results and there were no cases of aseptic loosening.[16]
- Early outcomes with highly porous metaphyseal cones used in large tibial defects for revision TKA have been reported by multiple authors.[11,13] Meneghini et al[13] reported a series of 15 revision knee arthroplasties that were performed with a porous metal metaphyseal tibial cone and were followed for a minimum of 2 years. All tibial cones were found to be osseointegrated radiographically and clinically at final follow-up with no reported failures in this initial series.
- In a series of 16 revision TKAs with severe tibial defects, Long and Scuderi[11] reported good results with osseointegration of the porous tantalum cone in 14 of 16 cases at a minimum 2-year follow-up. Two metaphyseal cones required removal for recurrent sepsis and were found to be well-fixed at surgery.[11] These early results appear equivalent to those obtained with bulk allograft, custom implants, or large modular metal augments at the same time interval. Further clinical and radiographic follow-up will provide insight into the long-term durability of these highly porous augments.
- Recently, short-term results of porous metal titanium metaphyseal sleeves have been reported in revision TKA.[1,2] Barnett et al[2] reported on 36 revision TKAs using stepped metaphyseal sleeves at a mean of 38 months. At final follow-up, all metaphyseal sleeves demonstrated radiographic osseointegration without loosening or migration.[2]

COMPLICATIONS

- Complications of revision TKA with metallic tibial augmentation can be divided into two categories: early and delayed.
- Perioperative or early complications can include intraoperative damage to neurovascular structures, extensor mechanism and collateral ligamentous disruption, and early postoperative infection.
- Delayed complications most commonly include osteolysis, aseptic loosening, and late septic prosthetic arthropathy.

REFERENCES

1. Alexander GE, Bernasek TL, Crank RL, et al. Cementless metaphyseal sleeves used for large tibial defects in revision total knee arthroplasty. J Arthroplasty 2013;28(4):604–607.
2. Barnett SL, Mayer RR, Gondusky JS, et al. Use of stepped porous titanium metaphyseal sleeves for tibial defects in revision total knee arthroplasty: short term results. J Arthroplasty 2014;29(6):1219–1224.
3. Chen F, Krackow KA. Management of tibial defects in total knee arthroplasty. A biomechanical study. Clin Orthop Relat Res 1994;(305): 249–257.
4. Collier MB, Engh CA Jr, McAuley JP, et al. Osteolysis after total knee arthroplasty: influence of tibial baseplate surface finish and sterilization of polyethylene insert. Findings at five to ten years postoperatively. J Bone Joint Surg Am 2005;87(12):2702–2708.
5. Engh GA, Ammeen DJ. Bone loss with revision total knee arthroplasty: defect classification and alternatives for reconstruction. Instr Course Lect 1999;48:167–175.
6. Engh GA, Ammeen DJ. Classification and preoperative radiographic evaluation: knee. Orthop Clin North Am 1998;29(2):205–217.
7. Fehring TK, Odum S, Calton TF, et al. Articulating versus static spacers in revision total knee arthroplasty for sepsis. The Ranawat Award. Clin Orthop Relat Res 2000;(380):9–16.
8. Fehring TK, Odum S, Griffin WL, et al. Early failures in total knee arthroplasty. Clin Orthop Relat Res 2001;(392):315–318.
9. Figgie HE III, Goldberg VM, Heiple KG, et al. The influence of tibial-patellofemoral location on function of the knee in patients with the posterior stabilized condylar knee prosthesis. J Bone Joint Surg Am 1986;68(7):1035–1040.
10. Haas SB, Insall JN, Montgomery W III, et al. Revision total knee arthroplasty with use of modular components with stems inserted without cement. J Bone Joint Surg Am 1995;77(11):1700–1707.
11. Long WJ, Scuderi GR. Porous tantalum cones for large metaphyseal tibial defects in revision total knee arthroplasty: a minimum 2-year follow-up. J Arthroplasty 2009;24(7):1086–1092.
12. Lotke PA, Ecker ML. Influence of positioning of prosthesis in total knee replacement. J Bone Joint Surg Am 1977;59(1):77–79.
13. Meneghini RM, Lewallen DG, Hanssen AD. Use of porous tantalum metaphyseal cones for severe tibial bone loss during revision total knee replacement. J Bone Joint Surg Am 2008;90(1):78–84.
14. Ninomiya JT, Dean JC, Goldberg VM. Injury to the popliteal artery and its anatomic location in total knee arthroplasty. J Arthroplasty 1999;14(7):803–809.
15. Patel JV, Masonis JL, Guerin J, et al. The fate of augments to treat type-2 bone defects in revision knee arthroplasty. J Bone Joint Surg Br 2004;86(2):195–199.
16. Rand JA. Modularity in total knee arthroplasty. Acta Orthop Belg 1996;62(suppl 1):180–186.
17. Smith DE, McGraw RW, Taylor DC, et al. Arterial complications and total knee arthroplasty. J Am Acad Orthop Surg 2001;9(4):253–257.
18. Smith PN, Gelinas J, Kennedy K, et al. Popliteal vessels in knee surgery. A magnetic resonance imaging study. Clin Orthop Relat Res 1999;(367):158–164.
19. Vessely MB, Frick MA, Oakes D, et al. Magnetic resonance imaging with metal suppression for evaluation of periprosthetic osteolysis after total knee arthroplasty. J Arthroplasty 2006;21(6):826–831.
20. Younger AS, Duncan CP, Masri BA. Surgical exposures in revision total knee arthroplasty. J Am Acad Orthop Surg 1998;6(1):55–64.

Revision Total Knee Arthroplasty with Femoral Bone Loss: Distal Femoral Replacement

41

CHAPTER

B. Sonny Bal

DEFINITION

- During revision of the femoral component in total knee arthroplasty (TKA), some bone loss from the distal femur is nearly inevitable when the femoral component is removed.
- Distal femoral bone loss can be repaired by bone cement (polymethylmethacrylate), metal augments fixed to the revision femoral component, particulate bone graft or substitutes, bulk allograft to augment one or both femoral condyles, porous metal cones designed for structural support, and complete distal femoral replacement with allograft or metal.

ANATOMY

- The anatomy relevant to bone loss during revision TKA are the metaphyseal femur, the medial and lateral epicondyles, and the medial and lateral femoral condyles.
- The femoral condyles support the revision femoral component. Accordingly, one goal of distal femoral reconstruction in revision TKA is to restore the condylar anatomy so that it can support a new component.

PATHOGENESIS

- The pathogenesis of distal femoral bone loss in revision TKA is related to removal of the previous implant and bone cement. Previous implants fixed to bone with cement or by porous ingrowth require dissection for mobilization and extraction; this process incurs a finite amount of bone loss.
- Even fine osteotomes and saws used to develop a plane between the implant and bone occupy space and cause bone loss from the distal femur. Aggressive extraction of well-fixed femoral components without first developing a plane between exposed metal and bone can result in avulsion of one or both femoral condyles, thereby compounding bone loss.
- Correction of internal rotation of the previous femoral component will result in bone loss both anteriorly and posteriorly as the new component is oriented in the proper rotation.
- Osteopenia from stress shielding of the periprosthetic femur, as well as osteolysis related to wear debris particles, can result in cavitary lesions in the distal femur that lead to significant bone loss.

NATURAL HISTORY

- Distal femoral bone loss, if severe, can result in the loss of the structural integrity of the femur. When this occurs, the existing femoral component can migrate into the varus or valgus position relative to the femoral shaft.
- Surgical treatment is directed at augmenting this bone loss following removal of the previous loose, unstable femoral component.
- If left untreated, continued particulate debris and motion between loose components and bone can lead to persistent symptoms and further bone loss in the distal femur of a failed TKA.

PATIENT HISTORY AND PHYSICAL FINDINGS

- The diagnosis of a failed TKA with loss of bone in the distal femur is best made by plain radiographs.
- Findings in any of the following categories can alert the surgeon to the possibility that significant bone loss may be encountered during revision surgery: the time elapsed since the index arthroplasty, the type of implant and fixation used, and any history of diseases such as osteoporosis, advanced age, corticosteroid use, use of cytotoxic drugs, irradiation, rheumatoid arthritis, and periprosthetic femoral fracture.
  - Patients who have loose femoral components with associated bone loss will present with knee pain, swelling, and instability that is usually worsened by activity.
- Failed TKA femoral components with bone loss will have tenderness to palpation over the distal femur.
  - An effusion may also be evident on physical examination.
  - A grossly unstable component may result in ligamentous instability of the knee that is elicited on careful examination.

IMAGING AND OTHER DIAGNOSTIC STUDIES

- High-quality radiographs of the knee can help identify and classify a bone defect in the distal femur. The true lateral view of the knee joint can demonstrate the location and extent of osteolysis and bone loss in the distal femur. Oblique views of the knee often result in obscuring of bony detail by the metal implants. Therefore, a true lateral view of the knee should be obtained in 90 degrees of knee flexion by placing the entire leg, including the knee and ankle joints, flat on the radiograph table.
- Other imaging modalities such as computed tomography scans and metal subtraction magnetic resonance imaging scans may prove useful in defining the extent of bone loss in the distal femur, although the efficacy of these imaging studies in routine revision TKA is not established.
- Intraoperative observation of bone loss after previous component removal and thorough débridement of osteolytic lesions and inflammatory membrane is the best determinant of the nature and extent of bone loss.
- The surgeon should be prepared for the worst-case scenario because preoperative radiographs will often underestimate the extent of bone loss adjacent to the existing femoral component.

- Accordingly, allograft bone, a wide range of revision implants, metal augments, porous metal reconstructive cones, and revision equipment should be available.
- The diagnostic workup of femoral bone loss in revision TKA should include a thorough evaluation to exclude the possibility of knee sepsis.
  - Preoperative nuclear medicine imaging, laboratory data, knee aspiration, and intraoperative frozen sections of periprosthetic tissues can assist in excluding sepsis.

DIFFERENTIAL DIAGNOSIS

- Deep knee sepsis can result in periprosthetic bone loss and is a relative contraindication to distal femoral reconstruction. Infection must be ruled out before reconstructing the distal femur in anticipation of implanting a revision femoral component.
- Stress shielding of bone adjacent to the femoral component can result in bone loss from the distal femur. When the existing femoral component is extracted, severe loss of bone may be discovered in such cases.
- Osteopenia of the distal femur from osteoporosis, lytic lesions of bone such as benign bone cysts, neuropathic changes, and malignancy can also result in distal femoral bone loss, thereby complicating femoral reconstruction in TKA.

NONOPERATIVE MANAGEMENT

- Nonoperative management of severe distal femoral bone loss in a failed TKA should be reserved for debilitated patients in whom surgery is otherwise contraindicated.
- Severe medical comorbidities, integrity of the extensor mechanism, poor condition of the soft tissue, radiation necrosis of adjacent bone, immunosuppression, and metabolic bone disorders should be evaluated carefully to determine whether reconstruction of the distal femur is a reasonable option.
- Where major knee surgery is contraindicated, nonoperative measures such as analgesics, limited ambulation, assistive devices such as a walker or wheelchair, and knee bracing are alternative considerations.
- Chronic suppressive antibiotics may be an option in patients with bone loss from severe deep sepsis in whom operative treatment is otherwise contraindicated.

SURGICAL MANAGEMENT

- Distal femoral bone loss can be managed surgically using bone cement (augmented with screws driven into existing bone, if necessary), morselized bone graft, metal augments fixed to the revision implant, porous metal cones designed to reproduce distal femoral anatomy, bulk allograft reconstruction of uncontained defects of the medial or lateral condyles, and bulk allograft replacement of the distal femur with allograft or a special customized prosthesis.

Preoperative Planning

- Preoperative planning includes making sure the patient is medically optimized for major elective surgery and excluding the possibility of deep sepsis in the knee. The surgeon should carefully assess existing scars, leg vascularity, nerve function, and the patient's overall medical condition.
- Pre- and intraoperative assessment of collateral ligament integrity will help the surgeon choose appropriate implants and plan the reconstruction.
  - In grossly unstable knees, constrained implants or even rotating hinge revision TKA implants may be indicated.
- The surgeon should prepare for the worst-case scenario so that the correct equipment, implants, and personnel will be available to address any circumstance. However, outside of straightforward TKA revision cases with minimal femoral bone deficiency, such procedures are limited to hospitals that have the necessary equipment and expertise due to the specialized procedures that are needed.
- A preoperative planning session with key personnel (ie, surgeon, assistants, and implant manufacturer representative) is invaluable for discussing the problem and considering all possible solutions for efficient execution of the procedure.
- Structural allografts to rebuild deficient distal femoral condyles should include several allograft femoral heads.
  - Fresh frozen prepared specimens are usually favored because of their superior mechanical strength.[7]
- Preoperative radiography and sizing of allograft tissue is desirable but may not be practical or feasible.
  - Instead, intraoperative preparation of the grafts with special equipment such as the Allogrip system (DePuy Synthes, Warsaw, IN) can shape the graft to proper dimensions so that wound closure is not a problem with an oversized graft.[4]
- A full set of revision TKA instruments is essential, consisting of fine osteotomes to develop the plane between metal and bone, curettes, punches, reamers, Gigli saws, and instruments to clean out the intramedullary femoral canal.
  - High-speed burrs attached to a pneumatic power driver can assist in loosening well-fixed implants while preserving bone.
  - A typical revision TKA instrument set from any major implant manufacturer has these instruments conveniently packaged in a single set.
- Porous tantalum metal cones (and similar cones made of porous titanium metal) are available for proximal tibia reconstruction in revision TKA as well as for distal femoral reconstruction.[6] The advantage of this type of metal reconstruction is the rapid healing of structural metal support to living host bone. Initial mechanical stability is achieved by impacting these cones into residual, viable bone of the distal femur. These metal cones offer a custom reconstruction option that permits load bearing and supports cement fixation of the revision implant. Depending on the extent of bone loss, the surgeon can choose the type of metal cone that will best address the deficiency, including replacement of both femoral condyles if necessary. Intermediate-term clinical outcomes with this type of reconstruction have been favorable.

Positioning

- The patient is placed supine, with a small pad under the ipsilateral buttock to ensure neutral position of the flexed knee. A Stulberg footrest or equivalent device is used to control knee flexion during surgery.
- The leg is scrubbed circumferentially and as far proximal as feasible to allow access to the thigh.

- In our practice, we do not use a tourniquet during any total knee procedure, but most surgeons exsanguinate the extremity with gravity or an Esmarch bandage before inflating and applying a well-padded tourniquet to the proximal thigh.
  - The surgeon must remain vigilant of the duration of tourniquet time, particularly if a long and complex reconstruction is anticipated.

Approach

- If several previous scars are present, choose the one closest to the midline that will allow extensile exposure proximally or distally. The most laterally based incision is the wisest as it preserves blood supply to the overlying skin. For most revision TKA that involves distal femoral reconstruction, a standard medial parapatellar arthrotomy will adequately expose the distal femur.
- Exposure can be facilitated by avoiding patella eversion in knee flexion. After the patellar component is addressed in knee extension, the patella can be pushed into the lateral gutter and retracted safely.
  - In our experience, exposure of the distal femur is improved if patella eversion is avoided.
- To understand the extent of bone loss, inflammatory membranous tissue overlying the femoral bone after removal of the previous component must be dissected away. The electrocautery knife works well for this purpose. Previous membrane and granulomas must be débrided thoroughly to appreciate the amount of distal femur available for reconstruction.
- Anteriorly, a proximal quadricepsplasty,[3,9] tibial tubercle osteotomy,[2] or other specialized dissection may be needed to mobilize the extensor mechanism safely and expose the distal femoral cortex.
  - The exposure chosen depends on the difficulty in exposing the distal femur and the extent of débridement and preparation for bone reconstruction required.

TECHNIQUES

Morselized Allograft or Bone Cement

- Small, contained defects in the femoral condyles can be filled with bone cement or morselized autograft or allograft.[10] These grafts are not load bearing and are suitable only for focal cystic lesions that are surrounded by intact structural bone (**TECH FIG 1**).
  - A burr or curette is effective in cleaning out such defects.
- To optimize allograft–host bone contact, excise the inflammatory membrane, remove previous metal and cement particles, and create a viable and healthy host bone bed.
- Morselize an allograft femoral head using small acetabular reamers. Pack graft into the defects and cement the revision implant in place.
  - Alternatively, bone cement or a synthetic bone graft substitute filler can be used to pack small, contained defects between the revision implant and host bone.

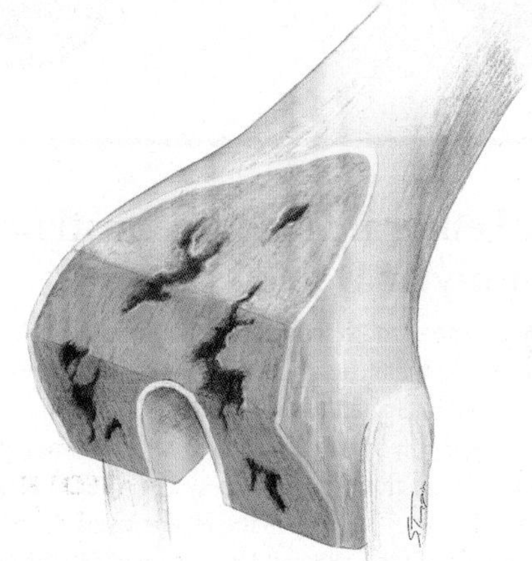

TECH FIG 1 • Cavitary, contained defects that do not affect the structural integrity of the distal femur can be packed with cement, morselized autograft or allograft, or synthetic bone fillers.

Metal Augments on Revision Femoral Component

- After excision of previous cement and inflammatory granulomas, remove the minimum amount of bone from the distal and posterior femoral condyles to expose viable host bone (**TECH FIG 2A,C**).
  - Small defects in the distal and posterior femoral condyles can be reconstructed by using metal augments on the revision femoral component[8] (**TECH FIG 2B,D**).
- Determine the joint line by examining the position of the epicondyles, the existing femoral component, position of the patella relative to the femur, contralateral knee radiographs, and the contour of the posterior femoral condyles projected laterally.
  - A combination of these variables makes it possible to accurately estimate and recreate the joint line.
  - Removal of additional bone from the distal femur will move the joint line more proximally.
- Impact the trial femoral component on the distal femur and measure the defects between metal and host bone distally, anteriorly, and posteriorly after determining proper external rotation of the component.
  - Reinsert the trial implant after installing trial augments of the appropriate thickness and check the fit.
- Augments in revision TKA systems come in a variety of thicknesses to accommodate femoral bone loss from the anterior cortex, posterior condyles, and distal femoral condyles.
  - The goal of revision component augmentation is stable contact between metal and host bone without resorting to a custom implant.
- If metal augments are used on the revision femoral component, an intramedullary rod extension should be attached to the revision femoral component to achieve initial implant stability.[8]

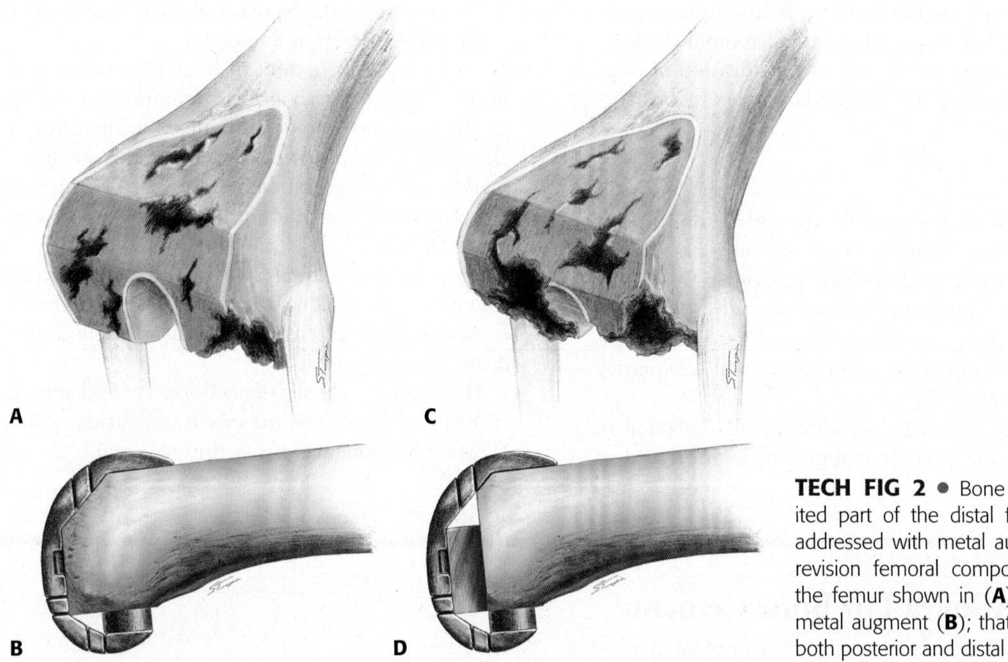

TECH FIG 2 • Bone loss that affects a limited part of the distal femoral condyle can be addressed with metal augments attached to the revision femoral component. Reconstruction of the femur shown in (**A**) will require a posterior metal augment (**B**); that shown in (**C**) will need both posterior and distal metal augments (**D**).

Bulk Femoral Head Reconstruction of Condylar Defects

- If one or both femoral condyles are not amenable to reconstruction with metal augments, structural deficiencies can be addressed with allograft tissue (**TECH FIG 3A,B**).
- The condylar defect is reamed with small diameter male acetabular reamers from the Allogrip system (**TECH FIG 3C**).
- Matched diameter female reamers are used to prepare the convex surface of the allograft femoral head (**TECH FIG 3D**).
- The allograft femoral head is placed in the reamed defect. Either a whole or a half femoral head allograft will fill the cavitary defect where it is attached to host bone with cancellous screws (**TECH FIG 3E**).
- Then the allograft–host bone composite is cut to match the size of the revision femoral component.
- Metal augments may be needed for residual bone defects that remain after femoral head allograft reconstruction of the femoral condyles or to recreate the joint line.
  - The technique of using metal augments on the revision femoral component is described earlier.
- Attention must be maintained throughout to ensure recreation of the joint line and the appropriate external rotation of the femoral component needed for patella stability.

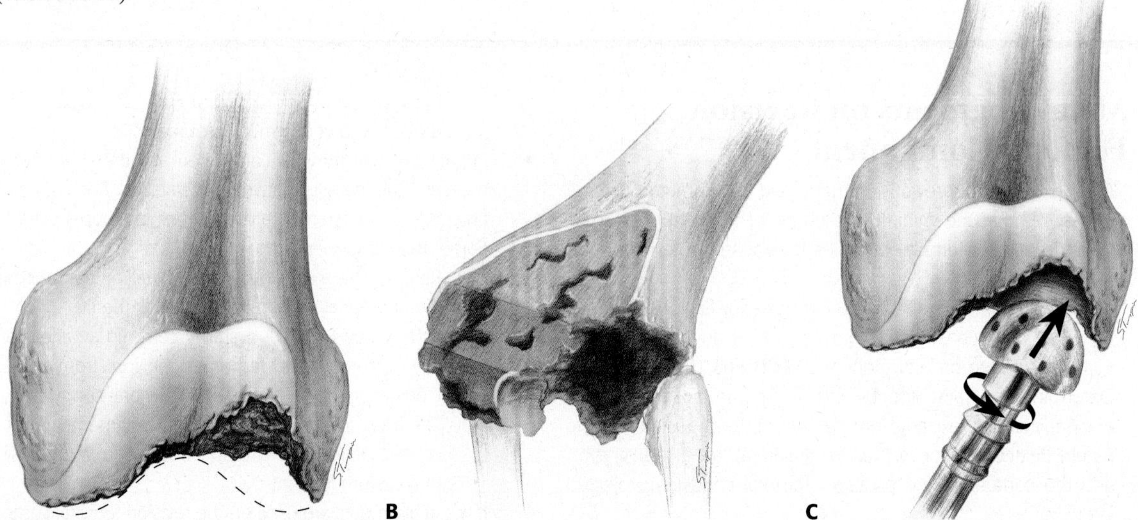

TECH FIG 3 • **A,B.** Severe and complete loss of structural bone in the condyle of the distal femur can be addressed with bulk femoral head allograft to rebuild the deficient bone. **C.** Acetabular reamers are used to prepare the host condyle for a matching allograft. *(continued)*

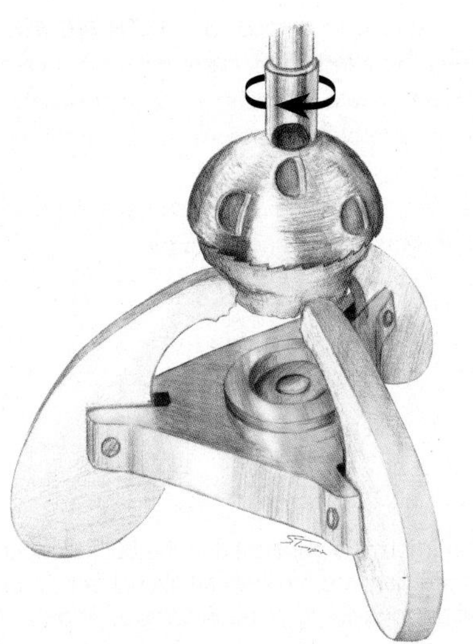

D

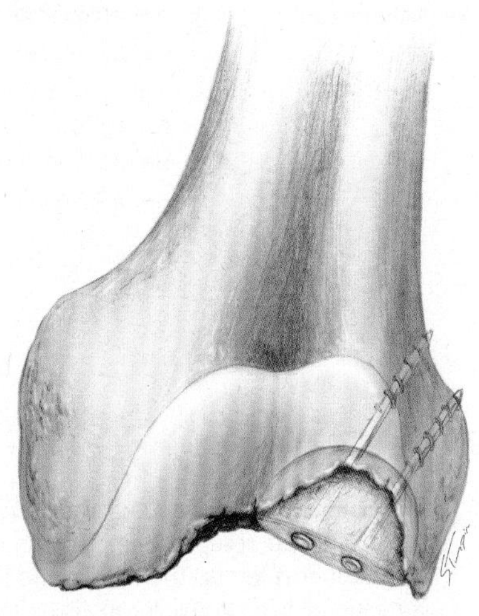

E

TECH FIG 3 ● *(continued)* **D.** The Allogrip system is illustrated, with a femoral head allograft held tightly in the vise while female acetabular reamers expose cancellous bone and size the graft to match the condylar defect. **E.** The cavitary defect in the femur is filled with a bisected femoral head allograft, which is flush against host bone and stabilized with two compression screws.

Bulk Allograft Replacement of the Distal Femur

- For extensive loss of the distal femur, reconstruction with bulk allograft replacement of deficient bone is a proven option.[1]
- If extensive bone loss leaves only an intact cortical shell in the distal femur, an undersized distal femur bulk allograft matched to the operative side can be stabilized within the host cortical shell (**TECH FIG 4A**).
- The proximal end of the graft should rest against viable host bone, with mechanical stability and maximum host bone–allograft contact to promote healing.
  - Conservative resection of the distal femur to match the end of the allograft will accomplish contact between host bone and allograft.
- Once stabilized, the allograft distal femur within the host cortex is sized and cut to match the revision femoral component.
  - Collateral ligaments, if present, are preserved on the outer shell of host cortical bone.
- An alternative to this technique is osteotomy of the epicondyles and replacement of deficient bone by a bulk femoral allograft (**TECH FIG 4B,C**).
  - The graft–host bone junction can be cut in a step cut configuration to ensure rotational stability.
- In all cases of allograft reconstruction of the distal femur, offloading of the graft and rotational stability should be ensured by using an intramedullary rod attached to the revision femoral component.
- If necessary, the rod can be cemented into the allograft and host bone for stability, although extrusion of cement at the host bone–allograft junction must be avoided to allow healing.

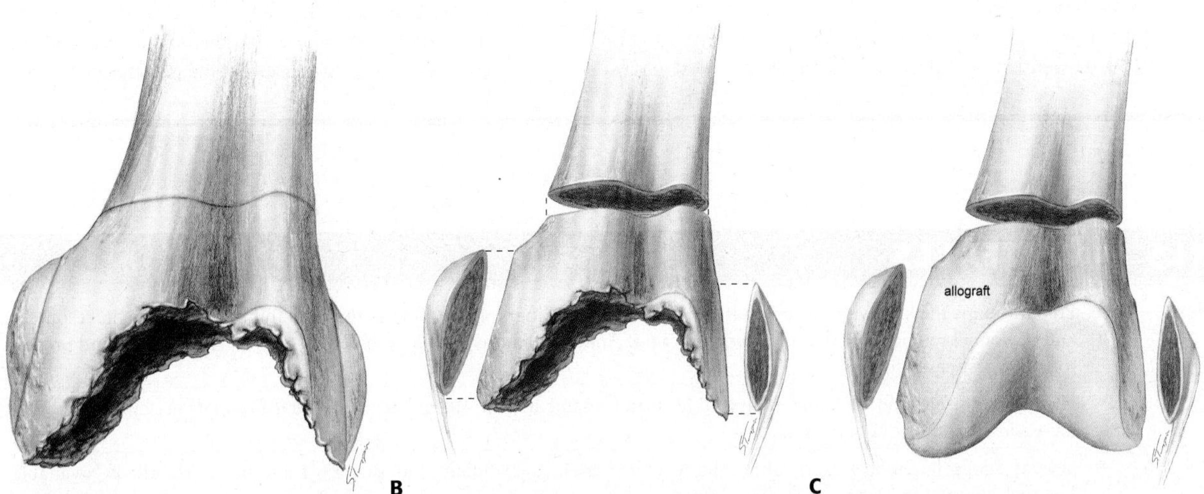

A B C

TECH FIG 4 ● **A.** Severe deficiency of both femoral condyles can be addressed by pressing an undersized distal femoral allograft into this void while retaining the host cortical bone around it. After stabilization to surrounding host bone with screws, the allograft–host composite is shaped to receive the revision femoral component. **B.** To replace the distal femur, existing epicondyles are osteotomized and the deficient distal femur is cut to expose viable, stable host bone. In this case, a bulk distal femoral allograft will be used to rebuild the femur. **C.** The allograft femur is in place with host epicondyles and distal femur shown. *(continued)*

TECHNIQUES

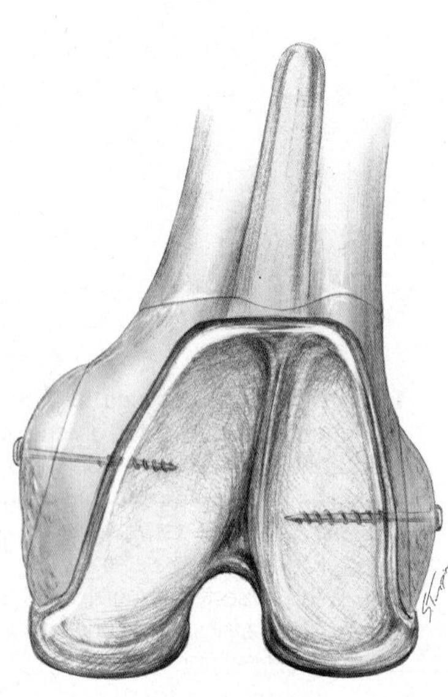

- After implantation of the revision component (**TECH FIG 4D**), the epicondyles should be attached to the allograft with cancellous screws augmented with washers. To accomplish this step, the epicondyles on the bulk allograft must be cut off and removed.
- Before final implantation, check the soft tissue envelope to make sure inadvertent oversizing has not occurred.

TECH FIG 4 • (continued) D. The revision implant is positioned in the bulk allograft that was cut to accept the implant. An intramedullary rod provides additional fixation in the distal host femur. The medial and lateral epicondyles have been screwed into their corresponding anatomic locations on the bulk allograft.

Replacement of Distal Femur with a Tumor Reconstruction Prosthesis

- For severe loss of the metaphyseal and diaphyseal femur (such as in tumor resection), modular implants designed for limb salvage may be the only option for reconstruction.[5]
  - This option is reserved for cases in which the extent of bone loss precludes reconstruction with bulk allograft.
- Template radiographs and have appropriate reconstruction systems with varying modular lengths available to rebuild the deficient femur.
- Perform an osteotomy of the femur to expose viable bone that is suitable for weight bearing.
- Prepare the femur retrograde for cementing, using techniques similar to those for cementing a femoral implant in total hip replacement surgery.
- Use trial and error to reproduce the appropriate limb length, soft tissue tension, and implant rotation. This is most easily accomplished by reconstructing the tibial side first, so that all trial reductions can be assessed by changing the femoral side only, thereby simplifying the procedure.
- When correct rotation and length are determined, mark the host bone and implant to reproduce this rotation, and cement the implant into the distal femur to the appropriate depth and in the desired rotation.
  - Uncemented fixation into the distal femur may be an option with some reconstruction systems.
- Assemble the knee articulation (these designs usually rely on a rotating hinge articulation with multidirectional constraint built into the articulation).
- In severe cases, or if the proximal femur is unsuitable for mechanical fixation with an intramedullary rod, the entire femur can be bypassed with metal.
  - In cases of complete femoral replacement, a rotating hinge knee reconstruction is done at the distal end and a constrained hip replacement at the proximal end.

PEARLS AND PITFALLS

Preparations	■ Preparation is the key, with a team conference to review radiographs and assess the availability of equipment, resources, and personnel required for femoral reconstruction. Anticipate more bone loss than that seen on radiographs and prepare for the worst-case scenario.
Implants	■ Have a wide selection of implants available: metal augments, intramedullary rod extensions, offsets, and those with increasing amounts of constraint.
Grafts	■ Several allograft femoral heads and equipment for milling, grinding, and shaping these heads should be available. Fixation of grafts to host bone requires interfragmentary screws and small plates, which should be readily available. Two or more graft specimens must be available for distal femoral allograft replacement so that the closest size can be chosen.
Sizing	■ Graft sizing can be judged by preoperative radiographs of the graft superimposed on the patient's knee or by intraoperative assessment. Oversized grafts will present problems with wound closure; check soft tissue tension before final fixation of the graft to host bone.

Experience and resources	▪ Be realistic about surgeon experience, support, equipment, and resources available to perform complex distal femoral reconstruction. Specialized training, intensive equipment, and personnel demands effectively prevent surgeons at smaller institutions from doing such surgery.
Operative time	▪ Either avoid using a tourniquet or be wary of the tourniquet time in lengthy total knee reconstructions. If necessary, the tourniquet can be let down for selected parts of the procedure to minimize limb ischemia time.

POSTOPERATIVE CARE

- The goal of distal femoral reconstruction is to achieve initial mechanical stability. Accordingly, the surgeon should aim for weight bearing as soon as possible after surgery.
- If allograft reconstruction of the femur is necessary, healing to host bone occurs over a prolonged time. Therefore, protected weight bearing will be required for an extended period of time.
- Assistive devices such as a cane, walker, or crutches should be prescribed for all patients who undergo revision TKA with distal femoral reconstruction to protect them against accidental falls or twists on the reconstructed knee and to allow healing of graft tissue.
- Range of motion should be assessed intraoperatively following distal femur reconstruction. Usually, range of motion will depend on the quality of the soft tissues and integrity of the extensor mechanism, assuming that mechanical stability of the reconstruction has been achieved. If knee range of movement must be limited for a period of time, a knee brace that allows movement only through a prescribed range of motion may be necessary.
- Straight-leg raises, isometric exercises, and ankle and calf rehabilitation should be possible soon after all distal femoral reconstructions.
- A multimodal deep venous thrombosis prevention regimen should be instituted after surgery and the patient monitored appropriately.

OUTCOMES

- Radiographs at regular intervals and patient interviews will allow assessment of outcomes. Radiographs should be assessed for stability of the reconstruction and for healing of bone at the allograft–host bone junction.
- Bulk allografts heal to living host bone, and allograft bone away from this healed junction remains nonviable over the long term. In load-sharing configurations, where the allograft is supported by host bone or by metal implants, the long-term outcomes are excellent.
- If allograft bone is used in load-bearing configurations, late failure of the nonviable bone from repetitive loading is predictable.
  - Allograft bone cannot remodel in response to stress; therefore, intramedullary stems that bypass the graft completely and transfer loads to living host bone are essential during the reconstruction.
- In some complex reconstructions involving distal femur replacements with bulk allograft or limb salvage implants, the patient should be counseled to use protected weight bearing for a prolonged time, such as 6 months or longer.

COMPLICATIONS

- Postoperative infection is a devastating complication following complex distal femoral reconstruction with allograft bone. Early diagnosis and aggressive wound débridement may salvage the situation in some instances, but removal of all allograft, cement, and implants in preparation for a staged reconstruction is usually necessary.
- Late deep infections with a virulent organism in a knee with massive bone loss and allograft reconstruction of deficient host bone may necessitate a limb amputation.
- Mechanical failure of distal femoral reconstructions usually occurs if the surgeon fails to achieve initial mechanical stability. Repeat surgery is necessary to rebuild the femur and achieve rotational and axial stability to permit protected weight bearing after the procedure.
- Because anticoagulation for prophylaxis against deep venous thrombosis is necessary after distal femoral reconstruction in revision TKA, the surgeon should monitor the patient for postoperative bleeding.
- If a tense hematoma develops or new wound drainage is encountered, aggressive surgical decompression should be considered early to avoid the risk of infection.

REFERENCES

1. Bezwada HP, Shah AR, Zambito K, et al. Distal femoral allograft reconstruction for massive osteolytic bone loss in revision total knee arthroplasty. J Arthroplasty 2006;21:242–248.
2. Clarke HD. Tibial tubercle osteotomy. J Knee Surg 2003;16:58–61.
3. Della Valle CJ, Berger RA, Rosenberg AG. Surgical exposures in revision total knee arthroplasty. Clin Orthop Relat Res 2006;446: 59–68.
4. Engh GA, Herzwurm PJ, Parks NL. Treatment of major defects of bone with bulk allografts and stemmed components during total knee arthroplasty. J Bone Joint Surg Am 1997;79A:1030–1039.
5. Harrison RJ Jr, Thacker MM, Pitcher JD, et al. Distal femur replacement is useful in complex total knee arthroplasty revisions. Clin Orthop Relat Res 2006;446:113–120.
6. Levine BR, Sporer S, Poggie RA, et al. Experimental and clinical performance of porous tantalum in orthopedic surgery. Biomaterials 2006;27:4671–4681.
7. Pelker RR, Friedlaender GE. Biomechanical aspects of bone autografts and allografts. Orthop Clin North Am 1987;18:235–239.
8. Radnay CS, Scuderi GR. Management of bone loss: augments, cones, offset stems. Clin Orthop Relat Res 2006;446:83–92.
9. Trousdale RT, Hanssen AD, Rand JA, et al. V-Y quadricepsplasty in total knee arthroplasty. Clin Orthop Relat Res 1993;286: 48–55.
10. van Loon CJ, de Waal Malefijt MC, Verdonschot N, et al. Morsellized bone grafting compensates for femoral bone loss in revision total knee arthroplasty. An experimental study. Biomaterials 1999;20: 85–89.

Revision Total Knee Arthroplasty with Tibial Bone Loss: Bone Grafting

Emmanuel Thienpont

DEFINITION

- Substantial bone loss and bone defects are among the most challenging problems faced by surgeons performing revision knee arthroplasty. Tibial bone loss in failed total knee arthroplasty (TKA) is a complex and difficult problem.
- Awareness and proper management of bone loss through cement fill, metal augments, or bone grafting are crucial for achieving stability and longevity of the newly implanted revision components.

ANATOMY

- Tibial bone loss during revision TKA is common. The most common areas of deficiency involve the posterolateral and medial tibial plateau.
- Bone loss is typically inconsequential and contained; even after component removal, bone loss can be restricted to discrete cancellous defects.
- Smaller, contained defects can often be addressed with morcellized autografts from bone cuts (or allograft if unavailable) or with bone cement alone. Larger, uncontained defects may require the use of metallic wedges or structural allografts.

PATHOGENESIS

- The etiology of bone loss after TKA is usually multifactorial. Bone stock deficiency may result from any of the following causes:
  - Aseptic loosening. Secondary to component malposition or ligament imbalance, aseptic loosening can cause collapse of the tibia plateau on the compression side as well as lift-off on the tension side.
  - Periprosthetic osteolysis. Wear debris following TKA is frequently due to high-contact stresses secondary to poor implant design or poor component alignment or ligament balance[12] and can result in lysis of the bone.
  - Infection
  - Removal of well-fixed implants. Even using proper technique, implant removal can result in some degree of bone loss, particularly from the implant-adherent region.[7]

NATURAL HISTORY

- Regardless of the mechanism of bone loss, it is likely that continuing progression, leading to eventual failure of the TKA, will occur once significant bony destruction is visible on plain radiographs.
- In this spiral toward implant failure, patients may be asymptomatic initially. However, pain, swelling, and instability, including hyperextension due to loss of tibial height, can be expected and are likely sequelae of a failing TKA with significant tibial bone loss.

PATIENT HISTORY AND PHYSICAL FINDINGS

- Preoperative evaluation begins with a detailed history and clinical examination.
- It is paramount that the cause of failure is determined in the preoperative assessment to reduce the risk of repeating mistakes that may have led to failure of the initial TKA.
- Other causes of pain, such as spinal or hip pathology, should be ruled out.
- Contraindications for surgery, such as infection, poor general condition, Charcot arthropathy, or neuromuscular disorders, must be ruled out.
- Reports of previous surgeries must be obtained to gather information on prior soft tissue releases performed as well as the type and size of the current prosthetic components.

IMAGING AND OTHER DIAGNOSTIC STUDIES

- A thorough clinical and radiographic evaluation is a prerequisite for revision TKA. The extent and location of bone loss, the quality of the remaining bone, the degree of cortical continuity, and the absence of infection must be determined.
- Full-length standing anteroposterior radiographs should be taken to assess coronal limb alignment and the presence of diaphyseal deformities or hardware.
- Weight-bearing anteroposterior, lateral, and Merchant patellar views allow the femoral and tibial implant size to be evaluated and current bone stock, implant position and fixation, and patellar height and coronal position to be assessed (**FIG 1**).
- The true magnitude of bone loss is often underestimated on radiographs. Computed tomography (CT) scans may estimate the degree of bone loss more accurately, particularly when there is massive bone loss or abnormal anatomy, as

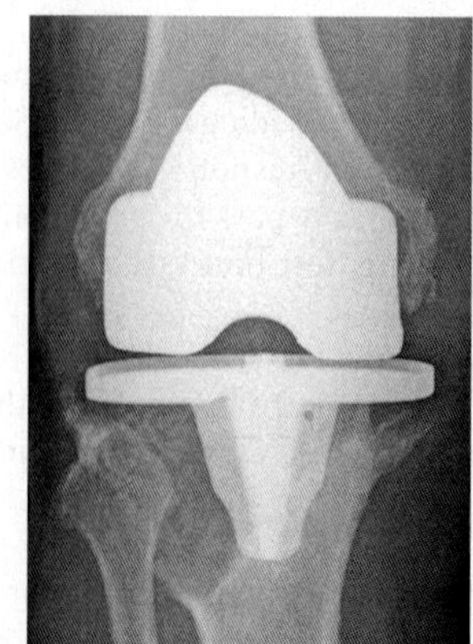

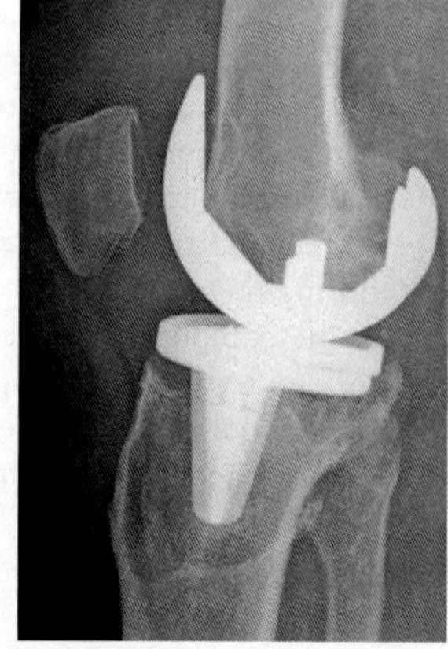

FIG 1 • **A,B.** Anteroposterior (AP) and lateral preoperative radiographs showing a failed TKA with tibial component subsidence and loosening.

well as help in identifying malrotation of the femoral or tibial component.[14]

- All patients should have the appropriate infection laboratory studies (ie, complete blood count, C-reactive protein, erythrocyte sedimentation rate). Knee aspiration should be considered in order to obtain culture specimens as well as a cell count with differential. Synovial fluid aspirates with leukocyte counts greater than or equal to 2500 per mm^3 in conjunction with a neutrophil percentage of 60% are indicative of infection.[11]

DIFFERENTIAL DIAGNOSIS

- Extremity pain in a patient with a TKA can have several possible nonsurgical diagnoses, including the following:
  - Referred pain from the hip, thigh, or calf
  - Complex regional pain syndrome
  - Pes anserine bursitis
  - Patellar or hamstring tendinitis
  - Crystal deposition disease (ie, gout or pseudogout)
  - Neurovascular problems: neuropathy, radiculopathy, spinal stenosis
  - Tumor (should eventually be considered)
  - Vascular claudication
  - Thrombophlebitis or deep vein thrombosis
  - Fibromyalgia

NONOPERATIVE MANAGEMENT

- Nonoperative management of a painful TKA with tibial bone loss is often not indicated. However, if revision is not deemed safe for medical, psychosocial, or other reasons, management is similar to that for a patient with end-stage knee arthritis.
- Treatment options are symptom-based and can include activity modification, walking aids, nonsteroidal pain medications, and bracing.

SURGICAL MANAGEMENT

- Various joint reconstruction techniques have been described for dealing with bone loss. The choice of reconstruction depends largely on the type of bone loss (ie, contained or uncontained) and the location and size of the defect (Table 1).
  - Cement and screw reconstruction
  - Morcellized autograft or allograft with impaction grafting[16]
  - Prosthetic augments
  - Modular hinged prosthesis
  - Metaphyseal sleeves or cones
  - Structural allograft
- A contained defect is surrounded by intact bone and has an intact peripheral cortical rim that allows treatment with morcellized bone graft or cement and screws.[2,12]
- An uncontained defect has no peripheral cortical rim and typically requires modular block augments, bulk allograft, or metal metaphyseal sleeves or cones for reconstruction.[2]

Preoperative Planning

- Bone loss around a knee implant should be assessed systematically and include both femoral condyles, both tibial plateaus, and the patellofemoral joint.
- Location of the joint line is marked. Reference points include the fibular head and the epicondyles of the femur. The joint line typically sits 20 to 25 mm distal of the lateral epicondyle.[4]
- The magnitude of bone loss has significant implications for decisions regarding the use of bone graft or prosthesis augmentation, choice of prosthesis sizing, selection of articular constraint, and need for supplemental stem fixation.[5]

Positioning

- Revision TKA is usually performed with the patient in the supine position.

Approach

- Sufficient surgical exposure is of critical importance in revision TKA. With revision surgery, the soft tissue planes are often blurred by extensive scar tissue. The incision should therefore be lengthened as necessary to allow adequate exposure and visualization and the surgeon should work from normal tissue to recreate the tissue planes.
- A standard medial parapatellar arthrotomy of the knee is routinely performed; however, for some cases, the subvastus approach could still be used.
- Next, a thorough intra-articular synovectomy is performed to expose the implants and recreate the lateral gutters.

Table 1 Anderson Orthopaedic Research Institute Bone Defect Classification Guidelines

Type	Description	Preoperative Radiographic Appearance	Treatment Options[15]
I	Intact metaphyseal bone	Metaphyseal bone intact above the tibial tubercle No component subsidence	Cement alone Metal augments Morcellized allografts
II	Damaged metaphyseal bone	Component subsidence or position up to or below the tip of the fibular head	Cement in conjunction with other options Metal augments Morcellized allograft Impaction grafting Structural allograft Metaphyseal sleeves Porous metal cones
III	Deficient metaphyseal bone	Bone damage or component subsidence to the tibial tubercle	Impaction grafting Structural allograft Metaphyseal sleeves Porous metal cones Composite allograft Custom prostheses

- Additional exposure is often required if a metal wire mesh is needed for unconstrained defects. The proximal portion of the tibia must be well exposed to ensure fixation of the wire mesh onto the bone. External rotation of the tibia and elevation of the medial sleeve often help with exposure of the cortical margins.
- The surgeon should assess the stability of the collateral ligaments prior to removal of the implants.
- Following medial release, the knee is dislocated and the polyethylene insert removed. The patella is sublimated rather than everted to minimize tension on the extensor mechanism. A quadriceps snip can be performed if needed, which reduces the risk of iatrogenic disruption to the extensor mechanism without exacerbating postoperative restrictions for the patient.[3]
- Once the components are adequately exposed, they are evaluated and implant removal is initiated. The implant–bone or cement–bone interface should be disrupted with a combination of flexible osteotomes and thin saw blades on an oscillating saw.
- Cavitary defects need to be contoured. In case of multiloculated defects, they need to be cleaned from the cavitary defects. In addition, sclerotic areas need to be decorticated. This is best accomplished with a high-speed burr.
- When removing the components, the degree of iatrogenic bone loss can be minimized with a careful and methodologic surgical technique.

TECHNIQUES

Morcellized Allograft

- Morcellized grafting is indicated in Anderson Orthopaedic Research Institute (AORI) type 1 and type 2 defects, in which the metaphyseal rim is intact.[15]
- The primary advantage is a restoration of bone stock without the need for donor bone. This is of particular importance in young patients in whom further revision procedures can be expected.
- As a part of the débridement process, a high-speed burr/reamer or a curette is typically used to remove sclerotic bone down to the underlying bleeding bed.
- After thorough débridement, allograft bone is placed within the contained defect before placement of the final components.

Impaction Grafting

- Indications for impaction grafting are AORI type 2 and type 3 defects.[9]
- Impaction grafting is an attempt to reconstitute bone stock and avoid problems associated with excessively large or long uncemented stems.
- It is particularly indicated in younger patients.
- Unlike augments, impaction grafting can use irregular-shaped areas of bone loss. It is typically employed in contained defects, although the addition of a wire mesh to enclose any metaphyseal defects extends its application to uncontained defects.
- The impaction of the different layers of graft is time-consuming.
- Impaction grafting is associated with an increased risk of iatrogenic intraoperative fracture or perforation of metaphyseal or diaphyseal bone.

Contained Defects

- A trial stem is inserted into the tibial canal to determine the proper size and stem length. The stem could be larger than the anticipated stem. Care should be taken to align the stem properly.
- Contained defects require impaction of bone directly into the defect (**TECH FIG 1**).
- Morcellized bone graft is progressively impacted in layers around the stem until the metaphysis has been filled.
- The surgeon should be prepared to fix or bypass, as appropriate, iatrogenic fractures or perforations of the metaphyseal or diaphyseal bone.
- Once the impaction process is complete, the trial stem is carefully removed. The final components are cemented into place and excess cement removed.

Uncontained Defects

- Uncontained defects call for a wire mesh to reproduce the cortical anatomy (**TECH FIG 2**).
- The wire mesh is molded to estimate the normal contours of the proximal tibia and is held in place with small cortical screws.
- A central intramedullary guide rod with cement restrictor is inserted to allow a gap of 2 cm from the anticipated end of the final tibial stem component.
- A trial tibial stem is inserted into the tibial canal in neutral alignment. The final chosen stem should be smaller to allow for a 2-mm circumferential cement mantle.
- Thawed fresh frozen morcellized cancellous allograft is introduced into the tibial canal and impacted tightly around the stem using either cannulated or standard tamps and a mallet.
- The trial stem is removed, leaving a restored mantle of cancellous bone.
- The stemmed tibial prosthesis is cemented in standard fashion.

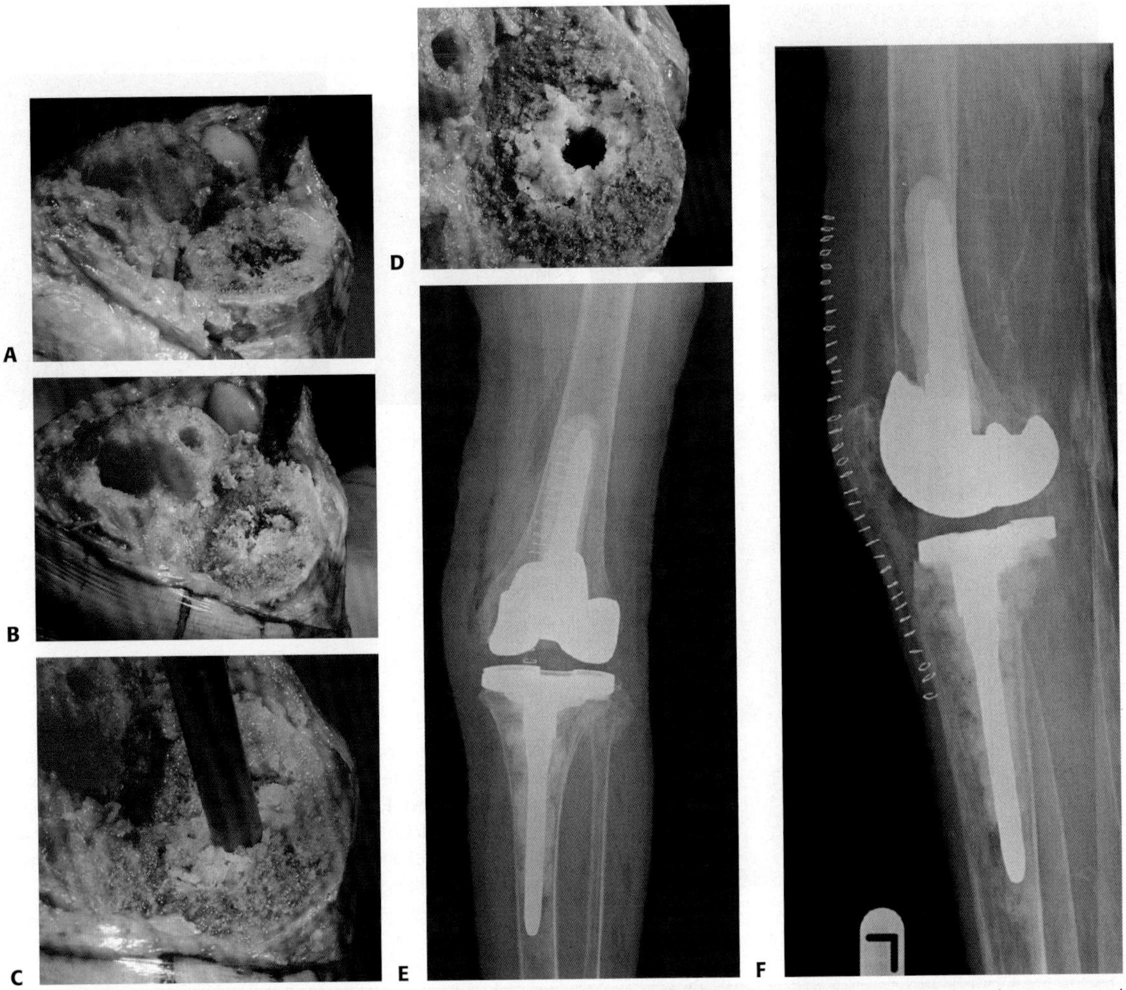

TECH FIG 1 • Contained tibial defect in the same patient shown in **FIG 1 A,B**. **A.** Primary components have been removed and the lesion has been found to have intact cortices. **B.** Cancellous allograft is introduced into the tibial canal. **C,D.** A trial stem is inserted into the tibial canal in proper alignment and bone graft is impacted around the stem. When the bone graft has filled the defect, the stem is removed. **E,F.** Postoperative anteroposterior (AP) and lateral radiographs after completion of the tibial impaction grafting and cementing of the final components.

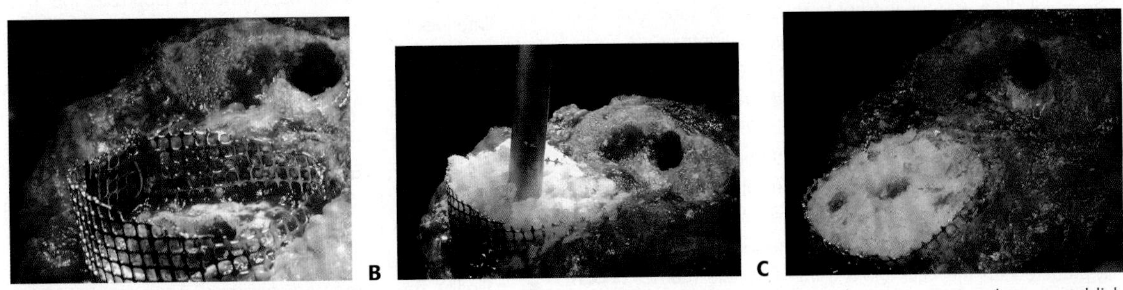

TECH FIG 2 • Uncontained tibial defect. **A.** Intraoperative photograph showing a wire mesh cage contoured to reestablish approximate proximal tibial anatomy and held in place with small cortical screws. **B.** The trial tibial stem is inserted in proper alignment and bone graft is impacted surrounding the stem. (The trial used is larger than the actual stem to allow for several millimeters of cement mantle.) **C.** The trial tibial stem is removed. *(continued)*

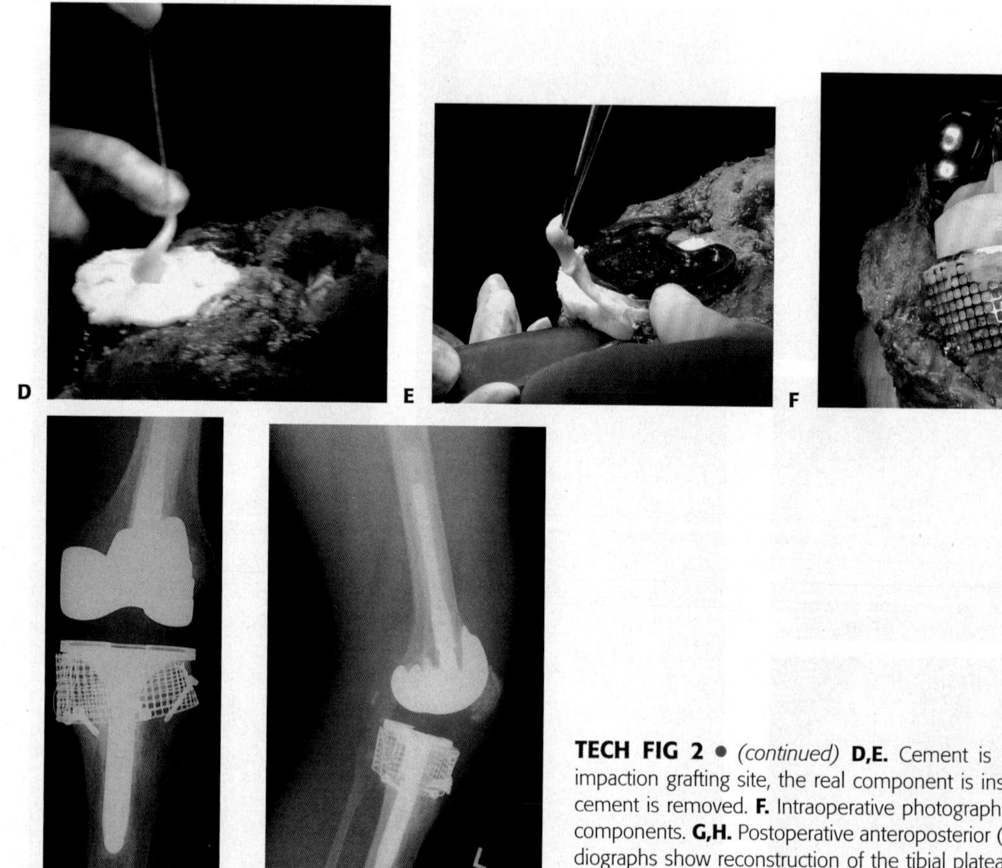

TECH FIG 2 • *(continued)* **D,E.** Cement is introduced in the impaction grafting site, the real component is inserted, and excess cement is removed. **F.** Intraoperative photograph showing the final components. **G,H.** Postoperative anteroposterior (AP) and lateral radiographs show reconstruction of the tibial plateau with wire mesh and impaction grafting.

Structural Femoral Head Allograft

- Indications for structural, or bulk, allograft are AORI type 2 and type 3 defects.[5]
- Structural allograft is typically used for defects larger than the metal augments available for use in revision TKA.
- Structural allograft is an attempt to reconstitute bone stock. It is therefore particularly indicated in younger patients.
- Preoperatively, estimate the size of the defect and order appropriate-sized femoral head allografts. The size of the graft should match as closely as possible with the size of the defect.
- Following débridement, the metaphyseal bone is hemispherically reamed. Reaming through the thin metaphyseal cortical bone, with the creation of an uncontained defect, must be avoided.
- Once the recipient bed is prepared, the femoral head allograft is prepared on the back table using a female reamer (**TECH FIG 3A**). The graft should be irrigated using a pulsatile irrigator and, depending on the size of the graft, 2 or more liters of saline.
- The allograft is usually reamed to one size larger than the male reamer used to prepare the metaphyseal bone (**TECH FIG 3B**). The host bone is reamed to expose healthy, bleeding cancellous bone, with removal of all fibrous tissue and cement.
- Sclerotic bone may cause the reamer to wander. In these cases, a high-speed burr may be used to remove sclerotic bone.
- The allograft is prepared to maximize the contact surface area across the allograft–host junction, optimize the mechanical interlock between the graft and host, allow rigid implant fixation, and restore anatomy.
- The allograft is placed into the defect and provisionally secured with Kirschner (K) wires or Steinmann pins. These should be placed so that they do not interfere with the stemmed prosthesis insertion (**TECH FIG 3C,D**).
- Revision cutting guides are used to trim the allograft for component implantation. Tibial component preparation should follow standard revision principles.
- Finally, the K-wires are removed. They can be replaced with partially threaded 4.0- or 4.5-mm cancellous screws, and the tibial component is press-fitted or cemented in the standard fashion (**TECH FIG 3E–G**).

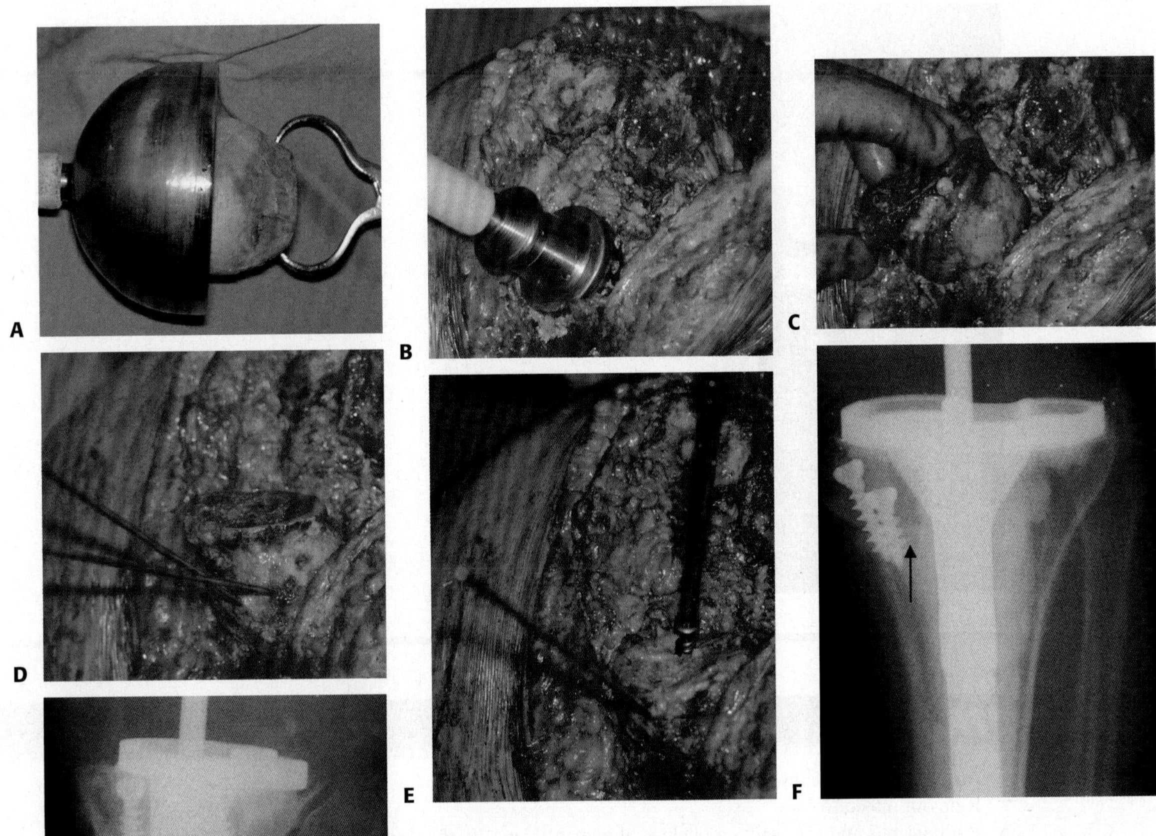

TECH FIG 3 • Femoral head allografting. **A.** The femoral head allograft is secured into a grip device and a female-type cheese grater reamer is used to denude the allograft of cartilage and subchondral bone. **B.** A male-type reamer of appropriate size is used to create a socket for the allograft. **C,D.** The allograft is impacted into place and secured with K-wires. **E.** The allograft is cut to the appropriate height and fixed with cancellous bone screws. **F,G.** Final anteroposterior (AP) and lateral radiographs of the medial tibial plateau reconstruction with femoral head allograft secured with screw fixation (*arrows*). (From Hanssen A. Managing severe bone loss in revision knee arthroplasty. In: Lotke PA, Lonner JH, eds. Knee Arthroplasty, ed 2. Philadelphia: Lippincott Williams & Wilkins, 2003:321–344.)

Massive Tibial Allograft

- The indication for massive tibial allograft is AORI type 3 defects with or without extensor mechanism failures (**TECH FIG 4**).[8]
- Implantation of an allograft prosthetic component (APC) is a challenging salvage procedure in the presence of uncontained circumferential defects that involve a large part of the proximal tibia and cannot be treated with cement, augments, or structural allograft alone.
- It can be considered as an alternative to a tumor prosthesis.
- The APC of the tibia is fashioned to the correct size based on careful measurements of the host tibia after thorough débridement.
- After careful measurement (and following débridement) of the host tibia, the graft should be slightly oversized in length. If necessary, it should be trimmed down to size.
- The allograft–host junction should be bypassed by a press-fit stem by approximately 5 cm.
- To optimize rotational stability of the implant, the host bone and graft bone should be shaped with oblique or step cuts.
- Positioning of the graft should be carried out with the trial implants already in place to verify that anatomic positioning and good patella height and tracking has been obtained.
- The final position should be marked with a cautery or marking pen to assist appropriate overall orientation in final implantation of the APC.
- If the extensor mechanism is deficient secondary to bone loss, or in the presence of tendon rupture or erosion of the extensor mechanism, the procedure can be performed in conjunction with reconstruction of the extensor mechanism.

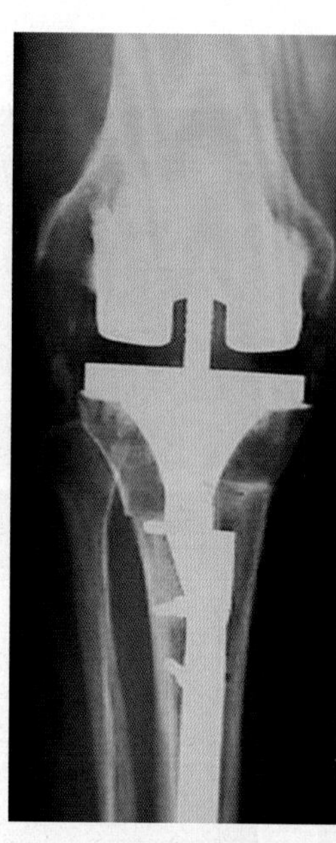

TECH FIG 4 • Proximal tibial allograft with step cuts combined with a condylar constraint knee (CCK)-type implant.

PEARLS AND PITFALLS

Preoperative planning	▪ Attempt to define cause of tibial bone loss. ▪ Rule out infection. ▪ Radiographs and CT scans can help evaluate and quantify the degree of bone loss.
Débridement	▪ All defects must be thoroughly débrided. Use of a high-speed burr often is helpful in removing old cement, bony sclerosis, and fibrous membranes.
Mechanical contouring	▪ The goal should be to restore the normal contour and anatomy of the proximal tibia to provide a stable platform for the revision tibial component. ▪ Structural allografts and mesh wires should be sized and contoured to match the patient's anatomy and secured with screws.
Impaction grafting	▪ Use a larger trial stem during canal preparation to allow for a circumferential 2 mm of cement mantle. ▪ The morcellized bone graft should be impacted as tightly as possible.
Morcellized allograft	▪ Carefully remove sclerotic bone down to the underlying bleeding bed.
Impaction grafting	▪ Use a larger stem during canal preparation to allow for a circumferential 2 mm of cement mantle. ▪ Morcellized bone graft is progressively impacted in layers around the stem. ▪ The morcellized bone graft should be impacted as tightly as possible.
Structural allograft	▪ Attempt to match the size of the uncontained defect with the allograft bone. ▪ Avoid oversizing the allograft to prevent overhang and soft tissue irritation. ▪ Provisionally fix the allograft in place using K-wires during tibial preparation. If necessary, replace wires with cancellous screws following insertion of the definitive implant.
Massive tibial allograft	▪ Extremely challenging procedure ▪ Use anatomic landmarks, such as the tibial tubercle, patellar tendon, and patellar tracking, to place the APC in the correct rotation.

POSTOPERATIVE CARE

- Postoperative management should be tailored to the individual patient and depends on the degree of bone loss, the primary stability of the implant and graft, soft tissue quality, and extensor mechanism compromise.
- The priority should be wound healing and incorporation of the graft. With large allograft techniques, weight bearing is restricted until graft incorporation has occurred. Partial weight bearing is typically recommended for a minimum of 6 to 8 weeks and continued until radiographic signs of union at the graft–host interface are present.[1]

OUTCOMES

- Lotke et al[10] reported prospectively on 48 consecutive patients treated with impaction allograft for substantial bone loss in revision TKA. They found no mechanical failures and all radiographs showed incorporation and remodeling of the bone graft. Six complications (14%) were reported, including two infections and two periprosthetic fractures.

- Engh and Ammeen[6] reported outcomes at a mean of 7.9 years postoperatively in 49 knees with severe tibial bone defects requiring revision arthroplasty. Three patients could not be assessed. Four revision procedures had failed and required reoperation. No instance of graft collapse or aseptic loosening associated with the structural graft were found.
- Naim and Toms[13] published prospective findings on 11 patients with large tibial defects treated with knee impaction bone grafting and a short cemented stem. Over a minimum follow-up of 2 years, there were no mechanical failures, all radiographs showed incorporation and remodeling of the graft, and none of the patients required secondary procedures or further revisions. One complication—superficial dysesthesia around the operative scar—was recorded.

COMPLICATIONS

- Bone graft resorption
- Graft collapse
- Infection
- Instability
- Joint line elevation
- Stiffness
- Periprosthetic fracture
- End-of-stem pain[1]
- Allograft nonunion[2]

REFERENCES

1. Barrack RL, Rorabeck C, Burt M, et al. Pain at the end of the stem after revision total knee arthroplasty. Clin Orthop Relat Res 1999;(367):216–225.
2. Daines BK, Dennis DA. Management of bone defects in revision total knee arthroplasty. Instr Course Lect 2013;62:341–348.
3. Della Valle CJ, Berger RA, Rosenberg AG. Surgical exposures in revision total knee arthroplasty. Clin Orthop Relat Res 2006;446: 59–68.
4. Dennis DA. A stepwise approach to revision total knee arthroplasty. J Arthroplasty 2007;22:32–38.
5. Elia EA, Lotke PA. Results of revision total knee arthroplasty associated with significant bone loss. Clin Orthop Relat Res 1991;(271): 114–121.
6. Engh GA, Ammeen DJ. Use of structural allograft in revision total knee arthroplasty in knees with severe tibial bone loss. J Bone Joint Surg Am 2007;89:2640–2647.
7. Engh GA, Parks NL. The management of bone defects in revision total knee arthroplasty. Instr Course Lect 1997;46:227–236.
8. Kuchinad RA, Garbedian S, Rogers BA, et al. The use of structural allograft in primary and revision knee arthroplasty with bone loss. Adv Orthop 2011;2011:578952.
9. Lonner JH, Lotke PA, Kim J, et al. Impaction grafting and wire mesh for uncontained defects in revision knee arthroplasty. Clin Orthop Relat Res 2002;(404):145–151.
10. Lotke PA, Carolan GF, Puri N. Impaction grafting for bone defects in revision total knee arthroplasty. Clin Orthop Relat Res 2006;446: 99–103.
11. Mason JB, Fehring TK, Odum SM, et al. The value of white blood cell counts before revision total knee arthroplasty. J Arthroplasty 2003;18:1038–1043.
12. Morrison JC, Reilly DT. Allograft in revision total knee arthroplasty. In: Bono JV, Scott RD, eds. Revision Total Knee Arthroplasty. New York: Springer Science+Business Media, Inc, 2005: 81–96.
13. Naim S, Toms AD. Impaction bone grafting for tibial defects in knee replacement surgery. Results at two years. Acta Orthop Belg 2013;79: 205–210.
14. Nicoll D, Rowley DI. Internal rotational error of the tibial component is a major cause of pain after total knee replacement. J Bone Joint Surg Br 2010;92:1238–1244.
15. Stock GH, Austin MS, Meneghini RM. Management of bone loss in revision total knee arthroplasty. In: Parvizi J, ed. Principles and Techniques in Revision Total Knee Arthroplasty. Rosemont, IL: American Academy of Orthopaedic Surgeons, 2012:49–60.
16. Stulberg SD. Bone loss in revision total knee arthroplasty: graft options and adjuncts. J Arthroplasty 2003;18:48–50.

CHAPTER

Revision Total Knee Arthroplasty with Removal of Well-fixed Components

Adeel Husain, Matthew S. Austin, and Charles L. Nelson

DEFINITION

- Estimates indicate that by the year 2030, the volume of primary total knee arthroplasty (TKA) cases will increase to 3,480,000 and the number of revision procedures is expected to rise to 268,200 per year.[1]
- Indications for removing well-fixed total knee components include infection, malalignment, malpositioning, instability, periprosthetic fracture, stiffness, or aseptic loosening of other part(s).
- Achieving the goal of safe removal of well-fixed components during revision TKA depends on meticulous surgical technique and availability of appropriate instruments. In many ways, these are the most important portions of the revision TKA procedure because careless technique may lead to damage of the remaining bone stock, iatrogenic fracture, and disruption of soft tissues, ultimately compromising the quality of the revision construct and the outcome for the patient.

ANATOMY

- Removal of well-fixed TKA components necessitates good exposure.
- Protection of neurovascular structures and the extensor mechanism is essential. A medial parapatellar arthrotomy allows extensile exposure, and when combined with synovectomy, lateral retinacular release and quadriceps snip provide the necessary exposure required for safe component removal and subsequent reconstruction in most cases. Extensile exposure techniques using a quadriceps snip, tibial tubercle osteotomy, or V-Y quadricepsplasty allow enhanced exposure when necessary and are described in Chapters 37 and 39.

PATHOGENESIS

- Indications for removal of well-fixed TKA components include infection, malalignment, malpositioning, instability, periprosthetic fracture, stiffness, or aseptic loosening of other component(s).

PATIENT HISTORY AND PHYSICAL FINDINGS

- The history and physical examination should determine whether the patient's pain is extrinsic or intrinsic to the TKA.
- Extrinsic sources of pain (eg, lumbar radiculopathy, referred hip pain) should be considered for differential diagnosis.
- Pain that is determined to be intrinsic to the TKA should be correlated with history, physical examination, and radiographic findings to confirm that the cause of the pain can be corrected with revision TKA.
- Failure to identify a cause for the patient's pain before performing the revision TKA portends a poor outcome.
- Physical examination includes the following:
  - Visual inspection of the previous incision and the surrounding skin. The most lateral anterior-based incision is selected to avoid wound necrosis and maximize healing potential.
  - Passive and active range of motion (ROM) is assessed. Normal ROM after TKA ranges from full extension to 120 to 135 degrees. It is important to inform patients that revision TKA may not improve their ROM. Stiff knees may require extensile exposure techniques.
  - The medial and lateral collateral ligaments are tested in full extension and at 30 degrees of flexion. Coronal plane instability may make it necessary to remove well-fixed components and implant appropriately sized and positioned components, occasionally with more constraint.
  - The anterior and posterior stability of the knee is assessed. Sagittal plane instability may make it necessary to remove components to improve flexion–extension gap balancing or to compensate for a deficient posterior cruciate ligament (PCL) in patients with a cruciate-retaining design.
  - The coronal plane alignment is assessed with the patient standing. The femorotibial angle is measured; it is usually 5 to 7 degrees of valgus. It may be necessary to remove well-fixed components to correct malalignment.

IMAGING AND OTHER DIAGNOSTIC STUDIES

- Standard radiographic views include standing anteroposterior (AP), lateral, and tangential patellofemoral (Merchant) views.
- Full-length standing AP radiographs are useful to determine the overall mechanical alignment of the lower limb.
- The radiographs should include the diaphysis above the femoral prosthesis and well below the tibial prosthesis.
- The radiographs are assessed for alignment, component positioning and size, joint line position, loosening, bone stock, and osteolysis.
- Computed tomography (CT) scans are useful to assess for presence and severity of osteolysis or to assess femoral and tibial component rotation.
- Erythrocyte sedimentation rate (ESR) and C-reactive protein (CRP) are obtained to screen for the presence of infection.
- Aspiration of the knee is indicated if either the ESR or CRP is elevated or if there is clinical suspicion of infection.

DIFFERENTIAL DIAGNOSIS

- Lumbar radiculopathy
- Hip pathology
- Neuropathy
- Complex regional pain syndrome
- Vascular claudication

- Primary bone tumors
- Metastatic disease
- Inflammatory arthritis
- Infection

NONOPERATIVE MANAGEMENT

- Nonoperative management of failed TKA may consist of activity modification, physical therapy, bracing, and consultation with pain management specialists.

SURGICAL MANAGEMENT

- Surgical management begins with preoperative planning.
- The patient's history, physical examination, radiographs, and laboratory studies are reviewed well in advance of the surgery to allow for adequate preparation time.
- The cause for failure of the TKA is determined.
- The surgical plan is delineated, a primary plan is formulated, and contingency plans are developed.
- The appropriate instrumentation, implants, and bone graft (if necessary) are ordered.
- The knee is exposed, with extensile approaches if necessary.
- Disruption of the prosthesis–cement interface is targeted in cemented components.
- Disruption of the prosthesis–bone interface is targeted in noncemented components.
- The components are removed carefully with meticulous attention paid to preservation of bone stock and the soft tissues.
- The knee is subsequently reconstructed.
- Layered closure is performed carefully.

Preoperative Planning

- The key to any successful revision TKA is preoperative planning. The reason for failure of the original TKA is determined from study of the preoperative history, physical examination, imaging studies, and laboratory results.
- It is decided whether removal of the femoral, tibial, and/or patellar component is necessary.
- Previous operative reports are reviewed, with particular attention paid to the surgical approach, releases performed, and implants that were used.
- Careful review of the operative report or implant stickers allows planning and availability of compatible implants or tibial polyethylene liners when partial revisions are planned. It should be determined whether the tibial polyethylene component is modular and what sterilization method was used. If some of the index TKA components are to remain in situ, the surgeon must determine whether compatible parts are available. In addition, for some implants, implant-specific extraction devices may facilitate implant removal.
- Radiographs are reviewed for bone stock quality and quantity.
- Particular attention is paid to the fixation method of the components. Ultrasonic cement removal tools may facilitate cement removal, particularly in the setting of previously cemented stemmed implants.

Surgical Instruments to Have Available Intraoperatively

- Generic or implant-specific femoral and tibial extraction tools
- Flexible and rigid osteotomes
- Narrow and wide osteotomes
- Oscillating, reciprocating, and microsagittal power saws
- Gigli saw
- Moreland cement and noncement removal instruments
- High-speed burr
- Vice grips
- Ultrasonic cement removal device

Positioning

- The patient is positioned supine on the operating table.
- Two paint rollers are placed in locations to stabilize the foot as the knee is held at both 90 degrees of flexion and hyperflexion.
- The knee is draped to allow for an extensile surgical exposure.
- The knee is ranged through a full ROM and stressed in all directions to assess stability.

Approach

- The preferred surgical approach is a standard medial parapatellar approach, although an extensile approach may be necessary (see Chaps. 45 and 46).
- Medial subperiosteal exposure with tibial external rotation decreases tension on the patellar tendon. Patella subluxation is preferred over eversion to decrease the risk of patellar tendon avulsion.
- Good exposure is important to allow unimpeded access to interfaces between components and bone or cement, allow axial extraction of existing implants, and protect key structures.
- Implant removal proceeds in the following order (if all components are being removed): tibial polyethylene, femoral component, tibial tray, and patellar component.
  - Removal of a modular tibial polyethylene creates more space, enhancing exposure of all components.
  - Removal of the femoral component initially creates more space for axial extraction of the tibial component.
  - If the trajectory of removal of the tibial tray is not obstructed by the femoral component, the tibial tray can be removed prior to the femoral component.

Exposure

- The extensor mechanism must be subluxed laterally, with careful attention to avoid detaching the insertion of the patellar tendon. We protect the extensor mechanism by using an A-cup Hohmann retractor along the lateral tibial plateau to retract the quadriceps tendon.
- A thorough synovectomy is performed and the medial and lateral gutters are recreated.
- If there is lateral scarring or retinacular tightness compromising lateral patellar displacement, a lateral retinacular release is helpful in improving lateral patellar translation.
- A quadriceps snip may also decrease proximal lateral tightness and facilitate exposure.
- The collateral ligaments are identified and protected.
- The prosthesis–cement interface of the femoral, tibial, and patellar implants must be adequately visualized and unimpeded exposure must be achieved.

Tibial Component Polyethylene Removal

- The tibial polyethylene is removed first. This allows a larger working space to ease removal of the components.
- If a modular implant was used, it is removed by inserting an osteotome at the interface of the polyethylene and the tray and then levering the polyethylene out. This can also be accomplished with a nonmodular design (**TECH FIG 1**).
- One must be aware that certain posterior-stabilized designs have a reinforcing metal pin in the post which fixes the polyethylene insert to the tray. Other inserts can be secured to the tray with clips or screws. These may need to be removed before the polyethylene can be levered out.
  - Special instruments from the implant manufacturer may need to be ordered to facilitate removal of the polyethylene.
  - If special instruments are unavailable, a saw can be used to divide the post, and the pin can be removed with a rongeur.
  - As a last resort, the tibial tray and polyethylene insert can be removed together as a single unit. However, additional care must be taken to clear the trajectory for two-component extraction.

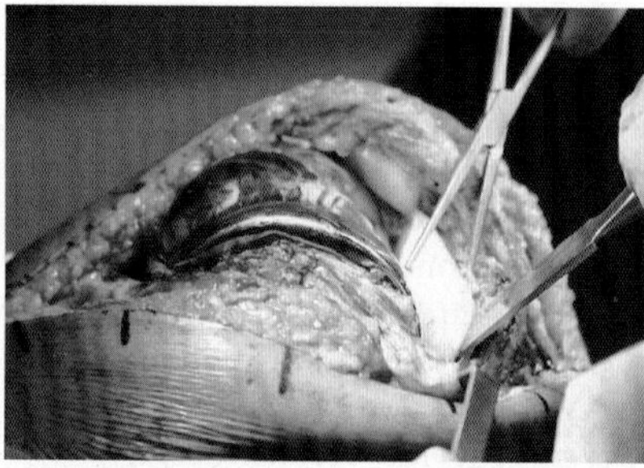

TECH FIG 1 • Method of removing the tibial polyethylene from the tray. The osteotome is inserted between the polyethylene and the tray, and the insert is levered out.

Femoral Component Removal

- Initially, a clear visualization of the interface is achieved by removing scar tissue, bone, and cement using an osteotome, curette, rongeur, or burr.
- Methods to disrupt the prosthesis–cement interface are listed in the following text:
  - A thin saw can be used initially with careful protection of the soft tissues.
  - We typically use a reciprocating saw in the interface along the anterior surface around the femoral component as well as along the anterior chamfer and distal surface (**TECH FIG 2A**).
  - We then use osteotomes to continue to disrupt these interfaces for the posterior chamfer and the posterior condylar interface (**TECH FIG 2B,C**).
  - Thin osteotomes are preferred for well-fixed cementless implants to minimize bone loss.

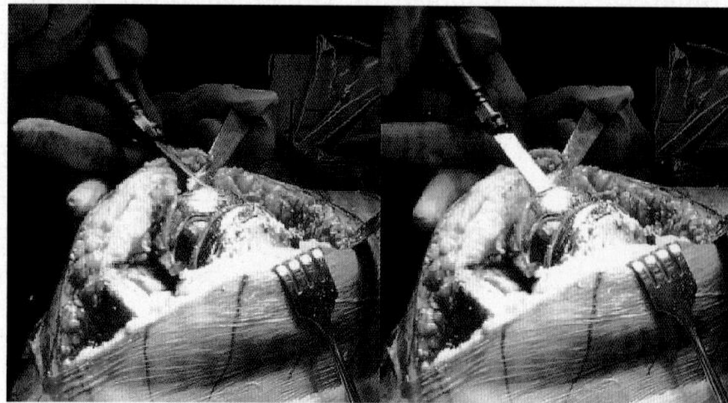

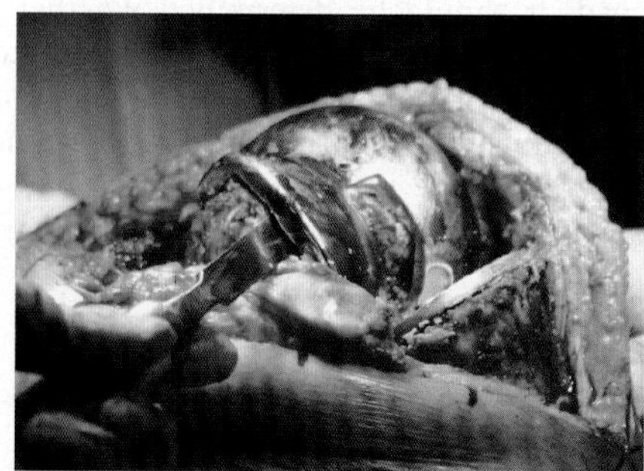

TECH FIG 2 • **A.** We typically use a reciprocating saw in the interface along the anterior surface around the femoral component as well as along the anterior chamfer and distal surface. **B.** The femoral component–cement interface is disrupted with an osteotome. The osteotome should be inserted parallel to the component. Smaller width osteotomes can be used at the interface of the chamfer cuts and around distal pegs. Curved or angled osteotomes are helpful to work the interface of the posterior condyles. *(continued)*

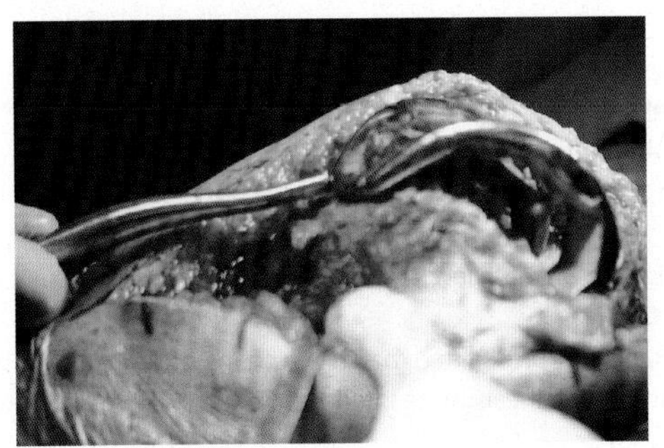

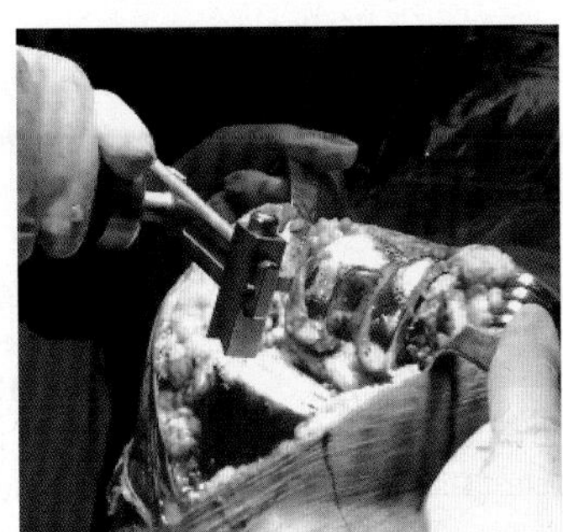

TECH FIG 2 • *(continued)* **C.** It should be possible to remove the femoral component easily by hand or with light taps from a punch. If the component is not extracted with gentle force, then further work with the osteotomes is needed. **D.** A femoral extractor that grasps the distal aspect of the femoral component can be used to gently remove the implant. Excessive force should be avoided. If the component cannot be extracted with gentle force, then further work is needed.

- Rigid osteotomes are easier to control and often work better for cemented implants when properly placed in the interval between the implant and cement and often displace the implant from the cement. However, care must be taken, as excessive levering can impact or fracture the bone of the distal femur.
- Straight osteotomes are suitable for clearing the anterior flange and posterior condyles as well as the outer portion of the medial and lateral condylar "runners."
- Narrow osteotomes are used for the chamfer cuts and for prostheses where there are pegs at the distal aspect of the component.
- The posterior condylar interface can be disrupted with a curved, angled, or offset osteotome.
- It may be necessary to use a metal-cutting instrument if certain implants, specifically PCL-sacrificing implants with a central housing, do not come out easily after releasing all available surfaces. This allows exposure of the inner interfaces of the runners, which can be disrupted with osteotomes.
- Care must be taken with the use of Gigli saws, as they can result in the removal of more bone than is seen with the meticulous use of osteotomes.

- The interfaces should be worked from the medial and lateral sides rather than attempting to traverse the entire prosthesis with the instruments. This allows a more controlled division of the interface and minimizes iatrogenic bone loss.
- It is important to direct the removal instruments parallel to the component to avoid removing additional bone unnecessarily.
- After the prosthesis–cement interface is disrupted, it is possible to remove the implant easily by hand, with light taps from a punch set on the anterior flange or with an extraction device.
  - Alternatively, a femoral extractor that grasps the distal aspect of the femoral component can be used to gently remove the implant (**TECH FIG 2D**). Excessive force may result in unnecessary bone loss or fracture.
  - If it is difficult to extract the implant, the surgeon must reassess and ensure all interfaces have been disrupted. Axial extraction is important in these cases.
- The remaining cement is then removed with saws, burrs, osteotomes, and curettes. Cement gouges and splitters can break the cement plug or mantle.
- Ultrasonic instruments facilitate bone preservation during cement removal, especially with cemented, stemmed implants. Ultrasonic instruments are occasionally useful in disrupting the prosthesis–bone interface in noncemented implants.

Tibial Component Removal

- Methods to disrupt the prosthesis–cement interface are listed below.
  - The prosthesis–cement interface is initially disrupted with an osteotome or saw to separate the interface. If the component does not separate readily from the cement mantle–bone portion, then further work with saws or osteotomes is necessary. Excessive force will lead to unnecessary bone loss or fracture.
  - A thin oscillating saw blade, with careful protection of the soft tissues, can also be used initially to disrupt the interface medial to the patellar tendon (**TECH FIG 3A**). Oscillating saws can be the easiest way of disrupting the interface, but care must be taken to protect the patellar tendon and collateral ligaments.
  - The area under the tray posterior and lateral to the patellar tendon is not safely accessible to an oscillating saw and can be disrupted with a narrower reciprocating saw or osteotome (**TECH FIG 3B**).
  - Narrow and broad osteotomes are effective but care must be taken to avoid impaction or fracture of the underlying bone when levering is used to extract the implant (**TECH FIG 3C**).
  - Stacking of osteotomes can disrupt the interface between the prosthesis and cement and facilitate tibial component extraction. When stacking osteotomes, it is important that the widest osteotome be adjacent to tibial bone to distribute force over a large surface area and decrease the risk of tibial bone compression or fracture (**TECH FIG 3D**).
- Once the interface is disrupted prior to extraction, a clear trajectory for egress of the tibial component must be achieved.
- The tibia can be externally rotated to provide access to the posterior aspect of the component. Care must be taken to protect the neurovascular structures posteriorly.

- The tibia can be hyperflexed and anteriorly subluxed or dislocated to provide access to the posterolateral aspect of the tibia. The tibial component must clear the posterolateral femoral condyle. Care must be taken to avoid injury to the patellar tendon and medial collateral ligament.
- Once the implant interface is entirely disrupted, it can be removed by hand with a punch or generic or implant-specific extractions devices.
  - We prefer to use a femoral extractor to extract the tibial component if hand removal is inadequate (**TECH FIG 3E,F**). This allows even force distribution while elevating the tibial component, preserving bone stock around the keel.
- The remaining cement is then removed with saws, burrs, osteotomes, and curettes. Cement gouges and splitters can break the cement plug or mantle (**TECH FIG 3G**). Cement drills can create a central hole in the cement plug and reverse scrapers can be useful in removing cement from the canal (**TECH FIG 3H**).
- If the implants are press-fitted, a similar means of removal can be used at the prosthesis bone interface.

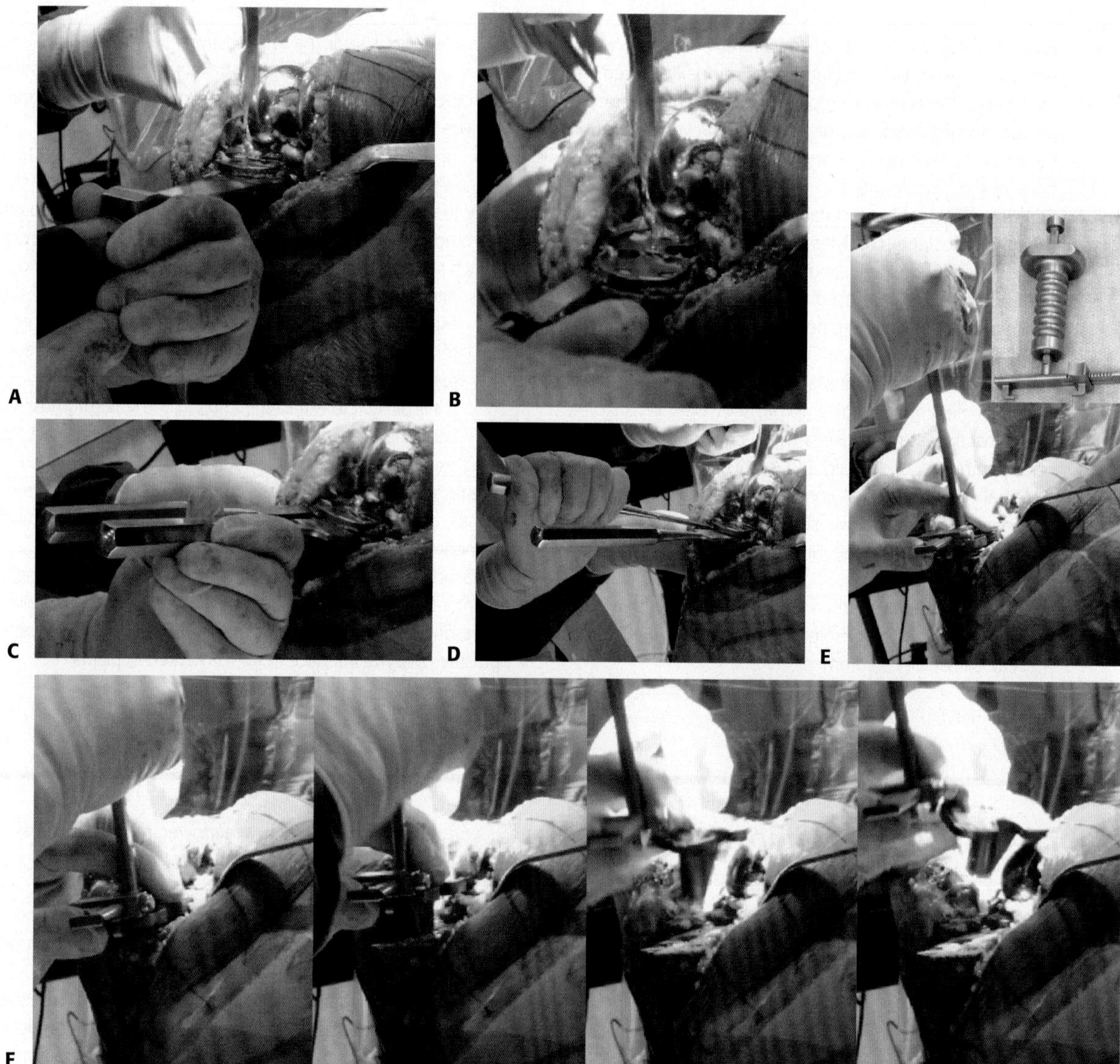

TECH FIG 3 ● **A.** The tibial prosthesis–cement interface is initially disrupted with a thin oscillating saw blade, with careful protection of the soft tissues. **B.** A narrow reciprocating saw can be used lateral to the keel of the tibial component, being careful to protect the patellar tendon. **C.** Interruption of the prosthesis–cement interface using broad osteotomes to cover a large tibial surface area medially and narrow osteotome placed between the tibial keel and the patellar tendon. **D.** Stacking broad osteotomes can be more effective in maintaining the bony structure, as the force is distributed across a greater surface area of bone, minimizing impaction and fracture. **E.** Once the interface has been disrupted, the femoral extractor with an attached slap hammer easily extracts the tibial component if hand removal is inadequate. Hyperflexion, external rotation, and anterior dislocation of the knee facilitate access to the posterior aspect of the tibial component. **F.** Sequential images of tibial component extraction with a generic femoral extractor. This can be used if implant-specific instrumentation is unavailable. *(continued)*

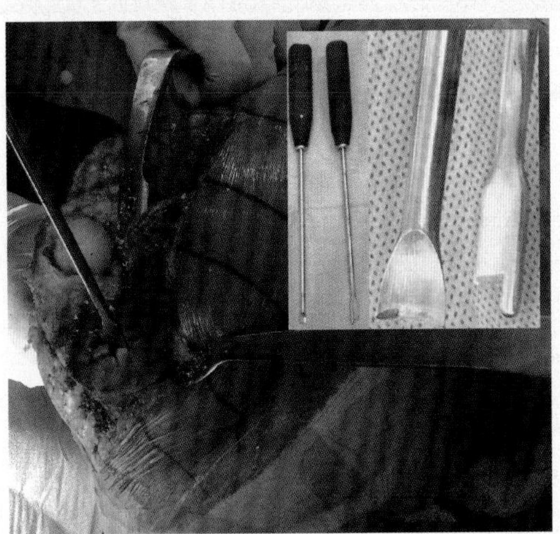

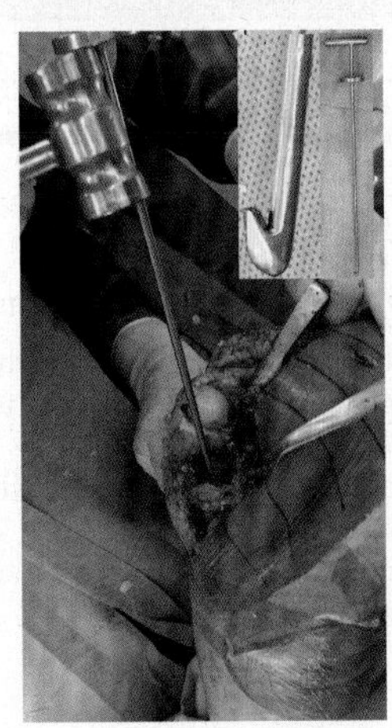

TECH FIG 3 • *(continued)* **G.** The remaining cement is then removed with saws, burrs, osteotomes, and curettes. Cement gouges and splitters can break the cement plug or mantle. **H.** Reverse scrapers can be useful in removing cement from the canal safely without excessive bone loss.

Patellar Component Removal

- The removal of a well-fixed polyethylene patellar component should be done only after thoughtful consideration.
- The remaining patella bone stock is often thin and osteopenic with one or several stress risers from previous fixation pegs. It is usually covered with a scar that should be débrided prior to finalizing the decision for removal or retention of the component (**TECH FIG 4A**).
- The target interface is disrupted with a thin saw blade.
- All polyethylene components can be removed with a saw blade and the pegs subsequently burred. Cementless components may require the use of a metal-cutting diamond wheel to sever the pegs from the plate. A pencil-tip burr can then be used to remove the pegs (**TECH FIG 4B,C**).
- Any remaining cement is removed with curettes, saws, and burrs.

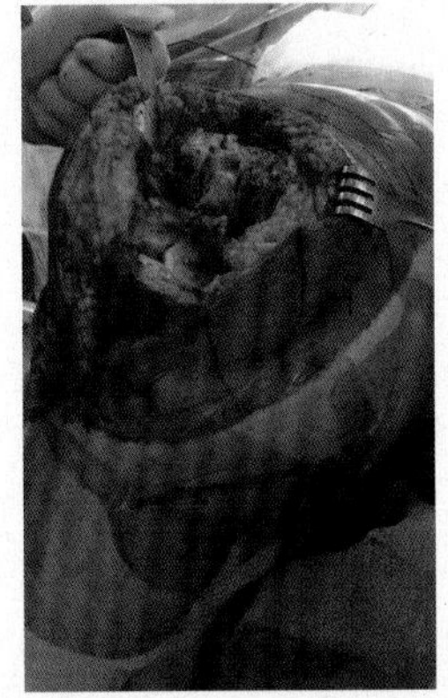

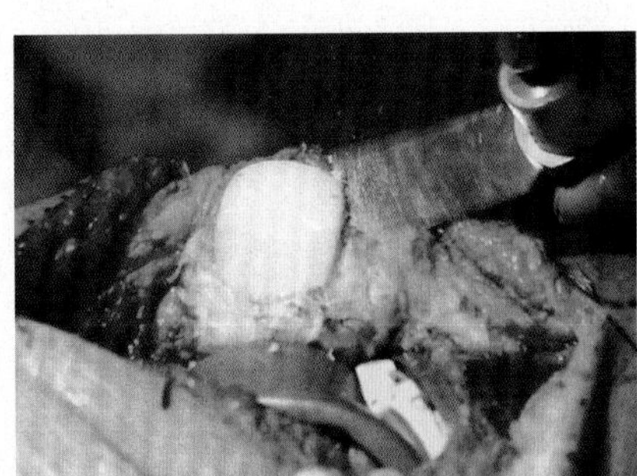

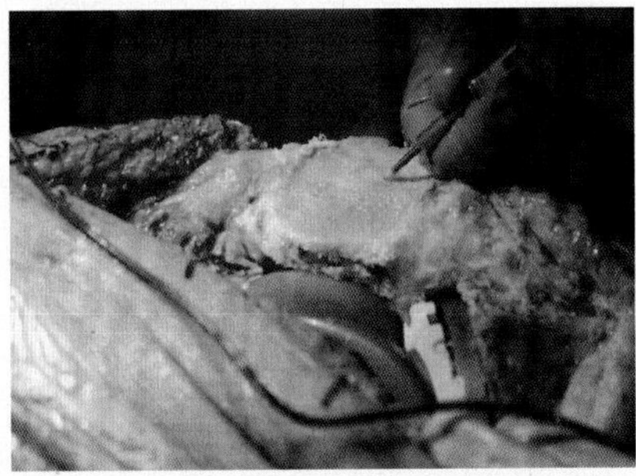

TECH FIG 4 • **A.** The femoral and tibial components have been removed with the patellar component covered by scar tissue. This scar tissue will need to be débrided before a decision to revise the patellar component can be made. **B.** The patella button is removed with a thin saw blade. The pegs remain embedded in the cement. **C.** A pencil-tip burr is used to lever the polyethylene pegs out of the cement mantle. The burr is advanced into the polyethylene and stopped; the polyethylene is then easily levered out of the cement mantle. A larger burr is then used to remove the remaining cement mantle.

Stemmed Implant Removal

- Stemmed implants can usually be removed once the fixation between the condylar portion of the femoral component and the tray portion of the tibial component has been separated from the bone.
- Preoperative planning should take into consideration the use of stemmed implants, which may complicate extraction of the component.
- Some modular designs allow for disassembly of the stem from the remainder of the implant.
- Metal-cutting burrs may be necessary to separate the condylar portion of the femoral implant or the keel portion of the tibial implant from the stem. The stem can then be removed with trephine reamers, burrs, or ultrasonic tools. Some companies may make special extraction devices available to assist in removal of the stem.
- Rarely, it may be necessary to perform a tibial tubercle osteotomy to extract well-fixed stems.

PEARLS AND PITFALLS

Preoperative planning	■ Thorough preoperative planning makes it possible for the surgeon to have the appropriate instrumentation, implants, bone graft, staff, and assistants available.
Preoperative workup	■ Infection must be excluded. ■ The patient's medical status must be optimized. ■ The patient must be compliant. ■ Information regarding previous surgical procedures and implants must be obtained.
Intraoperative technique	■ Good exposure must be achieved to avoid iatrogenic bone and soft tissue damage. ■ The extensor mechanism should be treated with care to avoid avulsion of the patellar tendon insertion. ■ The tibial polyethylene is removed first. ■ The femoral component or tibial component is removed next. ■ If necessary, the patellar component is removed. ■ Stemmed implants may require special instrumentation, metal-cutting burrs or discs, or ultrasonic tools to remove.

COMPLICATIONS

- Bone loss
- Fracture
- Ligament disruption
- Tendon disruption

REFERENCE

1. Kurtz S, Ong KL, Schmier J, et al. Future clinical and economic impact of revision total hip and knee arthroplasty. J Bone Joint Surg Am 2007; 89A:144–151.

Revision Total Knee Arthroplasty with Extensile Exposure: Tibial Tubercle Osteotomy

44

CHAPTER

Gregg R. Klein and Mark A. Hartzband

DEFINITION

- Obtaining adequate anterior exposure of the knee can be difficult using standard approaches during revision total knee arthroplasty (TKA).
- The options available for dealing with difficult exposure include quadriceps snip (done 5 to 8 cm proximal to the superior pole of the patella), V-Y quadriceps turndown, and tibial tubercle osteotomy.
- Tibial tubercle osteotomy is performed to obtain an extensile exposure of the knee during difficult revision TKA.
- An osteoperiosteal segment—which includes the tibial tubercle and upper tibial crest—is elevated to relax the extensor mechanism and allow safe subluxation of the patella.
- The technique was first described by Dolin[6] in 1983 but subsequently was modified and popularized for exposure in revision TKA by Whiteside.[10]

ANATOMY

- The extensor mechanism consists of the quadriceps muscles (ie, rectus femoris, vastus lateralis, vastus medialis, and vastus lateralis), quadriceps tendon, patella, and patellar tendon.
- The quadriceps muscle inserts into the patella via the quadriceps tendon and then into the tibial tuberosity via the patellar tendon.
- Tendinous fibers of the vastus medialis and vastus lateralis form the medial and lateral patellar retinaculae, respectively, which together reinforce the capsule of the knee joint anteriorly (**FIG 1A**).
- The tibial tuberosity forms the truncated apex of a triangular area at the proximal end of the tibia. It has a distal "rough" area, which is subcutaneous and palpable, and a proximal "smooth" area attached to the patellar ligament (**FIG 1B**).

PATHOGENESIS

- Adequate anterior exposure of the distal femur and tibial plateau during revision TKA is crucial for gentle soft tissue handling, safe implant removal, recognition of bone defects, and correct placement of revision components.
- During revision TKA, adhesions and fibrosis within the extensor mechanism restrict subluxation of the patella and limit exposure.
- A medial parapatellar arthrotomy, combined with intra-articular excision of the fibrous pseudocapsule, allows subluxation of the patella in most cases.
- Inadequate exposure with continued forceful retraction of the extensor mechanism risks avulsion of the patellar ligament from the tibial tubercle.

NATURAL HISTORY

- Avulsion of the patellar tendon is a serious complication during revision TKA because it results in prolonged immobilization, extensor lag, and a poor functional outcome.
- To avoid this complication, an extensile exposure is required to relax the extensor mechanism and allow safe eversion of the patella.

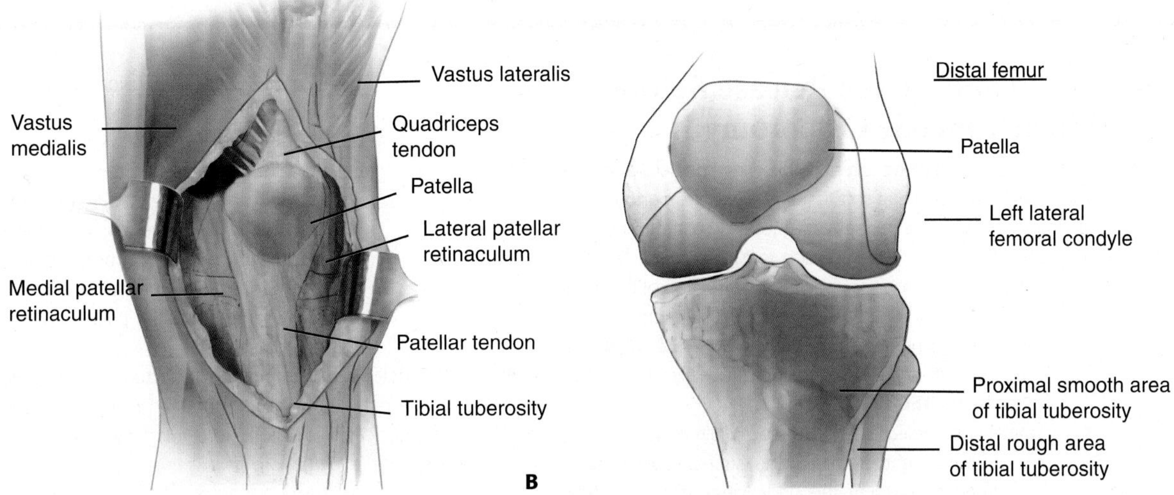

FIG 1 • **A.** The extensor mechanism of the knee. Note that the medial and lateral patellar retinaculae originate proximally from the tendinous fibers of the vastus medialis and lateralis muscles, respectively. **B.** The tibial tuberosity. The distal rough area is subcutaneous and palpable. The patellar ligament is attached to the proximal smooth area.

- Three options for obtaining such an extensile exposure during revision TKA are quadriceps snip, V-Y quadriceps turndown, and tibial tubercle osteotomy.
- Tibial tubercle osteotomy is preferred to a V-Y quadriceps turndown because it has a lower incidence of extensor lag and quadriceps weakness.[1,7]

PATIENT HISTORY AND PHYSICAL FINDINGS

- A history of joint stiffness and complications after primary TKA (eg, arthrofibrosis, infection, hematoma) should alert the surgeon regarding potential difficulties with exposure during revision TKA.
- Physical findings indicating possible difficulty with exposure during revision TKA include multiple scars, reduced active and passive knee range of movement, a tight posterior cruciate ligament, and patella baja.

IMAGING AND OTHER DIAGNOSTIC STUDIES

- Standing anteroposterior and lateral radiographs of the knee usually are adequate in planning for extensile exposures during revision TKA.
- The radiographs are specifically inspected for tibial osteopenia (especially around the tibial tuberosity) and osteolysis, both of which are relative contraindications for tibial tubercle osteotomy.

SURGICAL MANAGEMENT

- A tibial tubercle osteotomy is indicated when there is any concern regarding patellar tendon avulsion despite adequate initial soft tissue release, as discussed later in this chapter.

Preoperative Planning

- Exposure should be thought about preoperatively: The history and physical findings should alert the surgeon regarding the potential need for extensile exposures during revision TKA.
- Previous operative records and radiographs are studied to identify the initial approach during primary TKA, design of the implanted components to be removed, and potential problems during implant removal.
- The quality of skin overlying the tibial tubercle should be assessed. In patients with multiple scars, the most recent, appropriate, healed scar is used, but in many situations where tibial tubercle osteotomy is indicated, it may be necessary to consult with a plastic surgical team to plan soft tissue coverage (**FIG 2**).

Positioning

- The patient is positioned supine on the operating table.
- A tourniquet is sited around the upper thigh, and the leg is exsanguinated before inflation.

Approach

- A medial parapatellar approach is used whenever possible because extensile exposures are most easily incorporated proximally (V-Y quadriceps turndown) and distally (tibial tubercle osteotomy).

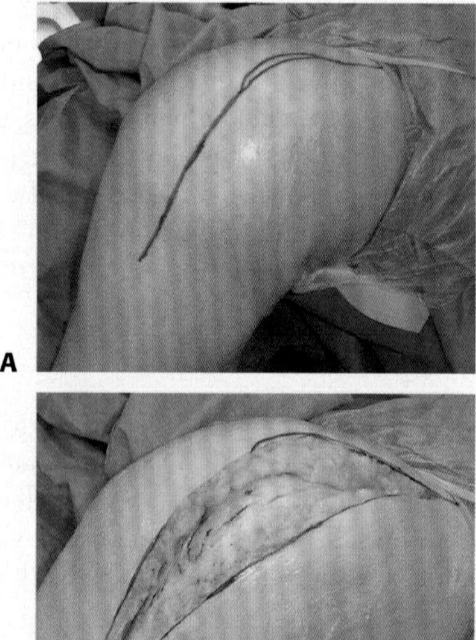

FIG 2 • Skin incisions. **A.** Previous skin incisions marked. **B.** Midline incision through most recent, healed scar.

TECHNIQUES

Initial Soft Tissue Release Before Tibial Tubercle Osteotomy

- If the patella cannot be everted following medial parapatellar arthrotomy, the following soft tissue releases are performed sequentially before considering a tibial tubercle osteotomy.
  - Medial release: The dissection is carried medially around the proximal tibia with subperiosteal elevation of the medial retinaculum and deep medial collateral ligament around to the semimembranosus insertion (**TECH FIG 1A,B**). This allows external rotation of the tibia and relaxes the extensor mechanism (**TECH FIG 1C,D**).
  - Lateral gutter release and pseudocapsule excision
    - Superior to the patella, the suprapatellar pouch is freed by dividing the underlying adhesions tethering the extensor mechanism to the anterior femur (**TECH FIG 1E**).
    - Lateral to the patella, adhesions in the lateral gutter tethering the extensor mechanism are divided (**TECH FIG 1F**).
    - Inferior to the patella, the interval between the patellar tendon anteriorly and fat pad posteriorly is identified and the intervening pseudocapsule excised distally to the insertion of the patellar tendon (**TECH FIG 1G,H**). The interval between the posterior patellar tendon and the tibia should be freed of scar and adhesions.
- If the patella still cannot be retracted appropriately, a tibial tubercle osteotomy is performed to reduce the risk of patellar tendon avulsion from forceful retraction of the extensor mechanism.

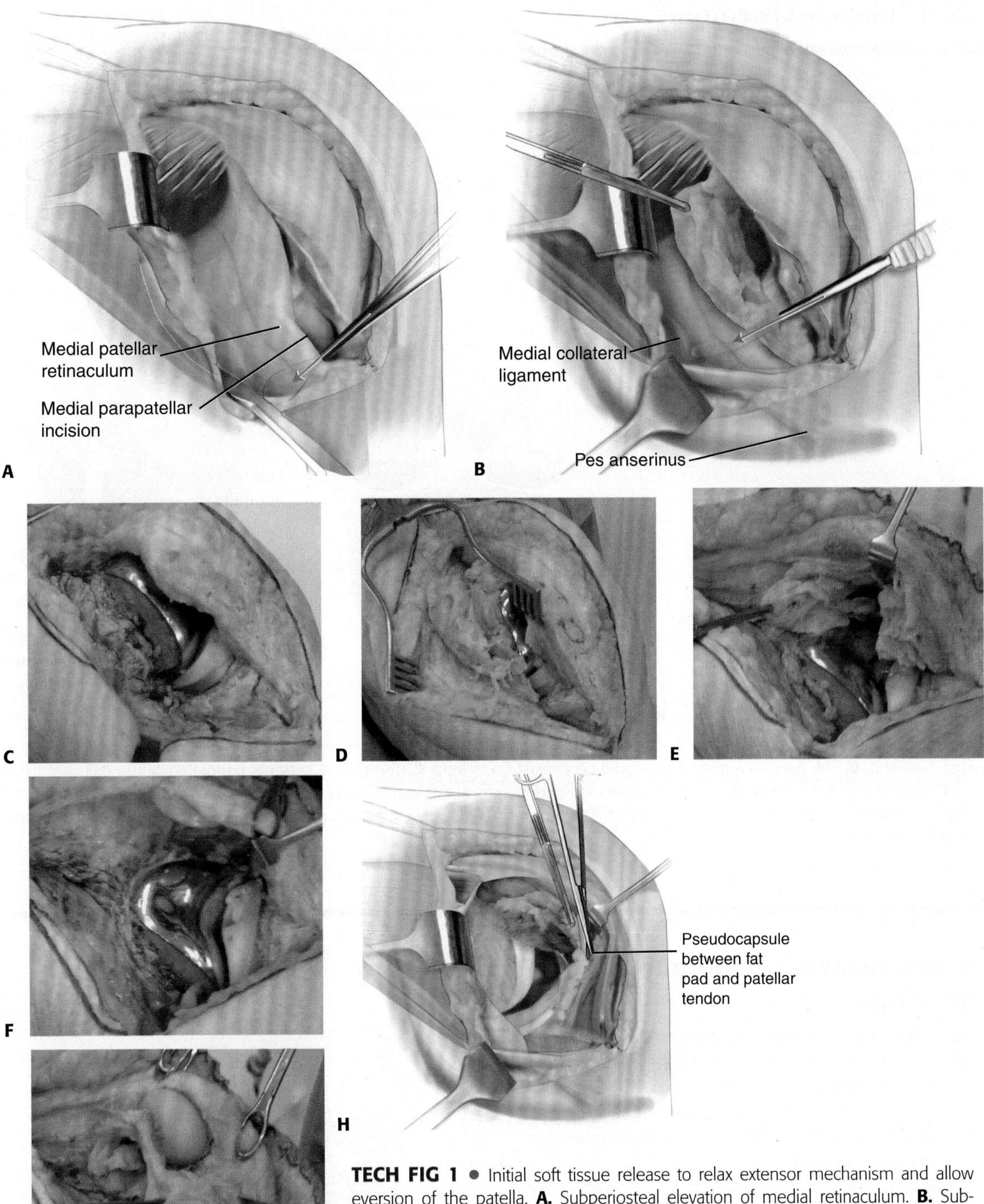

TECH FIG 1 • Initial soft tissue release to relax extensor mechanism and allow eversion of the patella. **A.** Subperiosteal elevation of medial retinaculum. **B.** Subperiosteal medial release to semimembranosus insertion. **C,D.** The pseudocapsule is completely excised medially to free the medial gutter. **E,F.** First, the suprapatellar pouch with the lateral gutter is freed from underlying adhesions. **G,H.** Next, the pseudocapsule inferior to the patella is excised.

Tibial Tubercle Osteotomy

- The skin incision is extended 8 to 10 cm below the tibial tubercle.
- The periosteum is vertically incised 1 cm medial to the tibial tubercle.
- An osteotomy site measuring 6 cm long, 2 cm wide, and 1 cm thick,[5,7] which includes the tibial tubercle and anterior tibial crest, is marked with electrocautery (**TECH FIG 2A,B**).
  - The 6-cm medial, vertical limb of the osteotomy is tapered distally to prevent a stress riser.
  - The 2-cm horizontal limb proximal to the insertion of the patellar tendon resists proximal migration of the osteotomized segment.
- The proposed medial, lateral, and proximal osteotomy cuts are perforated using a drill (**TECH FIG 2C**).
- Sequential osteotomes are used to transect the medial tibial crest and separate the osteotomized segment from the tibia.
- The lateral cortex is transected through the osteotomy, but the lateral periosteum and soft tissues are left attached to the elevated segment to act as a "hinge," allowing eversion of the extensor mechanism.

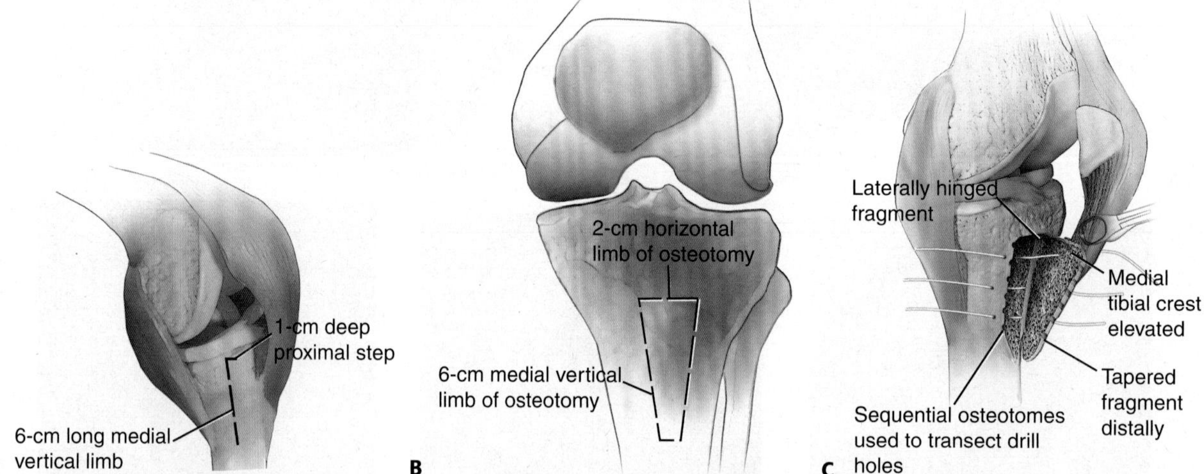

TECH FIG 2 • Tibial tubercle osteotomy. **A.** The distal cut is tapered to prevent a stress riser. Proximally, the step cut reduces the risk of proximal migration. **B.** The medial, vertical limb should be at least 6 cm long. **C.** The medial cortex is perforated with a drill, and the drill is passed through the lateral cortex to create corresponding perforations in the lateral cortex that will allow the osteoperiosteal segment to be "hinged" around the lateral soft tissue attachments. The proximal osteotomy cut is perforated, and sequential osteotomes are used to elevate the osteotomy.

Reattachment of Osteotomy with Wires

- In our preferred technique, three 18-gauge stainless steel wires are inserted and left untied before the final components are implanted.
  - The most proximal wire is passed through the osteotomized segment and through a drilled hole in the medial tibial cortex. Placement of a wire through the fragment prevents proximal migration.
  - The two distal wires are passed around the osteotomized segment and through drilled holes in the medial and lateral tibial cortices (**TECH FIG 3**).
- The wires are twisted until tight, cut, and angled 45 degrees posteromedially to prevent soft tissue irritation.[10]

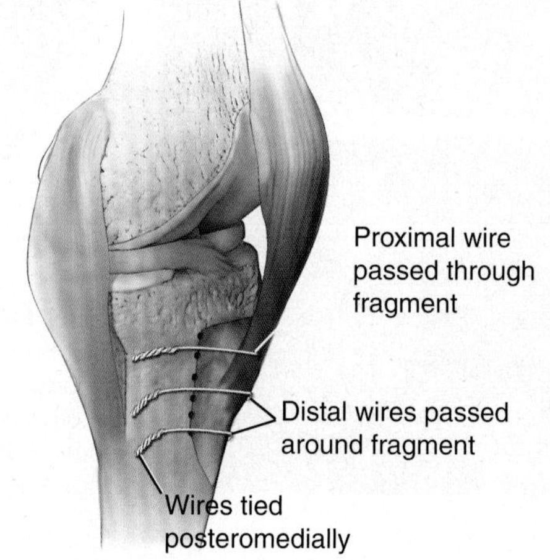

TECH FIG 3 • Reattachment of osteotomy with wires. The most proximal wire is passed through the osteotomized segment to prevent proximal migration; the two distal wires are passed around the osteotomy segment. Wires are cut and angled posteromedially to prevent soft tissue irritation.

Reattachment of Osteotomy with Screws

- At least three cortical screws are inserted after implantation of the tibial component (**TECH FIG 4**).
- The screws are passed posteromedially and posterolaterally around the tibial component using the triangular cross-section of the proximal tibia.[3,9]

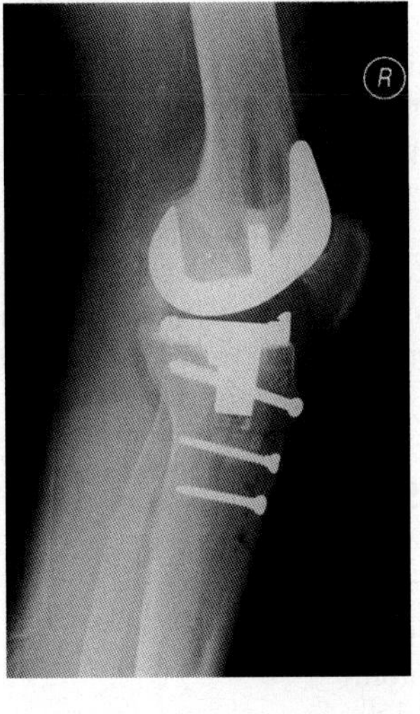

TECH FIG 4 ● Lateral radiograph of the knee after revision TKA with reattachment of the tibial tubercle osteotomy using screws.

PEARLS AND PITFALLS

Indications	■ Anticipate need for extensile exposure preoperatively. ■ Anticipate need for soft tissue coverage with plastic surgery.
Initial exposure	■ Medial parapatellar approach ■ Medial release, meticulous lateral gutter release, and excision of pseudocapsule before tibial tubercle osteotomy
Tibial tubercle osteotomy	■ Use a long (6–8 cm) osteoperiosteal segment. ■ Use a proximal step cut to prevent proximal migration. ■ Taper distally to avoid stress risers. ■ Use sequential osteotomes, not an oscillating saw.
Reattachment of osteotomy	■ Anatomic fixation of the osteotomized segment is critical to ensure union of the osteotomy. ■ At least one wire is passed through the osteotomy fragment to prevent proximal migration.

POSTOPERATIVE CARE

- If fixation of the tibial tubercle osteotomy is adequate, weight bearing is permitted as tolerated with unrestricted range of movement in a hinged knee brace.
- If fixation is not adequate, the patient can bear weight as tolerated with the knee locked in full extension in a brace until there is radiologic evidence of union.

OUTCOMES

- Whiteside[10] reported good results using a tibial tubercle osteotomy to gain extensile exposure during 136 TKAs, of which 110 were revision procedures. At 2-year follow-up, the mean postoperative range of movement was 94 degrees, with a 1.5% incidence of extensor lag. Three tibial shaft fractures and two avulsions of the tibial tubercle were reported in this series but no nonunions.
- Mendes et al[8] reported 87% good-to-excellent results (based on the Knee Society Score [KSS]) in 64 patients in whom a tibial tubercle osteotomy was used for extensile exposure during revision TKA. At an average follow-up of 30 months, the mean postoperative range of movement was 107 degrees, with a 4.5% incidence of extensor lag. One fracture of the tibia, no tibial avulsions, and two nonunions of the osteotomy were reported in this series.
- Barrack et al[1] reported a significantly lower incidence of extensor lag following tibial tubercle osteotomy when compared to V-Y quadriceps turndown, although outcome scores were similar for both groups at the 4-year follow-up.
- Biomechanical studies show that although reattachment of an osteotomy with screws has greater fixation strength than cerclage wires, placement of screws around revision tibial component stems is difficult.[3] Cerclage wires are easier to place and still provide solid fixation, especially when combined with a proximal step cut osteotomy.
- High rates of fixation failure with tibial tubercle osteotomy most likely are due to the use of small (<3 cm) osteoperiosteal fragments and failure to maintain lateral soft tissue attachments in continuity with the osteotomized segment.[11]

- Bruni et al[2] prospectively randomized patients being treated with two-stage exchange to either receive a quadriceps snip or a tibial tubercle osteotomy. The tibial tubercle osteotomy group showed a higher mean KSS score and a higher mean maximal flexion and a lower incidence of extension lag than the quadriceps snip group.
- Choi et al[4] has reported on the outcome of sequential repeated tibial tubercle osteotomy performed in two-stage revision in 13 patients and found satisfactory clinical and radiographic outcomes. However, there were three cases of proximal migration of the osteotomy fragment and one case of partial avulsion of the osteotomy fragment.

COMPLICATIONS

- Extensor lag[1,8,10]
- Tibial fracture[8,10]
- Tibial tuberosity avulsion[9,10]
- Nonunion of osteotomy[8]
- Metalwork removal[9,10]

ACKNOWLEDGEMENT

The authors wish to gratefully acknowledge the contributions made by Drs. Anish K. Amin and James T. Patton, authors of the previous chapter. Their material is incorporated into this chapter.

REFERENCES

1. Barrack RL, Smith P, Munn B, et al. The Ranawat Award. Comparison of surgical approaches in total knee arthroplasty. Clin Orthop Relat Res 1998;356:16–21.
2. Bruni D, Iacono F, Sharma B, et al. Tibial tubercle osteotomy or quadriceps snip in two-stage revision for prosthetic knee infection? A randomized prospective study. Clin Orthop Relat Res 2013;471(4):1305–1318.
3. Caldwell PE, Bohlen BA, Owen JR, et al. Dynamic confirmation of fixation techniques of the tibial tubercle osteotomy. Clin Orthop Relat Res 2004;424:173–179.
4. Choi HR, Kwon YM, Burke DW, et al. The outcome of sequential repeated tibial tubercle osteotomy performed in 2-stage revision arthroplasty for infected total knee arthroplasty. J Arthroplasty 2012;27(8):1487–1491.
5. Clarke HD. Tibial tubercle osteotomy. J Knee Surg 2003;16:58–61.
6. Dolin MG. Osteotomy of the tibial tubercle in total knee replacement: a technical note. J Bone Joint Surg Am 1983;65A:704–706.
7. Kelly MA, Clarke HD. Stiffness and ankylosis in primary total knee arthroplasty. Clin Orthop Relat Res 2003;416:68–73.
8. Mendes MW, Caldwell P, Jiranek WA. The results of tibial tubercle osteotomy for revision total knee arthroplasty. J Arthroplasty 2004;19:167–174.
9. Ries MD, Richman JA. Extended tibial tubercle osteotomy in total knee arthroplasty. J Arthroplasty 1996;11:964–967.
10. Whiteside LA. Exposure in difficult total knee arthroplasty using tibial tubercle osteotomy. Clin Orthop Relat Res 1995;321:32–35.
11. Wolff AM, Hungerford DS, Krackow KA, et al. Osteotomy of the tibial tubercle during total knee replacement. J Bone Joint Surg Am 1989;71A:848–852.

Revision Arthroplasty with Extensile Exposure V-Y Quadricepsplasty

45 CHAPTER

Thomas C. Emmer, Jonathan Salava, and Ali Oliashirazi

DEFINITION

- Gaining exposure during revision total knee arthroplasty (TKA) and primary TKA for the ankylosed knee can be challenging.
- Patients undergoing revision TKA are at particular risk for wound healing problems, extensor mechanism rupture, and infection.[17]
- Although over 90% of revision TKA procedures can be performed through a standard surgical approach, the surgeon should be familiar with more extensile techniques in case one must be used to avoid extensor mechanism disruption.[6]
- If adequate exposure is not obtained through a standard surgical approach, a graduated approach is necessary:
  - Quadriceps snip is used most commonly, followed by tibial tubercle osteotomy, and, rarely, a V-Y quadriceps turndown.
  - The quadriceps snip has the advantage of requiring no postoperative immobilization or changes to postoperative rehabilitation but may not give adequate exposure in very stiff knees.[17]
- Although it may be possible to perform a prosthetic implantation without using an extensile exposure in the ankylosed knee, quadriceps contracture can limit extensor mechanism excursion, leading to poor postoperative flexion.
  - V-Y quadricepsplasty may be performed after prosthetic insertion to improve flexion.[13]

STANDARD APPROACH

- Any skin incisions from previous procedures are clearly marked before skin preparation begins.
- Although a straight, midline anterior incision is preferred because the vascular supply to the anterior skin of the knee comes primarily from the medial side, the most lateral usable incision is chosen to preserve blood supply to the lateral flap.
- It is recommended that a minimum of 6–7 cm distance between the previous and any new incisions be maintained if possible to prevent skin bridge necrosis.[7,11]
- Previous skin incisions are ideally crossed perpendicular to the scar. If this is not possible, they should be intersected at an angle of no less than 60 degrees.
- Transcutaneous oxygen tension studies have shown that following skin incision, the inferolateral portion of the skin incision has the lowest oxygen tension, resulting in a decrease in wound healing potential.[2,9,10]
- Thick flaps are developed that include the superficial fascia. Dissection superficial to the fascia should be avoided as the blood supply to the anterior skin of the knee comes from perforating vessels which traverse this fascia and the subcutaneous tissue.[2,7,17]
- A medial parapatellar arthrotomy is made at the junction of the medial and central thirds of the quadriceps tendon.
- Subperiosteal dissection of the tibia is extended from the tibial tubercle to the posteromedial corner.
- The suprapatellar pouch and the medial and lateral gutters are reestablished, all adhesions are released, and a thorough synovectomy is performed.
- All peripatellar scar tissue is removed.
- Prior to flexion of the knee, the patellar tendon may be stabilized with a pin, towel clip, or small staple placed into the tibial tubercle to prevent patellar tendon avulsion.[11]
- The knee is gently flexed while the tibia is externally rotated and subluxed laterally. These maneuvers reduce tension on the extensor mechanism.
- If the extensor mechanism is still under too much tension, a lateral retinacular release may be performed from inside out, making sure to preserve the lateral superior genicular artery, which is now the primary blood supply to the patella.
- If adequate exposure is still not possible, a quadriceps snip is performed.
- In most revision TKAs, adequate exposure can be obtained with these maneuvers.[11]

Tibial Tubercle Osteotomy

- Tibial tubercle osteotomy (see Chap. 44) is chosen in cases with difficulty in stem or cement extraction or in patients with patella baja.[5]
- Potentially serious complications of this procedure include proximal migration of the tibial tubercle as well as tibial tubercle nonunion.[14,16]
- Other common complications include tibial tubercle pain and prominent hardware following fixation. These are often successfully treated with removal of hardware following tibial tubercle union.[4,14]

Quadriceps Turndown

- The quadriceps tendon is exposed proximal to the insertion of the vastus lateralis and medialis muscles.
- The medial parapatellar arthrotomy is extended proximally to the insertion of the vasti.
- The quadriceps is then incised distally and laterally at an angle of about 45 degrees along the insertion of the vastus lateralis (**TECH FIG 1**).
  - This inverted V incision creates a distally based flap that includes the patella. Essentially, the medial arthrotomy is connected to the lateral release.
- Care should be taken to preserve the lateral superior geniculate artery.
- The patella is now "turned down" anterolaterally, providing excellent exposure to the joint.

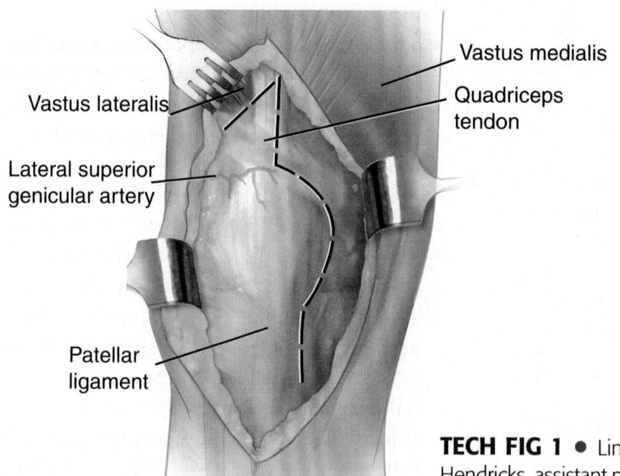

TECH FIG 1 • Line of incision. (Based on drawing by Dr. Greg Hendricks, assistant professor, Department of Orthopaedics, Joan C. Edwards School of Medicine, Marshall University, Huntington, WV.)

V-Y Quadricepsplasty

- This procedure is indicated to increase postoperative flexion.
- The quadriceps is repaired in situ with multiple interrupted no. 2 nonabsorbable sutures and range of motion (ROM) is assessed.
- If ROM is acceptable, closure is completed, leaving the lateral retinacular release open.
- If increased passive ROM is desired, the V is converted to an inverted Y.
- The knee is flexed and sutures or clamps are placed along the apex of the Y.
- Once appropriate lengthening is established, no. 2 nonabsorbable sutures are used to close the medial side of the quadriceps mechanism.
- The lateral retinacular release (lateral limb of the Y) is left open.
- The lateral limb of the quadricepsplasty is covered by closing the quadriceps mechanism to the superficial fascia of the vastus lateralis (**TECH FIG 2**).
- The maximum flexion of the knee that will not put undue tension on the repair is recorded prior to routine skin closure.

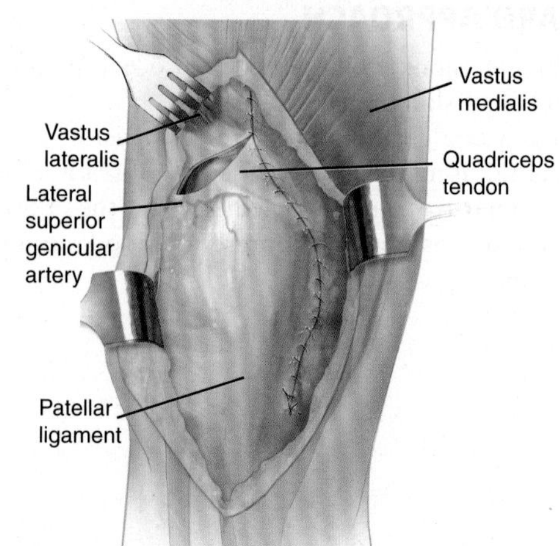

TECH FIG 2 • Closure. (Based on drawing by Dr. Greg Hendricks, assistant professor, Department of Orthopaedics, Joan C. Edwards School of Medicine, Marshall University, Huntington, WV.)

PEARLS AND PITFALLS

- The patient and family members should be counseled preoperatively regarding the possibility that this approach may be required and prepared for the subsequent need for postoperative bracing.
- Intraoperatively, a graduated approach is necessary, starting with a medial parapatellar approach with lateral release, advancing to quadriceps snip, and lastly to tibial tubercle osteotomy or rarely a V-Y turndown as needed.
- Preserve the superior lateral geniculate artery.
- Do not be aggressive with ROM, particularly during the first 2 weeks postoperatively.

POSTOPERATIVE CARE

- One disadvantage of V-Y quadricepsplasty is the necessity to modify postoperative rehabilitation.
- Maximum passive flexion to avoid tension on the repair is determined intraoperatively after capsular closure. This is not exceeded in the first 2 weeks.
- The patient is place in a knee immobilizer immediately postoperatively.
- A hinged knee brace is fitted after the first dressing change. A flexion stop is used for the first 2 weeks.
- Passive knee extension and active knee flexion are done for 6 weeks.
- Partial weight bearing is required for 6 weeks.
- The brace is locked in extension at night and with ambulation until the extensor lag is less than 15 degrees.

OUTCOMES

- Knee scores are similar to those of patients who have had revision TKA and reflect the difficulty of knees that need this procedure.[1,15]
- A study comparing patients who underwent quadriceps turndown and tibial tubercle osteotomy to patients whose revision TKAs were performed with routine exposure found patients in the quadriceps turndown and tibial tubercle osteotomy groups had equivalent postoperative scores, which were significantly lower than those of patients in the routine exposure revision TKA group. The turndown group had a higher increase in ROM than the osteotomy group, but they also had a higher degree of extensor lag. The turndown group also had a lower percentage of patients who considered their surgery unsuccessful in relieving pain and return of function and a lower percentage of patients who had difficulty with kneeling and stooping.[3]
- A prospective randomized controlled trial with 8 years minimum follow-up comparing quadriceps snip to tibial tubercle osteotomy for revision TKA cases for prosthetic knee infection found patients undergoing tibial tubercle osteotomy had significantly higher Knee Society Scores, higher postoperative knee flexion, and lower postoperative extension lag. All patients in the tibial osteotomy group showed radiographic evidence of tibial tubercle healing, 11 patients had pain over the tibial tubercle at 6 months, and 8 elected to undergo removal of fixation hardware and were pain free at 1 year.[4]
- One study evaluating the effectiveness of V-Y quadricepsplasty found an average increase in postoperative flexion of 49 degrees, with an overall increase in postoperative ROM to 52 degrees. The patients also had average postoperative extensor lag of 8 degrees.[13]
- Trousdale et al[15] evaluated functional outcomes following V-Y quadricepsplasty found a trend toward knee extension weakness, but this only reached statistical significance at knee extension test speeds of 120, 180, and 240 degrees per second. Overall, the extensor weakness did not appear to be clinically significant.[15]
- In a mixed population of primary and revision TKA, Cybex testing revealed that the quadriceps was weaker on the V-Y quadricepsplasty side, but this did not reach statistical significance. Only 5 of 14 patients had extensor lag greater than 5 degrees, with active extension lag averaging 4 degrees (range 0 to 20 degrees).[15]
- A study of patients undergoing TKA with preoperative knee stiffness (defined as preoperative ROM <50 degrees) found that patients requiring the V-Y quadricepsplasty intraoperatively to increase ROM had a significantly higher rate of postoperative extensor lag greater than 10 degrees. However, these patients also had significantly lower preoperative knee function scores and ROM and higher incidence of flexion contracture.[8]

COMPLICATIONS

- As detailed and referenced above. Mainly extensor lag and mild extensor weakness of questionable clinical significance.
- Additionally, patellar osteonecrosis was observed in 8 of 29 patients with quadriceps turndown in one study.[12]
- One case of minor wound dehiscence was also reported in a hemophiliac patient during manipulation under anesthesia after TKA using V-Y quadricepsplasty.

REFERENCES

1. Aglietti P, Buzzi R, D'Andria S, Scrobe F. Quadricepsplasty with the V-Y incision in total knee arthroplasty. Ital J Orthop Traumatol 1991;17(1):23-29.
2. Aso K, Ikeuchi M, Izumi M, et al. Transcutaneous oxygen tension in the anterior skin of the knee after minimal incision total knee arthroplasty. Knee 2012;19(5):576–579.
3. Barrack RL, Smith P, Munn B, et al. The Ranawat Award. Comparison of surgical approaches in total knee arthroplasty. Clin Orthop Relat Res 1998;(356):16–21.
4. Bruni D, Iacono F, Sharma B, et al. Tibial tubercle osteotomy or quadriceps snip in two-stage revision for prosthetic knee infection? A randomized prospective study. Clin Orthop Relat Res 2013;471(4):1305–1318.
5. Clarke HD, Scuderi GR. Revision total knee arthroplasty: planning, management, controversies, and surgical approaches. Instr Course Lect 2001;50:359–365.
6. Della Valle CJ, Berger RA, Rosenberg AG. Surgical exposures in revision total knee arthroplasty. Clin Orthop Relat Res 2006;446:59–68.
7. Garbedian S, Sternheim A, Backstein D. Wound healing problems in total knee arthroplasty. Orthopedics 2011;34(9):e516–e518.

8. Hsu CH, Lin PC, Chen WS, et al. Total knee arthroplasty in patients with stiff knees. J Arthroplasty 2012;27(2):286–292.
9. Johnson DP. Midline or parapatellar incision for knee arthroplasty. A comparative study of wound viability. J Bone Joint Surg Br 1988;70(4):656–658.
10. Johnson DP, Houghton TA, Radford P. Anterior midline or medial parapatellar incision for arthroplasty of the knee. A comparative study. J Bone Joint Surg Br 1986;68(5):812–814.
11. Laskin RS. Ten steps to an easier revision total knee arthroplasty. J Arthroplasty 2002;17(4)(suppl 1):78–82.
12. Parker DA, Dunbar MJ, Rorabeck CH. Extensor mechanism failure associated with total knee arthroplasty: prevention and management. J Am Acad Orthop Surg 2003;11(4):238–247.
13. Scott RD, Siliski JM. The use of a modified V-Y quadricepsplasty during total knee replacement to gain exposure and improve flexion in the ankylosed knee. Orthopedics 1985;8(1):45–48.
14. Tabutin J, Morin-Salvo N, Torga-Spak R, et al. Tibial tubercule osteotomy during medial approach to difficult knee arthroplasties. Orthop Traumatol Surg Res 2011;97(3):276–286.
15. Trousdale RT, Hanssen AD, Rand JA, et al. V-Y quadricepsplasty in total knee arthroplasty. Clin Orthop Relat Res 1993;(286):48–55.
16. Young CF, Bourne RB, Rorabeck CH. Tibial tubercle osteotomy in total knee arthroplasty surgery. J Arthroplasty 2008;23(3):371–375.
17. Younger AS, Duncan CP, Masri BA. Surgical exposures in revision total knee arthroplasty. J Am Acad Orthop Surg 1998;6(1):55–64.

Revision Total Knee Arthroplasty with Extensor Mechanism Reconstruction

46

CHAPTER

Alvin Ong and Fabio Orozco

DEFINITION

- Extensor mechanism disruption following total knee arthroplasty (TKA) is a devastating complication, with a prevalence of 0.17% to 2.5%.[1,3]
- The patella tendon is involved more commonly (0.22%) than the quadriceps tendon (0.1%).
- Despite reports of encouraging results following direct repair in native knees, primary repair in TKA rarely results in successful restoration of extensor function.
- Augmentation or reconstruction with allograft tissue is recommended to increase success of repair.

ANATOMY

- The patella tendon connects the tibia and the patella. It originates from the inferior pole of the patella and inserts onto the tibial tuberosity. It is about 5 to 6 cm long and 3 cm wide.
- Anteriorly, the fibers of the rectus femoris traverse the patella and insert on the tibial tubercle inferior to the patella as the patella tendon.
- The fibers of the vastus lateralis muscle expand to the superolateral border of the patella and proximal tibia to form the lateral retinaculum.
- The fibers of the vastus medialis muscle insert into the superomedial border of the patella and tibia to form the medial retinaculum.

PATHOGENESIS

- The etiology of extensor mechanism disruption is multifactorial.
- Factors associated with patella tendon rupture include the following:
  - Difficult exposure in stiff knees
  - Extensive release of the patella tendon at the time of surgical exposure
  - Manipulation for treatment of limited motion
  - Revision TKA
  - Malrotation of the components
  - Overly aggressive postoperative physical therapy
  - Distal realignment procedures
- Factors associated with quadriceps tendon rupture include the following:
  - Steroid use
  - Systemic diseases such as diabetes mellitus, chronic renal failure, Parkinson disease, or gout
  - Morbid obesity
  - Multiple intra-articular injections
  - Lateral release
  - Quadriceps snip

NATURAL HISTORY

- Only partial ruptures, where active extension is intact, can be treated with observation.
- The majority of full-thickness ruptures require surgical intervention.
- Direct repair following TKA rarely results in successful restoration of extensor function.
- Augmentation with autograft or allograft tissue often is required.

PATIENT HISTORY AND PHYSICAL FINDINGS

- The patient presents with weak or no active extension of the knee.
- Quadriceps tendon rupture
  - An injury is often associated with tear, such as a fall or vigorous activity.
  - Patient presents with severe pain and weakness.
  - There is difficulty with weight bearing.
  - Pain is localized just above the patella.
  - On examination, there is swelling of the knee with tenderness in the quadriceps tendon. There may be a palpable defect above the superior pole of the patella.
- Patella tendon rupture
  - Patients may or may not report a history of injury.
  - Often occurs intraoperatively or in the perioperative period.
  - Presents with pain at the region of the tibial tubercle
  - It may be difficult to distinguish normal surgical pain from patella tendon rupture.
  - On examination, the most common finding is a high-riding patella. There is swelling and pain below the patella.
  - There may be a palpable defect at the level of the patella tendon.

IMAGING AND OTHER DIAGNOSTIC STUDIES

- Anteroposterior (AP) and lateral radiographs of the knee should be obtained.
- Comparison with immediate postoperative or preoperative films is helpful.
- Patella alta may be present in complete patella tendon rupture (**FIG 1**).
- Patella baja or distal position of the patella may be present in quadriceps tendon rupture. However, a normal patella position does not rule out rupture of the quadriceps tendon.
- Bony fragments may be seen superior or inferior to the patella at/or near the tibial tubercle, indicating avulsion of the tendon.

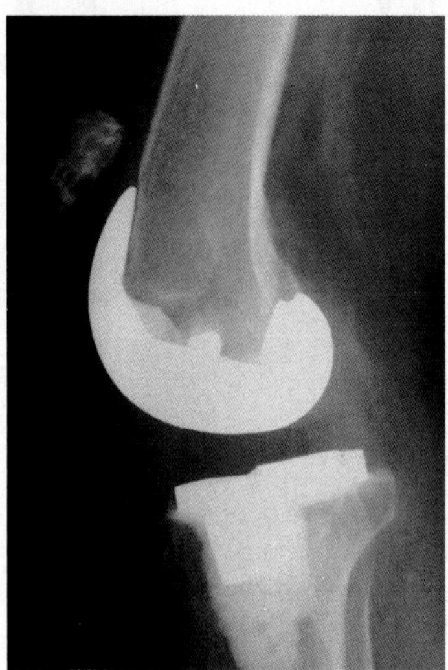

FIG 1 • Knee lateral radiograph demonstrating characteristic patella alta seen in patella tendon rupture.

DIFFERENTIAL DIAGNOSIS

- Patella tendon rupture
- Quadriceps tendon rupture
- Patellar fracture
- Patellar contusion
- Patellar tendonitis
- Prepatellar bursitis

NONOPERATIVE MANAGEMENT

- Nonoperative management of extensor mechanism disruption is uncommon.
- For the rare person with partial tendon rupture where active extension is preserved, consideration for cast or brace immobilization in full extension for 8 to 10 weeks followed by physical therapy to regain motion. Progress should be slow; regaining functional range of motion (ROM) should be the primary goal after immobilization. Strengthening exercises should be delayed for 3 months.
- Contraindications for surgical reconstruction include the following:
  - Active infection
  - Inability to comply with postoperative immobilization and the physical therapy program

SURGICAL MANAGEMENT

- A deficient extensor mechanism in patients with a TKA poses a very challenging problem.
- Direct suture or staple repair alone is often unsuccessful.
- Options for management of extensor mechanism disruption after TKA include direct repair with augmentation using autogenous hamstrings tendon (semitendinosus tendon), allograft Achilles tendon or whole quadriceps-patella-patellar tendon allograft, or a synthetic graft or mesh.
- This chapter will describe the use of Achilles tendon allograft tissue in the reconstruction of complete disruption of the extensor mechanism after TKA. Calcaneal bone block may be used if allograft needs to be extended past the tibial attachment of the patella tendon, such as in avulsion injuries of the patella tendon.

Preoperative Planning

- Initial evaluation of the patient should include the following:
  - History
  - Physical examination
  - Radiographs
- Previous operative reports should be reviewed. The surgeon should be prepared to perform revision surgery of any of the components of the TKA, specifically to address malrotation or malalignment.
- Make certain that optimal allograft tissue is available.
  - Fresh frozen allograft is preferable to freeze-dried allograft tissue.
  - The allograft should be inspected to ascertain it is of adequate size and quality.
  - A calcaneal bone segment of at least 3 cm attached to the patella tendon is preferred.

Positioning

- The patient is positioned supine on a radiolucent table.
- A regular pneumatic tourniquet is used proximally around the thigh.
  - Alternatively, a sterile tourniquet can be employed if there is concern for the proximal extent of the incision.
- The leg is prepared and draped in the standard, sterile fashion for joint replacement surgery.
- Fluoroscopic equipment is in the room with the technician in case imaging is necessary intraoperatively; for example, to aid in proximal tibial osteotomy, placement of fixation screws, judgment of joint line, and patellar height.
- The pneumatic tourniquet is inflated (usually to 250 to 300 mm Hg) after the limb has been exsanguinated with an Esmarch bandage.

Approach

- The previous incision should be used. In cases with more than one incision, the most midline (extensile) incision should be chosen (**FIG 2**).

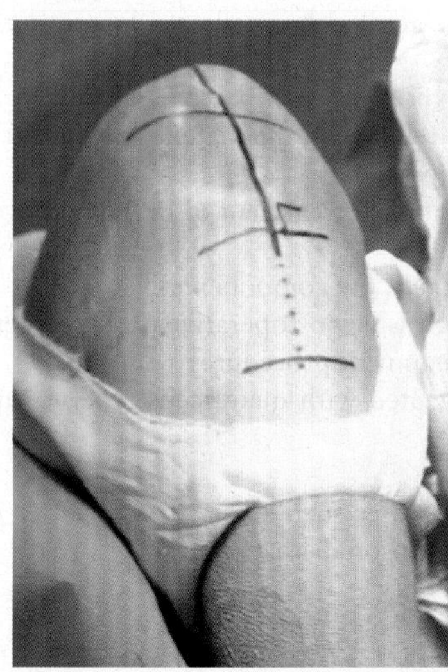

FIG 2 • Patient in supine position, with previous incision marked.

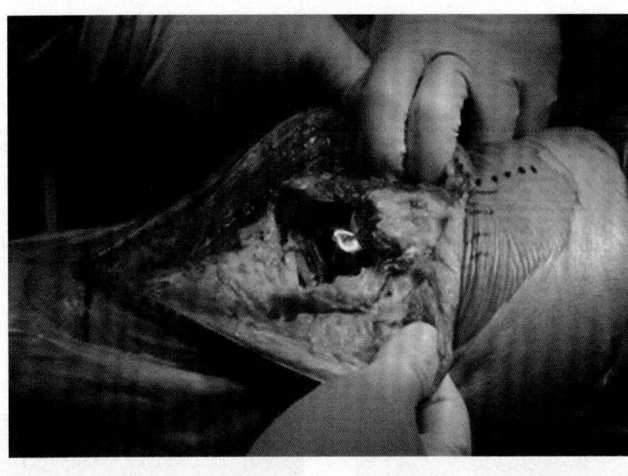

FIG 3 • Medial and lateral sleeves have been created, allowing direct exposure to the anterior aspect of the tibia and tibial tubercle.

- The dissection is carried down the midline, elevating medial and lateral skin and subcutaneous flaps.
- The extensor mechanism and retinacular tissue is exposed. Often, the incision is extended proximally and distally to expose normal tissue.
- The tendon rupture is exposed and identified (**FIG 3**).
- To aid in dissection, a medial peripatellar approach can be incorporated for better exposure or access to the joint.
- The joint is drained of any hematoma and irrigated using pulsatile lavage.

Primary Repair

- Primary repair of the ruptured tendon is always attempted.
- In case of patella tendon rupture, two parallel drill holes are created longitudinally into the patella (**TECH FIG 1A**).
- Use a no. 5 nonabsorbable suture (FiberWire [Arthrex, Naples, FL] or Ethibond) in a running, locked fashion into the remnant native tendon (**TECH FIG 1B**).
- The suture is then passed into the drill holes and tied over bony bridge. The repair is performed with the knee in full extension (**TECH FIG 1C**).
- The repair is augmented with no. 1 Vicryl to achieve end-to-end repair as best as possible.

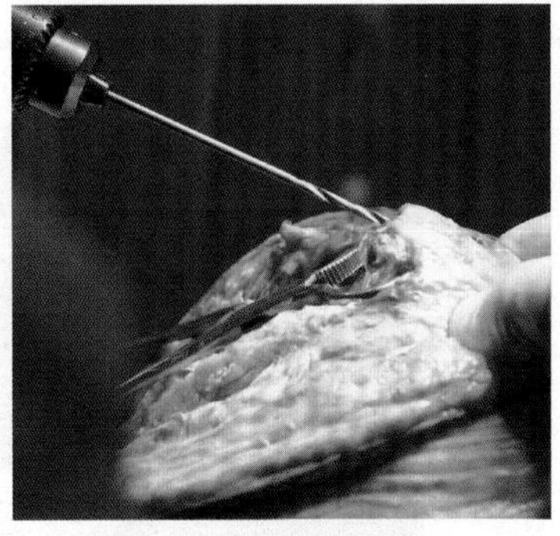

A

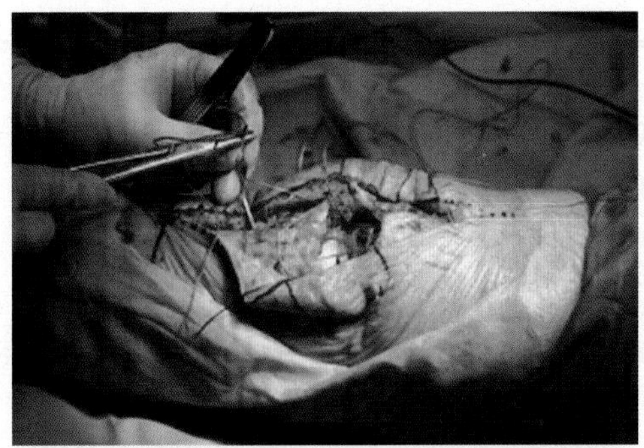

B

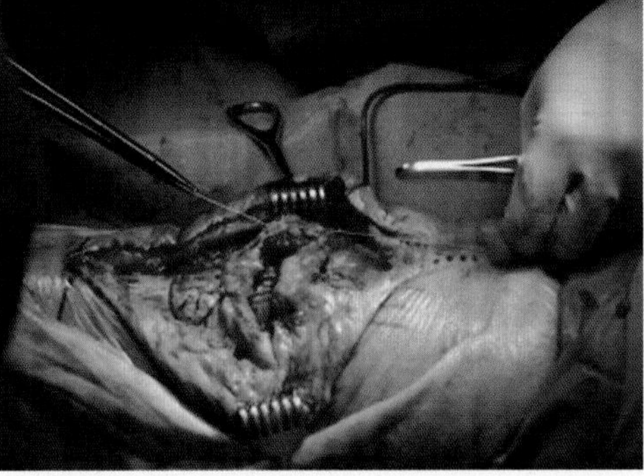

C

TECH FIG 1 • **A.** Two parallel tunnels are made through the patellar bone. **B,C.** A heavy no. 2 nonabsorbable suture is used to perform the primary repair in a running, locked fashion. The repair is augmented with the use of no. 1 Vicryl in an interrupted figure-8 technique.

Preparation of the Tibia and Allograft

- A small oscillating saw is used to make a rectangular cavity 2.5 × 1.5 × 1 cm in the proximal tibia slightly distal to the insertion of the patella tendon. Care should be taken to prevent iatrogenic fracture of the proximal tibia (**TECH FIG 2A–C**).
- The allograft tendon is thawed and soaked in antibiotic-impregnated saline.
- The allograft calcaneal bone is contoured to the desired shape on the back table. The goal is to form a trapezoidal bone block that will be press-fit into the tibial osteotomy site. Tight fit is preferred to get good bony stability and bone contact (**TECH FIG 2D,E**).

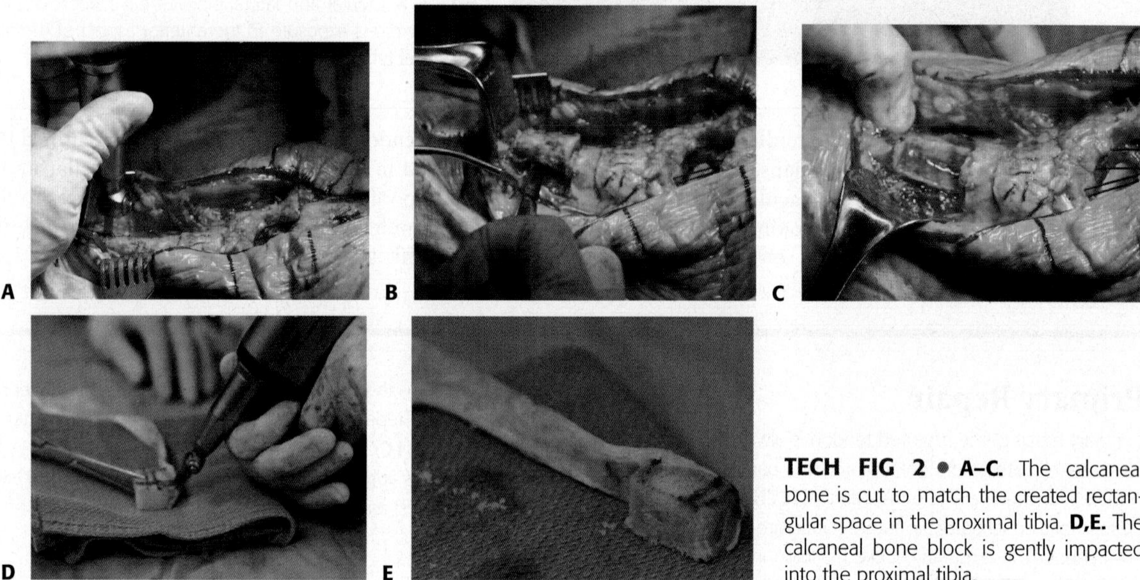

TECH FIG 2 • A–C. The calcaneal bone is cut to match the created rectangular space in the proximal tibia. **D,E.** The calcaneal bone block is gently impacted into the proximal tibia.

Reduction and Fixation of Calcaneal Bone Block

- The calcaneal bone block is gently impacted into the proximal tibia (**TECH FIG 3A**).
- Two 3.5-mm screws, angled to avoid the tibial component, are used to secure the bone block to the tibia (**TECH FIG 3B**).

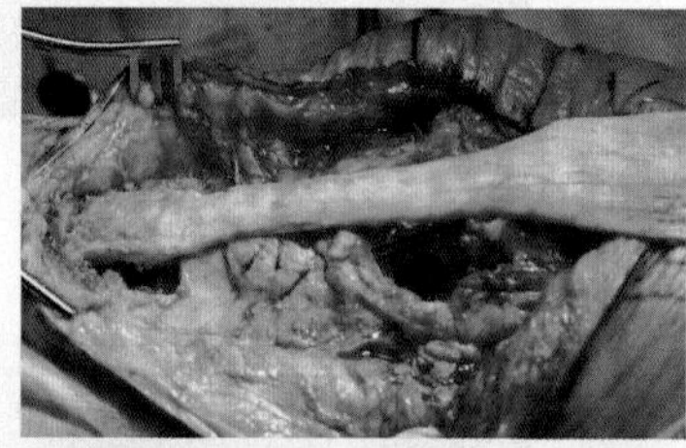

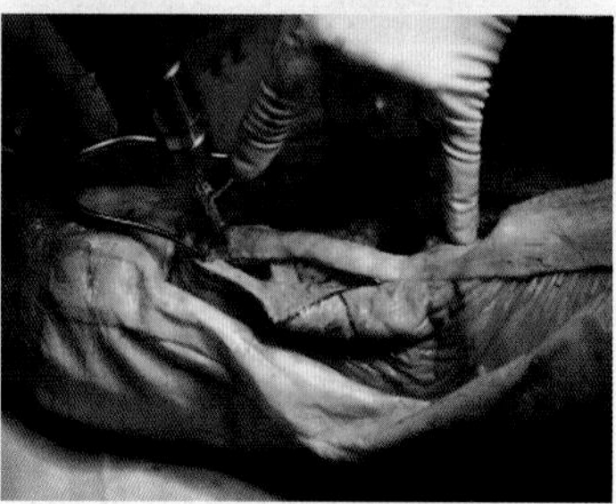

TECH FIG 3 • A. The calcaneal bone block is gently impacted into the proximal tibia. **B.** The calcaneal bone block is fixed to the proximal tibia with the use of two 4.5-mm screws.

Placement and Fixation of the Allograft Tendon

- The Achilles tendon is draped over the anterior tibia and patella while the knee is in full extension.
- Tension is applied to the graft to keep it taut.
- There is often excess allograft tendon. This proximal portion is trimmed to size and used to reinforce the reconstruction (**TECH FIG 4A**).
- This excess patch of allograft is used to reinforce the repair at the rupture site (**TECH FIG 4B**).
- The Achilles graft is attached to the underlying native extensor tissue using no. 1 and no. 2 nonabsorbable sutures (Ethibond or FiberWire) (**TECH FIG 4C,D**).
- Care must be taken to keep graft under tension during the repair. Likewise, the knee is kept in full extension during the reconstruction.

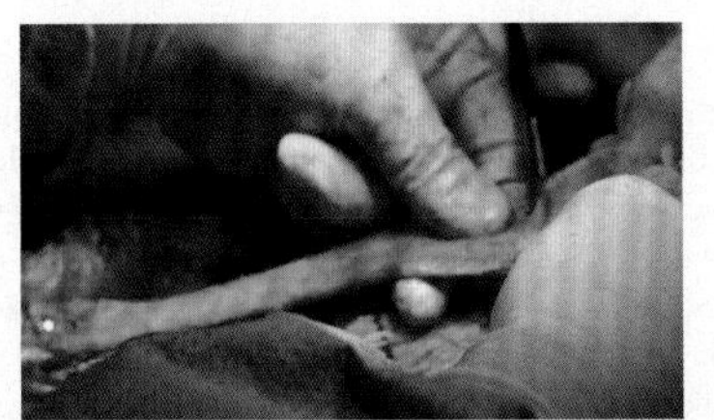

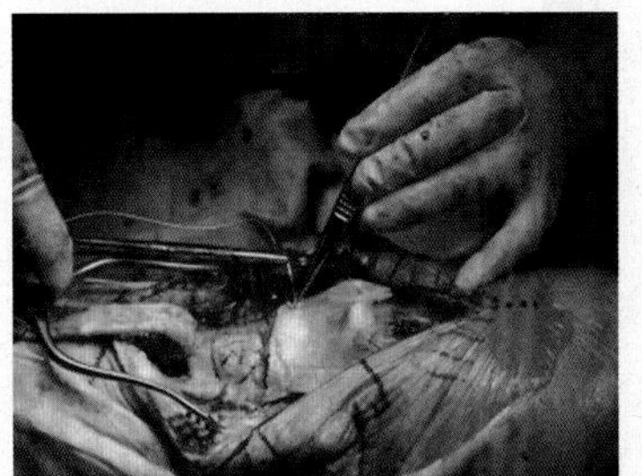

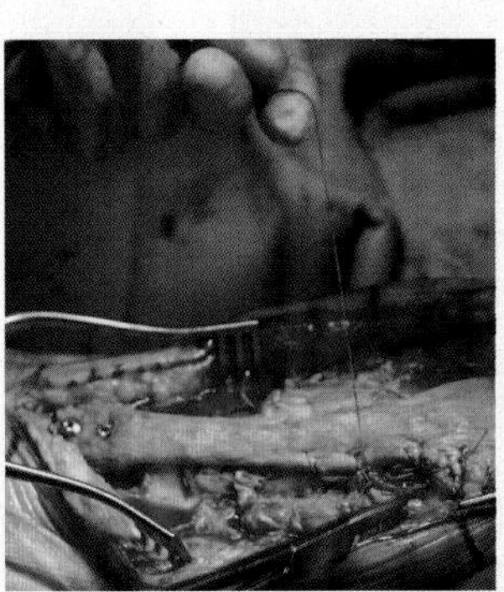

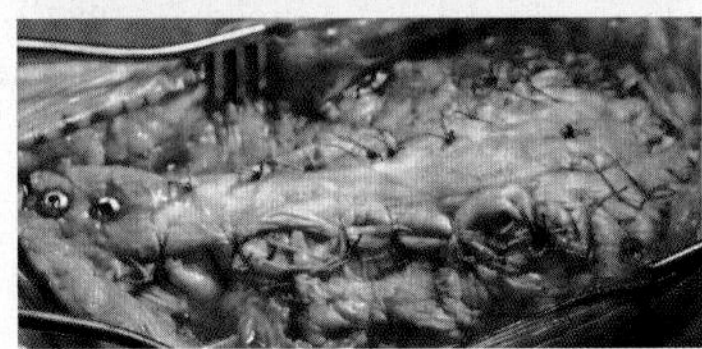

TECH FIG 4 • **A.** The Achilles tendon allograft is cut to obtain a rectangular patch. **B.** The rectangular patch is used to augment the attempted primary repair. **C,D.** The Achilles graft is attached to the underlying extensor mechanism.

Wound Closure

- The subcutaneous flap is closed in the routine fashion using a combination of no. 1 Vicryl and 2-0 Vicryl sutures.
- The skin is closed using skin staples, and a compression dressing is applied. The tourniquet is deflated after dressing is applied.
- A knee immobilizer is applied to keep the knee in full extension.

PEARLS AND PITFALLS

Indications	■ Primary repair of extensor mechanism disruption following TKA is rarely successful, and in most instances, augmentation with autograft or allograft tissue is necessary.
Graft	■ A fresh frozen, nonirradiated Achilles allograft with calcaneal bone block is preferred. ■ Visually inspect the graft to make sure it is of adequate size and quality. There should be at least 3 cm of calcaneal bone attached.
Reconstruction	■ Intraoperative fluoroscopy can help ensure correct position of the tibial osteotomy and placement of fixation screws. ■ Attachment of graft to the native tissue is accomplished with nonabsorbable sutures. ■ Repair is performed with graft in tension and the knee in full extension.
Revision of total knee comparison	■ Be ready to perform revision surgery to correct malrotation or malalignment.
Postoperative care	■ The knee is kept in full extension in a brace for 8–10 weeks. ■ Initially, non–weight bearing (NWB) is prescribed for 6 weeks. ■ ROM is delayed for a full 8–10 weeks.
Failure	■ Graft failure ■ Infection

POSTOPERATIVE CARE

- Postoperative AP and lateral radiographs are obtained in the postoperative care unit (**FIG 4**).
- The knee is immobilized in full extension for 8 to 10 weeks using a hinged knee brace.
- Staples are removed 3 weeks postoperatively.
- At 8 to 10 weeks, a brace with 30 degrees of flexion is used for 2 weeks and progressed to 60 degrees for an additional 2 weeks.

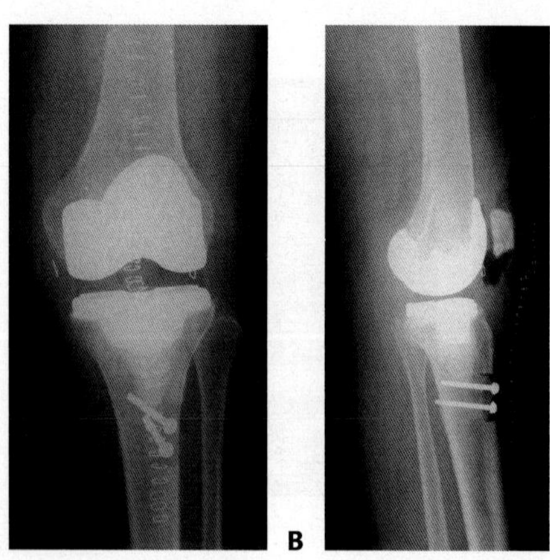

FIG 4 • Postoperative AP (**A**) and lateral (**B**) radiographs of the knee.

- Flexion past 90 degrees is delayed until 14 to 16 weeks postoperatively.

OUTCOMES

- Short-term results are encouraging, but residual extensor lags of 5 to 20 degrees are common.[2,4]
- The patient is encouraged to stay in the brace for 8 to 10 weeks postoperatively. Prolonged immobilization decreases the risk of extensor lag postoperatively.
- Longer term follow-up of patients with Achilles tendon reconstruction for extensor mechanism disruption is required.

COMPLICATIONS

- Graft failure
- Infection

REFERENCES

1. Cadambi A, Engh GA. Use of a semitendinosus tendon autogenous graft for rupture of the patellar ligament after total knee arthroplasty: a report of seven cases. J Bone Joint Surg Am 1992;74(7):974–979.
2. Crossett LS, Sinha RK, Sechriest VF, et al. Reconstruction of a ruptured patellar tendon with Achilles tendon allograft following total knee arthroplasty. J Bone Joint Surg Am 2002;84(8):1354–1361.
3. Lynch AF, Rorabeck CH, Bourne RB. Extensor mechanism complications following total knee arthroplasty. J Arthroplasty 1987;2:135–140.
4. Rand JA. Extensor mechanism complications after total knee arthroplasty. Instr Course Lect 2005;54:241–250.

Revision Total Knee Arthroplasty to Correct Stiffness

47
CHAPTER

Craig J. Della Valle

DEFINITION

- At less than 90 degrees of active knee flexion, a total knee arthroplasty (TKA) has inadequate range of motion (ROM) for performing many activities of daily living. The required ROM for daily activities are as follows[4,12]:
  - Sixty-seven degrees of flexion for normal gait on level ground
  - Eighty-three degrees of flexion to climb stairs
  - Ninety to 100 degrees of flexion to descend stairs
  - Ninety-three degrees of flexion to stand from a standard-height chair
  - One hundred five degrees of flexion to tie a shoe
- Flexion contractures can be equally disabling: A flexion contracture of more than 15 degrees is usually considered pathologic because it greatly inhibits normal gait.

ANATOMY

- The primary impediments to exposure of the revision TKA, particularly a stiff TKA, are the extensor mechanism and the patella. The exposure can be thought of as a progressive release or "unleashing" of the extensor mechanism.
- The four tethers of the extensor mechanism (**FIG 1**) are the following:
  - Proximal: quadriceps tendon and musculature
  - Medial: medial joint capsule and retinaculum with the insertion of the vastus medialis
  - Lateral: lateral joint capsule and retinaculum with the insertion of the vastus lateralis
  - Distal: patellar tendon
- The blood supply to the patella is provided by an anastomotic ring of vessels supplied by the geniculate arteries. It is important to try to avoid complete devascularization of the patella because avascular necrosis can occur.
- The blood supply to the skin overlying the knee travels from the deeper tissues up through the superficial fascia and does not run superficially. If skin flaps are required at the time of surgery, they must be full thickness to avoid skin necrosis.

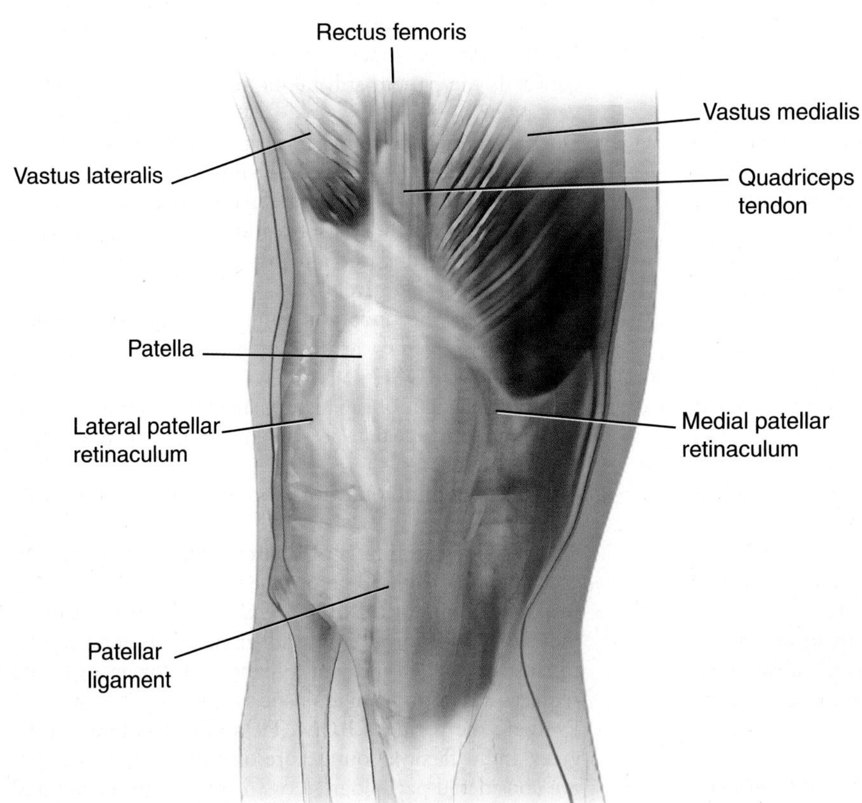

FIG 1 • Anterior view of the knee showing the patella, patellar tendon, quadriceps tendon, vastus medialis oblique muscle, and vastus lateralis.

PATHOGENESIS

- Many potential causes for stiffness following TKA exist and multiple mechanisms may act in concert in a given patient, resulting in suboptimal ROM.
- Poor perioperative pain control or suboptimal physical therapy. In rare cases, a chronic regional pain syndrome develops, characterized by severe pain, cutaneous hypersensitivity, vasomotor disturbance, and stiffness.
- Technical issues related to the original surgical procedure may play a role.
  - Femoral component
    - Oversized: leads to tightness in flexion
    - Internally rotated: leads to patellar maltracking or an asymmetric flexion gap
    - Inadequate distal femoral resection: leads to tightness in extension and a potential flexion contracture, or alternatively, a knee that is stable in extension but loose in flexion
    - Overresection of the distal femur: requires a thicker polyethylene insert to obtain stability in extension, thereby leading to tightness in flexion
    - Inadequate removal of posterior femoral osteophytes: leads to tenting of the posterior capsule and flexion contracture or osteophytes that can impinge on the tibial polyethylene insert, limiting flexion
    - Anterior placement of the femoral component: can lead to "overstuffing" of the patellofemoral joint
  - Tibial component
    - Most commonly, inadequate or reverse slope of the tibial cut, which leads to tightness in flexion
    - Internal rotation of the tibial component, which leads to patellar maltracking
    - Oversized tibial component, which can lead to soft tissue impingement and pain
    - Inadequate resection of the tibia: leads to tightness in both flexion and extension
  - Patellar component
    - Under-resection of the patella: can lead to overstuffing of the patellofemoral articulation. The native patella–prosthetic composite in most cases should be equivalent in thickness to the patella before resection.
    - Excessive patellar resection: leads to weakness of the extensor mechanism with initial extensor lag and eventual flexion contracture
    - Inadequate medialization of the component: can lead to patellar maltracking
    - Inadequate removal of lateral patellar osteophytes: can lead to impingement and pain
  - Ligamentous imbalance: flexion–extension mismatch (typically too tight in flexion, particularly with a cruciate-sparing design) or varus–valgus instability
  - Elevation of the joint line (particularly if >1 cm): leads to poor ROM secondary to altered patellofemoral joint mechanics
  - Poor component fixation: failed ingrowth of cementless components or inadequate cement mantle around cemented components, resulting in persistent pain that inhibits physiotherapy
- Patient-related factors
  - Poor preoperative ROM (the best predictor of postoperative ROM is preoperative ROM)
  - Genetic predisposition to scarring and stiffness
  - A history of previous surgery on the knee that has led to stiffness or a patella baja (shortening of the patellar tendon)
  - Noncompliance with physical therapy
  - Obesity (soft tissue envelope of the posterior thigh and leg limits flexion)
  - Stiffness or arthritis of the ipsilateral hip
- Deep infection must always be considered in the differential diagnosis.
- Heterotopic ossification

NATURAL HISTORY

- The natural history of stiff TKA is poor. Even with time, patients' ROM rarely improves enough to positively impact their gait pattern, and chronic pain develops.
- Flexion contractures are equally poorly tolerated. Flexion contractures greater than 15 degrees limit the ability to stand up straight and cause substantial fatigue when walking.
- Patients with only mild stiffness (ie, ROM near 90 degrees) may improve slightly (5 to 10 degrees) in the first 2 years after surgery, reaching a level of flexion that is tolerable for most activities of daily living.

PATIENT HISTORY AND PHYSICAL FINDINGS

- The history is a critical part of the evaluation to determine which of the factors listed under Pathogenesis have led to stiffness; in most cases, more than one factor is at work.
- Direct questions should be asked to determine whether pain control was adequate in the postoperative period.
  - Did the patient have severe pain postoperatively that limited his or her ability to perform physical therapy?
  - For how long postoperatively did the patient require narcotics? Is the patient still taking narcotics and still in severe pain?
  - Does the patient have hypersensitivity of the skin overlying the incision or other complaints that suggest neurogenic pain or a chronic regional pain syndrome?
  - How was the patient's stiffness addressed postoperatively?
    - Did he or she undergo a manipulation under anesthesia (MUA) postoperatively?
    - Has he or she undergone any other operative procedures (eg, open or arthroscopic release) in an attempt to improve ROM?
  - Does any element of the history suggest infection?
    - Wound drainage that persisted for more than a few days after surgery
    - The use of antibiotics for more than 24 hours postoperatively
    - Persistent pain that is of a different character than the pain the patient had before the surgery
  - Inspect the skin for the presence of a past or present sinus, indicating infection. Densely adherent skin is much harder to close and may represent a higher risk for necrosis and requires attention from a plastic surgeon.
  - Evaluate the patient's ROM. Flexion of less than 90 degrees and a flexion contracture of more than 15 degrees are considered pathologic. Loss of ROM affects gait and ability to perform activities of daily living.

IMAGING AND OTHER DIAGNOSTIC STUDIES

- Standing anteroposterior, lateral, and patellar radiographs should be obtained to identify component loosening, malposition, or improper sizing (**FIG 2A**).
  - Patella baja and joint line position also should be noted (**FIG 2B**). Severe ligamentous imbalance may be readily apparent on the plain radiographs. Patellar maltracking can also be identified (**FIG 2C**), as can an unresurfaced patella, which may cause pain that leads to stiffness.
  - Serial radiographs often are helpful in confirming component loosening.
- A computed tomography (CT) scan to determine femoral and tibial component rotation is often performed (**FIG 2D–F**). If component malposition is identified (eg, internal rotation), the components are revised.[3]
- Erythrocyte sedimentation rate (ESR) and C-reactive protein (CRP) level are obtained before every revision TKA.
  - If either is elevated, or if the history is very suspicious for an infection, an aspiration of the knee joint is obtained and sent for a cell count with differential and cultures. A synovial fluid white blood cell count above 3000 WBC/μL is considered consistent with infection, as is a differential of greater than 80% neutrophils.
  - Patients must have been off antibiotics for at least 2 weeks before the knee aspiration to avoid falsely negative cultures.
- At the time of revision, additional tissue or fluid cultures are taken from within the joint and an intraoperative frozen section is taken from the synovial tissues. An average of more than 10 polymorphonuclear cells identified within tissue (and not fibrin) is consistent with infection.
- Nuclear medicine studies, such as a triple-phase bone scan, are occasionally helpful in identifying subtle loosening but are not routinely obtained.

DIFFERENTIAL DIAGNOSIS

- Deep infection
- Component malposition (eg, internal rotation of the femur or tibia)
- Patellar maltracking or overstuffing of the patellofemoral joint
- Improper component sizing
- Ligamentous imbalance (eg, tightness in flexion)
- Component loosening
- Chronic regional pain syndrome

NONOPERATIVE MANAGEMENT

- If the patient is seen early in the postoperative period (<6 to 12 weeks postoperatively), he or she can be managed with a combination of the approaches discussed in this section.
- Aggressive pain management, supervised by a physician with expertise in this area—usually an anesthesiologist who specializes in pain management
  - If chronic regional pain syndrome is considered, a sympathetic blockade is often administered.
  - Intensive physical therapy, stressing active and passive ROM exercises
  - In cases of flexion contracture, dynamic splinting or the use of serial casts can be tried in an attempt to obtain full extension
- MUA can also be performed. When performing an MUA, the author prefers to place an indwelling epidural catheter at

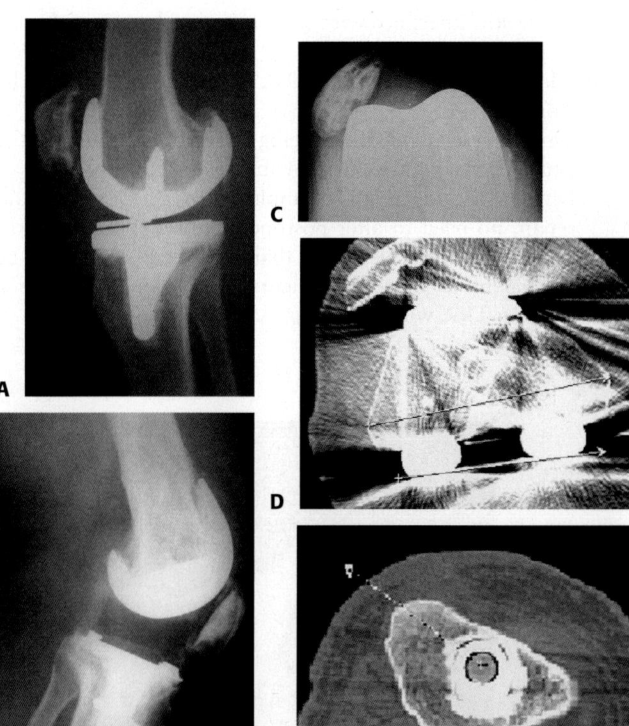

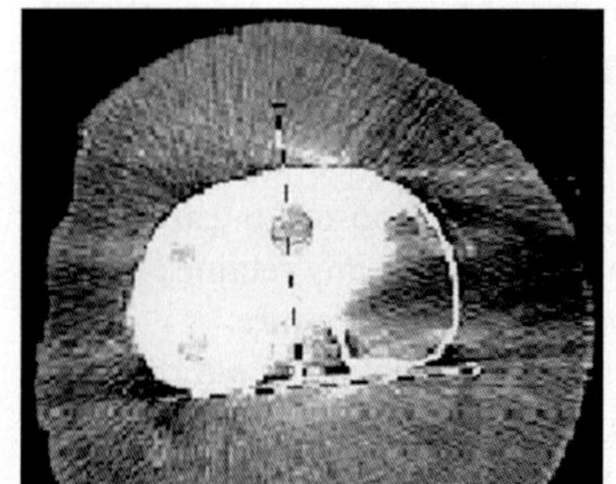

FIG 2 • **A.** Lateral view of a stiff TKA showing an oversized femoral component. **B.** Stiff TKA with joint line elevation and patella baja. **C.** Lateral dislocation of the patella. **D.** CT scan of the distal femur of a right knee. The top line marks the epicondylar axis and the bottom line marks the posterior condylar line; the component in this case is internally rotated. Note the dislocated patella. CT scans of the proximal tibia identifying the apex of the tibial tubercle (**E**) and alignment of the tibial component (**F**). These images are overlaid to determine the rotation; normal is 18 degrees of internal rotation. The component in this case is internally rotated 16 degrees.

the same time, which will remain in place for several weeks after the procedure to assist with administration of medication for pain control. Patients are sent home with a pump to administer the medication and are carefully monitored by a pain control specialist.

- MUA seems to be most effective and is associated with a lower rate of complications (eg, periprosthetic fracture) if performed within 3 months of the index procedure.
- The literature is unclear as to the magnitude of benefit derived. Most studies show that patients improve after MUA, but that their final ROM is less than that of their nonmanipulated counterparts.
- Other potential complications of MUA include rupture of the patellar or quadriceps tendon, periprosthetic fracture of the femur or tibia, and wound dehiscence. The manipulation should be performed using a short-lever arm with the patient completely relaxed until a firm end point is reached. X-rays should be obtained following the manipulation to ensure that a fracture has not occurred.

SURGICAL MANAGEMENT

- The decision to proceed with revision TKA for stiffness should be considered carefully and only after a full investigation as to the cause or causes of stiffness. The patient must be fully informed of the risks of the procedure and that the ROM may not improve, even with further surgery. It is crucial to work with a pain management specialist and a physical therapist to ensure that stiffness does not recur postoperatively.
- Options for surgical management include the following:
  - Arthroscopic débridement with manipulation[2,5,7,15]
    - This can be performed in patients with well-fixed, appropriately aligned components. The procedure is technically demanding and the results reported in the literature are variable, with most studies showing mild improvements in ROM (15 to 30 degrees, on average).
    - The technique includes release of the posterior cruciate ligament (if present), clearing of scar from the suprapatellar region, and typically MUA once the scar has been cleared.
    - Flexion contractures are harder to address arthroscopically, but a posterior release can be performed using small, open, medial and lateral incisions.
  - Open arthrolysis with exchange of the modular polyethylene liner.[1,9,10,13]
    - This procedure can also be performed in selected patients with well-fixed, appropriately aligned components. However, it often is difficult to fully release the posterior capsule to treat flexion contractures, and it is unclear whether this technique has any benefit over arthroscopic release. This option should be performed rarely.
  - Revision TKA[6,8,10,11,14]
    - Revision TKA is the most appropriate treatment for most patients. It allows for optimization of component alignment, size, and rotation while providing the opportunity to restore the joint line and optimize ligamentous balance.
    - It affords complete access to the posterior capsule to perform a capsulectomy and remove any retained osteophytes from the previous surgical procedure.
    - An additional benefit is the option of using a more constrained polyethylene insert, if desired, to optimize stability if extensive releases are performed.
    - If a large flexion contracture is being addressed, a flexion–extension mismatch often is present (ie, extension space smaller than the flexion space) and constrained and even hinged implants may be required.

Preoperative Planning

- The history, physical examination, plain radiographs, and CT scan (if obtained) are reviewed before a definite decision is made whether the components are to be removed or retained.
- The ESR, CRP, synovial fluid white blood cell count with differential, and culture results are reviewed to determine whether a deep infection is present.
- If any of the prosthetic components are to be retained, the operative note from the previous procedure must be reviewed to definitely identify manufacturer, model, and size so that appropriate matching replacement implants and trials are available on the day of surgery.
- An examination under anesthesia confirms the limits of motion.

Positioning

- The operative extremity is draped free from the hip to the ankle and a tourniquet is placed on the upper thigh.
- A bump, placed underneath the ipsilateral hip, assists in keeping the leg upright.
- A leg holder keeps the leg in the desired position for surgery.
- An elastic bandage placed on the lower leg defines the malleoli, which are used as a reference for tibial cut alignment (**FIG 3**).

Approach

- The workhorse method for exposure in revision TKA is the medial parapatellar approach with complete excision of intra-articular scar tissue. This approach is useful for most revision TKAs.
  - In the stiff knee, however, a more extensile approach may be required.
- If additional exposure is needed, a quadriceps snip can be performed.
  - This maneuver assists in freeing the proximal tether of the extensor mechanism, thereby improving exposure.
  - Benefits include relative simplicity of performance and repair, no need to alter postoperative rehabilitation protocols, and clinical results that have been shown to be equivalent to those in patients who have undergone a revision TKA without a snip.

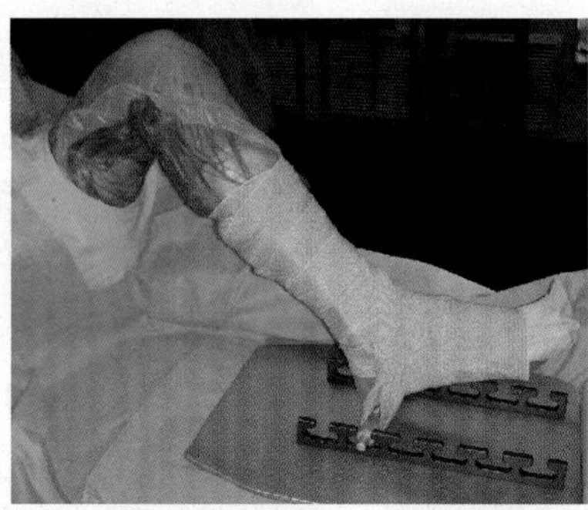

FIG 3 • The lower extremity is draped free with a bump underneath the hip. A leg positioner holds the extremity in the desired position.

- If a more extensile exposure is needed, the extensor mechanism can be completely released proximally with a V-Y quadricepsplasty (see Chap. 45) or distally with a tibial tubercle osteotomy (see Chap. 44). However, these maneuvers may be rarely required, and as their performance may in many cases lead to limitations in postoperative physical therapy, they should be avoided if possible when revising the stiff TKA.

Medial Parapatellar Arthrotomy with Complete Intra-articular Release

- Skin incision
  - Previous skin incisions are used whenever possible.
  - Avoid parallel incisions. If choosing among multiple previous incisions, the most lateral one is selected because the blood supply is derived predominantly from the medial side.
  - Full-thickness flaps are raised, if required.
- The arthrotomy extends from the apex of the quadriceps tendon, around the medial aspect of the patella and just medial to the tibial tubercle (**TECH FIG 1A**).
- On entering the joint, large amounts of scar are typically encountered (**TECH FIG 1B**); these prevent proper exposure and contribute to stiffness.
- A medial release is performed with electrocautery by subperiosteally releasing a continuous soft tissue sleeve all the way to the posteromedial corner of the tibia and the semimembranous insertion (**TECH FIG 1C**).
  - This allows for external rotation of the tibia, which relaxes the extensor mechanism and improves exposure.
- The junction between scar and the extensor mechanism is identified (**TECH FIG 1D**). The scar is meticulously removed from underneath the extensor mechanism laterally (**TECH FIG 1E**) and from underneath the joint capsule medially until the medial and lateral gutters have been reestablished (**TECH FIG 1F**).
  - A thin layer of soft tissue is left on the distal femur to prevent excessive bleeding and the extensor mechanism from becoming readherent in this area.
- The scar tissue is carefully cleared from the interval between the patellar tendon and the scar behind it to release it from the proximal tibia.
- At this point, the modular polyethylene liner is removed to allow for patellar eversion or subluxation. In most cases, patellar subluxation is preferred because it places less tension on the extensor mechanism and provides adequate exposure in most cases.
- If difficulty is encountered, soft tissue can be peeled off the lateral border of the patella to make it more mobile, and any osteophytes that are present can be removed.
- If exposure still cannot be accomplished, a formal lateral retinacular release may be required.
  - This release involves a full-thickness division of the capsule along the lateral border of the patella from the proximal tibia (just lateral to the patella tendon) to the vastus lateralis.
  - A lateral release performed from the inside out eliminates the need to raise additional skin flaps.

A
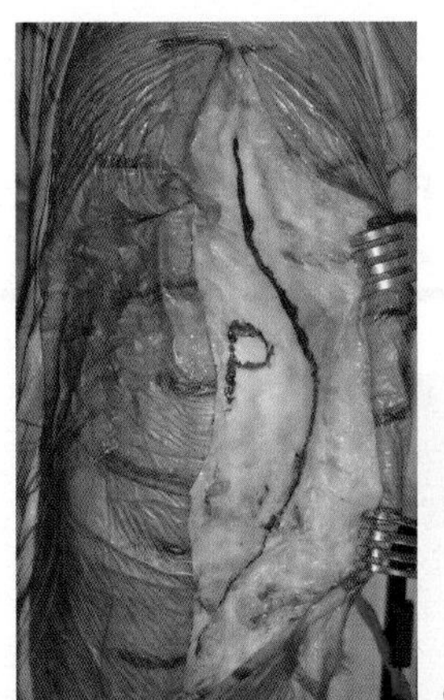
C
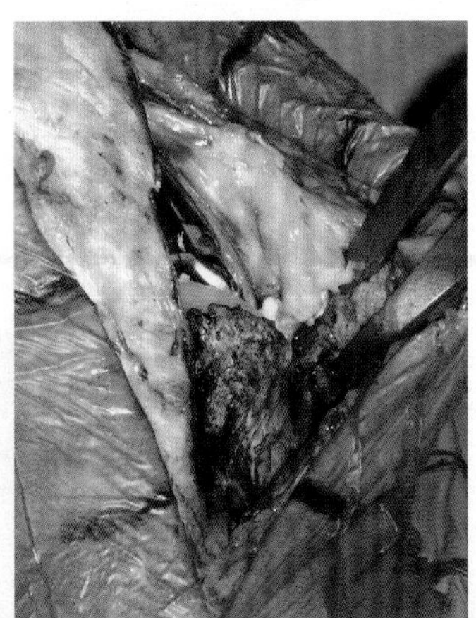
F
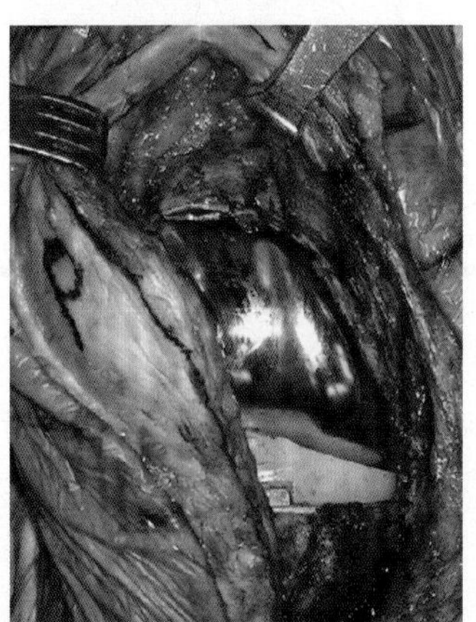
B
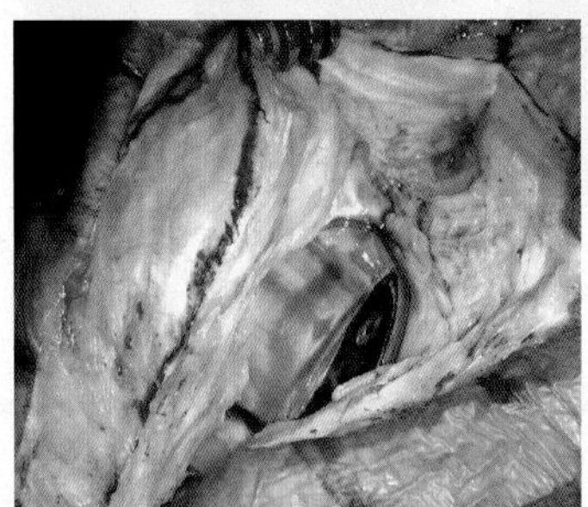
D
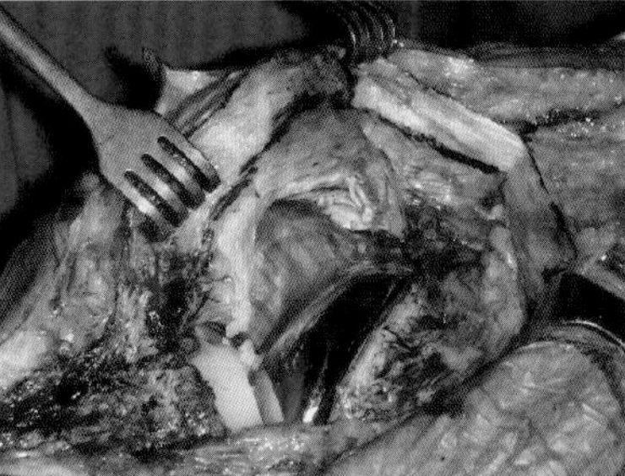
E
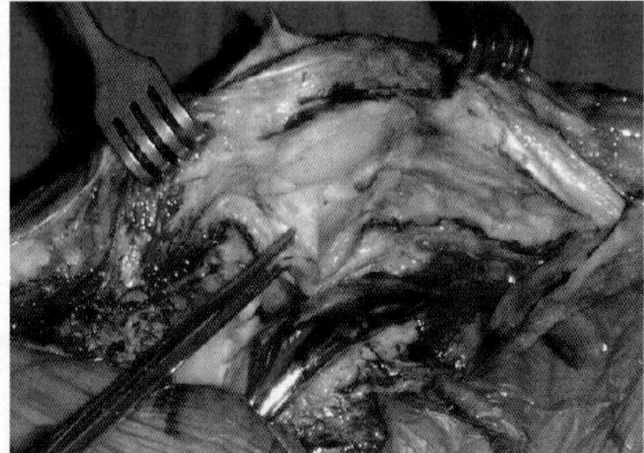

TECH FIG 1 • **A.** Arthrotomy for the medial parapatellar approach. *P* marks the patella. **B.** Large amounts of scar in the suprapatellar pouch. **C.** A medial release has been performed. **D.** The line identifies the boundary between the scar and the extensor mechanism. Everything below the extensor mechanism is resected. **E.** Scar tissue is dissected out from underneath the extensor mechanism using a knife, scissors, or electrocautery. **F.** Scar has been completely cleared from the suprapatellar pouch and the medial and lateral gutters have been reestablished.

Quadriceps Snip

- If inadequate exposure has been afforded by the medial parapatellar arthrotomy and a complete intra-articular release, a quadriceps snip often provides enough additional exposure to complete the procedure safely.
- The snip is made at the apex of the arthrotomy, obliquely across the quadriceps tendon at a 45-degree angle in line with the fibers of the vastus lateralis (**TECH FIG 2**).
- At the end of the procedure, the snip is closed side-to-side using nonabsorbable suture.
- The postoperative therapy protocol is not altered if a quadriceps snip has been performed.

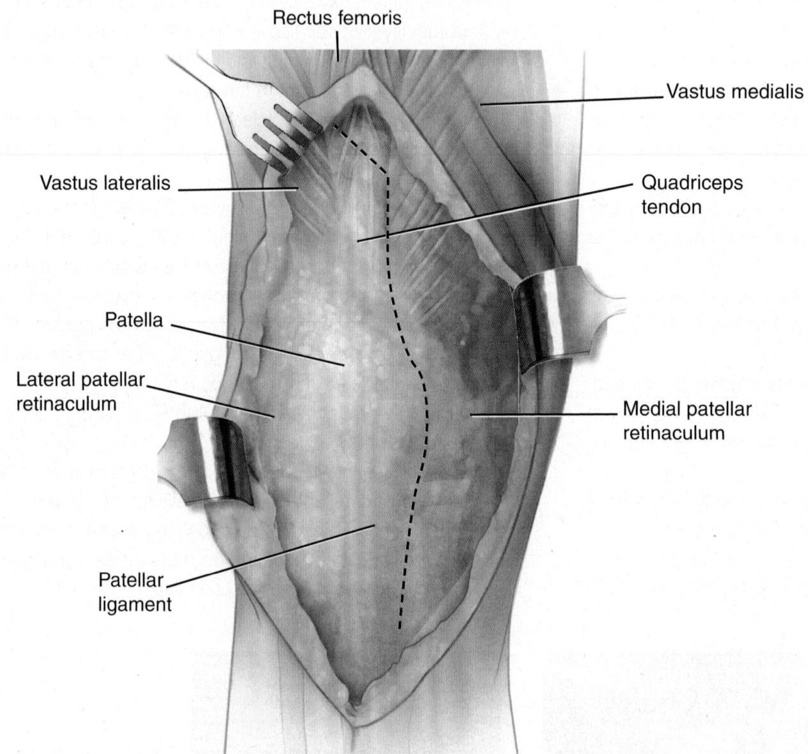

TECH FIG 2 • Quadriceps snip.

Component Removal

- The femoral and tibial components are then carefully removed as described in Chapter 44.
- The patella then is assessed. Its thickness is determined (**TECH FIG 3**), and if the composite is considered to be too thick (ie, >25 mm for women and >30 mm for men) or in an otherwise suboptimal position (eg, lateralized), the component is removed.
- If the component is to be retained, any osteophytes or unresurfaced sections of the native patella are removed.

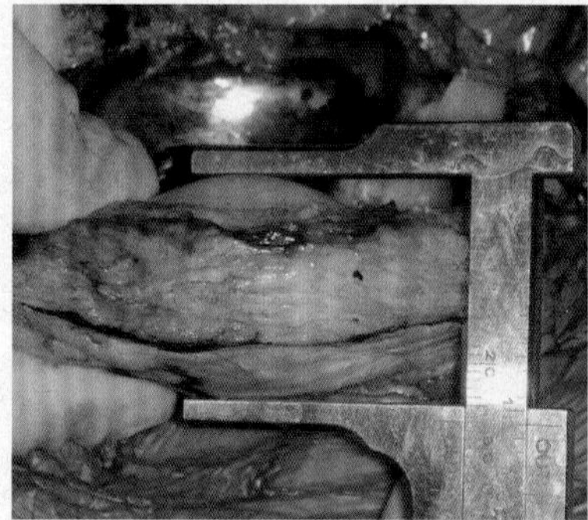

TECH FIG 3 • Patellar thickness is assessed. In this case, the patella was 27 mm thick in a female patient and the component was revised.

Recutting the Upper End of the Tibia and Performing a Posterior Release

- The proximal tibia is recut perpendicular to its mechanical axis with neutral slope. Either an intra- or extramedullary guide may be used. A neutral slope is recommended; rotation of the cut is not important at this point. The revision component often has an appropriate amount of slope built in (5 to 7 degrees) so that rotation in the optimal position can be set later.

- A laminar spreader is then inserted both medially and laterally, and the scar tissue in the posterior aspect of the knee along with any remnant of the posterior cruciate ligament, if present, is removed completely to reestablish the flexion space and restore full extension (**TECH FIG 4A**).
  - At this point, ligamentous balance is assessed and appropriate releases are performed until the flexion gap is of equivalent size medially and laterally.
- A curved osteotome is then used to release any remaining capsule from the posterior aspect of the femur and to clear any residual osteophytes retained at the time of the original TKA (**TECH FIG 4B**).
  - Given the tendency to elevate the joint line in revision TKA, a complete posterior capsular release is performed in all cases.

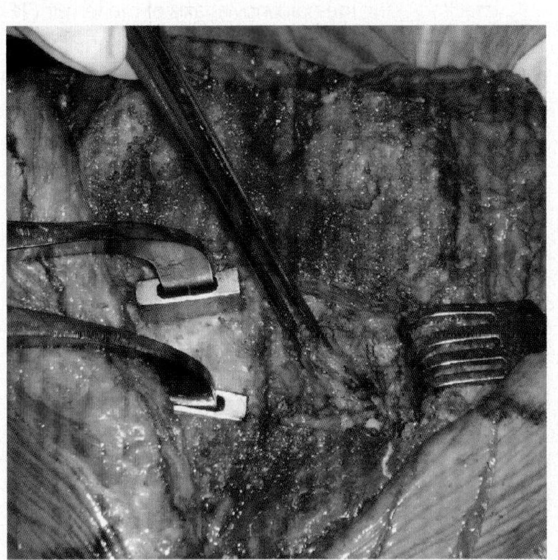
A

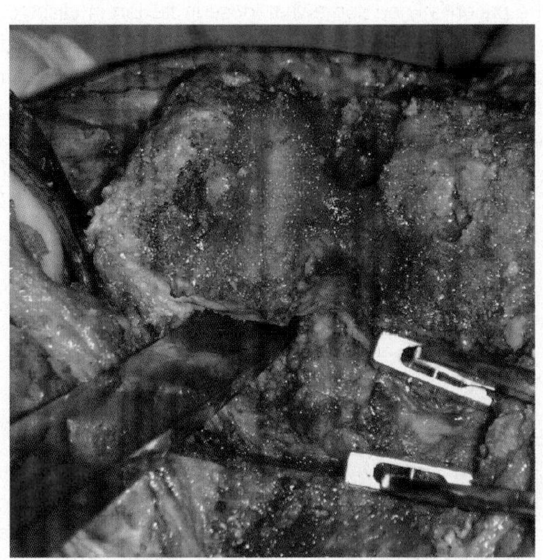
B

TECH FIG 4 • **A.** Performance of a posterior release and capsulectomy. The posterior capsule has already been removed on the lateral side. **B.** A curved osteotome is passed subperiosteally behind the femur to complete the posterior release, reestablishing the flexion space and restoring full extension. The patella has been subluxed laterally but not everted.

Creating the Tibial Platform

- The tibia is prepared first, as tibial height affects both the flexion and extension gaps.
- The tibial component is sized to maximize coverage of the upper end of the tibia.
- A stem typically is used to provide support for the revision component. Stems also assist with component alignment, particularly if a cementless diaphyseal engaging stem is selected. It is necessary to remember that the tibial shaft is offset posteromedially in relation to the center of the upper end of the tibia, and a stem that allows for offset is often required to optimize coverage of the upper end of the tibia (the stem is used to bring the component anterior and lateral in most cases).
- The tibial trial component is then placed in the appropriate amount of external rotation; typically, the center of the component is aligned with the junction of the medial and middle thirds of the tibial tubercle (**TECH FIG 5**).
- See Chapters 41 and 43 for additional details.

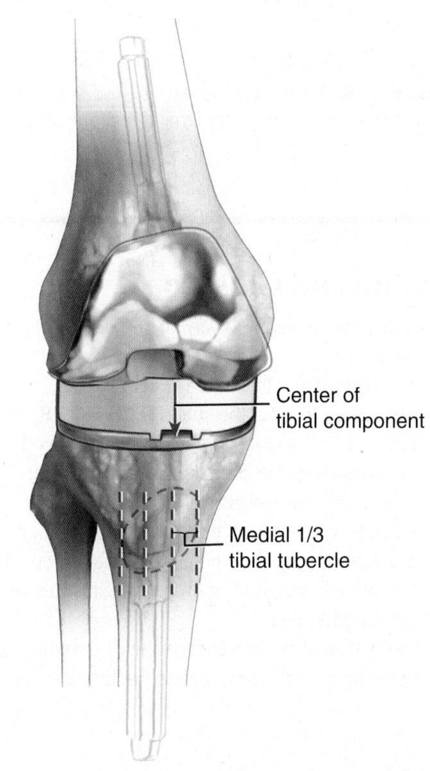

TECH FIG 5 • The center of the tibial component is placed in line with the medial third of the tibial tubercle to be in appropriate external rotation.

Choosing the Femoral Trial Size and Augments

- Sizing of the femoral component can be difficult, but it is a critical portion of the procedure. If the original component is thought to have been too large, a smaller trial component is selected; however, in some cases, a larger femoral component will be needed to balance the flexion gap.
- The surgeon must keep in mind that although it is desirable to leave the patient's knee somewhat loose in flexion in cases of stiffness, this does risk flexion instability. Consideration should be given to using a more constrained insert in cases of revision TKA for stiffness.
- The knee is initially trialed with a long intramedullary stem to assist with determining appropriate valgus alignment; a shorter stem can be substituted later if desired. Stems are used routinely, both to support the revision component and to assist with alignment.
- The initial augments typically used include a posterolateral augment to encourage appropriate external rotation of the revision component and distal augments placed both medially and laterally to distalize the femoral component in response to the tendency of revision TKA to elevate the joint line.
- Appropriate external rotation of the femoral component is checked using the epicondylar axis of the femur (**TECH FIG 6A**). The surgeon also can check to make sure that a "piano" or "boot" sign is present when the cut surface of the femur is viewed from above (**TECH FIG 6B**). This sign indicates that the cut on the lateral side is deeper than that on the medial side, confirming appropriate external rotation of the femoral cut.

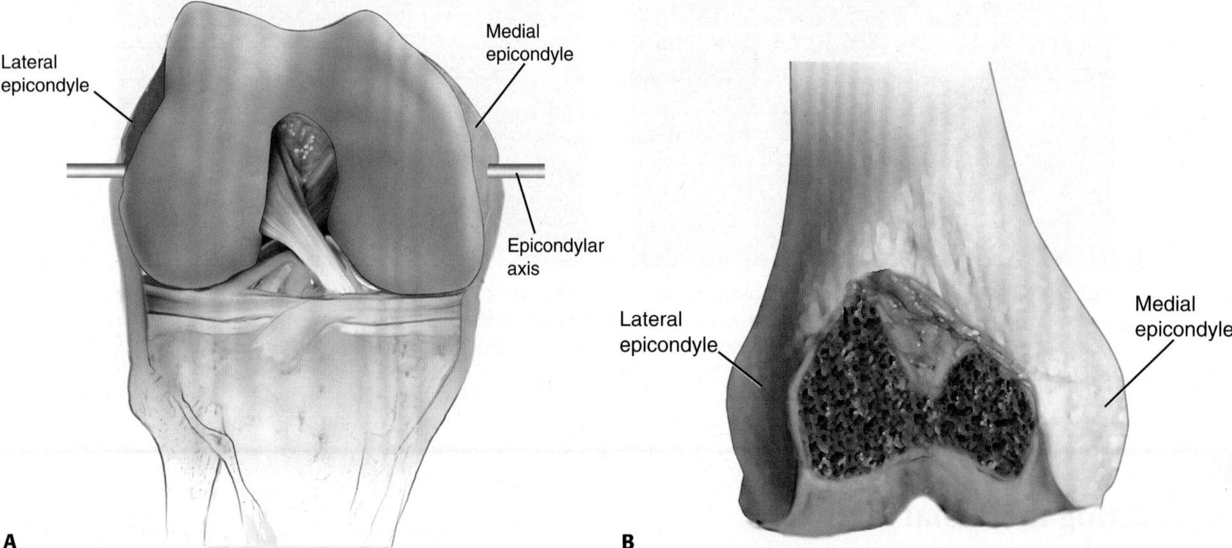

TECH FIG 6 • **A.** The epicondylar axis is used to ensure appropriate external rotation of the femur. **B.** View of the distal femur from above showing the piano or boot sign, confirming appropriate external rotation of the femoral component.

Trialing and Closure

- The knee is now trialed with varying thicknesses of polyethylene liners to ensure
  - Full extension of the knee (**TECH FIG 7A**)
  - Adequate flexion of the knee (**TECH FIG 7B**). A good predictor of postoperative flexion is that achieved at the time of surgery with the knee flexed against gravity.
  - Adequate varus–valgus stability
  - Good patellar tracking. If patellar tracking is not acceptable, the rotation of the femoral and tibial components must be carefully assessed and changed if necessary until the patella tracks well.
  - Restoration of the joint line to within 1 cm of its normal position. The easiest way to assess the joint line is to compare the superior pole of the patella to the superior flange of the revision femoral component with the knee fully extended.
  - Various combinations of augments and polyethylene liners should be tried until the optimal combination is found; this may take a considerable amount of time to achieve.
- The revision components are now assembled on the field. The stems can be either firmly press-fit into the diaphysis, with cement placed only around the metaphyseal segment of the component (**TECH FIG 7C**), or fully cemented, depending on the surgeon's preference. Antibiotic-loaded cement is recommended, given the higher risk of infection in the setting of revision TKA.
- The knee is closed in at least 90 degrees of flexion because this has been shown to increase final flexion. Following closure of the arthrotomy, ROM and patellar tracking are carefully assessed once again.

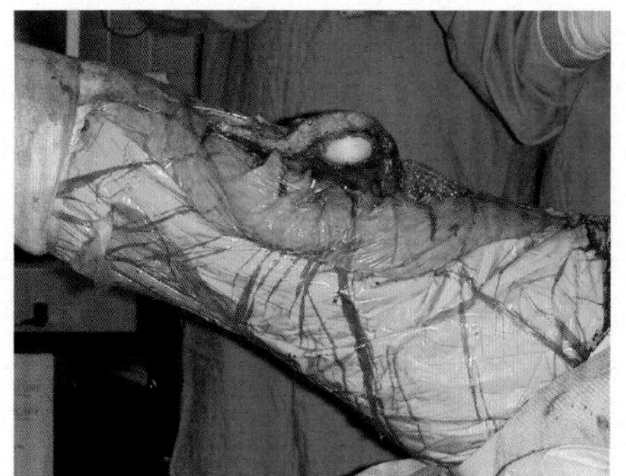
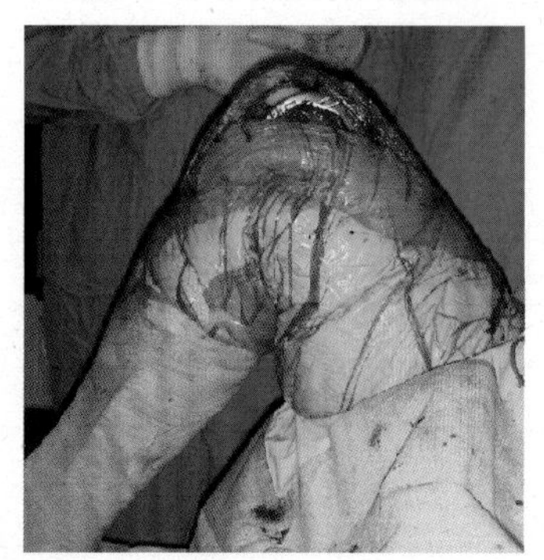
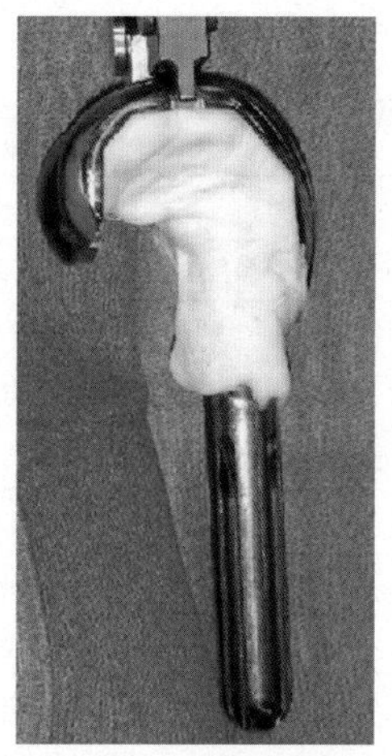

TECH FIG 7 • A. Full extension of the knee. **B.** More than 120 degrees of knee flexion. The patella is tracking centrally. **C.** The components are cemented in the metaphyseal region of the revision component (just distal to the modular junction between the revision component and the stem), and the stem is press-fit tightly into the canal.

PEARLS AND PITFALLS

Indications	■ Patients must be assessed carefully before surgery and must have realistic expectations about the procedure. ■ Patients must be willing to be active participants in their postoperative therapy.
Pain management	■ The assistance of a specialist in pain management is essential to ensure that patients can participate in their physical therapy. ■ An indwelling epidural catheter is a useful adjunct to this goal.
Preoperative planning	■ Ensure that operative notes from previous procedures have been reviewed and that replacement parts and trials are available if necessary.
Perioperative evaluation for sepsis	■ All patients should have a thorough perioperative evaluation for deep infection.
Retention of components	■ An arthroscopic or open arthrolysis should be attempted only after the surgeon is sure that the components are well fixed, appropriately sized, and aligned. ■ If not, a full revision should be performed.
Patellar tendon avulsion	■ Great care should be taken to protect the insertion of the patellar tendon at the time of surgery. ■ More extensile approaches, such as the quadriceps snip or tibial tubercle osteotomy, should be used if deemed necessary.

POSTOPERATIVE CARE

- Perioperative care must be monitored closely in conjunction with a pain management specialist and a physical therapist.
- Patients are placed on a continuous passive motion (CPM) machine starting at 0 to 90 degrees in the recovery room, advancing the setting as tolerated. CPM is used for 4 to 6 hours per day and patients must understand that it is an adjunct to, not a substitute for, active and passive ROM exercises.
- The indwelling epidural catheter is continued for up to 6 weeks. The patient is seen by the surgeon and the pain management specialist weekly for the first 6 weeks to monitor progress.
- Patients are engaged in an aggressive physical therapy program emphasizing ROM, gait training, and strengthening.
- If the patient has not achieved 90 degrees of flexion by 6 weeks, MUA is performed.

OUTCOMES

- Table 1 summarizes the results of arthroscopic release, open arthrolysis, and revision TKA for the treatment of stiffness.
- Most of the literature suggests that revision for stiffness is associated with improvements in ROM, pain, and function, but that these gains are modest and, in a certain percentage of patients, stiffness will recur. Our own experience with a cohort of 35 patients showed that although 75% of patients had an improvement of at least 30 degrees of motion, the complication rate was high; nearly 50% of patients required some additional intervention to achieve that ROM.
- An arthroscopic release seems most appropriate for select patients with well-fixed, appropriately positioned and rotated components.
- Flexion contractures are particularly difficult to correct.

Table 1 Results of Arthroscopic Release with Manipulation, Open Arthrolysis, and Revision Total Knee Arthroplasty for the Treatment of Stiffness

Procedure/Author Arthroscopy	Year	No. Knees	Mean Length of Follow-up (mo)	Mean Increase in ROM (degrees)
Bae et al[2]	1995	13	12	42
Campbell[6]	1987	8	12	11
Diduch et al[9]	1997	8	20	26
Williams et al[18]	1996	10	20	31
Lysis and liner change				
Babis et al[1]	2001	7	51	19
Hutchinson et al[12]	2005	13	87	36
Keeney et al[13]	2005	12	37	26
Mont et al[16]	2006	18	30	31
Femoral component revision				
Ries and Badalamente[17]	2000	6	33	50
Revision TKA				
Bedard et al[3]	2011	34	22	38
Christensen et al[7]	2002	11	38	56
Haidukewych et al[10]	2005	16	42	33
Hartman et al[11]	2010	35	55	45
Keeney et al[13]	2005	11	37	18
Kim et al[14]	2004	56	43	28

ROM, range of motion; TKA, total knee arthroplasty.

COMPLICATIONS

- Recurrent stiffness
- Extensor mechanism disruption (particularly patellar tendon avulsion)
- Infection
- Instability
- Neurovascular injury
- Deep venous thrombosis

REFERENCES

1. Babis GC, Trousdale RT, Pagnano MW, et al. Poor outcomes of isolated tibial insert exchange and arthrolysis for the management of stiffness following total knee arthroplasty. J Bone Joint Surg Am 2001;83:1534–1536.
2. Bae DK, Lee HK, Cho JH. Arthroscopy of symptomatic total knee replacements. Arthroscopy 1995;11:664–671.
3. Bedard M, Vince KG, Redfern J, et al. Internal rotation of the tibial component is frequent in stiff total knee arthroplasty. Clin Orthop Relat Res 2011;469:2346–2355.
4. Berger RA, Crossett LS, Jacobs JJ, et al. Malrotation causing patellofemoral complications after total knee arthroplasty. Clin Orthop Relat Res 1998;356:144–153.
5. Bong MR, Di Cesare PE. Stiffness after total knee arthroplasty. J Am Acad Orthop Surg 2004;12:164–171.
6. Campbell ED Jr. Arthroscopy in total knee replacements. Arthroscopy 1987;3:31–35.
7. Christensen CP, Crawford JJ, Olin MD, et al. Revision of the stiff total knee arthroplasty. J Arthroplasty 2002;17:409–415.
8. Della Valle C, Parvizi J, Bauer T, et al. American Academy of Orthopaedic Surgeons clinical practice guideline on the diagnosis of the periprosthetic joint infection. J Bone Joint Surg Am 2011;90: 1355–1357.
9. Diduch DR, Scuderi GR, Scott WN, et al. The efficacy of arthroscopy following total knee replacement. Arthroscopy 1997;13:166–171.
10. Haidukewych GJ, Jacofsky DJ, Pagnano MW, et al. Functional results after revision of well-fixed components for stiffness after primary total knee arthroplasty. J Arthroplasty 2005;20:133–138.
11. Hartman CW, Ting NT, Moric M, et al. Revision total knee arthroplasty for stiffness. J Arthroplasty 2010;25(6 suppl):62–66.
12. Hutchinson JR, Parish EN, Cross MJ. Results of open arthrolysis for the treatment of stiffness after total knee replacement. J Bone Joint Surg Br 2005;87:1357–1360.
13. Keeney JA, Clohisy JC, Curry M, et al. Revision total knee arthroplasty for restricted motion. Clin Orthop Relat Res 2005;440: 135–140.
14. Kim J, Nelson CL, Lotke PA. Stiffness after total knee arthroplasty: prevalence of the complication and outcomes of revision. J Bone Joint Surg Am 2004;86:1479–1484.
15. Laubenthal KN, Smidt GL, Kettelkamp DB. A quantitative analysis of knee motion during activities of daily living. Phys Ther 1972:52: 34–43.
16. Mont MA, Seyler TM, Marulanda GA, et al. Surgical treatment and customized rehabilitation for stiff knee arthroplasties. Clin Orthop Relat Res 2006;446:193–200.
17. Ries MD, Badalamente M. Arthrofibrosis after total knee arthroplasty. Clin Orthop Relat Res 2000;380:177–183.
18. Williams RJ III, Westrich GH, Siegel J, et al. Arthroscopic release of the posterior cruciate ligament for stiff total knee arthroplasty. Clin Orthop Relat Res 1996;185–191.

Knee Arthrodesis

Rajit Chakravarty, Bhaveen H. Kapadia, Julio J. Jauregui, and Michael A. Mont

48

CHAPTER

DEFINITION

- Knee arthrodesis offers an excellent salvage option for an infected total knee arthroplasty (TKA), periarticular tumor, posttraumatic arthritis, and chronic sepsis in the knee. It is a viable solution that allows for stable and painless lower extremity ambulation.
- The energy expenditure for an arthrodesed knee is 30% higher than required for normal walking. Nevertheless, walking with a knee fusion requires 25% less energy expenditure than walking with an above-the-knee amputation (AKA). This is an important consideration particularly for elderly patients with associated comorbidities who are often unable to walk with an amputation.[14,18]
- In the younger, posttraumatic population, knee fusion may allow for participation in more physically demanding activities as opposed to AKA.
- Relative contraindications are marked contralateral limb dysfunction, marked back pain and arthritis, contralateral knee amputation, and severe ipsilateral hip or ankle degenerative changes.

ANATOMY

- The relevant anatomy depends on previous surgical procedures that the patient has undergone. For example, in the case of an infected TKA-required knee arthrodesis, the extensor mechanism is often no longer present and a soft tissue defect may occur anteriorly.
- To obtain the best bone contact for a knee arthrodesis, elevating the posterior capsule off of the distal femur and the proximal tibia allows the knee to be brought into full extension and allows achievement of the best bony contact between the femur and tibia.
- The structures in the popliteal region, posterior to the posterior capsule, are the popliteal artery, popliteal vein, and sciatic nerve as it branches into the posterior tibial and peroneal nerve (**FIG 1**).
- When using a long intramedullary rod for a knee fusion, the recommended landmark for nail entry is the piriformis fossa.

PATHOGENESIS

- At present, the most common indication for knee arthrodesis is a failed, unrevisable TKA. These conditions may be secondary to persistent infection, gross instability, massive bone loss, inadequate soft tissue coverage, deficient extensor mechanism, or when the patient is unwilling to consider revision arthroplasty. Additionally, other conditions necessitating knee arthrodesis include periarticular tumors and severe posttraumatic degenerative joint disease.[11,18]
- Trauma, aggressive periarticular tumor destruction, or débridement as a result of infection can lead to extensive bone loss of the distal femur and proximal tibia.
- The most common method to fill bony defects is by acutely shortening the limb.
  - The mean limb shortening associated with knee arthrodesis is 4 cm, which can be addressed with a shoe lift to equalize the limb lengths.[12]
  - In cases with marked shortening (5 to 6 cm), concomitant lengthening can be performed in the proximal femur.
  - In cases with substantial bone loss (7 to 10 cm) with adherent soft tissues and vessels that do not allow acute compression, gradual compression of 2 mm/day with an external fixator is an option for knee arthrodesis. However, even with this procedure, the limb may remain markedly shortened.

NATURAL HISTORY

- The underlying pathology of severe traumatic and infectious processes occurring within the knee is poor. Without a stable lower limb, the patients are unable to bear weight.
- Survivorship of a knee arthrodesis is generally for the duration of the patient's lifetime.[3]
  - As patients with knee arthrodesis age, increased pelvic tilt, hip abduction, and ankle dorsiflexion on the ipsilateral side may lead to degenerative changes of the contralateral joint.

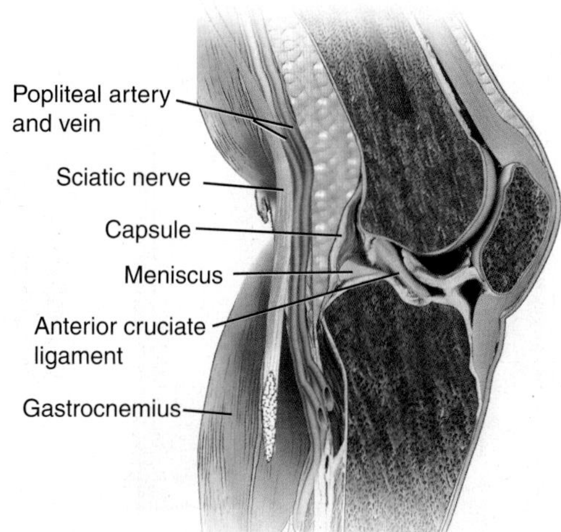

FIG 1 • Proximity of the posterior neurovascular bundle to the posterior aspects of the femur and tibia at the level of the residual knee joint. Also, the bones are very subcutaneous anteriorly and do not have good blood supply secondary to the relatively avascular quadriceps and patellar tendons and lack of good muscle with good blood flow to the bones anteriorly.

- The alternative to knee fusion is AKA, which allows the young, healthy posttraumatic population to walk with an above-the-knee prosthesis.
  - However, AKA in the elderly population with infected TKAs may result in a patient becoming nonambulatory.[14]

PATIENT HISTORY AND PHYSICAL FINDINGS

- Preoperative assessment for knee arthrodesis should include an evaluation of all surgical and traumatic events relating to the patient's knee.
- An evaluation of comorbidities, including peripheral vascular disease, smoking, diabetes, ambulatory status, social resources, and corticosteroid use, are also important as they may affect the patient's ability to heal following arthrodesis.
- Physical examination of the knee joint should consist of assessing the alignment, range of motion, extensor lag, fixed deformities, and ligamentous stability. Assessment of other joints such as the hips and ankles is important to assess the integrity of the remaining joints that will be compensating for the resultant lack of knee motion.
  - The presence of any equinus contracture can be addressed at the time of surgery with Achilles tendon lengthening or gastrocsoleus recession.
- Dorsalis pedis and posterior tibialis pulses should be palpated; if they are poor, a vascular evaluation may be obtained.
- The cutaneous integrity over the anterior knee is assessed for scars, previous flaps, and any defects. If the skin condition is poor, the surgeon should consider alternative wound closure techniques postoperatively, such as a wound vacuum or preoperative plastic surgical consultation.

IMAGING AND OTHER DIAGNOSTIC STUDIES

- The most important imaging studies are long-standing anteroposterior (AP) and long lateral view radiographs of the lower limbs (**FIG 2**).
  - These radiographs allow the surgeon to assess the present as well as predicted limb length discrepancy after knee fusion.
  - Due to the risk of bony defects greater than 5 or 6 cm leading to vascular compromise from vessel kinking, radiographs are essential for determining the method of fusion.[4]
  - Any residual bone cement in the medullary canals can also be visualized on these views, allowing the surgeon to plan for proper removal at the time of surgery.
- Magnetic resonance imaging may be helpful in determining the extent of any infection in the distal femur or proximal tibia. Care must be taken when interpreting the images because bone edema can be misinterpreted as osteomyelitis and result in an aggressive resection.
- Furthermore, if the dorsalis pedis and posterior tibialis pulses are weak or cannot be palpated, a Doppler ultrasound may permit the visualization of the blood supply of the limb. If this cannot be done, a computed tomographic (CT) angiogram may be a better alternative.

INDICATIONS FOR KNEE FUSION

- Infected revision TKA
- Severe trauma to the knee, preventing reconstruction
- Reconstruction after tumor resection

NONOPERATIVE MANAGEMENT

- Nonoperative management of a knee with a marked bone defect following trauma or joint infection is quite difficult. These patients typically have an unstable limb for weight bearing and require a cast or brace for support.
- Resection arthroplasty is usually reserved for patients who are not able to ambulate or are too medically ill to undergo a major surgical procedure.
- The presence of advanced degenerative changes to the ipsilateral hip/ankle or an amputation of the contralateral knee should preclude undergoing a knee arthrodesis. Additionally, the presence of an arthrodesis of the contralateral hip or knee is a contraindication.

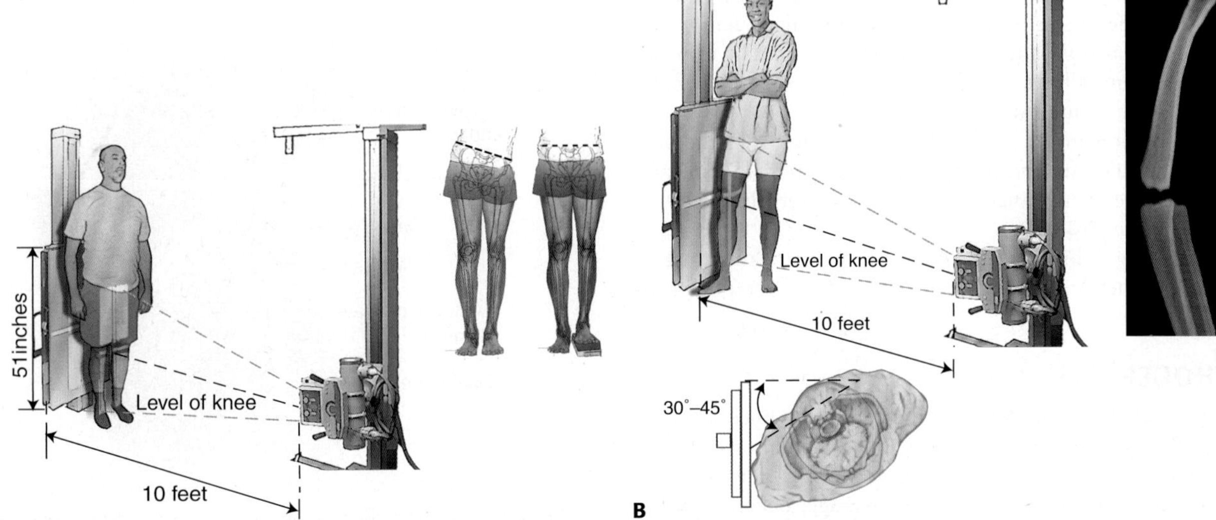

FIG 2 • A,B. AP view erect lower limbs radiograph and a long lateral view radiograph. These figures also demonstrate how to obtain the radiograph. Valuable information regarding alignment and limb length discrepancy is determined by using these films. The pelvis is leveled with blocks before the radiograph is obtained to ensure accurate measurements. With the pelvis leveled, the patient cannot compensate for the limb length discrepancy with equinus of the short limb or knee flexion of the long limb. The radiographs are obtained from 10 feet away by using a 51-inch cassette.

SURGICAL MANAGEMENT

- Knee arthrodesis requires a patient who is medically stable enough to undergo a 2- to 6-hour procedure with a potential blood loss of 500 to 2500 mL.[4]

Preoperative Planning

- Proper preoperative planning begins with the critical points outlined in the Patient History and Physical Findings and Imaging and Other Diagnostic Studies sections.
- Employing sound fracture fixation principles can help achieve a successful arthrodesis. Thus, it is imperative that good bony contact is achieved with rigid fixation while preserving vascularity.
- It is also paramount that proper alignment is obtained. The aim should be to achieve an overall limb alignment of the knee in 5 to 7 degrees of valgus and 15 ± 5 degrees of flexion.[6,18] TKA cutting instrumentation may help facilitate achieving the desired alignment, but its usefulness is limited in the presence of extensive bone loss.[11,18]
- Essential to preoperative planning is the determination of the resultant gap that will be present at the site of the knee fusion, especially with the presence of infection (Table 1).
  - Acute compression of any bony loss with an intramedullary rod fusion should be reserved for bony gaps of no more than 5 to 6 cm. Acute compression greater than that degree can cause vessel kinking and ischemia of the lower extremity.
  - Bony gaps greater than 5 to 6 cm can be managed with gradual compression or bone transport to fill in the defect. Bone transport with a fixator allows the limb to remain at a desired length (ideally 1 cm shorter than the contralateral limb) and fills the gap with healthy bone from the proximal tibia or femur.
  - In cases with large gaps, gradual compression without lengthening, achieved by using an external fixator, will eliminate vessel kinking. However, the resultant limb length discrepancy might require the use of a 2- to 3-inch shoe lift, which could become uncomfortable for ambulation.
  - Discussions with the patient regarding the goals of knee arthrodesis before surgery are vital. The surgeon must be sure that the patient is willing to accept a large shoe lift; if not, they must be willing to undergo additional steps to ensure that the limb is of acceptable length.
  - The strategy for knee fusion is patient dependent. The lengthening can be performed at a second surgical setting or during the same surgical setting. It is important to realize that with concomitant lengthening, the rate-limiting step in the complete healing process is typically the fusion site, not regenerate bone formation.
- Knee arthrodesis after infected TKA requires bone grafting. This is used to address loss of bone stock from the distal femur or proximal tibia. However, this is performed when there is no evidence of infection.
  - At the time of surgery, bone loss can be classified according to the system proposed by Klinger et al[10] and Somayaji et al[18]:
    - Mild: Full bony contact is possible.
    - Moderate: There is incomplete bony contact.
    - Severe: There is minimal or no bony contract.
  - In cases of extensive bone loss, a vascularized fibular graft may be used to bridge the gap from the distal femur to the proximal tibia. In situations of marked bone loss (≥10 cm) from the femur, a free fibular graft is often needed. This fibular graft is used as an onlay graft and is fixed via plate and screws.[10,11,18]
  - Knee arthrodesis in the setting of infection can be performed either as a single-stage or a two-stage process. Single-stage fusion consists of adequate débridement of infected tissue and insertion of a fixation device.
  - In cases of failed infected TKA, a two-stage knee fusion is preferred. A thorough surgical débridement with removal of components and insertion of an antibiotic-impregnated cement spacer should comprise the first stage. This is followed by a course of antibiotics for multiple weeks. When eradication of infection is confirmed, progression to the second stage commences and consists of performing the knee arthrodesis with the chosen fixation in mind.
  - For patients undergoing two-stage procedures (infection eradication and spacer plus clean fusion with intramedullary rod or plates), bone grafting is performed at the time of fusion.
  - In patients who have external fixation and in whom fusion is initiated at the time of the infection eradication surgery, bone grafting is performed at a second surgical setting.
  - Regardless of the method used, fusion after infection typically requires two or more surgical procedures.

Table 1 Strategy Based on Size of Segmental Defect

Size of Gap	Treatment Strategy
<5 cm	Intramedullary rod, external fixator, lengthening optional
5–10 cm	External fixator with bone transport of one segment (femur or tibia) Transport over nail; gradual compression and fusion with lengthening at second surgical setting
>11 cm	Double-level transport over rod; double-level transport with circular frame Bone graft to all docking/knee fusion sites when infection is eradicated

Hardware Considerations

Long Knee Arthrodesis Rods

- Intramedullary rods allow for early mobilization, rigid fixation, and shorter times to fusion and can be either short or long nails. The long intramedullary rod is an excellent method of fixation for knee arthrodesis. It is well tolerated by patients and provides good neutralization of the forces generated by the muscles around the knee.
- Common complications are the risk of infection and, specific to intramedullary nails, the risk of nail migration.
- There are three companies that offer long knee fusion rods: Biomet Trauma (Warsaw, IN), Smith & Nephew (Memphis, TN), and Stryker Orthopaedics (Mahwah, NJ).
- The Stryker intramedullary rod offers 5 degrees of valgus to counteract the mild varus mechanical axis of the limb with insertion of the straight rod. It also has the ability to compress the fusion site after rod insertion and locking.

- Compression is performed by a proximal compression bolt end cap inserted in the proximal rod. The compression bolt end cap sinks into the rod and engages the proximal interlocking screw in the dynamic slot, which allows for an additional 1 cm of compression at the fusion site.

Short Intramedullary Fusion Rods

- Short intramedullary devices function as a modular system that form a stable couple at the arthrodesis site.
- This system avoids a surgical approach at the piriformis fossa of the hip. Additionally, the surgical site at the knee offers an advantage of débridement followed by insertion of the nail and bone grafting, employing the same surgical incision.
- The Wichita Fusion Nail (Stryker) device (**FIG 3**) has two separate segments of different diameters for the femur and tibia to allow for a more accurate intramedullary canal fit. Each segment is fixed with interlocking screws, and a coupling device is used to engage and compress the bone ends.
- The device works quite well for a primary knee arthrodesis that has good metaphyseal bone.[2]
  - However, with poor metaphyseal bone and tight-fitting rods in the femoral and tibial canal, this system does not provide enough stability to neutralize the long lever arms across the knee.
- Preoperative planning is essential to ensure that the tibial and femoral rods will achieve good fit in the bone. The femoral rod is 14 cm long and the tibial rod is 16 cm long.

External Fixation

- In the setting of a failed infected TKA, external fixation offers a viable option for knee arthrodesis.
- Many systems are available for external fixation: monoplanar, biplanar, and circular frames.
- Monoplanar fixators consist of two femoral and two tibial pins. They allow for good bony contact between the femoral and tibial segments but offer minimal stability.
- Circular frames modify alignment of the arthrodesis and provide mechanical stimulus for bone formation while also providing rigid fixation. However, they require considerable surgical skills while applying this fixation device and the bulkiness of the frame can become cumbersome for daily activities.
- The biplanar Orthofix LRS external fixator (Verona, Italy; **FIG 4**) system has two long, smooth rails (65 and 80 cm) that are mounted anteriorly and laterally from the hip to the ankle to adequately neutralize the long lever arms across the knee.
- The advantages of external fixation are that at the completion of the fusion, no hardware remains as a nidus for recurrent infection and the external fixator can be applied at the same surgical setting as the removal of infected TKA components or débridement of osteomyelitis. This allows for immediate initiation of bone contact and knee fusion.
- It is not recommended to perform bone grafting at this time but to wait until the soft tissue envelope is stable and there is minimal concern for infection at the knee fusion site. This is often done 6 to 8 weeks after the application of external fixation.
- With a circular or biplanar system, external fixation can be set up so that as the fusion occurs, the resultant limb length discrepancy can be diminished by performing an osteotomy of the proximal femur or distal tibia at the same surgical setting.
- Circular fixation, with the rings sitting at the medial aspect of the thigh, can be cumbersome for large or elderly patients; therefore, the biplanar Orthofix external fixator can be a good choice.

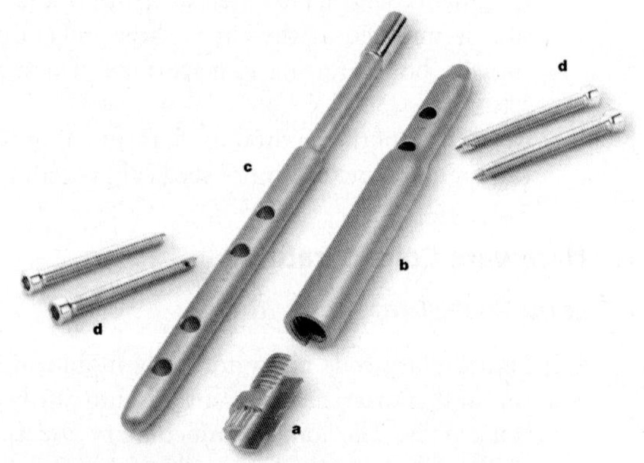

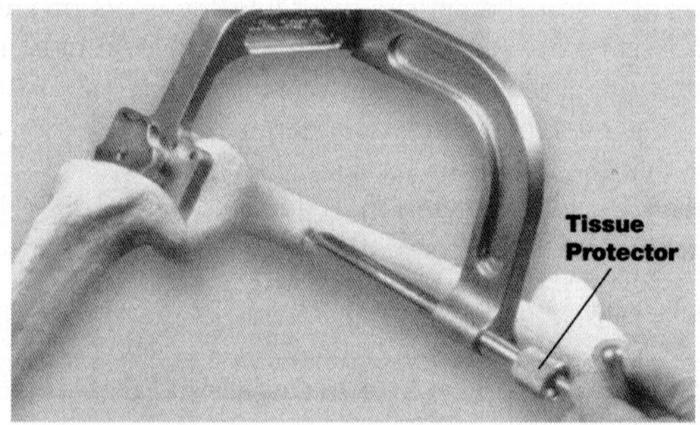

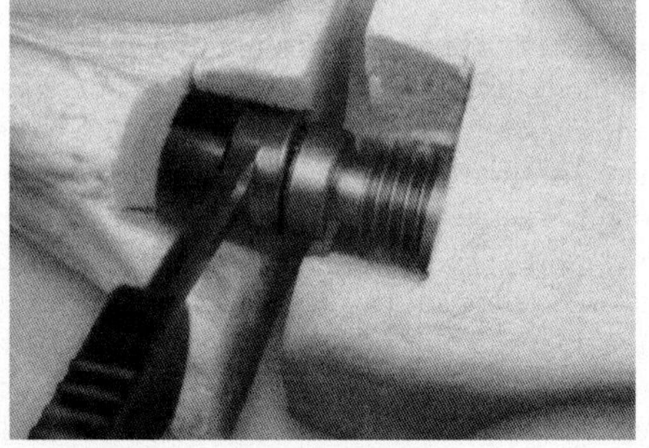

FIG 3 • **A–C.** The Wichita Fusion Nail. Several figures from the technique guide depict the separate components, insertion handle, and compression mechanism. Note the separate femoral and tibial components with the coupling device.

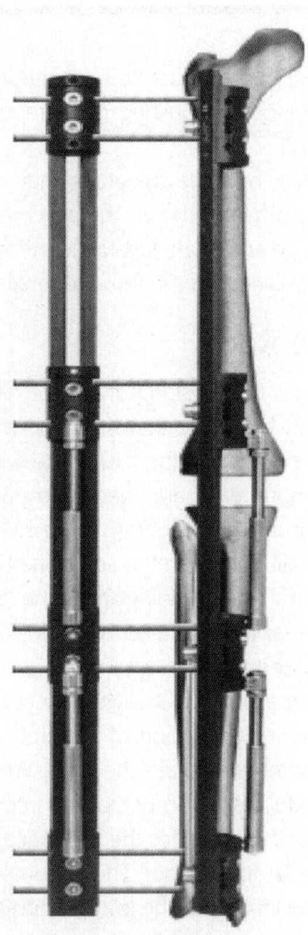

FIG 4 • Biplanar mounting of the external fixator for fusion of the knee.

- Any monolateral system can be set up in a biplanar fashion. The system used must span the length of the femur and tibia to achieve rigid fixation.

Plates

- Plates are not commonly chosen implants for knee fusion because of their bulkiness and the lack of soft tissue envelope in the anterior aspect of the knee. However, plates might be preferred for patients with a total hip arthroplasty above the desired fusion site.
- The ideal construct for plates should be 90-90 in which an anterior plate is used to counteract the flexion–extension forces and a medial or lateral plate is used to counteract the varus–valgus forces.
- The plates should initially be used in compression mode and the remaining screw holes should be inserted in a locking manner into a locked plate.
- Many plating systems with locking capability are commercially available (eg, Synthes, Smith & Nephew).

Arthrodesis Prostheses

- Prostheses consisting of cemented tapered femoral and tibial stems that couple with a cam and post mechanism that lock at the joint line preclude the need for bony contact at the distal femoral/proximal tibial joint. The Stanmore Knee Arthrodesis Prosthesis (Middlesex, United Kingdom) is a commercially available implant.[1]
- It is helpful for cases with massive bone loss due to a failed tumor endoprosthesis or after multiple failed revision TKA, where conventional arthrodesis techniques are not able to establish adequate bone contact for a successful fusion.
- It serves as an alternative to vascularized fibular grafts, allografts, and bone transport techniques.
- This prosthesis incorporates a 6-degree valgus angle, has customizable augments, and allows recreation of the desired limb alignment and length.

Positioning

- A bump is placed under the buttock to allow for visualization of the femoral neck and head on the lateral radiograph.
- The entire limb, including the foot, needs to be visualized to ensure proper rotation of the limb and assess pulse during surgery (**FIG 5**).

Approach

- The most common approach to knee fusion is anterior.
  - It should be noted that a longitudinal incision can become difficult to close once the bone ends are shortened.
- If knee fusion is performed as a solution for infection, the fusion can often be performed within the same surgical setting as the débridement.
- The preferred technique is to use a separate area for the débridement.
  - When débridement is completed, this "dirty" area is moved away, the limb is reprepared, and clean drapes and new gowns are used.
- A high-speed burr with continuous cooling irrigation is used for débridement of clean, healthy, bleeding bone and to obtain good bone surfaces for maximum bone contact during compression.
- A VersaJet hydroscalpel (Smith & Nephew, London, United Kingdom) can be used to achieve thorough débridement of the soft tissue, especially the posterior capsule.
- The back of the capsule is freed from the posterior aspect of the bone to allow good bone contact without compromising vasculature behind the capsule. This is usually done very carefully with a Cobb elevator.
- Once the bone ends are prepared, any of the methods described in the following discussion can be used to stabilize the fusion.

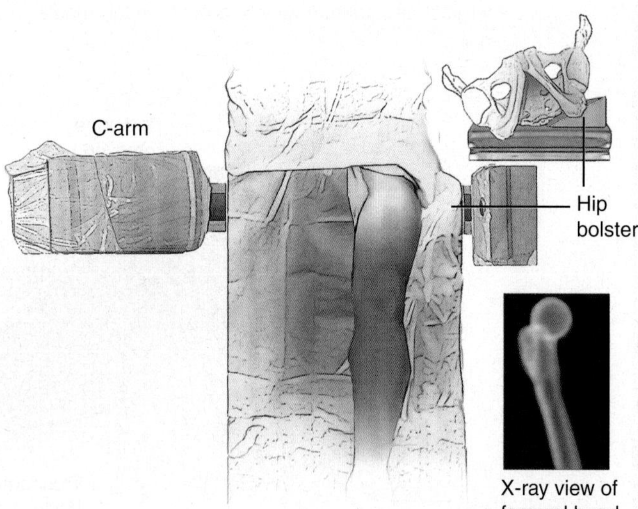

FIG 5 • Intraoperative patient positioning used for all knee fusion cases. The entire limb is prepared, with a bump placed under the ipsilateral buttock. The bump allows for access to the proximal femur for intramedullary rodding or placement of external fixator pins.

Long Intramedullary Rod Insertion

Incision and Exposure

- This technique begins with an incision at the knee, centered between the tibia and femur as determined using fluoroscopy.
- All soft tissue tethering the bone ends' ability to compress must be released without compromising the blood supply to the fusion site.
- As mentioned earlier, this includes freeing the capsule from the posterior aspects of the femur and tibia in a very careful fashion with an elevator to allow direct contact of the bone ends.
- Bone is resected, particularly necrotic bone, in a careful manner to minimize resultant shortening of the limb and to achieve the maximum bone contact possible.

Reaming the Tibia and Femur

- Once the bone ends are prepared, the tibia is reamed first.
- The femur must be reamed to the same diameter as that of the tibia so that maximum stability of the fusion can be achieved with the nail.
- Overreaming the femur will prevent the best tight fit of the nail into the femoral canal.
  - Previous generation knee fusion rods had different diameters for the femur and tibia but are no longer commercially available. If this type of rod were available, the femur would be reamed to 1 mm more than the available diameter for the femur (**TECH FIG 1**).
- The tibia and femur are reamed separately over a guide rod.
  - The tibia is reamed in an antegrade fashion, whereas the femur is reamed in a retrograde fashion.
- The guide rod is tapped out of the proximal femur through the piriformis fossa, which facilitates visualization of the nail insertion site at the proximal femur.
- However, care must be taken to ensure that the starting point is not too medial. If this seems to be the case, the proximal starting point is found with a Steinmann pin proximally to ensure that femoral neck fracture will not occur from too medial a starting point.
- The guide rod that was inserted in a retrograde fashion through the piriformis fossa is pushed out through the skin through a small incision.
- The proximal 8 cm of the antegrade knee arthrodesis nail is usually 13 to 14 mm in diameter. The proximal portion of the femur is reamed in an antegrade fashion to preserve the tight fit of the nail in the remainder of the femoral canal.

Inserting the Rod

- Rod insertion is the most important part of the case.
- It is important to ensure that the bone ends are lined up and there is compression at the fusion site with insertion. It is critical that the bone ends are lined up evenly with the guide rod inserted the entire distance from the femur to the ankle because the rod can still deviate in the soft bone with insertion and violate the cortical wall. Holding the bone ends compressed will also ensure maximum contact at the fusion site after the nail is completely inserted.
- Following proper rotational alignment of the limb at this stage is critical. The initial position of the limb when prepared is on a bump to internally rotate the limb. When inserting the rod, the limb is adducted. Because of the internal rotation from the bump, the final position for the foot once the limb is adducted is perpendicular to the floor. This ensures that there is external rotation of the limb once the bump is removed (**TECH FIG 1B**).
- The rotation is fixed once the nail has engaged the tibia and should not be manually rotated. Due to the tight fit of the nail in the tibial canal and the anterior bow of 5 to 7 degrees, rotating the tibia once the rod is fully engaged in the tibia can lead to tibial fracture.
- Once the rod is inserted and locked proximally with a guide arm, additional compression can be achieved at the knee fusion site by holding the foot and driving the rod in further.
- The limb is taken out of adduction and locked distally with the use of a fluoroscopy-guided freehand technique.
- It is important to make sure that adequate compression is maintained until the locking screws are inserted.
- Some knee arthrodesis rods have a compression screw that can be inserted proximally and allow up to 1 cm of additional compression after the distal interlocking screws are inserted.

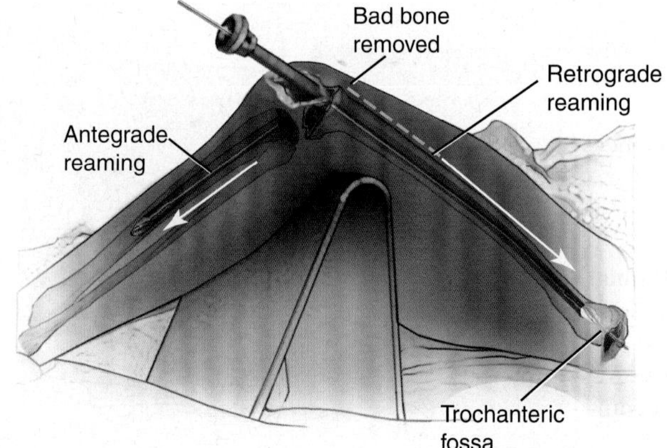

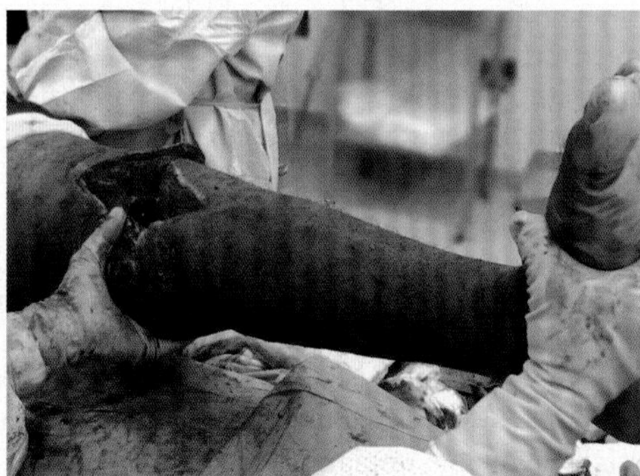

TECH FIG 1 • **A.** Lateral depiction of antegrade reaming of the tibia and then retrograde reaming of the femur. The trochanteric fossa is also known as the *piriformis fossa*. **B.** Position of the limb as the intramedullary rod is inserted at the hip. The critical portion of the procedure is to set the rotation with the foot perpendicular to the floor to obtain some final external rotation when the bump underneath the buttock is removed.

Wound Closure

- After nail insertion, the incisions are closed with absorbable monofilament sutures.
- If minor gapping is present at the fusion site, bone graft, bone morphogenic protein, or both can be added to the fusion site before closure.

Short Intramedullary Rod Insertion

- The surgical approach can be a standard medial parapatellar approach.
- Once the bone ends are exposed, an intramedullary guide is used to align the distal femoral and proximal tibial cuts in about 5 degrees of flexion and neutral varus–valgus alignment.
- A trial reduction of the bone ends is performed after the bone cuts to check the bone position and alignment.
- Another factor to keep in mind is the resultant limb shortening. The mean knee arthrodesis is 4 cm shorter. Too aggressive a resection will result in more shortening and the patient will need to wear a larger shoe lift.
- An additional way to ensure some flexion in the system is to ream the femur from distal posterior to proximal anterior. Because the tibial canal is smaller, it is more difficult to ream the tibia in a fashion similar to the femur.
- Once the femur is reamed, the femoral rod is inserted and locked with the targeting arm, with the placement of two screws in a lateral to medial fashion.
- A slot is then cut into the tibia to allow for a coupling mechanism between the two rods and the tibial guide arm for the interlocking screws.
- The bone plug may be saved for grafting at the end of the case.
- There are two options for the tibial screws. It is preferred to use screws that will capture the best bone.
- The tibia is inserted and locked in a medial to lateral fashion.
- When inserting the screws, placing a bump underneath the knee will ensure that the femur and tibia are locked with the rods in some flexion, ideally 5 degrees.
- Once the rods are placed and locked, an additional femoral slot can be removed to allow further visualization of the coupling mechanism. This bone plug can also be saved for grafting at the end of the case.
- It is important to make sure that the rotational alignment is in neutral to 5 degrees external before completely engaging the tibial rod in the femoral rod and screwing down the compression mechanism. Tighten the screw to get good compression at the bone ends. However, overtightening may fracture the bone.
- Once the fusion site is compressed, the bone plugs are replaced as bone graft and the incision is closed.
- Full weight bearing is allowed after this procedure if the surgeon is satisfied with the amount of bone contact at the fusion site.

External Fixation

Application of the Lateral Rail

- The first step after adequate exposure of the bone ends and débridement of any residual infection is the application of the lateral rail.
- The lateral rail is set up with four clamps: two for the tibia and two for the femur.
- The most proximal clamp is placed at the level of the lesser trochanter, perpendicular to the femoral shaft on the AP view, and in the midshaft of the femur.
- When placing the proximal femoral pins, ensure that they are not positioned too anteriorly in the femoral shaft. This is a major stress riser and can cause a femoral fracture.
- Once one proximal pin is inserted, the most distal tibial pin is inserted perpendicular to the shaft of the tibia in the AP view. Rotation of the limb is set with this pin insertion.
- After the pin insertions, the middle clamps are positioned (**TECH FIG 2A–D**).
- Positioning of the clamps is variable and based on the bone quality at the proximal tibia and distal femur. Better fixation is usually achieved with a greater span of the clamps.
- A lateral view radiograph is obtained to check the middle clamps.
- The clamps are often too posterior to hit the bone and need to be moved proximally or distally accordingly.
- The clamps can also be adjusted by adding a half or full "sandwich" to the clamps to raise the pin insertion site more anteriorly. It is preferable to use the sandwiches to raise the pin insertion sites as opposed to moving the clamps further away from the knee joint.
- It is at this stage that flexion of the knee can begin. More flexion will necessitate raising the middle lateral two clamps more anteriorly to hit the bone.
- Positioning at 5 degrees of flexion minimizes any additional limb shortening from excessive flexion. In this position, the two middle clamps need one full sandwich to hit the bone.
- After the insertion of one pin in each clamp, the remaining pins are inserted for a total of eight half-pins (two pins per clamp).
- The preferred half-pins are hydroxyapatite-coated and inserted so that the thread distance is the same as the diameter of the bone.
- If the threads remain outside the bone, the pin is weaker than if the threads were buried to the shank.

Alignment and Mechanical Axis

- Once all the pins are inserted, the mechanical axis of the limb is checked. The limb is first placed in the "patella forward" position. Under fluoroscopic guidance, a straight line from the center of the femoral head to the center of the ankle indicates mechanical alignment. After confirming these points, fluoroscopy is used to check where this line or mechanical axis lies at the knee.

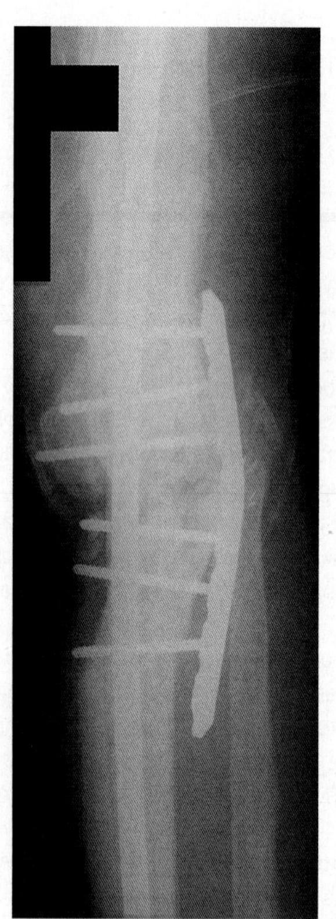
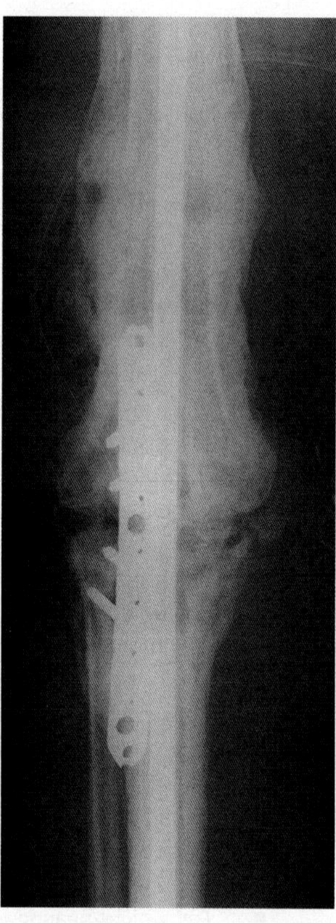
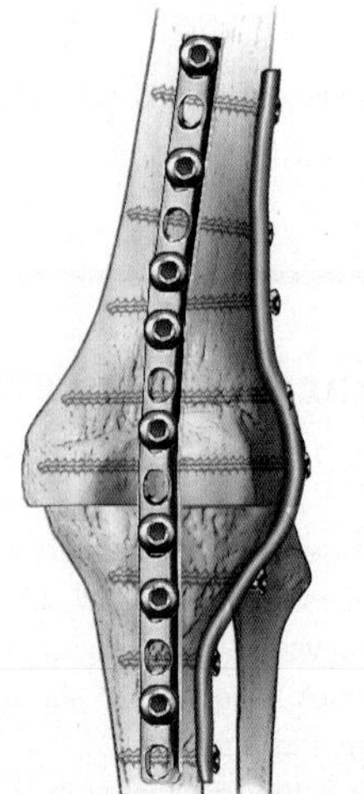
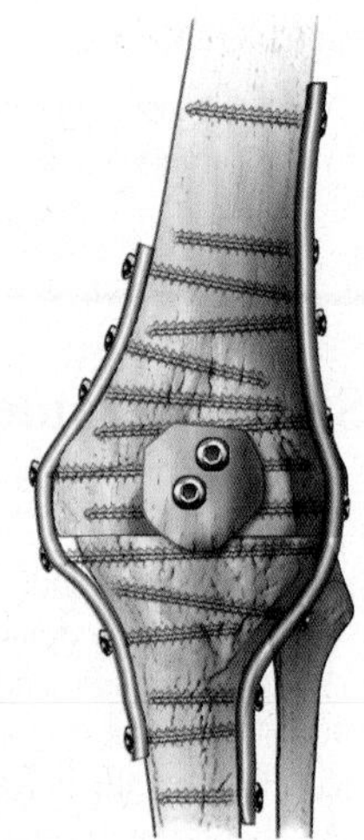
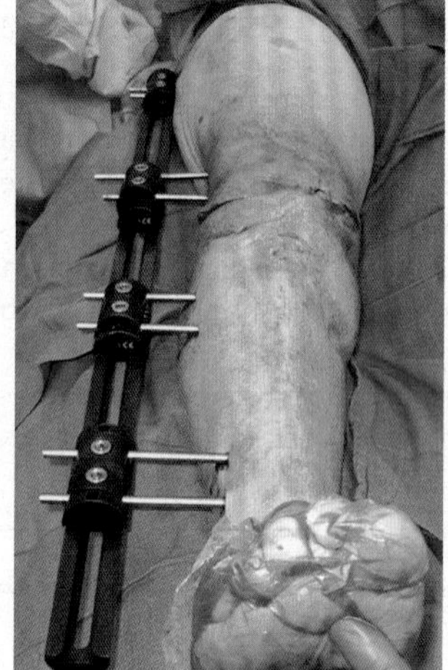

TECH FIG 2 • **A,B.** Radiographs of a posterior plate in a patient with scarring of the anterior soft tissue envelope. **C,D.** Ideal positioning for the plates (90-90) and alternative plating positions (ie, medial and lateral). **E.** The mounted rail after the lateral fixator is applied. (**C,D:** Adapted from Conway JD, Mont MA, Bezwada HP. Arthrodesis of the knee. J Bone Joint Surg Am 2004;86:835–848.)

It should be at the center of the knee or slightly medial. If not, the tibial pins can be moved in the clamps more medial or more lateral until the mechanical axis is acceptable.

- Once this has been performed, the pins are secured in the clamps and the tibial clamps are linked with a compression–distraction device. The proximal femoral clamps are secured to the rails.
- A second compression–distraction device is placed between the tibial and femoral clamps and compressed.
- The knee fusion site is visualized during the compression to ensure good bone contact and make sure that there is no soft tissue interposition at the bone ends.

Wound Closure

- Once the bone ends are opposed and compressed, the anterior knee wound is closed, usually over a drain.
- Once the lateral rail is applied and the wound is closed, an anterior fixator is applied. The long rail is placed anteriorly with four clamps set up in the same fashion as the lateral rail. The clamps are placed so as not to hit the other pins upon insertion of the anterior pins (**TECH FIG 2E**).
- Additional compression can be obtained at the knee fusion site in the office by using the compression–distraction device between the femoral and tibial clamps.

Plating

Plate Size

- The number of holes in the plates chosen depends on the bone available for fusion in the tibia and femur.
- If a total hip arthroplasty was performed, stopping the plate immediately distal to this can be a stress riser. In such cases, sliding the plate a few holes past the total hip arthroplasty stem and using unicortical screws in the region is helpful.
- The ideal number of holes is 11:5 for femoral fixation, 4 for tibial fixation, and 2 left empty at the fusion site.

Exposure

- The surgical technique begins with the same exposure as previously mentioned.

- The plates can be inserted percutaneously in both the anterior and mediolateral plane.
- Fluoroscopy is used to ensure that the plates are securely fastened to the bone.
- The important step is preparation of the bone ends and good bone contact.
- When using plates, the area must first be sterilized with the two-stage approach of using an antibiotic-coated cement spacer followed by 6 weeks of antibiotics.
- Once this stage is completed, the plates are inserted as a "clean procedure." This allows autogenous bone graft to be inserted at the fusion site with bone morphogenic protein.
- After preparation of the bone, the alignment is assessed.

Anterior Plate

- When good bone contact and good alignment are achieved, the plates are applied.
- The first step is ensuring that the proximal and distal ends will be well approximated to the bone. This is done with a provisional fixation pin at both ends.
- Great care must be taken to ensure that the rotational, sagittal, and coronal alignments are maintained while the plate is applied.
- A four-pin temporary lateral fixator can be helpful to achieve alignment and to hold the alignment while the anterior plate is applied.
- Once the alignment is good and the plate is applied with the provisional pins, the next pins to be inserted are close to the fusion site—one on the femoral side and one on the tibial side—placed in compression mode.
- This compresses the fusion site and pulls the plate down to the bone.
- Once the two screws are inserted, the remaining screws can be placed in a locked mode.
- This allows for maximum rigidity of the construct so that some weight bearing can be initiated immediately postoperatively.

Medial or Lateral Plate

- After anterior plate insertion, the medial or lateral plate can be applied. This is the easier of the two plates to be inserted because the alignment is rigid.
- Medial or lateral is best determined by the amount of soft tissue coverage, with the plate applied where there is the chance for the best soft tissue envelope.
- Occasionally, a posterior plate can be applied on the lateral side of the knee when the anterior soft tissue is too deficient to cover the plate (**TECH FIG 3**).
- This requires repositioning the patient in a prone position to apply the plate.

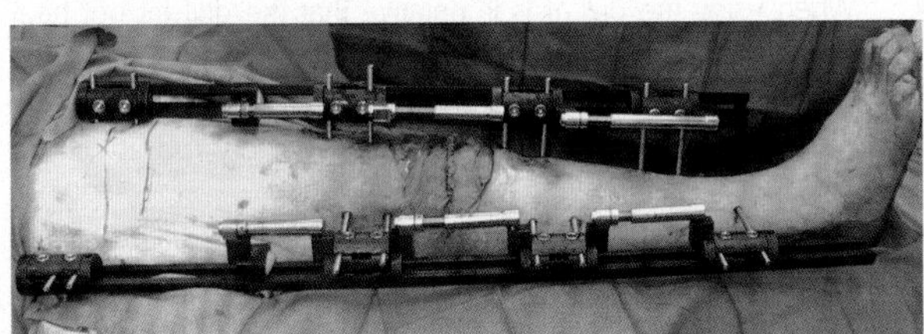

TECH FIG 3 • The mounted rail with the completed frame.

Strategy for Substantial Bone Loss: Transport over a Nail

- For bone loss of more than 5 cm and noncompressible soft tissue defects at the knee secondary to extensive scarring, bone transport is the best option to fill the defect.
- The technique begins with determining the extent of the gap. If the gap at the knee will be more than 10 cm, a double-level transport can be performed.
- The first step for transport over a nail is to insert the long intramedullary rod as described earlier.
- When inserting the rod, make sure that the limb does not inadvertently lose any length. This can best be accomplished by preoperatively determining the rod length to be used with an erect lower limb radiograph. The length of the normal side can be used as a reference as long as significant shortening of the affected limb is not also present. The affected limb cannot be acutely lengthened because the soft tissues near the knee are not compliant.
- Ideally, the affected limb should be 1 cm short to allow clearance of the foot when ambulating. The mean knee fusion shortening is 4 cm and is tolerable. Any limb shortening more than this can be addressed with the lengthening over a nail technique at the completion of the transport.
- The rod diameter chosen for the transport is 10 mm. This allows the transport segment to slide over the rod when the canal is reamed to 12 mm.
- Determine the segment to be transported.
- When determining which segment to be transported, the femur is preferred because of the need to perform only one osteotomy and because of the detrimental effects that proximal tibial transport can have on the ankle (equinus).
  - If proximal tibial transport is necessary because of the large segmental defect, the fibula should also be osteotomized at the midshaft and a distal syndesmotic screw should be placed to prevent any proximal fibular migration.
- Mark out the osteotomy site of the transported segment.
- Once the guide rod is inserted into the femur and tibia, the rod is backed out past the level of the osteotomy, which is predrilled with multiple holes before reaming. This allows the reamings to exit out the osteotomy site and for bone graft of the regenerate site.
- The first step is reaming the intramedullary canal of the tibia and femur to 12 mm.
- This can be done through the knee, reaming the tibia and femur separately, or from the hip using long, 80-cm reamers.
- Once the rod is inserted and locked at the desired length, the monolateral external fixator is applied.
- Applying the monolateral frame to move the transported segment over the nail requires inserting the pins so that there is no contact between the rod and the pins. With this technique, because the rod and pins are so close, there is a 5% chance for infection of the rod.[13]

- The cannulated wire technique starts with a 1.8-mm wire inserted perpendicular to the rod on the AP view fluoroscopic projection but away from the rod by a few millimeters on the lateral view projection.
- The most common location in the femur for these pins is proximally and posteriorly at the level of the lesser trochanter (**TECH FIG 4**).
- Once the wire is inserted, it is visualized using fluoroscopy. This is to confirm that when the pin is drilled and placed, it will not be touching the rod.
- Fluoroscopy must be used frequently to confirm that the pins are placed away from the rod.
- Once the wire is in a satisfactory position on the AP and lateral view projections, a 4.8-mm cannulated drill bit is used to drill the near cortex. This drill bit and the wire are removed and a solid 4.8-mm drill bit is used to complete the tract for the pin.
- Drilling with the cannulated drill bit and the solid drill bit is important because the cannulated drill bit is not end-cutting and sharp enough to go through the cortical bone of the far cortex. Often, these pins are placed entirely in the cortical bone.
- When using the drill, it is imperative that the drill bit not heat up and cause osteonecrosis of the bone. If this happens, the pin will become infected and a ring sequestrum will develop. Also, an infected pin places the intramedullary rod at risk for contamination.
- To prevent this, the drill bit is removed at regular intervals while the drill is cooled and cleaned with a wet, cool laparotomy sponge.
- Once the bone is drilled, a 6-mm hydroxyapatite-coated pin is inserted.
- After insertion of the pins with use of the clamp as a guide, the frame is removed and the bone is cut with an osteotome.
- A small incision is used laterally at the level of the femur. Often, the bone cannot be completely cut through one incision around the rod. A second incision is placed anteriorly to complete the osteotomy along the medial femur.
- If the tibia is chosen, the incisions are placed anteriorly and medially to obtain access to the lateral cortex and posteromedial cortex, respectively.
- Once the bone is cut, the pins are used to carefully rotate the bone and determine that the osteotomy is complete.
- When the osteotomy is complete, the fixator is reapplied and the osteotomy site distracted to ensure that the bone ends will separate. This is confirmed by using fluoroscopy, and the osteotomy site is reapproximated.
- Postoperatively, the pins are cleaned daily with saline and redressed with a Kerlix dressing wrapped tightly around each set of pins.
- The dressing prevents skin pistoning around the pins and limits soft tissue trauma, which leads to pin tract infections.
- Postoperatively, minimal weight bearing for balance only is permitted.
- Full weight bearing is permitted once two cortices are present at the regenerate site on the radiographs and the consolidation phase of bone healing has begun.
- Distraction is begun at postoperative day 5 and is continued until the gap is closed at the knee region.
- When the gap has closed, the patient is brought back to the operating room for insertion of bone graft at the docking site and percutaneous locked plating at the docking site. The locked plating is essential to prevent the transported bone end from migrating.
- Custom rods with predrilled holes to lock the transported segment weaken the rod and are not recommended.
- Once the bone graft and locked plate are inserted, the external fixator is removed.
- If the limb is still markedly short after the docking of the transported segment, the distal interlocking screws are removed from the rod and the external fixator is left in place to continue lengthening.
- Once the desired length is achieved, the patient is returned to the operating room for insertion of the locking screws and removal of the external fixator.
- The patient is allowed full weight bearing once two to four cortices are present on the radiographs.

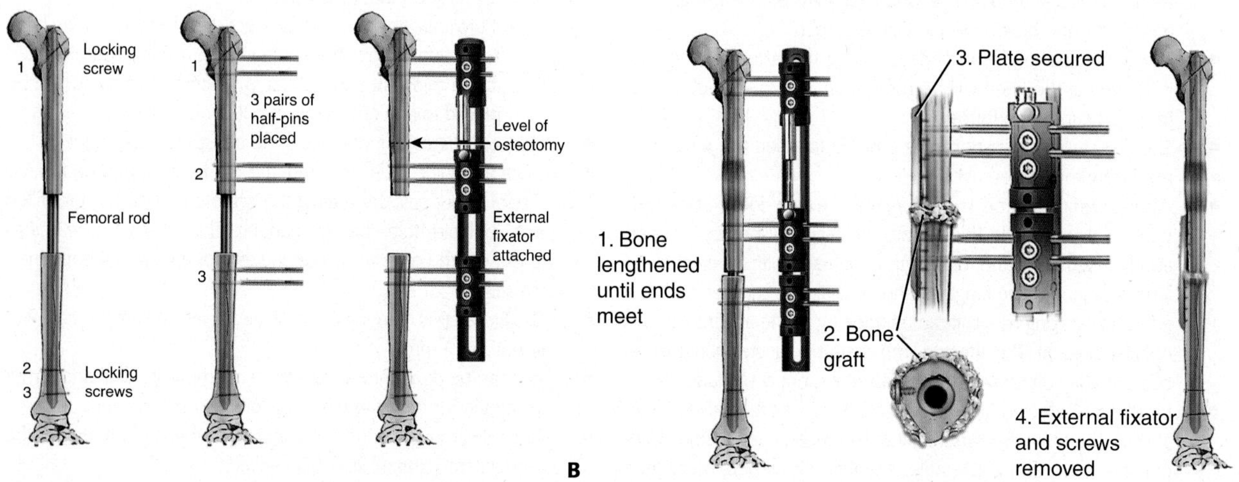

TECH FIG 4 • **A,B.** Steps involved in the transport over a nail technique. Bone graft and a plate are applied to the docking site and the fixator is removed at the final surgical setting.

PEARLS AND PITFALLS

Poor bone approximation on one side of the fusion or anteriorly	▪ This is common anteriorly with good approximation of the medial, lateral, and posterior bone ends. As much as 50% of the diameter of the bone is approximated at the time of fusion; if those bone ends are viable and healthy, the fusion will be successful. Secondary bone grafting can be performed at the defect site. More bone contact is preferred but not at the expense of massive limb length discrepancy. If massive limb length discrepancy occurs, a different strategy for fusion should be used.
Difficulty holding the position of the knee fusion with rod insertion	▪ Temporary use of an external fixator (one or two pins proximally and one or two pins distally) with the pins placed out of the path of the nail will hold the fusion in a compressed and properly rotated position when inserting the rod. This application is quite helpful but not frequently needed for straightforward fusion.
Femoral neck fracture	▪ Too medial a starting point for insertion of the antegrade long knee fusion rod can result in femoral neck fracture. This is very difficult to treat and is best treated with exchange rodding to a long custom knee fusion cephalomedullary nail with screws into the femoral neck and head.

POSTOPERATIVE CARE

- Regardless of the surgical technique, the patient is encouraged to undergo physical therapy for muscle strengthening of the hip postoperatively.
- For patients with external fixators, pin tract infections that may occur are initially treated with orally administered antibiotics.
  - All patients are given a prescription for an antibiotic, most commonly cephalexin, to be taken orally before discharge and are instructed to start the antibiotic at the first sign of redness, increased tenderness at the pin site, or drainage.
- Follow-up office visits are every 2 weeks for patients who undergo bone transport or lengthening. Once the consolidation phase starts, only monthly follow-up visits are required.
- For patients with external fixation, once the bone has consolidated, the frame is then dynamized in the office 1 month before removal.
  - Dynamization of the frame is usually performed by taking the tension off the compression–distraction devices. This allows the bone to accommodate more loads and become stronger before the frame is completely removed.
- For patients with external fixation, if bone graft was not performed at the time of fusion, a second-stage bone grafting procedure can be performed once there is no longer any evidence of infection, approximately 6 to 8 weeks after the index procedure.
- Most patients will need shoe lifts added to the outside of their shoe during the postoperative period.

OUTCOMES

- Harris et al[6] compared the function of knee arthrodesis after tumors with that of constrained TKA and found that knee arthrodesis patients had better stability and performed more physically demanding activities.
- Rud and Jensen[16] examined 23 knee arthrodesis patients and found that 18 had returned to normal physical activities and returned to work.
- Most patients should expect to have difficulty with stairs, rugs, and ladders[17]; patients who performed strenuous work before the arthrodesis rarely resume that strenuous work postoperatively.
- Rand et al[15] reported that seven patients with knee arthrodesis could walk one to three blocks and nine successful knee arthrodesis patients were able to walk more than six blocks.
- Compared with AKA, knee fusion offers a stable, painless, and uninfected limb for weight bearing. Most knee arthrodesis patients are able to ambulate normally, whereas according to Pring et al,[14] of 23 patients who underwent an AKA for infected TKA, only 7 were able to ambulate.
- The best way to achieve optimal patient satisfaction for those with difficult problems is to be thorough during preoperative discussions regarding what knee arthrodesis can achieve for them.
  - Realistic patient expectations are critical in achieving successful outcomes.
  - Although revision TKA might be the more attractive alternative, many patients are not proper candidates secondary to poor soft tissue envelope, bone loss, or recurrent infections.
  - Hanssen et al[5] documented that 50% of patients with infected revision TKA eventually went on to undergo knee arthrodesis.
- Conversion from arthrodesis to a TKA is fraught with complications such as infection, ligamentous instability, and the need for refusion.[7,9,11]

COMPLICATIONS

- The complications associated with knee arthrodesis are related to the increased stress placed on the hip, back, and ankle. Concomitant osteoarthritis of these joints can often occur.
  - Takedown of the knee fusion in these circumstances is not recommended secondary to the extensive complications reported in the literature.[8]
- Other complications that occur include recurrent infection and nonunion.
  - These complications can be extremely difficult to treat, considering the many medical comorbidities in the older population.

REFERENCES

1. Bartlett W, Vijayan S, Pollock R, et al. The Stanmore knee arthrodesis prosthesis. J Arthroplasty 2011;26:903–908.
2. Christie MJ, DeBoer DK, McQueen DA, et al. Salvage procedures for failed total knee arthroplasty. J Bone Joint Surg Am 2003:85(suppl 1):S58–S62.
3. Conway JD, Mont MA, Bezwada HP. Arthrodesis of the knee. J Bone Joint Surg Am 2004;86:835–848.
4. Enneking WF, Shirley PD. Resection-arthrodesis for malignant and potentially malignant lesions about the knee using an intramedullary rod and local bone grafts. J Bone Joint Surg Am 1977;59:223–236.

5. Hanssen AD, Trousdale RT, Osmon DR. Patient outcome with reinfection following reimplantation for the infected total knee arthroplasty. Clin Orthop Relat Res 1995;321:55–67.
6. Harris IE, Leff AR, Gitelis S, et al. Function after amputation, arthrodesis or arthroplasty for tumors about the knee. J Bone Joint Surg Am 1990;72:1477–1485.
7. Henkel TR, Boldt JG, Drobny TK, et al. The knee arthroplasty after formal knee fusion using unconstrained and semi-constrained components: a report of seven cases. J Arthroplasty 2001;16: 768–776.
8. Kim YH, Kim JS, Cho SH. Total knee arthroplasty after spontaneous osseous ankylosis and takedown of formal knee fusion. J Arthroplasty 2000;15:453–460.
9. Kim YH, Oh SH, Kim JS. Conversion of used knee with use of a posterior stabilized total knee prosthesis. J Bone Joint Surg Am 2003;85:1047–1050.
10. Klinger HM, Spahn G, Schultz W, et al. Arthrodesis of the knee after failed infected total knee arthroplasty. Knee Surg Sports Traumatol Arthrosc 2006;14:447–453.
11. MacDonald JH, Agarwal S, Lorei MP, et al. Knee arthrodesis. J Am Acad Orthop Surg 2006;14:154–163.
12. Oostenbroek HJ, van Roermund PM. Arthrodesis of the knee after an infected total knee arthroplasty using the Ilizarov method. J Bone Joint Surg Br 2001;83:50–54.
13. Paley D, Herzenberg JE, Paremain G, et al. Femoral lengthening over an intramedullary nail. A matched-case comparison with Ilizarov femoral lengthening. J Bone Joint Surg Am 1997;79(10):1464–1480.
14. Pring DJ, Marks L, Angel JC. Mobility after amputation for failed knee replacement. J Bone Joint Surg Br 1988;70:770–771.
15. Rand JA, Bryan RS, Chao EY. Failed total knee arthroplasty treated by arthrodesis of the knee using the Ace-Fischer apparatus. J Bone Joint Surg Am 1987;69:39–45.
16. Rud B, Jensen UH. Function after arthrodesis of the knee. Acta Orthop Scand 1985;56:337–339.
17. Siller TN, Hadjipavlou A. Knee arthrodesis: long-term results. Can J Surg 1976;19:217–219.
18. Somayaji HS, Tsaggerides P, Ware HE, et al. Knee arthrodesis—a review. Knee 2008;15:247–254.

Exam Table for Joint Reconstruction Surgery

Examination	Technique	Illustration	Grading & Significance
Anterior impingement test	The examiner simultaneously flexes (90 to 100 degrees), adducts (10 to 20 degrees), and internally rotates (5 to 20 degrees) the hip.	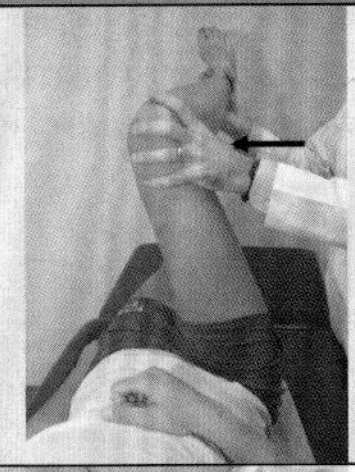	A positive test elicits hip pain that reproduces symptoms and is frequently associated with guarding. Absence of pain indicates a negative test. The test is specific for intra-articular pathology and is present in the majority of patients with a labral tear.
Apprehension test	The hip is externally rotated in an (over-) extended position.	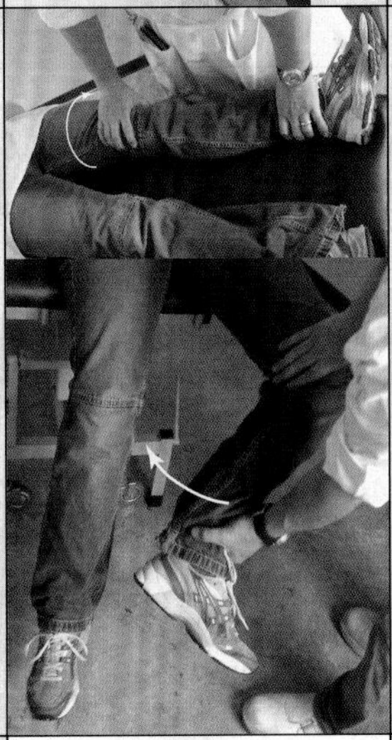	Test is positive if the patient complains about the feeling of imminent joint luxation. Indicates an insufficient coverage of the femoral head.
Gait	Legs should be exposed. Gait is observed with and without the use of walking aids.	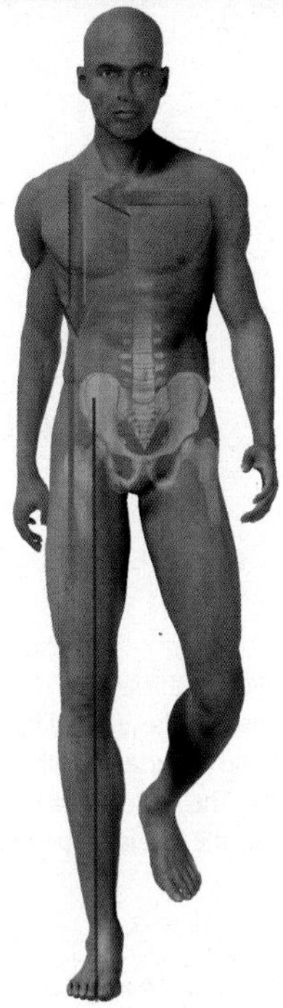	Trendelenburg gait suggests abductor weakness or hip discomfort. Coxalgic gait suggests hip pain of any cause. Stiff hip gait may be present with hypertrophic osteoarthritis. Short limb gait may be present with developmental dysplasia of the hip. No limp is normal. A slight abductor lurch or antalgic gait is abnormal. Intra-articular hip disease (labral tear or chondral flap) can produce an early limp. As secondary osteoarthritis progresses, a limp is common. The examiner should look for varus thrust. Painful total hip arthroplasty may result in shortened stance phase or stride length, or abnormal pelvic rotation. May confirm hip pathology or indicate extrinsic source of pain. May raise concern regarding hip abductor function that can limit success of revision. Pain or muscle weakness may cause limp. Trunk may shift over affected hip.

(continued)

Examination	Technique	Illustration	Grading & Significance
Hip abductor strength	In the lateral decubitus position, the patient is asked to elevate the limb and the examiner applies manual resistance.	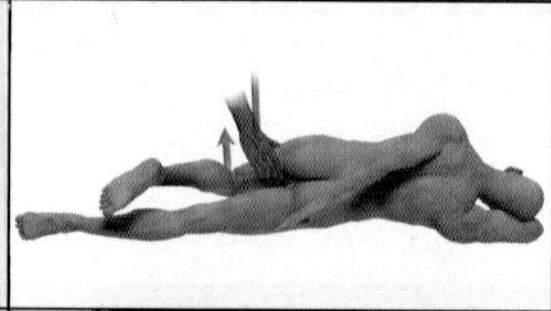	Graded using traditional manual muscle testing five-point scale. May indicate abductor weakness, trochanteric bursitis, abductor avulsion, or loose femoral component.
Leg length, apparent	With the patient supine, the examiner measures the distance from the umbilicus to each medial malleolus.	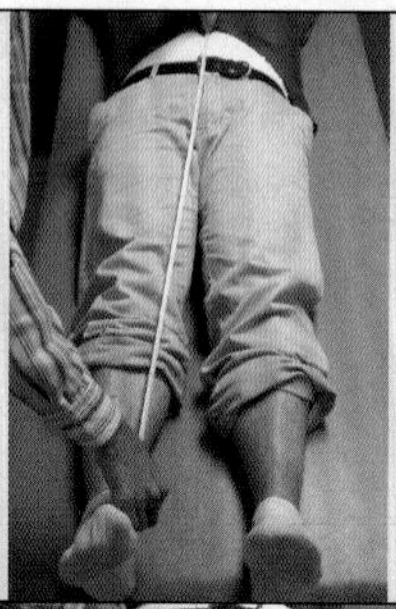	Values may be affected by atrophy, obesity, or asymmetric positioning of the legs. May indicate abductor or adductor contractures, or pelvic obliquity due to scoliosis.
Leg length, true	The patient is supine with feet 15 to 20 cm apart. The examiner measures the distance from the anterior superior iliac spine to the medial malleolus of each leg. In obese patients with poor pelvic landmarks, the examiner should line up the medial malleoli to get an approximation of leg lengths. It is important to assess the patient while standing as well to observe for pelvic obliquity and scoliosis.	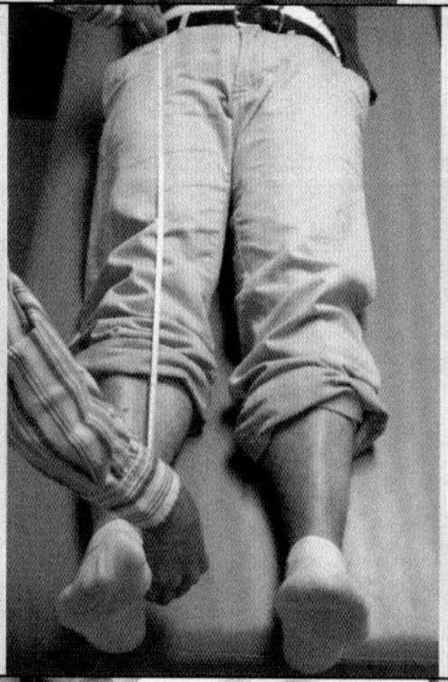	A slight difference of <1 cm is considered normal but may be symptomatic in some patients. Progressive leg-length discrepancy suggests implant subsidence. Adduction contracture may cause apparent shortening when supine, but may elevate the hemipelvis when standing. Pelvic tilt from spinal deformity may contribute to functional leg-length inequality.
Logroll	The lower extremity is rolled side to side at the proximal thigh.	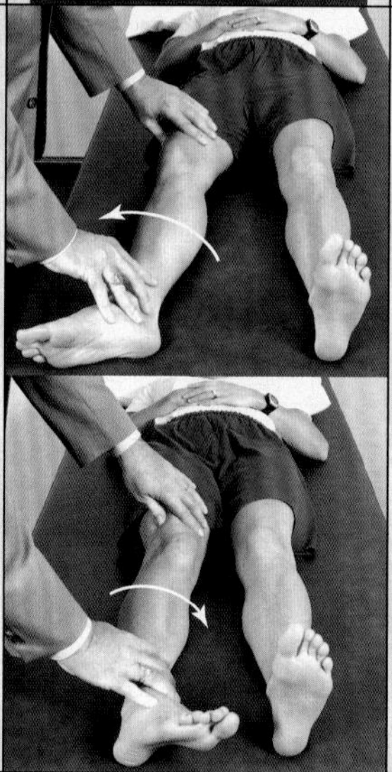	Positive if maneuver elicits pain at groin. Most sensitive physical finding. Side-to-side movement of the lower extremity creates shear forces across a femoral neck fracture, leading to exquisite pain.
Ober Test	With the patient in the lateral decubitus position, the affected hip is extended and abducted and the knee is flexed. The thigh is then released while the foot is supported.	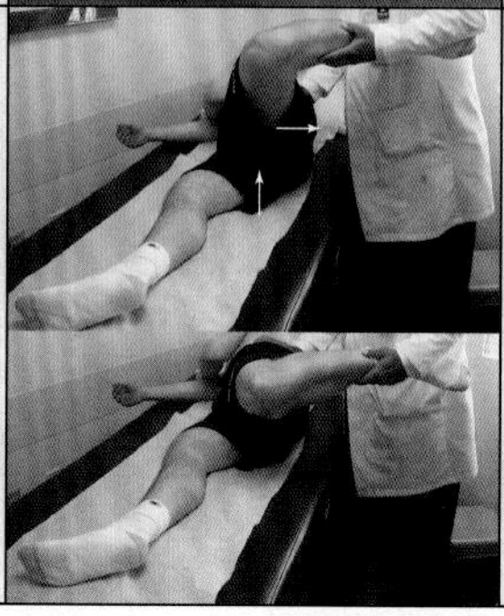	Persistent abduction of the hip reveals tightness of the iliotibial band. This finding is important to note preoperatively so it is not misinterpreted as overlengthening intraoperatively.

Examination	Technique	Illustration	Grading & Significance
Patrick test	Hip discomfort is assessed with the hip in flexion, abduction, and external rotation with the ipsilateral foot placed on the contralateral knee.		Negative test is no discomfort. Positive test produces groin pain that mimics the patient's symptoms. This is a sensitive screening examination for hip joint irritability and intra-articular hip disease.
Posterior impingement test	The hip is extended, externally rotated, and adducted. This can be tested in the supine or prone position.		Pain perceived posteriorly in the buttock corresponds to a positive impingement test. The absence of pain indicates a negative test. Normal internal rotation is considered to be about 15 to 20 degrees. In femoroacetabular impingement, internal rotation is decreased. Normal test is no pain. Positive test is groin or buttock pain that reproduces symptoms. Uncommonly, patients have associated structural posterior impingement. The posterior impingement test assists in identifying the presence of associated posterior disease.
Straight-leg raise	The presence of radicular pain with a passive straight-leg raise should be noted. The examiner assesses active straight-leg raising.		The angle of elevation at which straightleg raising induces radicular pain is measured. Radicular pain suggests lumbar pathology. May be limited by pain from infection or loose implants.
Trendelenburg test	The examiner observes and palpates the pelvis from behind while the patient performs a single-legged stance.		Level pelvis in single-legged stance is normal. The test is positive if the contralateral hip drops inferiorly. A positive test may indicate that the hip abductors are compromised. Dropping of the contralateral hemipelvis indicates abductor weakness of the symptomatic hip. Abductor weakness is common in patients with early intra-articular hip disease and impingement. May indicate abductor dysfunction; may be positive because of pain or neurologic problem (superior gluteal nerve or L5 nerve root).
Arc of rotation, hip	This is performed in the prone position, starting with the knee flexed to 90 degrees. Starting with the hip in neutral rotation, the hip is internally rotated and externally rotated.		The arcs of internal and external rotation from the midline are measured in degrees with a goniometer. Normal arc of rotation is age-dependent. External rotation usually exceeds internal rotation. When the arc of internal rotation exceeds the arc of external rotation, the presence of increased anteversion can be inferred.

(continued)

Examination	Technique	Illustration	Grading & Significance
Barlow maneuver	The examiner's hand is on the proximal femur, fingers over the greater trochanter, and the leg is in a flexed position. The leg is adducted with gentle posterior pressure to see if the hip can be dislocated.	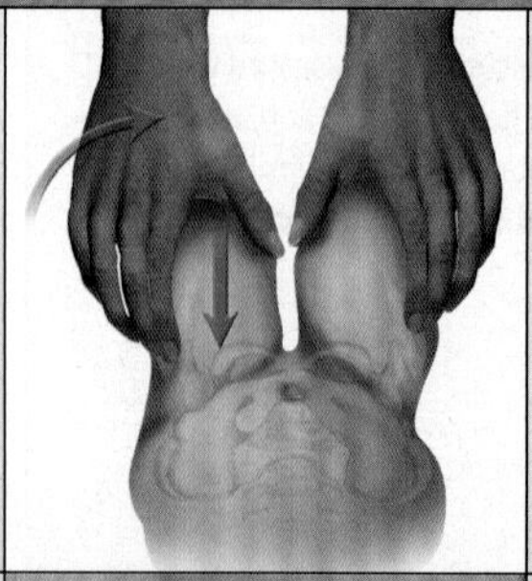	Positive or negative. Positive Barlow sign represents the ability for a reduced hip to be dislocated due to instability. Disappears as fixed dislocation develops.
Galeazzi sign	On a flat surface, the thigh lengths are assessed with the knees flexed. The examiner flexes the hips to 90 degrees and notes the height of the knees.	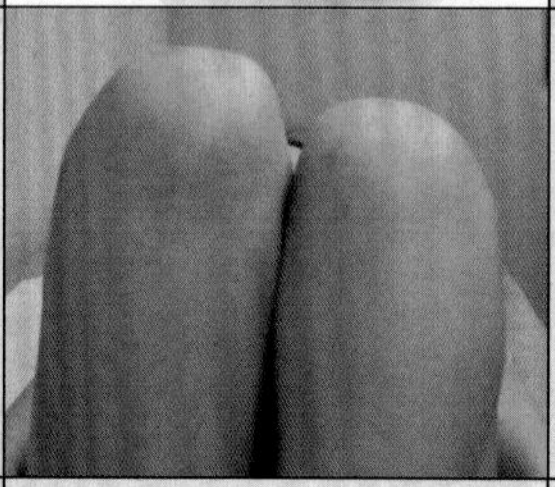	Positive if there is a difference in thigh length. A positive Galeazzi sign can indicate a dislocated hip, a short femur, or a congenital hip deformity. The apparent femoral lengths will be equal in bilateral dislocations.
Hip abduction	On a flat surface, the patient's hips are flexed to 90 degrees and abducted and the anterior superior iliac spines palpated to make sure the pelvis remains level. Abduction of the hips should be checked in both the flexed and extended positions.	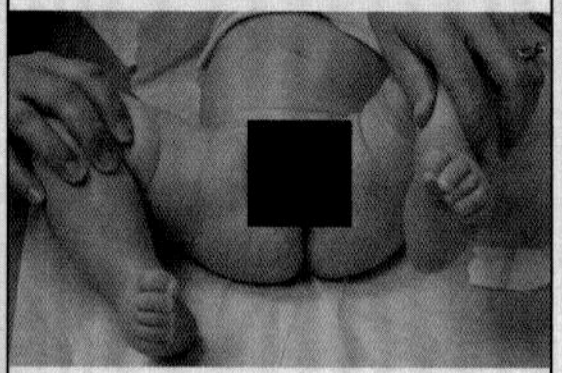	In a normal hip, abduction should be >60 degrees and symmetric. May be the only abnormal sign in infants. A difference of 10 degrees or more is significant. Decreased hip abduction is the most common physical finding in patients with hip pathology. A marked loss of abduction in extension is particularly important in Perthes disease, suggesting hinge abduction.
Ortolani sign	With a hand on the proximal femur, fingers over the greater trochanter, and the leg in a flexed position, the examiner abducts the leg with gentle traction to see if the hip can be reduced. The hip is flexed 90 degrees. The hip is abducted gently with the thumb on the medial femoral condyle and the third finger on the greater trochanter. The examiner lifts with the third finger and feels for a "clunk."	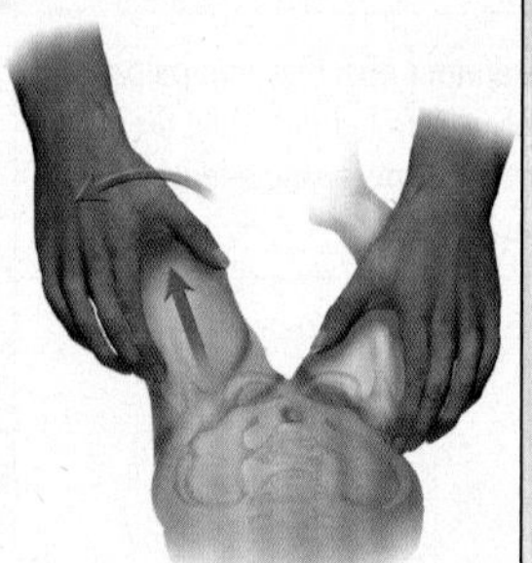	Positive or negative. A positive Ortolani sign represents the reduction of a dislocated hip. Usually present in the newborn with developmental dysplasia of the hip, but disappears as the dislocation becomes fixed. The test is positive if a clunk is felt as a dislocated hip reduces.
Pelvic obliquity	Examiner sits or stands behind patient. Fingers are placed on the iliac crests and the thumbs are placed on the posterior superior iliac spines. Presence of asymmetry is noted.	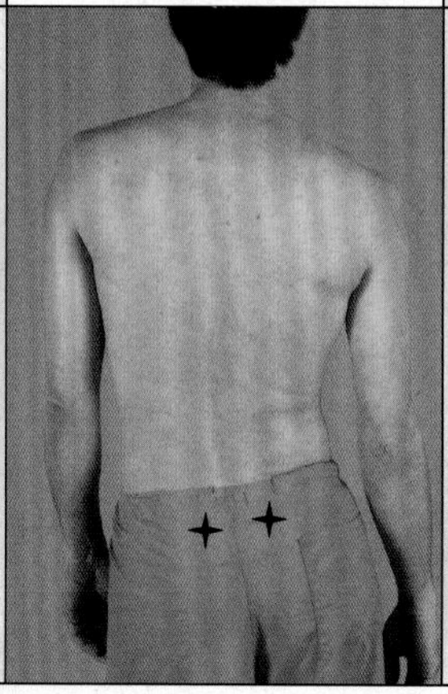	Can indicate a possible leg-length discrepancy that can mimic a lumbar scoliosis

Examination	Technique	Illustration	Grading & Significance
Range of motion (ROM), hip	Abduction–adduction and flexion ROM is examined in the supine position. Fixed flexion deformity of the hip is measured. Hip internal rotation–external rotation is measured in prone position, together with the thigh–foot angle. Muscle length tests include popliteal angle (hamstring length) and prone knee bend (rectus femoris muscle length).	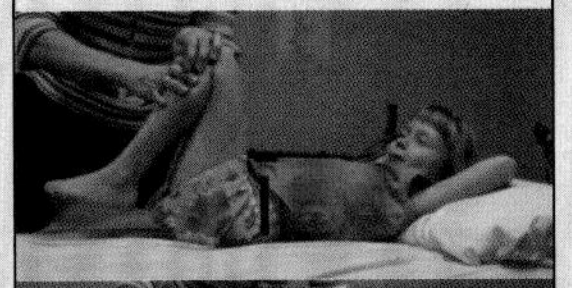 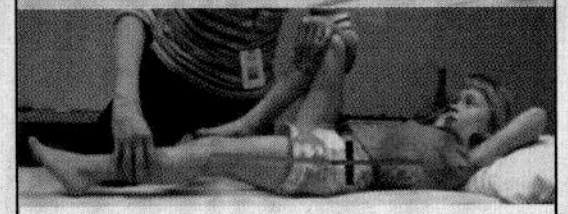	ROM is measured and contractures are identified and quantified in degrees. A popliteal angle >0 degrees and prone knee bend less than supine knee bend indicates tightness of hamstring and rectus femoris muscles, respectively. Contractures need to be treated in preparation for lengthening. Lengthening of rectus femoris and hamstring muscles is recommended for positive muscle tightness. Normal extension range of motion is from 10 degrees beyond horizontal. Maximum flexion is limited by the abdomen and the trunk. Normal walking function requires 7 degrees extension beyond neutral pelvic position. Therefore, even small contractures limit functional range of motion, shorten step length, and induce compensatory movements. Restricted ROM can indicate a joint abnormality, capsular contracture, or spasticity of the internal or external rotators of the hip. Excessive ROM indicates relative ligamentous laxity. Shifted ROM (eg, excessive internal ROM) indicates excessive femoral anteversion.
ROM	The hip is flexed to its maximum extent and the examiner records the degrees of flexion. The hip is then flexed to 90 degrees and passively internally and externally rotated.	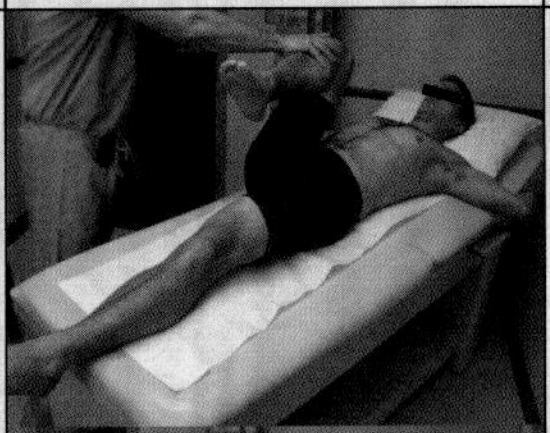 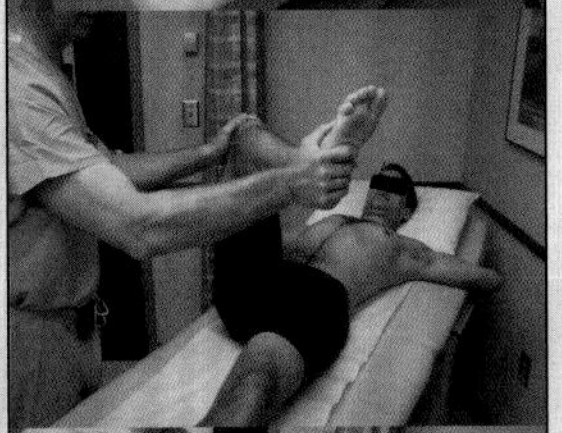 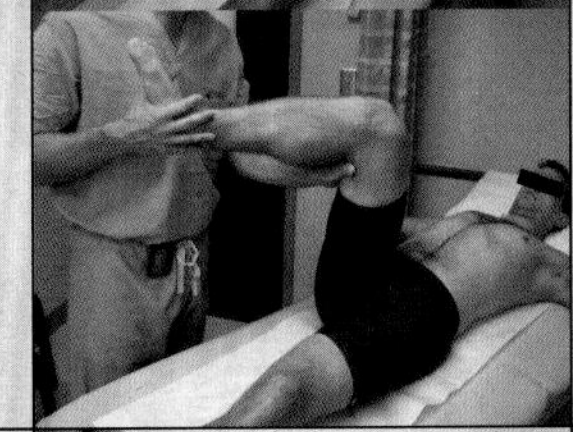	Loss of motion is often associated with arthritis.
Abduction external rotation test	The hip is passively forced into maximal abduction with external rotation.	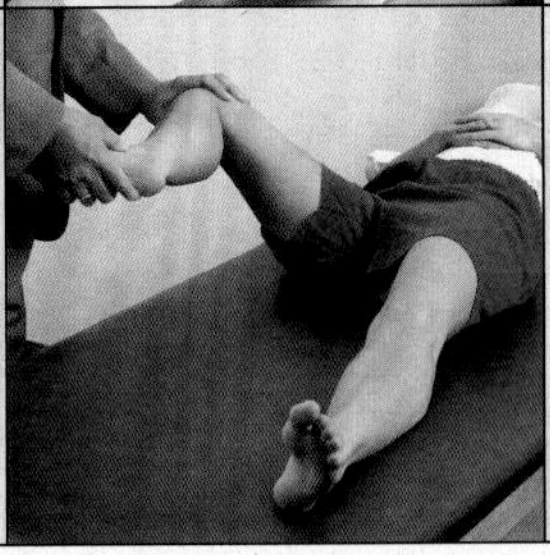	May create symptoms associated with posterior joint pathology by compression, or anterior pathology by anterior translation of the femoral head.

(continued)

Examination	Technique	Illustration	Grading & Significance
C sign	Patient cups hand above greater trochanter, gripping fingers into groin.	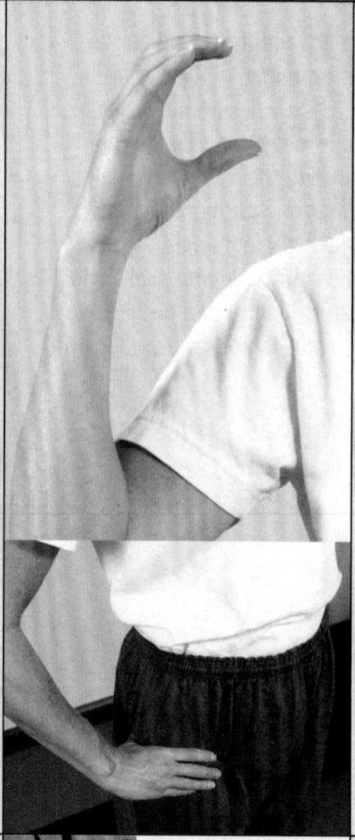	Common observation with patients describing interior hip pain.
Impingement test	The hip is passively forced into maximal flexion, adduction, and internal rotation.	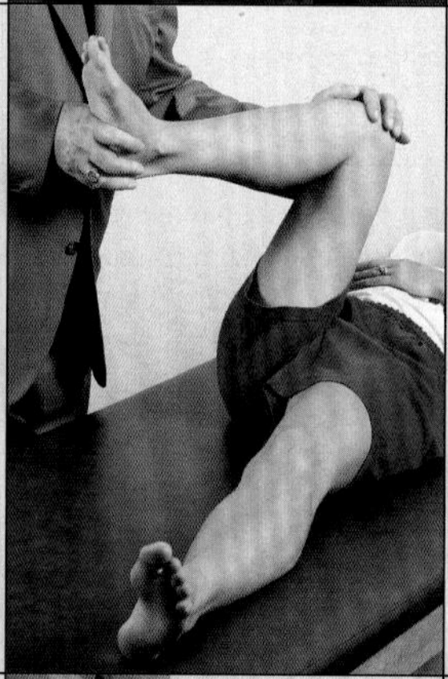	A more sensitive test for detecting hip joint irritability. This is associated with impingement findings but is positive with most sources of hip pathology.
Anterior compression of the iliopsoas tendon	Firm digital pressure over the anterior hip capsule may block the snapping.	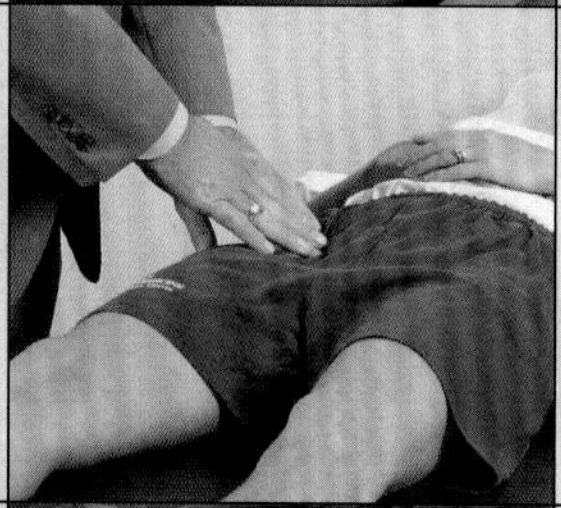	Applying pressure to block the snapping of the tendon substantiates the diagnosis. However, often this maneuver is uncomfortable and not well tolerated by the patient.
Squeeze test	Supine subject actively attempts adduction by squeezing legs against resistance provided by examiner.	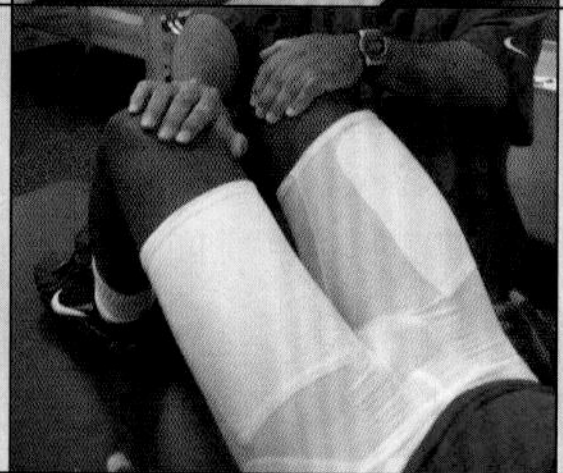	The presence or absence of pain is noted. Strength is graded as mild (minimal loss of strength); moderate (clear loss of strength); or severe (complete loss of strength). Pain with or without a strength deficit implies adductor-related groin pain.
Hamstring strength	Patient lies prone. Patient attempts knee flexion against resistance.	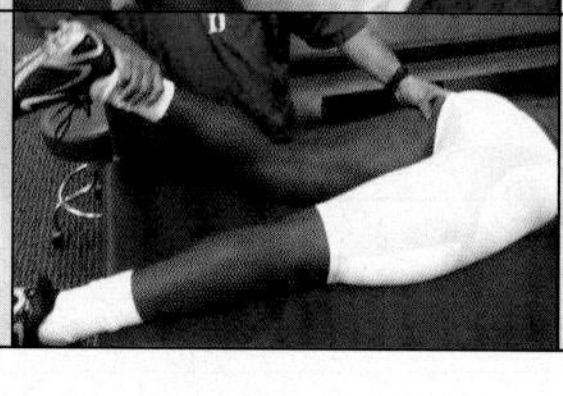	Mild: minimal loss of strength; moderate: clear loss of strength; severe: complete loss of strength. Severe injury implies proximal avulsion.

Examination	Technique	Illustration	Grading & Significance
Passive hamstring stretch	Patient performs a hurdler's stretch.		Apparent hamstring flexibility is compared to the uninjured side. An obvious increase in apparent hamstring flexibility of injured extremity implies proximal avulsion.
Passive adductors stretch	The subject lies supine. The examiner either abducts the leg or places the leg in a figure 4 position.		The presence or absence of pain is noted. Pain localized to the adductor implies adductor-related groin pain.
Inspection for Effusion	The examiner palpates and performs ballottement of the patella. Smaller effusions can be detected by compressing fluid from the suprapatellar pouch.		Trace, mild, moderate, or large. Presence of an effusion is indirect evidence of intra-articular injury. Most commonly graded subjectively as mild, moderate, or larger. New onset of effusion after injury localizes injury to within the capsule of the knee.
Heel strike	Light blows of the fist or heel of hand to the heel of the injured leg		Groin pain that did not exist at rest implies hip fracture.
Lower extremity rotation	In a patient with a suspected femoral neck fracture, gentle internal and external rotation at the leg is all that is needed to elicit pain.		Pain in the groin is concerning for femoral neck fracture but may also be caused by fractures of the anterior pelvic ring.
Midfoot joint palpation	Direct palpation of each of midfoot joints, particularly the medial column of the foot		Presence or absence of pain. The presence of pain at the midfoot with palpation suggests a Lisfranc injury.
Midfoot stability	Gentle passive dorsiflexion and plantarflexion of each of the metatarsal heads; gentle passive abduction and adduction through the forefoot		Presence or absence of pain. The presence of pain at the tarsometatarsal joint region with passive forefoot range of motion suggests a Lisfranc injury.

(continued)

Examination	Technique	Illustration	Grading & Significance
Patellar palpation	The patella, quadriceps tendon, and patellar tendon are palpated for defects. The examiner notes inferior or superior patellar displacement in comparison to the unaffected side.		Patella baja is an inferiorly displaced patella seen with quadriceps tendon rupture; patella alta is a high-riding patella associated with patellar tendon rupture. The placement of the patella and palpation of defects with the patella, quadriceps tendon, or patellar tendon can help differentiate between patellar fracture and ligamentous extensor disruption.
Iliac wing compression	The examiner can test for stability of the pelvic ring by placing the palms of the hands on the outside of the iliac wings and pushing the two wings together.		This should be avoided if radiology demonstrates displacement.
Pelvic instability: external rotation	Legs are positioned flexed, abducted, and externally rotated. Hands are placed on the iliac crests and an AP force is applied.		Palpable widening of the pelvis or increased sacroiliac joint space or symphyseal widening is seen on simultaneous fluoroscopic images with the C-arm.
Pelvic instability: internal rotation	Legs are positioned extended and internally rotated. Hands are positioned lateral to iliac crests and a lateral-to-medial compressive force is applied.		Palpable instability of the pelvis or a decrease in sacroiliac joint space or symphyseal diastasis is seen on simultaneous C-arm images.
Pelvic instability: vertical instability	Legs are positioned extended. While one extremity is supported at the heel, traction is applied to the other.		A visual change in leg-length discrepancy can be seen in some cases. Otherwise, simultaneous C-arm images may disclose one acetabulum or iliac crest at a different level than the other.

Index

Page numbers followed by *f* and *t* indicate figures and tables, respectively.

S

T

U

V

W

Y

Z